Diagnostic and Therapeutic Cardiac Catheterization

Third Edition

Diagnostic and Therapeutic Cardiac Catheterization

Third Edition

Edited by

Carl J. Pepine, M.D.

Professor of Medicine
Co-Director, Division of Cardiology
University of Florida
Gainesville, Florida

and Associates

James A. Hill, M.D.

Professor of Medicine
Department of Medicine
University of Florida
Gainesville, Florida

Charles R. Lambert, M.D., Ph.D.

Professor of Medicine
Department of Medicine
University of Florida
Director, Health First Heart Institute
Melbourne, Florida

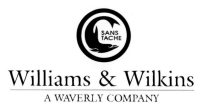

Williams & Wilkins
A WAVERLY COMPANY

BALTIMORE • PHILADELPHIA • LONDON • PARIS • BANGKOK
BUENOS AIRES • HONG KONG • MUNICH • SYDNEY • TOKYO • WROCLAW

Editor: Jonathan W. Pine, Jr.
Managing Editor: Molly L. Mullen
Marketing Manager: Daniell T. Griffin
Production Coordinator: Danielle Hagan
Book Project Editor: Karen M. Ruppert
Illustration Planner: Ray Lowman
Typesetter: Maryland Composition Co., Inc.
Printer/Binder: Mack Printing

Copyright @ 1998 Williams & Wilkins
351 West Camden Street
Baltimore, Maryland 21201–2436 USA

Rose Tree Corporate Center
1400 North Providence Road
Building II, Suite 5025
Media, Pennsylvania 19063–2043 USA

Accurate indications, adverse reactions and dosage schedules for drugs are provided in this book, but it is possible that they may change. The reader is urged to review the package information data of the manufacturers of the medications mentioned.

Printed in the United States of America

First Edition, 1989
Second Edition, 1994

Library of Congress Cataloging-in-Publication Data

Diagnostic and therapeutic cardiac catheterization / edited by Carl J.
  Pepine and associates, James A. Hill, Charles R. Lambert.—3rd ed.
      p.   cm.
    Includes bibliographical references and index.
    ISBN 0-683-30125-X
    1. Cardiac catheterization.   I. Pepine, Carl J.   II. Hill, James
A., 1950–   .   III. Lambert, Charles R., 1951–   .
    [DNLM: 1. Heart Catheterization—methods.   2. Heart Diseases—
diagnosis. 3. Heart Diseases—therapy.   WG 141.5.C2 D536   1997]
RC683.5.C25D53   1997
616.1'20754—dc21
DNLM/DLC
for Library of Congress   97-21511
                                                              CIP

The publishers have made every effort to trace the copyright holders for borrowed material. If they have inadvertently overlooked any, they will be pleased to make the necessary arrangements at the first opportunity.

To purchase additional copies of this book, call our customer service department at **(800) 638–0672** or fax orders to **(800) 447–8438.** For other book services, including chapter reprints and large quantity sales, ask for the Special Sales department.

Canadian customers should call **(800) 665–1148,** or fax **(800) 665–0103.** For all other calls originating outside of the United States, please call **(410) 528–4223** or fax us at **(410) 528–8550.**

Visit Williams & Wilkins on the Internet: http://www.wwilkins.com or contact our customer service department at **custserv@wwilkins.com.** Williams & Wilkins customer service representatives are available from 8:30 am to 6:00 pm, EST, Monday through Friday, for telephone access.

98 99 00 01 02
1   2   3   4   5   6   7   8   9   10

To our wives and families
The time that was taken from them
enabled us to develop this book.
In this way, they are
very special contributors to this work.

Preface
to the
Third Edition

Cardiac catheterization comprises a number of specific procedures that require introduction of special catheters into the central arterial and/or venous circulation to obtain information or to apply treatment related to the heart and vascular system. Very few procedures in medicine have provided more excitement and contributions to research, diagnosis, and treatment of disease than those encompassed by cardiac catheterization. This benchmark has brought about substantial change in the approach to patients with either known or suspect cardiovascular disease of all types.

Specifically, cardiac catheterization procedures, such as coronary angiography, left ventriculography, pressure and flow recordings, and oximetry give graphic descriptions of the anatomy and physiology of the heart and great vessels, and of circulatory function. Catheter obtained endomyocardial biopsy provides tissue for histologic diagnosis of a variety of disease states and is an objective method to document responses to specific treatment. The rapid growth of a number of therapeutic procedures has given the cardiovascular catheterization specialist a direct method of intervention in the treatment of many patients with a variety of cardiac disorders. These interventions range from dilation of vascular obstructions to creation of atrial septal defects, and from ablation of arrhythmias

to introduction of prosthetic devices. These cardiac catheterization-based procedures, their theory, and clinical application are the subject of this text. The framework for this approach to the field of cardiac catheterization was set in the first edition of this text in 1989.

PURPOSE

The general aims of this book are to provide the reader with an in-depth look at the general and specific areas of cardiac catheterization with the background material needed to make appropriate decisions concerning the role, value, and application of diagnostic cardiac catheterization (e.g., right and left heart catheterization, coronary angiography) and therapeutic interventions (e.g., percutaneous transluminal coronary angioplasty, atherectomy, valvuloplasty, stenting).

The approach is divided into six specific sections.

Section 1 reviews the historical background of diagnostic and interventional cardiac catheterization.

Section 2 describes catheterization laboratory organization, administration, and such related issues as training and possible conflicts of interest.

Section 3 addresses the practice of general catheterization procedures that have application to both diagnostic and interventional work: preparation of patients for various procedures, patient risks, and the general background and technical information needed to use catheterization, radiologic techniques, and special procedures used in the catheterization laboratory.

Section 4 focuses on diagnostic catheterization, such as the practical aspects of various physiologic measurements made in the catheterization laboratory.

Section 5 addresses interventional techniques and includes both basic and complex coronary angioplasty, as well as atherectomy, laser angioplasty, and stents. Balloon valvuloplasty and antithrombolytic therapy are addressed.

Section 6 represents a unique feature of this text. These chapters are designed to guide the reader in selecting the approach needed to address specific clinical states through an integration of cardiac catheterization data. Each clinical state is reviewed in terms of natural history and clinical presentation in view of the cardiac catheterization data, stressing correlation or lack of correlation. The noninvasive laboratory data obtained to supplement the clinical data that aids in either selecting patients for catheterization or obviating the need for cardiac catheterization are reviewed. Catheterization data critical to providing optimal management are discussed in detail. Finally, the use of specific cardiac catheterization data in de-

termining medical, surgical, or catheter directed interventional treatment plans is evaluated. From this information, dealing with specific patient and clinical subsets, the reader will learn what to expect from diagnostic and therapeutic catheterization procedures when applied to patients with suspected or known disease states. The reader will also learn how to use this information in the optimal management of these patients.

Last, the Appendix contains some useful tables, equations, and nomograms presented in summary form for quick day-to-day reference.

This book is a complete text on all aspects of the practice of cardiac catheterization. It is intended for physicians at all levels of training or follow-up training who care for patients with cardiovascular disease, refer patients for cardiac catheterization, and/or perform catheterization. Nonphysicians (e.g., nurses, physician assistants, technicians, students) working in cardiovascular care areas (catheterization laboratories, coronary care units, critical care units, etc.) will also find this text very useful. Those working in health care policy and related areas should find this book helpful in understanding catheter laboratory planning and procedure. Workers in reimbursement areas, managed care planning, and related fields will also find this text useful in better comprehension of catheterization procedures and patients undergoing these procedures.

With an appreciation of this information, the reader should be able to make appropriate decisions concerning the precise role, value, and application of the diagnostic and interventional techniques that comprise the field of cardiac catheterization.

ACKNOWLEDGMENTS

We are indebted to our collaborators for their invaluable contributions to this book. Special thanks are directed to those individuals who have helped to provide the opportunity for each of us to develop a career in the catheterization laboratory and the environment that enabled us to write about it. We have made unreasonable demands upon the time and temperament of these individuals so that this book might reflect what we feel represents the current state of cardiac catheterization.

Contributors

George S. Abela, MSc, M.D.
Professor of Medicine
Chief, Cardiology Division
Michigan State University
East Lansing, Michigan
Director, Cardiology Fellowship Program
  MSU/Sparrow Hospital
Lansing, Michigan

Michael E. Assey, M.D.
Professor of Medicine
Medical University of South Carolina
Director, Adult Cardiac Catheterization
  Laboratories
Director, Division of Cardiology
Charleston, South Carolina

Thomas M. Bashore, M.D.
Professor of Medicine
Duke University
Division of Cardiology
Duke University Medical Center
Durham, North Carolina

Barry D. Bertolet, M.D.
Assistant Professor of Medicine
Division of Cardiology
University of Florida
Director, Coronary Care Units
Shands Hospital
Gainesville, Florida

John A. Bittl, M.D.
Associate Professor of Medicine
Harvard Medical School
Director of Interventional Cardiology
Brigham and Women's Hospital
Boston, Massachusetts

Lawrence R. Blitz, M.D.
Cardiovascular Division
Hospital of The University of
  Pennsylvania
Philadelphia, Pennsylvania

Jeffrey A. Brinker, M.D.
Professor of Medicine and Radiology
Johns Hopkins University
School of Medicine
Johns Hopkins Hospital
Director of Interventional Cardiology
Director of Adult Pacemaker Laboratory
Division of Cardiology
Baltimore, Maryland

Kimberly Brown, R.N., B.S.N.
Manager
Intensive Care Unit, Catheterization
  Laboratory
Cardiac Rehabilitation
Columbia Alaska Regional Hospital
Anchorage, Alaska

Robert M. Califf, M.D.
Associate Vice Chancellor for Clinical
  Research
Professor of Medicine
Duke University
Director, Duke Clinical Research Institute
Duke University Medical Center
Durham, North Carolina

Blase A. Carabello, M.D.
Professor of Medicine
Division of Cardiology
Medical University of South Carolina
Director, Non-Invasive Laboratory
Director, Clinical Cardiology Fellowship
  Training Program
Charleston, South Carolina

C. Richard Conti, M.D.
Palm Beach Heart Association
    Eminent Scholar, Cardiology
Professor of Medicine
Chief, Division of Cardiology
University of Florida
Gainesville, Florida

Jamie Beth Conti, M.D.
Assistant Professor of Medicine
Division of Cardiology
University of Florida
Gainesville, Florida

John S. Douglas, Jr., M.D.
Associate Professor of Medicine
Emory University School of Medicine
Co-Director, Cardiovascular Laboratory
Emory University Hospital
Atlanta, Georgia

Joel D. Eisenberg, M.D.
Associate Professor of Medicine
Division of Cardiology
Michigan State University
East Lansing, Michigan

Eric L. Eisenstein, DBA
Assistant Research Professor
Duke University
Duke Clinical Research Institute
Durham, North Carolina

Stephen G. Ellis, M.D.
Professor of Medicine
Ohio State University
Director, Sones Cardiac Catheterization
    Laboratories
The Cleveland Clinic Foundation
Cleveland, Ohio
Columbus, Ohio

David L. Fischman, M.D.
Assistant Professor of Medicine
Division of Cardiology
Jefferson Medical College
Philadelphia, Pennsylvania

F. Jay Fricker, M.D.
Professor and Chief of Pediatric
    Cardiology
University of Florida
Gainesville, Florida

Sheldon Goldberg, M.D.
Director, Center of Excellence in
    Interventional Cardiology
Visiting Professor in Medicine,
    Harvard Medical School
Massachusetts General Hospital
Boston, Massachusetts

Christopher B. Granger, M.D.
Assistant Professor of Medicine
Duke University
Director, Cardiac Care Unit
Duke University Medical Center
Durham, North Carolina

Robert A. Harrington, M.D., MBA
Assistant Professor of Medicine
Duke University
Duke University Medical Center
Durham, North Carolina

Howard C. Herrmann, M.D.
Associate Professor of Medicine
University of Pennsylvania
Director, Interventional Cardiology
University of Pennsylvania Medical
    Center
Philadelphia, Pennsylvania

Frederick A. Heupler, Jr., M.D.
Director, Quality Assurance
Sones Cardiac Catheterization
    Laboratories
Department of Cardiology
The Cleveland Clinic Foundation
Cleveland, Ohio

James A. Hill, M.D.
Professor of Medicine
Division of Cardiology
University of Florida
Gainesville, Florida

L. David Hillis, M.D.
James M. Wooten Chair in Cardiology
Vice Chairman, Department of Medicine
University of Texas Southwestern Medical
    Branch
University of Texas Southwestern Medical
    Center
Dallas, Texas

John W. Hirshfeld, M.D.
Professor of Medicine
University of Pennsylvania
Director, Cardiac Catheterization
  Laboratory
Cardiovascular Division
Hospital of the University of Pennsylvania
Philadelphia, Pennsylvania

David R. Holmes, Jr., M.D.
Professor of Medicine
Mayo Medical School
Director, Adult Cardiac Catheterization
  Laboratory
Division of Cardiovascular Diseases and
  Internal Medicine
Mayo Clinic and Mayo Foundation
Rochester, Minnesota

Paul R. Julsrud, M.D.
Associate Professor
Department of Radiology
Mayo Medical School
Department of Diagnostic Radiology
Mayo Clinic and Mayo Foundation
Rochester, Minnesota

Paul Kelly, M.D.
Senior Registrar in Cardiology
Department of Invasive Cardiology
Royal Brompton Hospital
London, United Kingdom

J. Ward Kennedy, M.D.
Robert A. Bruce Professor of Medicine
Director, Division of Cardiology
Department of Medicine
University of Washington
Seattle, Washington

Richard A. Kerensky, M.D.
Assistant Professor of Medicine
Division of Cardiology
University of Florida
Gainesville, Florida

Morton J. Kern, M.D.
Professor of Medicine
Department of Internal Medicine
Saint Louis University Health Sciences
  Center
St. Louis, Missouri

Spencer B. King III, M.D.
Professor of Medicine
Division of Cardiology
Director of Interventional Cardiology
Emory University Hospital
Atlanta, Georgia

Daniel M. Kolansky, M.D.
Assistant Professor of Medicine
Cardiovascular Division
Hospital of the University of Pennsylvania
Philadelphia, Pennsylvania

Michael Kutryk, M.D., Ph.D., F.R.C.P.
Department of Interventional Cardiology
University Hospital Rotterdam
Rotterdam, The Netherlands

Charles R. Lambert, M.D.
Professor of Medicine
Division of Cardiology
University of Florida
Director, Health First Heart Institute
Melbourne, Florida

Richard A. Lange, M.D.
Associate Professor of Medicine
Division of Cardiology
University of Texas Southwestern Medical
  Branch
Director, Cardiac Catheterization
  Laboratory
Parkland Memorial Hospital
Dallas, Texas

Jannet F. Lewis, M.D.
Associate Professor of Medicine
Director, Clinical Echocardiography
Division of Cardiology
University of Florida
Gainesville, Florida

Robert G. MacDonald, M.D., F.R.C.P.
Assistant Professor of Medicine
Dalhousie University
Halifax, Nova Scotia
Director, Cardiac Catheterization
  Laboratory
New Brunswick Heart Centre
Saint John Regional Hospital
St. John, New Brunswick
Canada

Kenneth W. Mahaffey, M.D.
Assistant Professor of Medicine
Division of Cardiology
Duke University Medical Center
Durham, North Carolina

Daniel B. Mark, M.D., M.P.H.
Associate Professor of Medicine
Duke University
Director, Outcomes Research and
   Assessment Group
Duke Clinical Research Institute
Durham, North Carolina

Tomas D. Martin, M.D.
Associate Professor of Surgery
Chief, Adult Thoracic and Cardiovascular
   Surgery
University of Florida
Gainesville, Florida

David C. Mayer, M.D.
Assistant Professor of Pediatrics
University of South Alabama
Mobile, Alabama

Roger M. Mills, Jr., M.D.
Professor of Medicine
Clinical Director, Division of
   Cardiovascular Medicine
University of Kentucky College of
   Medicine
Lexington, Kentucky

Wilmer W. Nichols, Ph.D.
Associate Professor, Medicine and
   Physiology
Division of Cardiology
University of Florida
Gainesville, Florida

Francesca A. Nicolini, M.D.
Director, Experimental Thrombosis
   Laboratory
Department of Cardiology
The Cleveland Clinic Foundation
Cleveland, Ohio

Steven E. Nissen, M.D.
Professor of Medicine
Ohio State University
Vice Chairman
Department of Cardiology
Director, Clinical Cardiology
The Cleveland Clinic Foundation
Cleveland, Ohio

E. Magnus Ohman, M.D.
Associate Professor of Medicine
Duke University
Coordinator of Clinical Trials in
   Interventional Cardiology
Duke University Medical Center
Durham, North Carolina

Hercules Panayiotou, M.B.B.Ch., M.Med
Associate Professor of Medicine
Division of Cardiology
University of South Alabama
Mobile, Alabama

Carl J. Pepine, M.D.
Professor of Medicine
Co-Director, Division of Cardiology
University of Florida
Gainesville, Florida

Scott J. Savader, M.D.
Associate Professor of Radiology and
   Surgery
Division of Cardiovascular &
   Interventional Radiology
Johns Hopkins University School of
   Medicine
Johns Hopkins Hospital
Baltimore, Maryland

Michael P. Savage, M.D.
Associate Professor of Medicine
Division of Cardiology
Thomas Jefferson University
Director, Cardiac Catheterization
   Laboratory
Thomas Jefferson University Hospital
Philadelphia, Pennsylvania

Patrick J. Scanlon, M.D.
Professor of Medicine
Loyola University
Director, Cardiovascular Institute/
   Medicine
Loyola University Medical Center
Maywood, Illinois

Norberto S. Schechtmann, MD
Attending Cardiologist
Holmes Regional Medical Center
Melbourne, Florida

Jay D. Schlaifer, M.D.
Instructor of Medicine
Division of Cardiology
University of Florida College of Medicine
Pittsburgh, Pennsylvania

Patrick W. Serruys, M.D., Ph.D.
Professor of Cardiology
Eramus University Rotterdam and
    Interuniversity Cardiology Institute of
    the Netherlands
Catheterisation Laboratory, Thoraxcenter
Erasmus University Rotterdam
Rotterdam, The Netherlands

Florence H. Sheehan, M.D.
Research Professor
Division of Cardiology
University of Washington
Seattle, Washington

Ulrich Sigwart, M.D.
Director, Department of Invasive
    Cardiology
Royal Brompton National Heart and
    Chest Hospital
London, United Kingdom

Barbara E. Tardiff, M.D.
Assistant Professor of Anesthesiology
Division of Cardiothoracic Anesthesia
Duke University
Duke Clinical Research Institute
Durham, North Carolina

Bruce W. Usher, M.D.
Charles Ezra Daniel Professor of
    Cardiology
Department of Medicine
Medical University of South Carolina
Charleston, South Carolina

George W. Vetrovec, M.D.
Professor of Medicine
Chairman, Division of Cardiology
Virginia Commonwealth University
Medical College of Virginia Hospital
Richmond, Virginia

Ronald E. Vlietstra, M.B., Ch.B.
Clinical Professor of Medicine
Division of Medicine
University of Florida
Gainesville, Florida
Clinical Cardiologist
Watson Clinic
Lakeland, Florida

Andrew Wang, M.D.
Division of Cardiology
Duke University
Duke University Medical Center
Department of Medicine
Durham, North Carolina

Michael D. Winniford, M.D.
Professor of Medicine
Department of Internal Medicine
University of Iowa
Associate Director, Cardiovascular
    Division
Director, Cardiac Catheterization
    Laboratory
University of Iowa Hospitals & Clinics
Iowa City, Iowa

Merrill A. Wondrow, M.D.
Associate, Division of Cardiovascular
    Diseases and Internal Medicine
Mayo Clinic and Mayo Foundation
Rochester, Minnesota

James B. Young, Jr., M.D.
Professor of Medicine
Ohio State University
Chief, Section of Heart Failure and
    Cardiac Transplant Medicine
The Cleveland Clinic Foundation
Cleveland, Ohio

Contents

Section **5**
Coronary and Noncoronary Therapeutic (Intervention) Cardiac Techniques **541**

Section **6**
Specific Clinical States and Their Assessment and Intervention by
Catheter Techniques . . . .

Section

1

INTRODUCTION

1
Development and Application of Cardiac Catheterization and Interventional Procedures: Historical Background

Carl J. Pepine, MD
James A. Hill, MD
Charles R. Lambert, MD, PhD

HISTORICAL BACKGROUND

In order to practice cardiac catheterization and make use of the results of the procedure to its full extent in managing patients, some knowledge of its development is useful. Like many diagnostic and therapeutic techniques, cardiac catheterization evolved through several phases before it reached the position that it now occupies in the practice of medicine. The development and application of cardiac catheterization can be traced through four distinct phases: (*a*) development of a technique for measuring intracardiac and intravascular physiologic variables in animals; (*b*) application of these techniques to patients; (*c*) development of techniques for selective coronary angiography; and (*d*) application of catheter-based therapeutic procedures.

DEVELOPMENT OF A TECHNIQUE FOR MEASURING INTRACARDIAC AND INTRAVASCULAR PHYSIOLOGIC VARIABLES IN ANIMALS

Claude Bernard is given credit for developing a technique for catheterization of the heart of living animals from the peripheral vessels (1). His initial work in this area began in 1844, when he inserted a mercury thermometer into the carotid artery of a horse and advanced it through the aortic valve into the left ventricle. He also advanced a thermometer from the jugular vein to the right ventricle. The purpose of these experiments was to determine the temperature difference between blood returning from the lungs and that returning from the remainder of the body. His work continued for almost 40 years. During this period, he described in great detail the procedures for venous and arterial catheterization of many animals, crossing the aortic valve and measuring intracardiac pressures. He refined these techniques and then used them as tools to gather data and to solve many scientific problems. From his work, the catheter became the accepted reference standard by physiologists for cardiovascular hemodynamic study.

The next important milestone came with Adolph Fick's brief but famous single-page note on the calculation of blood flow in 1870 (2). Thus, with the measurement of intracardiac pressures and blood flow by cardiac catheterization, detailed studies of the heart and circulation of animals followed.

3

APPLICATION OF CATHETERIZATION TECHNIQUES TO PATIENTS

Credit for human cardiac catheterization is not as easily assigned. Several years before Claude Bernard, J.F. Dieffenbach published his experience with an elastic catheter used to remove extra blood from the central circulation of a patient dying of cholera (3). He described introduction of the catheter into the brachial artery approximately as far as the heart, but we do not know if the heart chambers were actually entered. Frizt Bleichroeder, E. Unger, and W. Loeb published descriptions of human catheterization as early as 1912 and were among the first workers to insert catheters into the blood vessels without x-ray visualization (4). They assigned no specific purpose to these experiments other than to document that catheters could be passed through human veins from the forearm to axilla and from the thigh to the vena cava without problems. During one attempt, Unger and Loeb catheterized Bleichroeder, who reported a stabbing pain in his chest, suggesting that they may have reached his heart.

The advent of chemotherapy apparently stimulated interest in catheterization for the purpose of injecting drugs directly into the central circulation. Bleichroeder and colleagues examined the effects of inserting catheters into dog arteries and leaving them in place for several hours (4). They reported no clot formation or other complications. A clinical trial was done in four patients with puerperal sepsis. They were injected with collargol through a catheter inserted into the femoral artery and advanced to the bifurcation of the aorta.

In 1923, Sicard and Forestier (5) were investigating the use of lipiodol (as iodized poppy seed oil) for studies in man. In these studies, they described injecting 4 mL into an anticubital vein and observing it by x-ray flow into the right heart and out into the pulmonary circulation. Berberich and Hirsch (6) used a solution of strontium bromide and, for the first time, produced angiograms of the peripheral vessels in living man. These angiograms were done in the arteries and veins of the arms.

In 1924, Brooks (7) used a solution of sodium iodide to perform an angiogram in the leg of a live patient. In the United States, Carnett and Greenbaum (8) used lipiodol for intra-arterial injection to demonstrate local occlusions.

In 1929, Werner Forssmann, a 25-year-old surgical trainee in Germany, apparently unaware of Bleichroeder's work, became interested in catheterization of the heart (9). After experimenting on a human cadaver, Forssmann realized how easy it was to guide a urologic catheter from an arm vein into the right atrium (10). Apparently he had the same objective as Bleichroeder et al.—intracardiac injection of drugs—but Forssmann also recognized the potential for diagnosis. Against the advice of his colleagues, he dissected the veins of his own forearm and guided a urologic catheter into his right atrium using fluoroscopic control and a mirror. He then walked to the x-ray department with the catheter in place, without discomfort or other ill effects, to have chest radiographs filmed. Thus, Forssmann was the first to document right heart catheterization using radiographic techniques in humans. Over the next 2 years, Forssmann studied a technique in which radiographic contrast material was injected directly into the right atrium through a catheter for radiologic examination of the right heart (11, 12). He also injected 40% uroselectan through a catheter that he had positioned in his own right heart (12, 13).

In 1929, Renaldo dos Santos and colleagues performed abdominal aortography using sodium iodide and a compressed air pressure injector (14). In 1930, Jimenez Diaz and Sanchez-Cuenca advanced a urethral catheter through a cannula into an arm vein of a moribund patient and provided x-ray confirmation of its location in the right atrium. They also suggested cardiac catheterization's many diagnostic and therapeutic possibilities (15). In the same year, they measured the oxygen content in peripheral veins and the right atrium and also the arteriovenous difference (16). At about the same time, in Prague, O. Klein sampled venous blood from the right ventricle and applied the Fick principle to determine cardiac output in several patients with chronic disease (17) (see Chapters 21 and 23). Similar studies were done in 1932 by Padilla and associates in Buenos Aires (18). Except for the development of pulmonary angiography, these cardiac catheterization procedures were done sporadically over the next decade. This limbo status was possibly the result of severe criticism stemming from a lack of understanding of the full clinical and research applications of the information that could be obtained from cardiac catheterization. Undoubtedly, another reason was related to fear about serious reactions to the early contrast media, "blind punctures" and other sequelae.

Finally, in the early 1940s, Andre Cournand and Hilmert Ranges (19), working in New York with Dickinson Richards, began a systematic and comprehensive investigation of cardiac function in normal and diseased patients using **right heart catheterization.** They made many technical advances, which included catheter design and construction with features resembling those used today. These features included balance between flexibility and rigidity to enhance maneuverability, coating with a nonwettable radiopaque material and a preformed tip. They also designed a special needle cannula with the assistance of Richard Riley. This needle could be inserted percutaneously into the brachial or femoral artery and left in place for long periods of time. They even developed a mobile recording system capable of recording multiple pressures from fluid-filled manometers along with the electrocardiogram (ECG). They clearly popularized the procedure of right heart catheterization by demonstrating that it was safe and useful; and, it subsequently won widespread application.

Cournand and his collaborators and trainees advanced cardiac catheterization to a level where it became a reference standard for precise anatomic and physiologic studies for the evaluation of heart disease. Andre Cournand, Dickinson Richards, and Werner Forssmann shared a Nobel Prize (1956) in physiology and medicine in recognition of their contributions to cardiac catheterization. By 1947, Zimmerman, working in Cleveland, had developed a completely intravascular technique for human **left heart catheterization** (20). This carefully-planned procedure involved retrograde catheterization of the left ventricle from the ulnar artery in a patient with severe aortic insufficiency. This condition was chosen to allow relatively easy retrograde passage of the catheter across the incompetent aortic valve. Soon after, Zimmerman and colleagues performed simultaneous catheterization of both the right and left heart. They are thus credited with the development of **combined heart catheterization** (21).

In 1953, Seldinger described a percutaneous approach to introduce catheters for either right or left heart catheterization (22). An extension of this approach led to the atrial **transseptal approach** (Chapter 9) to the left heart from the right femoral artery using a long needle that was developed independently in 1959 by John Ross Jr (23) and Constantin Cope (24). Later, Brockenbrough and Braunwald (25) modified the apparatus so that the last centimeter of the transseptal needle was narrower (21-gauge instead of 18-gauge). Thus, if the needle puncture was done in the wrong place, the resulting hole was not as large. By 1960, Charles Dotter and Goffredo Gensini had adapted the Seldinger technique to special catheters that were more practical for left heart catheterization (26) (see Chapter 9). With the introduction of cardiopulmonary bypass, which made open heart surgery possible, diagnostic catheterization became established for confirmation of clinical findings before cardiac surgery for valvular or congenital heart disease.

DEVELOPMENT OF A TECHNIQUE FOR CORONARY ANGIOGRAPHY IN PATIENTS

During the late 1940s and early 1950s, many investigators were working to develop non-selective techniques to visualize the coronary arteries (27). These inc'·rect methods included simply flooding the aortic root with a large quantity of contrast material that flowed into the coronary arteries in diastole. In most instances, only the proximal portions of the left and right coronary arteries were adequately visualized using conventional cineradiographic techniques.

Opacification of distal vessels and collaterals was poor, and assessments of coronary obstruction based on this method of visualization were limited. Because most coronary blood flow occurs in diastole, attempts to develop a method of injecting contrast material during diastole were made using electronic devices to activate pressure injectors at selected phases of the cardiac cycle (28, 29). These methods improved opacification, but there were still limitations in visualizing the mid and distal portions of major coronary vessels.

Another example of the indirect method was advanced by Arnulf and Chacornac (30). They observed excellent opacification of coronary arteries in dogs with contrast material injected during cardiac arrest, which was produced accidentally as a complication of anesthesia. This prompted them to arrest an animal's heart deliberately, using acetylcholine. Resumption of the heart beat was usually spontaneous but, if necessary, could always be induced by atropine. In animal experiments in the United States, Lehman and colleagues used this technique to visualize most of the left coronary system (31). It is interesting to note that intracoronary acetylcholine injection has recently been used in humans during coronary angiography to evaluate endothelial function and to provoke coronary artery constriction in patients with variant angina and other conditions (32) (see Chapters 17 and 36).

Another novel, indirect method was advanced by Boerema and Bickman (33). They caused tamponade of the superior vena cava to limit right heart filling by intrabronchial pressure elevation to levels above venous pressure. This maneuver reduced both cardiac output and coronary flow, and improved opacification of coronary vessels with nonselective injections. The technique was standardized by Nordenstrom et al. and applied clinically in the early 1960s (34). In further attempts to improve opacification of coronary arteries, Dotter and Frische used a double-lumen balloon occlusion catheter (35). The soft balloon on this catheter occluded the ascending aorta above the coronary ostia, and a port was provided for contrast material injection below the balloon and just above the aortic valve. General anesthesia was used, and the catheter was introduced through the surgically exposed right brachial artery. Gensini and associates combined this method with either acetylcholine arrest or intrabronchial pressure elevation to improve coronary artery visualization (28).

Bellman and colleagues introduced a specially-designed catheter to direct the stream of injected contrast material laterally toward the walls of the aorta to improve opacification of coronary arteries (36). The catheter was preformed into a loop configuration and slightly smaller in diameter than the aortic root diameter, which was judged by chest x-ray. Side holes along the outer periphery of the loop were oriented to point toward the coronary ostia. Success in dogs prompted Williams and co-workers to apply this technique to human coronary angiographic studies (37).

In 1958, Mason Sones, working in Cleveland, began to develop a **selective coronary angiography** procedure that used electronic image amplification and optical amplification with high-speed cine technique. In 1959, while Sones was developing these methods for use in animals, he and his colleagues accidentally injected approximately 40 mL of 90% Hypaque into the right coronary artery of a patient with aortic valve disease during a planned aortogram (38). Although asystole occurred, the patient was resuscitated using coughs and had an uneventful recovery. Sones and Shirey then developed a catheter to selectively enter the coronary arteries. The catheter body was relatively rigid for good torque control but tapered at the tip to facilitate formation of a curve as the tip was advanced against the left aortic valve leaflet (39). They also demonstrated that the selective procedure using this type of catheter was very safe. Thus, selective coronary angiography became the reference standard to assess the coronary arteries for both diagnostic and research purposes (see Chapter 17).

In 1962, Ricketts and Abrams introduced a **percutaneous technique for selective coronary angiography** (40). By 1967, Melvin Judkins (41) and Kurt Amplatz et al. (42) had applied preformed catheters that actually "sought" each coronary ostium from the percutaneous femoral artery approach.

A single-catheter technique, using a modified Sones-type catheter for use from the percutaneous femoral approach, was introduced in 1966 by Schoonmaker and King (43). Again, with introduction of a safe and effective surgical procedure for coronary artery bypass by Favalaro (44) in 1968, selective coronary angiography grew to become the most frequently performed cardiac catheterization procedure.

Originally a technique to assess only the relatively static anatomy of the coronary artery lumen, coronary angiography has evolved to include many other areas. Introduction of nitroglycerin and some vasoconstrictors like ergonovine have become standard in the evaluation of patients with suspected coronary artery spasm (see Chapters 17 and 36). More recently, the use of intracoronary acetylcholine infusion permits identification of coronary artery endothelial dysfunction that characterizes early arterial wall damage before the lumen is significantly narrowed, as in atherosclerosis. Application of miniature intravascular ultrasonic Doppler devices, to either a coronary artery catheter or a guidewire, has facilitated measurement of phasic coronary blood flow velocity and direct estimates of flow reserve during coronary angiography (see Chapters 17, 21, and 24). Most recently, detection and quantification of coronary atherosclerosis has been validated by adding ultraminiature intracoronary ultrasound transducers to the coronary angiographic evaluation (see Chapter 17). This addition permits assessment of intimal thickness to detect early atheromatous lesions, dissection, and lumen size (45). Angioscopic evaluation of the lumen surface provides a method for detecting and quantifying intravascular thrombus.

DEVELOPMENT AND APPLICATION OF THERAPEUTIC CATHETERIZATION

Although clearly in the mind of early workers for the purpose of delivering drugs and withdrawing blood, using catheterization for therapeutic purposes was delayed until 1950, when Rubeo-Alvarez and Limon-Lason suggested that a catheter method might be used to treat pulmonic stenosis (46). Practical therapeutic catheterization was then realized with the work of William Rashkind, working in Philadelphia, who developed a successful procedure to enhance pulmonary blood flow by creation or enlargement of an atrial septal defect using a balloon (47). Since then, **balloon atrioseptostomy** has enjoyed widespread acceptance.

The **catheter embolectomy technique** was developed using a small balloon catheter, which is now popular for routine clinical use. Catheter-mounted balloons were also used to test-occlude the pulmonary artery for preoperative evaluation of separate lung function (48, 49). Pressure recordings distal to the pulmonary artery balloon occlusion suggested the potential for obtaining pulmonary-capillary pressure from the balloon-occlusion pressure. Lategola and Rahn used this technology to develop a **"self-guiding" catheter** for cardiac and pulmonary artery catheterization and occlusion in dogs (50). Swan and Ganz then adapted the concept into a fast, safe, and reliable technique to monitor left ventricle filling pressure and cardiac output in the critical care setting using a **balloon flotation catheter** (51) (see Chapters 9 and 10). Moulopoulos et al. (52) adapted catheter-mounted balloon technology in the form of an **intra-aortic balloon pump** (IABP) for use as a circulatory assist device.

Independently, several groups developed methods to close congenital cardiac defects with devices delivered by catheters. The first double-umbrella device for intracardiac use received little attention when introduced by King and Mills for closure of secundum atrial septal defect in 1976 (53). Steady progress has been made, however, since Rashkind and Cuaso (54) developed their double-umbrella device for transcatheter closure of patent ductus. This device has also been used as an alternative to surgery for closure of aortopulmonary collaterals, aortopulmonary windows, and venous connections (55, 56). Recently, the clamshell double umbrella has resulted in enlargement of this list of conditions to include atrial and ventricle septal defects, as well as patent foramen ovale in children and adults (57–59). Most recently, Hourihan and colleagues (60) have adapted these techniques to extend the transcatheter umbrella delivery for closure of valvular and paravalvular leaks. With further advances in technique, some of the devices are now in use (see Chapter 40). Likewise, techniques evolved to partially interrupt the inferior vena cava with catheter-delivered devices (umbrellas, caval filters, etc.) to prevent recurrent pulmonary embolization.

In 1964, Dotter and Judkins were the first to extend interventional catheter techniques to the area of atherosclerosis (61). Intraluminal catheter angioplasty was first performed using serial coaxial catheters to puncture soft thromboatheroma and stretch the lumen of peripheral arteries. Balloons were later applied to the peripheral angioplasty technique by Portsmann (62) and Zeitler et al. (63), in the early 1970s. The balloon technique was further modified and subsequently popularized by Andreas Gruentzig (64). He developed cylindrical, thin-walled, relatively nondistensible balloons for peripheral angioplasty. The balloon was mounted on a double-lumen catheter with equipment for high-pressure inflation of the balloon with fluid. Several years later he constructed miniaturized balloons on very small double-lumen catheters for application in the proximal coronary arteries. In 1977, Gruentzig applied this technique for the first time to a patient in Zurich (65, 66). His concept of protecting the artery by flexible, small guidewires and using balloons that maintained a relatively uniform preselected size and shape resulted in high success rates and very low occlusion rates. Over the course of several years, Gruentzig and others refined the balloon catheter approach to coronary arteries that is now firmly established as **percutaneous transluminal coronary angioplasty (PTCA)** (see Chapters 27 and 28). Its success has stimulated the development of many other catheter-based interventional vascular procedures, including atherectomy devices (see Chapter 20), lasers (see Chapter 30), rotating drills, and balloon-delivered endovascular stents (see Chapters 29–33). Further evolution of the interventional coronary artery

techniques referred to above is discussed in detail in the noted chapters.

In 1982, the balloon catheters used for peripheral angioplasty were enlarged and modified for dilatation of stenotic pulmonary valves in children and adults (67, 68). These balloons were later applied to stenotic mitral and aortic valves (69, 70), and also are now used to create pericardial windows (see Chapter 42). **Balloon valvuloplasty** techniques continue to evolve (see Chapter 35).

Numerous implantable devices for continuous intravascular drug infusion, **cardiac pacing,** and **control of arrhythmias** also have been developed. The latter depends on insertion of catheter-mounted electrodes. Since the introduction of a technique for His' bundle recording in 1969 (71–72), the diagnostic application of catheter techniques to sense intracardiac electrical activity and induce arrhythmias has advanced rapidly. Electrical application has developed into a catheter laboratory-based field of **clinical electrophysiology.** This field now also includes catheter-directed His' bundle and arrhythmia foci ablation procedures using radio frequency current.

SUMMARY

Cardiac catheterization was developed and applied to humans more than 5 decades ago. Over these years, it has evolved through four major phases. Each phase has led to far-reaching advances in our knowledge and practice of medicine. In its current phase, catheterization is a highly specialized discipline encompassing more and more therapeutic procedures that promise to further expand our abilities to manage many problems. Continued advances in the fields of material science, miniaturization, and digital technology are only likely to yield new applications.

References

1. Buzzi A. Claude Bernard on cardiac catheterization. Am J Cardiol 1959;4:405–409.

2. Fick A. Uber die Messung des Blutquantums in den Herzventrikeln'. Phys-med Ges Wurzburg, July 9, 1870.

3. Dieffenbach JF. Physiologish-chirurgish beobachtigen bie cholera-kranken. Cholera Arch 1832;1:86–105.

4. Bleichroeder F, Unger E, Loeb W. Intraterielle therapy. Klin Wochenschr 1912;49:1503.

5. Sicard J, Forestier J. The use of lipiodol. Oxford: Oxford University Press, 1932.

6. Berberich J, Hirsch S. Die rontgenographische darstellung der arterien und venen am lebended menschen. Klin Wochenschr 1923;2:2226.

7. Brooks B. Intra-arterial injection of sodium iodide; preliminary report. JAMA 1924;82:1016.

8. Carnett JB, Greenbaum SS. Blood vessel visualization. JAMA 1927;89:2039.

9. Forssmann W. Die sondierung des rechten Herzens. Klin Wochenschr 1929;8:2085–2087.

10. Benatt AJ. Cardiac catheterization: an historical note. Lancet 1949;746–747.

11. Forssmann W. Uber Kontrastdarstellung der Hohlen des lebenrden rechten Herzens und der Lungenschlagader. Munchen Med Wochenschr 1931;78:489–492.

12. Forssmann W. Experiments on myself. Memoirs of a surgeon in Germany. New York: Saint Martin's Press, 1974:84–85.

13. Cournand A. Cardiac catheterization: development of the technique, its contributions to experimental medicine and its initial applications in man. Acta Med Scand 1975;579:7–32.

14. dos Santos R, Lamas AC, Pereira-Caldas J. Arteriografia da aorta e dos vasos abdnominais. Med Contemp 1929;47:93–96.

15. Jimenez-Diaz C, Sanchez-Cuenca B. El sondage del corazon derecho. Arq Cardiol Hemat 1930;11:105–108.

16. Jimenez-Diaz C, Sanchez-Cuenca B. Estudios de insuficiencia circulatoria: investigaciones sobre los gases en la sangra arterial y venosa en reposo y en el esfuerzo. Arq Cardiol Hemat 1930;11:531–550.

17. Klein O. Determining human cardiac output (minute volume) using Fick's principle (extraction of mixed venous blood by cardiac catheterization). Med Wochenschr 1930;77:1311–1312.

18. Padilla T, Cossio P, Berconsky I. Sondeo del Corazon: determinacion del volumen minuto circulatorio. Semana Medica 1932;2:445–448.

19. Cournand A, Ranges HA. Catheterization of the right auricle in man. Proc Soc Exp Biol Med 1941;46:462–466.

20. Zimmerman HA, Scott RW, Becker NO. Catheterization of the left side of the heart in man. Circulation 1950;1:357–359.

21. Zimmerman HA, ed. Intravascular catheterization. Springfield, IL: Charles C Thomas, 1959.

22. Seldinger SI. Catheter replacement of the needle in percutaneous arteriography. Acta Radiol 1953;39:368–376.

23. Ross J. Transseptal left heart catheterization: a new method of left atrial puncture. Ann Surg 1959;149:395–401.

24. Cope C. Technique for transseptal catheterization of the left atrium: preliminary report. J Thorac Surg 1959;37:482–486.

25. Brockenbrough EC, Braunwald E. A new technique for left ventricular angiocardiography and transseptal left heart catheterization. Am J Cardiol 1960;6:1062–1064.

26. Dotter CT, Gensini GG. Percutaneous retrograde catheterization of left ventricle and systemic arteries of man. Radiology 1960;75:171–184.

27. Radner S. An attempt at the roentgenologic visualization of coronary blood vessels in man. Acta Radiol 1945;26:497–502.

28. Gensini GG, Di Giorgi S, Black A. New approaches to coronary arteriography. Angiology 1961;12:223–238.

29. Richards LS, Thal AP. Phasic dye injection control system for coronary arteriography in the human. Surg Gynecol Obstet 1958;107:739–743.

30. Arnulf G, Chacornac R. L'arteriographie methodique des arteres coronaires grace a l'utilisation de l'acetylcholine. Donnees experimentales et cliniques. Bull Acad Natl Med (Paris) 1958;25, 26:661–673.

31. Lehman JS, Boyer RA, Winter FS. Coronary arteriography. Am J Roentgenol 1959;81:749–763.

32. Yasue H, Horio Y, Nakamura N, et al. Induction of coronary artery spasm by acetylcholine in patients with variant angina: possible role of the parasympathetic nervous system in the pathogenesis of coronary artery spasm. Circulation 1987;74:955–963.

33. Boerema I, Blickman JR. Reduced intrathoracic circulation as an aid in angiocardiography: an experimental study. J Thorac Surg 1955;30:129–142.

34. Nordenstrom B, Ovenfors C, Tornell G. Coronary angiography in 100 cases of ischemic heart disease. Radiology 1962;78:714–724.

35. Dotter CT, Frische LH. Visualization of the coronary circulation by occlusion aortography: a practical method. Radiology 1958;71:502–523.

36. Bellman S, Frank HA, Lambert PB, et al. Coronary arteriography. I. Differential opacification of the aortic stream by catheters of special design—experimental development. N Engl J Med 1960;262:325–328.

37. Williams JA, Littmann D, Hall JH, et al. Coronary arteriography. II. Clinical experiences with the loop-end catheter. N Engl J Med 1960;262:328–332.

38. Sones MF, Shirey EK, Proudfit WL, et al. Cine coronary arteriography. Circulation 1959;20:773. [Abstract]

39. Sones FM, Shirey EK. Cine coronary arteriography. Mod Concepts Cardiovasc Dis 1962;31:735–738.

40. Ricketts HJ, Abrams HL. Percutaneous selective coronary cine arteriography. JAMA 1962;181:620–624.

41. Judkins MP. Selective coronary arteriography. I. A percutaneous transfemoral technic. Radiology 1967;89:815–824.

42. Amplatz K, Formanek G, Stanger P, et al. Mechanics of selective coronary artery catheterization via femoral approach. Radiology 1967:89:1040–1047.

43. Schoonmaker FW, King SB. Coronary arteriography by the single catheter percutaneous femoral technique. Experience in 6800 cases. Circulation 1974;50:735–740.

44. Favalaro RG. Saphenous vein autograft replacement of severe segmental coronary artery occlu-

sion: operative technique. Ann Thorac Surg 1968; 5:334–339.

45. St. Goar FG, Pinto FJ, Alderman EL, et al. Detection of coronary atherosclerosis in young adult hearts using intravascular ultrasound. Circulation 1992: 86(3):756–763.

46. Rubeo-Alvarez V, Limon-Lason J. Treatment of pulmonary valvular stenosis and tricuspid stenosis with a modified cardiac catheter. Washington, DC: Proceedings of the First National Conference on Cardiovascular Diseases, 1950.

47. Rashkind WJ, Wagner HR, Tait MA. Historical aspects of interventional cardiology: past, present and future. Tex Heart Inst J 1986;13:363–367.

48. Carlens E, Hanson HE, Nordenstrom B. Temporary unilateral occlusion of the pulmonary artery. J Thorac Surg 1951;22:527–536.

49. Dotter CT, Lukas DS. Acute cor pulmonale. An experimental study utilizing a special cardiac catheter. Am J Physiol 1951;164:254–262.

50. Lategola M, Rahn H. A self-guiding catheter for cardiac and pulmonary arterial catheterization and occlusion. Proc Soc Exp Biol Med 1953;84:667–668.

51. Swan HJC, Ganz W, Forrester JS, et al. Catheterization of the heart in man with use of a flow-directed balloon-tipped catheter. N Engl J Med 1970;283: 447–451.

52. Moulopoulos SD, Topaz S, Kolff WJ. Diastolic balloon pumping (with carbon dioxide) in the aorta: mechanical assistance to the failing circulation. Am Heart J 1962;63:669–675.

53. King TD, Mills NL. Secundum atrial septal defect: nonoperative closure during cardiac catheterization. JAMA 1976;235:2506–2509.

54. Rashkind WJ, Cuaso CC. Transcatheter closure of a patent ductus arteriosus: successful use in a 3.5-kg infant. Pediatr Cardiol 1979;1:3–7.

55. Lock JE, Cockerham JT, Keane JF, et al. Transcatheter umbrella closure of congenital heart defects. Circulation 1987;75:593–599.

56. Rashkind WJ. Transcatheter treatment of congenital heart disease. Circulation 1983;67:711–716.

57. Lock JE, Rome JJ, Davis R, et al. Transcatheter closure of atrial septal defects. Experimental studies. Circulation 1989;79:1091–1099.

58. Rome J, Keane J, Perry S, et al. Double umbrella closure of atrial defects. Circulation 1990;82: 751–758.

59. Lock JE, Block PC, McKay RG, et al. Transcatheter closure of ventricular septal defects. Circulation 1988;78:361–368.

60. Hourihan M, Perry SB, Mandell VS, et al. Transcatheter umbrella closure of valvular and paravalvular leaks. J Am Coll Cardiol 1992;20(6): 1371–1377.

61. Dotter CT, Judkins MP. Transluminal treatment of arteriosclerotic obstruction: description of a new technique and a preliminary report of its application. Circulation 1964;30:654–670.

62. Porstmann W. Ein neuer korsett-ballonkatheter fur transluminalen rekanalisation nach dotter unter besonderer berucksichtigung von obliterationen an den beckenarterien. Radiol Diagn (Berlin) 1973; 14:239–244.

63. Zeitler E, Schmidtke J, Schoop W. Die perkutane Behandlung von arteriellen Durchblutungsstorungen der extremitaten mit katheter. Vasa 1973;2: 401–408.

64. Gruentzig A. Die perkutane Rekanalisation chronischer arterieller Verschlusse (Dotter-Prinzip) mit einem doppellumigen Dilatations-katheter. Fortschr Roentgenstr 1976;124:80–86.

65. Gruentzig A, Senning A, Siegenthaler WE. Nonoperative dilatation of coronary-artery stenosis: percutaneous transluminal coronary angioplasty. N Engl J Med 1979;301:61–68.

66. Gruentzig A. Transluminal dilatation of coronary-artery stenosis. Lancet 1978;I:263. [Letter to Editor]

67. Kan JS, White RI, Mitchell SE, et al. Percutaneous balloon valvuloplasty: a new method for treating congenital pulmonary valve stenosis. N Engl J Med 1982;307:540–542.

68. Pepine CJ, Gessner IH, Feldman RL. Percutaneous balloon valvuloplasty for pulmonic valve stenosis in the adult. Am J Cardiol 1982;50:1442–1445.

69. Cribier A, Saoudi N, Berland J, et al. Percutaneous transluminal valvuloplasty of acquired aortic stenosis in elderly patients: an alternative to valve replacement? Lancet 1986;1:178–179.

70. Inoue K, Owaki T, Nakamura T, et al. Clinical application of transvenous mitral commissurotomy by a new balloon catheter. J Thorac Cardiovasc Surg 1984;87:394–402.

71. Damato AN, Lau SH, Berkowitz WD, et al. Recording of specialized conducting fibers (A-V nodal, His bundle, and right bundle branch) in man using an electrode catheter technique. Circulation 1969; 39:435–447.

72. Scherlog BJ, Lou SH, Helfont RH, et al. Catheter technique for recording His bundle activity in man. Circulation 1969;39:13.

Section

2

CATHETERIZATION LABORATORY ORGANIZATION, ADMINISTRATION, AND RELATED ISSUES

2
Cardiac Catheterization Laboratory Settings

Thomas M. Bashore, MD
Andrew G. Wang, MD

INTRODUCTION

Continuing Expansion of Cardiac Catheterization Facilities

Cardiac catheterization procedures are growing steadily in the United States. As the mean age of the population continues increasing, the expression of ischemic heart disease becomes ever more evident. Aging of the baby boomers will soon result in many individuals experiencing heart disease for the first time. Coronary artery disease is and will likely remain the number one killer. Six million Americans have either had an acute myocardial infarction or have angina pectoris. There are 1.5 million heart attacks each year (one-third of them fatal). In addition, 8 of every 1000 children are born with congenital heart disease, and by the year 2000, an estimated 500,000 patients with congenital heart disease will require cardiac services. Rheumatic heart disease affects an estimated 1.3 million people despite the virtual disappearance of acute rheumatic fever. Approximately 20,000 patients are hospitalized with endocarditis each year. The incidence of degenerative aortic and mitral valvular disease also increases as the population ages. Thus, the expansion of cardiac catheterization laborato-

ries is a result, at least in part, of the **high prevalence of cardiac disease** in the population (1).

Other factors are operative, however. The **safety of cardiac catheterization has improved** impressively in the last decade (2), leading to a decline in the threshold for recommending cardiac catheterization. Even while extremely ill patients (including those in cardiogenic shock from acute myocardial infarction) can now be studied at an acceptable risk, selected stable cardiovascular patients can readily undergo cardiac catheterization as an outpatient procedure without adverse consequences.

Both the success and failure of revascularization procedures has further driven the expansion. The number of coronary interventional procedures performed has skyrocketed to more than 400,000 yearly, approximately the same number as that for coronary bypass procedures (3). The declining risk for coronary angioplasty and the introduction of a variety of novel coronary interventional procedures have fostered this increase. The realization, however, that coronary artery grafts have a finite life span (4) and that there remains a humbling 30 to 40% restenosis rate following coronary angioplasty (5) means that many patients now undergo multiple cardiac catheterizations. Although the initial vessel lumen is larger and there is clearly less abrupt closure following interventional procedures such as coronary stents (6), the actual long-term restenosis rates with coronary stents remain under investigation (7). Thus, repeat procedures will continue to have an impact on the increased volume of procedures now being observed.

It has become clear to health care providers that cardiac services represent a "cash cow" in an ever-competitive medical marketplace. Cardiac services tend to be well compensated, and income from these services often support many other areas of a hospital. In the lay press, this phenomenon has been referred to as the "cardiac money machine" (8). With the general decline in the certificate-of-need process in many states, those states without rigid regulatory agencies have experienced a virtual explosion in the number of facilities offering invasive cardiac services, at least in part to maintain "market share." This unprecedented expansion has resulted in an increase in the number of cardiac catheterization facilities in the United States to well over 1300 (9). Many of the newer catheterization laboratory facilities are in what would be considered "nontraditional" settings, such as in a freestanding building unattached to a hospital or in a mobile cardiac catheterization laboratory. The wisdom of these nontraditional catheterization laboratory settings is a matter of great concern to the cardiology community (10–12).

Another factor in the expansion of services has been the result of a quirk in the **regulatory system.** Because of federal, state, and regional regulatory requirements, many cardiac catheterization laboratories are initially developed without cardiovascular surgical backup. Indeed, approximately one-third of all laboratories do not perform in-house cardiovascular surgery (9). Cardiovascular surgery is permitted only after a certain arbitrary volume of diagnostic cardiac catheterizations has been achieved per year. This policy creates a marketplace that further urges the hospital and physicians to expand services to achieve the necessary volume to keep the laboratory in compliance with such requirements. Because it has generally been accepted that surgical backup should be available before interventional procedures are allowed, the

pressure to provide interventional services further drives the facility to expand the cardiac catheterization program.

Recent evidence of the clinical benefit from **primary percutaneous angioplasty** in acute myocardial infarction has fueled the fire (12A). Less than 20% of hospitals in the United States have adequate facilities for percutaneous transluminal coronary angioplasty (PTCA), and fewer are able to perform primary PTCA (13). Arguments are being made that the availability of interventional procedures must be expanded if primary PTCA is to be available as first-line therapy in acute myocardial infarction. If this trend is justified in the future, a great debate will undoubtedly be staged. It will be argued that not only should diagnostic facilities be brought closer to the patient, but also that these facilities should provide interventional coronary capabilities as well!

Concerns Fostered By This Expansion

Many issues need resolution before the current expansion of cardiovascular services can be readily embraced by either the medical community or the patients these facilities are designed to serve. **Patient safety** must always be foremost in the development of any cardiovascular services. Other operational issues must be addressed, such as staffing, ownership, quality control, reimbursement, and credentialing. Some of these nontraditional settings may lead to at least the perception of physician conflict-of-interest. In addition, there is little data available regarding the impact of these services on local and regional fixed cardiac catheterization services and on overall medical costs.

Regardless of the laboratory setting, certain basic guidelines must apply. For optimal laboratory usage and cost effectiveness, the cardiac catheterization laboratory should not be used as a multipurpose facility but should be reserved for cardiovascular procedures only. It is generally accepted that a minimum caseload of 300 adult (14) and 150 pediatric (15) procedures a year should be done in any laboratory. A minimum of 150 adult or 75 pediatric procedures a year should be done per physician to maintain skills. A cardiologist performing PTCA should do at least 50 per year, and electrophysiologists should participate in no less than 100 cases annually (11).

These physician and laboratory minimums could be problematic in some of the new cardiac catheterization laboratory settings. For instance, a local cardiologist performing studies in a smaller hospital or in a mobile van may not always meet these minimal guidelines. In addition, even in a traditional catheterization laboratory setting, many cardiologists perform PTCA only when they are on call, and thus do not come close to achieving the minimum suggested. With the expansion of invasive services to smaller hospitals and communities, the wisdom of allowing for arrangements where less than minimal procedures are performed should be seriously questioned.

Importance of Minimal Patient and Procedural Volumes

Several recent reports have focused on whether minimum volumes are relevant in determining the need to expand catheterization laboratories. This relevancy is perhaps best exemplified by examining outcome data relative to volume of procedures in facilities performing PTCA. Jollis et al. examined the relation between the volume of PTCA procedures performed by individual hospitals and subsequent short-term mortality in a Medicare database (16). A strong inverse correlation between the volume of procedures and short-term mortality (as well as coronary artery bypass procedures after PTCA) was found. Extrapolation of these findings led to the author's suggestion that an annual volume of 200 to 400 PTCA procedures per hospital is the minimum necessary to reduce the risk of negative outcomes from these procedures. This volume is higher than that recommended by the current American College of Cardiology/American Heart Association (ACC/AHA) guidelines but is supported by analysis of the 1992 and 1993 Society for Cardiac

Angiography and Interventions (SCAI) registry data (17). In these latter registries, no significant difference in outcome was found in laboratories performing less than 200 interventions per year compared with those performing a larger number, but a significant decrease in major complications in those performing more than 400 cases versus those performing less than 200 was noted.

The inverse relationship between procedure volume and outcome is also evident when the volume of procedures performed by the individual interventional cardiologist is considered. Recent findings from the Medicare database have shown that lower physician PTCA volumes (less than 50 Medicare cases per year) were associated with higher rates of bypass surgery or death after controlling for a variety of baseline patient characteristics (18A, 18B). The minimum number of cases per physician thus translates into approximately 100 to 150 Medicare cases per year for any one individual physician. If interventional procedures are allowed to expand to remote sites, it seems unlikely that minimal numbers could be achieved by most of the practicing cardiologists in these areas.

The issue is currently even more topical because of the ploy applied by some centers to justify the development of an interventional laboratory to support primary angioplasty requirements. Recent randomized trials comparing primary PTCA with thrombolytic therapy for the treatment of acute myocardial infarction have shown a significant reduction of recurrent ischemic events with direct PTCA (12A, 19–21). However, in the Myocardial Infarction, Triage, and Intervention (MITI) Registry, the advantages of primary PTCA over thrombolytic therapy were less apparent when the procedures were compared on a community-wide level (22).

The discrepancy between randomized trial data and the community-based registry results may be the result of many factors, including the experience of the physicians performing primary PTCA, adherence to the strict protocol for primary PTCA, and the ability and dedication of the personnel to perform primary PTCA in a timely fashion. These factors may not be uniformly present or reproducible in the community setting or for all patients suffering acute myocardial infarction. Indeed, there is evidence from a number of community-based registries demonstrating greater time delays to primary PTCA (door-to-balloon inflation) compared with thrombolytic therapy (door-to-needle) (22–24). The apparent influence of these factors on the role of primary PTCA has led the ACC/AHA Committee on Management of Acute Myocardial Infarction to recommend that primary PTCA be performed "as an alternate to thrombolytic therapy only if performed in a timely fashion by individuals skilled in the procedure and supported by experienced personnel in high-volume centers" (i.e., physicians performing more than 75 PTCA procedures per year in centers that perform more than 200 PTCA procedures per year) (25). Otherwise, clearly the highest risk patients (those with acute myocardial infarction and often with hemodynamic instability) will have emergent PTCA performed by operators with the least experience.

Concern over the potential delay in achieving vessel patency in patients with acute myocardial infarction undergoing primary PTCA (the ACC/AHA guidelines recommend balloon dilatation within 60 to 90 minutes of diagnosis of an acute MI) has prompted questions of whether this procedure should be performed in hospitals without on-site cardiac surgery. Obviously, to meet the stringent time guidelines for efficacy, transfer between hospitals becomes almost impossible. Data from the MITI registry suggested that primary PTCA could be performed in hospitals without cardiothoracic surgical backup (26). Overall procedural success rates were 88% in this registry, and only 1.4% of patients so treated underwent emergency surgery. Furthermore, in comparing patients treated at centers without surgical backup with those treated at centers with on-site surgery, no significant difference in mortality as evaluated during the procedure, at the time of discharge, or at one year follow-up was found.

The limiting caveat in the MITI trial that might not make it universally applicable, however, was that the cardiologists at the centers without on-site surgery were all high-volume interventionalists. Additionally, the mechanisms for transfer to a tertiary center were well-defined, and the surgical centers were close by. This scenario may be a workable one in isolated settings but would not be universally applicable.

CARDIAC CATHETERIZATION LABORATORY SETTINGS

Cardiac catheterization is associated with well-defined risks to the patient. Although these risks have declined in the last decade, there remains a finite risk of death from diagnostic catheterization of approximately 1 to 1.5 per thousand. Other patients at highest risk for morbidity or mortality include the very young and very old, those with left main coronary artery disease, those with significant congestive heart failure and reduced left ventricular function, those with renal insufficiency, and those with significant valvular disease, especially aortic stenosis (2, 27) (Table 2.1).

Patients undergoing interventional procedures are at even greater risk because of the very nature of the procedure. Although overall mortality is similar to that for diagnostic catheterization in patients with stable

Table 2.1.
High-Risk Patients for Diagnostic Cardiac Catheterization

Patient Characteristic	Mortality Rate (%)
Overall mortality	0.14
Age-related mortality	
<1 yr	1.75
>60 yr	0.25
Severity of coronary artery disease	
Single or double vessel disease	0.03
Three vessel disease	0.16
Left main disease	0.86
Severity of congestive heart failure	
NYHA FC I or II	0.02
NYHA FC III	0.12
NYHA FC IV	0.67
Symptomatic valvular heart disease	0.28

NYHA FC, New York Heart Assoc. Functional Class.

Table 2.2.
High-Risk Patient Clinical Characteristics
for Coronary Interventional Procedures

Advanced age
Female gender
Diabetes mellitus
Congestive heart failure
Unstable angina
Inadequate antiplatelet therapy
PTCA immediately following thrombolytic
   therapy
PTCA at the time of initial catheterization for
   unstable angina

Adaptd from Ryan TJ, Bauman WB, Kennedy JW, et al. Guidelines for percutaneous transluminal coronary angioplasty. J Am Coll Cardiol 1993;22:2033–2054.

symptoms (presumably because of a selection bias regarding what patients undergo interventional procedures), abrupt closure remains a problem in approximately 5% and urgent coronary artery bypass surgery for acute complications is required in 1 to 3% (28). Even though high-risk procedures often can be anticipated, the *only "easy" case is in retrospect* (Table 2.2).

Cardiovascular surgery is, therefore, an important adjunct to invasive procedures whenever high-risk patients are studied or interventional procedures are contemplated. While most interventional facilities no longer have a standby operating room or surgeon except in unusually high-risk situations, such facilities must be available in-house if even diagnostic catheterization is to be performed on the highest risk patients. Facilities that have such approved cardiovascular surgical backups can obviously offer the full range of invasive services.

"Traditional" Adult Cardiovascular Laboratory with In-House Cardiovascular Surgery

Definition

The traditional cardiac catheterization laboratory is organized, operated, and administrated in a hospital setting. Depending on hospital size, number of cardiologists, types of procedures, and financial constraints, many hospitals have more than one such laboratory. In-house cardiovascular surgery implies that a cardiac operating facility is accessible from the catheterization laboratory by gurney. Thus, in-house surgical suites may be located in a building directly connected or adjacent to the cardiac catheterization suite.

Operational Concerns

The operation of the traditional laboratory should be in accordance with the most recent guidelines from the ACC/AHA Task Force report (11). Complication rates should be carefully recorded and a prospective registry maintained. This registry should be regularly reviewed, and scheduled conferences should be held to review major complications. If research protocols are combined with diagnostic catheterization, these studies must not increase procedural risk; and all research-related procedures must be reviewed and approved by a committee established by the local institution review board.

Cardiac catheterization laboratories are changing rapidly. There is continuing movement away from cinefilm as a review media and toward digital methods. Many laboratories have made the move prematurely, before the complete development of the transfer media and archival methods has been resolved (29). Recent efforts by the American College of Cardiology, the European Society of Cardiology, the American Radiological Society, and NEMA have led to the acceptance of the DICOM (Digital Imaging and Communications in Medicine) standards as the format for all digital imaging. This group has approved the use of recordable discs (CD-R) as a transfer media among laboratories. A variety of solutions for archival storage are now available that allow for the complete conversion from cinefilm to digital imaging. Most fixed laboratories will move to incorporate these new technologies. Because laboratories with in-house surgery will continue providing interventional services to patients catheterized in outside laboratories that may be slow to convert to digital imaging, the full-service laboratory must be equipped to handle a variety of media until the transition to all-digital laboratories is complete. The tertiary facility provides an opportunity for some quality assessment of these referral sites, and every effort should be made to relate any problems observed to the referring site to improve the quality of these facilities.

High-risk procedures should always be done in consultation with cardiovascular surgery. This is especially true when support devices, such as percutaneous cardiopulmonary bypass, are used (30). Cardiac anesthesia may also be helpful in some instances. A few facilities now have a cardiac catheterization laboratory room that can be urgently converted into a surgical suite. This type of facility is generally unavailable to most physicians, however. In general, interventional procedures are performed at a setting separate from the diagnostic procedure, although time and money may be saved by using a combined approach (31). If a combined approach is planned, patient consent for both procedures should be obtained before the catheterization. It is inappropriate to ask the patient to consent to an interventional procedure while he or she is still on the catheterization table.

Because of the specialized nature of pediatric and electrophysiologic procedures, separate technical staffing for those procedures is desirable whenever possible. If too few procedures of this nature are done in one facility to allow for such specialized staffing, the institution should review the appropriateness of performing such procedures. This helps to ensure that specialized studies are consistently performed in the highest manner possible.

Patient Types

The full-service facility provides an environment for interdisciplinary interaction among the adult and pediatric cardiologists, radiologists, anesthesiologists, and surgeons. Certain procedures, including PTCA or other coronary interventions, valvuloplasty, myocardial biopsy, transseptal catheterization, and left ventricular punc-

ture, should be performed only where cardiovascular surgical support is available. Both inpatients and outpatients may be studied. Because of a growing trend toward outpatient cardiac catheterization, facilities should be made available to appropriately house these ambulatory patients and any accompanying family members both before and after the procedure. Table 2.3 summarizes the patients appropriate for study in a facility with cardiovascular surgical backup if appropriate equipment, clinical competence, and expertise are present. Basically, most types of cardiovascular patients may be studied in this setting. Obviously, many traditional facilities with surgical backup should not perform certain complex studies if these types of patients present problems that are beyond the capabilities of either the facility or the physicians involved.

Specialized Cardiovascular Laboratory with In-House Cardiovascular Surgery

Pediatric Cardiac Catheterization Laboratory

Definition

The pediatric cardiac catheterization laboratory is a specialized laboratory for children that should be supervised by a pediatric cardiologist and supported by both pediatric cardiac surgery and anesthesia. Its mission is the study of complex congenital heart disease in the neonate, infant, and adolescent. As the role of pediatric cardiac catheterization has expanded to include many interventional procedures, such as closure devices, septostomy, and vascular coils, the pediatric catheterization program should be developed in close cooperation with pediatric surgery. Adult patients with congenital heart disease are usually best studied in the adult cardiac catheterization laboratory, with both an adult and a pediatric cardiologist in attendance. When this is not possible, it is sometimes better for the adult patient with congenital heart disease to be studied

Table 2.3.
Patients Eligible for Catheterization Procedures when In-house Cardiovascular Surgery Is Available

Adult Patients	
Most facilities:	All diagnostic cardiovascular procedures within competence of operators
	All therapeutic coronary procedures within competence of operators
Specialized facilities:	Complex diagnostic procedures
	Transseptal catheterization, patients with complex congenital heart disease
	Complex therapeutic procedures
	Highest risk angioplasty, atherectomy or stents, balloon valvuloplasty, adult congenital intervention
Pediatric Patients	
Most facilities:	All diagnostic procedures within competence of operators
	Limited therapeutic procedures
	Balloon septostomy, pulmonic valvuloplasty
Specialized facilities:	Complex diagnostic procedures
	Therapeutic procedures
	Blade septostomy, coil embolization, coarctation, angioplasty, occluder applications (ASD, PDA, VSD closure), aortic or mitral valvuloplasty, pulmonary arterial and other stents, other investigational methods
Electrophysiology Patients	
Most facilities:	Diagnostic procedures within competence of operators
	Limited therapeutic procedures
	Permanent pacemaker implantation, drug evaluation
Specialized facilities:	Complex diagnostic problems
	Therapeutic procedures
	Implantable defibrillators, arrhythmia ablation, antitachycardia devices

ASD, atrial septal defect; PDA, patent ductus arteriosa; VSD, ventricular septal defect.

in the pediatric facility where there is familiarity with the problems involved.

Operational Concerns

The pediatric cardiac catheterization laboratory should have biplane cineangiography available. Digital angiography is also desirable. Temperature regulation equipment is important if neonates are to be studied. A large and complete inventory of specialized catheters and emergency devices is important. The pediatric cardiologist must be proficient in pediatric invasive cardiology and should meet requirements suggested by the ACC/AHA Task Force on pediatric therapeutic intervention if such procedures are contemplated (15). Close cooperation with

a cardiovascular surgeon familiar with congenital disease is critical to ensure that adequate data is obtained.

Patient Types

A diagnostic pediatric cardiac catheterization laboratory should be able to tackle all diagnostic procedures and perform balloon atrial septostomy. Table 2.3 outlines appropriate patient types depending on the commitment of the laboratory and personnel. The more complex the interventional procedure, the greater the commitment must be by the institution and pediatric cardiologists involved. The most complex procedures should be performed only in active therapeutic catheterization centers, by cardiologists who have had specific training in the use of these devices and who are participating in active investigational protocols (15).

Invasive Electrophysiology Laboratory

Definition

The invasive electrophysiology laboratory is a dedicated facility with provisions for pacing, defibrillation, and resuscitation. A trained and experienced clinical electrophysiologist must supervise it. It is designed for both a diagnostic and a therapeutic approach to arrhythmia identification and management.

Operational Concerns

The dedicated electrophysiologic laboratory should have high-resolution fluoroscopy available for localization of catheters within the heart and should be equipped to perform a complete electrophysiology study of any type of cardiac conduction disturbance. A minimal facility would include a programmable stimulator and recording devices. The electrophysiology laboratory should be an integral part of a complete electrophysiology program that includes noninvasive capabilities such as routine ECG, ambulatory and exercise ECG, and signal-averaging capabilities. A pacemaker program, including a follow-up system, should also exist. As the opportunities for interventional procedures continue advancing, the laboratory must review its capabilities in depth to ensure that the facility and personnel can adequately and safely perform procedures such as radiofrequency ablation, transseptal puncture, and defibrillator implantation (32).

A surgical program is highly desirable and should be considered mandatory in a training environment (33). Surgery provides not only effective therapy for selected ventricular or supraventricular tachyar-

rhythmias but also backup for potential complications in the laboratory. Complication rates during electrophysiologic studies are surprisingly low, however, partly because primary access is venous. Perforation (often through the right ventricle or coronary sinus) occurs in 1 of 1000 patients, with death occurring in 1 of 2000 (34).

Patient Types

Clinical electrophysiologic testing is useful in a variety of conduction disorders. Most electrophysiologic laboratories should be equipped to evaluate the common bradyarrhythmias and tachyarrhythmias by use of intracardiac electrograms and programmed stimulation. Both temporary and permanent pacemaker implantations should be part of the program. The use of the newer implantable arrhythmia devices and the performance of arrhythmia ablation are best left to a center where the expertise and volume warrant this therapeutic approach. Training guidelines recommend that at least 10 implantable defibrillators, 10 transseptals, and 50 radiofrequency ablations be performed for certification (32). Although there are no established minimums for sustaining competency at this time, clearly only a large center with a wide referral base could sustain enough volume to ensure the safety and adequacy of studies performed.

Cardiac Catheterization in a Facility Without Cardiothoracic Surgical Support

Performance of cardiac catheterization in a facility without cardiovascular surgical support is now commonplace in the United States. Patients undergoing procedures in this type of facility need very careful screening to minimize risks. Patients can be studied in many settings, including the more traditional in-hospital fixed laboratory, the mobile unit attached to either a hospital or a freestanding facility, or an entirely separate freestanding facility. In the mobile and freestanding facilities, the majority of patients are ambulatory.

Traditional Fixed Cardiac Catheterization Laboratory in a Hospital Without Cardiovascular Surgical Support

A random survey of cardiac catheterization facilities in 1989 by the SCAI revealed that 453 of 1302 (35%) of all catheterization laboratory facilities were located in hospitals without surgical support (9). Since the publication of that report, the number of such laboratories has likely increased substantially. There is little data available to compare the patient populations and results from these laboratories with programs with in-house cardiovascular surgery.

In a preliminary review of two such programs associated with Duke Medical Center, certain observations are summarized in Table 2.4. One of the fixed laboratories reviewed is in a rural hospital with 388 beds; the other is in a suburban hospital with 457 beds. The data presented is compared with that of Duke Medical Center, with 1125 beds and cardiovascular surgical backup. Using appropriate screening, complication rates in facilities without surgical backup appear acceptably low. Of interest, however, is that one would expect much less severe illness in these fixed laboratories without backup surgery; but the data suggest that this is not necessarily so. Although fewer patients with severe heart failure were seen, a high number of patients with unstable angina (34–54%) were studied. In fact, 32 to 41% of patients were on the local coronary care unit at the time of the procedure. The breakdown in the extent of coronary disease discovered is not dissimilar to that seen at a tertiary center with surgical backup. This clearly suggests that guidelines need to be developed for these hospitals to reflect the practice being performed. Unfortunately, guidelines specific for such a setting have yet to be explicitly defined. It also means that some patients at high risk will be studied at these facilities regardless of the best intentions. For this reason, careful quality control measures must be included when establishing these programs.

Operational Concerns

Cardiac catheterization procedures in a hospital without surgical backup require that a meticulous and careful screening procedure be in place to avoid situations that might require urgent cardiac surgery. A formal review process should be instituted, and for-

Table 2.4.
Comparison of Patient Populations Undergoing Diagnostic Cardiac Catheterization in Differing Laboratory Settings

	No On-site CV Surgery			On-site CV Surgery	
	Rural Lab n = 155	Suburban Lab 235	Mobile Lab 237	Outpatient 570	Inpatient 1277
Complication rates					
All patients	3%	1 %	3 %	2%	9 %
Severe	1%	0.4%	0.3%	0%	0.7%
Relevant patient characteristics					
Unstable angina	54%	34%	3%	4%	49%
Patients on CCU	41%	32%	8%	0%	42%
NYHA FC 3–4 CHF	1%	1%	<1%	1%	6%
Severity of coronary artery disease					
None/insignificant	33%	30%	46%	44%	27%
None + prior PTCA	3%	<1%	3%	22%	2%
Left main disease	7%	3%	4%	1%	6%

CV, cardiovascular; NYHA FC, New York Heart Assoc. Functional Class; CHF, congestive heart failure; CCU, coronary care unit.

mal relationships with a nearby tertiary hospital should be established. Screening criteria should be published and enforced to reduce the risks of serious complications. The fixed laboratories should be of a quality similar to those where surgical programs exist. The safety, quality assurance, staffing, and utilization requirements for such laboratories should adhere to published guidelines (11). Minimal caseloads must be maintained for the laboratory and the physicians performing procedures. Each laboratory should have appropriate hemodynamic support devices available (such as balloon aortic counterpulsation devices) and the expertise to quickly stabilize the patient with a complication until arrangements for transfer to a referral center are underway.

Patient Types

Intuitively it seems that patient screening at any site without in-house cardiovascular surgery should mimic that described for the ambulatory patient. In reality, however, many patients with serious disease are being studied in fixed laboratories without surgical backup. While the data do not yet support such an aggressive approach, patients are obviously being safely cared for in such facilities. Table 2.5 shows which patients should be considered for diagnostic catheterization in these facilities. Clearly, *no* data support interventional procedures

such as PTCA, myocardial biopsy, or transseptal catheterization in any setting without cardiovascular surgical support. Putting the patient at unnecessary risk by performing coronary interventions in a facility where cardiovascular surgery is not readily available is not an accepted standard of care, despite anecdotal reports of its safety. Generally, no pediatric patient procedure and only basic diagnostic electrophysiologic procedures should be done in such a facility. In most situations, the volume of pediatric and electrophysiology procedures do not support such programs in this environment.

Mobile Cardiac Catheterization

Mobile cardiac catheterization laboratories have increased in number since their inception in 1987. These laboratories were initially developed in the Midwest, and their expansion to other states has led to controversy among members of the cardiology community (10–12). Attempts at collecting important data on these units have been limited, unfortunately.

Mobile cardiac catheterization facilities provide several potentially positive features that make them attractive to the hospital using the service. For the patient, they provide a means of undergoing an invasive diagnostic procedure while remaining at home or in the local hospital. The units may

Table 2.5.
Patients Eligible for Cardiac Catheterization when In-House Surgery is Not Available

Type of Patient	Diagnostic Procedures	Therapeutic Procedures
Adult	All patients except those at greatest risk for mortality or morbidity. Includes stable patients following myocardial infarction, those without NYHA FC III or IV CHF and those with low risk for left main disease	None approved at this time
Pediatric	None approved at this time	None approved at this time
Electrophysiology	Routine evaluation of both supraventricular and ventricular arrhythmias; drug evaluations	Permanent pacemaker implantation, cardioversion

NYHA FC, New York Heart Assoc. Functional Class; CHF, congestive heart failure.

also provide access to care that the patient might not receive otherwise. It may also be less risky for the patient to undergo cardiac catheterization with an experienced cardiologist who normally performs many procedures and comes to the rural hospital than it would be with a local cardiologist who may perform only a few procedures on the mobile unit. For the local hospital, mobile catheterization provides a visible symbol to the public that the facility is able to provide a more comprehensive cardiovascular evaluation. By affiliating with a major tertiary center, the hospital also can market a credibility that might not be possible otherwise. Importantly, the hospitals can generally profit from mobile laboratory usage—both in keeping cardiovascular patients at home and in receiving the fees for service generated. For the local physician, the patient remains in town instead of being potentially lost to a tertiary care center. The patient also remains under the care of the local physician, who undoubtedly knows the patient's overall medical problems in the greatest degree. For the referral cardiologist, mobile laboratories provide access to a referral base in which they might otherwise not have a presence. Because these procedures are performed on a fee-for-service basis, the time commitment is generally justified. For the referral hospital, mobile services provide a means of increasing market share for cardiovascular services. If the hospital owns the mobile service, there are also direct profits to be realized, not only from increased referrals but also from the recovery of technical fees.

Several caveats exist however. There is no clear evidence that current use of mobile laboratories provides service for remote areas—an argument fostered by many. In actuality, recent data from Health Care Financing Administration (HCFA) suggests that there are few underserved areas. Plotting the home zip codes of 212,000 patients who had undergone cardiac catheterization against the zip codes of the catheterization laboratories revealed that 95% of the United States population lives less than 50 miles from an established catheterization laboratory and 80% live less than 25 miles away (Carl Pepine, MD, unpublished data).

Safety is a major concern. The data accumulating, however, shows that procedures done in the mobile laboratory can be done safely if screening procedures are rigorously enforced (35). How well these procedures are followed is unknown, however, and there are many unresolved problems inherent in the use of these facilities. These problems include self-referral of patients, physician ownership, and the potential for fee splitting or fee sharing between the local physician and the cardiologist (11). Minimal data is available regarding the cost effectiveness of the service and the impact these laboratories have on established cardiac catheterization facilities in the same area. Emergency transportation can also be problematic, especially in poor weather, or when there is only an all-volunteer ambulance service without EMS training available for transporting a critically ill patient.

Oversight remains an issue, especially when a mobile laboratory is not directly affiliated with a tertiary hospital. These units may foster the unnecessary expansion of services for financial reasons rather than for patient care ideals. Currently, no mechanisms are in place to ensure that patients are being studied for appropriate medical reasons and not for convenience or profit. In an era in which many local hospitals are in financial jeopardy, there is certainly an opportunity for direct or indirect pressure to be applied to local physicians to support a mobile program in an effort to help the hospital's bottom line. There is little penetrance of managed care in many areas of the United States, despite its gradual spread. The financial advantages or disadvantages of mobile programs in a heavily managed care environment need to be addressed.

Some of the general issues surrounding mobile cardiac catheterization have been reviewed by the SCAI (36). The Society stresses that (a) the mobile laboratory should not be used solely to expand market share; (b) the need should be determined by an objective governmental authority (although this is unspecified); (c) formal agreements should be made for ambulance support and emergency backup to ensure patient safety; (d) screening procedures should be specific, and a local vascular surgeon's involvement should be included in the program; (*e*) the cardiologist should be on the staff of the tertiary hospital and meet credentials outlined by the Society; and (*f*) cardiologists performing procedures should not have a financial interest in the mobile laboratory itself. These recommendations make common sense and should be considered whenever a mobile program is being initiated.

Definition

Mobile laboratories are transportable catheterization laboratories. They can be used temporarily at a hospital while a fixed laboratory is undergoing construction or repair. Occasionally this "temporary" status is transformed into a much more permanent arrangement. In this temporary role, they may be continuously left on site or intermittently used. When used in a temporary role, the laboratories may be at a hospital with or without cardiovascular surgical backup. Mobile units can also be used to provide strictly mobile services as an outreach function of a major tertiary care physician group or hospital. As such, the units move periodically (usually daily) to a series of sites. These sites are usually rural hospitals, but the mobile units also can be used in an entirely freestanding situation in urban areas.

Operational Concerns

The proper operation of a mobile van for the performance of cardiac catheterization at a local hospital requires a major commitment on the part of local physicians, the local hospital, the cardiologists involved, and the tertiary care facility. The mobile van service should be operated by either the tertiary care center or a separate organization established to provide such services. Physicians should not become owners in these ventures to avoid conflict of interest. Neither the referring physician nor the cardiologist should profit from technical fees received.

Duke Medical Center has successfully operated a mobile program since 1989. In reviewing that experience, several issues appear important for the successful operation of such units. Motivation for the performance of a mobile service should come from the local community and not be driven by a tertiary facility wishing only to capture more market share. In the Duke Medical Center experience, the service is provided as part of an outreach program that involves consultative services in many areas. The mobile unit was also used as part of an effort to recruit local cardiologists for the community. The service is owned and staffed by Duke Medical Center. Two nurses and one or two technicians are in the van at all times. The second nurse provides important backup; if a patient needs urgent transportation from the van, this nurse would accompany the patient back to the hospital. The mobile van crew also spends considerable time teaching the staff at each hospital involved. Before the service is initiated, the local hospital nurses also spend time at Duke Medical Center learning how to care for the postcatheterization patient. Several meetings are held with the local medical staff to review selection criteria, establish a method of referral to the mobile laboratory, and outline procedures for the urgent removal and transfer to Duke via air or ground ambulance should a complication arise. Provisions for foul weather are arranged and in place. Periodic review of the program is provided to the local medical staff.

The mobile laboratory itself is equipped precisely as a fixed laboratory, although digital imaging has not yet been incorporated in the vans. The hospital has added an additional air conditioner and an emergency power backup for safety. The hospital has also developed a rapid, automated cardiac catheterization report generation system that allows for a graphical tree and full cardiac catheterization report to be generated, completed, and signed before the cardiologist leaves the local site (37). All hemodynamic, anatomic, and ventriculographic data, along with a complete demographic description of the patient and the procedure, are then entered on-line into a searchable permanent record for later data analysis (38). The referring physician is called after each procedure and the completed report is placed in his or her mailbox before the van departs.

These vans travel to sites as far as $2\frac{1}{2}$ hours away by automobile. Generally, the cardiologist and one or two staff members fly a fixed wing aircraft to these distant sites. The rest of the staff arrive by custom van. Each patient is seen, screened for appropriateness, and worked up by the catheterizing cardiologist while the crew prepares the mobile laboratory.

The cardiologist remains on-site until all patients are ambulatory. More than 90% of patients studied in the mobile van are ambulatory. The patients are given a copy of their report and a series of phone numbers to use if problems arise. In addition, a postcard is provided for comments and follow-up data. All patients are subsequently followed as part of the Duke Database for Cardiovascular Diseases. Follow-up is obtained at 6 months, 1 year, and then yearly.

The hospital that allows the mobile service charges for the procedure. A fixed technical fee is charged by Duke Medical Center. A single mobile van services only one hospital each day. Fees for professional services are billed separately. The mobile unit is moved at night between hospitals and does not operate if inclement weather would prohibit emergency transportation.

Patient Types

The type of patients eligible for cardiac catheterization in a mobile van depends on the facilities available at the local hospital. Table 2.6 reviews patient eligibility for the mobile laboratory when in-house cardiovascular surgery is present. These are similar to a fixed laboratory with adequate backup. If there is no in-house cardiovascular surgery, the criteria used are similar to those for ambulatory patients. These are summarized in Table 2.7.

We have limited experience in testing these criteria. Table 2.4 describes the initial 6-month mobile van data and compares it with our simultaneous in-house outpatient program. Complications were minimal using the screening criteria described; only one serious complication occurred (transient ventricular fibrillation that was cardioverted without sequelae). In general, the patient characteristics compared favorably with that observed in our outpatient program.

It does appear that a mobile service that operates safely can be developed when appropriate safeguards are built into the system. Patients studied in the mobile vans have generally had positive feelings toward the experience, and it generates income for both the tertiary hospital and the local community. In our own experience, the greatest financial benefit has been through establishment of important ties to the local community and through the identification of patients requiring further procedures. The service itself is run at a slight loss.

Several important observations have been noted. The number of patients without significant ($\leq$50% diameter narrowing) coronary disease is high—46% in our initial experience. There are several possible explanations for this, including the rigid

Table 2.6.
Patients Eligible for Cardiac Catheterization in a Mobile Van Facility when In-House Surgery is Available

Type of Patient	Diagnostic Procedures	Therapeutic Procedures
Adult	Patients within operator competence	None recommended; general suboptimal laboratory environment
Pediatric	Patients within operator competence	None recommended; general suboptimal laboratory environment
Electrophysiology	Selected low-risk patients within competence of operator	Temporary pacemaker implantation, cardioversion (chemical, electrical, or catheter)

Table 2.7.
Patients Eligible for Cardiac Catheterization in a Mobile Van at a Hospital Site when In-House Surgery is Not Available

Type of Patient	Diagnostic Procedures	Therapeutic Procedures

Adult	Exclusionary criteria:
	  High risk for severe CAD
	    Unstable or progressive angina
	    Recent MI (<7 d) with any postMI symptoms
	    Pulmonary edema felt as a result of ischemia
	    High risk based on noninvasive tests
	  Congestive heart failure symptoms
	    NYHA FC III or IV
	  Certain valvular heart diseases
	    Severe AS
	    Severe AI (pulse pressure >80 mm Hg)
	  Congenital heart disease
	    Suspected severe pulmonary artery hypertension (>½ systemic)
	    Any complex congenital heart disease patient
	  High-risk resulting from systemic problems
	    Severe peripheral vascular disease, advanced age, anticoagulation, uncontrolled systemic hypertension, poorly controlled diabetes mellitus, renal insufficiency
		None

Pediatric	Not recommended at this time, although data is not available	None
Electrophysiology	None	Temporary pacemaker implantation, cardioversion

NYHA FC, New York Heart Assoc. Functional Class; CHF, congestive heart failure; AS, aortic stenosis; AI, aortic insufficiency.

screening criteria and a high prevalence of minorities. Others have reported that perhaps because of the higher prevalence of left ventricular hypertrophy in blacks, cardiac catheterization in the black population often reveals less severe coronary disease (39). When coronary disease is present in the black population, however, the survival data suggests a particularly harsh outcome—possibly related to the associated effects of hypertension and smoking (40). An alternative explanation for the high rate of insignificant disease or normal coronaries is that the threshold for cardiac catheterization has been reduced to a level wherein studies are being performed that might not have been ordered otherwise. Medicine does not tend to be a supply–demand business; the availability of a procedure tends to result in its use. This latter area clearly needs monitoring to assure that unnecessary expansion of invasive cardiovascular services is not occurring.

Freestanding Cardiac Catheterization Facilities

A freestanding facility is one that provides cardiac catheterization services but is not physically attached to a hospital. It may be located adjacent to a hospital or be a considerable distance from the hospital. "Adjacent" has been defined as so close that patients could be transported by gurney to the hospital. The unit may be within an established building, within an attached modular building, or a mobile laboratory. A 1989 survey revealed 21 of 1302 (1.6%) cardiac catheterization facilities were freestanding at that time. The number of freestanding facilities has likely grown minimally since then, although there are no definite data describing the current prevalence of this type of facility.

Freestanding facilities are saddled with the same concerns expressed for mobile units, with the added skepticism that such a facility will lend itself to even less regulation than a mobile laboratory associated with a hospital. The HCFA defines these freestanding units as independent ambulatory surgical centers (41). Data from such freestanding facilities is sparse (40–44). In a review of outpatient and freestanding facilities, Kahn (41) could find no data comparing complications between hospital-affiliated and freestanding units. Beauchamp (43) reported in 1981 that approximately $360 could be saved by using freestanding facilities, but there is a paucity of recent data available to interpret current cost effectiveness.

A freestanding facility must be developed in a manner similar to that described for mobile units, with the added responsibility of reassuring the public that procedures are being carefully monitored. It should be the responsibility of the tertiary hospital used for backup to ensure that quality assurance measures are followed. These freestanding facilities should therefore be part of the JCAHO (Joint Commission on Accreditation of Healthcare Organizations) regulations applied to the supporting tertiary facility. **Because of the lack of data and the concern regarding such units, a freestanding facility cannot be recommended at this time.** In general, patient criteria would be expected to be the same as with a mobile facility.

AMBULATORY CARDIAC CATHETERIZATION

Outpatient cardiac catheterization for stable patients at low risk for complications has

Table 2.8.
Patients Eligible for Outpatient Cardiac Catheterization

Type of Patient	Diagnostic Procedures	Therapeutic Procedures
Adult	Exclusions (similar to Table 2.7) High risk for severe CAD Unstable or progressive angina Recent MI (<7 d) with any postMI symptoms Pulmonary edema as a result of ischemia High risk based on noninvasive testing Congestive heart failure NYHA FC III or IV Advanced age or the very young Certain valvular heart diseases Severe AS or AI Congenital heart disease Any complex congenital heart disease problem High risk for catheterization as a result of other problems Severe peripheral vascular disease Morbid obesity Anticoagulation Uncontrolled systemic hypertension Poorly controlled diabetes mellitus Renal insufficiency (>1.9 creatinine) General debility, mental confusion, cachexia Recent stroke (<1 mo)	None recommended at this time
Pediatric	Stable symptoms whose diagnostic problems are within competence of operator	None recommended at this time
Electrophysiology	Simple diagnostic problems within competence of operator	Cardioversion

NYHA FC, New York Heart Assoc. Functional Class; CHF, congestive heart failure; AS, aortic stenosis; AI, aortic insufficiency.

repeatedly been shown to be cost-effective (43) and safe in selected adult (45, 46) and pediatric (47) populations. This seems to be true regardless of whether the brachial or femoral artery approach is used (48).

There have been few rigorously controlled trials, however. In one early study by Block et al. (49), even after eliminating almost 80% of eligible patients, 12% required urgent hospitalization. These results are sobering and emphasize that one must always be aware that serious complications can occur even in the apparently lowest risk patient populations. Table 2.8 reflects the highest risk diagnostic patients (2, 27, 50), and these patients should obviously not be treated, if possible, in an ambulatory setting or in one in which there is no surgical backup.

Table 2.8 summarizes the additional major exclusions one should utilize in screening patients for ambulatory cardiac catheterization (9). Patients with unstable coronary syndromes often have associated thrombus or vasoactive coronary disease; a more prolonged monitoring period after such a procedure seems only prudent. Similarly, those patients with significant left or right heart failure, with suspected severe aortic stenosis or aortic insufficiency, or symptomatic patients with complex congenital heart disease are at greater risk for early postcatheterization hemodynamic complications and should not be studied in an outpatient setting. Ambulatory patients are also at risk for vascular problems, delayed metabolic derangements, or bleeding complications. Patients with renal insufficiency are at risk for contrast nephrotoxicity and should be hydrated before the procedure and watched afterward. They should not be studied as outpatients. Despite those extensive-appearing lists, many patients are clearly eligible for ambulatory cardiac catheterization. An internal review at Duke Medical Center prior to the development of mobile services suggested that 45 to 50% of all patients previously studied as inpatients would have been eligible for an outpatient procedure using these criteria. In fact, since the inception of the Duke outpatient program in 1985, the percentage of diagnostic catheterizations performed as outpatients has increased from 16 to 36%.

SUMMARY

In the two reviews of cardiac catheterization laboratories by task forces from the ACC and AHA (9, 36), the conclusions have been similar. There is a general feeling within the cardiology community that freestanding and mobile units should not be condoned. In fact, the most recent Task Force recommended that **"the development of new facilities must be based on patient need. When a need can be documented, a traditional laboratory with cardiac surgical support is recommended.** Without supporting data from appropriate clinical trials, the development of new laboratories without cardiovascular surgical backup cannot be recommended at this time" (11). The reality is that there is continued pressure to expand services. Most recently, effort is underway not only to expand diagnostic laboratory development but also to develop—under the guise of needing a local facility to support primary angioplasty—interventional laboratories without proper cardiovascular surgical backup. It behooves us all to ensure that the expansion of both traditional and nontraditional cardiac catheterization laboratory facilities does not contribute to an expansion of services that cannot be supported by patient need. The potential for abuse requires that expansion be carefully monitored. It is in everyone's interest that the cardiology community controls the process before unnecessary governmental regulations are forced upon us. As hospital consolidations, mergers, and managed care measures continue increasing in the United States, the use of cardiac catheterization facilities in all of the settings described will continue to be carefully scrutinized.

References

1. Report of the Task Force on the availability of cardiovascular drugs to the medically indigent. Circulation 1992;85:849–860.
2. Johnson LW, Lozner EC, Johnson S, et al. Coronary arteriography 1984–1987: Report of the registry of the Society for Cardiac Angiography and Interventions. Cathet Cardiovasc Diagn 1989;17:5–10.

3. Baim DS. Angioplasty as a treatment for coronary artery disease. N Engl J Med 1992;326:56–58. [Editorial]
4. Loop FD, Lytle BW, Cosgrove DM, et al. Influence of the internal mammary artery graft on 10-year survival and other cardiac events. N Engl J Med 1986;314:1–6.
5. Califf RM, Ohman EM, Frid DJ, et al. Restenosis: the clinical issues. In: Topol E, ed. Interventional cardiology. Philadelphia: WB Saunders, 1990: 363–394.
6. Serruys PW, de Jaeger P, Kiemeneij F, et al. A comparison of balloon-expandable stent implantation with balloon angioplasty in patients with coronary artery disease: Benestent Study Group. N Engl J Med 1994;331:489–495.
7. Eeckhout E, Kappenberger L, Goy J-J. Stents for intracoronary placement: current status and future directions. J Am Coll Cardiol 1996;27:757–765.
8. Consumer Reports. Wasted health care dollars. July 1992:435–448.
9. Scanlon PJ and the Board of Trustees. Society for Cardiac Angiography and Interventions. List of U.S. cardiac catheterization laboratories. Cathet Cardiovasc Diagn 1989;16:39–77.
10. Conti CR. Cardiac catheterization laboratories: hospital-based, freestanding, or mobile? J Am Coll Cardiol 1990;15:748–750.
11. Pepine CJ, Allen HD, Bashore TM, et al. ACC/AHA guidelines for cardiac catheterization and cardiac catheterization laboratories. J Am Coll Cardiol 1991;84:2213–2247.
12. Holmes DR Jr and the Trustees of the Society for Cardiac Angiography and Interventions. The mobile cardiac catheterization laboratory: should we pick it up and move it? Cathet Cardiovasc Diagn 1992;26:69–70. [Editorial]
12A. The Global Use of Strategies to Open Occluded Coronary Arteries in Acute Coronary Syndromes (GUSTO IIb) Angioplasty Substudy investigators. A clinical trial comparing primary coronary angioplasty with tissue plasminogen activator for acute myocardial infarction. N Engl J Med 1997;336: 1621–8.
13. Lange RA, Hillis LD. Should thrombolysis or primary angioplasty be the treatment of choice for acute myocardial infarction? N Engl J Med 1996; 335:1311–1312.
14. Friesinger GC, Adams DF, Bourassa MG, et al. Optimal resources for examination of the heart and lungs: cardiac catheterization radiographic features. Circulation 1983;68:893A–930A.
15. Allen HD, Driscoll DJ, Fricker FJ, et al. Guidelines for pediatric therapeutic cardiac catheterization. A statement for health professionals from the Committee on Congenital Cardiac Defects of the Council on Cardiovascular Disease in the Young. Circulation 1991;84:2248–2258.
16. Jollis JG, Peterson ED, DeLong ER, et al. The relation between the volume of coronary angioplasty procedures at hospitals treating Medicare beneficiaries and short-term mortality. N Engl J Med 1994;331:1625–1629.
17. Kimmel E, Berlin JA, Laskey W. The relationship between angioplasty procedure volume and major complications. JAMA 1995;274:1137–1142.
18. Jollis JG, Peterson ED, Nelson CL, et al. Relationship between physician and hospital coronary angioplasty volume and outcome in elderly patients. Circulation 1997;95:2485–2491.
18A. Ellis SG, Weintraub W, Holmes D, et al. Relation of operator volume and experience to procedural outcome of percutaneous coronary revascularization at hospitals with high interventional volumes. Circulation 1997;95:2479–2484.
18B. Teirstein PS. Credentialing for coronary interventions: practice makes perfect. Circulation 1997;95: 2467–2470.
19. Zilstra F, deBoer MJ, Hoorntje JC, et al. A comparison of immediate coronary angioplasty with intravenous streptokinase in acute myocardial infarction. N Engl J Med 1993;328:680–684.
20. Gibbons RJ, Holmes DR, Reeder GS, et al. Immediate angioplasty compared with the administration of a thrombolytic agent followed by conservative treatment for myocardial infarction: the Mayo coronary care unit and catheterization laboratory groups. N Engl J Med 1993;328:685–691.
21. Grines CL, Browne KF, Marco J, et al. A comparison of immediate angioplasty with thrombolytic therapy for acute myocardial infarction: the primary angioplasty in myocardial infarction study group. N Engl J Med 1993;328:673–679.
22. Every NR, Parsons LS, Hlatky M, Martin JS, and Weaver WD. A comparison of thrombolytic therapy with primary coronary angioplasty for acute myocardial infarction. Myocardial Infarction Triage and Intervention Investigators. N Engl J Med 1996;335(17):1253–1260.
23. Rogers WJ, Dean LS, Morre PB, et al. Comparison of primary angioplasty versus thrombolytic therapy for acute myocardial infarction. Am J Cardiol 1994;74:111–118.
24. Tiefenbrunn AJ, Chandra NC, French WJ, et al. Experience with primary PTCA compared to alteplase in patients with acute myocardial infarction. Circulation 1995;92(suppl I):1–138. [Abstract]
25. Ryan TJ, Anderson JL, Antman EM, et al. ACC/AHA guidelines for the management of patients with acute myocardial infarction: a report of the American College of Cardiology/American Heart Association Task Force on practice guidelines (committee on management of acute myocardial infarction). J Am Coll Cardiol 1996;28:1328–1428.
26. Weaver WD, Litwin PE, Martin JS, et al. Use of direct angioplasty for treatment of patients with acute myocardial infarction in hospitals with and without on-site cardiac surgery. Circulation 1993; 88:2067–2075.
27. Folland ED, Oprian C, Giacomini J, et al. Complications of cardiac catheterization and angiography in patients with valvular heart disease. Cathet Cardiovasc Diagn 1989;17:15–21.
28. Forrester JS, Eigler N, Litrack F. Interventional cardiology: the disease ahead. Circulation 1991;84: 942–944. [Editorial]
29. Nissen SE, Pepine CJ, Bashore TM, et al. Cardiac angiography without cine film: erecting a "Tower of Babel" in the cardiac catheterization laboratory. J Am Coll Cardiol 1994;24:834–837.
30. Cohn LH, Chitwood WR Jr, Jones RH, et al. Interventional catheterization procedures and cardio-

thoracic surgical consultation. Cardiovascular Surgery Committee. J Am Coll Cardiol 1992;19:1363.

31. O'Keefe JH Jr, Gernon C, McCallister BD, et al. Safety and cost effectiveness of combined coronary angiography and angioplasty. Am Heart J 1991; 122:50–54.

32. Josephson ME, Maloney JD, Barold SS, et al. Training in specialized electrophysiologic cardiac pacing and arrhythmia management. J Am Coll Cardiol 1995;25:1–35.

33. Flowers NC, Abildskov JA, Armstrong WF, et al. Recommended guidelines for training in adult cardiac electrophysiology. J Am Coll Cardiol 1991;18: 637–640.

34. Horowitz LN, Kay HR, Kutalek SP, et al. Risks and complications of clinical cardiac electrophysiologic studies: a prospective analysis of 1,000 patients. J Am Coll Cardiol 1987;9:1261–1268.

35. Elliott CM, Bersin RM, Elliott AV, et al. Mobile Cardiac Catheterization Laboratory, Cathet Cardiovasc Diagn 1994;31(1):8–15.

36. Goss JE, Cameron A. Mobile cardiac catheterization laboratories. Cathet Cardiovasc Diagn 1992; 26:71–72.

37. Spero LA, Fortin DJ, Cusma JT, et al. A computerized method for the application of coronary artery disease risk classification models to a large patient population. IEEE Comput Cardiol 1992:211–214.

38. Hlatky MA, Lee KL, Harrell FE Jr, et al. Tying clinical research to patient care by use of an observational database. Stat Med 1984;3:375–384.

39. Simmons BE, Castaner A, Mar M, et al. Survival determinants in black patients with angiographically defined coronary artery disease. Am Heart J 1990;119:513–518.

40. Maynard C, Fisher LD, Passamani ER. Survival of black persons compared with white persons in the coronary artery surgery study (CASS). Am J Cardiol 1987;60:513–518.

41. Kahn KL. The efficacy of ambulatory cardiac catheterization in the hospital and freestanding setting. Am Heart J 1986;111:152–167.

42. Baird CL. The trend to outpatient care: ambulatory cardiac catheterization. VA Med Mon 1980;107: 621–629.

43. Beauchamp PK. Ambulatory cardiac catheterization cuts costs for hospitals and patients. Hospitals 1981;55:62–67.

44. Jackson MN. Cardiac catheterization in a standing setting. Health Technol Assess 1989;6:1–8.

45. Klinke WP, Kubac G, Talibi T, et al. Safety of outpatient cardiac catheterizations. Am J Cardiol 1985; 56:639–641.

46. Clements SD Jr, Gatlin S. Outpatient cardiac catheterization: a report of 3,000 cases. Clin Cardiol 1991; 14:477–480.

47. Cumming GR. Cardiac catheterization in infants and children can be an outpatient procedure. Am J Cardiol 1982;49:1248–1253.

48. Oldroyd KG, Phadke KV, Phillips R, et al. Cardiac catheterization by the Judkins technique as an outpatient procedure. Br Med J 1989;298:875–876.

49. Block PC, Ockene J, Goldberg RJ, et al. A prospective randomized trial of outpatient versus inpatient cardiac catheterization. N Engl J Med 1988;319: 1251–1255.

50. Kennedy JW and the Registry Committee of the Society for Cardiac Angiography. Complications associated with cardiac catheterization and angiography. Cathet Cardiovasc Diagn 1982;8:5–11.

3
Training and Training Requirements for Cardiac Catheterization

Patrick J. Scanlon, MD

INTRODUCTION

The cardiology fellowship program has been and continues to be the main arena for training in cardiac catheterization. Although the emergence of new interventional procedures and technologies requires that some training occurs postfellowship, it is never appropriate to initiate the learning of basic catheterization skills outside a fellowship program. Thus, this chapter will mainly emphasize the fellowship training of cardiac catheterization.

There are no objective data available regarding the best method of training a cardiologist in cardiac catheterization, including the number of months or the number of cases needed. Guidelines for training are based on expert consensus in the field of catheterization and continue to evolve (especially in interventional cardiology) as new procedures emerge. Until objective data become available, training recommendations should stand as guidelines only, not as standards.

The 17th Bethesda Conference Report established the most widely accepted guidelines for training in adult cardiology (1). The Task Force on training in cardiac catheterization of that conference defined three levels of training for three types of cardiologists: level 1, the cardiologist not doing cardiac catheterization or angiography; level 2, the cardiologist performing diag-

nostic cardiac catheterization and angiography; and level 3, the cardiologist performing diagnostic cardiac catheterization, angiography, and other advanced cardiac catheterization procedures such as angioplasty or similar procedures as they develop (2). Guidelines were updated in 1995 by the Core Cardiology Training Symposium (COCATS) (3). Task Force 3 of COCATS specifically dealt with training in cardiac catheterization and interventional cardiology (4). Much of the information in this chapter is based on that group's report.

FELLOWSHIP TRAINING IN CARDIAC CATHETERIZATION

Little has been written about the appropriate process for selecting young physicians into cardiology training programs. All too often a program will take an applicant mainly to fill a manpower service need, with little concern for the trainee's education. This type of program may accept an applicant based more on availability than on his or her qualifications to learn the broad range of knowledge and skills required to become an effective cardiologist. This practice must be condemned. **Inevitably, even well-intentioned programs will have a trainee who is unsuited for the rigors of cardiology training;** the program director must "weed out" that person. More commonly, there are fellows who are suited to the broad field of cardiology but who lack the technical or cognitive facility to become adequate invasive cardiologists. Such individuals should be dissuaded from continuing in the catheterization laboratory or actually prevented from doing so by the laboratory director. There are already too many cardiologists doing invasive procedures, and some of them are potentially dangerous to their patients. To allow for further proliferation of invasive cardiologists with less than excellent skills is unacceptable.

Training in cardiac catheterization should be only one part of a well-rounded cardiology fellowship experience (3, 5–7). Just as a fellow uninterested in practicing catheterization must gain a clear understanding of the indications, limitations, complications, and implications of catheterization and angiography findings, a fellow planning to practice catheterization must learn not only all the above but also as much as possible about all of cardiology, with special emphasis on general clinical skills and on the knowledge and use of pathophysiology in evaluating and managing cardiac patients (5).

The Society for Cardiac Angiography and Interventions recently published core curricula for training both adult and pediatric invasive and interventional cardiologists (8, 9). Training in invasive cardiology begins with an understanding of the anatomy and physiology of the cardiovascular system (2). Although it is assumed that the fledgling cardiologist has gained some of this knowledge as a student and resident, appropriate texts should be available and teaching conferences should be held to fill in the gaps. Similarly, books and conferences should be provided to teach more specific aspects of invasive cardiology, including historical data, equipment need and use, pathophysiology, hemodynamic interpretation, angiographic technique and interpretation, procedural process, radiation physics and safety, and the indications, contraindications, limitations, complications, and implications of the findings at catheterization (2). Ideally, this information will be available to and used by the trainee

before he or she first enters the catheterization laboratory.

Diagnostic Cardiac Catheterization—Procedural Training

Hands-on training in catheterization includes knowledge regarding the preprocedural events, the procedure itself, and the postprocedural course. The pre- and postprocedural periods are just as important as the procedure itself and should be stressed equally in the teaching process.

Preprocedure Events

A thorough history and physical by the fellow is often the single most important aspect of a cardiac catheterization. One learns not only the physical problem at hand but also the patient's emotional state, particularly in relation to the threat of an invasive procedure. The interchange between fellow and patient sets the stage for the safe conduct of the procedure and the comfort of the patient during it. This interchange also leads to a patient consent that is as fully informed as possible and necessary.

With the knowledge gained from the history and physical examination, the fellow will be able to write appropriate precatheterization orders. He or she must learn that orders should not be routine but will have to be as specific as necessary for the individual patient. For example, a patient with a history of contrast allergy will need medications ordered that most patients will not require. Also, based on the findings of the history and physical examination, the fellow will learn to plot a course for the procedure itself. He or she will decide on the type of contrast, whether to do a right heart catheterization, the size and type of catheters to use, access site for catheter introductions, and many other features of the procedure that will vary from patient to patient.

Many patients undergoing cardiac catheterization have been through the procedure before, and many have had previous cardiac surgery. As part of the preparation, the fellow must review previous catheterization data and angiograms and previous surgical summaries to have the knowledge needed to properly plan for the procedure. Before every procedure, the responsible attending cardiologist should have a discussion with the fellow about the patient's history and physical examination, emotional state, indications for the procedure, and special needs, concerns, and risks expected for that particular patient. Together they should finalize the plans for the course of the procedure. If the fellow has concerns about the indications and/or risks, he or she must feel free to express them to the attending cardiologist.

Procedural Events

Proper training in performance of an invasive cardiovascular procedure demands constant interaction between attending physician and fellow throughout the procedure. The attending physician should be present or immediately available throughout the procedure. In some cases, a more senior fellow can substitute for the attending; but, the ultimate responsibility for patient safety, appropriate performance of the procedure, and fellow training remains with the attending cardiologist.

Procedural training should begin by having the trainee observe at least several procedures without direct participation. He or she should observe every aspect of the procedure, from the time the patient arrives in the laboratory until the patient returns to his or her hospital bed. The fellow should watch the technicians prepare, drape, and monitor the patient, set up the sterile table with the necessary in-laboratory equipment, and arrange and use the transducers, camera, tape recorder, injector, and all physiologic recording equipment required to successfully perform cardiac catheterization. He or she should observe the proper equipment and methods of cine film processing; be exposed to laboratory methods for equipment preventive maintenance and film quality assurance.

During the procedure itself, the fellow should observe the attending and/or senior fellows as they anesthetize the entry site, and place needles, wires, dilators, sheaths, and catheters of various types into the veins and arteries. The interaction between the fluoroscope and table movement, as the wires and catheters are advanced through the circulation to their final destinations, should be noted. He or she should observe the safe use of catheters and the prevention of clot formation or air entry into catheters and eventually the body of the patient. The fellow should watch as blood is drawn for oxygen and Fick cardiac output determinations, as thermodilution cardiac outputs are performed, as pressures are measured and recorded in various cardiac chambers and blood vessels, and as radiographic contrast is injected for angiography and arteriography. He or she should observe the process of removing the catheters and sheaths, and of establishing hemostasis at the entry site.

Direct fellow participation should begin with less difficult and lower risk elements of the procedure, continuing on to more difficult and higher risk elements only when the trainee has developed some basic technical facility and confidence; overconfidence must be watched for and carefully stifled, if necessary. The fellow should be allowed to do as much as he or she is qualified to do in every teaching situation and should not be abused by being used as an assistant only. The fellow eventually should be directly involved in and perform each and every aspect of the procedure.

He or she must be taught that **the major concerns during the study are twofold: (*a*) the safety and welfare of the patient are paramount and (*b*) the procedure should be carried out in an organized and efficient manner** to obtain all information necessary for making a complete diagnosis, unless the patient's condition prevents one from doing so. Flexibility is mandatory, and changes in procedural order and type are often necessary based on the findings of the procedure or the changing condition of the patient. The fellow should learn that patient safety and comfort require ongoing communication between physician and patient. This can be handled directly by the fellow and attending physician or, less ideally, indirectly via nurse or technician.

The fellow should learn not only from the attending cardiologist but also from the nurses and technicians working in the laboratory, especially if he or she intends to eventually supervise a catheterization laboratory. These individuals perform duties ancillary to the case that can be overlooked easily during one's training but that are integral to the success of the individual procedure, as well as to the laboratory as a whole.

During the course of invasive cardiovascular training, the fellow should be exposed to and learn to perform a wide array of procedures, including vascular entry by cutdown and percutaneous approaches, right and left heart catheterization, temporary pacemaker insertion, pericardiocentesis, endomyocardial biopsy, and angiography of many types, including pulmonary, ventricular, aortic, coronary, aortocoronary bypass graft, and internal mammary artery bypass graft (2). From the number of procedures listed, obviously this kind of knowledge cannot be obtained in a short time or in a small number or limited variety of patients (10).

During the course of training, fellows intending to practice invasive cardiology should be given the opportunity to act as teachers in the catheterization laboratory, under the ultimate direction of an attending cardiologist. The role of teacher requires a higher level of attention to detail than that gained as a student, resulting in a broader understanding of the procedure as a whole.

Finally, the fellow must learn when to stop. Some cases are too difficult to complete without jeopardizing the patient. Others require greater skill and experience than one can provide and require that another physician be called in to the laboratory to safely complete the procedure. This can happen to anyone, whether new in the laboratory or very experienced, and one's ego should not jeopardize patient welfare.

Postprocedure Events

The two main elements of the postprocedural period are the care of the patient, and the interpretation and use of the data acquired during the procedure. The fellow must be directly involved in both elements.

The immediate postprocedure concern is the care of the patient. The fellow, along with the laboratory nurses, should evaluate and take care of the wound created by the procedure. Attention is given to the cardiac status (particularly as it may have been altered by the stress of the procedure) and to the general condition of the patient (particularly relating to vital signs, pain, anticoagulation, hydration, vascular competency, and renal function). The fellow should learn to write thorough postprocedure orders so that proper care will continue after the patient leaves immediate care and observation. He or she should be taught to follow the patient's progress in the hospital setting and learn that he or she has some responsibility for posthospital events, especially as they relate to the entry site and its vascular distribution, and to any procedure-related complications. **Clear communication of postprocedure instructions to the patient and family is most important.**

After the procedure, the fellow should be involved in processing, interpreting, reporting, and communicating the data acquired. As a part of information processing, the fellow wishing to practice invasive cardiology should learn about the equipment used for recording and analyzing hemodynamic information, for obtaining angiographic images, and the use of video recorders and film processors. The fellow cannot simply accept computerized hemodynamic data (such as valve gradients and areas); he or she must learn to process this information independently. The fellow should know how to make shunt calculations and how to perform every aspect of hemodynamic measurement.

Learning to properly interpret physiologic and hemodynamic data requires not only the use of standardized texts and articles on the subject but also the personal attention of the attending cardiologist. Hemodynamic data and films should be read together by the attending fellow. Too often a fellow analyzes data without the direct oversight of the teacher, and too often the attending cardiologist reviews and reports the data and films alone to save time. Ideally, the fellow learns to complete the official postprocedure report and then the attending cardiologist critiques the report; together they create the final version.

Not uncommonly, the fellow is left out of the process of communicating the results of the cardiac catheterization to either the patient and his or her family or to other physicians. The trainee should be taught not only the importance of this type of communication but also how to do it. Additionally, the fellow should learn the importance of adding individual patient data to a local hospital database, not only in the interests of any organized laboratory research but also for quality assurance for the laboratory.

Regular cardiac catheterization conferences should be held. A wide variety of cases should be presented over time. Complications and quality assurance data should be discussed. Each trainee should present his or her cases at this conference, and should be ready to defend his or her decisions and actions.

Each invasive trainee should keep a log of all cases performed. This log should include not only the name of the patient, the type of procedure, and the diagnosis, but also the outcome and complications. The log provides the trainee with evidence of his or her case volume and its breadth and depth, and becomes an excellent resource to which he or she may refer when faced with a difficult patient problem that has been seen previously.

Minimum Caseload and Duration of Diagnostic Catheterization Training

As stated above, no objective studies have been done regarding the duration of training or the minimum number of cases required to adequately train one to learn cardiac catheterization. Task Force 3 of COCATS (4) recommends that all trainees have 4 months of training in the catheterization laboratory, with participation in at least 100 cases in which they are involved from precatheterization clinical evaluation to final disposition (level 1). The Task Force recommends that, for a trainee planning to practice diagnostic catheterization and angiography, a minimum of 12 of his or her 36 months of required cardiology training should be spent in the catheterization laboratory, during which time a minimum of 300 procedures must be performed, including 200 or more as primary operator (level 2).

The Report of Bethesda Conference #23 (Access to Cardiovascular Care) recommends that fewer cardiologists be trained in invasive cardiology and more in clinical and preventive cardiology (11). It suggests, but does not explicitly state, that not all cardiology fellows should spend time training directly in the cardiac catheterization laboratory.

The author believes that a fellow not planning a career in an invasive field of cardiology should be allowed to spend less than the COCATS recommended 4 months of training in the catheterization laboratory and, in some cases, should be able to omit such training completely. Much of the nontechnical aspects of catheterization (including the indications, analysis of data, and data utilization in patient management) could be acquired by a combination of reading, clinical service rotations, and attendance at catheterization conferences. This would allow these trainees to spend more time learning on aspects of cardiology, including research. Clearly this would result in a smaller pool of half-trained angiographers who, in the interest of economics, might eventually practice invasive cardiology despite their lack of adequate invasive training during fellowship. **Adequate training to practice invasive cardiology should include 12 months in the catheterization laboratory with documented performance of at least 300 cases, with at least 200 as primary operator.**

Fellowship Training in Interventional Cardiology

Interventional training should not be undertaken except during specialized fellowship training. By 1997, any invasive physician trained prior to the coronary angioplasty era has had plenty of opportunity to learn to perform coronary angioplasty if so desired. The Cardiac Catheterization Committee of the American College of Cardiology has recommended that any invasive cardiologist desiring to learn interventional procedures after July 1995 be required to have an additional year of fellowship training in interventional cardiology (12). Therefore, the author recommends that from this point on, basic interventional training should be undertaken only at the fellowship level, and further credentialing for interventional cardiology should take that into account.

Interventional training is not a "God-given right." Not all cardiologists are suited for the stress of interventional procedures or have the technical coordination to perform them with a high level of expertise. Others who have technical skill but demonstrate a lack of good laboratory judgment should also not practice in this area of cardiology. Thus, fellowship training in interventional cardiology should be highly selective.

Percutaneous Transluminal Coronary Angioplasty

Although a wide array of cardiac interventional procedures is now being performed, **percutaneous transluminal coronary angioplasty (PTCA) remains the cornerstone of interventional training.** Interventional training should begin with PTCA and not move to other procedures until the trainee has developed some technical skill and confidence with PTCA. The trainee could then go on to those other procedures that are most commonly performed in the specific training laboratory (e.g., directional atherectomy). Interventional fellows should be exposed to uncommonly performed procedures, such as balloon valvuloplasty, but should not directly participate in or be primary operator for these procedures until they have become very knowledgeable and quite facile in interventional procedures as a whole.

The ACP/ACC/AHA Task Force on

Table 3.1.
Cognitive Skills Needed to Perform Percutaneous Transluminal Coronary Angioplasty Competently

---

Knowledge of current indications for the procedure and likelihood of success in individual cases (class I, II, and III)

Knowledge of contraindications to the procedure

Knowledge of preprocedural evaluation, including reasons for selecting percutaneous transluminal coronary angioplasty over potential alternatives (i.e., coronary artery bypass surgery; medical therapy alone)

Knowledge of the anatomy, normal physiology, and pathophysiology of the coronary circulation

Knowledge of ventricular physiology

Ability to recognize complications of cardiac catheterization and percutaneous transluminal coronary angioplasty promptly

Knowledge of and experience in the management of complications

Ability to communicate the risk, benefits, and results of the procedure to the patient, to the medical record, and to others involved in the care of the patient so that appropriate informed consent can be obtained

---

Reprinted with permission from Ryan TJ, Klocke FJ, Reynolds WA, et al. Clinical competence in percutaneous transluminal coronary angioplasty. A statement for physicians from the ACP/ACC/AHA Task Force on clinical privileges in cardiology. Circulation 1990; 81:2041–2046.

clinical privileges in cardiology issued a position statement on competence in PTCA that clearly enunciated both the **cognitive and technical skills needed to perform PTCA competently** (13). These skills form the basis for training in interventional cardiology and are shown in Tables 3.1 and 3.2.

Newer Interventional Procedures

Each new intervention developed will require a standard approach relating to teaching and learning. The trainee should acquire as much basic knowledge as possible from didactic sessions and by reading available literature. Part of this knowledge should come from assigned materials. The knowledge base should include the technique

Table 3.2.
Technical Skills Needed to Perform Percutaneous Transluminal Coronary Angioplasty Competently

Manual dexterity

Operational skill in the use of x-ray, video, and other required equipment

Seasoned experience with cardiac catheterization, coronary arteriography, and radiation safety

Additional demonstrated competence in percutaneous transluminal coronary angioplasty

Technical aspects of management of complications of percutaneous transluminal coronary angioplasty

Demonstration of continued technical competence in the procedure over time

Reprinted with permission from Ryan TJ, Klocke FJ, Reynolds WA, et al. Clinical competence in percutaneous transluminal coronary angioplasty. A statement for physicians from the ACP/ACC/AHA Task Force on clinical privileges in cardiology. Circulation 1990; 81:2041–2046.

itself, the specialized equipment for the specific technique, and the indications, expected outcome, and risks inherent with that technique.

Some cardiology programs are now performing peripheral transluminal angioplasty and other peripheral vascular interventions. If these programs are going to provide training to fellows in this interventional type of procedure, the curriculum of the program should include regular instruction on the natural history of and the anatomic changes occurring with peripheral vascular disease; on noninvasive peripheral vascular assessment; on the indications for, as well as the risks and benefits of, different treatment modalities (including conservative measures, angioplasty, other interventional techniques, and surgery); and on the indications for and use of thrombolytic agents in peripheral vascular disease (14).

Interventional Procedural Training

Preprocedure Events

For any intervention, the preprocedure contact between fellow and patient should include a discussion regarding available interventions, why one may be selected over another, the expected outcome, and the risks—particularly the possible need for emergency surgery. Before each procedure, the fellow should meet with the responsible attending physician, discuss the clinical presentation of the patient, review the diagnostic angiogram, and plan the procedure itself, especially relating to specific equipment, balloon sizes, and the reason to approach one artery or lesion before another.

Procedural Events

Teaching during the procedure should first consist of an in-depth demonstration of the specialized equipment and a thorough explanation of how it works. After at least a few cases as an observer, the fellow should begin direct hands-on experience performing the procedure, first as an assistant and later as the primary operator. It is particularly important for the trainee to be exposed to a range of equipment options, including guiding catheters, wires, balloon catheters, interventional devices, and stents. With this exposure, the fellow should gradually become involved in the selection of the proper equipment for a specific patient and should be involved in the decision to change from one piece of equipment to another as the need arises.

Any interventional procedure can go awry, and emergency surgery may become necessary. A fellow must develop good judgment in deciding when a situation is getting out of hand and a surgeon should be called, and he or she must learn how to manage the complicated patient while awaiting transfer to the operating room. Because emergency surgery is now necessary in less than 2 to 3% of interventions, the fellow must be part of a relatively large number of interventional cases during his or her training to gain experience with this problem.

Postprocedure Events

Postprocedural care of the interventional patient is much more complicated than that of the average diagnostic catheterization patient. The fellow must learn to anticipate and recognize postinterventional complications, especially vascular problems, bleeding, and early coronary reclosure. He or she must become adept in the management of the vascular sheath, anticoagulation, and subtle and overt symptoms and signs of myocardial ischemia. The trainee should be taught that ongoing follow-up observation is particularly important and that education of the nurses caring for the postinterventional patient is critical. The postprocedural orders should take all the above into consideration. Ideally, the fellow should participate in late postdischarge follow-up of interventional patients.

The trainee should be taught to properly analyze and report the results of each interventional procedure, just as when performing diagnostic catheterization. He or she should also be involved in communicating the results to the patient and referring physician. The fellow should keep a log of all interventional cases performed—their indications, course, outcome, and complications.

Weekly interventional conferences should be held, and the fellow should actively participate. Open discussion and criticism should be encouraged, both by and of the fellow. In interventional cardiology, as in other fields, one learns by one's mistakes, especially when they are pointed out by others.

Although it is not mandatory that a fellow attend an Interventional Seminar at one of the nation's centers of excellence, it should be encouraged. Ongoing education in this ever-changing field is a must.

Every laboratory training fellows to perform interventional cardiac procedures should have some ongoing research in this field. The fellow should actively participate in this research as a significant part of his or her educational process.

Minimum Caseload and Duration of Training

Most authorities in this field, and particularly COCATS (3, 4), recommend that interventional training require one full year beyond basic cardiology and cardiac catheterization training—a total of 4 years of cardiology fellowship. COCATS recommends that during that 4th year an interventional fellow should directly participate in at least 300 interventional cases and in at least 125 cases as primary operator (3, 4). They assume that most of these 125 primary cases will utilize balloon angioplasty. For training in other interventional procedures, they recommend formal didactic training plus at least 10 additional cases focused on each specific procedure.

Nonangiographic Invasive Imaging

Currently there are three forms of nonangiographic invasive imaging that are conducted in the cardiac catheterization laboratory: coronary intravascular ultrasound, intracoronary Doppler ultrasound, and coronary angioscopy. The first two procedures are now practiced clinically; coronary angioscopy remains essentially a research tool. These nonangiographic imaging techniques require specialized training, which is usually given as part of an interventional training program (4th year). Although many centers employ intravascular ultrasound during diagnostic catheterization, most laboratories limit credentialing for intravascular imaging procedures to personnel with interventional training (15). In the unlikely event of internal coronary disruption caused by these techniques, this safety measure ensures that the necessary personnel and equipment are immediately available to initiate appropriate corrective actions.

There are no published guidelines regarding the number of cases required for adequate training in these procedures. After first gaining significant experience performing PTCA as part of an interventional training program it seems reasonable that a trainee should participate in at least 10 cases focused on each specific nonangiographic invasive imaging procedure.

POSTFELLOWSHIP TRAINING IN CARDIAC CATHETERIZATION

Diagnostic Catheterization

As stated above, basic diagnostic cardiac catheterization should be learned during fellowship training only and should never occur during the postcardiology fellowship years.

Occasionally, a physician trained to perform catheterization during a fellowship stops performing catheterizations in practice and later wishes to return to the diagnostic catheterization laboratory. The ACC/AHA Ad Hoc Task Force on cardiac catheterization recommends that to be credentialed, this person must first be certified as adequately trained and competent by the director of his or her training program (16). If the time away from the cardiac catheterization laboratory has been from 1 to 3 years, the physician should undergo a period of preceptorship, working under the direct observation of the laboratory director until certifiable by the director as competent. This work should include at least 25 cases with a variety of diagnoses. In longer absences from the laboratory, credentials should not be granted until the physician fulfills at least 3 months of formal laboratory training at an institution with a fellowship training program and is certified by the program director.

The Canadian Cardiovascular Society recommends more stringent retraining guidelines, insisting on a minimum of 100 cases with 75 as primary operator. They believe that for an individual with a brief absence from catheterization practice, retraining could occur at his or her home institution, but with more prolonged absence, retraining should occur at an outside training center (17).

Interventional Training

As previously stated, basic interventional cardiology training—with training in PTCA as the cornerstone of interventional training—should occur only during a fellowship program. As new interventional procedures emerge, already trained and practicing interventional cardiologists will have a need for postfellowship training in those procedures. Postfellowship training in new procedures should be accessible only to those previously trained in and practicing interventional cardiology at an acceptable proficiency and volume (at least 75 cases/year) (13, 18). Currently, too many practicing interventional cardiologists are performing fewer than 75 PTCAs per year, the minimum number needed to maintain competence. The world does not need any more inadequately trained interventional cardiologists (19).

The postfellowship training of emerging interventional procedures should follow the same general course as that outlined for interventional training during fellowship. The preceptor for this training should expect the trainee to have the same level of commitment to learning as expected of the fellow. The trainee must read, attend conferences, and openly discuss his or her cases with the mentor and with others knowledgeable in the new technique. The trainee must be involved in all aspects of a patient's care, from preprocedure history and physical examination, through the procedure itself, to the postprocedure care of the patient, and in the analysis and reporting of the results of the procedure.

Little has been written regarding the number of cases needed for a trained and practicing interventional cardiologist to gain proficiency with a new interventional technique or a nonangiographic invasive imaging technique. One would think, however, that the case numbers would be the same as that required during formal fellowship training (i.e., at least 10 cases focused on each specific procedure). Special instruction in a new intervention or procedure should be obtained by participation in one or more formal courses that should include a minimum of 50 hours of CMI category I instruction.

It has been suggested that, to acquire skill in peripheral transluminal angioplasty, one should perform 100 diagnostic peripheral angiograms, 50 peripheral angioplasties with at least 25 as primary operator, and 10 peripheral thrombolytic therapy cases under the supervision of an experienced interventionalist (20, 21). Because peripheral angioplasty involves a part of the circulation outside the realm of the average cardiac interventionalist, these numbers are reasonable.

TRAINING LABORATORY

Fellowship Training

Fellowship training in diagnostic cardiac catheterization should only take place as part of a well-rounded fellowship program that leads to subspecialty board eligibility. The program's catheterization laboratory should have a full-time director recognized as an expert in cardiac catheterization. The laboratory should have at least one other full-time physician to provide training in the absence of the director and to offer another perspective. The laboratory should be adequately staffed and equipped to result in excellent diagnostic studies at low risk and should meet the 1991 ACC/AHA Guidelines for cardiac catheterization and cardiac catheterization laboratories (16). Laboratory case volume should be great enough to provide at least the minimum cases needed for adequate fellow training, as well as a variety of case types (10). An active in-hospital cardiac surgery program is mandatory.

The director of the laboratory must have a strong desire to teach and must instill the spirit of teaching in all physicians, fellows, nurses, and technicians in the laboratory. Catheterization teaching conferences should be held at least weekly. The teaching laboratory should maintain a registry of its cases, not only for quality assurance but also as a database for teaching and research. The teaching laboratory should have a commitment to some form of research, and fellows should be made a part of the research effort.

To provide training in interventional cardiology, a laboratory must provide all things necessary to teach diagnostic cardiac catheterization and must be a part of an American College of Graduate Medical Education (ACGME) approved cardiology training program (12). It must perform a minimum of 300 percutaneous coronary interventional procedures per year. It must also have at least one interventional cardiologist, primarily responsible for interventional training, who is full-time and recognized as an expert in this field. The laboratory must have all of the equipment required to perform safe and effective interventional procedures. A commitment to teaching must be pervasive in the laboratory, and there should be some commitment to research. Interventional teaching conferences should be held, ideally on a weekly basis. Each interventional instructor should have significant experience (greater than 500 cases) and a general caseload greater than 100 cases per year (12).

The laboratory director must prospectively evaluate the knowledge and skill of the fellow and identify and remove those fellows who lack cognitive or technical facility, those with poor laboratory judgment, and those who demonstrate a lack of concern for the safety and benefit of their patients.

References

1. Schlant RC, et al. 17th Bethesda Conference: Adult Cardiology Training. J Am Coll Cardiol 1986;7: 1191–1218.
2. Conti CR, Faxon DP, Gruentzis A, et al. 17th Bethesda Conference: adult cardiology training. Task Force III: training in cardiac catheterization. J Am Coll Cardiol 1986;7:1205–1206.
3. Core Cardiology Training Symposium (COCATS). Guidelines for training in adult cardiovascular medicine. J Am Coll Cardiol 1995;25:1–34.
4. Pepine CJ, Babb JD, Brinker JA, et al. Task Force 3: training in cardiac catheterization and interventional cardiology. J Am Coll Cardiol 1995;25:14–16.
5. Hurst JW. On the training of cardiologists. J Am Coll Cardiol 1986;7:1187–1190.
6. O'Rourke RA. Cardiology at a precipice. Circulation 1985;72:258–261.
7. Graduate Medical Education Directory, 1994–1995. Special requirements for residency education in internal medicine. Specialty requirements for residency education in cardiovascular disease. Chicago: American Medical Association, 1994:45–58.
8. Hodgson JM, Tommaso CL, Watson RM, et al. Core

curriculum for the training of adult invasive cardiologists: report of the SCAI Committee on training standards. Cathet Cardiovasc Diagn 1996;37: 392–408.

9. Ruiz CE, Mullins CE, Rochini AP, et al. Core curriculum for the training of pediatric invasive/interventional cardiologists: report of the Society for Cardiac Angiography and Interventions Committee on pediatric cardiology training standards. Cathet Cardiovasc Diagn 1996;37:409–424.

10. Ballal RS, Eisenberg MJ, Ellis SG. Training in cardiac catheterization at high-volume and low-volume centers: is there a difference in case mix? Am Heart J 1996;132:460–462.

11. Gunnar RM, Anderson TO, Cooper RS, et al. 23rd Bethesda Conference. Access to cardiovascular care. Task Force 2. Human and systems resources for cardiovascular care. J Am Coll Cardiol 1992;19: 1441–1492.

12. Douglas JS, Pepine CJ, Block PC, et al. Recommendation for development and maintenance of competence in coronary interventional procedures. American College of Cardiology Cardiac Catheterization Committee. J Am Coll Cardiol 1993;22: 629–631.

13. Ryan TJ, Klocke FJ, Reynolds WA, et al. Clinical competence in percutaneous transluminal coronary angioplasty. A statement for physicians from the ACP/ACC/AHA Task Force on clinical privileges in cardiology. Circulation 1990;81:2041–2046.

14. Spittell JA, Creager MA, Dorros G, et al. Recommendations for peripheral transluminal angioplasty: training and facilities. American College of Cardiology Peripheral Vascular Disease Committee. J Am Coll Cardiol 1993;21:546–548.

15. Scanlon PJ, Faxon DP, Audet A, et al. ACC/AHA guidelines for coronary angiography. J Am Coll Cardiol 1997 (in Press).

16. Pepine CJ, Allen HD, Bashore TM, et al. ACC/AHA guidelines for cardiac catheterization and cardiac catheterization laboratories. ACC/AHA Ad Hoc Task Force on cardiac catheterization. J Am Coll Cardiol 1991;18:1149–1182; Circulation 1991;84:2213–2247.

17. Miller RM, O'Neill B, Johnstone D, et al. Standards for training in adult cardiac catheterization and angiography. Catheterization and Angiography Subcommittee of the Canadian Cardiovascular Society Committee on Standards. Can J Cardiol 1996;12: 470–472.

18. Ryan TJ, Bauman WB, Kennedy JW, et al. Guidelines for percutaneous transluminal coronary angioplasty. A report of the American College of Cardiology/American Heart Association Task Force on assessment of diagnostic and therapeutic cardiovascular procedures (Committee on Percutaneous Transluminal Coronary Angioplasty). J Am Coll Cardiol 1993;22:2033–2054.

19. Scanlon PJ. The training for and practice of percutaneous transluminal coronary angioplasty: results of two surveys. Cathet Cardiovasc Diagn 1985;11: 561–570.

20. Wexler L, Dorros G, Levin D, et al. Guidelines for performance of peripheral percutaneous transluminal angioplasty. Interventional Cardiology Committee, Subcommittee on Peripheral Interventions SCAI. Cathet Cardiovasc Diagn 1990;21: 128–129.

21. Levin DC, Becker GJ, Dorros G, et al. Training standards for physicians performing peripheral angioplasty and other percutaneous peripheral vascular interventions. A statement for health professionals from the Special Writing Group of the Councils on Cardiovascular Radiology, Cardio-Thoracic and Vascular Surgery, and Clinical Cardiology, The American Heart Association. Circulation 1992;86: 1348–1350.

4
Aspects of Catheterization Laboratory Administration

James A. Hill, MD, MS
Charles R. Lambert, MD, PhD
Carl J. Pepine, MD

INTRODUCTION

Cooperation between the professional medical leadership and the administrative management is the key to successful function of a catheterization laboratory. People in these positions have different management tasks that are best separated. Most physicians do not have the skills, time, or inclination to handle many of the technical and personnel issues involved in a successful catheterization laboratory, and nonclinically based administrators often lack an understanding of patient care issues that arise. A good collegial relationship allows for effective problem solving, communication, efficient patient flow, and meeting physician and patient needs. This is true whether the laboratory is hospital-based or freestanding.

ADMINISTRATIVE STRUCTURE

All hospitals with catheterization laboratories must commit to maintaining high standards of professional practice, to providing adequate staffing and training, and to assuring the ability of operators to perform high-

quality invasive procedures. While it is neither desirable nor necessary to purchase the most expensive equipment or to replace it frequently, financial resources should be made available to maintain standards of safety and data quality. Occasionally equipment is purchased that is not ideal for the specific needs of cardiac imaging, such as when facilities also serve as peripheral vascular laboratories. Compromise in study quality often occurs. Sometimes equipment is allowed to become hopelessly out of date. And in many hospitals, personnel is shared with other areas of the institution for purely financial reasons. Cardiac catheterization requires special medical and technical skills unique to the environment. In any of the above circumstances, a hospital should strongly consider not offering catheterization services.

Medical Director

Every cardiac catheterization laboratory must have a medical director. Both the Society for Cardiac Angiography and Interventions (SCAI) and the ACC/AHA Task Force have provided guidelines regarding appropriate qualifications for such individuals (1, 2). As minimal requirements, the medical director should be board-certified in a specialty related to catheterization (such as adult or pediatric cardiology or cardiovascular radiology) and be a recognized expert in the field with at least 5 years of catheterization experience, performing at least 200 procedures per year during that time. He or she must also be thoroughly trained in radiation safety and imaging techniques.

The medical director has many responsibilities. These responsibilities include: (*a*) setting criteria for granting laboratory privileges; (*b*) periodically reviewing performance to renew privileges; (*c*) establishing and maintaining quality assurance (QA); (*d*) acting with the technical director to ensure efficient use of the laboratory including scheduling, equipment maintenance and replacement; and (*e*) acting with the technical director when preparing budgets and reports to ensure that relevant governing bodies are kept informed of laboratory activities. Specifically what role the medical director plays in these latter two functions will depend on the laboratory setting and on local institutional policy. Responsible physician input into these processes cannot be overemphasized, however, and should never be abdicated completely to purely administrative personnel.

Technical Director

The technical director is responsible for the efficient functioning of the day-to-day operations of the laboratory. These operations include most nonphysician personnel issues, equipment maintenance, inventory control, darkroom operation, film quality control, and staff training supervision. How much discussion with and joint supervision by the medical director occurs depends on the local environment, but close interaction is necessary. The size and complexity of the laboratory will dictate how much the director participates in patient management and procedure performance on a daily basis. The technical director should be familiar with all aspects of catheterization laboratory operation and should be able to perform virtually any function.

STAFFING

All catheterization laboratories must have well-trained technical staff to complement competent physician operators. Specific staffing patterns will depend on the types of procedures performed in the laboratory, caseload, and types of facilities present and their design (3). Types of staff background include nurses, cardiopulmonary technologists, radiology technologists, and emergency medical technicians. There is no ideal composition of staff, and how many of each type is available will depend on many factors. Generally, there should be enough staff available for each case to include someone to operate the physiologic recorder and record details of the procedure, to administer medications, etc. In addition, someone besides the physician should be able to administer medications in the laboratory. Finally, someone should be available to gather catheters and other equipment as necessary. Depending on local practice, one of the technical staff often scrubs, assists the operator, and operates the imaging equipment.

The cardiac catheterization laboratory is a unique setting in a field undergoing constant change; thus, substantial training is necessary for all personnel regardless of their background. The level of staff training necessary will vary, but some degree of cross-training in the various laboratory functions is desirable and is essential in laboratories with a small number of personnel and for the performance of procedures during off hours. Efforts should be made to ensure that all staff understand basic hemodynamics and arrhythmia recognition and have certification in life support techniques, preferably advanced cardiac life support. All staff should be familiar with sterile technique, the routine used for patient preparation and draping, and laboratory setup. Staff should be trained in the use of all the basic laboratory equipment, such as the physiologic recorder, digital imaging equipment, and power injector. For more specialized equipment such as intravascular ultrasound or Doppler flow wires, the authors have found that selecting staff members to focus in such areas as their "specialty" works well. This is especially true when usage is limited. Finally, it cannot be stressed enough that all technical personnel should know where all disposable equipment (e.g., catheters, contrast agents, and manifolds) is kept and have access to it quickly.

It is necessary to consider local regulations regarding specific staffing needs because some states require specific skill levels to perform certain tasks. This may mean a nurse to administer medication, a radiologic technologist to be responsible for radiation safety and equipment, or an individual trained in respiratory therapy to be responsible for blood gas analysis. Individual jurisdictions vary.

STAFF RADIATION EXPOSURE

Radiation exposure is a significant issue for physician and technical staff in cardiac catheterization laboratories, particularly with angioplasty and other interventional procedures. As noted in Chapter 11, the most potent source of radiation is from the x-ray tube, but there can be substantial scatter from the patient. The current recommendation for exposure limit is 5 rem/year for individuals exposed for occupational purposes. The three most effective ways to limit radiation exposure are barriers to radiation such as lead shielding, increased distance from the radiation source as the beam intensity changes inversely with the square of the distance, and limiting time of exposure. These procedures can and should be utilized in the laboratory. All personnel must wear lead aprons, lead glasses, and thyroid shields, as well as use the portable shields provided. All personnel also should be as far as possible from the x-ray imaging system, and the operator should refrain from using fluoroscopy when a staff person is in immediate proximity, such as adjusting intravenous lines, removing electrodes, and other patient care functions. Finally, although not uniformly enforced, personnel should be removed from exposure once they exceed their recommended allowance. This policy should be reviewed on an annual basis at minimum. More detailed discussion of this issue is available elsewhere (4, 5).

INVENTORY

Inventory management involves maintaining a supply of the various types of disposable equipment needed to perform procedures while reducing the costs of maintaining supplies and protecting against shortages. Large numbers of specially designed disposable catheters for virtually every use have been developed over the years. Inventory problems have been magnified by the number of products available, often with only subtle differences, for interventional procedures. In addition, percutaneous transluminal coronary angioplasty (PTCA) products are expensive compared with diagnostic equipment. There is no ideal number of each disposable item that should be stocked. The number depends on storage capacity, patterns of procedure volume, available budget, and other factors. Generally, a minimum 3 to 5 day supply of all equipment should be available at all times.

Several inventory management methods are currently used. Using a fixed time period to assess inventory entails physical counting and ordering, often by a person trained in the techniques of the catheterization laboratory. This is not efficient because shortages or extra inventory can occur when patterns of activity in the laboratory temporarily change. Another method is to use a continuous assessment of inventory change. This is done from procedure logs submitted to clerical personnel after procedures are performed or, alternatively, is computer-maintained. The latter aspect can be done using an automatic inventory management program that cues to the equipment entered for the clinical record or by the use of bar codes on the various disposable items. Use of a removable sticker with the bar code imprinted can help the laboratory staff maintain a reliable record at the time of the procedure. However, it requires that each disposable item be labeled with an inventory slip. In a computer-maintained system, orders can be automatically cued or generated when inventory reaches target limits. Whether such a system is integrated into an institution-wide system is best determined by local resources and ordering policies. But a personal computer-maintained system is inexpensive and efficient in the catheterization laboratory since many of the supplies needed are unique to the environment. The different policies of various vendors regarding shipping should also be considered. Increased cost and the need for advance procedure planning become major problems when excessive dependence on overnight shipping is a pattern in inventory management. With proper planning, second-day air or standard ground transport of 5 to 7 days will usually be adequate and prove more cost effective.

Other issues can affect inventory. Competitive bidding and volume purchases can be utilized to reduce cost. However, this is useful only if relatively long-term commitment can be made to a specific vendor, if agreement can be reached by the users regarding the types of equipment to stock, and if adequate storage space is available for volume delivery. Some vendors are willing to provide automatic trade-outs of outdated and unused equipment. This is particularly helpful with PTCA equipment, since new and "better" devices rapidly become available. Some vendors are also willing to put equipment into a laboratory on consignment. This is undesirable because bookkeeping, liability, and storage may be problems.

CREDENTIALING

Guidelines for training in catheterization procedures have been widely discussed and are generally determined within training programs. The reader is referred to Chapter 3 and to publications specifically addressing this (6–9). Each hospital has a different mechanism for credentialing physicians for various aspects of the practice of medicine. With regard to granting privileges to perform diagnostic cardiac catheterization procedures, it is the responsibility of the medical director in conjunction with the catheterization committee, when present, to ensure competence and compliance with staff bylaws. Various professional organiza-

Table 4.1.
Guidelines for Professional Staff Privileges in the Cardiac Catheterization Laboratory

Fully accredited member of professional staff
Licensed to practice
Board-certified or qualified in internal medicine/cardiology, radiology/catheterization and angiography, or pediatrics/pediatric cardiology
Willingness to participate in quality assurance and peer review
Maintain an annual caseload of at least 150 procedures except in special circumstances
Certified as competent in catheterization procedures by training director with at least 1 year of recent (within 1 yr) formal catheterization laboratory training. If formal training >1 and <3 years, preceptorship with the laboratory director with at least 25 cases and certification locally. If formal training >3 years, formal training of at least 3 months in a fellowship program with certification by the program director.
Considerations for addition of staff members:
  Needs of community served by laboratory
  Needs of hospital and its staff
  Demand for service
  Capacity of laboratory

Adapted from Guidelines for percutaneous transluminal coronary angioplasty: a report of the American College of Cardiology/American Heart Association Task Force on assessment of diagnostic and therapeutic cardiovascular procedures (subcommittee on percutaneous transluminal coronary angioplasty). J Am Coll Cardiol 1988;12:529–545. Guidelines for approval of professional staff for privileges in the cardiac catheterization laboratory. Cathet Cardiovasc Diagn 1984;10:199–201.

tions including the SCAI, ACC, and AHA have provided guidelines for granting privileges to perform procedures in the catheterization laboratory (2, 10). A composite of the recommendations is listed in Table 4.1.

Privileges to perform interventional procedures, specifically coronary angioplasty, should be granted according to the recommendations of the same organizations (8, 11, 12). As summarized in Table 4.2, these guidelines require significant experience in standard catheterization procedures and ongoing training in PTCA.

QUALITY ASSURANCE

The types and incidence of the different complications that occur with cardiac catheri-

Table 4.2.
Guidelines for Professional Staff Privileges in Coronary Angioplasty

Fully credentialed operator for diagnostic cardiac catheterization and angiography; and

Performed minimum of 300 coronary angiographic procedures with 200 as primary operator; and

Completion of formal 1-year training program, performing 125 PTCA procedures with 75 as primary operator
OR

2–3 years of independent catheterization experience with a minimum of 500 cases; and

Instruction in formal angioplasty courses with at least 50 hours of category 1 CME; and

Performance of 125 PTCA procedures with 75 as primary operator under the supervision of local laboratory director

Considerations for maintenance of privileges:
    Minimum of 50–75 cases per year
    CME in interventional procedures (25 hours/ 2 years is recommended)
    Participation in regular review of procedures and complications

---

Adapted from Guidelines for credentialing and facilities for performance of coronary angioplasty. Cathet Cardiovasc Diagn 1988;15:136–138. Ryan TJ, Klocke FJ, Reynolds WA. Clinical competence in percutaneous transluminal coronary angioplasty. Circulation 1990; 81:2041–2046. These are consistent with anticipated recommendations by the American Board of Internal Medicine.

---

zation procedures are discussed in detail in Chapter 8. Based on accepted norms, all laboratories should ensure that monitoring of complications occurs and that the laboratory is in compliance with various accrediting bodies, such as the Joint Commission on Accreditation of Health Care Organizations (JCAHO). The peer review function necessary for compliance to accepted standards is best carried out by individuals familiar with cardiac catheterization procedures, in conjunction with the medical director. **Ideally, these reviewers should not be directly involved in performing catheterization procedures in the institution being reviewed.** Although often impractical, peer review can take many forms, including: (*a*) outside review from an independent expert, such as a laboratory director from a noncompeting institution; (*b*) review by noncatheterizing cardiologists within the same institution; or (*c*)

review by an independent committee that includes radiologists, internists, surgeons, and other members of the medical staff, in consultation with both the medical and technical directors of the laboratory. It cannot be overemphasized that review of complications should be carried out in such a way that it is not perceived as representing either a process whereby one operator or group of operators uses it to gain competitive advantage or a conflict of interest (i.e., physicians reviewing their own complications). Included in any review process should be (*a*) complications; (*b*) appropriateness of indications; and (*c*) documentation of results, including record and report maintenance. **Some physicians advocate the establishment of catheterization laboratory committees for monitoring activities and setting policies.** Other aspects of this issue are discussed in the recent ACC/AHA Task Force (2) and in the SCAI guidelines (13).

Guidelines for quality assurance of PTCA were briefly discussed in a recent ACC/AHA Task Force report (8). With these procedures, the possibility of operator conflict of interest is even more prevalent, and consideration should be given to establishing a formal second opinion mechanism to protect against this. Briefly, a mechanism should exist in every laboratory for the assurance that both the indications and results of these procedures are monitored. Currently, in large and busy laboratories, this is often the responsibility of a separate director of interventional cardiology.

In recent years, QA has been reevaluated primarily as a result of the JCAHO Agenda for Change, which emphasizes a continuous monitoring of process using the continuous quality improvement (CQI), total quality management (TQM), and continuous quality management (CQM) approaches. The strengths of traditional QA relate as much to the historical perspective in which it was developed as it does to the actual assurance of quality that it provides. In the development of hospital accreditation, it was necessary to accomplish setting minimal standards of care at certain points. Standards were developed that required specific criteria that could be measured and documented, which were often retrospective, limited to small areas or departments of the hospital, and generally designed to capture outliers. Feedback was often lacking or not effectively delivered. Despite these limitations, QA programs set the stage for monitoring and evaluating medical practice and the provision of health care within hospitals. The newer CQM approach is designed as a much more collaborative effort to be applied across an organization. QA and CQM have several things in common. Both focus on particular areas of an organization, although the levels of involvement of the workers in those areas may differ. Both methods require the collection of data and use that data to evaluate the performance of outcomes. Both look at outcomes and use those outcome measurements to make improvements. Finally, both QA and CQM use collected data to assess improvement. The fundamental differences lie in the different way the processes are evaluated and the data utilized.

The focus of QA has traditionally been on high-risk services performed in clinical departments, with evaluation based on outcomes. The emphasis is on individuals and special causes for variance from the accepted minimal standard with a punitive nature to the process. Conversely, CQM focuses more on variation and consensus for multiple processes—not simply high-risk ones—across the organization with evaluation of both process and outcome. The emphasis is on systems and on common and special causes of variance rather than on people, with a resulting nonpunitive outlook. Finally, a constant emphasis on quality by the leadership of the organization is much more a factor in the success of CQM programs than was ever present with QA.

Jennison (14) discusses a number of fundamental differences between the QA and CQM approaches. She differentiates QA and CQM on the basis of the following characteristics:

—*Motivation to participate*
  Avoidance with QA and self-motivation with CQM
—*Notion of customers*
  External regulators for QA and multiple customers for CQM
—*Focus of data collection and analysis*
  Indicators of poor care for QA and examination of process for CQM
—*Evaluating why competent physicians make errors*
  Retrospective record review for QA and process problems with CQM
—*Methods used to analyze process performance*
  List of optimal practices with QA and study of process with CQM
—*Use of simple statistics*
  Wait for delineation of quality standards from outside sources with QA and following daily operations with CQM
—*Relationship of cost and quality*
  CQM encompasses cost as a factor in quality whereas QA does not
—*Scope of the quality program*
  QA emphasizes individual departments whereas CQM is more integrated and encompasses the entire organization
—*Impact on the work force*
  Punitive with QA, empowering with CQM

For those familiar with the JCAHO accreditation process, it is clear that **both traditional QA with the emphasis on sentinel events and CQM are necessary for the modern hospital and catheterization laboratory.**

FILM AND EQUIPMENT MAINTENANCE

A discussion of the various aspects of film and equipment maintenance is presented in Chapter 11. The same types of routine maintenance procedures should be policy in every laboratory for every piece of equipment. This is the responsibility of the technical director. It is best to follow vendors' recommended schedules, and usually a service contract is the best way to handle this. The authors' experiences suggest that the companies that make the equipment, although not necessarily the cheapest, often provide the most knowledgeable and effective service.

INFECTION PREVENTION

There is a great deal of variability among laboratories regarding appropriate dress for performing procedures. Some require full surgical clothing and sterile technique with gowns and gloves. In others, street clothes with gloves only is the rule. How this impacts on infection rates, which are generally very low, is unknown. A survey performed by Leaman and Zelis (15) that included more than 107,000 procedures showed an infection incidence of 0.35% at the entry site. Infection was much more common (approximately a tenfold higher incidence) in patients undergoing procedures that used a cutdown. With the percutaneous technique there was no relationship of dress to infection; but when a cutdown was performed, infection was less common when operators and observers wore a mask, cap, and gown.

A major problem with capturing the true incidence of infections resulting from cardiac catheterization procedures is that the mechanisms for capturing complications generally involve only the immediate 24- to 48-hour period after the procedure, which is inadequate to reliably recognize all infectious complications. The SCAI has published guidelines for infection prevention in the catheterization laboratory (16). Their report emphasized several important points. First, the catheterization laboratory should follow standard precautions for the prevention of surgical wound infections that would be followed anywhere such a wound is created. This includes surface preparation and hair removal, sterile draping, wound irrigation, and appropriate dressings. Second, the likelihood of an infectious complication is higher with a cutdown technique compared with a percutaneous one, and sterile precautions should be more stringent. However, with the frequent occurrence of leaving sheaths and catheters in place for periods longer than that required for the procedure and with the placement of permanent intravascular prostheses, it is reasonable to afford equal caution to every procedure. These precautions include wearing a cap and mask, scrub clothes and a sterile gown, and performing a vigorous hand scrub before putting on sterile gloves. Finally, the room and equipment should be kept clean for each procedure. The report also gives recommendations on protecting the staff from bloodborne infections, which should be identical in any operating room environment.

SUMMARY

The modern cardiac catheterization laboratory is a complex environment in which various types of diagnostic and therapeutic procedures are performed, often on critically ill patients. Proper administration is important if quality is to be maintained and appropriate care rendered. Physician and technical leadership and expertise provided in a collegial and communicative atmosphere are essential for successful operations.

References

1. Guidelines regarding qualifications and responsibilities of a cardiac catheterization laboratory director. Cathet Cardiovasc Diagn 1983;9:619–621.
2. ACC/AHA guidelines for cardiac catheterization and cardiac catheterization laboratories. J Am Coll Cardiol 1991;18:1149–1182.
3. Friesinger GC, Adams DF, Bourassa MG, et al. Optimal resources for examination of the heart and lungs: cardiac catheterization and radiographic facilities. Circulation 1983;68:893A–930A.
4. Johnson LW, Moore RJ, Balter S. Review of radiation safety in the cardiac catheterization laboratory. Cathet Cardiovasc Diagn 1992;25:186–194.
5. Curry TS, Dowdey JE, Murry RC, eds. Christensen's introduction to the physics of diagnostic radiology. Philadelphia: Lea & Febiger. 1984.
6. Conti CR, Faxon DP, Gruentzig A, et al. Bethesda Conference: adult cardiology training: Task Force III: training in cardiac catheterization. J Am Coll Cardiol 1986;7:1205–1206.
7. Standards for training in cardiac catheterization and angiography. Cathet Cardiovasc Diagn 1980; 6:345–348.
8. Ryan TJ, Klocke FJ, Reynolds WA. Clinical competence in percutaneous transluminal coronary angioplasty. Circulation 1990;81:2041–2046.
9. Hodgson JM, Tommaso CL, Watson RM, et al. Core curriculum for the training of adult invasive cardiologists: report of the Society for Angiography and Interventions Committee on training standards. Cathet Cardiovasc Diagn 1996;37:392–408.
10. Guidelines for approval of professional staff for privileges in the cardiac catheterization laboratory. Cathet Cardiovasc Diagn 1984;10:199–201.
11. Guidelines for credentialing and facilities for performance of coronary angioplasty. Cathet Cardiovasc Diagn 1988;15:136–138.
12. Guidelines for percutaneous transluminal coronary angioplasty: a report of the American College of Cardiology/American Heart Association Task Force on assessment of diagnostic and therapeutic cardiovascular procedures (subcommittee on percutaneous transluminal coronary angioplasty). J Am Coll Cardiol 1988;12:529–545.
13. Guidelines for organization and quality assurance in cardiovascular laboratories. Cathet Cardiovasc Diagn 1983;9:327–328.
14. Jennison K. Total quality management—fad or paradigmatic shift? In: Couch JB, ed. Health care

quality management for the 21st century. Tampa, FL: American College of Physician Executives, 1991:444–464.

15. Leaman DM, Zelis RF. What is the appropriate "dress code" for the cardiac catheterization laboratory? Cathet Cardiovasc Diagn 1983;9:33–38.

16. Heupler FA, Heisler M, Keys TF, Serkey J, and the Society for Cardiac Angiography and Interventions Laboratory Performance Standards Committee. Infection prevention guidelines for cardiac catheterization laboratories. Cathet Cardiovasc Diagn 1992;25:260–263.

5

Quality Assurance for Cardiac Catheterization Procedures: Continuous Quality Improvement, Clinical Pathways, and Scorecarding

Frederick A. Heupler Jr, MD
Kimberly Brown, RN
Stephen G. Ellis, MD

INTRODUCTION

The domain of quality assurance in the cardiac catheterization laboratory, as in medicine in general, has enlarged greatly in the last decade. Ten years ago, it was sufficient for the responsible catheterization laboratory director to provide for the collection of rudimentary nonphysician-specific complication statistics, to discuss major procedural complications at a morbidity and mortality conference, and to ensure that the laboratory met certain minimal radiation and infectious disease control specifications (1). **Angiographers have assumed that their individual conscientious efforts, with an occasional glance at their peers' performances, are sufficient to maintain quality.** These assumptions have been quashed by several developments over the last decade:

- Epidemiologic and administrative studies have revealed wide variations among physicians in indications for procedures, treatment methods, and outcomes of medical care. These studies create the impression that much medical treatment either lacks a scientific basis or is unnecessary (2–5).

- Changes in health care financing have empowered insurers and aggregate purchasers of health care to demand proof of the appropriateness and quality of medical care in return for reimbursement (6, 7).
- State and Federal government agencies have demanded risk-adjusted outcome information to ensure the quality of hospital services (6).
- Specialists in health services research and health science information management have developed improved tools for evaluating and improving the quality of medical care (8).

Previously, **quality assurance** in most laboratories meant searching out poor performers—defined as those with high mortality rates—and restricting their privileges ("getting rid of the bad apples"). In contrast, modern **continuous quality improvement** (CQI) techniques, based on industrial quality management procedures, employ an extensive database, organized methods of data collection and analysis, and constructive interventions directed at improving quality (9, 10). It is now necessary for physicians to establish and implement methods to measure and improve the quality of performance in the catheterization laboratory and to demonstrate objective results to skeptical third-party payors and government agencies. However, a commonly accepted uniform methodology has not yet been established (11), so individual laboratories must develop their own programs. It is the purpose of this chapter to offer practical suggestions for establishing and refining a catheterization laboratory CQI program.

ESTABLISHING A CQI PROGRAM

The process of establishing a CQI program can be divided into five steps: committee organization, database construction, data collection, data analysis, and interventions to improve performance.

Committee Organization

The laboratory director should organize a committee of catheterization laboratory physicians, nurses, and technicians to plan and implement the program. The chairperson of this committee should be an unbiased, respected individual who will ensure fair and objective evaluation. The committee should include representation from each group of physicians in the laboratory. Multiple reviewers improve the reliability and objectivity of the review process (12). One or more members of the committee must be familiar with the methodology of modern CQI techniques.

Database Construction

The CQI committee must establish a catheterization-specific database, which should include demographic, procedural, administrative, and quality-related information. It must include semi-quantitative performance attributes (quality indicators) that function as the "measuring sticks" of quality in the laboratory (13). The three major aspects of quality to be measured include:

1. **Catheterization laboratory infrastructure,** which includes laboratory personnel, equipment, and organization.
2. **Processes of medical care,** which assess how the patient was evaluated and treated. These are measured by clinical pathways, treatment algorithms, and clinical practice guidelines.
3. **Outcomes of medical care,** which indicate what happened to the patient after treatment. These are commonly expressed as a "scorecard" or "profile" of performance.

Each of these major aspects of quality measurement will be discussed in detail later.

Data Collection

A laboratory-specific computerized data collection system is a necessity for obtaining meaningful CQI data. Data obtained from insurance claims or other financial information sources are unreliable for CQI purposes but may be useful for evaluating the costs of medical care (14). Generic databases, which judge severity of illness independent of diagnosis, are also unreliable because process-of-care and outcomes analysis require diagnosis-specific information. A variety of catheterization laboratory-specific databases are available commercially. Many are too detailed and expensive for practical use in a busy clinical laboratory.

Reliable data collection is commonly the "weak link" in the CQI process. Ideally, data collection should occur concurrently at the time of the patient encounter. This helps ensure completeness and reliability of the data regarding events that occur within the laboratory, unbiased by procedural outcome. Follow-up data must be obtained by another method, such as chart review. **Several studies have shown that the physicians performing procedures cannot be expected to reliably report all adverse outcomes.** It takes great effort to train data collectors to extract information completely, accurately, and consistently. The data must be audited periodically to ensure validity (7).

Data Analysis

Data become most useful for CQI purposes when organized into graphic displays and clinical performance profiles. These profiles can be based on variability in processes of care; conformance with clinical pathways and clinical practice guidelines; outcomes (e.g., mortality and morbidity rates, procedural success rates); trends and patterns of care; and costs. These profiles must be analyzed carefully to prevent assigning the cause of an adverse event or an outlier position to an individual's performance when it is actually caused by random fluctuation or defects in the medical environment (15).

All serious adverse outcomes related to catheterization laboratory procedures should be subject to detailed scrutiny, including review of the chart, nursing notes, and cineangiograms. The goal is to evaluate the appropriateness of the indications, technical performance, and management of any complications of the procedure. This review may be performed by individual physicians, by a committee, or by a group of physicians at morbidity and mortality conferences.

Interventions to Improve Performance

The ultimate goal of CQI is to improve quality by changing the performance and environment in the catheterization laboratory. This can be accomplished by standard methods, discussed in detail later in the chapter. All interventions must be followed by repetition of data collection and analysis to determine if the intervention was successful.

INFRASTRUCTURE OF THE CATHETERIZATION LABORATORY

The infrastructure of a catheterization laboratory includes the personnel, equipment, and organization. These "structural" indicators are objective and easy to collect, but they provide only an indirect indication of the quality of care. They have been largely overshadowed by outcomes analysis and process-of-care evaluation (16).

Personnel Indicators

Personnel indicators reflect the qualifications of the physicians, nurses, and technicians who work in the laboratory (17). Establishment of minimum criteria for credentialing and recredentialing tends to prevent future problems with incompetent personnel. These criteria should be personnel-specific and procedure-specific (diagnostic coronary angiography, coronary interventions, peripheral angiography and interventions, myocardial biopsy, and electrophysiologic procedures).

Criteria for credentialing may include education, special training, procedural experience, previous employment history, and licensure. The American College of Cardiology (ACC) and the American Heart Association (AHA) have defined training requirements for angiographers. These include completion of a 3-year cardiology training program during which the physician performed at least 300 diagnostic procedures, with 200 as primary operator, and 125 coronary intervention procedures, with 75 as primary operator (18, 19) (see Chapter 3).

Recredentialing criteria include maintenance of adequate procedural volume, fulfillment of postgraduate education requirements, licensure, and maintenance of standards of quality. The American College of Cardiology, American Heart Association, and the Society for Cardiac Angiography and Interventions (SCAI) have suggested a minimum of 150 total angiographic procedures and 75 coronary interventional procedures per year to maintain competence (20, 21). The establishment of minimum annual procedural volume requirements for physicians has become widespread, but there is disagreement regarding the appropriate minimum numbers. Any requirements must take into consideration operator experience and performance in addition to numbers of procedures. The overall expected mortality for elective diagnostic coronary angiography should average no greater than 0.1 to 0.2%, and for elective coronary interventional procedures no greater than 1% (19). **The frequency of diagnostic coronary angiographic procedures yielding "normal" results should not exceed 20% (20).**

Equipment Indicators

Equipment indicators refer to the quality of medical equipment used in the laboratory. Maintenance of fluoroscopic and cineangiographic image quality can be accomplished by a preventive maintenance program and by continuing physician feedback to the engineers responsible for equipment repair. Radiation safety can be ensured by periodic evaluation of the radiation output doses of the equipment and by regular feedback of radiation dosimetry badge readings to personnel. All electric equipment must be evaluated for electrical safety on a regular basis (22). The acquisition of new equipment should be undertaken by physicians and others familiar with the technical aspects of the products to be obtained (11).

Organization Indicators

Organization indicators reflect the system in which the personnel and equipment function. Laboratory utilization can be evaluated by estimating hours of laboratory use per day, procedural volume per laboratory, turnover time between cases, and total procedure time per case. Average fluoroscopy time per diagnostic coronary angiography and left heart catheterization case should be less than 15 minute/case and should rarely exceed 30 minutes, even for complicated cases with valve disease or multiple coronary bypass grafts. Fluoroscopy times for coronary intervention procedures commonly reach 30 to 60 minutes, depending on complexity. Procedures that exceed 60 minutes of fluoroscopy time should be infrequent because they produce high radiation exposure to both patient and operator (23).

Efficiency can be estimated by quantifying delays caused by patient availability, laboratory personnel performance, and physician promptness. Cost accounting has become increasingly important in evaluating the financial status of the laboratory. This involves collecting information regarding costs per case of disposable equipment; nonionic contrast material; in-laboratory personnel; total laboratory time; postprocedural observation time; and image processing, distribution, and archiving.

The adequacy of surgical and anesthesia backup support for emergencies can be evaluated by estimating the delay between notification and arrival of personnel.

CLINICAL PATHWAYS: THE PROCESSES OF MEDICAL CARE

Purpose

The purpose of clinical pathways is to improve efficiency—thereby decreasing costs—and monitor outcomes. Other uses include defining and/or protecting practice standards, teaching tools for interns and nursing staff, and patient education. Many institutions have found clinical pathways useful in competing for managed care contracts.

Clinical pathways are not without limitations. They are costly to write, implement, evaluate, and maintain. It may take as much as 1137 hours of time and $36,000 to initiate the first clinical pathway, and $336 hours and $8,000 for each additional one (24). They can be cumbersome for complex situations. Some institutions have supplemented with algorithms in these situations (25). Some practitioners view them as "cookbook" medicine or fear legal ramifications and, therefore, are not receptive to the implementation. Finally, effectiveness should not be confused with efficiency. Clinical pathways can be effective and help achieve a stated organizational objective but might not always be efficient or balance the amount of resources used to achieve an objective against what was actually accomplished. For example, one may meet the organizational objective of decreasing length of stay (LOS) by offering catheterization services on the weekend, but inadvertently increase costs through the overtime needed to provide those services.

Effectiveness

American Health Consultants, a medical economics company, publishes monthly Hospital Case Management, which shares numerous anecdotal success stories of clinical pathways being associated with decreases in LOS. In a descriptive study, Strong found components (activity progression, telemetry usage, and inspirometer use) of coronary bypass clinical pathways to be significantly associated with postoperative LOS (26). Significant increases in patient satisfaction have been associated with the use of clinical pathways in obstetric patients (27, 28).

Efficiency

Statistically significant decreases in LOS *and* costs, without adverse effect on clinical outcomes attributed to the use of clinical pathways, have been described for vascular surgery, urology, and obstetric patients (27, 29–31).

Design and Implementation

Development of a clinical pathway for cardiac catheterization or coronary intervention should include the following team members: catheterization laboratory medical director and nursing manager, nursing unit manager, diagnostic testing (stress, echo) manager, financial analyst, and cardiology case manager or nurse specialist. The following steps should be followed in pathways development (32).

Step 1: **Define the population.** One pathway for all cardiac catheterization procedures may not be sufficient. For example,

patients may undergo coronary angiography to further evaluate unstable angina, for risk stratification postmyocardial infarction, or to screen for coronary artery disease (CAD) as an underlying cause of arrhythmias and cardiomyopathy. Several pathways may be needed for one procedure.

Step 2: **Define current practice and "best" practice.** Simply sequencing current practice will not improve efficiency or outcomes. Current practice should be identified first. The feasibility of other possible practices should be evaluated and considered.

Step 3: **Identify and sequence the clinical interventions.** Identify physician activities as well as those of nursing and support services. Sequence the order in which these events must occur. Many events are dependent on a prior event occurring. One might be unable to do a cardiac catheterization until a stress test has been completed. The stress test cannot be completed until cardiac enzyme results are known and the patient has had nothing by mouth for several hours.

Step 4: **Turn the clinical pathway into a critical pathway.** Minimize downtime between activities. Practitioners sometimes prefer to make treatment decisions on a day-by-day basis, resulting in increased downtime. A patient is admitted with chest pain and cardiac enzymes are ordered. They are negative the following morning and a stress test is scheduled for the following day. Forty-eight hours have passed since admission. Alternatively, a patient is admitted with chest pain, enzymes drawn, and a stress test scheduled for the following day, pending enzyme results. The LOS has been decreased by 24 hours.

Step 5: **Reengineer processes and support systems.** It may be necessary to change the catheterization laboratory hours, the turnaround time of laboratory test results, the nursing unit admission and discharge criteria, the timing of patient education, and many other processes. It is important that the financial analyst advise if the cost of reengineering is more than the cost savings achieved.

Step 6: **Specify outcomes and variances to be measured.** Commonly measured outcomes include complications, LOS, cost, and readmission. Examples of variances that might be measured include timely ordering and scheduling of tests and procedures, laboratory turnaround times, use of nonionic contrast or other costly medications or devices, and discharge orders.

Step 7: **Educate and coach physician and other pathways users.** Before implementation, discussion and consideration of users concerns are essential. Education should include the purpose for critical pathways as well as acknowledgment of the limitations, the development process, and the method of data collection and analysis of variances. Users should be reassured that the primary purpose of the pathways is not to monitor individual practices but to identify, via variance monitoring, system issues that prohibit "best" practices.

Initially, daily monitoring of the critical pathways is needed to remind users of the expected activities and to identify problems. Monthly LOS, cost, and variance reports should be provided to users to encourage practice changes and continued support.

Table 5.1 shows an example of a clinical pathway. It describes the process of care for patients admitted with unstable angina. The purpose of this pathway is to ensure that the patient progresses to cardiac catheterization with minimal downtime. This pathway is also used by registered nurses to document their plan of care, interventions, and evaluation for the day. Note that some of the key events described are the timing of scheduling tests and procedures and critical decision making regarding therapeutic options.

Variance Analysis

A variance is when an event occurs that is not in the pathway or when an event does not occur that is in the pathway. A variance has the potential to delay diagnosis or treatment, or result in negative outcomes. The causes of variances can be placed in three categories: patient, system, and practitioner. Comorbid conditions and complications are the most common patient causes of variances. Selker et al. identified nine categories of system and practitioner causes of delays (33). These categories are delays

related to test scheduling, test results, surgery, consultation, patients, physicians, education/research, discharge planning, and appropriate level of care.

Whenever a variance occurs, it is noted on the pathway. The cause of the variance is noted on the variance record (Table 5.2), which is turned over to the case manager/nurse specialist at discharge. The causes of variances are summarized, benchmarked, and examined for possible ways to minimize. Results as well as any plans should be shared with the pathway users on a regular basis. Tables 5.3, 5.4, and 5.5 show a summary of common variances associated with the catheterization laboratories at a large teaching institution for 1 year.

An examination of the causes of variances in Tables 5.3, 5.4, and 5.5 shows that the most frequent cause of delay days in this catheterization laboratory was because the catheterization laboratory was not open for patient service on the weekend. The 134 delay days caused by bleeding complications were also of concern. This was reduced to 80 days of delay in 1995 by sharing the information with practitioners, reviewing sheath removal practices, reviewing anticoagulation protocols, and implementing a bedside Partial thromboplastin time monitoring program. The 478 weekend delay days was a more complex issue. A sensitivity analysis demonstrated that a 25% reduction in weekend delays would only result in a $35,000 per year cost avoidance. The decision was made not to pursue weekend hours.

Every institution will have its unique variances. The clinical pathway is a tool that can be used to identify variances that result in inefficiencies. Careful analysis of the cause of the variances may lead to improved outcomes and a more efficient catheterization laboratory.

SCORECARDS: THE OUTCOMES OF MEDICAL CARE

The intent of "scorecarding" is to improve the overall quality of patient care by allowing the triage of patients to the best physi-

TABLE 5.1.
Example of Clinical Pathway[a]

Unstable Angina/Chest Pain/Evaluate for Possible Myocardial Infarction

Time Frame / Location	Hospital Day 0 Date .... Unit	Hospital Day 1 Date .... Unit	Hospital Day 2 Date .... Unit ....
Discharge planning	Assess discharge needs, psychosocial needs; consult Social Services (if needed)	Discharge needs met; follow-up care arranged; prescriptions/homegoing meds received / *If functional test (−), CK (−), & discharge criteria met, discharge pt.*	If treatment plan: medical, discharge today / PTCA, proceed to PTCA clinical path today / CABG, proceed to CABG clinical path today
Patient education	Instruction re: 1) CP/change in symptoms; 2) communication with RN; 3) ICU/telemetry environment; 4) unstable angina pamphlet; medication teaching initiated; risk factor modification; preprocedure education	Outpatient cardiac rehab arrangements; smoking cessation program arranged (if needed); evaluation of teaching: medications, diet, CAD, unstable angina	
Tests/procedures/consults	CK isoenzymes q8 hours × 3; ECG on admit/with CP; H/H; SMA-17; CXR / *Order functional test vs. catheterization for tomorrow*	*Functional test if serial CK (−) and painfree or cardiac catheterization; ECG in AM/with CP;* / *If functional test (+) schedule cath for tomorrow* / *If cath (+) decision re: medical tx vs. PTCA vs CABG & place appropriate consult*	
Nursing/medical interventions	Pulse oximetry; O$_2$ to keep O$_2$ Sat > 92%; ECG with CP; continuous monitoring 5-lead or telemetry	Discontinue O$_2$; ECG with CP; Discontinue telemetry	
Medications	ASA; nitrates; β-blocker (if no CHF); IV heparin; Ca channel blockers	ASA; nitrates; β-blocker, discontinue heparin; Ca channel blocker, avoid nonionic contrast material	Medication adjustment if medical therapy planned
Activity/nutrition	Bedrest/BSC NPO/clear liquid	BRP/Ambulate NAS/LAF; NPO before procedure	
Outcome criteria	Hemodynamically stable; rhythm stable; CP relieved; PTT 60–85 sec; O$_2$ Sat > 92; absence of bleeding; absence of heart failure	Hemodynamically stable; rhythm stable; absence of chest pain; O$_2$ Sat > 92%; sufficient urine output; knowledgeable about disease, meds, treatment; absence of heart failure; absence of bleeding; decision re: treatment plan by evening	Tests/procedures/surgery scheduled

[a] Directions: If pathway is followed, initial and date at the top. Any variation from pathway should be circled and noted on the variance record. May add comments if needed. CK, creatine kinase; CP, chest pain; CAD, coronary artery disease; H/H, hemoglobin/hemocritic; SMA-17, blood chemistry; CXR, chest x-ray; ASA, aspirin; BSC, bedside commode; NPO, nothing per mouth; BRP, bathroom privileges; PTT, partial thromboplastin time; RN, nurse; ICU, intensive care unit; ECG, electrocardiogram; O$_2$ Sat, arterial oxygen saturation.

TABLE 5.1. *(continued)*

Acute Myocardial Infarction

Time Frame Location	Hospital Day 1–24° after MI Unit	Hospital Day 24–48° after MI Unit	Hospital Day Transfer to Telemetry 48–72° after MI Unit
Discharge planning	Assess discharge, psychosocial needs; identify risk factors	Consult ASC/Social Service (if needed)	ASC evaluation/Social Service evaluation
Patient education	Instruction re: 1) CP/change in symptoms; 2) communication with RN; 3) ICU environment	Normal heart book/TV; heart attack book/TV	Medication and diet teaching initiated; instruction re: telemetry unit
Tests/procedures/consults	CK isos q8 hours × 3; ECG on admit/with CP; H/H; SMA-17; PTT; CXR; Echo; Respiratory consult; IABP; SG; aline if needed	*Order cath vs. functional test for day 5*; ECG in AM/with CP; PTT; H/H; KP6; CXR; D/C IABP; ?PT/OT consult	ECG in AM/with CP; PTT; KP6; D/C SG and arterial-line; *Upon transfer to floor:* Consult CHIRP; Dietary consult re: diet teaching
Allied health interventions	Respiratory	Respiratory	CHIRP; Dietary
Nursing/medical interventions	Pulse oximetry; O_2 to keep O_2 Sat > 92%; ECG with CP/BP; neuro checks q4 hours; ST segment monitor; Mechanical vent; IABP 1:1 if needed	Pulse oximetry; O_2 to keep O_2 Sat > 92%; ECG with CP/BP; neuro checks qs; ST segment monitor; Wean mechanical vent/extubate; Wean IABP/remove	O_2 to keep O_2 Sat 92%; ECG with CP/BP; Telemetry; Monitor for complications
Medications	ASA; IV nitrates; β-blocker (if no CHF); IV heparin	ASA; change to oral topical nitrates; β-blocker; IV heparin	ASA; oral/topical nitrates; β-blocker; IV heparin; ?Coumadin
Activity/nutrition	Bedrest/BSC; Nutritional assessment: NPO/clear liquid	BSC/BRP; assess ability to perform ADLs; Clear liquid; NAS/LAF	BRP/ambulate/shower; NAS/LAF
Outcome criteria	Hemodynamically stable; rhythm stable; therapeutic PTT 60–85 sec; O_2 Sat > 92%; absence of CP; absence of bleeding; absence of heart failure; ST segment trend unchanged; neurologically intact; renal function adequate	Hemodynamically stable; rhythm stable; absence of CP; PTT 60–85 sec; O_2 Sat > 92%; absence of bleeding; absence of heart failure; neurologically intact; renal function adequate	Hemodynamically stable; rhythm stable; CP relieved; PTT 60–85 sec; O_2 Sat > 92%; absence of bleeding; absence of heart failure; ST segment trend unchanged; neurologically intact; renal function adequate

[a] Directions: If pathway is followed, initial and date at the top. Any variation from pathway should be circled and noted on the variance record. May add comments if needed. CK, creatine kinase; CP, chest pain; CAD, coronary artery disease; H/H, hemoglobin/hemocritic; SMA-17, blood chemistry; CXR, chest x-ray; ASA, aspirin; BSC, bedside commode; NPO, nothing per mouth; BRP, bathroom privileges; PTT, partial thromboplastin time; RN, nurse; ICU, intensive care unit; ECG, electrocardiogram; O_2 Sat, arterial oxygen saturation.

TABLE 5.1. *(continued)*

Acute Myocardial Infarction (Continued)

Time Frame Location	Hospital Day Date . . . . Day 4 after MI Telemetry Unit	Hospital Day Date . . . . Day 5 after MI Telemetry Unit	Hospital Day Date . . . . Day 6 after MI Telemetry Unit . . . .
Discharge planning	If site placement needed, Gold Form completed	Anticipated d/c plan communicated to patient/family; homegoing meds ordered	Discharge needs are met; follow-up care arranged; prescriptions/homegoing meds received
Patient education	Risk factor modification Preprocedure instruction	Review/evaluate understanding of medications, risk factors, diet, MI	Outpatient cardiac rehab arrangements received
Tests/procedures/consults	ECG in AM/with chest pain; KP6; PT (if on Coumadin)	ECG in AM/with chest pain; KP6; PT (if on Coumadin) *Stress test vs. Cardiac cath* Consult interventional cardiology vs. CTS after cath if indicated	ECG in AM/with chest pain; KP6; PT (if on Coumadin)
Allied health interventions	CHIRP	CHIRP	CHIRP
Nursing/medical interventions	Evaluate need for O$_2$ to keep O$_2$ Sat > 92%; ECG with CP/BP; telemetry; monitor for complications	ECG with CP/BP; telemetry; monitor for complications	ECG with CP/BP; telemetry; monitor for complications
Medications	ASA; oral/topical nitrates; β-blocker; ?Coumadin *Start ACE inhibitor*	ASA; oral/topical nitrates; β-blocker; ?Coumadin ACE inhibitor	ASA; oral/topical nitrates; β-blocker; ?Coumadin ACE inhibitor
Activity/nutrition	Bedrest/BSC NPO prior to procedure; NAS/LAF	BSC/BRP; assess ability to perform ADLs NAS/LAF	BRP/ambulate/shower NAS/LAF
Outcome criteria	Hemodynamically stable; rhythm stable; CP relieved; O$_2$ Sat > 92%; absence of bleeding; absence of heart failure; neurologically intact; renal function adequate	Hemodynamically stable; rhythm stable; CP relieved; O$_2$ Sat > 92%; absence of bleeding; absence of heart failure; neurologically intact; renal function adequate	Hemodynamically stable; rhythm stable; CP relieved; O$_2$ Sat > 92%; absence of bleeding; absence of heart failure; neurologically intact; renal function adequate

Reprinted from Cleveland Clinic Foundation, copyright 1997.

[a] Directions: If pathway is followed, initial and date at the top. Any variation from pathway should be circled and noted on the variance record. May add comments if needed.
CK, creatine kinase; CP, chest pain; CAD, coronary artery disease; H/H, hemoglobin/hemocritic; SMA-17, blood chemistry; CXR, chest x-ray; ASA, aspirin; BSC, bedside commode; NPO, nothing per mouth; BRP, bathroom privileges; PTT, partial thromboplastin time; RN, nurse; ICU, intensive care unit; ECG, electrocardiogram; O$_2$ Sat, arterial oxygen saturation.

TABLE 5.2.
Acute MI/Chest Pain/Unstable Angina/Acute Intervention Patient Variance Record

	DATE___ NO VARIANCE		DATE___ NO VARIANCE	IMPRINT LABEL
P H Y S I O L O G I C V A R I A N C E S	CARDIOVASCULAR Cardiogenic shock/hemodynamic instability CHF/pulmonary edema Cardiac ischemia/CP Dysrhythmias MI Vascular complications PULMONARY Respiratory failure RENAL ARF/CRF/dialysis/—BUN/CREAT NEURO CVA/TIA ID Infection (area):_____ MEDICATION ADJUSTMENT Non-therapeutic INR/PTT	P H Y S I O L O G I C V A R I A N C E S	CARDIOVASCULAR Cardiogenic shock/hemodynamic instability CHF/pulmonary edema Cardiac ischemia/CP Dysrhythmias MI Vascular complications PULMONARY Respiratory failure RENAL ARF/CRF/dialysis/—BUN/CREAT NEURO CVA/TIA ID Infection (area): MEDICATION ADJUSTMENT Heparin due to thrombus Nontherapeutic INR/PTT Nonionic contrast used EVALUATION OHS work-up Noncardiac work-up	INSTRUCTIONS 1. Identify variances by circling *key item(s)* thought to cause delays in diagnosis, treatment, or length of stay 2. Variance = a deviation from expected plan of treatment or patient outcomes
S Y S T E M	Delays Test/OR M-F or WE (circle) Cath Echo OHS PTCA Stress Other Record retrieval/lab results Hospital transfer PT/family refusal	S Y S T E M	Delays Test/OR M-F or WE (circle) Cath Echo OHS PTCA Stress Other Record retrieval/lab results PT/family refusal	
PRACTI-TIONER	Delays MD schedule Transcription error Consultant _____ Clinical decision/management PT not sufficiently prepped Procedure/surgery cancelled	PRACTI-TIONER	Delays MD schedule Transcription error Consultant _____ Clinical decision/management PT not sufficiently prepped Procedure/surgery cancelled	
INITIAL		INITIAL		

Table 5.3.
Variance Analysis. Causes of System Delays: PTCA Patients

Cause of Delay	Number of Delay Days
Related to cardiology diagnostic test scheduling	
Busy schedule	19
Test not done on weekends	30
Test not done in evenings	1
Related to catheterization laboratory	
Busy schedule	104
Test not done on weekends	478
Test not done on day of patient transfer from outside facility	211
Patient undecided/refuses treatment	5
Related to research protocol	5
Related to unavailability of outside resources	7

Table 5.5.
Variance Analysis. Causes of Patient Variances: PTCA Patients

Cause of Delay	Number of Delay Days
Bleeding/vascular complications	134
Renal failure	107
Warfarin therapy needed	63
Additional heparin threapy required	53
Heart failure	52
Acute MI (Q and non-Q wave)	33
Continued chest pain	28
Neurologic event	20
Infection	19
Abrupt closure	17
Staged procedure	10

cian providers and by identifying "inferior" providers to allow them to improve their skills or no longer practice certain facets of medicine. The underlying assumptions are seemingly simple: (*a*) in the performance of certain patient care activities, all physicians do not perform equally; (*b*) patient outcome can be directly linked to physician performance. In reality, however, many complex problems must be overcome for this process to achieve its objective:

- Agree on clinically meaningful patient outcomes;
- Understand nonphysician codeterminants of these outcomes;

Table 5.4.
Variance Analysis. Causes of Practitioner Delays: PTCA Patients

Cause of Delay	Number of Delay Days
Conservative practice: beyond the clinical pathway standard	42
Delayed clinical decision making	
Cardiology services	26
CT surgery services	22
Other services	50

- Obtain unbiased data for these clinical parameters;
- Obtain sufficient data to apply appropriate statistical methods;
- Use the results to achieve the desired ends in a hospital and community setting, wherein multiple forces often conspire to resist implementation of the inferences of the results of such analyses.

It is in the procedural-related aspects of cardiology, such as coronary bypass surgery and angioplasty, where the linkage between physician expertise and patient outcome is most direct and scorecarding methodology is most advanced (34–37). For angioplasty, the outcomes of death, emergency bypass surgery, and myocardial infarction are undeniably adverse and meaningful. In the authors' experience, distinguishing cardiac from noncardiac causes of death is sometimes subjective; and, if comorbid conditions can be accounted for, all-cause mortality is preferable to cardiac mortality as an outcome variable. Although the adverse prognostic implications of small "non-Q wave" infarctions related to interventional procedures recently have become apparent (38), there is little agreement as to the lower threshold required for creatine kinase (CK) rise to become meaningful in terms of its outcome implications. For this and other reasons described below, the authors favor the composite adverse outcome of death, bypass surgery, or Q-wave infarction as the primary marker of in-hospital outcome (39). Appropriateness of the procedure itself (40–42) and long-term outcomes, such as freedom from death, infarction, further need for revascularization, and low cost (43), are also meaningful but at present are less well studied as response variables for "scorecarding" after coronary angioplasty.

The correlates of major adverse outcomes of angioplasty are well studied and, in general, predictive of their related outcomes (39, 44). The best common statistical marker of a model's correlation with outcome, the c-statistic, or area under the receiver operating characteristic (ROC) curve (45), is typically in either the 0.80–0.89 (very good) or the 0.70–0.79 (good) range for models of these outcomes. Models less well-associated with outcome or for which this type of correlation is not provided in a validation sample should be viewed with some scepticism for these purposes. Tables 5.1 and 5.2 define the correlates of death and death, bypass surgery, and Q-wave infarction in a recent comprehensive analysis (39). Other models, including that from the New York State Registry, are similar (44). Given the subjectivity of some potential end points and their key covariates, and the naturally strong impetus for physician and hospital "self-preservation," it is understandable that obtaining unbiased data sets from many catheterization laboratories may be difficult. The increase in complexity of patients treated in New York since the inception of that state's Registry is probably the result of both more complete ascertainment of risk factors and some "gaming," or over-coding, in the system (46). Clearly, all valid comparisons of physician–patient outcome must rest on the collection of data, where bias is minimized. The authors have found that this can be achieved only when data are collected by trained staff members who are not involved directly in the care of the patient in question. Appropriately, the ACC database will not make interhospital comparisons on unaudited data.

A proper statistical analysis to determine if one physician's results differ from those of a larger group of physicians requires data from a sufficient volume of cases to provide narrow confidence limits about the point estimate of his or her inci-

dence of the adverse outcome. The confidence limits depend directly on the incidence of adverse outcomes and indirectly on the square root of the number of procedures (39). The authors have termed the relationship between a somewhat greater likelihood of having a poor outcome with a low volume operator and the greater uncertainty of knowing exactly that low operator's outcome as "low volume operator paradox" (39). Practically, this relationship means that statistical detection of outlier results at the traditional $p < 0.05$ level requires either that an operator have dramatically worse results than his or her peers or that only large volume operators (or systems) be compared. The authors and others have noticed that other physician and nurse catheterization laboratory staff often suspect an operator of poor judgment and results before it becomes statistically apparent using the methodology described. Thus this methodology should be only one part of an overall CQI approach in the catheterization laboratory.

Third-party payors and administrators often look for "value" in medical care. Value may be increased by improving the quality of patient care, decreasing its cost, or increasing the ratio between the two.

Given the complexities of ascribing patient outcome to physician management or in essence determining the quality of care, even in procedure-based subspecialties, it is tempting to focus on medical cost or, as it is easier to obtain, medical charges. Most medical economists agree that **charges should not necessarily be equated with cost** because of cost shifting (47). That issue aside, the authors believe strongly that one must judge both parts of this equation to optimize the results of medical care for both patient and society.

Practical Application

How should a catheterization laboratory director or CQI committee deal with a physician whose results appear to be below standard? Clearly the approach depends on the procedure, outcome, and setting. In situations in which the methodology exists (such as with coronary interventions), the authors believe it is important to try to objectively define the relationship between that operator's results and an appropriate standard. For a large volume institution interested in maintaining high standards, a formal approach similar to that outlined (39) using internal standards is feasible and appropriate.

For a small-volume laboratory, insufficient volume or resources may prevent such an approach. In this instance, participation in the ACC Interventional Registry with data auditing may allow external comparisons with appropriate risk adjustment. If this is or a similar analysis is not available, demonstrating the outlier position becomes more problematic. If the operator's patients have characteristics similar to those reported from large contemporary series, and the operator volume is between 60 and 100 cases, the author's experience indicates that an incidence more than four times the average for death or more than two times that reported for death, Q-wave infarction, or bypass surgery, possibly indicates a problem. If the operator's patient's key characteristics differ from those reported, formal risk adjustment is advisable. Finally, all comparisons should be made using contemporary data sets because the overall risk-adjusted complication rate for percutaneous intervention has decreased considerably, even over the period 1993–1995 (48). This type of analysis should be used in conjunction with formal review of procedures with complications, with particular non-biased focus on the appropriateness of the indication for the procedure, on the technique(s) used, and on management of the complication.

INTERVENTIONS TO IMPROVE PERFORMANCE

After the data have been collected and analyzed regarding the processes and outcomes of medical care, it is necessary to institute interventions to improve the processes of care. A variety of interventional tools are available for this purpose

(11). These tools are most likely to be accepted by physicians when they are introduced in a nonthreatening manner and do not interfere unnecessarily with physicians' authority and judgment. Interventions imposed in an autocratic or punitive manner are likely to generate resistance, defeating the aims of the CQI program.

Education

The didactic educational conference traditionally has been considered the primary tool for improving physician performance. Postgraduate continuing education credits are required in virtually every state. However, because of the "knowledge–performance gap," education when used alone is an unreliable method for changing physician behavior. It is most effective when reinforced by other interventional tools (49, 50).

Clinical Practice Standardization

As described above, clinical pathways are an important tool for standardizing the practice of medical care. Other tools include algorithms and clinical practice guidelines (51, 52). Algorithms are schematic outlines of strategies for clinical evaluation or management. Clinical practice guidelines are detailed plans, usually developed by expert opinion, for evaluation and treatment of specific medical conditions.

Proposals for clinical practice standardization should be considered as flexible recommendations, not as rigid rules of practice (51). They may require modification as a result of evolving technology and new information gained from randomized clinical trials and personal experience.

Physicians are most likely to accept clinical practice standardization methods when they have input into developing and implementing the methods and when they have a free hand in modifying and updating them as needed. Physicians will balk at accepting pathways and guidelines forcefully imposed. Even if physicians agree with these practice standardization methods, it is necessary to reinforce them with other interventional tools to encourage adherence (51, 53).

Feedback

Feedback is the most important tool for reinforcing other interventional methods (54, 55). Even when used alone, information feedback regarding outcomes and processes of care will often suffice to change physician performance. Feedback is most effective when it is physician-specific and contains **benchmarking,** or comparison, data from that physician's previous experience, from other physicians in the peer group, and from other institutions (51). Most physicians do not want to be "outliers," and they will commonly change behavior when they realize that their performance does not match that of their peers.

Professional Interaction

Group interaction among physicians at mortality and morbidity and other clinical conferences is a powerful tool for improving physician performance and for reinforcing other interventions (51, 54, 56). These conferences have the advantage of providing the opportunity to discuss and obtain consensus on methods to improve the processes of care. Physician interaction at these conferences is most productive when it focuses on issues, not personalities (56–58). The most effective format is to have an objective moderator solicit input from staff members to ensure participation.

Decision-Support Systems

Rapid advances in information technology will continue to make more information available rapidly to physicians via computer in the office and hospital (59, 60). Eventually, medical information sources will be integrated with an electronic charting system to provide on-line computerized

support for physicians. This support can take many forms:

- Medical history, x-ray, and hospital laboratory information;
- Differential diagnosis and treatment of disease;
- Disease-specific drug therapy information;
- Patient-specific doses and drug interactions;
- Clinical pathways and practice guidelines;
- Patient-specific expected clinical outcomes.

Incentives

Positive and negative incentives are commonly used to change physician performance. Financial incentives may increase (e.g., fee-for-service systems) or decrease (e.g., HMOs with financial penalties for physicians) use of medical services (61–63). Competition among institutions for managed care contracts provides a strong financial impetus to change physician performance. **Apart from financial considerations, most physicians will respond to any positive incentive that is perceived as likely to improve the quality of medical care.**

Administrative Interventions

Administrative interventions are imposed externally to control physician behavior (62). An example is utilization review, by which insurers may restrict the use of diagnostic and therapeutic procedures. Other examples include removal of drugs from hospital formularies and devices from catheterization laboratory inventories. Although they are usually successful, these interventions are commonly viewed as a "hassle" by physicians, unless the physicians provide input into their formulation.

The ultimate administrative intervention is to "get rid of the bad apple"; i.e., to restrict or remove the professional privileges of a physician perceived as a substandard performer (15, 54). This intervention should constitute only a minor part of a properly organized CQI program because its application is limited; it does not improve the performance of other operators; and most catheterization laboratory directors want to avoid actions that may decrease procedural volume (64, 65).

Administrative interventions that result in restriction of privileges may produce an anticompetitive effect, thus violating antitrust laws. The 1986 Federal Healthcare Quality Improvement Act specifies the following guidelines for proper conduct of a "professional review action" that results in restriction of physician privileges:

- The motive is to improve the quality of care;
- Reasonable efforts are made to gather the appropriate facts;
- The review proceedings are conducted fairly;
- The resulting action was warranted by facts obtained after due process (66).

The Act requires that any professional review action resulting in restriction of professional privileges for more than 30 days must be reported to the National Practitioner Data Bank. When this kind of intervention is applied, the administrators of the catheterization laboratory should seek legal counsel.

SUMMARY

The introduction of industrial quality control methods into medical practice provides great potential for improving the quality of care in cardiac catheterization laboratories. In spite of the fact that third-party pressure has stimulated the quality movement in medicine, it is important that physicians not confuse the application of new CQI methods with attempts by insurers, HMOs, and government organizations to control and restrict the practice of medicine for strictly financial purposes. It would be "self-defeating to resist a revolution in quality assessment and management that has its roots in the scientific traditions on which the legitimacy of the medical profession rests" (67). Physicians and their co-workers are the ones best suited to select and apply the tools of CQI in the catheterization laboratory environment. If physicians neglect this responsibility, other parties will likely fill the gap with expensive, misleading, and counterproductive mandates that will interfere with the quality of care.

References

1. Quality management in the cardiac catheterization laboratory. Policies and guidelines established by the Society for Cardiac Angiography and Interventions. Cathet Cardiovasc Diagn 1993;30:1–190.
2. Brand DA, Newcomer LN, Freiburger A, et al. Cardiologists' practices compared with practice guidelines: use of beta-blockade after acute myocardial infarction. J Am Coll Cardiol 1995;26:1432–1436.
3. Di Salvo TG, Paul SD, Lloyd-Jones D, et al. Care of acute myocardial infarction by noninvasive and invasive cardiologists: procedure use, cost, and outcome. J Am Coll Cardiol 1996;27:262–269.
4. Epstein AM. Use of diagnostic tests and therapeutic procedures in a changing health care environment. JAMA 1996;275:1197–1198.
5. Pilote L, Califf RM, Sapp S, et al. Regional variation across the United States in the management of acute myocardial infarction. GUSTO-1 Investigators. Global utilization of streptokinase and tissue plasminogen activator for occluded coronary arteries. N Engl J Med 1995;333:565–572.
6. Berwick DM. The society for medical decision making: the right place at the right time. Med Decis Making 1988;3:77–80.
7. Topol EJ, Block PC, Holmes DR, et al. Readiness for the scorecard era in cardiovascular medicine. Implications for cost effectiveness. Am J Coll Cardiol 1995;75:1170–1173.
8. Berwick DM. Health services research and quality of care. Assignments for the 1990s. Med Care 1989; 27:763–771.
9. Kritchevsky SB, Simmons BP. Continuous quality improvement: concepts and applications for physician care. JAMA 1991;266:1817–1823.
10. Laffel G, Blumenthal D. The case for using industrial quality management science in health care organizations. JAMA 1989;262:2869–2873.
11. Heupler FA, Al-Hani AJ, Dear WE, and Members of the Laboratory Performance Standards Committee of the Society for Cardiac Angiography and Interventions. Guidelines for continuous quality improvement in the cardiac catheterization laboratory. Cathet Cardiovasc Diagn 1993;30:191–200.
12. Goldman RL. The reliability of peer assessments of quality of care. JAMA 1992;267:958–960.
13. Berwick DM. Toward an applied technology for quality measurement in health care. Med Decis Making 1988;8:253–258.
14. Jollis JG, Ancukiewicz M, DeLong ER, et al. Discordance of databases designed for claims payment versus clinical information systems. Implications for outcomes research. Ann Intern Med 1993; 119:844–850.
15. Carey RG, Lloyd RC. Data collection. In: Carey RG, Lloyd RC, eds. Measuring quality improvement in

health care. New York, NY: Quality Resources, 1955:27–52.

16. Donabedian A. Quality assessment and assurance: unity of purpose, diversity of means. Inquiry 1988; 25:173–192.

17. Berwick DM. Measuring health care quality. Pediatr Rev 1988;10:11–16.

18. Alpert JS. Guidelines for training in adult cardiovascular medicine. Core cardiology training symposium (COCATS). J Am Coll Cardiol 1995;25: 1–34.

19. Ryan TJ, Bauman WB, Kennedy JW, et al. Guidelines for percutaneous transluminal coronary angioplasty. A report of the American Heart Association/American College of Cardiology Task Force on assessment of diagnostic and therapeutic cardiovascular procedures (Committee on percutaneous transluminal coronary angioplasty). Circulation 1993;88:2987–3007.

20. Pepine CJ, Allen HD, Bashore TM, et al. ACC/AHA guidelines for cardiac catheterization laboratories. J Am Coll Cardiol 1991;18:1149–1182.

21. Cowley MJ, Faxon DP, Holmes DR. Guidelines for training, credentialing, and maintenance of competence for the performance of coronary angioplasty: a report from the Interventional Cardiology Committee and the Training Program Standards Committee of the Society for Cardiac Angiography and Interventions. Cathet Cardiovasc Diagn 1993;30: 1–4.

22. Friesinger GC, Adams DF, Bourassa MG, et al. Optimal resources for examination of the heart and lungs: cardiac catheterization and radiographic facilities. Examination of the chest and cardiovascular system study group. Circulation 1983;68: 893A–930A.

23. Johnson LW, Moore RJ, Balter S. Review of radiation safety in the cardiac catheterization laboratory. Cathet Cardiovasc Diagn 1992;25:186–194.

24. Comried L. Cost analysis: initiation of HBMC and first CareMap. Nurs Econ 1996;14(1):34–39.

25. Schriefer J. The synergy of pathways and algorithms: two tools work better than one. Jt Comm J Qual Improv 1994;20(9):485–499.

26. Strong AG, Sneed NV. Clinical evaluation of a critical path for coronary artery bypass surgery patients. Prog Cardiovasc Nurs 1991;6(1):29–37.

27. Blegen M, Reiter RC, Goode CJ, et al. Outcomes of hospital-based managed care: a multivariate analysis of cost and quality. Obstet Gynecol 1995;86(5): 809–814.

28. Goode C. Impact of a CareMap and case management on patient satisfaction and staff satisfaction, collaboration, and autonomy. Nurs Econ 1995; 13(6):337–348.

29. Calligaro KD, Dougherty MJ, Raviola CA, et al. Impact of clinical pathways on hospital costs and early outcome after major vascular surgery. J Vasc Surg 1995;22(6):649–657.

30. Cohen EL. Nursing case management: does it pay? J Nurs Admin 1991;21(4):20–25.

31. Palmer JS, Worwag EM, Conrad WG, et al. Same-day surgery for radical retropubic prostatectomy: is it an attainable goal? Urology 1996;47(1):23–28.

32. Horne M. Involving physicians in clinical pathways: an example for perioperative knee

arthroplasty. Jt Comm J Qual Improv 1996;22(2): 115–124.

33. Selker HP, Beshansky JR, Paulker SG, et al. The epidemiology of delays in a teaching hospital. Med Care 1989;27(2):112–129.

34. Hannan EL, Kilburn H Jr, O'Donnell JF, et al. Adult open heart surgery in New York State: an analysis of risk factors and hospital mortality rates. JAMA 1990;264:2768–2774.

35. Hannan EL, Kilburn H Jr, Racz M, et al. Improving the outcomes of coronary artery bypass surgery in New York State. JAMA 1994;271:761–766.

36. Ritchie JL, Phillips KA, Luft HS. Coronary angioplasty: statewide experience in California. Circulation 1993;88:2735–2743.

37. Jollis JG, Peterson ED, DeLong ER, et al. The relation between the volume of coronary angioplasty procedures at hospitals treating Medicare beneficiaries and short-term mortality. N Engl J Med 1994;331:1625–1629.

38. Abdelmeguid AE, Topol EJ, Whitlow PL, et al. Significance of mild transient release of creatine kinase-MB fraction after percutaneous coronary interventions. Circulation 1996;94:1528–1536.

39. Ellis SG, Omoigui N, Bittl JA, et al. Analysis and comparison of operator-specific outcomes in interventional cardiology: from a multicenter database of 4860 quality-controlled procedures. Circulation 1996;93:431–439.

40. Leape LL, Hilborne LH, Park RE, et al. The appropriateness of use of coronary artery bypass graft surgery in New York State. JAMA 1993;269: 753–760.

41. Hilborne LH, Leape LL, Bernstein SJ, et al. The appropriateness of use of percutaneous transluminal coronary angioplasty in New York State. JAMA 1993;269:761–765.

42. Lauer MA, Ziskind AA, Lemmon CC, et al. Prospective assessment of revascularization appropriateness scoring systems: a comparison of RAND Expert Panel Ratings, ACC/AHA guidelines, and the University of Maryland Revascularization Appropriateness Score. J Am Coll Cardiol 1995;25: 344A.

43. Ellis SG, Miller DP, Brown KJ, et al. The in-hospital cost of percutaneous coronary revascularization: critical determinants and implications. Circulation 1995;92:741–747.

44. Hannan EL, Arani DT, Johnson LW, et al. Percutaneous transluminal coronary angioplasty in New York State. Risk factors and outcomes. JAMA 1993; 268:3092–3097.

45. Metz CE. Basic principles of ROC analysis. Semin Nucl Med 1978;8:283–298.

46. Green J, Wintfeld N. Report cards on cardiac surgeons. Assessing New York State's approach. N Engl J Med 1995;332:1229–1232.

47. Mark DB. Economic analysis methods and endpoints. In: Califf RM, Mark CB, Wagner GS, eds. Acute coronary care. 2nd ed. St. Louis, MO: Mosby Yearbook, 1995:167–182.

48. Ellis SG, Brown K, Howell G, et al. Two-year cardiac cost after cardiac catheterization—profound impact of revascularization after first PTCA compared with initial medical or surgical therapy. J Am Coll Cardiol February 1996:72A.

49. Davis DA, Thomson MA, Oxman AD, et al. Changing physician performance. A systematic review of the effect of continuing medical education strategies. JAMA 1995;274:700–705.
50. Pinkerton RE, Tinanoff N, Willms JL, et al. Resident physician performance in a continuing education format. Does newly acquired knowledge improve patient care? JAMA 1980;244:2183–2185.
51. James BC, Eddy DM. CPI and practice guidelines. In: Horn SD, Hopkins DSP, eds. Clinical improvement: a new technology for developing cost-effective quality health care. New York: Faulkner & Gray, 1994:127–140.
52. Eddy DM. Clinical decision making: from theory to practice. Designing a practice policy. Standards, guidelines, and options. JAMA 1990;263:3077–3084.
53. Chassin MR. Practice guidelines: best hope for quality improvement in the 1990s. J Occup Environ Med 1990;32:1199–1206.
54. Schoenbaum SC, Murrey KO. Impact of profiles on medical practice. In: United States Physician Payment Review Commission, ed. Physician Payment Review Commission Conference of Profiling. Washington, DC: Physician Payment Review Commission, 1992:72–102.
55. Restuccia JD. The effect of concurrent feedback in reducing inappropriate hospital utilization. Med Care 1982;20:46–62.
56. Thompson JS, Prior MA. Quality assurance and morbidity and mortality conference. J Surg Res 1992;52:97–100.
57. James BC, Horn SD, Stephenson RA. Management by fact: what is CPI and how is it used? In: Horn SD, Hopkins DSP, eds. Clinical practice improvement: a new technology for developing cost-effective quality health care. New York: Faulkner & Gray, 1994:39–54.
58. O'Connor GT, Plume SK, Olmstead EM, et al. A regional intervention to improve the hospital mortality associated with coronary artery bypass graft surgery. JAMA 1996;275:841–846.
59. Clemmer TP, Gardner RD. Medical informatics in the intensive care unit: state of the art 1991. Int J Clin Monit Comput 1992;8:86–92.
60. Shortliffe EH. Clinical decision-support systems. In: Shortliffe EH, Perreault LE, eds. Medical informatics: computer applications in health care. Reading, MA: Addison-Wesley, 1990:466–502.
61. Berwick DM. Controlling variation in health care: a consultation from Walter Shewhart. Med Care 1991;29:1212–1225.
62. Greco PJ, Eisenberg JM. Changing physicians' practices. N Engl J Med 1993;329:1271–1273.
63. Elson RB, Connelly DP. Computerized patient records in primary care. Arch Fam Med 1995;4:698–705.
64. Califf RM, Jollis JG, Peterson ED. Operator-specific outcomes. A call to professional responsibility. Circulation 1996;93:403–406.
65. Ellis SG, Omoigui N, Bittl JA, et al. Analysis and comparison of operator-specific outcomes in interventional cardiology. From a multicenter database of 4860 quality-controlled procedures. Circulation 1996;93:431–439.
66. Snelson E. Quality assurance implications of federal peer review laws. The Health Care Quality Improvement Act and the National Practitioner Data Bank. Qual Assur Util Rev 1992;7:2–11.
67. Blumenthal D. Quality of health care. 4. The origins of the quality-of-care debate. N Engl J Med 1996;335:1146–1149.

6

Conflicts of Interest in the Catheterization Laboratory: Strategies for Identification and Avoidance

Barry D. Bertolet, MD
Ronald E. Vlietstra, MB, ChB
Carl J. Pepine, MD

"Medicine is not merely a science but an art. The character of the physician may act more powerfully upon the patient than the drugs employed."—Paracelsus, c. 1525

INTRODUCTION

With physicians coming under the increasing scrutiny of government, business, and the public, invasive cardiologists face more ethical challenges than ever before (1). Where research was once the invasive cardiologist's most significant ethical concern, today one must also be concerned with self-ownership of catheterization laboratory facilities, self-referral of patients for catheterization-related procedures, self-reporting of outcomes, advertising, industry relationships, billing practices, managed care, cost cutting, and performance of ad hoc procedures, all of which can contribute to adverse public perception. Moreover, **patients often refer themselves directly to cardiologists, eliminating input from another treating physician.** The ethical physician must therefore balance the rights of patients and the responsibilities of physicians with the rights of physicians and the responsibilities of patients at a time when societal values and expectations are changing (2). In this chapter, potential ethical problems arising in the catheterization laboratory and invasive cardiology practice are discussed, along with recommendations for avoiding certain problems that could lead to ethical pitfalls.

SELF-OWNERSHIP OF FACILITIES

The emphasis on outpatient or ambulatory care in medicine and the entrepreneurial attitude that exists today have led to a proliferation of freestanding cardiology service centers, which often include cardiac catheterization laboratories. Some of these laboratories are owned by physicians, and some may be owned by physicians who either operate or refer patients to the same center. Particularly as catheterization services have expanded into rural areas at a time when public funds for expansion are decreasing, close association with and even ownership by group practices is probably inevitable. Some of these ventures may be in the form of limited partnerships, with the operating physician represented as the general partner and the referring physicians as limited partners. While many of these centers fill an obvious medical need and provide expedient, quality service to their patients, concerns may arise about the potential conflict of interest related to common ownership and operation. In other areas of medicine, some reports have suggested that the financial incentives of physician joint ventures may lead to an overuse of services, increased costs to consumers, reduced access for the poor, and diminished quality of service (3–6). Interestingly, although medical need is usually given as the justification for developing facilities, none of these physician-owned service centers seem to be located in the areas where indigent patients reside. **And increased scrutiny now surrounds all physicians who seem to benefit financially in excess of the reasonable professional fee for service.**

Recommendations

Invasive cardiologists are strongly advised to avoid entering any business arrangements that might influence their decision in the care of patients. It is unethical for any physician to receive a "kickback" or commission for referring a patient to a particular facility. In fact, it is a federal offense for physicians to receive fees or other rewards for referral of Medicare and Medicaid patients (7). Presently, 36 states further extend this law to protect public and privately insured patients (6). The welfare of the patient must be the sole guide in a physician's decisions. With this principle in mind, the cardiologist *can* refer patients to a facility in which he or she has invested as a result of a lack of similar services in the community or when the capital funding to provide these services is not otherwise available (8). In such cases, disclosing this information to the patient will help to avoid any perception of a potential conflict of in-

terest (9). Investments in publicly traded securities (e.g., stocks, bonds) do not represent a conflict of interest as long as these investments do not have the potential to influence the medical practice of the physician (8). The American Medical Association Council on Ethical and Judicial Affairs recommends that **"in general, physicians should not refer patients to a health care facility outside of their office, at which they do not directly provide care or services, when they have an investment interest in the facility"** (10).

SELF-REFERRAL OF PATIENTS TO FACILITIES

In the evaluation of patients with known or suspected cardiac disease, it is not unusual for a cardiologist, after initial diagnostic studies, to recommend further testing with cardiac catheterization. Those cardiologists with ties to a particular cardiac catheterization laboratory may refer their patients to the laboratory for diagnostic procedures (3, 11–12). In fact, the same cardiologist, or a member of the group, may perform the diagnostic procedure and either recommend or perform a therapeutic procedure, such as percutaneous transluminal coronary angioplasty (PTCA). Therefore, a single cardiologist—or one from the same cardiology group that has financial ties to the primary cardiologist—may recommend and receive fees for the initial evaluation, the diagnostic procedure, and even the therapeutic procedure. However, this case does not necessarily represent a conflict of interest if (*a*) the evaluation and therapy are medically justifiable; (*b*) the reasons are documented; and (*c*) the patient is informed of the doctor's financial interest in the facility and told of available alternatives (e.g., a second opinion). As has been demonstrated in self-referral situations outside cardiology (e.g., chemistry laboratories and surgical facilities), concern exists that physician self-referral of patients may lead to higher patient costs and increased rates of testing when compared with similar patients managed in independent referral situations (4–6, 13). The Ethics in Patient Referral Act (Stark I

Law) was significantly expanded with the passage of the Omnibus Budget and Reconciliation Act. Effective January 1, 1995, this new legislation (Stark II Law) bans physicians from referring Medicare and Medicaid patients to a variety of "designated health services" (including radiographic diagnostic services) if the physician or an immediate family member has a financial relationship with the designated service. **A financial relationship includes ownership or investment interest in that service, or any compensation arrangement involving any means of remuneration.**

Recommendations

The practice of self-referral for services such as cardiac catheterization may not always be in the patient's best interest. The cardiologist must ensure that the planned procedure is medically appropriate and that the decision is made exclusive of any financial gain (11–12). If there is a question regarding the appropriateness of such a procedure (e.g., PTCA), the cardiologist has an ethical responsibility to ask for a second opinion from another cardiologist, preferably one who has no fiscal connections with the referring cardiologist (9). The practice of having regular open conferences to discuss difficult problems also helps to defuse these concerns. In general, conflicts in this area can be avoided by following published guidelines for performance of diagnostic and therapeutic procedures (9).

SELF-REPORTING OF OUTCOME

As government and business more closely scrutinize the medical community, more emphasis will be placed on patient outcome as an index of physician competence and appropriateness of care. There is potential concern about accurate reporting of catheterization results and outcomes (e.g., complications), particularly from a laboratory where the reporting physician may also have a business interest. This concern can

be compounded when the referring cardiologist is also the catheterizing cardiologist and owner or investor. With the growth of ambulatory cardiac service centers, intense local competition often occurs, providing an environment that could lead to suppressing accurate data on adverse events. In addition, if such a competitive setting were to exist, these centers may try to maintain unreasonably low costs to solicit patients and third-party contracts. Ultimately, these actions could lead to lower quality medical care. This situation may be exacerbated by possible governmental moves toward managed care and preferred care centers.

Recommendations

All catheterization laboratories should be responsible for collecting accurate data on procedure-related adverse outcomes. This is best done by those not immediately involved with the procedure and the business interests of the laboratory. Initial data should be gathered within 24 hours of the patient's procedure. Another mechanism should be available for recording data on late complications (e.g., those occurring within 1 week). These results should be reviewed by an independent quality control committee and be open to peer review.

ADVERTISING

With the increasing number of ambulatory cardiac catheterization centers and increasing competition for patients, the amount of advertising might also increase, especially since many of these centers represent small business ventures. Advertising can educate the public as well as describe available cardiac services for referring physicians. However, many are concerned that these advertisements could lead to misleading claims in efforts to entice patients to the center. Additionally, in attempts to increase patient referrals, advertisements may be used to promote unapproved investigational devices being used for a specific trial. The overall concern is that, as a result of such advertising, the indirect cost of medical care may increase, the quality of patient care may diminish, and the "image of medicine" may be tarnished (9).

Recommendations

Physician advertising is unethical if it contains statements that are unsubstantiated, false, deceptive, or misleading. This includes statements that mislead by omitting necessary information (e.g., not stating that a new device is not yet FDA-approved). Because a catheterization laboratory receives patients only by professional referral, the majority of advertising should come in the form of announcements of laboratory services and staff (8). Such announcements should be directed for the most part at other physicians, and not at the general public. Advertising unapproved investigational devices for the purpose of increasing patient interest or referrals is clearly unethical. Cardiologists are referred to the American Medical Association statement concerning media relations for further guidance (14).

INDUSTRY RELATIONSHIPS

The relationship between medically related industry and the physician, which can be either beneficial or damaging to the public, has also come under increasing scrutiny. The benefits are that industry can offer additional sources of research support for the physician and facility, can offer greater potential for increased scientific and commercial productivity, and can enhance the educational experience (15). The risks are that industry involvement may lead to channeling of research to purely applied areas, to publication of data from poorly planned or conducted research, or even to suppression of damaging, negative, or inconclusive research data. Some manufacturers have offered inducements to physicians and hospitals to capture market share (16), such as quantity discounts, cash rebates, and shares of company stock. Because of the pressures of managed care and capitation, many man-

ufacturers have offered to assume some of the financial risk. In exchange for market share, these manufacturers will offer a capitated equipment price for diagnostic and interventional procedures.

With regard to industry–cardiologist interaction as it relates to education, much of the technical information on new catheterization products comes directly from industry representatives. Although the manufacturer is clearly an expert source, there is the potential for a positive "slant" that may mislead the practitioner. This bias is of particular concern when industry representatives attend actual catheterization procedures, where they may even have input into what equipment is used. Special attention was drawn to the risks of this practice by the U.S. Senate investigation of the pacemaker industry (17). Nevertheless, in certain select situations and when closely examined, the benefits of industry relationship may constitute a persuasive argument for a continuing alliance. This union, however, demands constant and careful examination to document the benefit of its continued existence.

Recommendations

Industry support should be disclosed whenever a cardiologist speaks or writes about a company's or competitor's products. Accepting gifts, and subsidies of any type from medical equipment or pharmaceutical companies in exchange for product "evaluation" is strongly discouraged (8). Industry should be discouraged from placing investigational devices in nonresearch-oriented clinical practices purely as a marketing ploy. It is a conflict of interest for cardiologists to receive inducements of any type from any manufacturer for the use of their medical instruments, catheters, or drugs in the care of patients (9). Companies violating these guidelines should be reported to the Compliance Division of the Food and Drug Administration (FDA). Physicians receiving inducements are also subject to action by their state medical professional regulation agencies.

As a result of increasing financial stressors, physicians will likely enter into agreements with manufacturers to limit equipment costs. When these contracts are made, it is the physician's duty to assure that patient safety and the quality-of-care being delivered do not suffer. The physician should not receive any direct financial benefit from such arrangements.

The catheterizing cardiologist should balance educational information obtained from industry with that obtained from professional medical journals and continuing medical education accredited courses. Undue industry influence in the catheterization laboratory should be minimized. Industry representatives generally should not attend actual procedures except to give technical counsel on the physician's initial use of a complex device.

BILLING PRACTICES

From the onset of the patient–physician relationship, the patient must understand a physician's general fees and overall costs for medical care. Financial arrangements (unless in an emergency situation) should be clarified before the delivery of service. Once an agreement is reached, it is the physician's duty to charge appropriately for services rendered (8). Patients should expect and demand responsible, ethical billing from the cardiologist. Above all else, the final bill will leave the most lasting impression on the patient. There is concern that invasive cardiologists may perform unnecessary procedures (e.g., routine right heart catheterization, routine standby pacer insertion for coronary angiography), duplicate services (e.g., repeat arterial punctures when two procedures are planned in the same day), or bill for procedures that may not be directly performed (e.g., done by a physician assistant).

Recommendations

The cardiologist should bill only for services provided directly to a patient, assuring that the fee accurately reflects the degree of service rendered. No cardiologist should

bill for a service that he or she did not personally perform. When catheterization procedures are combined or performed in tandem, some economy of scale takes place relative to savings of time, additional injections, interpretations, etc. An example may be the combination of a diagnostic coronary angiogram and a PTCA at the same setting or within several hours using the same arterial sheath. In such instances, the bill should accurately reflect these economies (e.g., one preprocedure and one postprocedure visit, one arterial puncture, one groin tamponade, etc.). An operator assistant's fee should be charged only for those procedures requiring the direct involvement of more than one physician (i.e., mitral valvuloplasty) (9). It is unethical to receive fees or commissions as a result of patient referral for cardiac catheterization. Cardiologists should neither provide nor seek compensation for either duplication of services or performance of services that may be unnecessary.

MANAGED CARE

Eighty-three percent of physicians in the United States hold some form of managed care contract. With this dramatic growth and the impact of managed care agencies on health care, there is concern whether managed care can be ethical care. Initially, managed care represented managed cost. Now, managed care is evolving into rationed care, hence the reason for concern. Several questions need to be addressed immediately. Who makes medical decisions —do the doctor and patient decide on what should be done and the managed care agency decide on whether it will be done? Is similar service provided by going to a "preferred" hospital or physician? Is the quality of medical care the same for managed care and fee-for-service patients? Can the managed care agency stop a physician from performing the evaluation he or she deems necessary for a patient? Are physicians required to sign an "anticriticism" or gag clause? How are physicians paid—do doctors get financial incentives from the managed care agency through the performance of more/less procedures or through withholding referrals?

Recommendations

The American Medical Association Council on Ethical and Judicial Affairs recently published a set of ethical guidelines for managed care agencies to follow (18). These include:

1. Establishment of allocation guidelines with physician input. The physician should, after consultation with the patient, be able to decide on the proper course of action in a patient's illness.
2. Full disclosure of benefit restrictions and treatment options, even those not included in the health plan, to all patients.
3. Full disclosure of any incentives to limit health care. Physicians, however, need not disclose their personal financial arrangement with the managed care agency to the patient, but should make sure that these arrangements are fully disclosed in the patient's health plan.
4. Use of financial incentives only to promote cost-effective delivery of quality patient care.
5. Encouragement of physicians and patients *not* to participate in any plan that provides substandard health care.

Additionally, physicians should refuse to sign any anticriticism or gag clause. Congress has recently declined to outlaw gag clauses, despite protest by the American Medical Association. However, 30 states have already banned or are considering banning gag clauses. These clauses may motivate some physicians to not completely inform patients about their illnesses and all treatment options (19). Managed care is necessary so that medical care is affordable and accessible for the majority of Americans. It is the physician's responsibility to assure that patients receive quality medical care in a timely manner.

CUTTING COSTS

Market forces mandate tighter budgeting in the catheterization laboratory. There is potential for significant ethical conflict as car-

diologists strive to keep expenses to a minimum yet provide optimal care for their patients (20). Independent predictors of hospital costs for percutaneous coronary revascularization include physician choices, age of the patient, and urgency of the procedure. Independent predictors of catheterization laboratory costs include physician choices and lesion type. Physician choices in the catheterization laboratory impact both hospital and laboratory costs in a major way—an approximate 20% variation (21). The behavior of physicians in the catheterization laboratory can be influenced in many ways, and some are ethical, some are not.

Recommendations

Quality as well as cost needs to be considered when cardiac catheterization laboratory equipment is stocked. Each physician or laboratory should be able to negotiate to use quality products at competitive prices. However, cost should not be a factor in the one-on-one encounter with the patient (20). Practice guidelines can improve objectivity in decision making and standardize the delivery of care (i.e., selective use of ionic contrast) (22). These guidelines should be flexible to allow for exceptional cases. Education, not coercion, should be used to encourage cost-conscious decision making.

PERFORMANCE OF AD HOC PROCEDURES AND VARIATIONS FROM ESTABLISHED GUIDELINES

While the performance of therapeutic interventions at the same time as initial diagnostic catheterization—so-called "ad hoc" procedures—offers some economies, as noted earlier, when done routinely they may be costly, unnecessary, poorly planned, and potentially risky for patients. Before performing any catheterization procedure, the operating cardiologist plans a course of action that is in the patient's best interests. He or she speaks with the patient in a language that the patient can understand. The patient should be informed of the planned procedure(s) and potential risks. The *possibility* of performing another procedure (e.g., angioplasty) at the same time should also be discussed if the patient's condition suggests that it is medically appropriate. The statement "If I find something, do you want me to take care of it?" is not medically acceptable. The patient should give signed consent for all considered procedures that are indicated. Obviously, certain procedures not previously discussed with the patient will need to be performed in emergency situations to prevent morbidity. These procedures, however, are no longer considered ad hoc.

Guidelines have been published relative to performance of angioplasty that clearly call for objective evidence of myocardial ischemia during laboratory testing (23). Yet a recent practice survey found that only 29% of patients undergoing angioplasty had stress testing before the procedure. So clearly a deviation from these guidelines was present in the majority (24).

Recommendations

No procedure should be done without both specific medically accepted indication and fully informed consent (25). The cardiologist should perform no routine procedure purely for financial or other gain (11–12). It is not appropriate to first approach the patient during the course of the diagnostic catheterization to discuss proceeding with immediate therapeutic procedures when the situation is not urgent (i.e., ad hoc angioplasty). The performance of other unnecessary routine procedures such as right heart catheterization, pacemaker placement, or peripheral angiography during coronary angiography should be avoided.

Whenever there is reason to deviate from published guidelines, the reasons should be clearly documented in the patient record and the options discussed with the patient.

SUMMARY

There are many additional conflict-of-interest issues that challenge the cardiologist practicing in the catheterization laboratory. When clear guidance is not available from professional societies, a useful guiding principle is to ask oneself, "Would I feel comfortable if my position on this issue was widely known?"

The American Medical Association has reminded all physicians that "medicine is a profession, a calling," and "not a business" (26). Some believe that physicians can best serve the interests of their patients by absolving themselves from the financial interests in the medical marketplace (3). However, economic reality dictates that the establishment, management, and maintenance of a healthy medical practice requires sound financial support. This dilemma will continue to exist as long as our present form of health care exists. Until real change occurs, the recommendations outlined hopefully will assist the invasive cardiologist to practice with compassion and sound ethical behavior.

References

1. Thompson DF. Understanding financial conflicts of interest. N Engl J Med 1993;329:573–576.
2. 21st Bethesda Conference. Ethics in cardiovascular medicine: October 5–6, 1989, Bethesda, Maryland. J Am Coll Cardiol 1990;16:1–36.
3. Relman AS. Dealing with conflicts of interest. N Engl J Med 1985;313:749–751.
4. Hillman BJ, Joseph CA, Mabry MR, et al. Frequency and costs of diagnostic imaging in office practice—a comparison of self-referring and radiologist-referring physicians. N Engl J Med 1990; 323:1604–1608.
5. Hemenway D, Killen A, Cashman SB, et al. Physicians' responses to financial incentives: evidence from a for-profit ambulatory care center. N Engl J Med 1990;322:1059–1063.
6. Mitchell JM, Sunshine JH. Consequences of physicians' ownership of health care facilities—joint ventures in radiation therapy. N Engl J Med 1992; 327:1497–1501.
7. Kusserow RP. Financial arrangements between physicians and health care businesses. Washington, DC: Office of Inspector General, May 1989.
8. 1991–1992 American College of Physicians Ethics Committee. American College of Physicians ethics manual. 3rd ed. Ann Intern Med 1992;117:947–960.
9. Pepine CJ, Allen HD, Bashore T, et al. ACC/AHA Ad Hoc Task Force Report. ACC/AHA guidelines for cardiac catheterization and cardiac catheterization laboratories. J Am Coll Cardiol 1991;18: 1149–1182.

10. American Medical Association Council on Ethical and Judicial Affairs. Current opinions of the council of ethical and judicial affairs of the American Medical Association. AMA Council Report C/I-91: 6–7.
11. Todd JS, Horan JK. Physician referral—the AMA view. JAMA 1989;262:395–396.
12. Stark FH. Physicians' conflicts in patient referrals. JAMA 1989;262:397.
13. Swedlow A, Johnson G, Smithline N, et al. Increased costs and rates of use in the California Workers' Compensation system as a result of self-referral by physicians. N Engl J Med 1992;327: 1502–1506.
14. American Medical Association Council on Ethical and Judicial Affairs. AMA Council Report. C/A-89. Chicago: American Medical Association, 1980.
15. Blumenthal D. Academic-industry relationships in the life sciences: extent, consequences, and management. JAMA 1992;268:3344–3349.
16. Cataract surgery: fraud, waste, and abuse: a report by the chairman of the Subcommittee of Health and Long-Term Care of the Select Committee on Aging, House of Representatives. Ninety-ninth Congress, July 19, 1985. Washington, DC: Government Printing Office, 1985. Committee publication no. 99–506.
17. Fraud, waste, and abuse in the Medicare pacemaker industry. Special Committee on Aging, United States Senate. Washington, DC: Government Printing Office. September, 1982: 62–64.
18. American Medical Association Council on Ethical and Judicial Affairs. Ethical issues in managed care. JAMA 1995;273:330–335.
19. Editorial. Manipulated care: gagging doctors, blinding patients. Lancet 1996;348:903.
20. Kassirer JP. Managed care and the morality of the marketplace. N Engl J Med 1995;333:50–52.
21. Heidenreich PA, Chou TM, Amidon TM, et al. Impact of the operating physician on costs of percutaneous transluminal coronary angioplasty. Am J Cardiol 1996;77:1169–1173.
22. Berger JT, Rosner F. The ethics of practice guidelines. Arch Intern Med 1996;156:2051–2056.
23. ACC/AHA Task Force Report. Guidelines for percutaneous transluminal coronary angioplasty: a report of the American College of Cardiology/American Heart Association Task Force on assessment of diagnostic and therapeutic cardiovascular procedures (subcommittee on percutaneous transluminal coronary angioplasty). J Am Coll Cardiol 1988;12:529–545.
24. Topol EJ, Ellis SG, Cosgrove DM, et al. Analysis of coronary angioplasty practice in the United States with an insurance claims database. Circulation 1993;87:1489–1497.
25. Rodwin MA. Physicians' conflicts of interest: the limitations of disclosure. N Engl J Med 1989;321: 405–408.
26. House of Delegates of the American Medical Association. Commercialism in the practice of medicine: report of the Board of Trustees of the American Medical Association, June 1983.

GENERAL CARDIAC CATHETERIZATION: APPLICATION TO BOTH DIAGNOSTIC AND THERAPEUTIC PROCEDURES

7

Evaluation and Preparation of the Patient for Cardiac Catheterization

Hercules Panayiotou, MBBCh, MMed
Charles R. Lambert, MD, PhD
Norberto Schechtmann, MD
Carl J. Pepine, MD
James A. Hill, MD, MS

INTRODUCTION

Evaluation of the patient to undergo cardiac catheterization is an integral part of the procedure. It should ensure that (*a*) an appropriate indication exists, (*b*) contraindications are recognized, (*c*) timing of the procedure is appropriate, (*d*) high-risk patients and conditions are identified, (*e*) adequate explanation and discussion of the procedure, including risks and potential benefits, are provided to the patient and family, and (*f*) informed consent is obtained.

INFORMED CONSENT

It is the duty of the physician who will perform the catheterization to obtain informed consent from either the patient or a surrogate (e.g., parent or valid legal representative). Most states require that legal consent be obtained while the patient is lucid and has not received any sedative in the preceding 6 to 8 hours. Informed consent implies

that the physician has provided the patient or legal guardian with enough information or knowledge to allow an informed judgment as to how to proceed. This usually focuses on informing the patient about his or her condition; what is to be gained by performing the catheterization; how this procedure complements, confirms, or adds to other procedures already performed; alternative procedures available; and the risks involved (1). It is also important to discuss how findings from the procedure may change treatment and aid in formulating an estimate of prognosis. In some circumstances it may be necessary to compare the costs of various procedures.

Although the type of information imparted depends on the level of the patient's understanding, it is important to converse in clear language. We have found that illustrating the proposed procedure with simple diagrams, brochures, and videotapes is very helpful. When discussing risks, it is important to **state major and minor complications.** If operator-specific complication data are available, they should be discussed. It is also important to mention the universal inconveniences and discomforts involved with catheterization, including lying on a hard table, transient warm flush with large bolus contrast agent injection, pain in the groin area with local anesthetic, several hours of strict bed rest, and possible need to void while lying flat.

It is prudent that the physician's presentation be as **unbiased as possible** and that coercion not be used to obtain consent (1). A second opinion may be helpful to both patient and physician. In some situations assistance of courts may be sought if a patient refuses a particular procedure or treatment and there is concern about the patient's competence. The patient should not be abandoned if he or she rejects a recommended management plan. If alternative options cannot be agreed on, transfer of care to another physician, after providing adequate notice, may be best for both patient and physician. The final decision to accept or reject a particular procedure or treatment rests with the patient, whose right to self-determination must be respected.

On occasion the cardiac catheterization protocol may have to be changed because of findings (e.g., critical coronary stenosis and need to proceed with percutaneous transluminal coronary angioplasty [PTCA]), technical reasons (e.g., inability to cross critical aortic stenosis and need to proceed with transseptal technique), or complications. Such possibilities and potential complications should also be discussed when obtaining informed consent; however, it is important not to alarm patients. Appropriate consents should also be obtained if surgical intervention may be urgently required (e.g., bypass for failed PTCA). It is not appropriate to approach the patient for permission to institute additional procedures for the first time while diagnostic catheterization is in progress (2).

If a team of physicians is to participate in the procedure, such as in a teaching institution, it is important that the patient be told who is the *attending physician in charge* of the procedure and that fellows or other physicians may be participating in the procedure. The attending cardiologist's name should appear on the consent form. If a patient requests that a particular physician be present, participate, or perform the catheterization procedure, the patient's wishes must be respected. This sometimes requires referral to another invasive cardiologist.

If a portion of the study is to be performed or information gained for research purposes, the patient should be notified beforehand. It should also be made clear that the patient can refuse the research portion of the procedure and the clinically indicated portion will still be performed. The patient should not feel obliged to participate in research if he or she deems it unnecessary, considers that it adds unreasonable extra risk, or simply does not desire to participate (3, 4).

At the conclusion of the precatheterization interview an **appropriate note** should be written stating that the patient's records and data were reviewed, that the patient was interviewed and examined, that the anticipated procedure and its timing are appropriate, and whether the patient is at high or low risk in the proposed study. Also note that the procedure was explained to the patient (and family) or legal guardian, that the risks were listed, and whether the patient agreed to have the procedure. A standard checklist may be helpful.

Some patients have the impression that physicians perform unnecessary and expensive procedures. If a perception of a conflict of interest arises, especially if the physician owns the medical facility in which the catheterization is to be performed, a second opinion is recommended (4).

ISSUES REGARDING CONSENT FOR THERAPEUTIC OR INTERVENTIONAL PROCEDURES

Therapeutic procedures in the catheterization laboratory are usually performed electively but increasingly at the same sitting as the diagnostic procedure. Informed consent for the therapeutic procedure should be obtained beforehand rather than during catheterization. Occasionally emergencies arise while the study is in progress, but even then some form of verbal consent should be obtained from the patient or the family. When possible the referring physician should also be consulted, and this should be documented in the medical record.

For certain subgroups of patients, interventional therapy can be anticipated, and these patients should be appropriately prepared and asked for consent and surgical support scheduled if appropriate (5). These include (*a*) patients with unstable angina that cannot be stabilized who require urgent PTCA, (*b*) patients with signs or symptoms suggesting restenosis following PTCA within the previous 12 months, and (*c*) patients undergoing PTCA for an acute myocardial infarction with planned PTCA of only the infarct-related artery.

Apart from these subsets of patients, it can be problematic to perform interventional procedures at the time of initial diagnostic catheterization. Often **the most difficult aspect of patient selection for angioplasty is evaluation of the coronary anatomy**, and this is best done by the unhurried review of the cineangiograms, often in consultation with a cardiac surgeon or colleagues. Video images obtained at initial diagnostic cardiac catheterization can be inaccurate and can lead to increased risk for the patient. When one is performing angioplasty at time of diagnostic cardiac catheterization, it is imperative that high-quality fluoroscopic and video replay images or promptly developed cine films be available. Another group of patients who may be prepared for a therapeutic procedure at time of initial cardiac catheterization is candidates for percutaneous balloon valvuloplasty. These patients usually have had extensive noninvasive evaluation, including echocardiography and Doppler studies, and the aims of diagnostic catheterization are usually to confirm the diagnosis of significant valvular stenosis and to document coronary anatomy. Proceeding to balloon valvuloplasty in the same sitting if no contraindications are present is reasonable. Chapter 35 discusses the indications, contraindications, techniques, and complications of valvuloplasty. If decisions about proceeding with therapeutic procedures are to be made, the invasive cardiologist should review all pertinent clinical and noninvasive data with the consulting surgeon.

PREPARATION FOR OUTPATIENT VERSUS INPATIENT CATHETERIZATION

Increasingly, cardiac catheterization procedures are being performed on an outpatient basis and both the American College of Cardiology and American Heart Association (ACC/AHA) (2) and the Society for Cardiac Angiography and Interventions (6) have provided guidelines for the performance of such procedures. The rationale for performing outpatient catheterization and angiography is that it reduces costs and causes less family inconvenience and patient discomfort while maintaining a high standard of care (7–9). Careful selection to include only low-risk patients is important. All high-risk patients and those in whom high-risk coronary anatomy or severe cardiac abnormality is suspected should be hospitalized formally. Patients with procedure-related complications should also be hospitalized. Additional and more detailed criteria have been provided by the ACC/AHA Ad Hoc Task Force on Cardiac Catheterization to exclude unsuitable patients from ambulatory cardiac catheterization. Indications for diagnostic and therapeutic procedures as well as further discussion of outpatient versus inpatient settings are included in Chapters 2 and 15.

Outpatients should have a complete history and physical examination. Preparatory laboratory work should include (*a*) electrocardiogram within a week of the procedure; (*b*) chest x-ray film within 6 months; and (*c*) blood work to include complete blood count with platelets, electrolytes, blood urea nitrogen, creatinine, and clotting studies within several days of the procedure.

Outpatients should make arrangements to be brought to the cardiac catheterization facility the morning of the procedure and taken home in the afternoon. Patients should not drive after the procedure and should restrict activity for at least 24 hours. The patient should also be forewarned that if severe cardiovascular disease is identified at cardiac catheterization or if complications occur, hospitalization may be needed. After the procedure the patient should be observed by personnel skilled in identifying and managing catheterization complications in an area equipped for acute medical care. If the arterial access site is stable for 4 to 6 hours, the patient can be walked with observation. When walking is uneventful for at least an hour, the patient can be discharged home after the access site is inspected by the procedural cardiologist or other trained professional. A responsible friend or relative should be available to help and should care for the patient for the first 24 hours after outpatient cardiac catheterization. The patient and family should have instructions and phone numbers to call in case any problem arises.

PREMEDICATION

Almost all patients are anxious and apprehensive about medical procedures, including cardiac catheterization. A complete, thorough, and reassuring explanation of the procedure can go a long way toward relieving anxiety and calming the patient. Although it is prudent to minimize use of sedation and analgesia, especially in the ambulatory setting, sedation and analgesia should not be withheld. Patients who show signs and symptoms of autonomic nervous system stimulation, such as tachycardia, hypertension, fine tremor, and sweating, should be given such medications. The objectives of premedication are to relieve anxiety and stress and to produce a relaxed, calm, and cooperative patient. Such a patient may be lightly asleep but easily aroused. Preventing pain and providing antegrade amnesia for the catheterization are also desirable.

Conscious sedation is the depressed level of consciousness in which the patient still can independently and continuously maintain an airway and respond appropriately to physical stimulation and verbal communication. The increasing use of sedation to enhance the patient's comfort during diagnostic and therapeutic procedures has been noted by the Joint Commission of Accredited Healthcare Organizations (10). Subsequently many institutions have developed guidelines for sedation by nonanes-

thesiologists that emphasize collaboration between anesthesiology and other departments, such as the cardiac catheterization laboratory, to ensure proper use of conscious sedation (11). We strongly urge such a collaborative effort to standardize conscious sedation for both inpatient and outpatient facilities.

An ideal agent should provide both sedation and anxiolysis and should have the following characteristics: (*a*) rapid absorption and onset of action, (*b*) a high therapeutic index, and (*c*) rapid recovery without prolonged psychomotor impairment (12, 13). No single regimen is suitable for all patients. Premedication must take into account the patient's age, level of anxiety, size (weight), concomitant medical problems, pain threshold, severity of illness, concurrent use of other medications, anticipated technical difficulty, and duration of the procedure and recovery time. Minimal sedation may be needed in an otherwise healthy young patient undergoing routine diagnostic left heart catheterization, and the regimen may be more complex, requiring use of several drugs, in an elderly patient undergoing staged angioplasty for multivessel disease. Some patients are so anxious that a hypnotic or an additional dose of oral sedative the evening before the procedure, to provide a good night's sleep, may be more effective than just the sedative or anxiolytic dose immediately before the procedure. Similarly, if the catheterization will occur late in the day, as is common for angioplasty procedures, an additional early morning sedative or anxiolytic dose may blunt buildup of anxiety.

Table 7.1 lists the most commonly used sedatives, anxiolytics, and analgesics used in patients undergoing cardiac catheterizations and angiographic procedures. If the premedication is to be given orally, it should be administered at least 60 minutes before the patient is taken into the catheterization laboratory. For inpatients sedatives are usually administered in the ward or intensive care unit as they are called to the catheterization laboratory. Sometimes, however, as with ambulatory patients or in emergencies, an injection route is more convenient and appropriate, as it provides adequate background sedation and anxiolysis,

Table 7.1.
Commonly Used Sedatives, Anxiolytics, and Analgesics for Adult Cardiac Catheterization

Medication	Oral	IM	IV	Comments
Antihistamines				
Diphenhydramine	25–50 mg	10–50 mg	10–50 mg	
Promethazine	25–50 mg	12.5–50 mg	12.5–50 mg	
Benzodiazepines				
Diazepam	0.15–0.3 mg/kg		0.1 mg/kg	
Lorazepam	0.5–2 mg	0.05 mg/kg	1–2 mg	
Midazolam	0.5–0.7 mg/kg	0.1–0.3 mg/kg	0.05 mg/kg	
Opioids				
Meperidine	1.5–3 mg/kg	1 mg/kg	1 mg/kg	
Morphine	0.5–1 mg/kg	0.1 mg/kg	0.1 mg/kg	Oral preparation is sustained release
Antagonists				
Naloxone (opioids)			0.01–0.1 mg/kg	Titrate to desired effect
Flumazenil (benzodiazepines)			0.01–0.02 mg 0.4–1.0 mg	Partial antagonism Complete antagonism

IM, intramuscular; IV, intravenous.

usually within minutes for intravenous medication and within 10 to 15 minutes for intramuscular medication.

Antihistamines

Both diphenhydramine and promethazine are H_1 blockers. The high incidence (75%) of sedation by these two drugs is clinically useful, and these are commonly used to provide preprocedure sedation. They also relieve apprehension and produce light sleep from which the patient can be easily aroused. Promethazine is particularly effective in the treatment of nausea and vomiting. Antihistamines antagonize and prevent the actions of histamine that may be released on administration of contrast or morphine. This may protect against anaphylactic bronchospasm, prevent vascular changes, reduce skin flare and itch, and reduce increases in capillary permeability. Their anticholinergic side effects, such as dry mouth and throat, palpitations, headache, and tightness in the chest, are not usually a problem, but urinary retention, frequency, and dysuria may occur. Although antihistamines produce central nervous system (CNS) depression in therapeutic doses, both small and large doses can stimulate the CNS.

With oral administration these agents are rapidly absorbed, with onset of action within 30 minutes, maximum effects in 1 to 2 hours, and duration of 3 to 6 hours. In some patients the action may last as long as 24 hours, so patients are advised not to drive a car or operate appliances or machinery for at least 24 hours after a dose of antihistamine. In older patients dizziness, sedation, and hypotension are more common.

Benzodiazepines

The benzodiazepines have replaced the barbiturates as the drugs of choice for oral and parenteral sedation and anxiolysis. The reasons for this are greater acceptance among patients, anxiolytic and amnesic properties, and very high therapeutic index. Benzodiazepines commonly used for sedation and anxiolysis are well absorbed from the gastrointestinal tract but have important variances in distribution and elimination. Intravenous administration of diazepam can cause venous irritation, and so it should be given slowly, allowing at least 1 minute for each 5 mg (1 mL). Intra-arterial injection of benzodiazepines should be avoided, as it may lead to arterial spasm and gangrene. Special care should also be taken to prevent extravasation into the perivascular tissues when benzodiazepines are administered intravenously. Although the benzodiazepines have a very high therapeutic index, these agents should be avoided in patients with certain medical conditions, including pulmonary disease, sleep apnea, porphyria, myasthenia gravis, hepatic or renal impairment, acute angle glaucoma, and alcohol intoxication.

Numerous drug interactions, including some in commonly used cardiac drugs, have been described. Metoprolol, propranolol, and digoxin increase the effect of benzodiazepines by reducing hepatic metabolism. Other commonly used drugs that may increase the effects of the benzodiazepine diazepam include anticonvulsants, alcohol, antihistamines, cimetidine, oral contraceptives, and tricyclic antidepressants.

The adverse effects of the benzodiazepines are usually an extension of their CNS actions and are most common in the elderly. It is recommended that for patients over age 60 years who are debilitated or chronically ill, including those with severe heart failure, dosage should be reduced by up to 50% and rate of administration should be slow. Children are also sensitive to the effects of benzodiazepines and should be dosed with extreme caution.

Paradoxic effects are occasionally seen, are most common with short-acting agents, and may be misinterpreted as indication for greater sedation. Paradoxic behavior usually presents as euphoria, restlessness, hallucinations, hypomanic behavior, anxiety, irritability, tachycardia, sweating, and talkativeness. When paradoxic effects occur, it is important to discontinue the drug and consider the administration of a competitive benzodiazepine antagonist, such as flumazenil (14) if symptoms are severe. The indication for this drug is to treat patients with benzodiazepine overdosage; however, it is useful to reverse conscious sedation. Because the half-life of flumazenil is relatively short (about 1 hour), resedation may occur, and additional doses (up to 3 mg cumulative) may be required. Flumazenil is relatively fast acting, and responses are usually

seen within 1 to 5 minutes. Flumazenil is usually well tolerated, with nausea and vomiting being its most frequent adverse effects.

Because benzodiazepine overdose may result in depressed respiration and coma, equipment necessary for airway management should be available before any benzodiazepine is administered intravenously. Patients should be continuously monitored for early signs of hypoventilation. The cardiovascular effects of benzodiazepines are usually minor, but in anesthetic doses all benzodiazepines decrease blood pressure and increase heart rate. The metabolism and excretion of benzodiazepines are usually slow in patients in congestive heart failure and low cardiac output states, and doses of benzodiazepines should be reduced appropriately. The dose of benzodiazepines should also be reduced in patients with significant liver and renal abnormalities. In addition to the reduced metabolism and excretion of these drugs resulting in prolonged and heightened effects, desensitivity of CNS receptors may make patients more sensitive to these agents (13). In these patients smaller doses of short-acting drugs and drugs that do not have active metabolites are preferable.

Although there are distinct pharmacokinetic differences among the various benzodiazepines, it is advisable that the cardiologist be familiar with one or two of these agents for combined oral premedication and intravenous sedation. The newer and shorter-acting agent midazolam (Versed) is probably the drug of choice for conscious sedation, and several studies suggest that this drug has important advantages over diazepam, including faster onset of action (within 1 to 2 minutes of intravenous injection), less pain during injection, profound antegrade amnesia lasting 20 to 40 minutes, shorter recovery time (60 to 70 minutes), and fewer postoperative complications (12). Diazepam is still widely used as an anxiolytic for outpatient procedures, as it rapidly crosses the blood-brain barrier, resulting in a fast onset of action. Because of the high lipid solubility it redistributes to the peripheral fat, and although clinical effects disappear within 2 to 3 hours, psychomotor impairment may be prolonged. Oral diazepam, with its long half-life and active metabolites, may be the premedication of choice when the preoperative waiting time may be several hours. Because it takes at least 1 hour to take effect, diazepam is not ideal to premedicate patients on call. Lorazepam is a potent short-acting agent available in both oral and parenteral preparations.

Narcotics

The two most commonly used narcotic drugs are morphine and meperidine. These agents are indicated for procedures that are long and known to cause discomfort. Narcotics are not recommended for outpatient premedication unless the patient is in pain before the catheterization. In man, morphinelike drugs produce analgesia, sedation, changes in mood, and mental clouding and decrease anxiety. Morphinelike drugs administered in therapeutic doses produce peripheral vasodilation, reduce peripheral resistance, and inhibit baroreceptor reflexes. Peripheral vasodilatory effects are usually not significant in the supine patient but may result in hypotension and fainting when the patient sits up. Hypotension is reversed by naloxone. Morphine also causes blunting of the reflex vasoconstriction caused by increased P_{CO_2}.

Morphinelike drugs do not have significant effects on the myocardium, cardiac output, or heart rate. In patients with acute myocardial infarction and pulmonary edema, morphine and morphinelike drugs produce a decrease in oxygen consumption, cardiac work, and left ventricular end diastolic pressure. Hypotension, a common side effect, may be troublesome in patients who are hypovolemic, and these agents can aggravate hypovolemic shock. Morphine should be used with great care in patients with decreased respiratory reserve such as severe obesity, chronic obstructive pulmonary disease, and kyphoscoliosis. The hypotensive and depressant effects of morphinelike drugs may be prolonged and exaggerated by the concomitant use of benzodiazepines, phenothiazines, monoamine oxidase inhibitors, and tricyclic antidepressants. Postoperative nausea and vomiting are common in patients receiving narcotic analgesics (morphine more than meperidine) and can prolong recovery time.

PREPROCEDURE MEDICATION CHANGES

To prepare the patient for cardiac catheterization certain medications may have to be discontinued, doses adjusted, or new medicines administered to minimize risks or aid in the successful completion of the study.

Anticoagulation

Oral anticoagulants, such as warfarin (Coumadin), should be discontinued for 2 to 3 days prior to scheduled procedures with the aim of decreasing the international normalized ratio to less than 1.5. Patients who are at high risk for thromboembolism, such as those with large mobile left ventricular (LV) or left arterial (LA) thrombi or embolic events while receiving adequate anticoagulation and those with prosthetic valves, can be given intravenous heparin. In emergencies, even if the prothrombin time is prolonged, cardiac catheterization can still be performed. If bleeding at the entry site or sites does not stop with pressure alone, anticoagulation can be reversed via fresh frozen plasma or a percutaneous closure device (15). Vitamin K is not recommended because it occasionally causes a hypercoagulable state. Some operators prefer to perform procedures by cutdown and arteriotomy in this circumstance. Patients who are receiving intravenous heparin for unstable ischemic syndromes or after thrombolytic therapy for acute myocardial infarction should probably continue taking the drug prior to catheterization to avoid a rebound phenomenon with varied adverse clinical manifestations.

Coronary Vasodilators

In patients in whom coronary artery spasm is suspected and ergonovine or acetylcholine provocation is planned, all drugs that interfere with coronary artery tone should be discontinued for at least five half-lives. This usually translates to five doses. Drugs with long half-lives, such as once-a-day calcium channel blockers, may have to be discontinued for at least a week. Patients who become hypertensive during drug withdrawal can be treated with β-blockers, ACE inhibitors, diuretics, methyldopa, or various α-blocking agents. Intravenous nitroglycerin should be discontinued for several hours prior to scheduled spasm provocation study.

Diabetic Control

In general, patients with diabetes mellitus should be scheduled early in the day. Patients receiving oral hypoglycemia agents should omit the morning dose, and the regular dose should be given once feeding has resumed. For patients who take their hypoglycemia drugs twice a day or in the evening, 5% dextrose in water solution may be infused at 70 to 100 mL/hour starting 3 to 4 hours after fasting begins. Hypoglycemia may occur in fasting patients even when a dose of oral hypoglycemic agent is omitted, as the half-life of some agents is long. Other sulfonylureas have much shorter half-lives and thus are less likely to cause late hypoglycemia. For individuals with high plasma glucose levels or chronic uncontrolled diabetes, it is advisable that glycemic control be improved before subjecting them to cardiac catheterization. Uncontrolled diabetes mellitus is not uncommon in patients who are critically ill or who recently had myocardial infarction. **Metformin should be discontinued several days prior to administration of contrast agents** because of the possibility of lactic acidosis.

For patients using short- (e.g., regular), intermediate- (e.g., NPH or lente), or long-acting (e.g., ultralente) insulin it is recommended that with fasting the dose of insulin be reduced by 50% or more. Hypoglycemia can, however, still occur, especially when large doses of insulin are used. Peak action of NPH insulin is 11 hours, with onset at 2.5 hours and total duration of action 25

hours. It is important to detect symptoms and signs of hypoglycemia early and to give appropriate treatment. An alternative regimen for fasting patients is to omit the usual insulin dose and administer regular insulin (0.5 to 1 IU/hour) in D_5W at 70 to 120 mL/hour. Obviously the aim in all diabetic patients is to get them back on their regular diet and insulin dose as soon as possible after cardiac catheterization. For diabetic patients in whom relatively heavy sedation is anticipated and reflexes blunted, it may be advisable to maintain slight hyperglycemia by glucose infusion. Patients taking NPH insulin are at increased risk for serious protamine sulfate reactions. Thus, protamine should be avoided or used only with great caution in patients with insulin-dependent diabetes mellitus.

Blood Pressure Control

Blood pressure should be normalized and controlled as closely as possible before cardiac catheterization. Hypertensive patients are at increased risk for pulmonary edema, aggravating ischemia, and bleeding complications, especially if thrombolytic therapy has been administered. Commonly used agents for rapid blood pressure control include sublingual nifedipine, intravenous metoprolol, intravenous labetalol, intravenous nitroglycerin, intravenous nicardipine, and sodium nitroprusside. Nitroprusside 0.25 to 10 mg/kg/minute is the drug of choice for patients with hypertension and known or suspected poor LV function.

Significant hypotension of cardiac or noncardiac origin, especially if there are signs of poor peripheral perfusion, should be treated to ensure a systolic pressure of at least 90 mm Hg before elective cardiac catheterization and angiography. Treatment, which depends on cause, may include discontinuation of negative inotropic or chronotropic drugs, intravenous fluids, and positive inotropic agents; use of a pacemaker; and improving ischemia pharmacologically or by intra-aortic balloon counterpulsation. Even in patients in whom urgent catheterization will be performed, all efforts should be made to improve hemodynamics prior to or during the study.

Ideally, all patients undergoing cardiac catheterization should be in normal sinus rhythm with a physiologic rate. This allows for more reliable hemodynamic data. Intravenous antiarrhythmics, such as lidocaine and procainamide, may be used to control or abolish frequent premature ventricular contractions (PVCs) or nonsustained ventricular tachycardia, at least for the duration of the cardiac catheterization. For patients in atrial fibrillation or other nonsinus rhythm, the ventricular response should be controlled with digitalis or other atrioventricular (AV) blocking drugs. Ideally, ventricular rate should be below 100 beats per minute. For supraventricular tachycardia intravenous adenosine, esmolol, verapamil, or diltiazem may be very effective. Other conditions that should be corrected or treated prior to elective cardiac catheterization include anemia (hematocrit below 30%), digitalis toxicity, potassium and other electrolyte abnormalities, acid–base disorders, febrile illness, dehydration, and severe heart failure.

PRETREATMENT FOR CONTRAST REACTIONS

Contrast reactions are covered in detail in Chapter 13. In general we pretreat all patients with oral or intravenous diphenhydramine prior to catheterization. **For contrast-allergic (real or suspected) patients a regimen of antihistamines and steroid premedication is strongly recommended.**

HEPARIN-RELATED THROMBOCYTOPENIA

Heparin should be withheld from patients with heparin-related thrombocytopenia during the procedure. Minimizing arterial time and frequent flushing of catheters is advised. Care must be taken to avoid heparin-containing flush solutions.

ALLERGY TO LOCAL ANESTHETICS

Allergic reaction to lidocaine hydrochloride may be manifested as urticaria, edema, or anaphylaxis. Such reactions may be the result of sensitivity to methylparaben, the preservative used in multiple-dose vials, or sulfite found in lidocaine with epinephrine solutions. Sulfite sensitivity is uncommon but more frequent in asthmatic than nonasthmatic people. In patients allergic to lidocaine or other aminoamide local anesthetic agents, an aminoester, such as bupivacaine HCl (Marcaine) 0.25%, can be used. There is no reported evidence of cross-sensitivity between the aminoamide and aminoester groups of local anesthetic, so most patients with bupivacaine allergy can receive lidocaine. Allergic reaction to the aminoester group of local anesthetics is rare but has been reported. It is due to either the local anesthetic itself, as with lidocaine, or formulation ingredients, such as methylparaben. Extremely rarely patients are allergic to both aminoamide and aminoester local anesthetics. In these patients, cardiac catheterization may be performed with heavy sedation and/or use of opioid analgesics without local anesthetic.

SPECIFIC PATIENT GROUPS AT HIGH RISK

Suspected Left Main Coronary Obstruction

The incidence of left main stenosis (more than 50% diameter reduction) varies from 6 to 13% of catheterization series (16, 17). Cardiac catheterization and coronary angiography of unsuspected left main obstruction is one situation in which a routine procedure can become catastrophic. The risk of death with left main stenosis is 27 times that of patients at low risk with no or minimal coronary artery disease (16) and 7 times that of patients with one, two, or three vessel disease (16, 18). In a study of 53,581 patients, cardiac catheterization mortality of patients with severe left main disease was 0.94% (19). Mortality was similar with the brachial and femoral approaches. Catastrophes may occur during vascular access if the patient has a vasovagal episode with marked hypotension and bradycardia; during coronary angiography with disruption of plaque, thrombosis, or dissection of the left main coronary artery; and during the early post-catheterization hours. Patients with ostial or proximal left main stenosis are at higher risk for dissection than patients with distal left main stenosis if the lesion is more than 6 mm from the catheter tip (20). Minor trauma during catheterization may initiate a dissection that extends slowly and may cause occlusion up to 7 hours later (19). Another cause of delayed hemodynamic collapse may be hypotension secondary to hypovolemia caused by contrast-induced diuresis. During ventriculography, hypotension and elevation of the left ventricular end diastolic pressure, caused by radiocontrast injection, especially if hyperosmolar agents are used, may reduce coronary perfusion pressure, exacerbate myocardial ischemia, and aggravate LV dysfunction, leading to cardiogenic shock and death.

Left main or severe triple vessel obstruction should be suspected from clinical, electrocardiographic, and other noninvasive testing. In patients with chest pain, the likelihood of severe coronary artery disease or significant left main stenosis is higher in older individuals (age over 70 years), in those with prior myocardial infarction, in the presence of multiple risk factors or a carotid bruit, and in patients with typical angina of long duration (21). Patients with rest angina, low effort tolerance, or pulmonary edema should also be suspected of having left main stenosis or severe triple vessel coronary artery disease. The exercise test suggests severe ischemia like that of left main or severe triple vessel stenosis if maximum work level is low (e.g., below 6.5 metabolic equivalent task score); if there is hypotension or failure of blood pressure to increase, marked ST segment depression (e.g., below 2 mm), early-onset (e.g., heart rate below 120 beats per minute) and late-offset ST depression (e.g., more than 6 minutes); or if resting ST depression is accentuated with exercise (22, 23). The magnitude of ST seg-

ment depression during or after exercise may be the most important if not the only variable with sufficient power to predict three vessel or left main obstruction with a high degree of confidence (24).

Thallium-201 scintigraphic findings suggesting left main stem stenosis include defects involving the anterior wall, septum, apex, and posterolateral walls (left main pattern). Severe triple vessel obstruction usually shows multiple redistribution defects (25). Occasionally thallium-201 scintigraphy in patients with severe triple vessel coronary artery disease or left main stenosis does not reveal the classical reversible defects if there is "balanced" ischemia in all three coronary artery distributions. These individuals, however, usually have markedly positive exercise ECG responses for ischemia. Increase in lung thallium-201 uptake and in transient left ventricular dilation are other markers of extensive myocardial ischemia (26). The use of radionuclide angiography and echocardiography during exercise or pharmacologic testing may reveal significant reduction in LV ejection fraction in addition to new wall motion abnormalities in patients with left main and triple vessel coronary artery disease (27). Detection and severity of left main coronary artery stenosis has been reported before catheterization using biplane transesophageal echocardiography and two-dimensional echocardiography with high sensitivity and specificity (28).

One objective of the precatheterization visit is identification of patients with possible left main disease or severe triple vessel disease so as to plan cardiac catheterization and angiography accordingly. In patients in whom left main stenosis is strongly suspected, it is prudent to obtain an estimate of LV function, regional wall motion, and valve function with echocardiography and/or nuclear studies before cardiac catheterization. Other suggestions are to perform coronary angiography before ventriculography and to use nonionic and/or low-osmolar agents to limit any hypotension and bradycardia. The first injection in such cases should be a cusp flush of the left coronary artery if possible. Although most patients with left main stenosis can tolerate left ventriculography, noninvasive assessment of wall motion may suffice.

Prior to cardiac catheterization it is important to avoid hypovolemia, hypotension, and hemodynamically significant arrhythmias and to treat any resting ischemia aggressively without inducing hypotension. Occasionally patients with left main stenosis and/or significant triple vessel disease remain ischemic despite maximal medical therapy. In these patients insertion of an intra-aortic balloon pump may be indicated. Patients with left main disease who have angina in the preceding 24 hours may have a much higher incidence of major complications than those without angina (20).

Unstable Ischemic Syndromes

Unstable ischemic syndromes include unstable angina, as well as Q- and non–Q-wave myocardial infarction. These patients have an increased incidence of catheterization complications, including death, which appears to be related to high incidence of left main disease (13%) and severe multivessel disease in up to 80%. In addition there is a tendency for such patients to have unstable lesions with superimposed thrombus and ulceration.

Prior to catheterization, early and aggressive treatment of unstable patients should include aspirin, heparin, nitroglycerin, and β-blockers as well as platelet glycoprotein IIb/IIIa receptor blockers. Calcium channel blockers may also be very helpful in relieving ischemia. Other extracardiac factors that may aggravate ischemia should be corrected promptly: blood transfusion for anemia, control of hyperthyroidism, and anxiolytic agents if indicated. Intra-aortic balloon counterpulsation may also be required. Other considerations relating to study and treatment of patients with unstable ischemic syndromes are covered in Chapter 37.

Severe Left Ventricular Dysfunction

Patients with severe LV dysfunction with ejection fraction below 30% have a tenfold

to fifteenfold higher death rate (0.3 to 0.54%) when undergoing cardiac catheterization and angiography than patients whose ejection fraction is above 50% (0.03 to 0.04%) (16, 19). The mechanism of procedure-related death in such series usually cannot be separated from the cause of the LV failure and reduced ejection fraction, most commonly severe coronary artery disease. Radiocontrast media have been blamed, as they can cause hypotension and arrhythmia, depress myocardial function, and elevate end diastolic pressure. Mortality in patients with severe LV dysfunction has fallen by more than 50% (from 0.67 to 0.29%) from an earlier (1979 to 1980) to a later (1984 to 1988) Society for Cardiac Angiography and Interventions report (16). This reduction may have been due to improved treatment of congestive heart failure, arrhythmias, and more frequent use of nonionic and low-osmolality contrast media. In preparing a patient to undergo cardiac catheterization and angiography, it is important to detect patients with severe LV dysfunction and to treat those in heart failure before the procedure is undertaken. Knowing the degree of LV dysfunction should prompt use of a low-osmolality or nonionic radiocontrast agent. Another reason to obtain an echocardiogram before cardiac catheterization is that patients with severe LV dysfunction have a higher incidence of mural thrombus. If the thrombus is highly mobile, entering the LV with a catheter should probably be avoided. **Treating symptoms of heart failure makes it easier to perform cardiac catheterization,** as patients can lie flat on the catheterization table and the hemodynamic data obtained are usually more reliable. In patients with acute severe pulmonary edema, such as is seen in patients with acute mitral or aortic insufficiency, aggressive treatment with diuretics, inotropic agents, or vasodilators for even a few hours may change a difficult and dangerous procedure into a smoother and safer one.

Valvular Heart Disease

Patients with severe aortic and mitral valvular disease have diagnostic catheterization mortality rate twice as high as that of patients without valve disease (19). Patients at particular risk are those with critical aortic stenosis (valve area less than 0.5 cm^2), severe aortic insufficiency, or mitral stenosis complicated by severe pulmonary hypertension. Most deaths in patients with aortic valve disease are associated with severe coronary artery disease (19). Patients with mitral regurgitation also have higher catheterization mortality. Further discussion of catheter-based evaluation and treatment of patients with valvular heart disease is included in Chapter 43.

Peripheral Vascular Disease

Patients with peripheral vascular disease (PVD) undergoing diagnostic catheterization and angiography, PTCA, and other more complex catheter-based intervention have increased vascular complications (29). These are probably related to multiple arterial punctures, use of larger sheaths, entry of vessels other than the common femoral artery, and atherosclerotic plaque and aneurysm. Complications that may occur at the arterial puncture site include hematoma formation, bleeding, AV fistula, pseudoaneurysm formation, infection, arterial laceration, and arterial occlusion due to thrombosis. Complications that may occur at a remote site include dissection, subintimal hematoma, remote perforation, and embolization. Although the femoral artery approach to cardiac catheterization carries a high technical success rate and is relatively safe, other anatomic approaches (usually brachial) are occasionally necessary for patients with PVD. Prosthetic graft catheterization is possible, but infection is a dreaded although uncommon complication, and some recommend prophylactic antibiotic administration when prosthetic graft catheterization is performed. Patients undergoing PTCA and more complex interventions have a much higher incidence of arterial injury at access sites than those having diagnostic studies (0.6 to 0.7% for diagnostic studies, 2.6% for PTCA, and 6% for complex interventions). With complex interventional procedures there is also more frequent need

to use intra-aortic balloon pumps and percutaneous partial cardiopulmonary bypass systems (29). Insertion of the intra-aortic balloon pump is associated with much higher incidence of local vascular complications in diabetic patients, women (smaller vessels), and in those with peripheral vascular disease. In one study (30), the incidence of major local complication (occlusive, embolic, and technical) was 60% in those with peripheral vascular disease (aneurysmal and occlusive disease) compared with 5% in those without PVD. Most patients with occlusive complications had preinsertion ankle-to-brachial indexes of less than 0.6 in the limb in which the intra-aortic balloon pump was inserted.

Cholesterol embolism is associated with high mortality (up to 90%), and as yet there is no effective treatment. Cholesterol embolism has been described in patients undergoing diagnostic catheterization (31, 32) and PTCA (33). The presentation of this complication may be delayed for several hours to several weeks after the arterial procedure. Patients usually present with acute hypertension, livedo reticularis, purple toes, gangrenous skin, progressive renal insufficiency (in most cases irreversible), bowel infarction, pancreatitis, myocardial infarction, neurologic abnormalities with agitation, and retinal artery occlusion. Many cases may be misdiagnosed initially as renal failure, and other signs develop 2 to 6 weeks after an uneventful retrograde cardiac catheterization. Almost all patients have extensive atherosclerotic disease and marked intimal ulceration of the aorta. In patients at high risk for cholesterol embolism, if cardiac catheterization is imperative, the brachial approach (upper limb arteries have less atheroma than the aorta or lower limb arteries) may be less hazardous than the femoral approach. Anticoagulants and probably thrombolysis should be avoided, as their use may initiate or exacerbate the syndrome.

Detection and assessment of the severity of peripheral vascular disease should be an integral part of the precatheterization visit. A thorough examination of all pulses, including palpitation, auscultation, and comparison of blood pressure in both upper and lower limbs, should be documented before the procedure. The dorsalis pedis pulse is congenitally absent in about 10% of normal persons, but the absence of the posterior tibial pulse is a very reliable marker of occlusive peripheral arterial disease. Occasionally severe aortoiliac disease (usually total occlusion) may be missed, as the femoral pulses may feel normal if adequate collaterals have developed. These patients may have radiofemoral delay. Normal systolic blood pressure at the ankle is slightly higher than at brachial level when a person is supine. A resting systolic ankle–brachial index less than 0.5 indicates severe arterial insufficiency, and less than 0.8, moderate insufficiency.

Patients with a history and physical examination consistent with significant PVD should undergo Doppler studies and pressure measurements, with documentation of ankle–brachial indexes and segmental waveforms (34). These studies may identify limbs at high risk for complications and may prompt the invasive cardiologist to use another vascular access site or another technique. Using a sheath (long sheath for tortuous or significantly atheromatous iliofemoral segment) and the smallest possible catheters to achieve the set objectives may also help reduce vascular complications. Patients with severe bilateral iliofemoral disease may present with unstable ischemic syndromes, including cardiogenic shock unresponsive to medical therapy. In these patients insertion of an intra-arterial balloon pump and urgent PTCA or coronary artery bypass graft (CABG) may be lifesaving. In the appropriate setting urgent angioplasty with or without stent implantation in the iliofemoral system may allow successful insertion of an intra-arterial balloon pump without occlusive complications (35) and the performance of cardiac catheterization and urgent PTCA. Rarely does a patient have both severe aortoiliac and axillary disease. In such a case the transseptal approach was adapted, allowing successful coronary angiography with Amplatz catheters (36). Obviously this should only be performed by those trained in the transseptal technique.

SUMMARY

At a time when health care is increasingly delivered in the outpatient setting, patients are older, and interventions more aggressive, preprocedure assessment is more important than ever. A thorough precatheterization evaluation aids the invasive cardiologist to prepare the patient, both emotionally and physically, to undergo cardiac catheterization with the least possible discomfort and risk. Such an assessment is an integral portion of modern quality control and risk management, as well as good medical practice.

References

1. Position paper. American College of Physicians Ethics Manual. Part 1: History; the patient; other physicians. Ann Intern Med 1989;111:245–252.
2. ACC/AHA Task Force Report. Guidelines for coronary angiography. J Am Coll Cardiol 1987, in press.
3. Brett A, Grodin M. Ethical aspects of human experimentation in health services research. JAMA 1991; 265:1854–1857.
4. Rodwin MA. Sounding board: physicians' conflicts of interest: the limitations of disclosure. N Engl J Med 1989;321:1405–1408.
5. ACC/AHA Task Force Report. Guidelines for percutaneous transluminal coronary angioplasty. J Am Coll Cardiol 1993;22:2033-2054.
6. Clark DA, Moscovich MD, Vetrovec GW, Wexler L. Guidelines for the performance of outpatient catheterization and angiographic procedures. Cathet Cardiovasc Diagn 1992;27:5–7.
7. Mahrer PR, Young C, Magnusson PT. Efficacy and safety of outpatient cardiac catheterization. Cathet Cardiovasc Diagn 1987;13:304–308.
8. Skinner JS, Adams PC. Outpatient cardiac catheterization. Int J Cardiol 1996;53:209–219.
9. Block PC, Ockene I, Goldberg RJ, et al. A prospective randomized trial of outpatient versus inpatient cardiac catheterization. N Engl J Med 1988;319:1251–1255.
10. Holzman RS, Cullen DJ, Eichhorn JH, et al. Guidelines for sedation by nonanesthesiologists during diagnostic and therapeutic procedures. J Clin Anesth 1994;6:265–276.
11. Joint Commission on Accreditation of Healthcare Organizations (JCAHO). Accreditation manual for hospitals. Oakbrook Terrace, IL: JCAHO. 1993:165–170.
12. Giacalone VF. Antianxiety/sedative drugs: the benzodiazepines. Pharmacology 1992;9:465–479.
13. Loeffler PM. Oral benzodiazepines and conscious sedation: a review. J Oral Maxillofac Surg 1992;50:989–997.
14. Brogden RN, Goa KL. Flumazenil: a preliminary review of its benzodiazepine antagonist properties, intrinsic activity and therapeutic use. Drugs 1988;35:448–467.
15. Kiemeneij F, Laarman GJ. Improved anticoagula-

tion management after Palmaz Shatz coronary stent implantation by sealing the puncture site with a vascular hemostasis device. Cath Cardiovasc Diagn 1993;30:317–322.

16. Lozner EC, Johnson LW, Johnson S, et al. Coronary arteriography 1984–1987: a report of the Registry of the Society for Cardiac Angiography and Interventions: 2. An analysis of 218 deaths related to coronary arteriography. Cathet Cardiovasc Diagn 1989;17:11–14.

17. Kowalchuk GJ, Siu SC, Lewis SM. Coronary artery disease in the octogenarian: angiographic spectrum and suitability for revascularization. Am J Cardiol 1990;66:1319–1323.

18. Yusuf S, Zucker D, Peduzzi P et al. Effect of coronary artery bypass graft surgery on survival: overview of 10-year results from randomised trials by the coronary artery bypass graft trialists collaboration. Lancet 1995;344:563–570.

19. Kennedy JW, Baxley WA, Bunnel IL, et al. Mortality related to cardiac catheterization and angiography. Cathet Cardiovasc Diagn 1982;8:323–340.

20. Gordon PR, Abrams C, Gash AK, Carabello BA. Pericatheterization risk factors in left main coronary artery stenosis. Am J Cardiol 1987;59:1080–1083.

21. Pryor DB, Shaw L, Harrell FE, et al. Estimating the likelihood of severe coronary artery disease. Am J Med 1991;90:553–562.

22. Aursnes I, Benestad AM, Sivertssen E, et al. Degree of coronary artery disease predicted by exercise testing. J Int Med 1991;229:325–330.

23. Ellestad MH. Stress testing: principles and practice. 4th ed. Philadelphia: FA Davis, 1996.

24. Ribisl PM, Morris CK, Kawaguehi T, et al. Angiographic pattern and severe coronary artery disease: exercise test correlates. Arch Intern Med 1992;152:1618–1624.

25. Dash H, Massie BM, Botvinick EH, Brundage BH. The noninvasive identification of left main and three vessel coronary artery disease by myocardial stress perfusion scintigraphy and treadmill exercise electrocardiography. Circulation 1979;60:276–284.

26. Chouraqui P, Rodrigues EA, Berman DS, Maddahi J. Significance of dipyridamole-induced transient dilation of the left ventricle during thallium-201 scintigraphy in suspected coronary artery disease. Am J Cardiol 1990;66:689–694.

27. Bolognese L, Rossi L, Sarasso G, et al. Silent versus symptomatic dipyridamole-induced ischemia after myocardial infarction: clinical and prognostic significance. J Am Coll Cardiol 1992;19:953–959.

28. Yoshida K, Yoshikawa J, Hozumi T, et al. Detection of left main coronary artery stenosis by transesophageal color Doppler and two-dimensional echocardiography. Circulation 1990;81:1271–1276.

29. Muller DWM, Shamir KJ, Ellis SG, Topol EJ. Peripheral vascular complications after conventional and complex percutaneous coronary interventional procedures. Am J Cardiol 1992;69:63–68.

30. Kvilekval KH, Mason RA, Newton B, et al. Complications of percutaneous intra-aortic balloon pump use in patients with peripheral vascular disease. Arch Surg 1991;126:621–623.

31. Hendel RC, Cuenoud HF, Giansiracusa DF, Alpert JS. Multiple cholesterol emboli syndrome: bowel infarction after retrograde angiography. Arch Intern Med 1989;149:2371–2374.

32. Applebaum RM, Kronzon I. Evaluation and management of cholesterol embolization and the blue toe syndrome. Curr Opin Cardiol 1996;11:533–542.

33. Tilley WS, Harston WE, Siami G, Stone WJ. Renal failure due to cholesterol emboli following PTCA. Am Heart J 1985;110:1301–1302.

34. Messina LM, Brothers TE, Wakefield TW, et al. Clinical characteristics and surgical management of vascular complications in patients undergoing cardiac catheterization: interventional versus diagnostic procedures. J Vasc Surg 1991;13:593–600.

35. Lewis BE, Sumida C, Hwang MJ, Loeb HS. New approach to management of intra-aortic balloon pumps in patients with peripheral vascular disease: case reports of four patients requiring urgent IABP insertion. Cathet Cardiovasc Diagn 1992;26:295–299.

36. Pearce AC, Schwengel RH, Simione LM, et al. Antegrade selective coronary angiography via the transseptal approach in a patient with severe vascular disease. Cathet Cardiovasc Diagn 1992;26:300–303.

8
Complications of Cardiac Catheterization and Strategies to Reduce Risks

Richard A. Kerensky, MD

INTRODUCTION

Cardiac catheterization as currently practiced includes a number of distinctly different diagnostic and therapeutic techniques. The risk of cardiac catheterization therefore depends on the procedure performed, the condition of the patient prior to the procedure, other therapeutic measures associated with the condition (e.g., anticoagulation), and the expertise of the operator. The decision to perform any diagnostic or therapeutic procedure should be determined by an estimate of the potential benefit versus risk. Accordingly, **an accurate assessment of risk must be made prior to any procedure** to determine whether the procedure is indicated. Also, informed consent can be obtained only if an accurate estimate of risk is communicated by the physician to the patient. Careful scrutiny of the complications associated with any particular procedure often leads to new techniques or strategies to prevent complications. The purpose of this chapter is to examine in detail the potential for complications of various cardiac catheterization procedures to assess the risks of current techniques and explore advances that may reduce complications.

GENERAL CONSIDERATIONS

Many of the general principles employed to reduce the risk inherent in catheterization are outlined in other chapters of this book, such as the chapters on training, catheterization techniques, and laboratory administration. In general **the expertise of the operator and the experience of the catheterization laboratory nurses and technologists are important determinants of risk** of whatever procedure is performed. Therefore, cardiac catheterization laboratory policies that ensure adequate qualifications and training of the physicians and staff are crucial to reducing complication rates to the lowest level possible (1).

The complications encountered during cardiac catheterization also relate specifically to the procedure being performed and the patient undergoing the procedure. Therefore, relatively few general remarks are relevant to all catheterization procedures. For example, the risk of endomyocardial biopsy in a patient who has undergone cardiac transplantation is completely different from the risk of rotational atherectomy in a patient with obstructive coronary disease. Therefore, most of this chapter focuses on the risk of specific procedures and data concerning the risk of each. Prospective data concerning complication rates are used whenever possible. However, much of the information is obtained from registry studies, and the limitations of this approach are highlighted when appropriate. The complications of diagnostic procedures, including right heart catheterization, endomyocardial biopsy, electrophysiologic procedures, coronary angiography, left ventriculography, and transseptal left heart catheterization, are reviewed first. The risks associated with therapeutic procedures, including percutaneous coronary interventional techniques, electrophysiologic pathway ablation techniques, and valvuloplasty, are reviewed separately. For each procedure we review complications arising from vascular access, unique complications related to the specific catheters or techniques used, and patient-related variables indicating high-risk patients.

DIAGNOSTIC PROCEDURES

Right Heart Catheterization

Excluding infectious complications due to indwelling catheters, approximately 1 to 2% of patients undergoing right heart catheterization have some type of complication related to the procedure (2). Major complications are rare. A number of case reports have highlighted the many rare complications of right heart catheterization (3–14). **The risk of right heart catheterization in the catheterization laboratory relates primarily to vascular access and manipulation of the catheter within the right heart and pulmonary artery.**

Vascular Access

Use of the proper technique for obtaining vascular access is imperative in reducing the risk of right heart catheterization. Each access site has unique landmarks and techniques, outlined in Chapter 9. In most patients having combined right and left heart catheterization in our laboratory the right femoral vein is used for access. It is a common misconception among relatively inexperienced operators that the venous access site is less likely to be a source of bleeding or other complications than the arterial site after catheterization. In our experience the venous site, especially if not entered carefully, can undergo significant bleeding, hematoma, pseudoaneurysm, or thrombosis (15). Important bleeding can occur if an artery is inadvertently punctured (puncturing too far laterally) or if the puncture is above the inguinal ligament (puncture too far superiorly). Bleeding may also occur if the subcutaneous tissue is not spread sufficiently, creating a burr at the end of the sheath that will injure the vein upon insertion.

For the internal jugular approach complications include pneumothorax and arterial puncture with hematoma formation (2). Arterial puncture occurs with a puncture site that is too medial, and pneumothorax occurs with a puncture too far inferior. We instruct our fellows to locate the jugular vein with the appropriate anatomic landmarks and insert the access needle into the proper position rather than searching for the vein with the needle. If the jugular vein can not be found, the landmarks should be reassessed and attempts at access repeated. The temptation to break the anatomic rules and search blindly for the vessel with the access needle should be resisted. Most inadvertent punctures occur after initial attempts to find the vessel fail and landmarks and correct technique are abandoned. If the vessel can not be located with the proper technique, a different access site should be tried. The use of a small-gauge finder needle prior to use of the 18-gauge access needle reduces complications.

With use of the subclavian vein for access the main complications are pneumothorax, hemothorax, or local hematoma formation due to inadvertent puncture of the subclavian artery. Because of its position beneath the clavicle, manual compression of the subclavian artery is impossible if it is inadvertently punctured during catheterization attempts. For that reason we avoid the subclavian approach if at all possible in patients receiving anticoagulation. The incidence of pneumothorax after attempts at subclavian vein access should be less than 1%.

The basilic vein is probably the safest access site for right heart catheterization if it is easily visible or palpable superficially near the antecubital fossa. Unfortunately, in more than 50% of patients the basilic vein is inadequate to accept a 7-F sheath. If the basilic vein is easily accessed, it is the approach we prefer for right heart catheterization in patients on anticoagulation, since the likelihood of inadvertent arterial puncture is very low.

Of the 283 isolated right heart catheterizations done in our laboratory over the past 2 years 60% were done via the internal jugular vein, usually the right; 34%, via the femoral vein, usually the right; and 6%, via the basilic vein, usually the right. The incidence of access site–related complications when the catheter is placed by an experienced operator in our laboratory is approximately 0.4%. There were no serious bleeding complications or pneumothoraces in this group.

Catheter-related Complications

After successful vascular access is obtained, the main risks of right heart catheterization are due to manipulation of the catheter within the cardiac chambers and pulmonary artery or infection if the catheter is left in place. Minor conduction disturbances and transient ventricular arrhythmias as the catheter moves through the right ventricle are common (11). The catheter should be advanced and withdrawn through the right ventricular outflow tract as quickly as possible to avoid sustained ventricular arrhythmias and heart block. The incidence of ventricular arrhythmias requiring treatment during right heart catheterization is less than 0.1% in our laboratory. The use of fluoroscopic guidance as the catheter passes through the right ventricle probably reduces the risk of serious arrhythmias. Patients with left bundle branch block are at risk for complete heart block during right heart catheterization. Prophylactic pacing is not required, however, since the incidence is low and complete AV block is often transient and does not require therapy. The physician and staff should be prepared, however, to institute temporary pacing quickly in a patient with left bundle branch block undergoing right heart catheterization.

Pulmonary artery rupture is a rare catastrophic complication of right heart catheterization (6, 7, 9, 12). It is caused by inad-

vertent inflation of the catheter balloon tip in a distal position where the vessel is too small to accommodate the balloon. Several precautions should be taken to prevent pulmonary artery rupture. First, only operators experienced at Swan-Ganz placement should perform right heart catheterization. Second, hemodynamic monitoring should be performed continuously during catheter advancement, and each waveform should easily identify the catheter location. When fluoroscopy is available, a central position of the catheter in the main pulmonary artery should be verified before the balloon is inflated. The distance the catheter is advanced into the pulmonary artery during the initial placement in the pulmonary capillary wedge position should be documented in the chart. The catheter usually softens over time and probably must be withdrawn somewhat after initial placement. The balloon of the pulmonary artery catheter should never be inflated unless a clear pulmonary artery tracing taken from the distal monitoring port is visible. Frequently a large V-wave in the wedge position resembles a pulmonary artery tracing. If the balloon is inflated with the catheter in the wedge position, the chances of pulmonary artery rupture are high. In many intensive care units policy restricts the inflation of the pulmonary artery catheter to experienced attending physicians. These policies, which are aimed at preventing pulmonary artery rupture, are appropriate in many situations.

Patient-related Variables

Patients with severe congestive heart failure, hypotension, massive cardiac enlargement, or cardiogenic shock present difficult management problems in the catheterization laboratory. If the respiratory status is impaired, elective intubation prior to right heart catheter placement should be strongly considered. This may allow a patient to lie comfortably on the catheterization table and safely undergo elective Swan-Ganz catheter placement. In critically ill patients we find that right catheter placement is safest in the catheterization laboratory because (*a*) technical support, (*b*) hemodynamic monitoring devices, (*c*) access to intra-aortic balloon placement, and (*d*) fluoroscopic capabilities are superior to those of most intensive care units. If the catheter is to be left in place for prolonged hemodynamic monitoring in the intensive care unit, the preferred access site is either the subclavian vein or the right internal jugular vein. A number of recent studies call into question the use of Swan-Ganz catheterization for diagnostic and monitoring purposes in the intensive care unit. (16, 17). These studies have shown no benefit in some cases and higher mortality in some cases when Swan-Ganz catheterization is used (17). No randomized trials comparing Swan-Ganz catheterization with less invasive monitoring techniques have been performed. Until randomized data are available, the use of Swan-Ganz catheters should be closely monitored for complications, and only experienced operators should perform insertion and interpret the hemodynamic data.

Endomyocardial Biopsy

The risk of endomyocardial biopsy varies greatly with the indication for the procedure. Patients undergoing biopsy for transplant rejection surveillance have the lowest risk, and those with dilated cardiomyopathy have the highest risk (18, 19).

Vascular Access

The same techniques for obtaining vascular access for right heart catheterization are used in endomyocardial biopsy, with similar risks. We use only the right internal jugular approach and the femoral venous approach for biopsy in our laboratory. The left internal jugular and subclavian approaches are not recommended because the stiffness of the bioptome makes entry into the right ventricle difficult with either of these access sites. The right internal jugular vein allows the easiest and straightest entry into the right ventricle. Some 51% of 542 the patients having endomyocardial biopsy for surveillance of transplant rejection in our laboratory in the past 2 years were sampled via the right internal jugular vein, 34% via the right femoral vein, and 15% via the left femoral vein.

Bioptome-related Injury

Cardiac perforation and arrhythmias are the most common complications associated with the use of the biopsy forceps during endomyocardial biopsy. The correct placement of the biopsy sheath near the apex of the right ventricle and directed toward the septum is critical to minimizing bioptome-related injury. We use fluoroscopic guidance and pressure waveforms to verify the correct position in the right ventricle in all cases. If the biopsy sheath is directed too superiorly toward the outflow tract of the right ventricle, arrhythmias or heart block can occur. Incorrect positioning, that is, toward the right ventricular (RV) free wall, right atrium, or within the coronary sinus, results in perforation. If the biopsy sheath is directed toward the ventricular septum, it has a posterior orientation on the left anterior oblique or lateral projection. The correct position of the biopsy sheath must be verified by fluoroscopy and pressure waveform prior to use of the bioptome. Sometimes the sheath appears to be in the correct position by fluoroscopy but actually is in the right atrium or coronary sinus. This situation is easily recognized by proper interpretation of the pressure tracings. Some transplant patients have extensive scarring after numerous procedures, and repositioning of the sheath several times may be required to obtain an adequate sample.

Patient-related Variables

Patients undergoing endomyocardial biopsy for detection of cardiac transplant rejection have a low incidence of bioptome-related cardiac injury. In fact, inadvertent cardiac perforation probably occurs in some patients but is clinically inapparent (18). Postsurgical scarring likely reduces the chances of significant intrapericardial bleeding or tamponade. In contrast, patients undergoing biopsy in the evaluation of dilated cardiomyopathy have a higher incidence of cardiac perforation and significant pericardial bleeding requiring pericardiocentesis. Decker et al. found a 6% incidence of complications during cardiac biopsy in adults with dilated cardiomyopathy, with two deaths from perforation in 464 patients (19). Because of the limited diagnostic information obtained from endomyocardial biopsy in patients with dilated cardiomyopathy and because of this risk, we do not routinely perform biopsy in these patients unless there is a specific indication (associated inflammatory illness such as sarcoid, suspicion of amyloid, and so on). The risk of cardiac perforation during biopsy is probably less in patients with restrictive cardiomyopathy, especially in those with a thickened right ventricle revealed by echocardiography.

Electrophysiologic Testing and Radiofrequency Catheter Ablation Techniques

Diagnostic electrophysiologic techniques require venous access, usually with multiple sheaths, and catheter manipulation with the right atrium and ventricle. Complications are uncommon and usually minor. Death and myocardial infarction are rare. In one recent study the complication rate for electrophysiologic testing was 1.1% (20). The risk is higher in older patients undergoing study for evaluation of possible ventricular tachycardia than in younger patients with supraventricular arrhythmias. Radiofrequency catheter ablation has a higher risk of cardiac perforation and other complications than diagnostic electrophysiologic studies. Left-sided pathway ablation is associated with a higher risk than right-sided pathway attempts. As with diagnostic studies, older age and systemic illness are associated with increased complication rates during radiofrequency ablation (20).

Left Heart Catheterization, Coronary Angiography, and Ventriculography

Left heart catheterization and coronary angiography are the most common diagnostic procedures performed in most cardiac catheterization laboratories. A number of prospective registries have examined the risks of these commonly performed procedures over the years (21–23). Improvements in techniques and equipment, potentially leading to decreases in risk of the procedure, have been at least partially offset by application of this technique to apparently higher-risk and older populations (23). The risks of left heart catheterization and coronary angiography relate to vascular access, ischemic complications in patients with severe coronary disease, catheter-related complications such as coronary dissection, embolic events, cerebrovascular accidents, and contrast-related risk.

Registry Data

In the past 15 years the Society for Cardiac Angiography and Interventions has published four reports from its catheterization registry on the safety of coronary angiography. The mortality of this procedure has remained constant at approximately 0.11% despite an older and sicker patient population. Interestingly, the incidence of major complications also has remained constant over the same period (Table 8.1). It appears that any technical advances, such as reduced catheter size and improved visualization in the laboratory, have been offset by an increasingly elderly population with more comorbid illness who keep the complication rates unchanged. In 1980 the percentage of patients over 60 years of age undergoing catheterization was approximately 33%, but by 1990 that percentage had risen to 58%. Alternatively, we may have reached a lower limit to some complications, such as embolic events. Also, registry data are often limited to events in the laboratory and do not include some of the

Table 8.1.
Complications of Cardiac Catheterization

	1979–1982 (53,581 pts)	1984–1987 (222,553 pts)	1990 (59,792 pts)	1991 (74,999 pts)
Death	0.14%	0.10%	0.11%	0.11%
MI	0.07	0.06	0.05	0.06
CVA	0.07	0.07	0.07	0.05
Arrhythmia	0.56	0.47	0.38	0.31
Vascular	0.57	0.46	0.43	0.44
Other	0.4	0.28	0.28	0.48

more common complications, such as vascular access problems, which often occur after the patient has left the cardiac catheterization laboratory.

Vascular Access

An extremely important risk of left heart catheterization is related to vascular injury at the arterial access site. As noted earlier, this risk is often underestimated in registry reports, since registry data are recorded in the catheterization laboratory and **access complications frequently occur late after the procedure** (21, 23). Major complications, including large hematoma formation, femoral artery pseudoaneurysm, arteriovenous fistula, arterial occlusion, bleeding requiring transfusion, and limb ischemia are recognized major complications of arterial catheterization (24–26). The vascular complications observed in a prospective study of 503 patients undergoing femoral arterial catheterization reported by Bogart et al. are shown in Table 8.2 (24). Using multiple logistic regression analysis, the authors found that **multiple procedures or punctures in the same femoral artery, reinstitution of heparin, and inability to comply with a standard bed rest program were strongly associated with an increase in risk of vascular complications.** Studies of patients undergoing surgical repair after catheterization reveal a high incidence of puncture in sites other than the common femoral artery (27). Age, body surface area, female gender, coronary angioplasty, and the use of thrombolytic agents have also been associated with complications following arterial puncture (22, 28–30). The size of the arterial

sheath does not appear to correlate with vascular complications (31, 32). Many patients in today's practice of interventional cardiology undergo diagnostic catheterization followed shortly thereafter by percutaneous coronary intervention. These patients are at increased risk for groin complications because of frequent reinstitution of anticoagulation and multiple arterial punctures if the ipsilateral site is used for the coronary intervention. Therefore, the timing of diagnostic catheterization in patients who may require subsequent intervention is crucial to reducing the risk of vascular complications. The use of newer anticoagulation and antiplatelet agents will likely further complicate this scenario. It may be appropriate to combine diagnostic and interventional procedures in some patients to avoid multiple arterial punctures and prolonged anticoagulation, but this strategy frequently leads to increased use of coronary interventions and other problems. One recent study shows that the use of a hemostatic device

Table 8.2.
Groin Complications in 503 Patients Undergoing Catheterization

Complication	N (%)
Small to moderate hematoma	51 (10.2)
Large hematoma (>10 cm)	5 (1)
Rebleeding	31 (6.2)
Limb ischemia	2 (0.4)
AV fistula	1 (0.2)
Thrombosis	2 (0.4)
Pseudoaneurysm	3 (0.6)
Transfusion	5 (1)

Reprinted with permission from Bogart DB, Bogart MA, Miller JT, et al. Femoral artery catheterization complications: a study of 503 consecutive patients. Cathet Cardiovasc Diagn 1995;34:8–13.

deployed via the sheath reduces bleeding after coronary intervention compared with manual compression, especially in patients receiving anticoagulation after the procedure (33). Further study is required to evaluate the efficacy of the many new hemostatic devices becoming available.

The assessment of patients with possible access site complications following catheterization includes physical examination, vascular ultrasound, and occasionally abdominal computed tomography (CT) to rule out retroperitoneal hematoma (25, 27, 34). Early hematoma formation may be obvious in the case of a pulsatile mass or fairly subtle, as is seen in slow retroperitoneal hemorrhage. Most centers performing diagnostic and therapeutic catheterization **rely heavily on intravascular ultrasound techniques** to evaluate patients with groin swelling after catheterization. Pseudoaneurysms, hematomas, and arteriovenous fistulas are all readily visualized by experienced sonographers. Hematomas and pseudoaneurysms can often be reduced with the ultrasound-guided compression (27, 35).

Surgical repair is infrequently required following arterial catheterization but is essential for patients with continued bleeding or large pseudoaneurysms. CT scanning can aid in the assessment of ongoing retroperitoneal bleeding (26, 27, 31, 36). Many

arteriovenous fistulas have no hemodynamic significance and close spontaneously, so surgery can be delayed. The morbidity of surgical repair of arterial complications is substantial, so that prevention of severe complications and treatment of hematomas and pseudoaneurysms with compression is preferable whenever possible (37).

A multifaceted approach is required to reduce the risk of groin complications and effectively manage access site bleeding. Table 8.3 lists risk factors for complications and important strategies we use in our laboratory to reduce risk.

Myocardial Ischemia and Infarction

Refractory myocardial ischemia during diagnostic cardiac catheterization, that is not due to thrombotic coronary obstruction, is relatively rare with modern techniques. Significant hemodynamic compromise is uncommon during coronary angiography with nonionic contrast agents. Severe ischemia may occur, however, in patients with left main coronary stenosis, severe three vessel coronary disease, and/or severe aortic stenosis. Intravenous anti-is-

Table 8.3.
Stategies to Reduce Groin Complications

Risk Factor	Strategy
Multiple arterial punctures	Combine diagnostic and therapeutic procedures when appropriate. Use intraarterial sheath.
Preprocedure thrombolytic therapy	Appropriate timing of diagnostic studies
Postprocedure anticoagulation	Anticoagulate for adequate duration before procedure
	Avoid heparin bolus post procedure
	Inspect groin prior to institution of heparin
Obesity	Experienced operator obtains access
	Prolonged compression and bedrest
	Frequent groin checks
	Minimize anticoagulation
Noncompliant patient or patient unable to comply with bedrest protocol	Consider delaying elective procedures in combative or confused patients
	More intensive postprocedure nursing (ICU)
	Restraints where appropriate
	Avoid unneccessary sedatives in elderly

chemic medications, intracoronary nitroglycerin, and capabilities for urgent intra-aortic balloon pumping should be available during all diagnostic left heart catheterizations. Early recognition of severe refractory ischemia is crucial to avoid more serious complications including hypotension and arrhythmias.

Most important ischemic events in the catheterization laboratory are likely due to atheroembolic or thromboembolic events. The incidence of thrombotic occlusion during coronary angiography is approximately 0.18% with nonionic or ionic contrast media (38). There is no evidence that 3000 to 5000 units of intravenous or intra-arterial heparin reduces thromboembolic or embolic complications, and we no longer routinely administer heparin for diagnostic catheterization. In our view meticulous technique of flushing catheters, wiping wires, and so on is the most important factor in reducing thrombotic complications. We do administer heparin during diagnostic catheterization to patients with aortic stenosis, to those in whom we use the brachial artery approach, and to those found to have significant left main coronary stenosis on the initial coronary injection. Of course, when there is use of any diagnostic intracoronary instrument (e.g., Doppler wire, intracoronary ultrasound), heparin should be administered.

Coronary Dissection

Dissection of the coronary artery, a rare complication during diagnostic catheterization, is usually due to trauma related to the position of the catheter. If vigorous injection is performed via an improperly placed catheter, a dissection may occur at the ostium of the artery where the catheter is positioned against an arterial plaque. A number of technical considerations are important in reducing the chances for coronary dissection during diagnostic catheterization.

Left Coronary Artery

Dissection of the left main coronary artery is a life-threatening complication of coronary angiography. The two most important technical considerations during left coronary injection are the position of the catheter within the left main and the appearance of the pressure tracing. The majority of left main angiograms are done with the Judkins type of catheter (see chapter 7). In 80 to 90% of cases minimal or no manipulation is required to engage the coronary artery. However, close attention should be paid to the orientation of the catheter within the artery. A Judkins catheter that is too short points superiorly, and one that is too large for the aortic root points inferiorly. If the catheter is severely missized, it should be changed before injections. Monitoring of the pressure tracing recorded from the tip of the catheter is crucial during coronary angiography. A good-quality tracing should be recorded prior to engagement of the coronary so that subtle changes in the pressure tracing can be noted after engagement. If dampening occurs, after engagement of the coronary, the operator must determine whether the dampening is due to incorrect position of the catheter or a stenosis of the left main coronary. Gentle test injections are often required to make this determination. If stenosis of the left main is present, some injections while the pressure tracing is dampened may be unavoidable. However, in the face of a dampened pressure tracing, injections should be kept to a minimum to minimize the chance of dissection. If dampening is thought to be due to catheter position, the catheter should be changed. If left main coronary dissection occurs, heparin should be administered, an intra-aortic balloon pump placed, and arrangements for emergency surgery made. Bailout stenting of the left main coronary artery has been performed successfully by experienced operators when the patient's condition is deteriorating too quickly to allow for emergency surgery (39). The use of emergency stenting for left main coronary disease requires further study.

Right Coronary Artery

Engagement of the right coronary artery generally requires manipulation of a Judkins or other type of catheter into the ostium of the artery. The appearance of the catheter within the artery varies with the takeoff and orientation of the artery. Again, as with the left coronary, careful monitoring of the pressure tracing is required to avoid injection with an improperly placed catheter. The right anterior oblique projection is often helpful in difficult-to-engage right coronaries to avoid directing the catheter too far posteriorly. Spasm at the ostium of the right coronary artery is common, and administration of intracoronary nitroglycerin may be necessary to relieve pressure dampening after engagement. Dissection of the right coronary does not always require emergency surgery, depending on the condition of the patient. If the patient has no ischemia, some dissections may be managed conservatively. **Urgent stenting is a reasonable treatment option for catheter-induced dissections of the right coronary artery if done by an experienced operator.**

Embolic Events and Cerebrovascular Accident

The risk of neurologic complications during diagnostic catheterization is approximately 0.07 to 0.3% (21, 23, 40). Common symptoms are visual disturbances, hemiparesis, and facial droop (40). Approximately two-thirds of patients have complete resolution with no residuum on long-term follow-up (40). The risk of cerebrovascular accident appears slightly higher with percutaneous transluminal coronary angioplasty (PTCA), in patients with tortuous aortas requiring multiple catheter exchanges, in the presence of left ventricular hypertrophy or depressed ejection fraction, and in women (40).

Contrast-related Complications

Complications arising from use of contrast agents may be anaphylactoid, toxic, or thromboembolic. Overall, some type of adverse event related to contrast administration occurs in approximately 2% of patients undergoing catheterization, most of these reactions being mild. Severe reactions requiring hospitalization occur in 0.007% of patients. A detailed review of the complications of contrast administration and selection of a contrast agent is presented in Chapter 13.

Cholesterol Emboli Syndrome

Multiple cholesterol emboli syndrome is an uncommon but important complication of catheterization and angiography (41–44). The syndrome is characterized by multiple organ dysfunction, usually following an invasive arterial procedure. The hallmarks are acute renal failure, hypertension, back, leg, and/or abdominal pain, eosinophilia, and livedo reticularis. The most worrisome feature in terms of prognosis is renal failure. Risk factors for this syndrome appear to include peripheral vascular disease, smoking, and advanced age. Diagnosis is sometimes difficult, and treatment is supportive. Anticoagulation is not beneficial but probably detrimental in this condition.

Transseptal Catheterization

The risk of transseptal cardiac catheterization relates to vascular access and complications arising from inadvertent puncture of cardiac structures other than the intraatrial septum. The improvement in echocardiographic techniques has greatly reduced the need for diagnostic transseptal catheterization. Most transseptal catheterizations today are done as part of mitral valvuloplasty or electrophysiologic catheter ablation of left-sided accessory pathways. Because of the small number of these procedures done in many cardiac catheterization laboratories, most cardiovascular fellows trained in the past 10 to 15 years are not experienced in transseptal catheterization. Competency in transseptal catheterization will be difficult to maintain for many cardiologists trained in recent years and probably can only be achieved in catheterization laboratories with an active mitral valvuloplasty program (see chapter 9).

Vascular Access

Complications of vascular access for transseptal catheterization are similar to that for right heart catheterization except that only the right femoral vein can be used. Special care must be taken to avoid injury to the inferior vena cava during advancement of the relatively stiff needle and stylet through the vascular sheath.

Needle- and Catheter-related Complications

The risk of cardiac perforation due to transseptal catheterization has been studied in patients with many indications for this technique. The risk of perforation is approximately 2.5% in patients undergoing transseptal catheterization for assessment of valvular heart disease, less than 1% in patients undergoing mitral valvuloplasty, and 2.2% in patients having ablation of left-sided accessory pathways (45–47). The use of transesophageal echocardiography probably reduces the risk of cardiac perforation, but many believe that fluoroscopic landmarks used by experienced operators are as important as or more important than transesophageal echocardiography guidance.

THERAPEUTIC CATHETERIZATION

Therapeutic cardiac catheterization includes the various coronary interventional revascularization techniques and valvuloplasty. Each of these techniques has unique risks that the operator must understand in detail prior to performing the procedure. Many of the specific risks of these interventions and technical considerations to reduce those risks are covered in the chapters concerning the specific procedures (e.g., rotational atherectomy, mitral valvuloplasty).

Complication rates for the newer coronary interventional techniques are often compared with the complication rates for standard PTCA. Table 8.4 shows the reported complication rates in two recent registries and two recent randomized trials for standard PTCA groups. In this section I review various risks and complications related to the practice of interventional cardiology.

Coronary Interventions

Common coronary interventions include PTCA, atherectomy, coronary stent placement, and intracoronary delivery of various pharmacological agents. The risks of these various techniques are related to vascular access, ischemic complications, anticoagulation, device-specific variables, and coronary anatomic features. The accurate assessment of each of these factors is crucial in determining (*a*) whether or not a patient should undergo percutaneous intervention and (*b*) which specific technique is safest and likely to be most effective.

Vascular Access

The risk of vascular access site complications is greater after PTCA than after diagnostic left heart catheterization (27, 30). This increased risk is probably due to more intense anticoagulation, more frequent anticoagulation after the procedure, and multiple procedures via the same site. Newer interventional devices are not necessarily associated with a higher risk of access site complications than standard PTCA, and the use of a larger vascular sheath than in diagnostic catheterization is probably not the cause of the increase in complications with PTCA or other devices (32). Coronary stenting followed by intense anticoagulation is associated with a markedly increased risk of peripheral vascular complications (32, 48, 49).

Ischemic Complications

Ischemic complications of percutaneous intervention include abrupt closure, threat-

Table 8.4.
Complications of PTCA Registries and Randomized Trials

Complication	SCAI 1990 N = 12,011	SCAI 1991 N = 17,073	PTCA arm BENESTENT 1994 N = 257	PTCA arm STRESS 1994 N = 202
Death	0.32%	0.3%	0%	1.5%
MI	0.61	0.5	3.1	5.0
CVA	0.05	*	0.4	0.5
Arrhythmia	0.81	*	*	*
Vascular	3.4	*	3.1	4.5
Perforation	0.11	*	*	*
Other	0.63	*	*	*
Emergency CABG	1.6	1.4%	1.6%	4.0%**

* Not available.
** 0–14 Days after procedure.

ened closure with prolonged ischemia, distal emboli, and the no-reflow phenomenon. The predictors of ischemic complications during or after percutaneous coronary interventions include clinical factors, pretreatment angiographic features, and immediate postprocedure assessment of results (50). The most consistent clinical predictor of ischemic complications during percutaneous intervention is an unstable ischemic syndrome prior to intervention. Other clinical factors associated with an increased risk of ischemic complications are diabetes and female gender. The angiographic feature most consistently associated with an increased risk of periprocedural ischemic complications is evidence of thrombus (50–52). Other angiographic features, such as severe angulation and calcification, have been associated with an increased risk of dissection, but with newer technologies higher success rates in these lesions can be achieved. The initial results after balloon dilation also predict ischemic complications. Dissection, a new filling defect, and post-PTCA residual stenosis predict acute ischemic complications (50, 52). Many laboratories have again begun to measure CK and CK-MB levels routinely following percutaneous coronary intervention. Further study is required to understand the mechanism responsible for and the implications of small rises in CK-MB following some coronary interventions (see chapter 38).

Anticoagulation

Before the Procedure   Although randomized trial data are lacking, it appears that prolonged administration of intravenous heparin prior to coronary intervention reduces the risk of ischemic complications during PTCA, especially in patients with angiographic evidence of thrombus at the time of diagnostic catheterization (53). The administration of **aspirin before the procedure is well known to reduce complications during PTCA,** and it should be administered to all patients except those with a history of true anaphylaxis after aspirin. **Patients with a history of possible severe aspirin allergy can be allergy skin tested and sometimes desensitized by experienced specialists** in allergy and immunology. We have used this approach in a number of patients with suspected aspirin allergy because of the strong evidence of the beneficial effects of aspirin. **Many aspirin "allergies" are not anaphylactic reactions,** and close questioning reveals no contraindication to the administration of aspirin before the procedure.

During the Procedure   Aggressive use of heparin during coronary interventions is generally accepted, although one study has shown that a less aggressive approach of a standard 10,000 unit dose without activated clotting time (ACT) measurement is acceptable in stable elective PTCA (54). Most laboratories now administer heparin during coronary intervention guided by the ACT. The most appropriate ACT is not known, but a target value of more than 300 or more than 350 seconds is reasonable. One recent study suggests that there is no minimum or maximum ACT but that the risk of acute closure decreases as the intraprocedural ACT increases (55). We generally aim for an ACT of more than 300 seconds for low-risk cases and an ACT of more than 350 for higher-risk cases if platelet glycoprotein IIb/IIIa receptor antagonists are not used. Lower target ACT values should be used when platelet glycoprotein IIb/IIIa receptor antagonists are administered (56, 57). The use of other anticoagulant regimens to prevent ischemic complications is reviewed in detail in Chapter 34.

Device- and Technique-specific Variables

Many of the complications of coronary interventions are related to the specific device used. The risk of standard angioplasty, for example, is quite different from the risk of rotational atherectomy. The no-reflow phenomenon, for example, is uncommon during routine PTCA but not during rotational atherectomy. Non–Q-wave infarction seems to be increased after directional atherectomy, and nose cone injury to the coronary artery can occur with this device. **When an interventional cardiologist begins to perform procedures using a new device or technique, the focus must be on understanding and minimizing the complications** of the new technique rather than attempting to employ the device as aggressively as possible. The complications of the various devices are discussed in more detail in the chapters dealing with each of these specific techniques.

Mitral Valvuloplasty

Balloon valvuloplasty of the mitral valve is effective therapy for selected patients with mitral stenosis (see chapter 35). The transseptal technique is used to gain access to the left atrium and left ventricle with the same risks as were previously discussed for diagnostic trans-septal catheterization. Because of dilation of the interatrial septum there is a greater risk of development of an atrial septal defect after valvuloplasty, but a hemodynamically significant atrial septal defect is quite uncommon, especially with the single balloon technique. The incidence of an iatrogenic atrial septal defect with more than 1:1.5 shunt after mitral valvuloplasty is 2% with the single balloon technique and 12% with the double balloon technique (58). The main risks of valvuloplasty are death, cardiac perforation, mitral regurgitation, and embolic events.

Mortality and Cardiac Perforation

The mortality with balloon mitral valvuloplasty ranges from 0 to 2.7% (47, 58). Most deaths occur with left ventricular perforation, usually with the double balloon technique. Cardiac perforation with the single balloon technique is rare. Transesophageal echocardiography during the procedure may help avoid cardiac perforation, but many operators perform valvuloplasty without transesophageal echocardiography guidance with low rates of cardiac perforation and other complications. Atrial perforation because of the transseptal puncture is tolerated much better than LV perforation and is usually not fatal. Other complications that may be fatal are coronary emboli and embolic stroke (discussed later in the chapter).

Mitral Regurgitation

Mitral regurgitation as assessed by left ventricular angiography increases by one or more grades in 4% of patients with the single balloon technique and 12% of patients after the double balloon technique (58). Some 3% of patients have severe mitral regurgitation after the single balloon technique and 4% after the double balloon technique (58). Severe mitral regurgitation complicating balloon commissurotomy usually requires urgent surgical intervention. Meticulous attention to the position of the guidewires within the left ventricle is important to minimizing the chance of severe mitral regurgitation or cardiac perforation when using the double balloon technique.

Emboli and Cerebrovascular Accident

Embolic stroke occurs in 1.1 to 5.4% of patients during balloon mitral commissurotomy (47). We administer 10,000 units of heparin immediately after successful transseptal puncture in hopes of decreasing the incidence of emboli. The **use of transesophageal echocardiography to eliminate patients with left atrial thrombus has almost certainly reduced the risk of emboli** during mitral valvuloplasty. We perform transesophageal echocardiography in all patients prior to mitral valvuloplasty, and we exclude patients with visible left atrial thrombus from balloon therapy, referring these patients instead for surgical correction.

SUMMARY

Understanding the risks of catheterization is essential for cardiologists performing invasive procedures and referring patients for them. With the variety of complex procedures now performed in the catheterization laboratory it is more difficult than ever to assess the various risks of these newer techniques. Complications related to vascular access are common and important with all catheterization techniques. Minimizing vascular complications requires expertise in catheter insertion and removal and with anticoagulation regimens. New devices aimed at sealing vascular insertion sites may be helpful in the future, but at this time proper catheter insertion appears to be the most important factor in reducing vascular complications. New techniques in the cardiac cath-

eterization laboratory are rapidly being developed and are employed with enthusiasm. A careful evaluation of the potential adverse events associated with any new technique is essential before it is accepted as an effective tool. Valid quality assurance reviews should be done regularly to identify recurrent problems within a catheterization laboratory. Finally, when any adverse event occurs in the cardiac catheterization laboratory, the case should be reviewed to determine whether the event could have been avoided. Only through careful critical review of our own techniques will we have continued improvement and fewer complications in the catheterization laboratory.

References

1. Kimmel SE, Berlin JA, Laskey WK. The relationship between coronary angioplasty procedure volume and major complications. JAMA 1995;274: 1137–1142 (see Comments).
2. Rosenwasser RH, Jallo JI, Getch CC, Liebman KE. Complications of Swan-Ganz catheterization for hemodynamic monitoring in patients with subarachnoid hemorrhage. Neurosurgery 1995;37: 872–875.
3. Benson J, Patla V. Real or apparent entrapment of a Swan-Ganz pulmonary artery catheter after cardiac surgery? Intensive Care Med 1994;20:309–310 (letter).
4. Bernardin G, Milhaud D, Roger PM, et al. Swan-Ganz catheter-related pulmonary valve infective endocarditis: a case report. Intensive Care Med 1994;20:142–144.
5. Davis MS. Hepatic vein obstruction due to Swan-Ganz catheter placement. Chest 1994;106:603–605.
6. Feng WC, Singh AK, Drew T, Donat W. Swan-Ganz catheter-induced massive hemoptysis and pulmonary artery false aneurysm. Ann Thorac Surg 1990;50:644–646.
7. Greeno E, Parenti C. Pulmonary artery rupture from Swan-Ganz catheter insertion: report of two cases. Crit Care Nurs Q 1992;15:71–74.
8. Jondeau G, Lacombe P, Rocha P, et al. Swan-Ganz catheter-induced rupture of the pulmonary artery: successful early management by transcatheter embolization. Cathet Cardiovasc Diagn 1990;19: 202–204.
9. Kearney TJ, Shabot MM. Pulmonary artery rupture associated with the Swan-Ganz catheter. Chest 1995;108:1349–1352.
10. Lee TS, Wu Y. Arterially misplaced Swan-Ganz catheter in a hypotensive and hypoxic COPD patient. J Clin Anesth 1995;7:320–322.
11. Lopez Sendon J, Lopez de Sa E, Gonzalez Maqueda

I, et al. Right ventricular infarction as a risk factor for ventricular fibrillation during pulmonary artery catheterization using Swan-Ganz catheters. Am Heart J 1990;119:207–209.

12. Pezzulli F, Goldberg N, Posner D. Pulmonary artery pseudoaneurysm secondary to Swan-Ganz catheterization: a case report. Australas Radiol 1992;36:59–61.

13. Unger P, Stoupel E, Berkenboom G. Misplacement of a Swan-Ganz catheter after insertion through the left internal jugular vein. Cathet Cardiovasc Diagn 1990;21:13–14.

14. You CK, Whatley GS. Swan-Ganz catheter-induced pulmonary artery pseudoaneurysm: a case of complete resolution without intervention. Can J Surg 1994;37:420–424.

15. Roizental M, Hartnell GG, Perry LJ, Kane RA. Pseudoaneurysm of the common femoral vein as a late complication of right heart catheterization. Cardiovasc Intervent Radiol 1994;17:301–303.

16. Zion MM, Balkin J, Rosenmann D, et al. Use of pulmonary artery catheters in patients with acute myocardial infarction: analysis of experience in 5,841 patients in the SPRINT Registry. SPRINT Study Group. Chest 1990;98:1331–1335.

17. Connors AF, Sperroff T, Dawson NV, et al. The effectiveness of right heart catheterization in the initial care of critically ill patients. JAMA 1996;276: 889–897.

18. Baraldi Junkins C, Levin HR, et al. Complications of endomyocardial biopsy in heart transplant patients. J Heart Lung Transplant 1993;12:63–67.

19. Deckers JW, Hare JM, Baughman KL. Complications of transvenous right ventricular endomyocardial biopsy in adult patients with cardiomyopathy: a seven-year survey of 546 consecutive diagnostic procedures in a tertiary referral center. J Am Coll Cardiol 1992;19:43–47.

20. Chen SA, Chiang CE, Tai CT, et al. Complications of diagnostic electrophysiologic studies and radiofrequency catheter ablation in patients with tachyarrhythmias: an eight-year survey of 3,966 consecutive procedures in a tertiary referral center. Am J Cardiol 1996;77:41–46.

21. Johnson LW, Krone R. Cardiac catheterization 1991: a report of the Registry of the Society for Cardiac Angiography and Interventions. Cathet Cardiovasc Diagn 1993;28:219–220.

22. Laskey W, Boyle J, Johnson LW. Multivariable model for prediction of risk of significant complication during diagnostic cardiac catheterization. The Registry Committee of the Society for Cardiac Angiography & Interventions. Cathet Cardiovasc Diagn 1993;30:185–190.

23. Noto TJ Jr, Johnson LW, Krone R, et al. Cardiac catheterization 1990: a report of the Registry of the Society for Cardiac Angiography and Interventions. Cathet Cardiovasc Diagn 1991;24:75–83.

24. Bogart DB, Bogart MA, Miller JT, et al. Femoral artery catheterization complications: a study of 503 consecutive patients. Cathet Cardiovasc Diagn 1995;34:8–13.

25. Cohen GI, Chan KL. Physical examination and echo Doppler study in the assessment of femoral arterial complications following cardiac catheterization. Cathet Cardiovasc Diagn 1990;21:137–143.

26. Babu SC, Piccorelli GO, Shah PM, et al. Incidence and results of arterial complications among 16,350 patients undergoing cardiac catheterization. J Vasc Surg 1989;10:113–116.

27. Lumsden AB, Miller JM, Kosinski AS, et al. A prospective evaluation of surgically treated groin complications following percutaneous cardiac procedures. Am Surg 1994;60:132–137.

28. Wyman RM, Safian RD, Portway V, et al. Current complications of diagnostic and therapeutic cardiac catheterization. J Am Coll Cardiol 1988;12: 1400–1406.

29. Muller DW, Shamir KJ, Ellis SG, Topol EJ. Peripheral vascular complications after conventional and complex percutaneous coronary interventional procedures. Am J Cardiol 1992;69:63–68.

30. Khoury M, Batra S, Berg R, et al. Influence of arterial access sites and interventional procedures on vascular complications after cardiac catheterizations. Am J Surg 1992;164:205–209.

31. Oweida SW, Roubin GS, Smith RBD, Salam AA. Postcatheterization vascular complications associated with percutaneous transluminal coronary angioplasty. J Vasc Surg 1990;12:310–315.

32. Waksman R, King SBr, Douglas JS, et al. Predictors of groin complications after balloon and new-device coronary intervention. Am J Cardiol 1995;75: 886–889.

33. Kussmaul WGR, Buchbinder M, Whitlow PL, et al. Rapid arterial hemostasis and decreased access site complications after cardiac catheterization and angioplasty: results of a randomized trial of a novel hemostatic device. J Am Coll Cardiol 1995;25: 1685–1692.

34. Trerotola SO, Kuhlman JE, Fishman EK. Bleeding complications of femoral catheterization: CT evaluation. Radiology 1990;174:37–40.

35. Sheikh KH, Adams DB, McCann R, et al. Utility of Doppler color flow imaging for identification of femoral arterial complications of cardiac catheterization. Am Heart J 1989;117:623–628.

36. Lilly MP, Reichman W, Sarazen AA Jr, Carney WI Jr. Anatomic and clinical factors associated with complications of transfemoral arteriography. Ann Vasc Surg 1990;4:264–269.

37. Ricci MA, Trevisani GT, Pilcher DB. Vascular complications of cardiac catheterization. Am J Surg 1994;167:375–378.

38. Davidson CJ, Mark DB, Pieper KS, et al. Thrombotic and cardiovascular complications related to nonionic contrast media during cardiac catheterization: analysis of 8,517 patients. Am J Cardiol 1990;65:1481–1484.

39. Garcia Robles JA, Garcia E, Rico M, et al. Emergency coronary stenting for acute occlusive dissection of the left main coronary artery. Cathet Cardiovasc Diagn 1993;30:227–229.

40. Lazar JM, Uretsky BF, Denys BG, et al. Predisposing risk factors and natural history of acute neurologic complications of left-sided cardiac catheterization. Am J Cardiol 1995;75:1056–1060.

41. Hauben M, Norwich J, Shapiro E, et al. Multiple cholesterol emboli syndrome: six cases identified through the spontaneous reporting system. Angiology 1995;46:779–784.

42. Colt HG, Begg RJ, Saporito JJ, et al. Cholesterol

emboli after cardiac catheterization: eight cases and a review of the literature. Medicine (Baltimore) 1988;67:389–400.

43. Freund NS. Cholesterol emboli syndrome following cardiac catheterization. Postgrad Med 1990;87: 55–60.

44. Hendel RC, Cuenoud HF, Giansiracusa DF, Alpert JS. Multiple cholesterol emboli syndrome: bowel infarction after retrograde angiography. Arch Intern Med 1989;149:2371–2374.

45. Folland ED, Oprian C, Giacomini J, et al. Complications of cardiac catheterization and angiography in patients with valvular heart disease. VA Cooperative Study on Valvular Heart Disease. Cathet Cardiovasc Diagn 1989;17:15–21.

46. Hahn K, Gal R, Sarnoski J, et al. Transesophageal echocardiographically guided atrial transseptal catheterization in patients with normal-sized atria: incidence of complications. Clin Cardiol 1995;18: 217–220.

47. Harrison JK, Wilson JS, Hearne SE, Bashore TM. Complications related to percutaneous transvenous mitral commissurotomy. Cathet Cardiovasc Diagn 1994; (Suppl 2):52–60.

48. Serruys PW, de Jaegere P, Kiemeneij F, et al. A comparison of balloon-expandable stent implantation with balloon angioplasty in patients with coronary artery disease. Benestent Study Group. N Engl J Med 1994;331:489–495.

49. Fischman DL, Leon MB, Baim DS, et al. A randomized comparison of coronary-stent placement and balloon angioplasty in the treatment of coronary artery disease. Stent Restenosis Study Investigators. N Engl J Med 1994;331:496–501.

50. Ellis SG, Roubin GS, King SBD, et al. Angiographic and clinical predictors of acute closure after native vessel coronary angioplasty. Circulation 1988;77: 372–379.

51. Cavallini C, Giommi L, Franceschini E, et al. Coronary angioplasty in single-vessel complex lesions: short- and long-term outcome and factors predicting acute coronary occlusion. Am Heart J 1991;122: 44–49.

52. Vaitkus PT, Herrmann HC, Laskey WK. Management and immediate outcome of patients with intracoronary thrombus during percutaneous transluminal coronary angioplasty. Am Heart J 1992; 124:1–8.

53. Kolansky DM, Shapiro TA, Laskey WK. Prolonged heparin therapy for occlusive intracoronary thrombus. Cathet Cardiovasc Diagn 1993;30:150–152.

54. Frierson JH, Dimas AP, Simpfendorfer CC, et al. Is aggressive heparinization necessary for elective PTCA?. Cathet Cardiovasc Diagn 1993;28:279–282.

55. Narins CR, Hillegass WB Jr, Nelson CL, et al. Relation between activated clotting time during angioplasty and abrupt closure. Circulation 1996;93: 667–671.

56. Moliterno DJ, Califf RM, Aguirre FV, et al. Effect of platelet glycoprotein IIb/IIIa integrin blockade on activated clotting time during percutaneous transluminal coronary angioplasty or directional atherectomy (the EPIC trial). Evaluation of c7E3 Fab in the Prevention of Ischemic Complications trial. Am J Cardiol 1995;75:559–562.

57. Use of a monoclonal antibody directed against the platelet glycoprotein IIb/IIIa receptor in high-risk coronary angioplasty. The EPIC Investigation. N Engl J Med 1994;330:956–961.

58. Multicenter experience with balloon mitral commissurotomy. NHLBI Balloon Valvuloplasty Registry Report on immediate and 30-day follow-up results. The National Heart, Lung, and Blood Institute Balloon Valvuloplasty Registry Participants. Circulation 1992;85:448–461.

9
Review of Techniques

James A. Hill, MD, MS
Charles R. Lambert, MD, PhD
Ronald E. Vlietstra, MD
Carl J. Pepine, MD

INTRODUCTION

Performing cardiac catheterization requires a great deal of technical skill, sophisticated instruments, and mature judgment to choose the appropriate procedures from among the various techniques available. Since the scope of cardiac catheterization has changed from primarily an elective diagnostic procedure in stable patients to a procedure often performed in combination with therapeutic interventions in the critically ill, the operator must be very familiar with disease processes and therapeutic alternatives to select the best technique and its timing.

The purposes of this chapter are to describe the various techniques available for catheter introduction; summarize their advantages, disadvantages, and uses; and briefly discuss some associated procedures that may provide additional information and therapeutic benefit in a given patient. Details of preparation and stabilization of patients are reviewed in Chapter 7.

METHODS USED TO INTRODUCE CATHETERS

There are two general methods in use for introduction of catheters regardless of the location of entry. These are (a) percutaneous introduction using needles and guidewires and (b) direct introduction after surgical isolation of the vessel. While either method may be used at any site, practical and anatomic considerations generally dictate which approach is appropriate.

Percutaneous Technique

The Seldinger technique or a modification of it is the method of most percutaneous catheter insertion (Fig. 9.1). When using this technique, the operator locates the vessel to be cannulated according to palpation or landmark identification and enters it with a needle through the skin. This may be preceded by a small nick in the skin using a #11 blade. An 18-gauge needle is generally adequate in adults, but any size into which a guidewire can be inserted will work. One of two general types of needles is used: (a) a sharp, long-pointed beveled needle with a cutting edge or (b) a less pointed beveled needle without a cutting edge containing an obturator (see Chapter 10). The techniques used for insertion vary somewhat in that the cutting needle ideally enters the front wall of the vessel as it is advanced. The bevel of the needle with an obturator is relatively blunt,

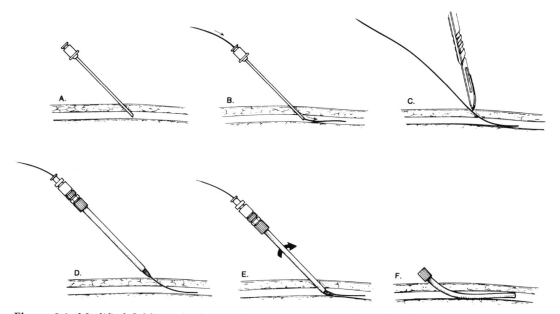

Figure 9.1. Modified Seldinger technique for percutaneous catheter sheath introduction. **A.** Vessel punctured by needle. **B.** Flexible guidewire placed in vessel via needle. **C.** Needle removed, guidewire left in place, and hole in skin around wire enlarged with scalpel. **D.** Sheath and dilator placed over guidewire. **E.** Sheath and dilator advanced over guidewire and into vessel. **F.** Dilator and guidewire removed while sheath remains in vessel.

so the needle often must be advanced more forcefully and deeply, especially with arterial puncture, and thus often enters both the front and back walls of the vessel. When the obturator is removed, the needle can only be withdrawn until blood flow results. This latter technique causes more trauma, particularly if the vessel is diseased and calcified. **We prefer to use a sharp 18-gauge needle without an obturator for all arterial and venous punctures.** Introduction of the needle should be nearly parallel to the vessel. A more nearly perpendicular angle makes passage of guidewires difficult and kinking of sheaths and catheters more likely.

Aspiration on the needle is often necessary with venipuncture to ensure vigorous blood return. Merely putting the needle into the vein and moving it back and forth to get blood flow risks lacerating the vessel needlessly, as flow is often not immediately evident, especially in those with low venous pressure. Blood should flow vigorously without aspiration when an artery is appropriately punctured. Once this occurs, a guidewire is inserted through the needle

into the vessel. We prefer an 0.035-inch Teflon-coated spring coil guidewire with a J-tip. If difficulty advancing this wire is encountered, an 0.025-inch wire or one with a very flexible tip that is more steerable, such as a Wholey (ACS) or 0.018-inch angioplasty guidewire is substituted. Skin pressure is applied proximal to the needle as it is removed to leave only the guidewire in place. The guidewire is wiped as the needle is removed. As skin pressure is maintained, the skin puncture site is enlarged with a scalpel blade followed by dilation of the skin entry site with a straight hemostat to create a percutaneous tunnel. This track must allow the catheter, dilator, or sheath to be inserted and move freely, so that its tip is not damaged as it traverses the skin and subcutaneous tissue. Otherwise a burr that can damage the vessel may be created on the tip of the catheter or sheath. If a sheath is not going to be left in place, a stiff, short dilator is necessary for dilating the subcutaneous tissue and vessel. The dilator is advanced over the guidewire after the needle is removed. After several passes into the vessel to make a tract, the dilator is removed as the wire is again wiped. The catheter is then advanced over the guidewire, and the guidewire is removed. If scarring or calcification makes entry difficult, a dilator several sizes smaller than the catheter to be used is first introduced. Serial dilations with successively larger dilators are made, with each introduced over the indwelling guidewire. **Sometimes it is also helpful to use a larger, stiffer guidewire (0.038 inch) when large dilators are needed in very heavily scarred or calcified vessels.** If the guidewire is bent in the subcutaneous tissue, it is extremely difficult to pass any dilator or catheter over it. The bent portion must be moved either into the vessel or preferably out of the skin to re-establish a straight segment in the subcutaneous tissue. When only the guidewire is in place, the operator should maintain finger pressure over the vessel to limit bleeding. We routinely use a short sheath with a hemostatic diaphragm to facilitate catheter exchanges.

The **advantages of the percutaneous technique make it the most popular method to introduce catheters** into the vascular system. It is fast, requires minimal surgical skill, and is more easily taught and mastered than other techniques. Repeat procedures can be more readily performed with less trauma than a cutdown.

The primary disadvantage of the percutaneous technique is that blind introduction does not allow one to avoid diseased portions of vessels where excessive damage may occur. This may be a disadvantage when arterial cannulation is performed in patients with peripheral vascular disease. Also, catheter control can be limited when there is a substantial amount of subcutaneous tissue, scar, or very tortuous vessel. A long sheath may help in this circumstance. Occasionally when catheters are removed, tamponade may be difficult in patients with clotting abnormalities, markedly widened pulse pressure, marked obesity, severe hypertension, calcified vessels, or deep punctures such as the subclavian.

Direct Surgical Cutdown

The cutdown is generally used only for the brachial approach. Cutdown in other sites is a more complex procedure and offers no particular advantage except in very select circumstances such as catheterizing small children. Femoral cutdown technique is not described in this chapter.

The aim of brachial artery cutdown is to mobilize about 1 to 2 cm of artery in an area of minimal branching prior to its bifurcation into radial and ulnar branches (Fig. 9.2). A 1.5- to 2-cm transverse skin incision along the skin lines is made for isolation of a vein and brachial artery. The incision is smaller and more medial if only a vein is needed. Some use a vertical incision, but this often leads to more obvious scarring. With the elbow extended, blunt dissection is performed with standard surgical instruments. In some this may require a pad under the elbow. The cutdown is best done approximately 1 cm proximal to the medial epicondyle directly over the brachial artery pulse, where the artery is becoming more superficial to cross the joint before it reaches the bicipital aponeurosis. This area is preferred because branches are limited, the artery is usually separated from the median nerve, and collateral flow is excellent, so that even with brachial artery obstruction in this area, ischemia of the forearm is uncommon. Also, in this area there is no need to cut through muscle or tendon to approach the artery. A vein is usually isolated in the brachial sheath or by exploring more medially for the median cubital vein. The vein is controlled with a short length of 3–0 or 4–0 suture placed on both sides of the planned venotomy site.

The artery should be handled and controlled with either umbilical tapes or sterile rubber bands placed proximal and distal to the planned arteriotomy site. The isolated area is mobilized to allow easy lifting of the segment to the level of the skin. This allows for more parallel entry of the catheter into the artery, permitting easier catheter manipulation and less arterial trauma. Traction is applied on the distal tape to distend the artery proximally, and after lifting the tape on the proximal segment to control bleeding, an incision large enough to allow introduction of the catheter tip is made. We use a pointed #11 blade and insert it slowly into the lumen. The hole is enlarged slightly as the blade is removed. A larger hole may

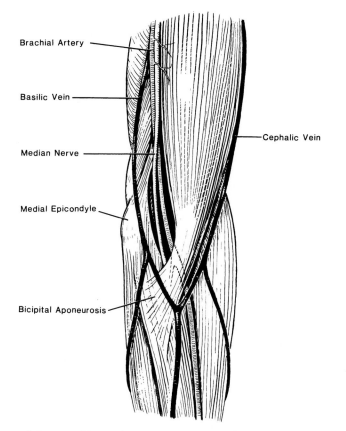

Brachial Artery

Basilic Vein

Cephalic Vein

Median Nerve

Medial Epicondyle

Bicipital Aponeurosis

Figure 9.2. Anatomy of the arm illustrating appropriate site for brachial artery cutdown. The ideal site is approximately 1 to 2 cm proximal to the bifurcation of the brachial artery in the triangle formed by the bicipital aponeurosis. This is generally less than 1 cm above the medial epicondyle of the elbow joint. Either the right or left arm (shown above) may be used.

permit substantial bleeding around the catheter. We consider a horizontal incision superior to a vertical one because the arteriotomy remains smaller rather than enlarging longitudinally with catheter manipulation. Some prefer a vertical incision, reasoning that its extension by catheter manipulation is longitudinal, involving less of the circumference of the vessel. The vertical incision is repaired horizontally. When the catheter is in the artery, we generally administer 5000 units of heparin. Placing a sheath in the artery in this situation is not necessary.

When catheters are exchanged or the procedure is complete and catheters are removed, the operator should allow bleeding from the vessel proximal and distal to the arteriotomy to establish adequacy of flow

and to wash out debris. **If flow is not brisk, balloon catheter thrombectomy should be performed.** Additional heparin may be administered to prevent further thrombus formation. Routine use of embolectomy catheters is not recommended because these catheters provide additional unnecessary trauma to the intima. After adequate flow has been established, vascular clamps are placed on both sides of the arteriotomy to occlude flow. The arteriotomy is inspected for thrombus and intimal damage. After debris is removed or damage is repaired, the arteriotomy is closed with 6–0 or 7–0 vascular suture. The suturing technique should be either horizontal mattress, starting at both sides and working toward the middle, or purse-string. Some prefer a continuous running suture, usually with a nonbraided suture. The goal is to evert the edges and provide intima-to-intima approximation to lessen potential for thrombus formation without compromising the vessel diameter. Veins should be ligated, making sure to isolate the venotomy site between the proximal and distal ties.

Brachial artery cutdown offers several advantages over the percutaneous technique. First, it provides direct visualization of the vessel in case of difficulty in catheter introduction. Second, it allows most local vascular problems to be corrected by the operator without surgical assistance, but if surgical intervention is necessary, it can generally be performed under local anesthesia. Finally, catheter control is better with direct exposure. Disadvantages of the technique include the greater surgical skills required, slightly increased procedure time, loss of venous access because of vein ligation, increased trauma required with repeat procedures, and limits on the catheter sizes that can be used (usually no larger than 8 or 9 F, in men and 7 or 7.5 F, in women [see chapter 10]).

CATHETER-RELATED PERIPHERAL VESSEL SPASM

Occasionally spasm of the artery or vein prevents the catheter from being easily removed or advanced, particularly with the brachial approach. This is rare with the femoral approach. Proper catheter sizing and not advancing catheters when they do not pass easily limit this problem. However, **if spasm occurs, the catheter should be replaced with a smaller size.** If this is not possible, intravenous or arterial vasodilators, such as nitroglycerin or low-dose tolazoline and even mild sedation usually provide enough local vasodilation to proceed. Sometimes oral or buccal nifedipine is very effective for arterial spasm. If after several minutes the catheter cannot be removed, it is best to keep the patient anticoagulated and try again about 30 minutes later, after more vasodilator is given. Some have suggested lightweight traction or even general anesthesia, but in our experience neither of these techniques has ever been necessary, and major arterial damage has not occurred.

SITES FOR CATHETER INTRODUCTION

The two most common sites used to enter the central arterial circulation and for performance of left-sided cardiac catheterization and angiography are the femoral and the brachial routes. **Recently the radial site is increasingly being used.** While venous access can be achieved via any of several routes, if both arterial and venous catheterization are to be performed, a single site is preferable for the patient's comfort and the operator's convenience. The well-equipped laboratory and skilled operator should be comfortable with both the femoral and brachial approaches.

Femoral Site

The percutaneous Seldinger technique in the femoral site is the most commonly used for left heart catheterization. The artery should be entered between the superficial femoral artery and inguinal ligament. Here it is relatively straight, without major branches, and is large enough for catheter passage. If the superficial femoral artery is punctured, the guidewire frequently does not traverse the bifurcation retrograde because of the acute angle at the origin of the common femoral artery. Furthermore, the superficial femoral artery may be too small for large catheters, and both spasm and trauma may result in occlusion. If venous catheterization is needed, the vein is punctured about 1 cm inferior or superior and directly medial to the artery to reduce the possibility of arteriovenous fistula formation.

In general **the percutaneous femoral approach is faster to perform and easier to master than the brachial cutdown.** There are several other advantages, including larger vessels to allow for the introduction of larger catheters; ease of abdominal, renal, and bilateral internal mammary artery angiography; ready access to virtually the entire central arterial circulation with the appropriate catheter; and the multitude of catheters available for adapting the procedure to the patient. Disadvantages of this approach are few. The primary one is the longer immobility required for recovery. However, the abdominal aorta and iliofemoral branches are generally more atherosclerotic and tortuous than upper-extremity branches and can present problems for catheter passage. Coronary sinus cannulation can be difficult when needed for coronary sinus flow measurement, blood sampling, atrial pacing, or electrophysiologic study. In addition, if there is a local vascular complication, repair generally requires surgery in the operating room under general anesthesia.

Brachial Site

The brachial site may be used either percutaneously or by cutdown. Both techniques have their advantages, and the way the brachial approach is used depends on the operator's experience and skill. If both arterial and venous catheterization are to be performed, a cutdown generally is necessary. The location for brachial catheter introduction was described previously.

In general, brachial catheterization is performed through less diseased vessels and is preferable in patients with severe abdominoiliac disease. With the left brachial approach preformed Judkins catheters can be used much as they are in the femoral artery. However, the left brachial approach is awkward for many operators, and many laboratories are set up to favor a right-sided approach. While some catheterization procedures, such as cannulation of the coronary sinus, are more easily performed from the arm, others, such as bilateral internal mammary artery angiography, are more difficult. In case of local vascular complications, need for extensive surgical intervention and general anesthesia is generally rare. Frequently there are excellent collaterals, so that surgical intervention may not be necessary, as limb ischemia is unusual even with arterial occlusion. With the brachial approach bleeding can easily be controlled if the patient is receiving uninterrupted anticoagulation therapy or has a clotting disorder or widened pulse pressure. Finally,

the brachial approach allows the patient to get up sooner, facilitating earlier discharge.

Radial Site

Jonsson used the radial artery in his pioneer studies of the coronary circulation 50 years ago (1). Today this approach may be preferred for selected patients with severe aortoiliac disease or marked obesity. It can also provide comfort and economic advantage to the patient by avoiding prolonged bed rest (2). It may be used for arteriography, balloon angioplasty, stenting, and small-burr rotational atherectomy (3). Suitable patients must have an easily palpable radial artery and a negative Allen test (4). The latter requirement is to avoid ischemia of the hand in case palmar arch and digital arteries are compromised by radial occlusion (Figure 9.3). Either the right or left arm may be used, with the right radial usually being preferred for easier access. Where possible, a femoral site is also prepared in case larger sheath access is required (e.g., for intra-aortic balloon pumping).

Typically the artery is punctured with a 2.75-inch 18-gauge needle or a 1.5-inch 21-gauge needle. A short 0.035-inch or 0.018-inch guidewire is followed by a 5-F (diagnostic cases) or 6-F (interventional procedures) sheath over an appropriately tapered dilator. Once the sheath is in place, additional lidocaine is injected around the sheath entry site. Nitroglycerin (200 μg) is administered into the radial artery through the sheath's side port. Lidocaine 50 to 100 mg may be used intra-arterially as prophylaxis against spasm.

Thin-walled Judkins or Amplatz shaped catheters are used for coronary intubation. Access to the ascending aorta may be facilitated by prebending the guidewire 2 to 3 inches proximal to its tip and imaging in the left anterior oblique projection. Gentle manipulation, sometimes leaving in the guidewire, often allows a size 3.5 or 4 Judkins left coronary catheter to enter both the left and right coronary ostia. Some operators prefer an Amplatz AL1 or AL2 as their primary catheter. At the conclusion of the procedure local pressure over the radial ar-

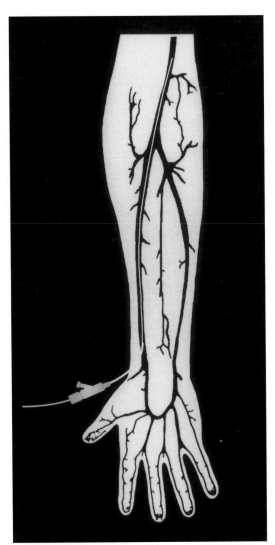

Figure 9.3. The palmar arch circulation is usually maintained by the ulnar artery if the radial artery becomes occluded. However, the Allen test must be done before radial catheterization to confirm that there is an adequate ulnar supply and a patent palmar arch.

tery is applied manually or with a custom tourniquet until the ACT is acceptably low (e.g., less than 150 seconds).

Special challenges with this approach include occlusion of the radial artery in approximately 5%; hence the importance of doing the Allen test before the procedure. The frequency with which this occurs may be underestimated because pulsation due to

collateral filling via the palmar arch may remain (5). Hematomas forming locally are infrequent and almost always superficial. Radial artery spasm limits free catheter manipulation in about 10% of cases. It is especially common in anxious subjects with small vessels. It is best prevented by adequate doses of sedation. Once it occurs, it can be overcome by further sedation and intraradial nitroglycerin and lidocaine.

Other Sites for Venous Access

Subclavian Vein

The subclavian vein (Fig. 9.4), an excellent access site to the central venous circulation, is used for a variety of procedures (e.g., cardiac pacemaker insertion, both permanent and temporary; pulmonary artery catheterization; parenteral hyperalimentation). The technique for subclavian catheterization is relatively simple but is associated with some important hazards, primarily pneumothorax and hemothorax. Patients who do not have engorged neck veins should be in head-down position to engorge the subclavian vein. It is helpful to place a small pillow or rolled sheet between the patient's shoulders to elevate the proximal and midclavicular area. The Seldinger technique, as previously described, should be used. After appropriate sterile preparation and local anesthesia, the needle is inserted perpendicular to the skin in the area just inferior to and between the middle and distal third of the clavicle to a depth even with the bottom of the clavicle. The hub of the needle is tilted, and the needle is aimed at a point 1 cm above the sternal notch. The needle is then advanced directly beneath the clavicle toward this point with constant negative pressure. When the vein is entered, the needle should be grasped and immobilized and the syringe removed. Just before and during the period when the hub of the needle is exposed, the patient should suspend breathing or perform a Valsalva ma-

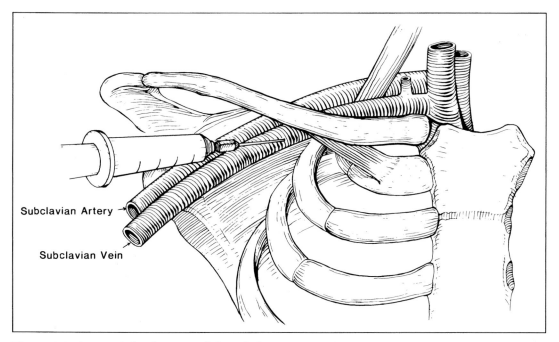

Subclavian Artery

Subclavian Vein

Figure 9.4. Anatomic localization of the subclavian vein. The appropriate site for puncture (in the middle to distal third of the clavicle) and the direction of the needle (toward a point just above the suprasternal notch) are illustrated.

neuver to minimize the chance of air embolus. A guidewire is then placed and the needle removed. The procedure is completed with whatever types of sheaths and catheters are required (see Chapter 10). General principles of central venous catheterization, regardless of route, are outlined in Table 9.1. Certain conditions make subclavian puncture somewhat more hazardous, and other approaches should be used in patients who have them. These include patients who would not well tolerate a pneumothorax, those with superior vena cava obstruction, and those with anatomic abnormalities that make the subclavian vein difficult to puncture. A recent study suggests that ultrasound guidance offers little benefit (6).

Jugular Vein

Internal. The internal jugular vein (Fig. 9.5) generally provides a straight pathway into the central venous circulation. Comparative data (7) suggest that approach through the external jugular vein is safer but less likely to be successful in reaching the superior vena cava than the internal jugular. The internal jugular approach is also less likely to be associated with the pneumothorax and hemothorax of the subclavian approach. In patients with carotid artery abnormalities on the contralateral side, superior vena cava obstruction, or distorted or difficult landmarks on the side of the neck to be used for puncture, internal jugular puncture should probably be avoided or **ultrasound localization used**.

Knowledge of the course of the internal jugular is essential to successful cannulation. After it enters the neck from the base of the skull, the internal jugular runs beneath and medial to the sternocleidomastoid muscle in its upper portion and medial to the lateral (clavicular) head of the sternocleidomastoid muscle in its lower portion. It joins the subclavian vein beneath the sternal end of the clavicle to form the innominate vein. The left internal jugular vein forms a

Table 9.1.
General Principles of Central Venous
Catheterization Technique

1. Choose the site for catherization with which you are most familiar and that carries the least risk in the clinical circumstance.
2. For cervical and subclavian punctures place the patient in a head-down position to engorge the central veins, increase the central venous pressure, and decrease the chance of air embolism unless obvious venous engorgement is present.
3. Ensure free-flowing blood before advancing any catheter or guidewire.
4. Always keep the tips of catheters and needles sealed and perform catheter or guidewire exchanges during forced expiration or Valsalva maneuver to limit the possibility of air embolism.
5. If arterial puncture is possible, use a relatively small-bore needle (no larger than 18 gauge) and the Seldinger technique to minimize trauma.
6. Maintain aspiration (negative pressure) when withdrawing the needle, as the initial pass may have perforated the vein, and free flow of blood and venous access may occur with withdrawal.
7. If a sheath without a catheter is left in place, make sure the diaphragm or some other hemostatic device provides an appropriate seal to prevent air leakage.

much more acute angle with the subclavian than the right does, making it somewhat more difficult to use for catheter manipulations. In addition, the thoracic duct enters the subclavian vein near the same place, adding another structure that can be inadvertently punctured.

The best location for puncture of the internal jugular vein depends on the operator's preference and experience (8–12). **There are at least three locations: central, anterior, and posterior.** The technique and equipment are the same for all locations. For all locations the patient's head should be turned approximately 45° off sagittal to the side opposite that of the puncture. Having a conscious patient gently lift the head allows better localization of the heads of the sternocleidomastoid muscle both visually and by palpation. The central approach uses a venipuncture near the apex of the triangle formed by the two heads of the sternocleidomastoid muscle. After local anesthesia the carotid artery is palpated beneath the sternal head of the muscle and gently retracted medially. The needle is advanced at approximately a 45° angle from the body's frontal plane and aimed laterally toward the ipsilateral nipple to the junction of the proximal and middle third of the clavicle. This approach directs the needle underneath the lateral (clavicular) head of the sternocleidomastoid muscle. Venipuncture should occur within 4 to 5 cm, or the needle should be withdrawn and redirected.

The anterior approach is similar except that the needle is placed at the midpoint of the sternocleidomastoid muscle and directed at a slightly more acute angle with the skin. Again, the needle is aimed under the clavicular head of the sternocleidomastoid muscle toward the ipsilateral nipple. Some operators advocate an even lower approach, just above the clavicle, using the notch on the medial clavicle as a landmark, and a more medially directed puncture.

The landmarks for the posterior approach are the lateral border of the clavicular head of the sternocleidomastoid muscle and the path of the external jugular vein.

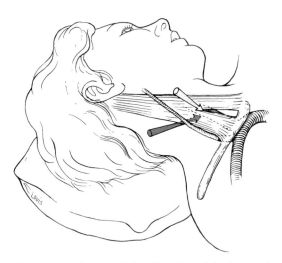

Figure 9.5. Anatomic localization of the internal and external jugular veins, *Arrows,* Appropriate location of internal jugular puncture. *Top arrow,* Anterior approach. *Lower arrow,* Posterior approach (just above the external jugular vein and under the sternocleidomastoid muscle).

The needle is introduced along the lateral border of the sternocleidomastoid muscle about 5 cm from the clavicle above the crossing point of the external jugular over the muscle. The needle is directed under the muscle caudally toward the suprasternal notch. Venipuncture should occur within approximately 5 cm, or the needle should be withdrawn and redirected. With any of these approaches, care should be given to avoid going through muscle. This is more painful and can lead to more bleeding. Catheters are introduced with standard percutaneous techniques.

With the internal jugular approach occasionally patients overrotate the neck, stretching the cervical nerves. This can cause temporary upper extremity paralysis. In addition, deep anesthetic infiltration can lead to prolonged numbness in the shoulder and neck. In our experience both conditions resolve within several hours without sequelae but can upset the patient.

External. When visible, the external jugular vein provides a convenient location for central venous access as it courses posteriorly across the lateral belly of the sternocleidomastoid muscle. As with subclavian and internal jugular cannulation, the patient is placed in a slight head-down position, and the vein is entered. Methods of catheter introduction are identical to those of other percutaneous techniques. The major problem with this route is that **occasionally the angle of entry of the external jugular into the subclavian is very acute** and does not allow for easy entry into the superior vena cava without guidewires and fluoroscopy. For this reason the external jugular is not frequently used for cardiac catheter introduction but only for fluid administration.

Direct Cardiac Puncture

Direct left ventricular puncture (13–16) still has application, particularly in patients with both mitral and aortic mechanical prosthetic valves (17, 18). Direct left ventricular puncture may be performed via either the subxiphoid or intercostal route in the apical area. Direct puncture should not be done in patients who are anticoagulated or have coagulation defects. Chronic anticoagulation should be discontinued and heparin begun so that normal clotting studies can be done just prior to the anticipated catheterization and for several hours afterward. It may help to place the patient in a shallow right anterior oblique position. Ascending aortic and pulmonary artery catheters should be placed first by standard approaches to monitor pressures. We use the technique described by Brock et al. (14). After appropriate local anesthesia, an 18-gauge needle is inserted at the apical impulse and directed toward the right second costochondral junction with a posterior angulation of approximately 35°. It is advanced until the heart pulsations are felt or ventricular ectopy is noted. We find it helpful to use fluoroscopy to note when ventricular contact is made. The needle is then advanced until blood flows freely. The pressure waveform should be inspected and recorded to ensure that the needle is within the left ventricle.

Occasionally an enlarged right ventricle is inadvertently entered. If this occurs, the needle should be removed and reinserted 1 to 2 cm to the left and redirected more posteriorly. If angiography is to be performed, it is preferable to place a 5 or 6 F high-flow pigtail catheter into the ventricle using a guidewire than to inject contrast material in high volumes through the needle. After the catheter is removed, the patient is asked to remain quiet on his or her back or left side and is sent to the coronary care unit for observation. After 3 hours heparin is restarted if needed. If any difficulty is suspected, an echocardiogram is done to evaluate for possible pericardial tamponade. Although this method is generally well tolerated, major complications, such as trauma to coronary arteries and pericardial tamponade, can occur. The procedure should therefore be done only in laboratories in hospitals with cardiac surgery available.

Transseptal Puncture

The transseptal catheter apparatus consists of a tapered needle designed to puncture

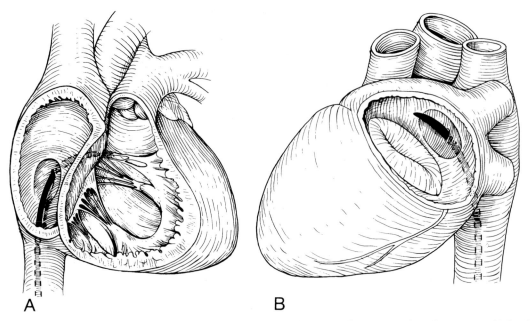

Figure 9.6. Anterior (**A,** front of the right atrium and right ventricle cut away) and posterior (**B,** back of the left atrium cut away) view of transseptal catheter in appropriate position across the atrial septum in the region of the foramen ovale.

the atrial septum and a tapered catheter that passes over the needle to enter the left atrium (Fig. 9.6). In addition, we prefer to use a long, curved sheath to facilitate catheter exchange. Use of the sheath eliminates the need for a tip occluder and other equipment formerly necessary for good quality angiography with a Brockenbrough catheter. Details of available transseptal equipment can be found in Chapter 10.

The most common diagnostic indication for transseptal catheterization is that left atrial or left ventricular pressure is needed and cannot be obtained by means of the retrograde technique. This may be in the rare patient with severe aortic stenosis whose valve cannot be crossed retrograde or with a mechanical (e.g., tilting disc) aortic valve prosthesis that cannot be safely traversed as a route to the left ventricle. Also the rare patient with aortic stenosis who has no arterial access can be evaluated using the transseptal approach with a flow-directed CO_2-filled balloon catheter floated to the aorta from the left ventricle. In hypertrophic cardiomyopathy, to avoid catheter entrap-

ment, left ventricular inflow and outflow pressures can be assessed by simultaneous transseptal left ventricular and retrograde aortic catheterization. Patients with severe pulmonary hypertension and mitral stenosis can be evaluated by means of transseptal technique when it is impossible to obtain a reliable wedge pressure. Diagnosis of cor triatriatum and pulmonary veno-occlusive disease may require the transseptal approach. Mitral and antegrade aortic valvuloplasty can be performed only via the transseptal approach. Finally, the transseptal approach may be used for atrial septostomy in patients with complete transposition.

Several anatomic considerations are important to patient selection for transseptal catheterization. Transseptal catheterization should not be done in patients with severe distortion of cardiac anatomy or cardiac position within the chest, including spinal deformities or abnormal heart position. The transseptal technique should not be used in the presence of thrombi or masses in the left atrium, recent systemic embolism, or suspicion of a left atrial myxoma or clot. If access to the right femoral vein and inferior vena cava is not available, the transseptal technique cannot be used. Finally, because of the stiff needle used, the patient must be cooperative and be able to lie still. General anesthesia may be necessary if transseptal catheterization is essential and the patient is unable to cooperate. Some other conditions may make the transseptal approach more hazardous but are not absolute contraindications. Giant right or left atria that distort the atrial septum, a markedly dilated aortic root with a small left atrium, and complex congenital heart disease that distorts either the inferior vena cava or the atrial septum are some of these conditions. Transseptal catheterization should not be done in patients who are anticoagulated or have a coagulation disorder. In those requiring anticoagulation, heparin should be started. When the prothrombin time normalizes, the procedure is scheduled and heparin discontinued several hours before the procedure is performed.

For transseptal catheterization, biplane fluoroscopy should be used when available. **We have found concomitant transesophageal two-dimensional echocardiography useful to help determine catheter position when there is some question.** Others have used an intracavitary electrogram (19). Some prefer to have a pigtail catheter in the ascending aorta as a landmark. Aortography used as a roadmap may also be useful (20). The right femoral vein is entered by percutaneous puncture. After the guidewire is in the inferior vena cava, the transseptal catheter and long sheath are passed as a unit over the wire, and the entire system is advanced into the superior vena cava. The sheath and dilator should move freely with good tactile perception. The guidewire is then removed, and the transseptal needle is advanced through the catheter with its stylet in place to approximately 1 cm from the end of the catheter but remaining inside the catheter. The stylet is then removed from the needle and the needle hub connected to a pressure transducer. The system is then withdrawn with the orientation of the needle and tip of the catheter rotated with clockwise torque to the four o'clock position, as gauged by the metal indicator arrow on the proximal end

of the needle. The catheter tip is upward and to the right as viewed by posteroanterior fluoroscopy. Because the atrial septum is oriented downward anteriorly and to the right, withdrawing the system with this orientation causes the catheter to orient itself toward and catch in the fossa ovalis after it is pulled back across the limbic ledge or ridge in the right atrium formed by the indentation of the aorta. Here the lateral view should confirm a slight posterior orientation of the needle. Care must be taken not to let the needle advance beyond the tip of the catheter until it is in the appropriate position in the fossa ovalis. Once this position has been reached, the catheter should be advanced to maintain contact with the fossa ovalis and kept in this position with some pressure exerted. In approximately 20% or more of cases the catheter crosses a catheter-patent foramen ovale to reach the left atrium without exposing the tip of the needle. If the catheter does not cross the foramen, the needle is advanced out of the catheter to a position across the septum and into the left atrium. Generally a popping sensation occurs with successful penetration of the atrial septum. Pressure measurement and oxygen saturation can be used to confirm that the needle is in the left atrium.

If the pressure tracing becomes damped and does not resemble left atrial pressure, contrast injection often reveals staining of the interatrial septum or posterior wall of the left atrium. If no other changes have occurred, the needle should be withdrawn and the system repositioned in the right atrium over a guidewire. The puncture is started again.

When left atrial pressure is obtained, the needle position is fixed against the patient's right thigh. Without advancing the needle further into the left atrium, the catheter and sheath are advanced over the needle and the needle removed, and heparin can be given. If the catheter does not go into the left ventricle as it assumes its preformed shape or with gentle advancing, the guidewire can be replaced and used to guide the catheter into the desired location. In addition, the tapered catheter can be removed and replaced by another catheter, such as a pigtail catheter, through the sheath for easier manipulation into the ventricle or angiography. A flow-directed balloon catheter may also be used through the sheath, but it should be filled with CO_2 as a safety precaution.

Complications of transseptal catheterization include aortic puncture, coronary sinus perforation, venous perforation, atrial puncture, and pericardial tamponade, as well as the other complications of the left heart catheterization. The complication rate is determined by the operator's experience but is usually higher than with all other catheterization techniques. Because of the risk of vascular perforation, systemic anticoagulation should not be performed until the actual transseptal puncture has been successfully completed. Further discussions of the transseptal technique and modifications of it (21) have been recently published (22, 23).

Other Sites of Arterial Access

Other sites have been used for arterial access for cardiac catheterization and angiography in very select circumstances. These include the translumbar (24) and axillary (25) approaches. The translumbar approach is appropriate in the rare case of occlusion of all peripheral arteries but requires a change in routine patient preparation, positioning, and laboratory setup. It is our opinion that with the advent of smaller catheters and the ease and safety of the percutaneous brachial technique, the axillary approach offers no particular advantage, and the lack of collaterals may make it riskier.

Regardless of the site or method of catheter introduction used, arterial sites and distal pulses should be assessed when the patient leaves the laboratory, again within 4 to 6 hours of the procedure, and several days after catheterization by either the catheterizing or referring physician. This should allow detection of both early and late arterial complications.

CATHETER MANIPULATION

A number of aspects of the manipulation of catheters into their desired locations be-

come part of the skills of a catheterizing physician but are not necessarily obvious to the beginner. Modern catheters are designed to make the techniques easier, but control of the catheter tip is still the key to its manipulation. The first and most important principle of successful catheter manipulation is to choose the correct catheter for the purpose. Preformed catheters assume their predetermined shape while in the patient. Body heat is generally not enough to alter the shape significantly but can make a small-bore polyethylene catheter softer after a few minutes, making it more difficult to control. Body heat can significantly change the shape of woven catheters. A good example of this is coronary catheterization with a woven Dacron Sones catheter.

Catheters should never be forced to move in a vessel. If advancement is not smooth and relatively effortless, generally something is wrong. It may be that the tip is pushed against the wall of a vessel, there is vasospasm, or the vessel is too narrow to permit further advancement. In any case, the catheter must be withdrawn, redirected, or replaced. Generally when the tip of the catheter is against a vascular structure, it is difficult and sometimes dangerous to advance it further. With soft or balloon-tip catheters and in certain cardiac chambers, such as the right atrium, forming a U-shaped loop in the catheter may be helpful or even necessary. This is true of coronary catheterization using the Sones technique in the aorta or right heart catheterization from the arm using a non–flow-directed catheter. It is important, however, not to force the tip against a vessel wall but to rotate the catheter gently as it is being advanced and to slide the tip up the vascular wall, not forcing it at a 90° angle. Also, loops should not be formed by pushing against the ventricular wall, as perforation can occur.

Maneuvers to form loops at the end of a catheter frequently create complex bends in the catheter in areas other than the end, particularly if the tip is not free to move. This can be a problem in catheters that are not preformed because of the tendency of the catheter to remember these bends. In the femoral site, if severe iliac tortuosity limits catheter control, a long sheath may be helpful. Rotating the catheter with a wire in place may also limit kinking. Catheters generally are easiest to manipulate when all of their angles are in the same plane. In this way coaxial pressure is transmitted to the tip. When using preformed catheters, the operator should take advantage of the curves in them. For example, a pigtail catheter with a 30° or 45° angle at the tip is designed to cross the aortic valve, pointing directly along the long axis of the left ventricle.

Because all catheters must pass through the skin, a sheath, or the wall of a vessel to enter the circulation, there is some resistance to that movement. Whenever a catheter must be rotated, this becomes a factor in maintaining control. Continuing to rotate a catheter without transmitting those turns to the tip does not allow for appropriate control of the catheter tip. Simple gentle movements of the catheter in and out, often only a very short distance, transmits torque to the tip as it is placed on the opposite end.

Finally, if a catheter is not doing what you want it to do because of shape, size, vascular abnormalities, or other factors, choose another one and start again. There is no advantage in trying to make a catheter do something it was not designed to do. This may be dangerous and frustrating. A well-equipped laboratory has a wide selection of catheters so that the operator can choose the most appropriate catheter design.

Approach to Catheterization of the Right Heart

Right heart catheterization is always performed antegrade from a systemic vein. It can be performed from either an upper or lower extremity or from the subclavian or jugular vein. Catheter manipulation is somewhat different with each approach. The type of catheter chosen also influences the type of manipulation performed.

Balloon flotation catheters (e.g., Swan-Ganz, Berman) are the most common types used for right heart catheterization. From the upper venous system, via the subclavian, jugular, or brachial vein, the catheter

is advanced into the superior vena cava or right atrium, and the balloon is inflated. Generally it floats into the pulmonary artery as it is advanced. Occasionally the catheter loops in the atrium and does not readily cross the tricuspid valve. In this circumstance deflating the balloon and redirecting the catheter prior to reinflation often allows it to pass. If this does not work, placing a guidewire in the central lumen usually stiffens the catheter enough to allow better manipulation, either with or without the balloon inflated. This is particularly helpful when there is significant tricuspid regurgitation or a very large right atrium. This latter technique should be performed with fluoroscopic guidance.

From the femoral vein two techniques may be used with a balloon catheter. The first involves forming a loop in the right atrium. The loop should enlarge as the catheter tip is directed laterally. Advancing the catheter should allow the tip to be directed inferiorly along the lateral wall of the right atrium and then medially toward the tricuspid valve and into the pulmonary artery. Once the catheter is in the pulmonary artery, the redundant loop should be removed. Another technique used to enter the pulmonary artery involves passing the catheter directly across the tricuspid valve. The tip of the catheter is positioned directly across the valve, pointing up toward the outflow tract. This often requires rotating the catheter, generally clockwise, while the patient inspires. Otherwise there is a tendency for the catheter to be directed toward the right ventricular apex, and from that position floating into the pulmonary artery is difficult. From the outflow tract, once the tip is directed toward the pulmonary artery, advancing the catheter allows it to float into the desired pulmonary artery location.

With a stiffer nonflotation catheter, such as a Cournand, Goodale-Lubin, or Zucker catheter, manipulation is very different. One should not generally attempt to pass these catheters from the upper extremity directly into the pulmonary artery without first forming a loop in the right atrium. Without a loop these catheters readily traverse the tricuspid valve to the right ventricular apex, where perforation may occur. The catheter is directed toward the lateral atrial wall until it is impeded by an irregular surface, usually the junction of the right atrium and the inferior vena cava. From here it is advanced to form a large loop with the tip pointing up. Then it is rotated, generally about 180° counterclockwise, to turn the loop and direct the tip toward the pulmonary artery, as the body of the catheter crosses the tricuspid valve first. Once this is accomplished and the catheter is not stuck on the right ventricular outflow region, advancing out into the pulmonary artery is straightforward. In general more catheter should be fed into the vein to help the tip move to the pulmonary artery. If the catheter starts to buckle in the right ventricle, however, it should be withdrawn and redirected because perforation of the outflow tract may occur readily. From the lower extremity a technique similar to that described for the direct passage of a balloon flotation catheter is performed. The tip of the catheter is placed across the tricuspid valve, with the tip turned up into the pulmonary valve as the catheter is advanced.

When a stiff catheter is directed toward the atrial septum, as with transseptal catheterization, it can often be advanced across a probe-patent foramen ovale. Left atrial position can be verified by noting left atrial pressure, by measuring systemic arterial oxygen saturation, or by a small contrast injection. In this same manner an atrial septal defect often can be crossed even with a balloon flotation catheter.

A brief note about coronary sinus catheterization is necessary. This is generally difficult from the inferior vena cava and should be performed from the upper extremity whenever possible. The ostium of the coronary sinus is inferior and medial to the tricuspid valve opening. If the catheter has pressure-monitoring capability, it should be pointed toward the tricuspid valve and directly passed into the right ventricle. After ventricular pressure is noted, the catheter is pulled back until atrial pressure is noted. The tip of the catheter should be facing inferiorly and to the patient's left. Rotating the catheter counterclockwise approximately 90° and advancing it should place it in the coronary sinus. Atrial pressure is still recorded, and the catheter appears as if it is going into the right ventricle. When pressure monitoring is not available,

as with electrophysiology catheters, catheter position, recorded electrical signals, and when necessary, lateral fluoroscopy confirm posterior catheter position. Absence of ventricular ectopy when the catheter looks as if it is directed into the right ventricular outflow tract also is a clue that the catheter is in the coronary sinus.

When performing right heart catheterization, **obvious areas of venous obstruction should be avoided, as in the patient with deep vein thrombosis in a femoral vein** or inferior vena cava obstruction. In individuals with a persistent left superior vena cava, venous drainage from the left upper extremity is into the coronary sinus. Occasionally this can be identified on chest x-ray film but often is first noted when a catheter takes an aberrant course from the left subclavian vein. In this situation manipulating a catheter into the right ventricle and pulmonary artery is usually quite difficult, and another site should be used.

Which catheter is chosen for right heart catheterization depends on the function it is to perform. Out of the catheterization laboratory setting, the only catheter generally used is the balloon flotation catheter. The specific model is chosen according to the capabilities that are necessary (e.g., pacing, cardiac output). In the catheterization laboratory either a stiff or balloon catheter may be used. For pressure measurements stiff catheters have a better frequency response and give a phasic pressure without the catheter whip that often accompanies softer balloon catheters. This is important when measuring pulmonary–capillary wedge pressure, particularly in patients with pulmonary hypertension. For this application an end-hole catheter, such as a Cournand, is most appropriate. Likewise, for determination of pressure gradients, as with pulmonic stenosis, an end-hole catheter should be used. For angiography of the right atrium, right ventricle, or pulmonary artery, a multiple side-hole catheter, such as a Berman angiographic, pigtail, or NIH, is necessary.

Approach to Catheterization of the Left Heart

Left ventricular catheterization is usually performed retrograde through the aortic valve. While it is usually performed with a pigtail catheter from the femoral approach, many other catheters can be used. Once the catheter has been flushed, it is advanced to the ascending aorta as pressure is monitored. Techniques used to cross the aortic valve include (*a*) the direct approach, in which the aortic valve is crossed with the tip of the catheter; (*b*) the indirect approach, in which a loop is formed so that the distal end of the catheter is backed across the valve; and (*c*) either of these two techniques combined with a guidewire. Ventricular ectopy upon entry to the cavity is common, and the operator must be ready to position the catheter quickly to find a stable position.

The direct approach is most often accomplished with relatively rigid catheters. These include the NIH, Lehman ventriculography, and Gensini catheters. All of these catheters have multiple holes and handle high flow rates; therefore, they can be used for ventriculography. Single-hole catheters, such as the right Judkins coronary catheters, can also be advanced directly into the left ventricle, but they are not suitable for the high-volume power injection necessary for adequate ventricular filling with contrast material, so this type of catheter must be exchanged for an appropriate ventriculography catheter. With the direct approach the catheter is advanced into the area just above the aortic valve and turned so that the tip faces left toward the valve orifice. The catheter is advanced gently until the valve is crossed or the left cusp stops forward motion of the catheter tip. If the cusp stops the catheter, it should be withdrawn slightly, redirected via either clockwise or counterclockwise rotation, and advanced again. Using this method, the operator explores the valve until the catheter tip advances easily into the left ventricle. In patients with aortic stenosis identification of the jet of blood ejected through the valve by observation of high-frequency vibrations of the catheter often can help recognize the location of the orifice. In addition, moving the fluoroscope into the left anterior oblique position or use of biplane fluoroscopy may be helpful. With some catheters, such as a large (8 F or larger) NIH catheter, the direct approach is the only appropriate method for crossing the aortic valve because the cathe-

ter is too stiff to form a loop safely, and guidewires cannot be advanced beyond the tip.

The indirect approach is most commonly used with pigtail catheters but is also suitable for any catheter that will easily form a loop within the ascending aorta, such as a Sones or multipurpose catheter. **The pigtail catheter is advanced to a position just above the aortic valve and rotated so that the tail is oriented toward the left coronary cusp.** The catheter is then advanced so that the loop of the pigtail is pushed firmly against the cusp. When the aortic valve is normal, the catheter often can be introduced into the ventricle by simply advancing it and forming a larger loop. If this does not cause the catheter to spring into the left ventricle, having the patient breathe as the catheter is withdrawn and rotated clockwise uncoils the loop, as the catheter easily crosses the valve in most patients. The right anterior oblique view may help in some patients. In the case of Sones and multipurpose catheters, a loop is formed by rotating and advancing the catheter simultaneously from either the left or the posterior cusp. Once the catheter is in the ventricle, the loop can be straightened by gentle retraction and rotation. Ventricular ectopy is usually controlled by these maneuvers.

Guidewires, often helpful for crossing the aortic valve, can be used in a number of ways, depending on the catheter. They can be advanced out of the end of an open-ended catheter and a loop formed either with the guidewire alone or with the catheter. The valve can be crossed indirectly with this loop. The catheter can also steer the guidewire directly across the aortic valve. This method is particularly useful with a straight guidewire in the case of either a stenotic valve or dilated root. When aortic valve stenosis is suspected, it is often helpful to start with a pigtail catheter and reinsert the guidewire to begin the crossing with the guidewire directed toward the center of the valve orifice. For this purpose many operators use a variety of catheters with the bend chosen to best reflect the specific anatomy of the aorta. These include pigtail catheters with and without preformed bends, right and left Judkins catheters, and Amplatz catheters. Guidewires can also be bent to reflect the specific anatomy to be negotiated. Again, if a single end-hole catheter is used, it must be exchanged for a more appropriate angiographic catheter prior to ventriculography using a 240- to 260-cm exchange wire of the largest diameter accepted by the catheter used. Creation of a large loop at the end of the exchange wire is helpful to keep the wire in a small left ventricular cavity with a minimum of ectopic beats. Guidewires can also be used to stiffen or straighten either an open- or closed-end catheter. Either the soft or hard end of the wire can be used for this purpose, but the hard end must never be advanced near or out of the end of the catheter tip. Crossing a stenotic valve can consume a considerable amount of time, so the amount of time the wire is in the catheter should be closely monitored. **The wire should be removed and wiped with heparinized saline and the catheter flushed every 2 minutes.**

ASSOCIATED PROCEDURES

Catheterization of the heart and vascular system is done to gain diagnostic information or to perform therapeutic procedures. The diagnostic procedures include angiography, pressure and function measurements, blood sampling for shunt detection and metabolic parameter determination, electrophysiologic measurements and stimulation, and other techniques that are discussed in other chapters. Therapeutic techniques such as angioplasty and valvuloplasty are likewise discussed elsewhere.

Endomyocardial Biopsy

Endomyocardial biopsy is unique among catheterization procedures in that it is performed only to remove a piece of tissue from the heart. This technique has undergone marked improvement since it was first attempted. Older techniques have been largely abandoned since development of

transvascular bioptomes of the Konno, King, and Stanford types. These instruments vary somewhat, but all can be introduced via a sheath placed in the internal jugular, brachial, or femoral vein for repeated sampling from the right ventricle. The brachial or femoral artery can be used for left ventricular biopsy. When transvascular myocardial biopsy is performed by experienced operators, the complication rate is very low. The complications include those related to the approach, such as vein thrombosis and hematoma, and air embolism. Arrhythmias are common with catheter manipulation, but it is rare to have sustained arrhythmia. Occasionally a patient develops transient right bundle branch or AV block, but permanent conduction abnormalities are rare. Cardiac perforation with tamponade has been reported in fewer than 0.05% in all series reported. The overall complication rate in most series is reported to be between 1 and 2%. In addition, it is rare not to obtain adequate tissue for examination (26).

The technique for obtaining biopsy specimens from the heart is relatively simple (Fig. 9.7). The right ventricular approach is described because it is the most commonly employed, but the technique is basically the same for the left ventricle. Either the internal jugular or femoral vein can be used. On occasion we have used the brachial approach. The short Stanford bioptome must be used only through the neck because of the length of the instrument, but other bioptomes (Cordis and Mansfield) come in lengths suitable for either the jugular or femoral approach. Regardless of the site or bioptome to be used, a sheath designed for this purpose is placed in the vein. These sheaths are made with a 45° angle on the terminal portion to allow for readier access to the right ventricle. After a long (145 cm) guidewire is placed in the vessel, a pigtail catheter inside the sheath is passed as a unit into the vessel. We prefer a pigtail with a 45° angle. If the bends in the sheath and the catheter are aligned to form one continuous bend in a single plane, maneuvering the system into the right ventricle is simple. Moreover, when the sheath is advanced over the pigtail, it follows a natural gentle curve directly into the desired location. The

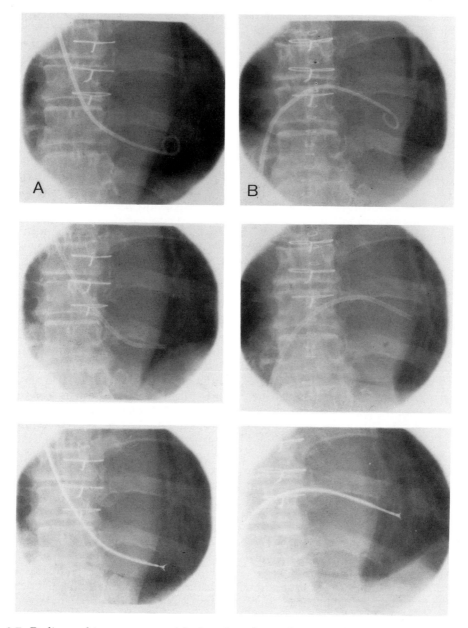

Figure 9.7. Radiographic appearance of the location of an endomyocardial biopsy apparatus in appropriate position. The sheath changes shape and position slightly with the catheter or biopsy forceps in it. **A,** Internal jugular approach. *Top,* Sheath and pigtail catheter in right ventricle. *Middle,* Sheath alone in right ventricle. *Bottom,* Biopsy forceps (open jaws) extended out of sheath and against the endocardium. **B,** Femoral vein approach. *Top,* Sheath and pigtail catheter in right ventricle. *Middle,* Sheath alone in right ventricle. *Bottom,* Biopsy forceps (open jaws) extended out of sheath and against the endocardium.

guidewire is used to help place the pigtail in the apex of the right ventricle, and the guidewire is removed. The pigtail catheter is fixed in this location as the sheath is advanced over it. When the sheath is in place, the catheter is removed, the sheath is flushed, and the side port is connected to a pressure transducer for monitoring. After right ventricular location is verified by pressure measurement, the bioptome is advanced into the sheath to a distance approximately 2 cm from the tip. This should be done while flush solution is flowing through the sheath to prevent infusion of air and thrombus formation. The sheath can then be rotated toward the ventricular septum, keeping in mind that the bioptome in the sheath tends to straighten it. The handle controlling the bioptome jaws should be moved to the open position so that the jaws will open immediately on exiting the sheath to limit the possibility of perforation. With the jaws open, the bioptome is pushed into the septal wall, and the jaws are closed and withdrawn with a jerking motion to remove a piece of the myocardium. Generally there are several premature ventricular beats during this portion of the procedure, but rarely are they sustained. This procedure can be repeated as often as necessary, and different locations in the septum can be sampled simply by moving the sheath. After each sample is taken, pressure should be checked to ensure that the sheath has not moved out of the ventricle. Three to five samples are adequate for most diagnostic purposes.

Some prefer to use a stiffer biopsy forceps that is introduced without the sheath in the ventricle but only in the superior vena cava. The forceps are slightly bent to allow easier passage into the right ventricle. There does not seem to be any advantage to this method, and lack of ability to measure pressure can be a disadvantage. It is also more time-consuming, particularly for those inexperienced in the technique.

The technique for left ventricular biopsy is very similar except that the approach is retrograde through the aortic valve. Extreme care must be used to avoid the introduction of air when advancing the bioptome into the sheath. Left ventricular biopsy should be avoided in patients with left ventricular thrombi and should not be considered in patients with right bundle branch block because of the chance of inducing complete AV block. Since there does not appear to be a substantial difference in yield between left and right ventricle sites, routine use of left ventricular biopsy is not justified (27–29).

Interpretation of the specimen is at least as important as the proper performance of the biopsy. Biopsy samples taken from a beating heart are not the same as specimens taken from autopsy material. Numerous artifacts related to the forceps, the size of the specimen, and the fact that the heart was actively contracting during the procedure can render accurate interpretation difficult.

Pericardiocentesis

Pericardiocentesis is occasionally necessary for the diagnosis and/or management of acute and chronic pericardial disease. It is essential for those performing cardiac catheterization to be skilled in pericardiocentesis, as it can be lifesaving in the event of tamponade due to cardiac perforation. Pericardiocentesis can be performed with fluoroscopic, two-dimensional echocardiographic, or electrocardiographic monitoring and guidance. Many use a combination of monitoring techniques. Except under the most urgent circumstances, pericardiocentesis should not be performed without monitoring, as cardiac damage can occur. Electrocardiographic guidance may be cumbersome and is occasionally misleading, as the right ventricle or right atrium may be punctured without registering a change in the readout, especially if a good signal cannot be obtained. We prefer direct fluoroscopic needle visualization with echocardiographic confirmation. Intravascular pressure monitoring is not essential but is important in some cases to confirm tamponade.

The only instrument absolutely necessary for this procedure is a needle of adequate size for fluid aspiration and a syringe. A long 16- or 18-gauge needle is appropriate, as it allows for the aspiration of even relatively viscous fluid and permits the introduction of a guidewire. The bevel on the

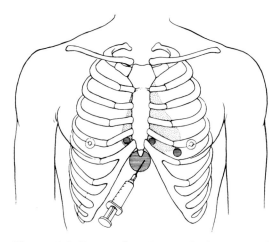

Figure 9.8. Proper location and direction of needle entry for pericardiocentesis from the subxiphoid area (*large stippled circle*). The needle is placed immediately under the xiphoid process and directed toward the left shoulder. Alternative sites are noted in the apical and left and right parasternal regions (*smaller stippled circles*).

needle should be relatively blunt. If catheters are to be placed for prolonged drainage or infusion, a large, soft multiple side-hole catheter, such as a pigtail catheter, should be inserted over a guidewire.

We prefer the subxiphoid route, but many other sites can be used, depending on the location and volume of the effusion (Fig. 9.8). The advantage of the subxiphoid approach is that it is extrapleural and avoids coronary and mammary arteries. The patient should be recumbent at an angle of approximately 30 to 45° to allow inferior pooling of fluid. Under local anesthesia the needle is inserted perpendicular to the skin in the subxiphoid region and advanced to just below the lower border of the ribs. This is usually approximately 5 to 8 mm, depending on the size of the patient. The hub of the needle is then angled inferiorly and the tip anteriorly by moving the barrel of the syringe toward the abdominal wall. If the patient is obese, considerable force may be necessary to force the syringe against the abdominal wall to direct the tip of the needle sufficiently anteriorly. Although the tip may be pointed in almost any cephalad direction depending on the size of the effusion, directing it toward the left shoulder has been most successful in our experience.

The needle is advanced while aspirating until fluid is withdrawn. Usually there is a distinct sensation of the needle popping through the parietal pericardium as the pericardial space is entered. Unless the fluid is under high pressure, it usually only drips out unless negative pressure is applied. As more fluid is withdrawn, the needle eventually comes into contact with the heart, and the operator feels the beating motion of the heart on the end of the needle. As a result, extensive cardiac trauma or perforation may occur, and it is prudent to replace the needle with a catheter before withdrawing large amounts of pericardial fluid.

If it is uncertain whether the fluid is from an intracardiac site, the quickest method of determining this is to inject a small amount of contrast material. This may be either a radiographic agent if the procedure is being performed with fluoroscopic guidance or saline to detect microbubbles by two-dimensional echocardiography. Contrast material either pools in the dependent part of the pericardial space or rapidly washes out into the vascular space if a cardiac chamber has been entered. In addition, performing a hematocrit on the fluid may be helpful but takes longer. Bloody pericardial fluid generally has a lower hematocrit than peripheral blood and does not clot because defibrination occurs when fluid has been in the pericardial space for a prolonged period.

Analysis of pericardial fluid generally does not yield much diagnostic information. While certain diseases, such as cholesterol pericarditis, rheumatoid arthritis, and hypothyroidism, may yield characteristic pericardial fluid profiles, most do not. Cytology and cultures may be useful, depending on the clinical circumstances.

Retrieval of Intravascular Foreign Bodies

Cardiologists and radiologists who perform invasive procedures are occasionally called on to remove intravascular foreign bodies. As catheter and guidewire systems change, the types of foreign bodies that get marooned in the vascular system also change, but usually it is a catheter or guidewire or some portion of them that necessitates retrieval. Most are in the venous system. Because of the type of catheter fragment concerned, most lie with their proximal end in the inflow area of the right atrium or completely in the pulmonary artery (20). Migratory patterns vary, but the distal ends of these right-sided catheters may be distributed in the right atrium, right ventricle, or pulmonary artery with a similar frequency, depending on length. A discussion of the different retrieval methods is beyond the scope of this chapter except for a brief description of some of the more commonly used techniques.

There are at least three basic methods for retrieval of intravascular foreign bodies: entangling, snaring, and grabbing. Often the foreign body must be shifted before any of these techniques is possible. Moving the foreign body may be necessary to dislodge the end to snare it or to get it into a position that is more easily approached. This can frequently be done with a soft standard catheter, such as a preformed coronary or pigtail catheter. Simply hooking the end of one of these catheters around some portion of the foreign body frequently dislodges or reorients it. The entangling technique is performed by carrying this one step further. A pigtail catheter can be turned in such a way as to tangle the foreign body around it. Once the catheter to be removed is securely around the pigtail catheter, the entire system is gently pulled back and removed. The difficulty with this technique is that the foreign body may be dislodged and embolize during removal, as there is no way to secure it.

The snare technique is the most commonly used. It entails passing a loop of exchange length guidewire into a catheter, which must have a large enough bore to accommodate the two wires without kinking. We usually use a 240-cm 0.025-inch guidewire in an 8-F, open-ended catheter. Removal of the movable core of standard guidewires softens the wire and limits kinking, but this is not essential. Commercial systems are variably elaborate but basically perform the same function. A catheter snare system similar to a urologic stone basket re-

trieval system provides several loops for snaring purposes. Basically, the snare is advanced with an open loop adjacent to the tip of the catheter to be removed. When the piece to be removed is in the loop, the snare is closed by retracting the guidewire ends. Tension is maintained on these ends, and the catheter snare is slowly removed with the foreign body.

Another technique is to grasp the foreign body directly with a biopsy instrument like that used for endomyocardial biopsy. This allows retrieval of a foreign body that does not have a readily free end by grasping it at any point. Once the foreign body is grasped, the biopsy forceps should be removed with any sheath used for its introduction while the grasp is maintained. Occasionally it is possible to use the biopsy forceps to free a catheter, particularly one that has been in place for a long period, such as a permanent pacemaker lead. Forceps can be used to remove small pieces of tissue near the lead to free it, allowing removal. Obviously, this should be done with great care, preferably in the ventricle only after more conventional methods have failed. These biopsy instruments are relatively rigid and difficult to maneuver, and perforation of a vascular structure is possible. Removal of a permanent pacemaker lead may require specialized equipment or surgery.

Several general rules should be kept in mind when planning removal of an intravascular foreign body. It is best to move the piece to be removed to a large chamber or vessel. The pulmonary artery and small peripheral vessels are the most difficult sites from which to retrieve a foreign body. A large venous sheath allows removal of the foreign body and retrieval device, occasionally without removing the sheath, thus maintaining venous access. If the body to be removed is in the arterial system, a cutdown and use of a large vessel such as the femoral artery lessens the chance of peripheral arterial injury on exit.

In our experience retrieval of intravascular foreign bodies has been fairly safe, and this has been confirmed by others (30). Each situation is different, however, and few general rules can be established as to the proper approach. This type of manipulation should be performed only by very experienced operators with a full array of catheters at their disposal and the ability to view the heart from a variety of vantage points fluoroscopically and echocardiographically, as serious adverse effects are possible.

SUMMARY

The various techniques of cardiac catheterization offer the physician a large number of options in terms of approach, site, procedures, and methods to aid in the diagnosis and treatment of a variety of conditions. The procedures are very safe when appropriately performed by trained individuals. Further improvements can be expected in both the techniques and the hardware available. However, as catheterization techniques and their indications expand, it is important to apply them with the knowledge that they are not without some degree of risk.

References

1. Jonsson G. Visualization of the coronary arteries. Acta Radiol 1948;29:536–540.
2. Kiemeneij F, Hofland J, Laarman G, et al. Cost comparison between two modes of Palmaz Schatz coronary stent implantation: trans radial bare stent technique vs. trans-femoral sheath-protected stent technique. Cathet Cardiovasc Diagn 1995;35: 301–308.
3. Keimeneij F, Laarman G. Percutaneous trans radial artery approach for coronary Palmaz-Schatz stent implantation. Am Heart J 1994;129:167–174.
4. Allen EV. Thromboangiitis obliterans: methods of diagnosis of chronic occlusive arterial lesions distal to the wrist with illustrative cases. Am J Med Sci 1929;178:237–244.
5. Hall JJ, Arnold AM, Valentine RP, et al. Ultrasound imaging of the radial artery following its use for cardiac catheterization. Am J Cardiol 1996;77: 108–109.
6. Mansfield P, Hohn D, Fornage B, et al. Complications and failures of subclavian-vein catheterization. N Engl J Med 1994;331:1735–1738.
7. Belani KG, Buckley JJ, Gordon JR, Castaneda W. Percutaneous cervical central venous line placement: a comparison of the internal and external jugular vein routes. Anesthesiology 1980;59:40–44.
8. English ICW, Frew RM, Pigott JF, Zaki M. Percutaneous catheterization of the internal jugular vein. Anaesthesia 1969;24:521–531.
9. Defalque RJ. Percutaneous catheterization of the internal jugular vein. Anesth Analg 1974;53: 116–121.
10. Seneff MG. Central venous catheterization: a comprehensive review. Part 1. J Intens Care Med 1987; 2:163–175.
11. Seneff MG. Central venous catheterization: a comprehensive review. Part 2. J Intens Care Med 1987; 2:218–231.
12. Rao TLK, Wong AY, Salem MR. A new approach to percutaneous catheterization of the internal jugular vein. Anesthesiology 1977;46:362–364.
13. Bjork VO, Cullhed I, Hallen A, et al. Sequelae of left ventricular puncture with angiocardiography. Circulation 1961;24:204–212.
14. Brock R, Milstein BB, Ross DN. Percutaneous left ventricular puncture in the assessment of aortic stenosis. Thorax 1956;2:163–171.
15. Greene DG, Sharp JT, Griffith GT, et al. Surgical application of anterior percutaneous left heart puncture. Surgery 1958;43:1–5.
16. Yu PN, Lovejoy FW, Schreiner BF, et al. Direct left ventricular puncture in the evaluation of aortic and mitral stenosis. Am Heart J 1958;55:926–941.
17. Baxley SW, Soto B. Hemodynamic evaluation of patients with combined mitral and aortic prostheses. Am J Cardiol 1980;45:42–47.
18. Cata C, Grassman E, Johnson S. Technique of apical left ventricular puncture revisited: a case report of double-valve prosthesis evaluation. J Invas Cardiol 1994;6:251–255.
19. Bidoggia H, Maciel, Maciel J, Alvarez J. Transseptal left heart catheterization: usefulness of the intracavitary electrocardiogram in the localization of the fossa ovalis. Cathet Cardiovasc Diagn 1991;24: 221–225.
20. Doorey A, Goldenberg E. Transseptal catheterization in adults: enhanced efficacy and safety by low-volume operators using a ''non-standard'' technique. Cathet Cardiovasc Diagn 1991;22:239–243.
21. Shaw TRD. Anterior staircase manoeuvre for atrial transseptal puncture. Br Heart J 1994;71:297–301.
22. Clugston R, Lau FYK, Ruiz C. Transseptal catheterization update 1992. Cathet Cardiovasc Diagn 1992;26:266–274.
23. Jung JS. Atrial septal puncture technique in percutaneous transvenous mitral commissurotomy: mitral valvuloplasty using the Inoue balloon catheter technique. Cathet Cardiovasc Diagn 1992;26: 275–284.
24. Marcus R, Grollman JH Jr. Translumbar coronary and brachiocephalic arteriography using a modified Desilets-Hoffman sheath. Diagnosis 1987;13: 288–290.
25. Valeix B, Labrunie P, Jahjah F, et al. Selective coronary arteriography by percutaneous transaxillary approach. Cathet Cardiovasc Diagn 1987;10: 403–409.
26. Fowles RE, Mason JW. Role of cardiac biopsy in the diagnosis and management of cardiac disease. Prog Cardiovasc Dis 1984;27:153–172.
27. Brooksby IAB, Jenkins S, Davies MJ, et al. Left ventricular endomyocardial biopsy: 1. Description and evaluation of the technique. Cathet Cardiovasc Diagn 1977;3:115–121.
28. Davies MJ, Brooksby IAB, Jenkins S, et al. Left ventricular endomyocardial biopsy: 2. The value of

light microscopy. Cathet Cardiovasc Diagn 1977;
3:123–130.

29. Davies MJ, Kennedy S, Brooksby IAB, et al. Left ventricular endomyocardial biopsy: 3. Ultrastructural characteristic of cardiomyopathy and cardiac hypertrophy with good or poor ventricular function. Cathet Cardiovasc Diagn 1977;3:131–137.

30. Bloomfield DA. The nonsurgical retrieval of intracardiac foreign bodies: an international survey. Cathet Cardiovasc Diagn 1978;4:1–14.

10
Catheters, Sheaths, Guidewires, Needles, and Related Equipment

Robert G. MacDonald, MD

INTRODUCTION

Invasive cardiology is a rapidly expanding and evolving subspecialty. Modern catheterization laboratories are equipped with an extensive inventory of catheters, wires, and other equipment for use in a wide variety of procedures. Technological advances produce increasing numbers of devices for monitoring the patient and the procedure itself. Development and marketing of equipment for cardiac catheterization is a major industry that is constantly providing new products for the catheterization laboratory. It is important that catheterizing physicians and technical personnel keep abreast of these developments. Since publication of the first edition of this textbook there have been many changes in catheter and sheath design and specialty products for catheterization. Regular interaction with manufacturers' representatives and attendance at product exhibitions at national scientific meetings provide familiarity with current equipment.

This chapter reviews some of the devices used for monitoring patients during cardiac catheterization and equipment used for the procedure, with brief commentary on technical considerations concerning different types of equipment and devices. This review is limited to items necessary for diagnostic catheterization and in general focuses on items common to most types of catheterization procedures (see Chapter 9). Highly specialized catheters and guidewires used for percutaneous transluminal coronary interventions and valvuloplasty are discussed in Chapters 27 to 31 and 35. An understanding of basic construction and design of these tools of the trade is important to selection of equipment for specific purposes, optimal manipulation of equipment, and avoidance of complications. This is further emphasized in selection of equipment in challenging cases when the first choice fails during a procedure.

Discussion of equipment and techniques for catheterization includes needles for percutaneous vascular access; guidewires, sheaths, and dilators for establishment and maintenance of a route for catheter insertion; timing and techniques for sheath or catheter removal and hemostasis; catheters for hemodynamic assessment and ventricular and selective coronary angiography; and new devices for periprocedural monitoring of the patient.

NEEDLES FOR PERCUTANEOUS VASCULAR ACCESS

Basic Design and Features

Choice of a specific needle for vascular access may seem to require little considera-

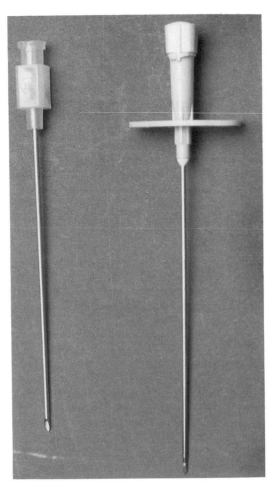

signed to prevent the lumen from being blocked with skin, subcutaneous tissue, and blood as the needle is inserted into the artery. Most contemporary designs have a single stylet or no stylet at all. The latter type is usually employed with the direct or modified Seldinger technique.

The hub of the needle must have several features. It must fit firmly onto the body of the needle and internally have a smooth funnel into the body to facilitate wire insertion. Some hubs have a short length of needle protruding back into the hub, necessitating use of a plastic wire tip–straightening device. Most hubs have a female Luer-Lok connector, allowing attachment to the male Luer connector on a syringe with an airtight seal. This is important for maintenance of negative pressure when withdrawing a needle into the lumen of a low-pressure vessel and observing blood return, as in the Seldinger technique. The hub section may have a winged baseplate or flange to allow gripping between the first two fingers and thumb, as used in the Seldinger technique, so that the needle can be controlled with one hand. During insertion the needle should always be controlled by the hand-held wing or hub rather than an attached

Figure 10.1. Two most commonly used needle types for vascular access. **Left,** A single-piece, thin-walled front wall needle. **Right,** A two-component thin-walled Seldinger needle.

tion. There are, however, two major differences in needle design suitable for different insertion techniques (Seldinger versus direct) and considerable variations in needle size and shape. A description of the components of a needle is necessary for further discussion. Figure 10.1 shows standard disposable Seldinger and direct front wall types of needles. Figure 10.2 shows a Seldinger needle with labeled components. Needles of this type, which are modifications of the older Riley and Cournand needles, have a blunted needle bevel and one or two stylets.

The innermost stylet is solid and de-

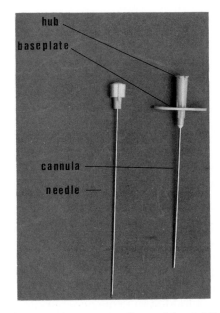

Figure 10.2. Two-piece disposable Seldinger needle with labeled components.

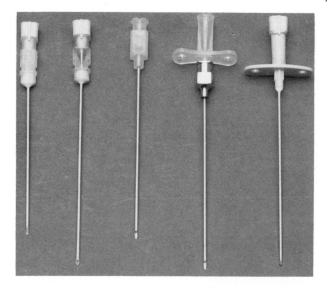

Figure 10.3. A selection of disposable arterial needles.

syringe to permit optimal ability to feel arterial pulsations transmitted from the needle tip. Numerous arterial needles are available, and some examples are shown in Figure 10.3.

Needles are sized according to their external diameter and an arbitrary gauging system (Table 10.1). The higher the gauge, the smaller the diameter.

Needles may be standard or thin-walled, for higher ratios of internal to external diameter. Most 18-gauge needles allow passage of a 0.035- or 0.038-inch standard guidewire, and these sizes are stocked in most laboratories. A needle must be long enough to pass through a considerable depth of subcutaneous tissue in obese patients and short enough to be manipulated

skillfully in puncturing the artery or vein. A standard length of 2.75 to 3 inches is acceptable for arterial needles in all but rare cases. The tip of the needle has a bevel that forms an angle less acute than that of standard injection needles. The needle must, of course, be sharp enough to avoid tearing the arterial wall on vessel entry and strong enough to pass through calcified arterial walls or subcutaneous fibrous tissue resulting from previous catheterizations or operations.

The technique of front wall puncture has become almost universal in percutaneous arterial access. It eliminates the risk of subcutaneous bleeding and hematoma formation via a puncture of the posterior wall of the artery, as occurs with the traditional Seldinger technique. This technical consideration is very important when catheterization is done under aggressive anticoagulation, immediately following or in conjunction with thrombolysis, or during infusion of glycoprotein IIB/IIIA inhibitors or other potent antiplatelet agents.

Needles for other uses, such as pericardiocentesis and direct percutaneous left ventricular puncture, are available in various designs and lengths up to 22 cm (Fig. 10.4). The bevels on these needles should be about 45°, and the point must be kept sharp,

Table 10.1.
Conventional Needle Sizing System

Stubs Needle Gauge	Outer Diameter (inches)
13	0.095
14	0.083
15	0.072
16	0.065
17	0.058
18	0.049
19	0.042
20	0.035

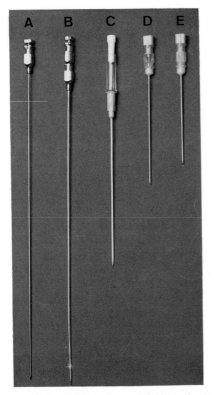

Figure 10.4. Variations in needle length. **A** and **B,** Reusable needles for pericardiocentesis or percutaneous left ventricular puncture. **C,** Intermediate length needle. **D** and **E,** Two shorter arterial needles.

as many special types are sterilized and reused.

The cost of standard arterial needles can vary as much as fivefold, depending on design and manufacturer. Since this amount is very small relative to the total cost of equipment used during a procedure, the quality and design of the needle, rather than cost, should dictate its selection. Needles for venous or arterial access that are designed for resterilization and reuse are no longer desirable from either a technical or financial point of view.

Needles for Bloodless Arterial Access

With increasing prevalence of patients carrying the human immunodeficiency virus

(HIV) and concern about contacting type B or C hepatitis or Jacob-Creutzfeldt disease, more rigid precautions are recommended for procedures involving direct contact with blood or blood products. Cardiac catheterization involves considerable contact with a patient's blood, so in most laboratories it is routine to wear masks, protective glasses, hats, and sterile gloves for the procedure. Gore-Tex sterile gowns have recently become popular in reducing blood contact with the operator's skin. In addition to exercising caution during every procedure, there are now devices—the bloodless needle and syringe—designed to reduce contact with blood during arterial puncture and guidewire insertion. Several manufacturers offer products to eliminate free exit of blood during arterial or venous puncture and wire insertion. AngioDynamics has introduced the SOS Bloodless Entry Needle, which is equipped with a hemostasis valve at the hub and a sidearm tubing to a collection bag via a three-way stopcock (Fig. 10.5). This allows for either blood withdrawal or contrast injection through the needle and guidewire insertion without permitting blood to leave the closed system. Arrow Inc. markets the Raulerson Syringe (Fig. 10.6), which has a hollow plunger and barrel with a hemostasis valve. When blood is aspirated, the needle is fixed and the guidewire is inserted through the syringe barrel without the syringe ever being disconnected from the needle. This system is claimed to

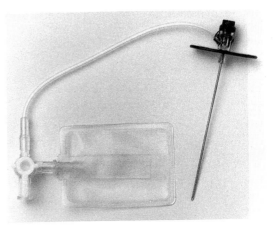

Figure 10.5. Angiodynamics SOS Bloodless Entry Needle.

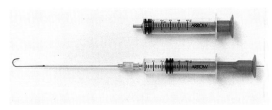

Figure 10.6. Raulerson Syringe marketed by Arrow. This system allows guidewire insertion directly through the barrel and plunger.

reduce blood exposure and risk of air embolism during venous access, and it may decrease the chance of needle displacement from the vessel during guidewire insertion.

Arrow has also developed a bloodless needle for arterial access. The Arrow-Fischell Evan vascular access needle has a capillary chamber with a hemostasis valve on the hub (Fig. 10.7). As the tip of the needle enters the artery, blood is seen to pulsate in the capillary chamber. The needle is then fixed and the guidewire inserted through the hemostasis valve.

These designs are claimed to reduce the surgical team's exposure to blood and may decrease the chance of needle displacement from the vessel during guidewire insertion. As with any arterial puncture, entry into the artery, even with an open-needle front wall approach, is not uniformly associated with visualization of blood pulsation. Thus, despite optimal equipment and technique, multiple arterial punctures are occasionally necessary for arterial access.

These needle systems for vascular access are new developments that may find regular use in some laboratories. Their use in patients known to have HIV or hepatitis appears prudent. Use of these more complicated needle systems, however, adds to the cost of the procedure.

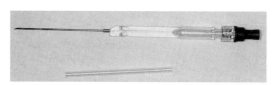

Figure 10.7. Arrow-Fischell Evan vascular access needle.

Ultrasound-guided Needles

A unique development by Peripheral Systems Group is a needle for vascular access that is guided by ultrasound (Fig. 10.8). The Smart Needle is designed to permit accurate location of the midpoint of the vessel and proper alignment of the needle. This requires connection to an ultrasonic amplifier and monitor via a small electrical cable. The ultrasonic stylet is easily removed from the needle to permit guidewire insertion. The monitor is relatively small and can be positioned on the catheterization laboratory table in a sterile clear plastic bag. This device may be useful in the occasional case of difficult arterial or venous access. The expense will likely limit regular use. It may be particularly useful if jugular vein or femoral artery puncture is required in the presence of thrombolytic therapy, to minimize the risk of bleeding related to suboptimal puncture of the vessel. Also, it should help to reduce inadvertent carotid artery puncture when the jugular vein is difficult to find with standard approaches.

GUIDEWIRES

Discussion of guidewires may be divided into a description of basic components and differences in length, size, and shape that are suited to specific uses.

Construction

Basic wire construction is illustrated in Figure 10.9. The coil is usually made by spinning a thin strand of round wire around a metal tube or rod. The coil is advanced over a core or mandrel and fixed at the ends by a soldered bond. A safety ribbon is soldered at the flexible end or tip and runs the length of the guidewire adjacent to the core. Another wire, designed by Schneider, has a flat strand of wire wrapped around a mandrel. This is claimed to reduce the surface area of the wire by 20%, hence reduce the irregular surface that predisposes to thrombus for-

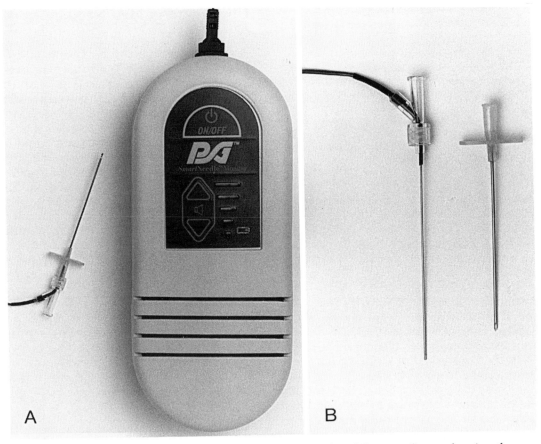

Figure 10.8. A and **B.** Smart Needle marketed by Peripheral Systems Group showing the ultrasonic stylet, needle, connecting cable and monitor.

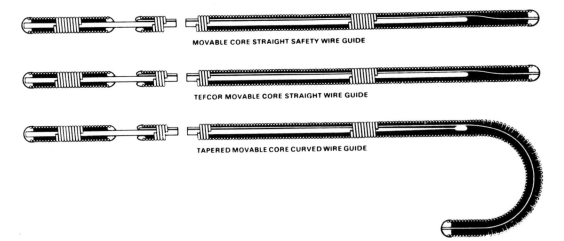

Figure 10.9. Movable-core wire guide construction. Diagram of basic construction of guidewires. (Reprinted with permission from Cook Products. Diagnostic and interventional products for radiology, cardiology and surgery. 1986;4.)

mation. Figure 10.9 shows that the length of the tip segment without a core determines how much wire can be advanced through a tortuous segment before the core meets a sudden bend. A gradually tapered core allows for a smoother transition from the very flexible end or tip to the stiffer body of the wire. One of the disadvantages of some movable-core wire designs is that with the core retracted, a very flimsy wire tip may be advanced around a sharp bend or complex atherosclerotic plaque, but the stiff core cannot follow. Gradual tapering of the core wire in both fixed and movable designs can overcome this problem.

Coatings

Another feature of certain wire designs is an external coating, most often Teflon. This is applied to the assembled wire as a bath or spray and bake-dried in an oven to ensure adequate bonding. In some designs the Teflon coating is applied to the wire strand before it is wound onto the mandrel rather than to the assembled guidewire. It is argued that this reduces flaking and cracking of the Teflon material during flexing of the wire. Wire coatings provide for lubricity (little friction between wire and catheter lumen) and reduced thrombogenicity. Despite Teflon coating the irregular surface of coiled guidewires continues to predispose to thrombus formation. All wires must therefore be left in the vessel for only the minimum time necessary for catheter positioning. Uncoated stainless steel wires are used mainly for venous access, not for catheter guidance or manipulation in the arterial system. The Radifocus Guidewire M, made by Terumo Corporation, is a more recent design consisting of an elastic alloy core coated with a polyurethane jacket and a hydrophilic coating (1). This provides for a pliable tip, a smooth outer coating, and excellent torque control. This design theoretically reduces thrombogenicity and resistance to wire advancement. This wire is very popular in many laboratories. The Terumo Glide Wire is now marketed in numerous diameters and tip configurations by Medi-Tech Inc. Other companies, such as

Arrow, market a wire of very similar design. This type of wire is very steerable and has good torque response. It can be supplied with a detachable multitorque vise or steering tool to enhance ability to steer the wire tip through tortuous and irregular vessels. The tip of the Arrow Truetorque guidewire is shapable, allowing modification for different types of vascular obstruction or anatomic variation. A major disadvantage of this type of wire is that it should not be pulled back through a needle because the polyurethane jacket can be sheared off (2).

New materials, such as polytetrafluoroethylene, may provide lubricity on both diagnostic and percutaneous transluminal coronary angioplasty (PTCA) wires. Recently Biocompatibles International Inc. has introduced a new hydrophilic coating, phosphorylcholine, that promises to be useful in coating many items to reduce adhesion of blood products and enhance lubricity.

Length

Guidewires are available in lengths from 35 to 260 cm and may be cut to any length. In general a guidewire should be at least 20 cm longer than the catheter for which it is to be used. The shorter length is used for the introduction of vascular sheaths, mainly into the venous system. A 145-cm wire is usually adequate for insertion or removal of catheters when only a short length of wire must remain in the artery. When difficulty is encountered crossing a tortuous arterial segment from either the leg or arm approach, an exchange wire approximately 240 to 260 cm long may be used. During change of catheters this avoids withdrawing the tip of the wire back through the tortuous segment already negotiated and thus minimizes trauma to the vessel at this region. An example of stainless steel wire for venous access and coiled Teflon-coated wire is shown in Figure 10.10.

Diameter

Guidewires most frequently used during diagnostic angiography have 0.035-inch or

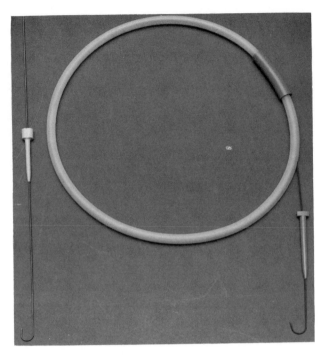

Figure 10.10. Safety guidewires. On the left is a 35-cm stainless steel J-tipped wire for venous sheath insertion. On the right is a 135-cm Teflon-coated J-tipped wire in its packaging ring.

0.038-inch external diameter. Both pass through an 18-gauge or larger needle and accommodate many angiographic catheters used in adults. The smaller 0.035-inch wire allows advancement of a catheter over it with less internal friction, hence greater ability to feel resistance when vascular obstruction or tortuosity is encountered. The wire itself is somewhat more flexible, softer, potentially less traumatic, and more easily manipulated through tortuous arterial segments. The stiffer 0.038-inch wire is less likely to bend when one is trying to advance a dilator through fibrotic subcutaneous tissue or a calcified arterial wall and when one is inserting a pigtail catheter over the wire through a distorted stenotic aortic valve via the retrograde approach. The 0.035-inch wire is perhaps better for routine use, and the 0.038-inch wire is best reserved for specific indications, such as those described here. The 0.025-inch wire is usually reserved for smaller-diameter catheters (4 F or less) or used when there is difficulty advancing a 0.035-inch wire. In the latter case the smaller wire is less traumatic to the vessel wall. Many manufacturers offer a selection of diameters, such as 0.016, 0.018, 0.025, 0.035, and 0.038 inch, allowing for virtually any purpose or challenge.

Configuration

Wires come with not only straight tips with a flexible or movable core but also curved tips or J-tips of several sizes (Fig. 10.11). J wires are described by the radius of curvature in the tip (e.g., 3-mm J). Sizes 1.5, 3, 6, and 15 mm are readily available.

The 3-mm J, indicated for routine use, has advantages over straight wires in its tendency to avoid entering side branches and to curve or glance off atherosclerotic plaques rather than dissect beneath them. With obstructive plaques in highly tortuous vessels, a larger J is sometimes helpful to avoid traumatic guidewire advancement. The only significant disadvantage of the J wire is that some physicians have difficulty introducing the tip through a needle or catheter hub. This is facilitated by a plastic tip introducer that is packaged with all J-tipped guidewires. Also, the operator can pinch the wire between the thumb and

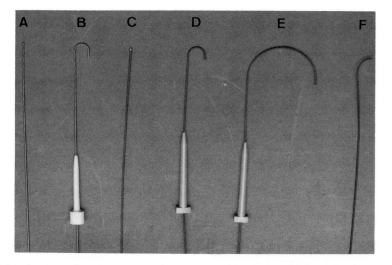

Figure 10.11. A selection of spring tip guidewires. **A.** Stainless steel straight tip. **B.** Stainless steel 3-mm J-tipped wire. **C** and **D.** Teflon-coated straight and 3-mm J-tipped wires. **E.** Teflon-coated 16 mm J-tipped wire. **F.** Terumo M wire.

index finger and retract a more proximal segment of wire between the palm and remaining fingers to straighten the spring tip. In rare cases a J-tipped wire with a movable core may be advanced through an arterial segment where a standard J-tip has been unsuccessful. Larger Js and other configurations are sometimes helpful for exchange purposes, particularly within the left ventricular cavity. Tip configurations can be changed by pulling the region to be curved between the thumb and the rounded edge of a hemostat.

Use of a straight-tipped wire is indicated when attempting to cross a stenotic aortic valve retrograde or when transversing a tight stenosis in the peripheral vascular system. In cases of aortic stenosis the J tip has too large a diameter to negotiate the narrow valve orifice, and the straight tip more readily penetrates the jet of blood exiting the valve and can better probe the valve orifice. Wires with a flexible J tip on one end and a flexible straight tip on the other are available from most manufacturers at slightly higher cost. A straight-tipped wire can also be shaped with the thumb and hemostat. Finally, a special movable-tip wire mated to a tip deflector may be used.

In summary, catheter guidewires are available in various designs, lengths, diam-

eters, and tip configurations. Knowledge of different wires allows a selection matched to particular needs, enhancing the success and safety of a procedure.

VASCULAR SHEATHS AND DILATORS

Techniques used to achieve and maintain vascular access have seen considerable refinement with advances in angiographic equipment. Previously, most arterial catheterization was done via the Seldinger technique with catheter insertion directly over a guidewire or by cutdown technique. With the Seldinger technique an arterial dilator was advanced over the wire to provide a tract through the subcutaneous tissue and vessel wall for catheter insertion. The dilator was generally at least 1 F smaller than the body of the catheter to be inserted, to reduce the possibility of leakage of blood around the catheter once in place. Thin-walled vascular sheaths offer a different approach, and in most laboratories their use has become common practice.

Current sheaths have a side port to allow for flushing of sheaths and pressure moni-

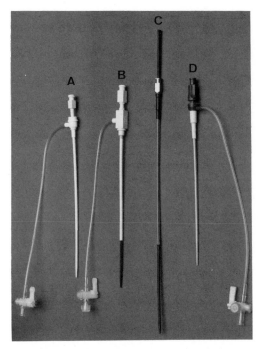

Figure 10.12. Various introducer sheath designs. **A.** Cordis 8 F. **B.** USCI 8 F. **C.** USCI Desilets-Hoffman sheath for venous access. **D.** Terumo Radifocus 8 F.

Dilators

Vascular dilators, which come in various lengths and French sizes, must meet certain requirements. The dilator must be of hard plastic, usually Teflon or polyethylene, to allow passage through fibrous tissue or atherosclerotic or calcified arterial walls. The tip must be tapered smoothly to minimize the possibility of tearing the arterial wall. The final tip taper and internal diameter of the dilator should closely fit the guidewire diameter to allow smooth advancement of the dilator over the wire, with little blood between the wire and dilator lumen and minimal trauma to the vascular wall. In cases of considerable resistance to dilator insertion, serial dilation with progressively larger dilators may be beneficial. Most dilators have a female Luer-Lok hub to allow secure attachment with the male Luer connector of a syringe. Ideally, the French size of the dilator should be imprinted on the hub, or different dilators may be color coded according to size to permit rapid identification.

toring from the sheath itself. Increasingly efficient backbleed valves provide a tight seal around the catheter, and even with the catheter removed or with only a guidewire inserted, there is little or no backbleeding. Yet they cause little resistance to catheter insertion and manipulation.

These features make catheterization easier for both the physician and patient. Catheter changes are rapid, and both arterial trauma and the possibility of bleeding into the subcutaneous tissues during the procedure are reduced. Following use of thrombolytic and anticoagulant agents, the sheath may be left in place until coagulation status has returned to baseline or has been actively reversed. A sheath may be left in place to allow for rapid repeat vascular access, as in unstable patients, or following PTCA, when reocclusion is a possibility and an emergency repeat dilation may be necessary. Detailed next are some of the features of different sheath and dilator designs. Figure 10.12 shows several vascular sheaths and introducers.

Sheaths

Vascular sheaths come in a variety of lengths and sizes (Fig. 10.13). Sizes 4 through 14 F are available, with the larger sizes used for insertion of intra-aortic balloons and valvuloplasty balloon catheters. Lengths as short as 6 cm may be used for percutaneous brachial entry, and longer sheaths (25 cm) for diagnostic catheterization or PTCA via tortuous iliac arteries with the femoral approach. For the percutaneous radial artery approach, sheaths of 4- to 6-F diameter may be used. There are differing individual preferences for short versus long sheaths, as some physicians prefer to avoid arterial spasm and kinking at the elbow by using a sheath up to 24 cm long. Arrow has packaged a kit that provides a unique needle and wire system for access through the radial artery. In these kits the sheaths are 11 cm long in 5 or 6 F and 24 cm in 6 F.

In sheaths with side extensions the tubing, which is polyethylene, extends to a

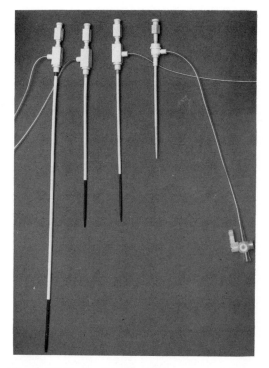

Figure 10.13. Various sheath lengths and diameters, ranging from a USCI 9-F PTCA sheath on the left to a Cordis 7-F short percutaneous brachial sheath on the far right.

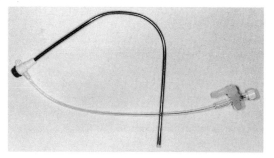

Figure 10.14. The Super Arrowflex sheath. The body of the long version is bent to illustrate resistance to kinking.

three-way stopcock, providing separate ports for pressure monitoring and flushing or administering medications. The sheath itself is made of a nonthrombogenic material, usually Teflon or polyethylene, which is extremely strong, thin, pliable, and radiolucent. The tip of the sheath is tapered by drawing (pulling) while it is hot during manufacture. This provides a taper that minimizes trauma as the sheath is advanced with the dilator into the vessel. The Cook Check-Flow Performer sheath has a radiopaque marker band at the tip to permit visualization and facilitate positioning of interventional devices in procedures in the periphery. This is also useful for retrieving stents and other material with snare devices on pulling the snare back into the sheath. Arrow has developed the Super ArrowFlex sheath (Fig. 10.14) to minimize the risk of sheath kinking. This design has coil wire construction to flex without kinking or collapsing. The coil wire is sandwiched between two layers of polyurethane with a

total wall thickness comparable to that of other sheath designs. In addition, an antibacterial coating is applied to the sheath surface, which theoretically reduces bacterial colonization when the sheath is left in place for long periods. This is particularly relevant for venous sheaths. This design is claimed to permit patients to sit upright in bed with a sheath in the femoral artery without risk of vessel trauma or bleeding (3). It should also be useful for avoiding sheath kinking in highly tortuous arterial anatomy.

Various hub designs are shown in Figure 10.15. One design, made by Arrow, has an accordionlike neck on the proximal end of the sheath to allow angulation of the hub

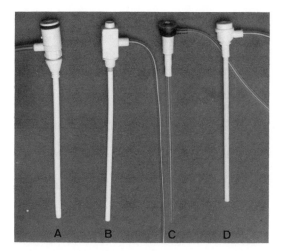

Figure 10.15. Various hub designs. **A.** Arrow 8.5 F. **B.** USCI 8 F. **C.** Terumo 8 F. **D.** Cordis 8 F.

without kinking the sheath itself. Others have a sleevelike support at the neck region. Some sheaths have a rotating suture collar in the hub region to permit easy suturing when sheaths are to be left in place for long periods.

If the sheath has no backbleed valve, it should have a Luer-Lok hub to allow attachment of a syringe or stopcock for aspiration or flushing. Separate backbleed valves are available for attachment to valveless sheaths when control of bleeding is necessary.

The hemostasis valve may have any of several designs. The Cordis Avanti sheath has a one-piece valve incorporating a biconcave spiral tricuspid (hexacuspid) design that will not backbleed even with a thin wire through it. The USCI input sheath has a Hemaquet valve that consists of a tricuspid valve, and other companies have valves with a diaphragm consisting of multilayered overlapping sheets of rubber. The Terumo Radifocus sheath has a valve consisting of a silicone plug with a crosscut for a tight seal with excellent lubricity. Longitudinal sections of a few sheaths are shown in Figure 10.16 to illustrate the complexity of different hub designs.

Selection of a particular sheath is most often based on the quality of the hemostasis valve. Valves that are too tight or do not maintain lubricity tend to grab the catheter, interfering with insertion, withdrawal, and rotation. This may significantly impair the operator's ability to safely position or manipulate a catheter. It is also important that the valve not be too loose, allowing bleeding through the insertion port after catheter removal or when only an exchange wire remains in the sheath. In addition, the depth of the recess of the hemostatic diaphragm can make catheter insertion difficult, such as with a pigtail catheter when straightening the tip is difficult. The less recessed the diaphragm, the better. Regardless of design, it is important to moisten the catheter frequently to keep the hemostasis valve lubricated during catheter insertion and manipulation.

Another weakness in some sheath designs is too great a step up in diameter at the junction of dilator and sheath tip, so that the sheath will not follow the dilator

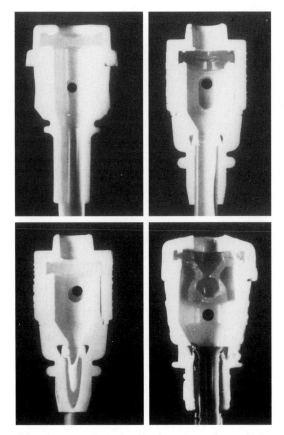

Figure 10.16. Longitudinal sections through the hubs of four sheaths showing the complexity of hub design.

through the arterial wall. This can result in failure to insert the sheath or burring of the edge of the sheath, causing arterial trauma. Several companies are pursuing design modifications to overcome this problem. More recent designs include sheath tips that are weakly bonded to the dilator, producing a very gradual transition from dilator to sheath, as in that by Daig Inc. The bond can be broken by rotating and withdrawing the dilator once the sheath is in the artery. Other designs have a depression in the dilator itself to allow the sheath tip to be flush with the dilator segment just distal to the sheath tip. Finally, some systems are coated with lubricant to permit easier passage through tissue. To avoid bleeding around the sheath, some have a slightly increasing diameter from tip to hub segment, which tightens the seal as the sheath is advanced into the vessel.

Selection of a catheter at least one size smaller than the sheath (e.g., 7-F catheter with an 8-F sheath) also permits blood sampling and pressure recording from the sheath sidearm (e.g., during dye dilution studies or for simultaneous pressure recording). In summary, although a vascular sheath may at first seem to be a very simple item, certain specific features lead to selection of a product from a particular manufacturer. A well-designed sheath markedly facilitates the catheterization procedure, while a poor design may not only make the procedure more difficult but also significantly increase the duration of the procedure and risk of bleeding and other arterial complications.

DEVICES FOR HEMOSTASIS AFTER SHEATH REMOVAL

With the advent of coronary interventional procedures and the increasing use of anti-platelet, anticoagulant, and thrombolytic agents, proper timing and removal of arterial sheaths is essential. The use of antiplatelet agents predisposes to delayed or recurrent bleeding after sheath removal. Performance of PTCA requires use of heparin; hence removal of the arterial sheath must be delayed until the heparin effect has greatly diminished. In these circumstances it may take considerably more time to achieve hemostasis. As a result, numerous devices to facilitate sheath removal are available. To clarify their use, it is necessary to review manual control of the puncture site.

Coagulation Status and Timing of Sheath Removal

The half-life of systemically administered heparin is approximately 1 hour. Routine practice has been to allow 4 half-lives (4 hours) before sheath removal after PTCA and in patients anticoagulated for other rea-

sons in whom reversal with protamine is not desirable. This empiric approach is usually successful. Earlier sheath removal reduces the potential for arterial thromboembolism but predisposes to prolong the time to achieve hemostasis and increased risk of rebleeding. Use of 5- or 6-F sheaths may reduce the time to hemostatis after sheath removal and permit earlier ambulation. Timing of sheath removal may be enhanced through monitoring of the activated clotting time (ACT) or activated partial thromboplastin time (APTT). Several companies provide portable monitors of these parameters for use in the catheterization laboratory, coronary care unit, or cardiology ward. Their use is commonplace for ensuring adequate anticoagulation during PTCA, but they are less often used for evaluating the ideal time for sheath removal. This is particularly important when sheath removal and early reanticoagulation are necessary, such as after PTCA, when there is significant coronary dissection, and in some cases after insertion of a coronary artery stent. Depending on the monitoring system used, an ACT of less than 150 seconds is generally associated with uncomplicated sheath removal.

Standard Technique for Vascular Compression

The traditional technique for catheter or sheath removal from the right femoral artery includes use of the first two fingers of the left hand applied to the groin. The middle finger is applied 2 cm above the puncture site, and the index finger is applied approximately 1 cm above the skin hole directly over the point of arterial puncture (Fig. 10.17). Firm, direct pressure is applied as the sheath is removed and then intensified to occlude the pulse for about 5 minutes. Pressure from the middle finger is then gradually reduced, leaving only the index finger pressing on the arterial puncture site. Pressure is gradually decreased over the next 15 minutes according to the bleeding response. If bleeding occurs, firmer pressure is applied until hemostasis is achieved.

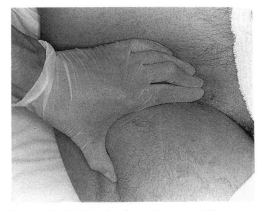

Figure 10.17. Standard positioning of fingers for manual technique for achieving hemostasis after arterial sheath or catheter removal from puncture site.

A given force from the arm can exert much more direct pressure to a small surface area; hence the advantage of only two fingers versus force applied over a much larger area (e.g., palm of hand). While the fingers of the left hand are applying pressure, the right hand can be used to examine the area around the puncture site to determine whether a hematoma is forming deep to the skin surface. This can often result from application of pressure to the skin puncture rather than to the area directly superficial to the arterial puncture site. In cases of removal of both arterial and venous sheaths from the groin, the right hand is used to apply pressure with a gauze bandage more diffusely and directly over the venous puncture site. Pressure on the groin above the hole used for venous puncture occludes the vein, increasing venous pressure distally, and can increase bleeding from the vein puncture site.

Groin Clamps

In absence of a wound closure device, direct manual pressure to an arterial puncture site continues to be the safest and most reliable way to achieve hemostasis while minimizing the patient's discomfort and the chance of hematoma. In many laboratories use of groin clamps to free up the laboratory staff

to perform other patient care has become commonplace. A standard groin clamp is shown in Figure 10.18. These are applied by putting the patient in a comfortable position close to the edge of the bed or stretcher, where the pressure applicator on the clamp arm can be properly positioned, as noted previously, for the index finger in the manual technique. The clamp is applied firmly at the outset to occlude the arterial pulse and then gradually released to permit increasing circulation to the leg without allowing bleeding from the puncture site. It is important that the patient be closely monitored during use of the clamp to avoid complications such as bleeding deep to the skin surface. Groin clamps are also very useful for nonoperative management of arterial pseudoaneurysms. Here, prolonged very firm pressure with or without ultrasonic guidance is used to obliterate the false channel and allow the sac to thrombose. This thrombus later resolves as the vessel remodels. The USCI FemoStop pneumatic compression system has also been advocated for this purpose (4, 5).

Pressure Bandages

After hemostasis at the arterial puncture site is achieved, it is desirable for patients to apply general pressure to the groin over the puncture site for approximately 20 minutes. In many laboratories pressure dressings of elastic tape and bandages or sandbags are applied and left in place for several hours. A number of commercial pressure bandages have also been used. All of these devices increase the risk of failing to observe bleeding deep to the skin surface and may give a false sense of security. They are, however, useful in selected cases when a degree of oozing after the procedure responds to light application of pressure.

Wound Closure Devices

Two factors led to the demand for devices that can seal the arterial puncture site at the end of an interventional procedure. With

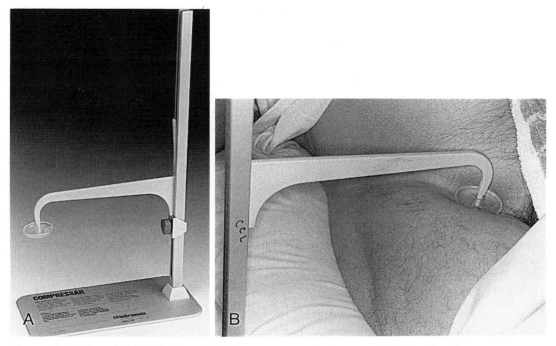

Figure 10.18. A and **B.** The Instromedix Compressar groin clamp equipped with a Compressar comfort disc showing proper application to the puncture site.

the intensive anticoagulation regimen previously associated with use of coronary stents, there was a desire to achieve hemostasis at the arterial puncture site in the face of continued anticoagulation. The use of potent platelet inhibitors such as those affecting the platelet glycoprotein IIB/IIIA receptor can increase groin complications after femoral arterial sheath removal. Also, there is increasing financial pressure to discharge patients early. With the risk of acute closure following angioplasty with high-pressure stent deployment reduced to as low as 1%, it is reasonable to discharge patients on the day of uncomplicated procedures. Wound closure devices fall into two categories: the collagen plug and the suture.

There are two collagen plug devices. The Angio-Seal Hemostatic Puncture Closure Device produced by Sherwood-Davis and Geck Inc. uses an absorbable 2 × 10 mm flat rectangular anchor plate within the arterial lumen. An attached absorbable suture is used to tie a small collagen sponge down into the subcutaneous tissue space, producing virtually immediate hemostasis without

manual pressure in most cases (6). Datascope Corporation has developed the Vaso-Seal Vascular Sealing Device. This is a purified bovine collagen plug that is injected subcutaneously down to the arterial surface via a guidewire and injector sheath system. With the plug in place, the time to achieve hemostasis by manual compression is reduced by 75% (7, 8).

The Perclose Corporation Prostar Percutaneous Vascular Surgical Device uses two polyester sutures to close the femoral arterial puncture site. This system is designed to allow immediate ambulation following an intervention in the face of full anticoagulation.

The price of these wound closure devices is an issue, and cost efficacy studies should be considered. With the use of much-simplified regimens following coronary stent deployment and virtual elimination of anticoagulation after stent procedures, the demand for these devices has diminished. There continues to be a need for such devices, particularly if nearly complete reliability can be achieved at acceptable cost.

CATHETERS

More than any other type of catheterization equipment, catheters are diverse in shape, design, and specific features. This section reviews some of the terminology used to describe catheters, principles of construction, and the wide selection of configurations and sizes available for cardiac angiography. In describing the merits and disadvantages of a specific catheter, the physician and manufacturer rely on specific terminology. Listed below is a short glossary of terms that are frequently encountered in product literature and may be used in discussions in the remainder of this chapter.

Axial control is the ability to transmit forces directly from the end of the catheter to the tip. The **body** is the segment of catheter between the tip and the hub. **Contrast medium delivery** or **maximum flow rate** is the ability to deliver high-contrast material within a specified injection pressure range. **Durometer** is the measure of degree of softness. **Flexibility** is the ability of a section of catheter to bend on contact with a resistant surface. The **hub** is the fitting on the proximal end of the catheter. **Internal diameter** is the diameter of the inside of the catheter; it determines which guidewires can be accommodated and expected contrast medium delivery. **Maneuverability** is the ability to advance a catheter around sharp bends or through tortuous vascular segments; it implies flexibility and torque control. **Memory** is the ability to recover and maintain a specific configuration after insertion and guidewire removal (shape retention). **Pliability** is the ability to bend and to be shaped. **Pressure monitoring characteristics** constitute the capacity to accurately transmit pressure from catheter tip to pressure transducer; they are a function of length, internal diameter, and stiffness. **Pushability,** or **power,** is the ability to directly transmit force applied to the hub of the catheter longitudinally to the tip; this has considerable importance in balloon angioplasty

catheters. **Radiopacity** is the ability to visualize the catheter under x-ray fluoroscopic control. **Softness,** the ability to bend, includes flexibility and implies poor stiffness and poor memory. **Stability,** the ability of a catheter to remain in position, is a function of stiffness, memory, and matching of catheter configuration to anatomy. **Stiffness** is the ability to resist bending; lack of flexibility. **Strength** is the ability to withstand high-pressure injections. It is generally applied to angiographic catheters, which must withstand high injection pressures associated with high-contrast flow rates. **Support, or backup,** the ability to remain in position despite resistance, refers to angioplasty guide catheters advancing a balloon catheter against resistance. It is a function of stiffness and configuration. **Tip** is the final taper or distal end of the catheter, the part inserted into the patient first. **Torque control,** the ability to directly transmit rotational forces from the end of the catheter to the tip, is synonymous with axial control. **Trackability** is the ability of a catheter to follow a guidewire along its course through the vascular anatomy. It is a function of the proper combination of size, flexibility, and pushability.

Catheter Components

A cardiac catheter is composed of several segments and parts (Fig. 10.19). The body of the catheter is generally straight over most of its length and may have any of various configurations toward the tip. The bends in a catheter are called curves, and the terms primary, secondary, and so on, are applied to the curves, beginning at the tip, as in Figure 10.19. Catheter tips may have a single end hole, closed end and any number of side holes, or end and side holes. Side holes allow for increased contrast delivery with less tendency for catheter recoil. Many end-hole catheters taper over a short segment to allow catheter insertion over a guidewire directly through the skin. Catheters designed for insertion through an arteriotomy or sheath do not necessarily have a tapered tip. Some newer designs have a

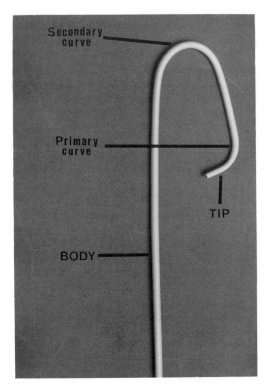

Figure 10.19. Sections of a catheter showing the different sections on a Judkins left 4 cm (JL4) coronary angiography catheter.

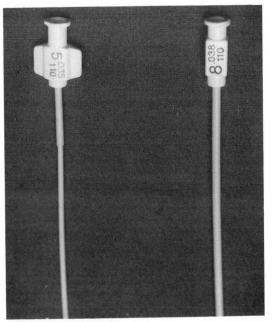

Figure 10.20. Catheter hubs from a Cordis 5 F and 8 F pigtail catheter demonstrating the winged hub design and reinforcing sleeve on the 5-F catheter and the specifications imprinted on the hub of both catheters.

grooved or soft tip, to be discussed in more detail later.

The hub of the catheter is bonded to the body and must have a strong, airtight seal. Specific design features include a female Luer-Lok for syringe or manifold attachment, winged tips or squared hubs for ease in rotation and handling, and imprinting of catheter specifications on the hub for easy identification (Fig. 10.20). The internal portion of the hub must have a smooth taper to facilitate guidewire insertion. In many designs the hub connection to the body of the catheter is reinforced by shrink tubing or a sleeve to decrease the chance of kinking or bending. Catheter specifications may also be imprinted on the sleeve. The internal design of a 5-F catheter hub is shown by scanning electron microscopy in Figure 10.21. This technique allows for assessment of possible compromise of lumen diameter at the hub.

Principles of Catheter Construction

Cardiac catheters may be composed of one or several layers. In most multilayered designs one tube is stretched or extruded over

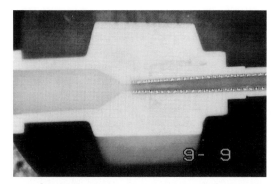

Figure 10.21. Internal design of braided catheter at point of hub attachment showing narrowing of the catheter lumen at point of insertion into the hub.

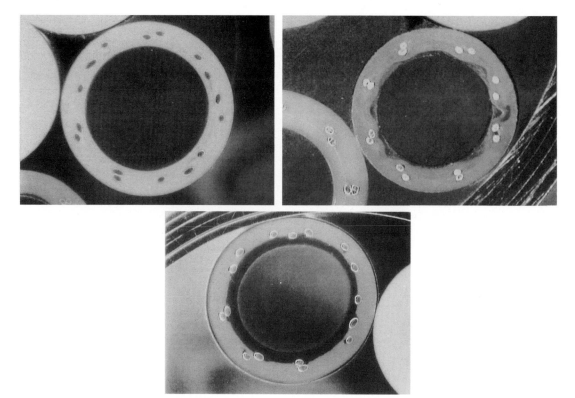

Figure 10.22. A–C. Scanning electron microscopic images of three catheter designs to illustrate how braiding is incorporated between catheter layers. **C,** Construction with layered materials.

another to form a bond. In catheters composed of several layers the components determine performance characteristics.

Most multilayered catheters consist of an inner tube of Teflon, over which is a layer of nylon, woven Dacron, or stainless steel braiding. A tube of polyethylene or polyurethane is heated and extruded over the two inner layers to bond firmly as a third external layer of the catheter. Others consist of a polyurethane core covered with stainless steel braiding and an external polyurethane jacket. Figure 10.22 illustrates scanning electron cross section micrographs of three catheter designs. Nonhomogeneity of material in the catheter layers can be assessed by this technique.

The inner layer, which provides a smooth surface through which guidewires and contrast agents may pass, should be nonthrombogenic. Quality control over surface irregularities can be readily checked by scanning electron microscopy as shown in

Figure 10.23. The thickness of the filaments and density of wire or nylon braiding in the middle layer and the type of plastic used determine the stiffness and torque control of the catheter. Some newer catheter designs have a much thinner wall, allowing

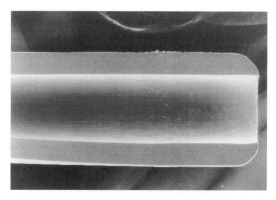

Figure 10.23. Scanning electron micrograph of internal surface of a catheter.

high flow characteristics but less flexibility and strength. This is accomplished by incorporating the braiding into the inner layer and reducing the number or thickness of layers in the catheter wall. A nylon layer or core imparting heat-resistant stiffness to the catheter is used in some 5- and 6-F designs and in some right heart and ventriculographic catheters.

Components of the external layer are also important determinants of catheter performance. The external layer must be impregnated with a radiopaque material, such as barium or bismuth, for easy fluoroscopic visualization. This process may soften the catheter material and may produce fine pitting of the surface of the catheter, increasing thrombogenicity. To overcome this materials may be incorporated into the middle layers of the catheter or a coating of silicone or other nonthrombogenic material may be applied to the outer catheter surface.

Polyethylene and polyurethane impart very different characteristics to a catheter. Both are thermoplastic materials. Polyethylene is relatively resistant to the softening effect of radiopaque materials but can be softened by heating to allow reshaping for special tip configurations. Polyethylene is more easily extruded over the inner two catheter layers. Because of its heat instability, polyethylene must be gas sterilized. Polyurethane, being less resistant to heating, is claimed to provide a catheter with better memory and yet is softer because it has more random molecular alignment. This softness is particularly desirable at the catheter tip, to reduce risk of arterial trauma during selective positioning. Now that most catheters are preformed in a large variety of configurations and intended for one-time use, reshaping by heating is rarely needed, and polyurethane is more commonly used in catheters for selective angiography.

Many companies now provide standard and high-flow designs for each diameter. The high-flow design has a thinner wall, hence a larger internal lumen for a given external diameter. This allows for higher-contrast flow rates at a specific injection pressure. High flow is particularly important in diagnostic catheters of small external diameter, that is, 4 to 6 F, and in guide catheters for coronary angioplasty, with which a large lumen is necessary for contrast injection around a balloon catheter or for placement of more than one dilating system or intracoronary guidewires. A very stiff catheter wall is necessary to maintain catheter strength in small-diameter high-flow designs. This provides fairly good torque response but sacrifices flexibility and pliability and increases the chance of kinking during advancement or rotation of the catheter.

Catheter Sizes

Diameter

Catheters for angiographic use are sized by external and internal diameter and length. The internal diameter is specified either by actual diameter in thousandths of an inch or millimeters or by the thickest guidewire that can be passed through the catheter. As noted previously, with newer thin-walled catheter designs, a much higher ratio of internal lumen to external diameter can be achieved. Thin-walled catheters can accommodate much faster contrast agent flow rates, allow the use of smaller-diameter catheters for angiography, and facilitates the radial artery approach to catheterization (9).

External diameter is expressed in French sizes; 1 F is 3 mm. French sizes 4 through 8 are used for diagnostic angiography. The differences in size are illustrated in Figure 10.24. Table 10.2 compares the internal and external diameters of some conventional thin-walled and high-flow designs in various French sizes. There may be as much as 0.013 inches greater internal diameter with a high-flow design. In general, braiding reduces the internal diameter by up to 0.007 inches. The table shows that the thin-walled design allows for faster contrast flow rates, enhancing opacification and improving potential for diagnostic-quality angiograms. It has also allowed for routine use of smaller-diameter catheters, hence smaller arterial punctures, less time to hemostasis after catheter removal, and less trauma to the vessel wall. Smaller catheters have been ad-

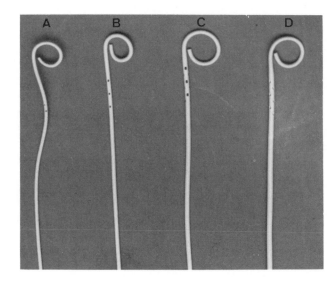

Figure 10.24. Four pigtail catheters of increasing size. **A.** 5 F. **B.** 6 F. **C.** 7 F. **D.** 8 F.

vocated for use in outpatient catheterization to reduce the time necessary for hemostasis, decrease the chance of rebleeding, and allow earlier ambulation and discharge after the procedure (10–12).

To maintain catheter control, as noted previously, the thin-walled designs incorporate much stiffer plastics, hence increase the potential for kinking during advancement or torquing. Reduced pliability of the catheter tip may decrease the ability to position catheters in anatomic orientations not perfectly matched to catheter configuration. In clinical trials comparing 7-F catheters with high-flow 5-F designs, the differences become apparent. The 5-F design more frequently fails to be manipulated to provide adequate seating in the coronary ostium,

and in about 10% of cases it fails to provide enough contrast flow to opacify the coronary artery sufficiently to evaluate stenoses. In patients with high coronary flow rates associated with conditions such as left ventricular hypertrophy and in large patients with high heart rates, 5- or 6-F catheters are often inadequate.

There is also concern that these stiffer catheter tips may increase the chance of arterial injury during selective coronary intubation. Many manufacturers have therefore included a flexible or soft tip in an attempt to overcome this problem while maintaining stiffness in the body and curvatures necessary for catheter tip placement (13) (Fig. 10.25). These tips, which are usually bonded to the end of the catheter, have several de-

Table 10.2.
Outer and Internal Diameter of Standard and High-Flow Diagnostic Catheters

French	OD	OD (millimeters)	Standard Minimum ID	High-flow Maximum ID
4	0.052	1.33	[a]	0.040
5	0.065	1.67	0.044	0.052
6	0.078	2.00	0.047	0.059
7	0.092	2.34	0.048	0.061
8	0.104	2.64	0.056	0.063
9	0.118	3.00	[a]	[a]

[a] No catheters made in this size/type.
All measurements in inches unless stated otherwise.
OD, outer diameter; ID, inner diameter.

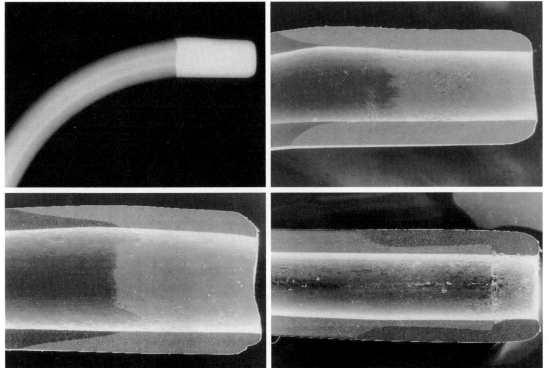

Figure 10.25. A–D. Softip design shown (**A**) externally and (**B–D**) internally.

signs. Because of concern that these thin-walled catheters are less radiopaque and difficult to visualize, some manufacturers incorporate radiopaque tips. This provides a soft and readily visible catheter tip to facilitate a traumatic coronary intubation. These concepts are theoretically attractive, and use of soft tips, particularly in thin-walled diagnostic and PTCA guiding catheters, has become common.

Length

Catheters vary in length, depending on configuration and purpose and on the route of insertion (brachial versus femoral). Most pigtail catheters are 110 cm long, and Judkins catheters are 100 cm long. Most brachial catheters are 80 or 100 cm long. Catheters for other specific designs and purposes vary in length.

Configuration

Numerous catheter configurations are available for ventriculography, large-vessel angiography, and selective coronary angiography. A detailed discussion of all of the many catheters used is not possible, but an overview of available catheters from the brachial and femoral approach is provided.

Specific Types

Central Venous Catheters

Catheters for central venous access are often routinely stocked not in catheterization laboratories but in critical care areas, where they are frequently used. These short (usually 20 to 30 cm) catheters are designed for insertion into the internal jugular, subcla-

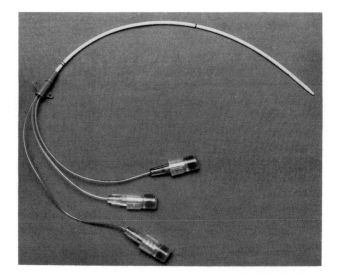

Figure 10.26. A 7-F triple-lumen central venous catheter 30 cm long (Cardiomed).

vian, or antecubital vein. They are intended for long-term access to the central venous system for measurement of central venous pressure and administration of nutrients or medications.

Catheters are made of soft material, such as polyurethane, Teflon, or Silastic, hence soften with body temperature in situ. Newer versions of central venous catheters have more than one lumen. Triple-lumen catheters (Fig. 10.26), now frequently used in critical care units, have a 16-gauge lumen for administration of blood products and two 18-gauge lumens for administration of crystalloids and medications. External size ranges from pediatric 4 to adult 7 F. These catheters are very useful in intensive care units, but they do carry a small risk of central venous or right heart perforation. Although new designs use softer materials, proper positioning and maintaining the tip at the superior vena cava right atrial junction are still essential. Because of risk of infection with catheters indwelling for long duration, some companies coat the surface with bacteriostatic agents.

Balloon Flotation Catheters

There have been numerous developments since the introduction of the balloon flotation catheter for clinical use by Swan and Ganz in 1970. The use of a flow-directed catheter for right heart catheterization without fluoroscopic control has significantly advanced management of patients in critical care areas.

In addition, when conventional right heart catheters cannot be directed into the pulmonary artery, a balloon flotation catheter is often successful. This fact and the ease of obtaining a pulmonary artery occlusion pressure, which approximates the capillary wedge pressure, have led to use of the flotation catheter as the first choice for right heart catheterization in some laboratories.

Most balloon flotation catheters are made of polyvinyl chloride (PVC) in a multiple extrusion, multilumen construction. The PVC is soft and becomes softer in situ when warmed by body heat. The balloon is usually composed of latex and has an inflated volume of 0.8 to 2.2 cc. The balloon is positioned within several millimeters of the tip to reduce contact of the tip with the myocardium during advancement. Catheters vary in length and diameter from 60 cm and 5 F for pediatric use to 110 cm and 7 F for use in adults. The catheter has one lumen for balloon inflation and may have additional lumens according to intended use. A Berman angiographic catheter (Fig. 10.27) has a second lumen for injection of radiographic contrast and has no end hole, but it has multiple side holes to prevent

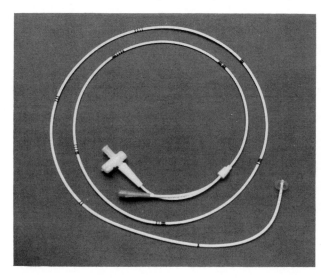

Figure 10.27. A 7-F Berman angiographic catheter (*arrow*).

catheter recoil during rapid injection of contrast material.

Balloon flotation pacing catheters may have a second channel for wires leading to the two electrodes at the catheter tip (Fig. 10.28). Balloon catheters for determining cardiac output by thermodilution technique (Fig. 10.29) have a lumen for pressure measurement from the tip, a thermistor about 4 cm from the tip, and a proximal port 20 to 30 cm from the tip for measurement of pressure in proximal chambers (right atrium) and injection of indicator. In some models two additional lumens and side ports allow for transcatheter placement of right ventricular and right atrial pacing wires for ventricular or atrioventricular sequential pacing.

Right Heart Catheters

Several right heart catheters are shown in Figure 10.30. The Cournand catheter is a woven Dacron and polyethylene or polyurethane single end hole catheter designed specifically for right heart catheterization. It can be used for selective blood sampling, and with its single end hole it can be used for obtaining pulmonary–capillary wedge

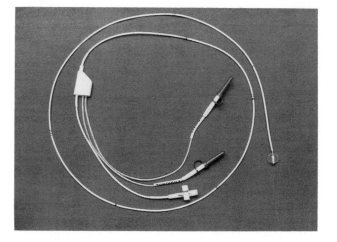

Figure 10.28. A 5-F Swan-Ganz bipolar pacing catheter (Edwards).

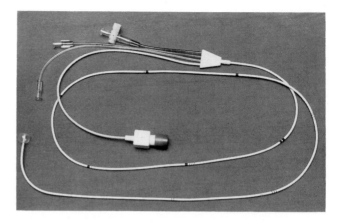

Figure 10.29. A 7-F Sorenson thermodilution catheter (Abbof).

pressure measurements with excellent pressure monitoring characteristics.

Gorlin and Zucker catheters have configurations similar to that of the Cournand catheter, but the Gorlin and Zucker have electrodes near the tip for optional cardiac pacing or simultaneous measurement of intracardiac pressures and electrograms. This makes them very stiff. The Goodale-Lubin catheter is very similar to the Cournand catheter except that it has two side holes close to the tip in addition to its end hole, making it very useful for blood sampling.

In many laboratories a multipurpose

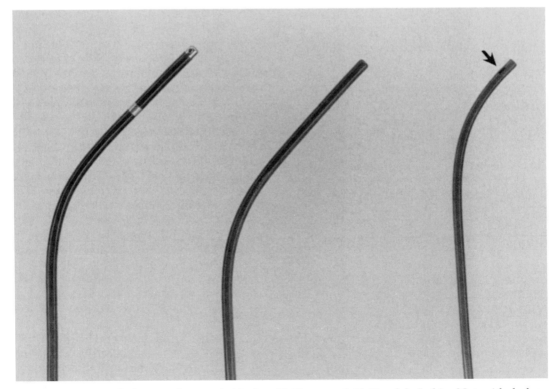

Figure 10.30. Right heart catheters. **A.** Zucker. **B.** Cournand. **C.** Goodale-Lubin. Note side holes near tip in Zucker and Goodale-Lubin catheters.

catheter similar to coronary angiographic catheters is used for right heart catheterization.

Transseptal Catheters

The transseptal catheter was developed specifically for crossing from right to left atrium through the interatrial septum at the fossa ovalis. The transseptal or Brockenbrough type of catheter is advanced over a Brockenbrough type of needle for left atrial catheterization. The catheter must then be manipulated from left atrium to left ventricle directly or assisted by a 0.035-inch guidewire (see Chapter 9). The Brockenbrough needle (Fig. 10.31) is 18 gauge in its shaft and tapers to 21 gauge at its tip. It has a central lumen for blood sampling and pressure measurement and at its proximal end has a flange with a pointer to indicate tip direction.

The Brockenbrough catheter is made of Teflon and is more rigid than conventional

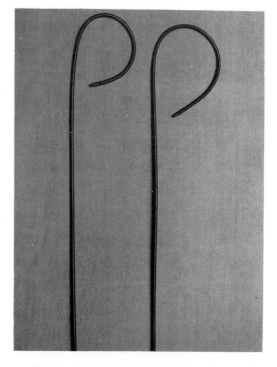

Figure 10.32. Brockenbrough transseptal catheters showing different tip curvatures.

catheters. It has a tapered tip with an end hole and two to six side holes for angiography. The catheter tip is curved to facilitate advancement from left atrium to ventricle. Catheters are available with various curves to accommodate variations in left atrial size. Standard radii of curvature of 2, 2.5, and 3 cm are available. Sizes are shown in Figure 10.32.

The transseptal catheter has been modified to a sheath design (Mullins sheath) to facilitate insertion of different catheters into the left atrium or ventricle. The Mullins sheath and introducer, along with the Brockenbrough needle, are shown in Figure 10.31. The introducer is advanced over the needle in a fashion similar to that of the transseptal catheter. The sheath is then advanced along with the introducer across the septum. Sheath sizes range from 6 to 8 F, with internal diameters of 0.078 to 0.104 inch, respectively. The 8-F sheath can accommodate a 7-F catheter of conventional or balloon flotation type.

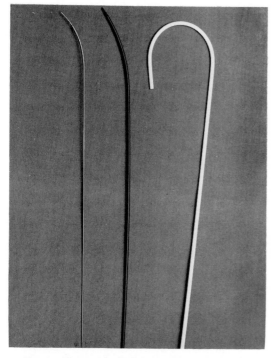

Figure 10.31. The Mullins sheath and dilator with Brockenbrough transseptal needle.

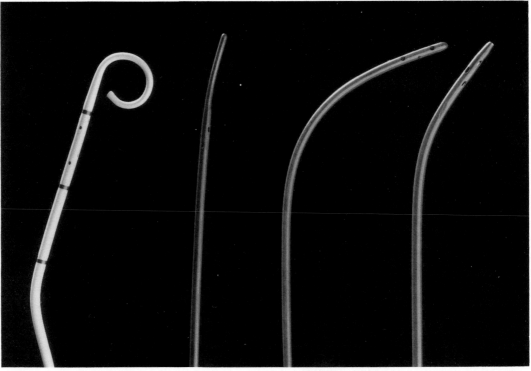

Figure 10.33. Ventriculographic catheters. **A.** Pigtail. **B.** Lehman ventricular. **C.** NIH. **D.** Gensini.

Angiographic Catheters

Numerous ventricular catheters are illustrated in Figure 10.33. The NIH catheter is a thick-walled, closed-end, rounded-tip catheter with four to six side holes at the tip. This catheter can be easily maneuvered and positioned directly through a sheath or cutdown. It is useful for crossing stenotic valves and with a closed end is stable during high-flow injections. It is frequently used from the brachial approach for right or left ventriculography and angiography in any of the major vessels. It has excellent pressure monitoring and angiographic characteristics.

The Gensini catheter is a thin-walled, woven Dacron catheter with an open end and six side holes. It is useful in crossing the aortic valve from the brachial approach, where guidewire assistance is necessary, and it is well suited to high-flow contrast studies. The Lehman ventriculography catheter has a woven Dacron core and a flexible, tapered, closed-end tip with four side holes. Its primary use is in crossing the aortic valve from the brachial approach; it can be used for left ventriculography and ascending aortography.

Pigtail catheters, which are primarily used for high-flow contrast studies, achieve stability through their curled-tip design and multiple side holes. The curled end may have a normal or tight radius. The distal catheter segment can be straight or angled to allow easier entry into the left ventricle from the aorta, particularly in cases of aortic stenosis in which the left ventricle is horizontal. These angles are generally 145 or 155°. The number of side holes, which varies considerably with different designs, influences the contrast flow rates at a given injection pressure. More than eight side holes provide little advantage and increase the chance of thrombus formation on the catheter. This catheter has to be flushed forcefully to ensure that the flush will include the end hole and not just the side holes. Newer cath-

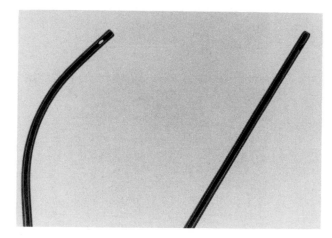

Figure 10.34. Sones catheters.

eter designs are constantly under development.

Coronary Angiography Catheters

Coronary angiography catheters can be grouped into several series: Sones, Judkins, Amplatz, multipurpose, and bypass graft. Sones catheters (Fig. 10.34) were initially designed for insertion via brachial artery cutdown, as described in Chapter 2 and more recently have been modified for percutaneous brachial insertion via a sheath system. Original construction was based on a woven Dacron design, but polyurethane and polyethylene may also be used. The percutaneous systems are frequently layered with external polyethylene or polyurethane coats.

Judkins catheters (Figs. 10.35 and 10.36) are intended for insertion over a wire from a femoral percutaneous approach. The principal advantage of Judkins catheters is that they naturally seek the coronary orifice when advanced into the sinus of Valsalva. The specifics of the Judkins technique are discussed in Chapter 17.

The Amplatz configurations and sizes for left and right coronaries are shown in Figures 10.37 and 10.38, respectively. Am-

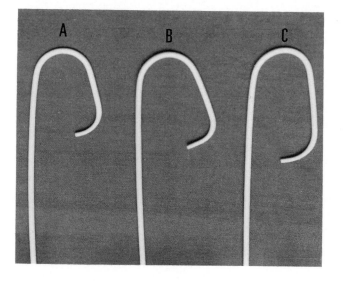

Figure 10.35. Judkins left coronary catheters. **A.** JL3.5. **B.** JL4. **C.** JL5.

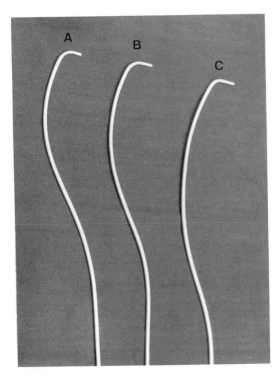

Figure 10.36. Judkins right coronary catheters. **A.** JR4. **B.** JR5. **C.** JR6.

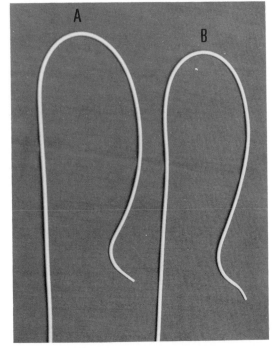

Figure 10.38. Amplatz right coronary catheters. **A.** ARI. **B.** ARII.

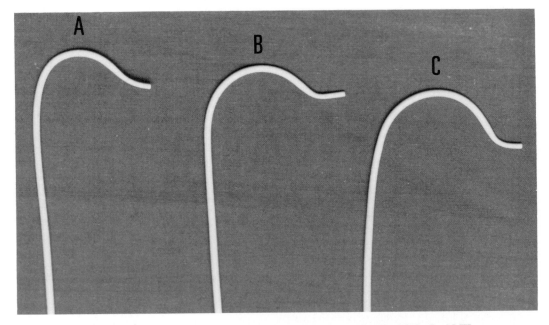

Figure 10.37. Amplatz left coronary catheters. **A.** ALI. **B.** ALII. **C.** ALIII.

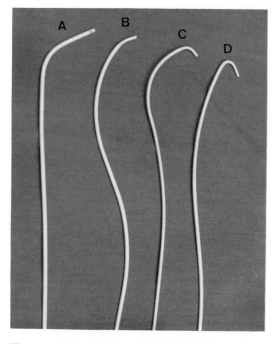

Figure 10.39. Multipurpose and bypass graft catheters. **A.** Multipurpose. **B.** Right bypass. **C.** Left bypass. **D.** Internal mammary artery.

platz catheters are particularly useful when Judkins catheters are not suited to a given anatomic conformation, particularly when the coronary artery originates posteriorly or from high in the sinus of Valsalva. The Amplatz configurations have also been adapted for use from the brachial approach when the Sones catheter cannot be manipulated into the coronary orifice.

The multipurpose catheter (Schoonmaker and King, single-catheter technique; Fig. 10.39) is unusual from the femoral approach in that it is used for both ventriculography and selective coronary angiography. It can also be used for aortography, although the jet of contrast from the end hole may artificially magnify the severity of aortic insufficiency as assessed angiographically. As Figure 10.39 shows, the multipurpose catheter is comparable with the Sones catheter in configuration and is manipulated in similar fashion.

Saphenous vein bypass graft and internal mammary artery catheters are available in several designs (Fig. 10.39). Separate configurations are available for venous bypass

grafts to the right and left coronary arteries and for selective internal mammary angiography. Use of these catheters requires considerable expertise for proper manipulation.

PATIENT MONITORING DEVICES

Catheterization laboratories are seeing increasingly aggressive interventional procedures in elderly and seriously ill patients. This has led to increased emphasis on monitoring the patient's physiologic status through the periprocedural period, particularly when using analgesic and tranquilizing agents that can profoundly depress respiration. Traditionally, patients were frequently monitored by nursing personnel before and after the procedure, but newer electronic devices provide for continuous and more extensive monitoring.

Standard Electrocardiographic Monitoring

Monitoring of the electrocardiogram (ECG) during diagnostic catheterization and interventional procedures is essential. The ECG provides evidence of change in heart rate and development of conduction disturbances or arrhythmias, and through ST segment analysis it alerts the physician to development or persistence of myocardial ischemia. For many diagnostic procedures it is reasonable to monitor only the limb leads. Leads I, II, and aVF provide adequate representation to detect most problems. During chest pain periods when coronary artery spasm or even acute ischemic injury is suspected, other leads must be examined and even recorded. During coronary interventional procedures, particularly involving the left anterior descending artery, monitoring the precordial leads is highly desirable. Radiolucent electrodes and wires can be used to avoid obscuring the fluoroscopic image. A single precordial lead is satisfactory in most cases. For lesions involv-

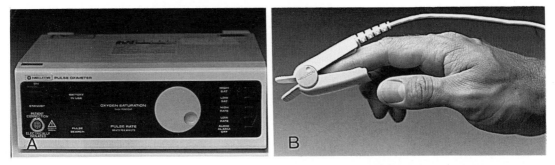

Figure 10.40. A and **B.** A Nellcor pulse oximeter showing oximeter connecting cable and sensor attached to tip of index finger.

ing the left anterior descending artery, a V_2 position is usually satisfactory, and for diagonal branch or intermediate branch distributions, a V_5 lead is preferable.

Bedside Noninvasive Pressure Monitoring

Continuous noninvasive arterial pressure monitoring devices used in intensive care units have recently been advocated for periprocedural monitoring of patients in the cardiac catheterization laboratory. A decline in blood pressure can occur in the absence of a significant change in heart rate in many patients. Availability of a pressure monitor increases the patient's safety and reduces need for continuous observation by nurses. These monitors are generally somewhat bulky and best limited to use before and after the procedure.

Bedside Pulse Oximeters

Increasingly compact modules for bedside pulse oximeters have made their use attractive for patient monitoring during cardiac catheterization. A model marketed by Nelcor is shown in Figure 10.40. Bedside pulse oximeters permit continuous monitoring of heart rate and have an alarm setting in addition to a continuous digital display. They can be hard-wired in the catheterization laboratory so that the moni-

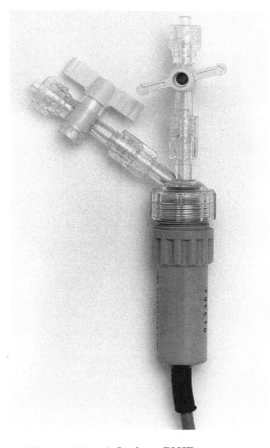

Figure 10.41. A Statham P23ID pressure transducer.

tor is kept in the hemodynamic recording area and the cable is tunneled to the base of the catheterization laboratory table. Alternatively, new portable monitors can be hung from an intravenous standard and used at the catheterization laboratory table itself. Continuous monitoring of oxygen saturation allows early detection of depression of respiration by narcotic analgesics and early development of pulmonary edema or other disturbances in oxygenation, although significant decline in P_{O_2} and alterations in pH and P_{CO_2} may occur before changes in oxygen saturation are detected. Use of these devices is relatively inexpensive, only slightly inconvenient, and therefore strongly recommended. They are often mandated by hospital policy regarding use of sedatives during procedures—so-called conscious sedation.

Hemodynamic Monitoring

Monitoring of pressure waveforms during cardiac catheterization is an integral component of the procedure. The details of physiologic measurement and recording are covered in Chapters 22 and 14 respectively. From these discussions it is clear that pressures may be recorded in many ways and that recording systems must be properly designed to provide optimal signals of diagnostic quality. These systems must also be convenient, safe, reliable, and inexpensive when used in laboratories assessing and treating large numbers of patients.

Some laboratories employ reusable pressure transducers. These are typically of the design of the Statham P23ID transducer shown in Figure 10.41. The fluid-filled catheter is connected to a manifold and then, by relatively rigid plastic tubing, to the transducer mounted at the side of the catheterization table. As noted in Chapter 22, the longer the fluid-filled tubing and the greater the number of connections, the greater the chance of a suboptimal pressure tracing. Reusable transducers require either repeated sterilization by gas or antiseptic bath or use of a dome equipped with a membrane or diaphragm to isolate the transducer from the fluid-filled system and blood elements. This type of system takes considerable time to prepare and has the potential for distortion of pressure signals if loose connections and air bubbles are not carefully eliminated. Even under ideal conditions, because of a length of fluid-filled tubing from the manifold to the pressure transducer, this type of system cannot accurately reproduce the pressure signal arriving at the proximal end of the catheter and manifold.

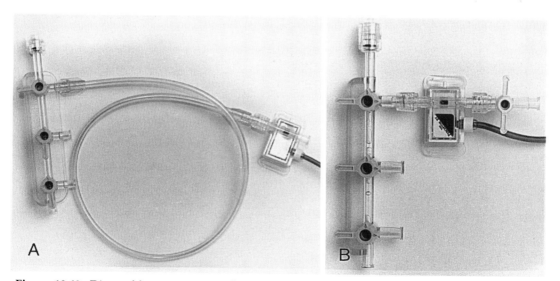

Figure 10.42. Disposable pressure transducer showing connection (**A**) to a manifold via pressure tubing or (**B**) directly via a stopcock.

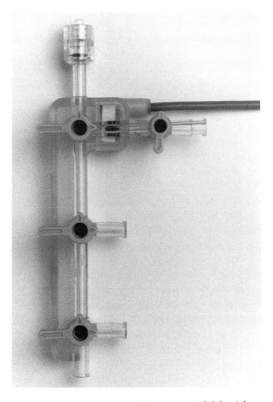

Figure 10.43. Perceptor Morse manifold with an integrated disposable manifold and pressure transducer.

Numerous companies have introduced disposable pressure transducers to overcome some inconveniences and problems of reusable systems. A system marketed by North American Instrument Corporation (NAMIC) is shown in Figure 10.42. This Perceptor system provides a disposable pressure transducer and electrical connector cable that can be mounted at the side of the table and connected either to a manifold via pressure tubing or directly to the manifold itself via stopcock (Fig. 10.42 *A* and *B*.). To eliminate the inconvenience of connecting the transducer to a manifold and possible pressure leak associated with loose connection, NAMIC has developed the Perceptor Morse manifold. This has a pressure transducer directly attached to a Morse manifold as a single unit (Fig. 10.43). This design eliminates a stopcock from the system, hence reduces the volume of fluid in the system and chance of air

bubbles and pressure leaks. The pressure waveform with this system has higher fidelity. In addition, pressure measurements are more reproducible from patient to patient, through elimination of errors induced by connecting independent components of other system designs.

SUMMARY

This chapter reviews many of the tools available to the catheterizing physician and comments on technical considerations pertaining to their use. It is essential for physicians performing invasive procedures to remain aware of new methods and technology that facilitate these procedures and enhance their safety.

References

1. Kikuchi Y, Graves VB, Strother CM, et al. A new guidewire with kink-resistant core and low friction coating. Cardiovasc Intervent Radiol 1989;12:107–109.
2. Siegel JB, Kim D, Porter DH. Embolization hazard of hydrophilic guidewires. Radiology 1989;171:582–583.
3. Waksman R, Scott NA, Ghazzal ZMB, et al. Randomized comparison of flexible versus non-flexible femoral sheaths on patient comfort after angioplasty. Am Heart J 1996;131:1076–1078.
4. Stables RH, Sigwart U. Post-stent management with a pneumatic groin compression device and self injected low molecular weight heparin. Heart 1996;75:588–590.
5. Dangas G, Mehran R, Duvvuri S, et al. Use of a pneumatic compression system (FemoStop^R) as a treatment option for femoral artery pseudoaneurysms after percutaneous cardiac procedures. Cathet Cardiovasc Diagn 1996;39:138–142.
6. Kussmaul WG, Buchbinder M, Whitlow PL, et al. Femoral artery hemostasis using an implantable device (Angio-Seal^{TM}) after coronary angioplasty. Cathet Cardiovasc Diagn 1996;37:362–365.
7. Aker UT, Kensey KR, Heuser RR, et al. Immediate arterial hemostasis after cardiac catheterization: initial experience with a new puncture closure device. Cathet Cardiovasc Diagn 1994;31:228–232.
8. Webb JG, Carere RA, Dodek AA. Collagen plug hemostatic closure of femoral arterial puncture sites following implantation of coronary stents. Cathet Cardiovasc Diagn 1993;30:314–316.
9. Kiemeneij F, Laarman GJ. Percutaneous transradial approach for coronary stent implantation. Cathet Cardiovasc Diagn 1993;30:173–178.

10. Molajo AO, Ward C, Bray CL, et al. Comparison of Superflow (5F) and conventional 8F catheters for cardiac catheterization by the femoral route. Cathet Cardiovasc Diagn 1987;13:275–276.

11. Brown RIG, Macdonald AC. Use of 5 French catheters for cardiac catheterization and coronary angiography. Cath Cardiovasc Diagn 1987;13:214–217.

12. Bush CA, VonFossen DB, Kolibash AJ, et al. Cardiac catheterization and coronary angiography using 5 French preformed (Judkins) catheters from the percutaneous right brachial approach: a comparative analysis with the femoral approach. Cathet Cardiovasc Diagn 1993;29:267–272.

13. Finci L, Meier B, Steffenino G, et al. Clinical evaluation of soft-tipped catheters for coronary angiography. Cathet Cardiovasc Diagn 1986;12:347–351.

11
Radiographic Techniques Used in Cardiac Catheterization

David R. Holmes, Jr., MD
Merrill A. Wondrow
Paul R. Julsrud, MD

INTRODUCTION

Cardiac catheterization continues to change rapidly as the field evolves from diagnostic imaging to an increasingly therapeutic arena (1–3). With the introduction of interventional therapeutic techniques such as percutaneous transluminal coronary angioplasty (PTCA), the demands on radiographic equipment have become more stringent. The pace of change has accelerated with the widespread use of stenting, which is performed in as many as 60 to 70% of interventional procedures. Given the need for precise placement of these stents and their lack of radiopacity, advanced radiographic capacities are required. These include roadmapping, digital enhancement, and subtraction and quantitative angiography. Quantitative coronary angiography has moved from an important scientific assessment technique to a required practical technique during this time because of the necessity to match specific device size to the arterial segment to be treated and to optimize the final result (4, 5–10). Achieving an optimal angiographic result as assessed by quantitative angiography has been found to enhance the chances of decreased angiographic and clinical restenosis and to decrease the potential for acute complications

such as subacute stent closure. To meet these demands there have been rapid improvements in both video and cine imaging capabilities (11–16). Also, major advances in computer techniques facilitate image analysis and processing. The invasive cardiologist must be familiar with radiographic techniques and principles to understand the benefits and limitations of the imaging chain, to relate to support personnel, to maximize room performance, and to enhance clinical decision making.

ANGIOGRAPHIC EQUIPMENT

In the past floating tabletop and rotational cradle combinations were used exclusively. These systems had the advantages of improved protection from radiation and short source-to-image distance (Fig. 11.1). Mechanically coupling the image intensifier and the x-ray tube facilitated cranial and caudal angulation to allow optimal assessment of different segments of the coronary anatomy (17, 18), particularly the proximal left anterior descending coronary artery. When the patient rather than the equipment was rotated into a left anterior oblique view, the heart shifted off the spine. This shift al-

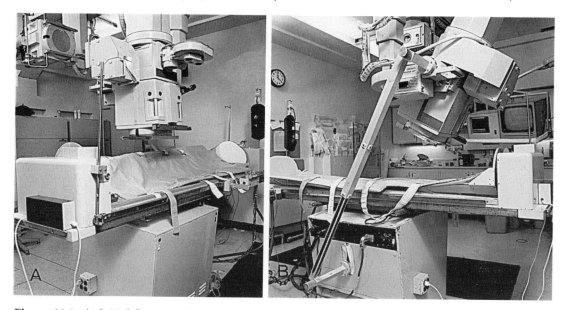

Figure 11.1. A. Initial floating tabletop with a rotational cradle. This system had the advantage of a short source-to-image distance. Cranial or caudal angulation was not possible without the use of a wedge. **B.** To obtain cranial or caudal angulation, the image intensifier and the x-ray tube were mechanically coupled.

lowed the proximal left anterior descending artery to be seen well and improved visualization of fine details. Another major advantage was easy access for a brachial approach. Other advantages were that the cradle could be rotated faster than the imaging equipment itself and access to the patient's head and airway was easier.

However, these systems had disadvantages: rotation was uncomfortable and disturbing for some patients; during rotation, catheter position, particularly with a brachial approach, could be lost; and the degree of angulation was limited to 30° cranial and 10 to 15° caudal.

The conventional floating tabletop and rotational cradle are no longer routinely available; instead cardiac laboratories have equipment that rotates around the patient. Various configurations from different vendors include, among others, an L–U arm combination, a U arm with a parallelogram, and a C arm with rotation around two axes (Fig. 11.2). These systems allow for maximal angulated views and excellent catheter stability because the patient is not turned. For some patients the flat table is also more comfortable than the rotating cradle. In ad-

dition, the operator can adjust the cranial and caudal angulations from the table itself.

The disadvantages to these newer systems include a longer source-to-image distance and increased radiation exposure (19).

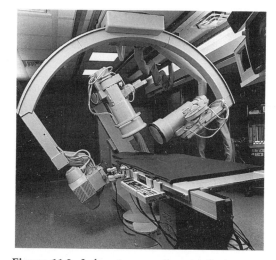

Figure 11.2. Laboratory equipment that rotates around the patient. Various configurations include the biplane L–U–C arm system shown here.

As interventional procedures become more complex and involve treatment of more vessels with more devices, radiation exposure to patient, physician, and technical personnel becomes more problematic. With these systems it is also more difficult to perform brachial procedures, particularly if biplane angiography is to be used. Other disadvantages include less than optimal access to the patient's head and airway. This is a substantial problem in critically ill patients who require ventilator support and in children. Another problem is that even though multiple angulated views can be achieved, the proximal left anterior descending coronary artery may not be seen as well because the heart does not move relative to the spine, as it does when the patient is rotated to the left anterior oblique position with a cradle. Because of the importance of this view, particularly with interventional procedures, we have combined a rotational equipment support system with a rotational cradle (Fig. 11.3). This cradle allows for table rotation up to 30°. This combination provides an excellent view of all aspects of the coronary arterial tree, particularly the proximal left anterior descending coronary artery in the left anterior oblique view. It also may decrease radiation exposure.

The choice between biplane and monoplane equipment depends on the purpose of the laboratory as well as on operator preference. Most cardiac catheterization laboratories rely on single-plane equipment; this is almost always related to the cost differential, but space considerations may also be important. In addition, the advantages of biplane imaging (discussed later) may be perceived as only potential and may not be considered cost-effective. For example, biplane left ventriculography is very helpful in assessing regional wall function. In laboratories without that capability, other imaging techniques, such as radionuclide or echocardiographic assessment, may be used. Biplane capability, however, does offer real advantages. It allows simultaneous orthogonal biplane angiography of the left ventricle, ascending aorta, and other cardiac structures. Biplane left ventriculograms recorded with 30° right anterior oblique and 60° left anterior oblique views allow assessment of more segments of the left ventricle than would be possible

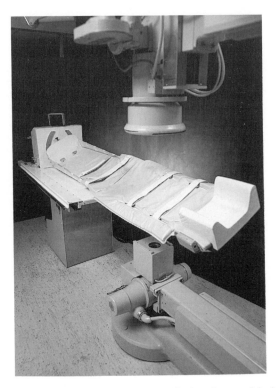

Figure 11.3. A modified cradle has been added to the system to improve cranial angulation images of the proximal left anterior descending coronary artery.

with single-plane right anterior oblique views alone.

Because coronary artery disease produces heterogeneous effects on regional left ventricular function, biplane views are important (20, 21), particularly for assessing the effect of reperfusion on ventricular function (20). In this situation improvement in regional function may be seen in either the right or the left anterior oblique view. The two projections are complementary, providing information about regional function not obtained by either view alone. Septal and posterolateral walls are not seen in the right anterior oblique view. If a biplane system is not available, the left ventricular angiogram may be recorded twice, once in the right anterior oblique view and once in the left anterior oblique view. This method has the disadvantages of increasing the amounts of contrast agent and radiation.

Biplane imaging is also being used with

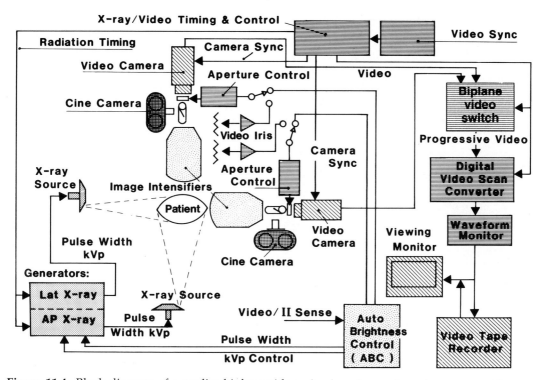

Figure 11.4. Block diagram of a cardiac biplane video–cine imaging system. A common video synchronizing generator drives a timing and control device. This is necessary for synchronization and progressive scanning. (From Julsrud PR, Wondrow MA, Stears JG, et al. X-ray equipment. In: Holmes DR Jr, Vlietstra RE, eds. Interventional cardiology. Philadelphia: FA Davis, 1989:30–41. By permission of Mayo Foundation.)

increasing frequency during other procedures. In transseptal catheterization it facilitates safe entry into the left atrium. It is also used with increasing frequency in dilation, although it is not essential. In this setting such biplane views are extremely helpful for crossing lesions, particularly chronic total occlusions. New approaches to chronic total occlusion, such as the laser guidewire systems, emphasize not only bilateral coronary injections but biplane imaging to optimize the result. Optimal views in each plane are frozen for review. Recording the angles used to obtain the diagnostic pictures is helpful in setting up these optimal views. During dilation it may not be necessary to move the imaging equipment at all except to switch from one video projection to the other. Biplane recordings cannot be used during dilation performed from the arm because the lateral tube interferes with the operator's position.

Biplane coronary angiography can be used to decrease the amount of contrast agent required for angiographic evaluation of patients with abnormal renal function. Biplane views are also used for interventional electrophysiologic procedures such as catheter ablation of accessory atrioventricular pathways.

In the future three-dimensional coronary angiography will be possible (Fig. 11.5). For this multiple biplane views obtained with a computer-controlled gantry will be used to construct a three-dimensional coronary arterial tree. The optimal number of biplane pairs required is yet to be determined. In addition, if transmyocardial revascularization is found to be effective, it may be adapted for cardiac catheterization. This will require multiplane imaging of the left ventricle to optimize procedural performance.

Biplane imaging does have some disad-

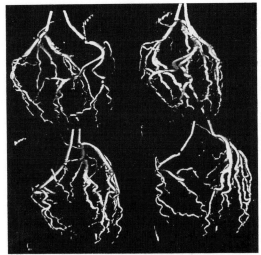

Figure 11.5. Angiogram obtained from a postmortem specimen with a computer-controlled gantry. Multiple views can be obtained and formatted for a more accurate representation of the three-dimensional structure of the coronary arteries.

vantages. **Typically a biplane system is twice as costly,** controlled blanking is required during angiography, and it makes access to the patient more difficult, particularly in emergencies when the airway must be secured. Finally, if biplane coronary angiography is performed, interpretation of the cine film is awkward because the orthogonal pairs are widely separated on the film and other views are interposed. This is particularly a problem for right coronary injections. As cine film is replaced, this will not be a problem because the image sequence will be movable electronically to facilitate review.

Image System

During imaging radiation produced by the x-ray tube is attenuated as it passes through the patient (Fig. 11.4). This attenuated radiation is detected by the image intensifier, which converts the x-ray energy (photons) to a light image that is coupled optically to the detector. An automatic brightness control that senses directly from the image intensifier output is used to maintain video output and cine film darkening over a wide range. In addition to the automatic brightness control, a manual iris can be used to optimize the video image (22). This manual iris will become more important as cine film is replaced.

Cardiac imaging places unique demands on the imaging system. Because the structures to be visualized, such as the coronary arteries, are moving rapidly, exposure times should be short to avoid motion blurring. If the catheterization suite is used for both children and adults, the demands are even greater. In children with rapid heart rates, an exposure time of 2 to 3 milliseconds is required; in adults, an exposure time of 5 milliseconds or less is satisfactory. Longer exposure times result in blurred images because of the motion artifact.

X-Ray Generation

X-Ray Generator

The x-ray generator produces the power that accelerates electrons in the x-ray tube. Various generators are available for cardiovascular applications. There are advantages and disadvantages to each type. Selection of the appropriate one depends on the equipment design, x-ray tube selected, and use intended for the room. Constant-potential and pulsed generators both are suitable. Important considerations include kilovoltage (kVp), milliamperage (mA), and kilowatt (kW) ratings and characteristics of timing. These specifications can be obtained from the manufacturers. Recommended minimal requirements are given in Table 11.1.

X-Ray Tube

There also is variation in x-ray tubes among different manufacturers. Selection of the appropriate one depends on the generator and on the major purpose of the room. Rooms designed for interventional procedures have somewhat different requirements

Table 11.1.
X-Ray Generators

Feature	Value
Kilovolt peak	
Minimum	40
Maximum	150
Milliamperes	
Maximum	200 (rms)
Timing	
Maximum exposure time (pulsed), milliseconds	5 (grid bias)
Kilowatt rating	
At 80 kVp	100
Automatic exposure control	Milliamperage and kilovolt peak combined

from those of rooms designed for diagnostic purposes only. Thus it has been suggested that there should be dedicated interventional rooms and other dedicated diagnostic rooms. However, few laboratories can afford a dedicated interventional room. In addition, there is increased emphasis on combined diagnostic and therapeutic procedures, such as PTCA, at the same time as initial diagnostic angiography. Therefore, given the expanding nature of interventional practice, it is reasonable that all new angiographic suites be suitable for both diagnostic and therapeutic procedures.

Various tubes are available. New advances include ceramic and graphite tubes and modified support structures. These tubes are significantly more expensive than conventional tubes, but they last longer and have high heat load capacity. The importance of sufficient heat load and cooling capacities must be emphasized. If these are insufficient, procedures must be prolonged to allow the units to return to normal, and tube life is shortened. Tubes with a heat load capacity of 1 million to 1.5 million heat units should be selected. Systems should also have a heat load readout. This is particularly important during stent placement when high-resolution features are selected. If the operator does not know about heat load, the procedure can be prolonged if the x-ray tube overheats, or the tube may be damaged, or both.

Focal spot sizes also vary. They should be between 0.5 and 1 mm for fluoroscopy and cineangiography. Smaller focal spots, 0.2 or 0.3 mm, may enhance TV resolution. Operating at smaller focal spots increases the demand for cooling because more heat is produced. **Heat capacity should be monitored during procedures.** If it decreases substantially, extra time between angiographic filming sessions may be required. Off-focal-spot radiation may be a significant problem. During acceptance evaluation, tubes should be tested to ensure that off-focal-spot radiation is absent.

Recommended specification minima for x-ray tubes are shown in Table 11.2. **These specifications should be obtained from the manufacturers before purchase** of new x-ray tubes.

The interface between x-ray generator and tube is undergoing considerable change (6, 8). In the past video images and pulsed cine images have been achieved by secondary electronic switching. The x-ray pulse produced by secondary electronic switching has a prolonged decay (Fig. 11.6). This is the result of the capacitance characteristics of the high-voltage cables between

Table 11.2.
Minimum Specifications of X-Ray Tubes

Feature	Value
Focal spot, millimeters	
Small	0.5
Large	1.0
Star measurements for testing	Yes
Rating, kilowatts	
Small focal spot	40–60
Large focal spot	80–100
Anode characteristics	
Angles	
Small focal spot	7°
Large focal spot	7°
Heat capacity	700,000 heat units
Cooling rate (maximum)	150,000 heat units/min
Housing characteristics	
Heat capacity	1.75 million heat units
Cooling capacity with liquid circulation system (maximum)	150,000 heat units/min

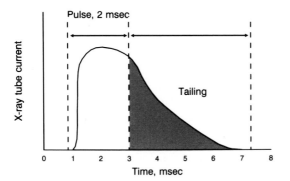

Figure 11.6. Secondary high-voltage electronic switching is often used to generate pulsed x-rays. The x-ray pulse produced in this manner has prolonged decay, the result of cable capacitance and varying x-ray tube current. (From Julsrud PR, Wondrow MA, Stears JG, et al. X-ray equipment. In: Holmes DR Jr, Vlietstra RE, eds. Interventional cardiology. Philadelphia: FA Davis, 1989:30–41. By permission of Mayo Foundation.)

the generator and x-ray tube, which must be charged and discharged during each exposure. Secondary electronic switching does not suffice for pulsed fluoroscopy or for cineangiography when the x-ray output per exposure is relatively small. To solve these problems, grid control of x-ray production may be preferred (Fig. 11.7). With this system the grid of the x-ray tube controls the length of the exposure. This eliminates prolongation of the x-ray rise and fall times at all exposure rates and pulse widths. A disadvantage of this design is that heat production is increased; these systems are more difficult to cool and thus may have shorter life expectancy and be more expensive.

Image Intensifier

The image intensifier converts an x-ray image into a visible light image. It is an evacuated bell-shaped glass tube or envelope that contains an input and an output phosphor. X-ray photons passing through the patient interact with the input phosphor, which produces light photons. These light photons are converted to electrons by the photocathode in the image intensifier to produce an electronic image. This image is focused by high-voltage potentials onto the output phosphor.

There have been major improvements in image intensifier technology (11, 14). Modern cesium iodide input phosphors and improved conversion factors allow lower cine exposure rates. The x-ray tube should deliver 20 to 40 μR per cine frame to the image intensifier in the 5- to 7-inch field of view, ideally at 75 to 85 kVp. Improved resolution has been achieved by use of columnar separation of phosphor crystals and low-absorption metallic input windows.

Veiling glare and detective quantum efficiency are important considerations that affect image intensifier performance. Veiling glare is caused by extraneous light from internal image intensifier light scatter; this extraneous light degrades the image. The use of gray glass at the output phosphor and fiberoptic coupling decreases veiling glare. Detective quantum efficiency is the efficiency with which the input phosphor absorbs x-ray photons. Improved detective quantum efficiency is characterized by a decrease in image noise at constant entrance exposure. Because keeping entrance x-ray exposure constant and low is important, im-

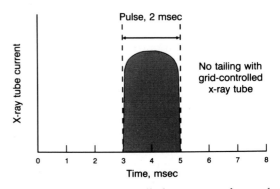

Figure 11.7. Grid-controlled system can be used to produce x-rays. A grid in the x-ray tube performs the switching. The high-voltage cables remain constantly charged. X-rays produced in this fashion have short duration and none of the tailing seen in Figure 11.6. With this system and progressive scanning a snapshot picture can be obtained. (From Julsrud PR, Wondrow MA, Stears JG, et al. X-ray equipment. In: Holmes DR Jr, Vlietstra RE, eds. Interventional cardiology. Philadelphia: FA Davis, 1989:30–41. By permission of Mayo Foundation.)

proved detective quantum efficiency has been achieved by finding an optimal cesium iodide input phosphor thickness. Although increasing the thickness of the input phosphor increases the absorption of x-rays, lateral light scatter is inversely proportional to input phosphor thickness. Therefore there must be a balance between increasing thickness to improve x-ray absorption and decreasing thickness to minimize lateral light scatter.

Contrast ratio is an important factor in assessing image quality. This ratio is measured by placing a lead disc in the x-ray field to block a portion of the field from radiation. The light level is measured in the blocked area. The ratio of the intensities measured with and without the lead disc in place is the contrast ratio. Both large-area and small-area contrast ratios are measured with a disc that covers either 10% of the input screen or a smaller area (10 mm). The contrast ratio should be at least 20:1.

As was true for pulse generators and x-ray tubes, image intensifiers can be rated with the information obtained from the manufacturers. The minimal specifications are shown in Table 11.3.

Optical Systems

The basic optical subsystem in an image chain consists of an objective lens and a camera lens. These lenses gather light generated in the image intensifier and focus it onto an image detector. To accomplish this the output screen of the image intensifier tube is located at the focal point of the objective lens. Therefore all light rays emerging from the objective lens are parallel. The camera lens collects the parallel light rays and forms an image at its focal plane.

Camera lenses of different focal lengths are available. The selection of the focal length depends on the degree of overframing used. Horizontal overframing is usually used to increase magnification and to eliminate marginal image area.

Optical systems are rated by their aperture size. Optical systems for cardiac imaging have apertures ranging from f-20 to f-75. The smaller the f-stop, the faster the lens. A fast lens with a large effective diameter allows more light to pass through it. However, the lens aperture determines the depth of the field, and if the aperture is large, the depth of the field in sharp focus is limited. As the aperture decreases, the range of image sharpness increases. If the f-stop is too small, however, more radiation is required to produce diagnostic images. Contrast and resolution can also be lost because of veiling glare in the optical subsystem. Use of an antireflective coating may minimize this.

Video Systems

The video system consists of a video camera, a monitor, and a recording system. These systems become more important as use of interventional procedures increases (15, 16). The ability to visualize the fine details of complex coronary anatomy is essential in planning and implementation of interventional procedures.

Video Camera

The television camera pickup tube is one of the most important components in the video chain. It consists of a target and an electron gun. The target itself has two layers, a photoconductive layer and a signal

Table 11.3.
Minimal Specifications for Image Intensifiers

Feature	Value
Input field size, inches (centimeters)	
Small	4.5 (11.4)
Medium	6.0 (15.2)
Large	9.0 (22.9)
Resolution, cycles/min	
Small field center	5.3
Medium field center	4.6
Large field center	4.0
Conversion factor	
Medium field	100
Contrast ratio	
Small area	20:1

plate. The metallic signal plate is applied to the inner surface of the faceplate. This layer must be thin enough to allow light photons to penetrate it but must be thick enough to hold an electrical charge. The photoconductive layer is applied to the signal plate. The electrical resistance of this layer changes in proportion to the intensity of the light transmitted through the signal plate. During operation the image from the output phosphor of the image intensifier is projected through the faceplate onto the target. The intensity of the light photons changes the resistance in the photoconductive layer. The electron gun beam scans the photoconductive layer, recharging the target to near equilibrium. The final video signal is proportional to the recharge current on the photoconductive layer.

Target material and design, faceplate, and gun structure determine the performance characteristics of the pickup tube. Important considerations include lag or image retention time, signal dynamic range, contrast, and sensitivity. Lag or image retention is the result of failure of the initial scan to neutralize the charge on the photoconductive layer completely. Minimal lag gives the sharpest image for viewing rapidly moving cardiac structures. Conventional Vidicon tubes are less efficient in neutralizing the charge on the photoconductive layer and thus have inherently more lag than Plumbicon tubes or tubes with newer target materials such as selenium arsenic tellurium (Saticon) and selenium tellurium arsenic (Primicon). These newer targets have the best lag characteristics: not more than 10% of the peak video signal in the third video field.

The signal dynamic range, a measure of image brightness, is expressed as the ratio of the logarithms of maximum brightness and minimum brightness. Contrast sensitivity also depends on target and faceplate design. Newer tubes have excellent contrast sensitivity in addition to good dynamic range and lag specifications.

In addition to lag, brightness, and noise, contrast is an important component of image quality. In the past the contrast in video systems has been higher than that with cine film. Current TV monitors have correction circuitry with extended dynamic range. These make the video image more similar to cine.

The widespread use of digital image processing allows dramatic improvements in image quality. With digital processing the video image can be zoomed and magnified. In addition, various filters can be used for edge enhancement and subtraction processing. Such systems have become essential in monitoring the outcome of interventional procedures on line and deciding what if any further treatments are required. It has become apparent that optimizing the initial result decreases the chance of acute complications and improves long-term results. Optimizing the initial result requires matching the correct device to the lesion, matching the correct device size to the arterial segment to be treated, and assessing the result, which should be a residual stenosis by measurement less than 20 to 30% for PTCA and less than 10% for stent implantation.

Image stabilization is as important during video imaging as during cine recording. Various approaches to this are available. Burnout, saturation, and blooming are specific problems, particularly during panning, when portions of the lung field are included in the field of view. During panning careful attention to minimizing the amount of lung in the field of view is essential. Use of radiation-absorbing filters also can help, particularly during digital image processing, when panning is not used but when there is overlap with the lung field. Automatic exposure and gain controls are useful. In addition, recent changes in amplifier design that prevent saturation may be helpful (13). These designs require adequate over-range capability in the pickup tube and preamplifier. An electron processing stage is used to compress the highlighted signals. In our system the video waveform is monitored and adjusted with a manual iris to give optimal images (Fig. 11.8) (22). Expert technical assistance is required for this approach to optimize the image.

A major factor affecting the optimal design of the video imaging system is selection of the video line rate. High–line rate (1024) systems have been given increasing attention, although few data compare 1024- and 525-line systems (23, 24). Some of the differences between these are subjective and

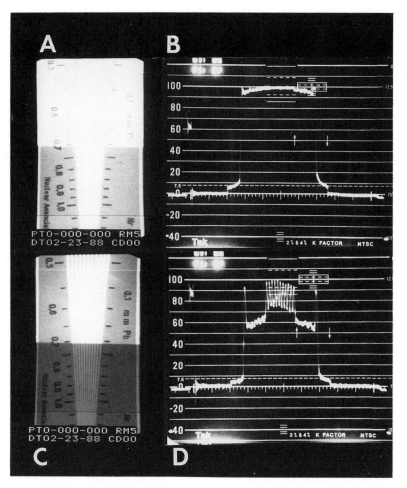

Figure 11.8. Adjustment of the video waveform is performed by an x-ray technician. Video image (**A**) and waveform (**B**) have improper manual iris settings and show saturation. The proper waveform and image are seen with optimal settings (**C** and **D**).

some are related to failure to optimize whichever system is in use (23). If a 1024-line system is used, the video bandwidth must be increased to keep vertical and horizontal resolutions equal: the video bandwidth must be 20 to 25 MHz compared with 10 to 15 MHz for a 525-line system. With this increase in video amplifier bandwidth, the signal-to-noise ratio falls significantly below the 45 to 50 dB recommended for cardiac imaging. In addition to a decrease in signal-to-noise ratio, quantum noise is more clearly seen and results in further image degradation. Some of this degradation is clearly subjective.

Upscan

Whether better visualization of the coronary arterial tree is achieved with a 525-line or 1024-line video image system is controversial. When a high-definition video acquisition system with a 525-line, 5-mHz bandwidth system was compared with a 1024-line, 10-mHz system, image degradation of low-contrast objects was documented with the 1024-line system (22, 23). This degradation was manifested by a noisier image caused by use of the 10-MHz bandwidth as opposed to the 5-MHz sys-

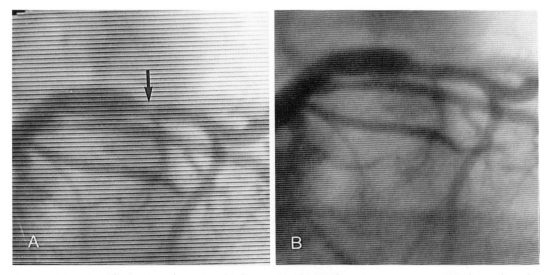

Figure 11.9. Magnified view of proximal left anterior descending coronary artery. With 525-line display (**A**), prominent raster lines obscure borders of stenosis (*arrow*); this was not a problem with the 1024-line display (**B**). (From Holmes DR Jr, Wondrow MA, Reeder GS, et al. Optimal display of the coronary arterial tree with an upscan 1,023-line video display system. Cathet Cardiovasc Diagn 1989; 18:175–180. Copyright 1989, Alan R. Liss. Reprinted by permission of Wiley-Liss, a division of John Wiley & Sons, Inc.)

tem, which significantly reduced both quantum and electronic noise. However, the raster lines of a 525-line display may interfere with the observer's perception of the image, particularly when the operator is close to the display monitor.

Electronic and computer advances allow for acquisition with the optimal 525-line progressively scanned image system and display of the image by upscanning to 1024 lines. The x-ray video signal generated by the video camera is filtered with a 6-MHz filter and digitized directly to produce a digital image (768 × 480 pixels with 256 [8

bit] gray level resolution) with an analog-to-digital converter. The image data are stored in a digital memory so that the memory read and write operations are independent and the images can be addressed separately. This digital technique provides for upscan capability, whereby each line of digital video data is read out of memory twice in one video frame time. The digital video data are converted to an analog video signal with a digital-to-analog converter at 256 (8 bit) gray level resolution for display on a high-resolution 1024-line video monitor. With this device a 525-line acquired video

Table 11.4.
Results of Assessment of Image Quality

Systems Compared	Best System	Investigator 1 Average Score	Investigator 1 P Value	Investigator 2 Average Score	Investigator 2 P Value
525-line display vs. 1023-line display	1023-line display	1.6	<.005	1.5	<.005
Video display (525- or 1023-line) vs. cine film	—	0.35	NSD[a]	0.25	NSD[a]

[a] NSD, no statistical difference.

frame is written to the high-resolution monitor as a field in a sixtieth of a second. During the following sixtieth of a second, the same image is once again written to the monitor, shifted so that it is placed between the scan lines of the previously written image. With this process an optimally acquired 525-line progressively acquired image can be displayed to produce a 1024-line interlaced display without the annoyance of raster lines.

In a study documenting this process the 525-line acquired and the 1024-line upscanned display were compared side by side on identical video monitors (Fig. 11.9). Cine images obtained during the same coronary injection were also compared with the video images. The results indicated that the upscan 1024-line display was better in image quality than the 525-line display. As seen in Table 11.4, with this system of acquisition and display there was also no statistical difference between this upscanned video and the cine image (25).

Results of this study indicate that the use of a high–line rate video system is an acquisition versus display issue. The use of upscan display allows image acquisition with a 525-line progressively scanned system and display in the 1024-line mode. The image quality of this system was judged better than that of the 525-line display and equal to that of state-of-art cineangiography.

Because important decisions in invasive cardiology are based increasingly on video images, these are important considerations. It is possible to obtain excellent images with a high-definition 525-line unit that achieves a signal-to-noise ratio of at least 45 dB (23). Newer video systems have the capability of both 525 and 1024 lines. The optimal configuration depends on the entire video image system. Our video system provides a 525-line EIA RS-170 signal with progressive scanning and a video bandwidth of 10 to 15 MHz (13, 22, 23, 26).

Progressive Versus Interlaced Scanning

Video fluoroscopy used interlaced scanning in the past (15, 16). This required radiation exposure at 60 x-ray pulses per second (pps). Each video frame is scanned from top to bottom in a thirtieth of a second. However, each frame is composed of two fields, each of which contains 262.5 horizontal lines. Alternate horizontal lines are scanned, starting with line 1 of the first field (Fig. 11.10). There is motion blurring because each frame is scanned twice. In the

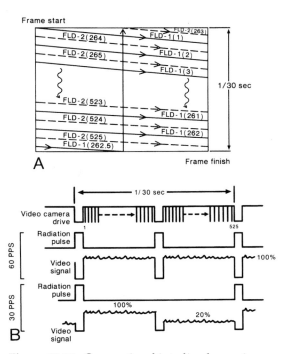

Figure 11.10. Conventional interlaced scanning. **A.** A 525-line video frame is scanned from top to bottom in a thirtieth of a second. Each frame is composed of two fields, each containing 262.5 horizontal lines. The starting point for scanning is line 1 of field 1 [FLD-1(1)]. The line scans from left to right on alternate lines until it reaches the middle of the image at the bottom [FLD-1(262.5)]. The scan then shifts back to the middle of the image at the top [FLD-2(263)]. For field 2 the remaining lines are scanned (*dashed lines*) to complete the frame. **B.** The radiation and video timing for interlaced scanning at 60 pps are shown in the second and third waveforms. If the radiation is pulsed at 30 pps (fourth waveform), image brightness is decreased. (From Holmes DR Jr, Bove AA, Wondrow MA, Gray JE. Video x-ray progressive scanning: new technique for decreasing x-ray exposure without decreasing image quality during cardiac catheterization. Mayo Clin Proc 1986;61:321–326. By permission of Mayo Foundation.)

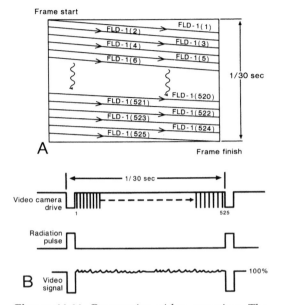

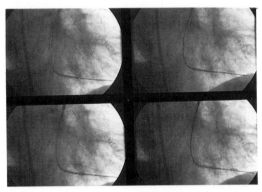

Figure 11.11. Progressive video scanning. The entire field is scanned in a thirtieth of a second. **A.** Each frame is composed of a single scan (field). **B.** Radiation can be pulsed at 30 pps with no degradation in image quality. (From Holmes DR Jr, Bove AA, Wondrow MA, Gray JE. Video x-ray progressive scanning: new technique for decreasing x-ray exposure without decreasing image quality during cardiac catheterization. Mayo Clin Proc 1986;61:321–326. By permission of Mayo Foundation.)

the advantages of improved image quality because it uses the short (3 to 5 milliseconds) snapshot mode, improved resolution because of the lack of interfield blurring that is inherent in interlaced scanning, and better signal-to-noise ratio than conventional interlaced scanning (Fig. 11.12). A major clinical advantage is that because 30 pps can be used, the radiation exposure is decreased by approximately 50% (Table 11.5). Progressive scanning can be used to enhance image quality for both cine and video recording. **Optimal decrease in radiation exposure and improvement in image quality are achieved with grid-biased x-ray generation** because of the short rectangular pulse waveform compared with the continuous wave from x-ray generators (Fig. 11.6 and 11.7). Various similar scanning systems have come into common use.

Video Monitor

The video image is becoming more important in the catheterization laboratory be-

Figure 11.12. Right anterior oblique images from a 74-kg patient undergoing dilation of the right coronary artery. The images were recorded at identical angles with interlaced scanning (*left*) and progressive scanning (*right*). Two distinct guidewires are seen with conventional recording. Because of the snapshot effect in progressive scanning, only a single wire is seen and image quality is improved. (From Holmes DR Jr, Bove AA, Wondrow MA, Gray JE. Video x-ray progressive scanning: new technique for decreasing x-ray exposure without decreasing image quality during cardiac catheterization. Mayo Clin Proc 1986;61:321–326. By permission of Mayo Foundation.)

past attempts were made to decrease the x-ray exposure by decreasing the x-ray pulses from 60 to 30 pps. This results in image degradation and increased flicker. With cine recording video flicker is also an annoyance at 30 frames per second.

One of the most important developments in cardiac imaging is progressive scanning (15, 16) (Fig. 11.11). This system is based on a different principle. A special video circuit sweeps the entire 525-line target once every 33.3 milliseconds. While the x-ray source is pulsed for 3 to 5 milliseconds, the image is written on the target. This specialized video signal is converted to standard video format by a real-time digital scan converter to produce a digital image (768 × 512 pixels with 256 [8-bit] gray level resolution). This image is then converted in real time to a composite standard EIA RS-170 video signal. Progressive scanning has

Table 11.5.
Radiation Entrance Exposure Rates at a Standard Vascular Phantom With Various Fluoroscopic X-Ray Systems

Mode	15-cm (6-in.) Image		23-cm (9-in.) Image	
	Rate, r/min[a]	Difference	Rate, r/min[a]	Difference
Conventional cineangiography at 60 pps	50.1	−52%	26.0	−53%
Cineangiography, progressive scanning at 30 pps	24.1		12.1	
Conventional fluoroscopy at 60 pps (30 fps)	3.7	−52%	1.3	−32%
Fluoroscopy, progressive scanning at 30 pps (30 fps)	1.78		0.88	

From Holmes DR Jr, Bove AA, Wondrow MA, Gray JE. Video x-ray progressive scanning: new technique for decreasing x-ray exposure without decreasing image quality during cardiac catheterization. Mayo Clin Proc 1986; 61:321–326. By permission of Mayo Foundation.
[a] 1 r = 0.258 mC/kg.
fps, frames per second.

cause it permits one to be certain that an adequate diagnostic study has been performed and it facilitates interventional procedures. **The configuration of the video monitor depends on the details of the laboratory suite and on personal preference.** The monitors should be as close as possible to the operator but not closer than 4 times the diagonal length of the monitor screen for optimal analysis and viewing. The stored freeze-frame video images should be displayed side by side with the live television images. In laboratories that use biplane video, a ceiling boom with four mounted video monitors may be optimal. The ability to move this along a ceiling support improves visualization. The video monitor should also be positioned so that the operator need not continually change visual field to see it. There is increasing concern about cervical disc disease in catheterization laboratory personnel. This may relate to angles of view required to see the video screen.

The video monitor displays the radiographic image in a visible form. It should be able to display all of the information acquired by the imaging chain and therefore should allow the operator to assess fine details of cardiac anatomy. This is true particularly for coronary interventions, during which decisions are based on the video images. The spatial resolution should match that of the imaging system and should have

a similar bandwidth (Table 11.6). The dynamic range should allow for reproduction of 10 levels of video gray scale. The monitor also should have circuitry that allows clamping of the black portion of the image to a reference level. The output phosphor used varies. We have found that a P-4 phosphor most closely matches the film color most physicians are accustomed to; it is the accepted standard.

Because video images are used to make important decisions, not only for diagnostic studies but even more important, also for interventional procedures, the video images must be clear. Quantum noise is an important consideration. **Quantum noise can be decreased by increasing radiation to the input phosphor of the image intensifier.** Because radiation exposure is usually less with fluoroscopy than with cine exposure and because quantum noise increases as the inverse of the square root of the exposure, fluoroscopic images may be noisier. With a manual video iris or an automatic brightness system in which the exposure rate behind the antiscatter grid is approximately 100 μR per second, fluoroimages can be optimized even over a wide range of patient sizes and angles of view.

Another approach to optimizing the fluoroscopic image is to increase the radiation exposure. A high-level control feature is available on many generators. This feature

Table 11.6.
Video Systems

Feature	Preferred Optimal
Video tube	
Type (e.g., vidicon, lead oxide vidicon, Plumbicon)	Plumbicon
Target voltage, V	45
Camera–video tube–amplifier chain	
Bandwidth, MHz at −3 dB	15
Signal-to-noise ratio (minimum), dB	50
Scan lines per frame	525
Shading correction	Yes
Gamma correction	No
Other signal processing (e.g., white clip or crush)	Extended dynamic range
Composite video signal, V	1.0
Sync pulse, V	0.3
RS-170 standard signal	Yes
Does video signal contain serrations and equalizing pulse?	Yes
AGC or ATC	AGC
Aspect ratio (e.g., 4:3, 1:1)	4:3
Pulsed progressive scanning	
X-ray pulsing, type	Grid-bias
Pulse width, msec	3–5
Frame rate/sec	30
Monitor	
Size (diagonal), in.	17–20
Bandwidth, MHz at −3 dB	15
Signal-to-noise ratio, dB	45
Black level clamping	Yes
Video tape recorder	
Format	1-in. type C (RS-170[2] 525 lines)
Bandwidth, MHz at −3 dB	5
Signal-to-noise ratio, dB	45

is variably known as fluoro boost, high contrast fluoro, image enhance, low noise, and turbo fluoro. This feature allows the operator of the x-ray equipment to produce fluoroscopic images without any limit on the x-ray exposure rate. The effect of changing x-ray exposure on image quality can be seen in Figure 11.13. At 64 mR it is not possible to see the details in the simulated 1- or 2-mm vessels. Details are readily visible at higher entrance exposure rates. Very high levels are unacceptable for procedures requiring many images. Recently a recommendation has been made to limit the maximum fluoroscopic exposure rate to 20 or perhaps 30 R per minute (typical fluoroscopic rates are approximately 2 R per minute, and cine exposure rates range from 15 to 30 R per minute). High-level control should be used only sparingly during procedures, not only to limit radiation exposure but also to avoid exceeding the heat load capacity of the x-ray tube if very high rates are used. All high-level control systems should have reset timers that draw attention to the increased exposure rates.

Video Recorder

Video disc, video cassette, and video tape recorders all are used. Video tape recorders range in format from 8-mm to 1-inch broadcast type. Minimal specifications for recording a 525-line video image include a bandwidth of 5 to 10 MHz and signal-to-noise ratio of 45 dB., Several factors must be kept in mind for optimal image recording: (*a*) sufficient bandwidth to reproduce the original image; (*b*) signal-to-noise ratio similar to that of the rest of the system; (*c*) precision

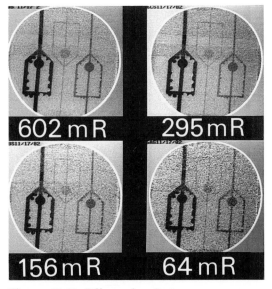

Figure 11.13. Effect of radiation exposure on image quality. At 64 mR, the fine details in the test pattern simulating 1- or 2-mm vessels are not distinct. At higher levels the details are apparent and the image is less noisy. (Photograph courtesy of Joel E. Gray, Ph.D.)

tracking during replay without misrepresentation; and (*d*) time base correction (22, 27, 28). This last feature allows absolute video registration. The ability to provide slow motion and freeze-frame without flicker or noise bars is also essential.

A broadcast standard helical scan 1-inch type C or digital D3 recorder is optimal. These have the bandwidth and signal-to-noise ratio sufficient to preserve the quality of the image. The image obtained with these recorders is similar to that of cine film.

Video disc recorders also can be used, particularly in combination with video tape recorders during interventional procedures. These devices, which can be used with either standard or high–line rate systems, operate with a signal-to-noise ratio of 40 to 45 dB and a bandwidth of 6 or 10 MHz.

QUALITY CONTROL

Quality control is an essential part of the operation of the catheterization laboratory. This includes preventive maintenance of the system, evaluation of proposed equipment additions, and continuing in-service education.

The aim of quality control is to obtain optimal cineangiograms at all times with the least possible radiation exposure. All parts of the system can be checked (Table 11.7). The effective kilovoltage, pulse width, and pulse waveform of the x-ray generator can change with time; these all can be monitored with a kilovoltage test device. The x-ray tube should be checked either at the factory (this is preferable) or after installation. The measured focal spot size should be compared with the manufacturer's specifications; a star resolution test pattern is used most frequently. In addition to the x-ray generator and tube, the x-ray beam collimation and filtration should be assessed. The collimator blades should be checked to see that they are just visible on the edge of the image.

An important area of quality control is the exposure rate. This must be measured periodically in all modes (Table 11.8). It should be measured under different conditions including direct readout with a dosimeter, with attenuators, and with a patient-equivalent phantom. Use of the phantom simulates clinical conditions and is helpful in evaluating patient entrance exposure rates.

The video imaging chain can be tested by viewing a resolution test target on the video display monitor (Fig. 11.14). In addition to resolution, the contrast and characteristics of the video signal are checked with either a waveform monitor or an oscilloscope. The waveform monitor is also used to measure the noise in the video image. The video viewing monitor also should be checked. For this the video signal generator is used. This has standard outputs so that the characteristics of the monitor, for example flat field resolution and gray scale, can be tested independently of the rest of the video imaging chain.

A final area of quality control is periodic testing of the cine film images. The focus characteristics of the image intensifier and optical lenses determine the sharpness of the cine images. This can be assessed with a step wedge and resolution pattern filmed as part of the identification marker at the

Table 11.7.
Quality Control Testing

Component Tested	Testing Frequency	Testing Equipment Used
Cine film processor	Daily	Sensitometer; densitometer
Cine film resolution	Daily	Visual assessment of resolution pattern
X-ray generator	Quarterly	kVp test device; high-voltage divider and oscilloscope
X-ray tube	Quarterly	Star resolution test pattern
Image intensifier	Quarterly	Assessed by observation of cine and video specification and recordings
Video system	Quarterly	Video signal generator; waveform monitor
Exposure rates	Quarterly	Dosimeter; half-value layer attenuator; patient-equivalent phantom
Cine projectors	Quarterly	Projection test film

start of each case. Other aspects of the cine film images deal with the cine film processor and cine projector, both of which need ongoing quality control assessment.

In addition to quality control, preventive maintenance with both mechanical and electrical inspection is essential for high-quality radiographic images, low numbers of equipment failures, early detection of failing equipment, and improved patient and operator safety.

IMAGE RECORDING AND STORAGE

Today 35-mm cine film remains the standard for recording and storage of coronary angiographic images. Depending on the specific circumstances, other modalities

may be used. For some pediatric cardiology applications large cut-film angiography is used in addition to cineangiography. For visualization of the details of the pulmonary arterial tree and thoracic aorta, cut film remains the standard medium. In addition, cut film is most commonly used for peripheral vascular angiography. Some coronary angiographic laboratories use 105-mm film in addition to 35-mm film. The 105-mm spot film images may be used as a permanent

Table 11.8.
Extrance Image Intensifier Exposure Rates

Modality	Exposure Rate, μR/Frame
Fluoroscopy	
6 in.	1–6
9 in.	0.5–2
Cine	
6 in.	25–35
9 in.	12–15
Video recording	
6 in.	16–30
9 in.	8–14

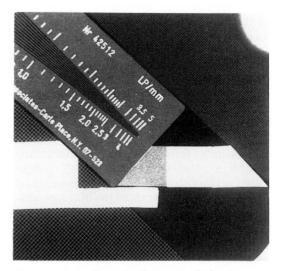

Figure 11.14. Cine resolution and density test pattern. (From Julsrud PR, Wondrow MA, Stears JG, Gray JE, Zahasky PE. X-ray equipment. In: Holmes DR Jr, Vlietstra RE, eds. Interventional cardiology. Philadelphia: FA Davis Company, 1986;30–41. By permission of Mayo Foundation.)

Table 11.9.
Cine Film

Advantages	Disadvantages
Industry standard	Capital costs
Unit record	Cine camera
Stable technology	Processor equipment
Longevity	Processor chemicals
Nondestructive	Developer personnel
	Storage
	Size
	Development processor
	dependent
	No postprocessing
	Data access delay

record in the patient's chart or sent to referring physicians for their records. In addition, the 105-mm spot film images may be useful in the operating room to remind the surgeons of the specific anatomy.

Cine Replacement (Digital Archiving) (29–32)

Cine filming techniques continue to play a major role in cardiovascular imaging (Table 11.9). However, cine film technology has remained virtually static. The needs of invasive cardiologists have changed with the advent of an increasing number of interventional cardiac procedures. Instant access to images during these procedures to assess outcome is essential. Cine filming does not meet these needs because of the requirements for development of the films, with its inherent delays. Another major factor is the relatively expensive medium and processing costs of cine film. In addition to the cost considerations, radiation exposure in the catheterization laboratory remains a significant problem. Cine film techniques use some of the highest levels of radiation in angiography, typically 15 to 70 R per minute. Reduction of radiation levels is important not only to the patient but also to the laboratory staff.

A final problem of cine filming is the inability to manipulate data after recording on the film, which prevents the use of computer techniques for image enhancement and quantification. A computer workstation can quantify the angiographic image and can indicate the extent of improvement after interventional procedures such as angioplasty. Densitometric analysis of cineangiograms is difficult because of variability of film processing, which can invalidate densitometric assessment and calibration. To overcome this problem some systems are configured to generate a video image from cine film; however, this technique is undesirable because image quality is lost when a video camera is coupled to the cine projector. Thus the image quality is poorer than that of the original video-generated images.

Because of these problems with cine film techniques, there has been great interest in replacing cine film, and requirements have been generated (Table 11.10). A number of alternatives explored in the early 1990s resulted in confusion and lack of standardization; they have been deemed the "Tower of Babel" (31). This resulted in some patients having coronary angiographic images recorded on substandard media, for example super VHS tape, so that the studies had to be repeated; in addition, some patients had angiographic studies performed on media that could not be reviewed at other institutions.

To address these problems, in 1992 the American College of Cardiology (ACC) (30, 32), American College of Radiology (ACR), and National Electrical Manufacturers Association (NEMA) began joint meetings. This group was later joined by the European Society of Cardiology (ESC). The goal of this working group was to plan and implement an approach to standardized cine film replacement. This complex procedure necessitates consideration of two main components: archive, or the ability to store images acquired during the angiographic study, and transport, or the ability to send or interchange the images within or outside of the institution where they are acquired. Cine film functioned both as an archive and the transport–interchange medium.

The committee focused on the latter, transport and interchange. This defined task has two components, the logical format, or the computer format by which information is laid down for subsequent retrieval and analysis, and the physical

Table 11.10.
Requirements for Cine Film Replacement

Absolute Requirements	Desirable Elements
Image quality equal to or better than cine	Low total costs relative to cine
Real-time motion reproduction ≥ 30 frames/sec	Modular components
Archive entire image run	Downloading time and cost efficiency
Patient unit record	Biplane recording
Off-line and random viewing access	Compatibility for playback images from other
Playback without time delay	diagnostic tests
Redundant transition capability	
Archival process that does not slow acquisition	

format, the actual medium. After a long series of meetings, the logical format selected was DICOM-3 (digital image communication in medicine), developed by the ACR for handling of radiographic images. Full implementation of this standard allows equipment from different manufacturers to transmit data; it also has potential for data to be integrated into hospital information systems (HIS) and radiology information systems (RIS).

Having settled on the logical format, the committee reviewed performance standards to be met for the physical format; both qualitative and quantitative requirements were evaluated. Availability, cost, potential for upward growth, and capacity were key features. After considerable deliberation, CD-R (compact disc, recordable) was chosen. This, the cine film of the future, is available now. This interchange medium has advantages as well as disadvantages but has been agreed on as the standard by ACC, ACR, ESC, and NEMA.

Other important aspects of cine film replacement have not yet been settled. Given the large amount of data in a coronary angiographic study, compression of data is an important consideration. It is commonly agreed that lossless compression (a mathematical formula that allows reconstruction of the full real data set) is optimal if compression is required. The other approach is lossy compression, which irretrievably loses data. At present a combined ACC–ESC study is being performed to evaluate whether compression affects decision making in evaluating coronary angiographic lesions. As computer and peripheral components continue to improve, the

need for compression may disappear. Compression may also affect quantitative coronary angiography. With conventional 512×512 systems, low-level lossless compression ratios may not affect results of quantitation coronary angiography; if systems evolve toward 1024×1024 approaches, compression may unfavorably affect results.

Although the ACC, ACR, NEMA, and ESC settled on the transport–interchange medium, it did not address the other essential part of cine film replacement, namely archiving. As previously mentioned, cine film functioned as both interchange and archive.

Archiving considerations, which include quantitative and qualitative issues, are very complex. They depend on the number of procedure rooms, case volume, need for interconnectivity between rooms, equipment from different manufacturers, the need for networking within an institution, and the rapidly changing technology. No single standard may be possible because of the variable requirements; each vendor will develop its own. Each system must be DICOM conformant and able to generate CD-R for interchange. A number of archival systems are available (Table 11.11). As previously discussed, super VHS videotape is inadequate and should not be considered. The other options are all being evaluated. For some smaller laboratories, CD-R and a manual or automatic library may be reasonable. Advancements in CD-R may enhance this option. For larger laboratories deep tape archival systems and an automatic tape library will be preferable. Continuing advances in the speed and capacity of digital

**Table 11.11.
Archival Media**

Super VHS videotape
Analog optical disk
D2 Digital videotape
8 mm Exabyte tape
CD-R
New modalities
   Compact tape archive
   IBM NTP
   Sony DTF
   Dec DLT
   DVD

tape will continue to make this an attractive option. Other options include large-capacity optical discs. A goal for catheterization laboratory archiving should be that a single archival system should serve the entire laboratory; that is, irrespective of how many vendors in a laboratory, there should be only a single archive. Otherwise a laboratory may have several archival systems, which would be less than satisfactory. No archival system will last as long as the cine standard did; computer improvements will render current archival systems more or less obsolete within approximately 10 years, whereas cine film lasted as a standard for 25 years.

A final important issue of cine film replacement is that of workstations that will of necessity change because of the shift to CD-R. Several workstations being developed and evaluated have variable complexity to allow the cardiologist options from basic viewing of the angiographic images to complex quantitative analysis. It is to be hoped that these complex work stations will also allow evaluation of images from other sources, such as fast cine computed tomography, echocardiographic studies, and magnetic resonance imaging.

RADIATION SAFETY (33, 34)

Radiation safety becomes increasingly important as the catheterization laboratory becomes more therapeutic. Coronary interventions are associated with increased radiation exposure because of longer fluoroscopy times, steep angulation, the system configurations with C and U arms and the use of high–dose rate, high-resolution systems to visualize the fine details of stent placement. These issues are magnified in interventional electrophysiology, when procedures may take several hours. Radiation skin damage following interventional procedures has been well documented. The magnitude of this problem is underreported because most radiation effects are not seen during hospitalization. In addition, it is difficult for the patient to evaluate mild radiation skin effects because they occur on the back when they present as erythema, and desquamation early and the potential for dermal atrophy and/or fibrosis late. Ulceration is extremely uncommon.

Data on specific radiation exposure are relatively limited. Dash and Leaman (33) found that mean cineangiographic times are similar for PTCA and diagnostic coronary angiography. However, fluoroscopy time is substantially longer. This prolonged fluoroscopy time resulted in a mean radiation exposure for PTCA procedures of 17 mrad per case per operator, compared with 9 mrad per case for routine coronary angiography. Overall there was a 93% increase in exposure of the operator to radiation. There is obviously also increased radiation exposure to patients during PTCA. Cascade et al. (34), using patient dosimeter probes, found that the average radiation exposure was 20 plus or minus 16 R for coronary angiography and 69 plus or minus 61 R for PTCA procedures. When procedures were attempted on two lesions, radiation exposure was significantly greater than when one lesion was involved (100 R compared with 47 R). As increased numbers of multivessel dilations and stenting are performed, this increased exposure has become more pronounced. These procedures with higher radiation exposure have important implications affecting not only physicians but also paramedical persons and patients.

In a study of the effect of new devices on radiation exposure, Federman et al. (41) found that on patients treated for single coronary arterial stenoses the duration of radiation exposure was not longer with directional coronary atherectomy, excimer laser, or elective stent placement as a stand-alone procedure than with conventional PTCA. However, when more than one procedure is performed, if there is a complication, or if multiple lesions are treated, there is a marked increase in radiation exposure. In addition, chronic total occlusion takes longer and entails more radiation exposure (42).

Although at present **coronary angiographic studies can be performed only with radiation exposure, exposure should be limited as much as possible.** The goal is to attain a dose as low as reasonably achievable (ALARA). The radiation risk to operators is low but is cumulative over a professional lifetime. The National Council on Radiation Protection and Measurement (NCRP) publishes guidelines on occupational effective dose received by radiation workers and recommends that it be limited to less than 10 m Sv (Sievert) per year (38).

The issue of radiation safety and protection is multifaceted. The potential for stray radiation is substantial. It has two sources: leakage from the x-ray tube and scatter from the patient. The radiographic equipment must be checked according to the preventive maintenance specifications to determine whether it is operating within accepted limits. **The goal is to deliver optimal images with the least amount of radiation.** Essential components are exposure rate, distance, exposure time, and shielding. The operators and room personnel should wear adequate shielding aprons, thyroid collars, and leaded glasses. For personnel who are exposed to radiation to the back—for example, technicians who are turned away from the imaging equipment—wraparound aprons are essential. The many kinds of equipment shields range from movable, free-wheeling full-length shields to ceiling-mounted clear shields and various lead beads (35). All of these can significantly decrease radiation exposure, but only if they are used routinely and properly. Careful avoidance of unneeded x-ray exposure is also essential. If the x-ray foot switch is turned on only when necessary, radiation exposure can be minimized.

Using last image hold and instant replay can reduce dose considerably. Proper columnation with shutters, using the largest field size possible (e.g., 7 versus 5 inches), ensuring that the distance from source to image is as low as possible, and optimizing the working angle are all essential. Steep caudal angulation markedly increases radiation exposure to the physicians. One of the most important considerations is distance. Because radiation exposure to the operator decreases by the square of the distance, the physician and technical people should position themselves as far as possible from the patient, although easy rapid access to the patient is essential.

Finally, improvements in video techniques, for example progressive scanning, can also significantly reduce x-ray exposure by changing x-ray pulsing from 60 to 30 pps. We evaluated the effect of this system on radiation exposure. During 3 years in our institution the caseload per physician increased by 63% and the number of coronary angioplasty procedures increased by 244%; despite these increases in both caseload and higher-radiation procedures, the coverage radiation exposure per physician decreased by 37% (43).

Every effort must be made to ensure that exposures to ionizing radiation are as low as reasonably achievable. Although the risk of development of a malignancy from exposure to ionizing catheterization radiation is low, it is cumulative. Given the repeated procedures that patients undergo, for example, for evaluation and treatment of restenosis and the prolonged procedure with either complex multivessel dilation or electrophysiologic ablation, exposure may be substantial. Similarly, lifetime exposures may be substantial for physicians and technicians in the cardiac laboratory. In addition to shielding and pulsed progression fluoroscopy, other procedures that may help include increasing the x-ray tube filtration, which reduces the soft radiation reaching the patient, and modification of the x-ray equipment to allow removal of the antiscatter grid during some prolonged fluoro procedures.

SUMMARY

Cardiovascular imaging is changing rapidly in response to the demands of the practice of interventional cardiology as well as the rapid advances in computer technology. The groundwork for cine film replacement has been laid, and the logical format and physical interchange medium selected and standardized. Remaining issues include the need for compression, specific compression ratio, identification of optimal archival approaches, and development of sophisticated workstations. In addition, networking strategies connecting catheterization laboratory databases with other satellites and with hospital information and radiology information systems must be developed and matured. With these changes cardiovascular imaging will become more multifaceted and sophisticated, with the potential to optimize outcome in an expanding number of patients and clinical settings.

References

1. Ellis SG and Holmes DR. Strategic approaches in coronary intervention. Baltimore: Williams & Wilkins, 1996.
2. Sewart U, Bertrand M, Serruys PW: Handbook of cardiovascular interventions. New York: Churchill Livingstone, 1996.
3. Topol EJ. Textbook of interventional cardiology. Philadelphia: WB Saunders, 1993.
4. Reiber JHC, Serruys PW. New development in quantitative coronary arteriography. Rotterdam: Kluver Academic, 1988.
5. Bell MR, Britson PJ, Chu A. Validation of a new Unix-based quantitative coronary angiographic system for the measurement of coronary artery lesions. In press.
6. Herrington DM, Siebes M, Sokol DK, et al. Variability in measures of coronary lumen dimensions using quantitative coronary angiography. J Am Coll Cardiol 1993;22:1068–1074.
7. Hausleiter J, Nolte CWT, Jost S, et al. Comparison of different quantitative coronary analysis systems: ARTREK, CAAS, and CMS. Cathet Cardiovasc Diagn 1996;37:14–22.
8. Keane D, Haase J, Slager CJ, et al. Comparative validation of quantitative coronary angiography systems: results and implications from a multicenter study using a standardized approach. Circulation 1995;91:2174–2183.
9. Reiber JH, van der Zwet PMJ, Koning G, et al. Accuracy and precision of quantitative digital coronary arteriography: observer-, short-, and medium-term variabilities. Cathet Cardiovasc Diagn 1993;28:187–198.
10. Haase J, van der Linden MM, Di Mario C, et al. Can the same edge-detection algorithm be applied to on-line and off-line analysis systems? Validation

of a new cine film–based geometric coronary measurement software. Am Heart J 1993;126:312–321.
11. Thompson TT, ed. A practical approach to modern imaging equipment. 2nd ed. Boston: Little, Brown, 1985.
12. Gray JE, Winkler NT, Stears J, Frank ED. Quality control in diagnostic imaging: a quality control cookbook. Baltimore: University Park Press, 1983.
13. Julsrud PR, Wondrow MA, Stears JG, et al. X-ray equipment. In: Holmes DR Jr, Vlietstra RE, eds. Interventional cardiology. Philadelphia: FA Davis, 1989:30–41.
14. Friesinger GC, Adams DF, Bourassa MG, et al. Optimal resources for examination of the heart and lungs: cardiac catheterization and radiographic facilities; examination of the chest and cardiovascular system study group. Circulation 1983;68:893A-930A.
15. Holmes DR Jr, Bove AA, Wondrow MA, Gray JE. Video x-ray progressive scanning: new technique for decreasing x-ray exposure without decreasing image quality during cardiac catheterization. Mayo Clin Proc 1986;61:321–326.
16. Wondrow MA, Bove AA, Holmes DR Jr, et al. Technical consideration for a new x-ray video progressive scanning system for cardiac catheterization. Cathet Cardiovasc Diagn 1988;14:126–134.
17. Aldridge HE. A decade or more of cranial and caudal angled projections in coronary arteriography: another look. Cathet Cardiovasc Diagn 1984;10:539–542 (editorial).
18. Lespérance J, Saltiel J, Petitclerc R, Bourassa MG. Angulated views in the sagittal plane for improved accuracy of cine coronary angiography. Am J Roentgenol Radium Ther Nucl Med 1974;121:565–574.
19. Balter S, Sones FM Jr, Brancato R. Radiation exposure to the operator performing cardiac angiography with U-arm systems. Circulation 1978;58:925–932.
20. Holmes DR Jr, Bove AA, Nishimura RA, et al. Comparison of monoplane and biplane assessment of regional left ventricular wall motion after thrombolytic therapy for acute myocardial infarction. Am J Cardiol 1987;59:793–797.
21. Cohn PF, Gorlin R, Adams DF, et al. Comparison of biplane and single plane left ventriculograms in patients with coronary artery disease. Am J Cardiol 1974;33:1–6.
22. Gray JE, Wondrow MA, Smith HC, Holmes DR Jr. Technical considerations for cardiac laboratory high-definition video systems. Cathet Cardiovasc Diagn 1984;10:73–86.
23. Holmes DR Jr, Smith HC, Gray JE, Wondrow MA. Clinical evaluation and application of cardiac laboratory high-definition video systems. Cathet Cardiovasc Diagn 1984;10:63–71.
24. Haendle H, Horbaschek HH, Alexandrescu M. High resolution x-ray television and the high-resolution video recorder. Electromedica 1977;3:83–91.
25. Holmes DR Jr, Wondrow MA, Reeder GS, et al. Optimal display of the coronary arterial tree with an upscan 1,023-line video display system. Cathet Cardiovasc Diagn 1989;18:175–180.
26. EIA Standard RS-170. Electrical performance standards: monochrome television studio facilities.

Washington: Electronics Industries Association, 1957.

27. Hathaway RA, Ravizza R. Development and design of the Ampex auto scan tracking (AST) system. J Soc Motion Picture Television Eng 1980;89: 931–934.

28. Fibush DK. SMPTE type-C helical scan recording format. J Soc Motion Picture Television Eng 1978; 87:775–760.

29. Holmes DR Jr, Wondrow MA, Gray JE. Isn't it time to abandon cine film? Cathet Cardiovasc Diagn 1990;20:1–4 (editorial).

30. ACC/ACR/NEMA Ad Hoc Group. American College of Cardiology, American College of Radiology and industry develop standard for digital transfer of angiographic images. J Am Coll Cardiol 1995; 25:800–802.

31. Nissen SE, Pepine CJ, Bashore TM, et al. Cardiac angiography without cine film: erecting a 'Tower of Babel' in the cardiac catheterization laboratory. J Am Coll Cardiol 1994;24:834–837.

32. Condit PB. Requirements for cardiac interchange media and the role of recordable CD. Int J Card Imaging 1995;11(suppl 3):153–157.

33. Dash H, Leaman DM. Operator radiation exposure during percutaneous transluminal coronary angioplasty. J Am Coll Cardiol 1984;4:725–728.

34. Cascade PN, Peterson LE, Wajszczuk WJ, Mantel J. Radiation exposure to patients undergoing percutaneous transluminal coronary angioplasty. Am J Cardiol 1987;59:996–997.

35. Gertz EW, Wisneski JA, Gould RG, Akin JR. Improved radiation protection for physicians performing cardiac catheterization. Am J Cardiol 1982; 50:1283–1286.

36. Handbook of selected tissue doses for fluoroscopic and cine angiographic examination of the coronary arteries. U.S. Department of Health and Human Services: HHS Publication FDA 1995:8289.

37. Johnson LW, Moore RJ, Balter S. Review of radiation safety in the cardiac catheterization laboratory. Cathet Cardiovasc Diagn 1992;25:186–1942.

38. National Council on Radiation Protection and Measurements. NCRP Report 116: limitation of exposure to imaging radiation. 1993.

39. Wu JR, Huang TY, Wu DK, et al. Radiation exposure of pediatric patients and physicians during cardiac catheterization and balloon pulmonary valvuloplasty. Am J Cardiol 1991;68:221–225.

40. National Council on Radiation Protection and Measurements. NCRP Report 107: implementation of the principle of as low as reasonably achievable (ALARA) for medical and dental personnel. 1990.

41. Federman J, Bell MR, Wondrow MA, et al. Does the use of new intracoronary interventional devices prolong radiation exposure in the cardiac catheterization laboratory? J Am Coll Cardiol 1994; 23:347–351.

42. Bell MR, Berger PB, Menke KK et al. Balloon angioplasty of chronic total coronary artery occlusion: what does it cost in radiation exposure, time, and materials? Cathet Cardiovasc Diagn 1992;25:10–15.

43. Holmes DR, Wondrow MA, Gray JE, et al. Effect of pulsed progressive fluoroscopy on reduction or radiation dose in the cardiac catheterization laboratory. J Am Coll Cardiol 1990;15:1:159–162.

12

Digital Angiography: Principles and Clinical Applications

Steven E. Nissen MD

INTRODUCTION

Since its introduction to the cardiac catheterization laboratory in 1982, digital angiography has grown steadily in importance. Although initially used only for review of angiograms during catheterization procedures, digital imaging has expanded in recent years to encompass both long-term archiving and network communication of angiographic studies (1–4). The expanding role of digital angiography reflects several of its inherent advantages. Digital angiography is unsurpassed as a means of immediate access to high-quality images during diagnostic or therapeutic catheterization, a feature that unquestionably improves the speed and efficiency of the operator. In recent years the value of digital angiography has been enhanced by the increasing importance of percutaneous interventions in clinical practice. During the era of diagnostic catheterization, operators were content to review films at a time of convenience, often minutes or hours following the procedure. However, in the setting of angioplasty, the instantaneous review provided by digital angiography has become an integral and indispensable feature of the modern catheterization laboratory. Accordingly, virtually all interventional laboratories have digital angiographic equipment and only a few diagnostic-only suites still lack it.

A working knowledge of the principles of digital angiography is essential to the safety and technical quality of catheterization. Cardiologists are often called on to determine the equipment configuration and vendor of choice for a digital catheterization laboratory. Indeed, most experts predict that digital imaging will replace both film and video recording systems during the next few years. Accordingly, invasive cardiologists must be reasonably familiar with the design and operational principles of digital imaging systems. However, most cardiovascular specialists receive little formal training in the principles underlying computer imaging techniques. This chapter is intended to introduce the practitioner to digital imaging in the catheterization laboratory and to prepare the reader to determine the optimal equipment for configuring a laboratory.

PRINCIPLES OF DIGITAL IMAGING

Image Acquisition

Current digital imaging systems employ a conventional television camera for image acquisition. Many laboratories record both cine film and digital angiography, employing the digital images primarily for in-room

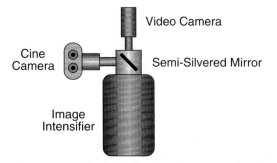

Figure 12.1. The light distribution system for simultaneous acquisition of cine film and digital angiography. A semisilvered mirror divides the light output of the image intensifier into two pathways. Typically 80 to 90% of the light is provided to the cine camera and 10 to 20% to the video camera.

guidance of the procedure. Film is used principally as a long-term archive but also functions as an exchange medium to allow other practitioners to review catheterization images. Simultaneous digital and cine film angiography are made possible through the use of a semisilvered mirror that divides into two parallel pathways the visible image formed on the output phosphor of the image intensifier (Fig. 12.1). Digital angiography systems usually provide 80 to 90% of the light output to cine film and 10 to 20% to the video camera. This unequal division is necessary because of the relative insensitivity of the cine film emulsions to visible light in comparison with modern video cameras. Contrary to a common misperception, this unequal light distribution does not materially influence image quality for either film or video-based techniques, because each device is operating efficiently within its normal range of sensitivity.

In a television camera the video signal is generated by an electron beam that scans a photoconductive material in the **target** of the video camera. The scanning results in a current that flows through a conductive **signal plate** in the camera. Circuitry in the video camera amplifies the current to produce a signal in which the voltage is proportional to the brightness of each point in the image. The camera scans the angiographic image to form a series of **raster lines** using one of two scanning patterns, **interlaced** or **progressive** (Fig. 12.2). Interlaced scanning generates 30 frames per second, each consisting of two **fields** of alternating scan lines obtained a sixtieth of a second apart, and progressive scan forms all lines of the image each thirtieth of a second. The number of raster lines, typically either 525 or 1024, is determined by the design of the video camera. In some cameras both modes are available.

The human eye has a **flicker fusion frequency** of 40 to 60 Hz (cycles per second). Therefore, images refreshed at 30 Hz appear to flicker, and images displayed at 60 Hz will appear smooth and continuous. Because interlaced video refreshes half the raster lines each sixtieth of a second, the annoying flicker is suppressed. In the initial development of digital imaging, nearly all acquisition systems used 525-line interlaced video, an approach identical to the scanning method used for broadcast television. Interlaced video was selected as the standard for broadcast television because it eliminates flicker while requiring the transmission of only half the data needed for 60-Hz progressive scan video. However, interlaced video has significant disadvantages for digital cardiac imaging, principally because images are composed of two fields separated in time by a sixtieth of a second (16 milliseconds). The right coronary can move across the image faster than 50 mm per second, resulting in unacceptable motion blur. Accordingly, nearly all digital imaging systems now employ progressive scan video cameras but avoid flicker by synthesizing an interlaced image during replay or using progressive scan faster than 60 Hz.

Several important characteristics of the video camera can be controlled by the designers of digital imaging systems. One important feature is **lag**, the persistence of the image on the target of the video camera. During fluoroscopy a very low radiation exposure results in images with considerable **quantum noise.** Video cameras with longer lag characteristics take advantage of image persistence to smooth the quantum noise prevalent during fluoroscopy. This approach is acceptable because still frames of fluoroscopy are rarely viewed for clinical diagnosis. However, for digital and cine film angiography, still-frame images are

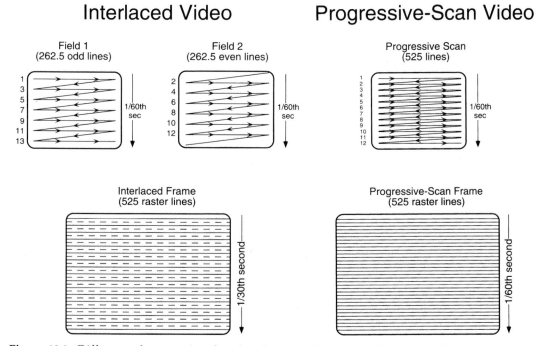

Figure 12.2. Differences between interlaced and progressive scan video. Interlaced video (*left panel*) is composed of two fields separated in time by a sixtieth of a second. Progressive scan video (*right panel*) reproduces all 525 lines in a single pass.

commonly reviewed, and excessive camera lag results in motion blur or double (ghost) images. Accordingly, the most sophisticated digital systems electronically control camera lag to optimize performance for both applications. During fluoroscopy the camera uses moderately long lag to smooth quantum noise, but during digital angiography the camera is electronically altered to produce low lag.

During coronary cineangiographic imaging, **pulse-mode** x-ray is employed to freeze coronary motion. Current digital systems electronically synchronize camera scanning with film transport to let each x-ray pulse simultaneously expose cineangiography and digital frames.

Analog-to-Digital Conversion

The principles underlying digital recording of video-generated images are relatively simple. The video camera output consists of an analog signal in which the voltage of the video signal is proportional to the brightness of each point in the raster line. For digital angiography the voltage-modulated video signal is **digitized** using an **analog-to-digital converter** consisting of a computer chip that samples the video signal and assigns a numeric value to the intensity (voltage). Because computers work in binary numbers, the number of possible gray levels is determined by the number of **bits** available for analog-to-digital conversion. In cardiac digital angiography this is typically 8 bits (1 **byte**), which in binary numbers corresponds to 256 possible gray levels. The digital representation of the original analog signal consists of a series of discrete steps that exhibit **quantitation error** (Fig. 12.3).

Resolution and Gray Scale

Mathematical calculations of the anticipated quantum statistical noise indicate that

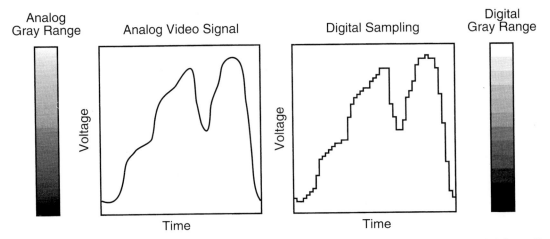

Figure 12.3. Differences between analog and digital video signals. The analog video signal (*left panel*) represents the gray range continuously so that the amplitude of the voltage is proportioned to the image brightness. Digital video is produced by sampling the analog video signal to yield a representation that consists of a series of discrete steps (*right panel*). The difference between the analog and digital signals is known as quantitation error.

an 8-bit gray scale (256 levels) is adequate for the typical exposures of 20 to 25 μR per frame used for coronary angiography. Thus for coronary angiography 256 gray levels are sufficient to render quantitation error clinically negligible. However, during certain critical imaging procedures, particularly the high-exposure techniques employed for peripheral vascular angiography, 10 or more bits of gray scale may be required to maintain image fidelity.

The horizontal and vertical sampling rates of the digital-to-analog converter determine the **matrix size** of the digital image (Fig. 12.4). Most systems for cardiac angiography generate 512 horizontal and 512 vertical samples, each called a picture element, or **pixel.** The **resolution** of the digital image is determined by the number of pixels, typically ranging from 256 rows by 256 columns (64,000 pixels) to 1024 × 1024 (more than 1 million pixels). As noted previously, coronary angiography is most commonly digitized at 8 bits per pixel (256 gray levels). Thus cardiac digital angiography most often consists of a 512 × 512 pixel acquisition with 1 byte gray scale per pixel.

This 512 × 512 matrix size is slightly below the optimum necessary to capture all the spatial information available from the best image intensifiers. At a 512 × 512 ma-

trix, the digital system generates 3.4 pixels per millimeter for a 15-cm (6 inch) field of view. However, a top-quality intensifier may resolve four to five line pairs per millimeter, and at least two pixels are required to reproduce each line pair. Thus a 512 × 512 digital image probably slightly undersamples the available diagnostic information. Accordingly, a strong and growing trend in system design is to replace 512 × 512 with 1024 × 512 or 1024 × 1024 matrices for digital coronary angiography.

Data Storage Requirements

The quantities of data generated by cardiac digital angiography are enormous. A single image at a 512 × 512 pixel matrix with an 8-bit gray scale contains 262,144 bytes of data (262 **kilobytes** [KB]) that must be stored in the computer (Table 12.1). Since full-motion imaging is typically performed at 30 frames per second, digital coronary angiography generates 30 × 262 KB per second, or about 7.5 million bytes (7.5 **megabytes** [MB]) of data per second. Thus an 8-second coronary injection requires about 60 MB and a full angiographic study in a single patient may

Table 12.1.
Data Requirements for Digital Storage of Cardiac Catheterization Images

Resolution	Single Image	8-sec Injection	Full Study
512 × 512	262 KB	63 MB	500 MB
1024 × 1024	1 MB	250 MB	2 GB

require up to 1 billion bytes (1 **gigabyte** [GB]) of data.

For a laboratory performing 1000 procedures annually, complete archiving of all angiographic studies would require storing approximately 1000 gigabytes (1 **terabyte)** of data. Because of these requirements, in current practice digital angiographic images are usually stored temporarily on a computer hard disk to enable immediate replay and review. In this application the size of the hard disk determines the capacity of the digital imaging system, typically 2500 to 25,000 images (2 to 14 complete patient studies). Unless digital long-term archiving is intended, the images recorded on the computer hard disk are erased within hours or days to make room for subsequent studies. In laboratories employing digital long-term storage, images recorded on the hard disk are transferred to another medium for archiving, a function usually performed between cases or at the end of the working day.

As noted previously, some digital imaging systems employ video cameras and monitors with 1024-line capability (high line rate video) and digitize the video signal at 1024 × 1024 × 8-bit resolution. Because the output monitor displays 1024 scan lines, not 525, the unpleasant effect of visible raster lines is significantly reduced. Despite several important advantages, 1024 digital systems do not yield images with twice the

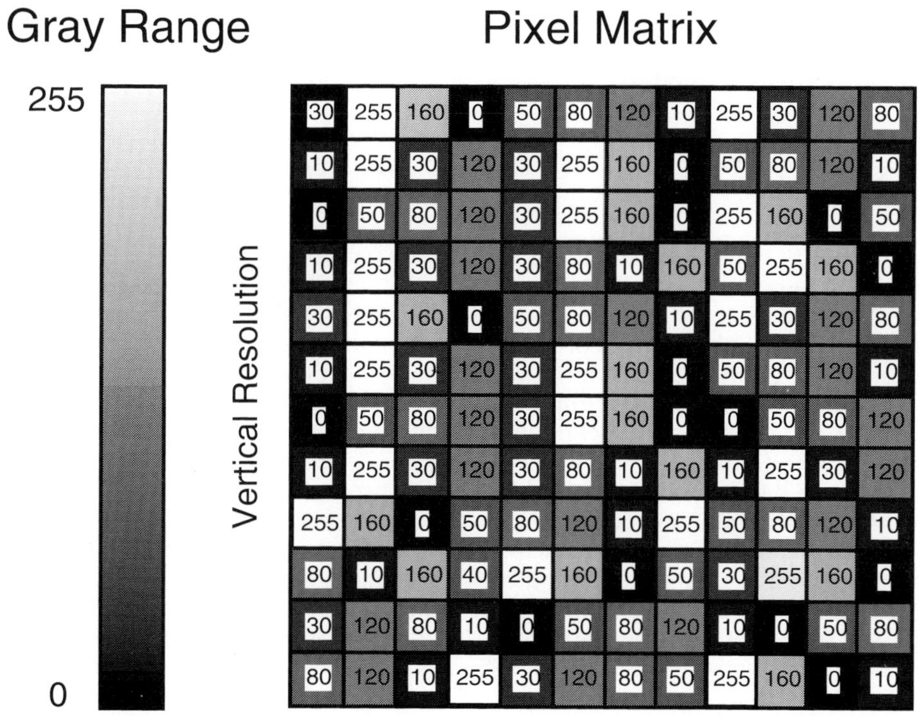

Figure 12.4. Schematic representation of digital imaging matrix. The image is divided into a series of picture elements (pixels). In typical coronary angiography the density of each pixel is represented with 256 discrete gray values (8 bits). The typical pixel matrix is 512 horizontal and 512 vertical pixels.

spatial resolution of 525-line systems. This disparity occurs because the low radiation doses used for cardiac imaging result in an image significantly degraded by quantum statistical noise. Accordingly, not all the potential for increased resolution (at 1024 matrix) translates into a usable improvement in image quality. In addition, high–line rate video cameras often generate more electronic noise than 525-line systems.

Several factors have limited the application of 1024 matrix digital imaging, most notably the increased storage requirements. Digital angiography at 1024 matrix requires four times as much data capacity as a 512 matrix. A compromise strategy for improving image quality is employed by several equipment vendors: the image is stored in a 512 matrix but displayed in the laboratory on a 1024-line monitor (**interpolated upscanning**). The visible effect of raster lines is suppressed, but the data storage requirements are identical to those of 512 matrix imaging. As computer storage technology evolves, it is likely that true 1024 matrix acquisition will eventually replace upscanning techniques, although the improvement in image quality will be modest.

Data Compression

The huge quantity of data storage required for digital angiography limits the number of images that can be stored cost-effectively on available computer hard disks or archival media. However, the numeric format of digital angiography is an ideal setting for application of data compression techniques. Nearly all current digital angiographic systems employ a compression algorithm, most commonly **Huffman encoding.** Huffman compression relies on the principle that many pixels have certain common gray values and that the gray value of a pixel is often similar to that of neighboring pixels. Hence some redundancy is produced by storing a full 8 bits to represent the gray value for each pixel. Huffman encoding reduces the number of stored bits by coding these common redundant values with fewer bits of data. Huffman encoding is **lossless;** that is, images compressed and decom-

pressed using this method are visually identical. Although the data storage required for each image is reduced, the numeric value for each pixel in the decompressed image is unchanged. The major limitation of Huffman coding is the modest degree of compression produced, typically not more than about 2.6 to 1.

Recent advances in computer technology have enabled much higher degrees of data compression with good to excellent image quality. These techniques are **lossy;** there is a measurable difference between original image and one that has been compressed and decompressed. The most important lossy compression technique was developed by an international committee, the Joint Photographic Experts Group (JPEG). The JPEG compression algorithm has been adopted for many computer and imaging applications outside of medicine and is beginning to achieve some popularity in medical imaging. Although lossy, JPEG encoding produces more compression than the Huffman method with minimal visible reduction of image quality at low compression ratios. The compression is variable, allowing system designers to determine the degree of image alteration acceptable for a given application.

The precise mathematics of JPEG compression are beyond the scope of this chapter, but it does not reduce the sharpness or contrast of compressed images. The most important compression step is performed on a subunit of the image consisting of small blocks of pixels, usually an 8×8 matrix. At low compression ratios (less than 4:1), when JPEG is used to encode coronary angiography, most observers cannot detect differences between compressed and uncompressed images, even in side-by-side comparisons (Fig. 12.5). At moderate compression ratios (less than 10:1), the only change in image content is a subtle shifting of gray values and occasionally a more objectionable artifact in which the 8×8 blocks become visible. At much higher compression ratios, visible deterioration in image quality is often evident.

A multicenter study organized by the American College of Cardiology (ACC) and European Society of Cardiology (ESC) is evaluating whether JPEG compression is

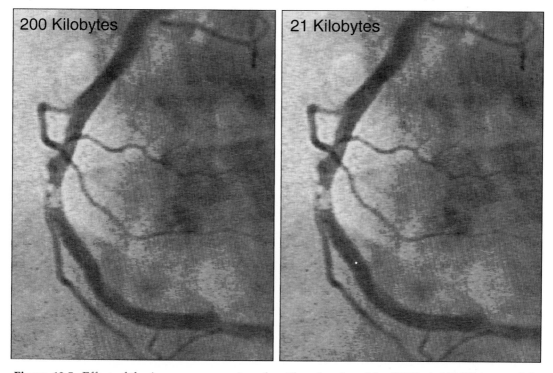

Figure 12.5. Effect of the image compression algorithm developed by JPEG. A 200-KB image (*left panel*) is reduced to 21 KB (*right panel*) with no apparent loss of image quality.

suitable for recording digital angiography, network transmission, or long-term archiving of images. If lossy compression is clinically acceptable, this approach is likely to accelerate the transition to filmless angiography and 1024 matrix recording by reducing the storage requirement to one-eighth or less, enabling large savings in the cost and bulk of storage media. Furthermore, compressed images could be transmitted to nearby or remote locations much faster than uncompressed images.

ADVANTAGES OF DIGITAL IMAGING

High-Speed Random Access Storage

Although the storage requirements are formidable, several practical advantages have prompted widespread acceptance of digital

angiography in the catheterization laboratory. Unlike film or video recording, digital angiography provides high-quality coronary images for immediate review during the procedure. Digital angiography allows the operator to examine the results of each contrast injection before proceeding to the next. During diagnostic angiography the immediate availability of images improves the confidence of the operators that they have obtained optimal views of the coronaries. Projections that best depict lesion geometry and side branches are produced more frequently and obtained with greater ease. The operator can avoid wasting time, contrast medium, and radiation to obtain unnecessary "routine views."

Because images are typically stored on a rapidly spinning hard disk platter, digital angiography permits **random access** to each imaging sequence during review. Thus any previous contrast injection can be replayed without reviewing all the intervening sequences. Digital angiography permits continuous review of each contrast injection in an endless **cine loop** to aid in identification of important anatomic or morphologic features. Following acquisition, digital image processing permits adjustment of image brightness, contrast, and sharpness. In some cases processing of suboptimal images obtained with steeply angled or unusual projections can in effect restore diagnostically useful images. In many digital systems review and processing are instantly available to the operator through a wireless hand-held remote control.

The immediate availability of high-quality images is particularly valuable in guiding serial interventional procedures. The instant replay of images enables the operator to examine the effects of each treatment before proceeding with the next. Efficient image review gives the interventional cardiologist the best accuracy in judging the adequacy of the revascularization and identifying complications such as thrombus, dissection, and side-branch occlusion. Areas of interest can be magnified and sharpened, and single frames can be selected for still viewing as a **roadmap** image. Most laboratories take advantage of instant imaging by proceeding with intervention immediately following diagnostic catheterization without waiting for film development in selected cases.

Digital Image Processing

Because computers employ a numeric format to store images, digital angiography readily permits computer-based manipulation of images. During the early development of cardiac digital angiography it was commonly believed that **digital subtraction** would be a valuable processing tool. Digital subtraction angiography (DSA) uses the imaging computer to acquire a **mask** consisting of one or more frames collected before the injection of iodinated contrast media (Fig. 12.6). The mask frame contains the digital gray scale values for all anatomic structures in the chest not opacified by iodinated contrast media. After contrast injection, the gray values for each pixel of the mask frame are mathematically subtracted from the corresponding pixel in the contrast-containing frame to yield a new image (Fig.12.6). Theoretically the subtraction should generate an image in which structures not containing contrast have been systematically removed. This process is often called **mask mode** subtraction.

In theory DSA should enhance **contrast sensitivity**, allowing lower doses of iodinated contrast media. Alternatively, the increased contrast sensitivity could be used to image poorly opacified structures such as the left ventricle or carotids following intravenous contrast administration. In practice, however, subtraction performs poorly for most cardiac applications, particularly coronary angiography. DSA is limited by **misregistration artifact**, a phenomenon produced by complex cardiac and respiratory motion during the interval between the acquisition of the mask and contrast frames (Fig 12.7). Misregistration artifact produces unpredictable effects that can significantly interfere with image interpretation. In addition, mask mode subtraction emphasizes quantum statistical noise because of the random nature of statistical fluctuations in density (quantum mottle) in both the mask and contrast frames. Subtraction of the mask frames from the contrast-containing frames summates these random density fluctuations, resulting in an increase in visible noise.

Current digital angiographic equipment commonly employs digital image spatial **filtration** rather than mask mode subtraction to improve image quality (Fig. 12.8). The mathematical concepts underlying filtration algorithms can be quite complex, although the results are easy to visualize. Filtration involves the modification of numeric pixel values with a predefined mathematical formula to generate a new and better image. Digital filtration is commonly employed to increase image contrast or enhance edge definition or both. This approach is generally sensible, because video-based methods typically produce images with lower contrast and reduced edge resolution than cine film. Thus filtration can restore an appearance that more closely mimics the characteristics of cine film.

Although edge enhancement filtration often produces visually appealing results, the process does not necessarily improve di-

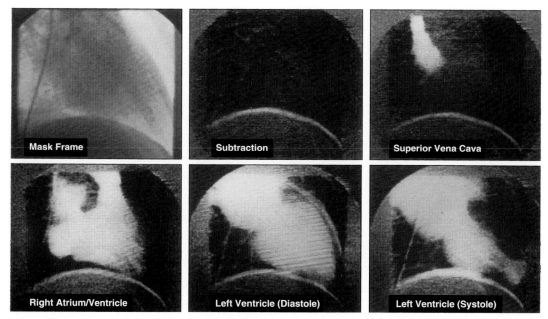

Figure 12.6. The process of digital subtraction angiography. A mask frame (*upper left*) is subtracted from all subsequent frames, a process known as mask mode subtraction. The increased contrast sensitivity produced by digital subtraction enables visualization of right and left heart structures following intravenous contrast administration. Movement of the diaphragm during this procedure results in a visible artifact.

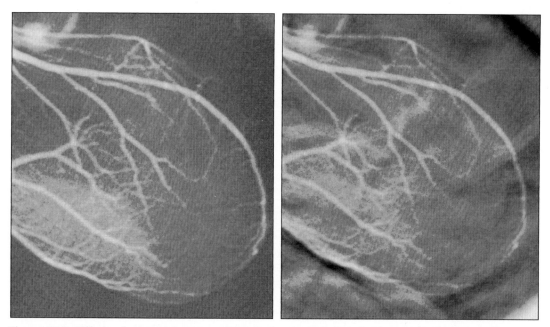

Figure 12.7. Effects of misregistration artifact. **Left panel.** A digital subtraction angiogram illustrates high image quality with excellent removal of background structures. **Right panel.** The subject has moved slightly, resulting in noticeable misregistration artifact that obscures recognition of coronary anatomy, particularly evident at the diaphragmatic surface of the heart.

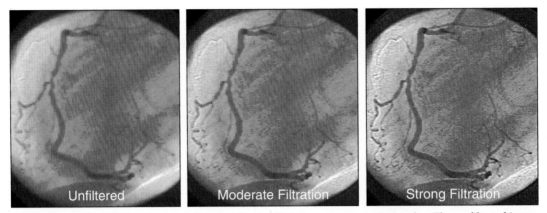

Figure 12.8. Effect of filtration on image quality in digital coronary angiography. The unfiltered image (**left panel**) appears somewhat blurred, and the filtered images (**middle** and **right panels**) show more sharpness and contrast.

agnostic accuracy. Indeed, there is potential for a strong edge enhancement filter to introduce imaging artifacts that may alter diagnostic interpretation. Most equipment vendors have not performed extensive clinical studies to examine the diagnostic effect of their filtration algorithms. Accordingly, caution is warranted in using heavily filtered images for decision making. Moderate degrees of filtration are reasonable because they improve subjective image quality with minimal risk of artifacts.

Additional image processing enhancements are commonly available on digital systems designed for the cardiac catheterization laboratory. These features include real-time magnification (**zoom**) of a selectable region with the ability to move the zoomed window dynamically during replay (**roam**). Because the pixel size during image acquisition is unchanged, magnification does not change resolution. However, the zoomed image can be more readily examined, an advantage most observers find helpful in evaluating lesion morphology. Some digital systems magnify the image with **pixel replication**, a technique in which every pixel in the original image is cloned to yield four pixels in the zoomed image (Fig. 12.9). Zoom by pixel replication generates a magnified image with a coarse texture in which pixels are easily seen. A more sophisticated approach uses an **interpolated zoom**, a technique in which the transitions between pixels are smoothed, yielding a less

pixelated image (Fig. 12.9). A further evolution is **acquisition zoom**, a technique in which the system records a 512 × 512 window from a 1024 × 1024 acquisition. Acquisition zoom increases actual pixel density and thereby improves resolution, but with the disadvantage of recording only a quarter of the image field.

CLINICAL APPLICATIONS OF DIGITAL IMAGING

Quantitative Angiography

Quantitative angiography is the application of computer-derived measurements to determine the severity of coronary stenoses (5–7). This approach was first proposed and validated in the 1970s, prior to development of digital angiography (5). Traditional quantitative angiography requires digitized cine film, usually via a projector equipped with a high-quality video camera. The digitized image is computer analyzed, typically with automated border detection and precise correction for radiographic magnification (Fig. 12.10). This technique yields measurements of both the minimum luminal diameter and percentage diameter stenosis. Under controlled conditions investigators have demonstrated excellent precision, low interobserver variability, and good repro-

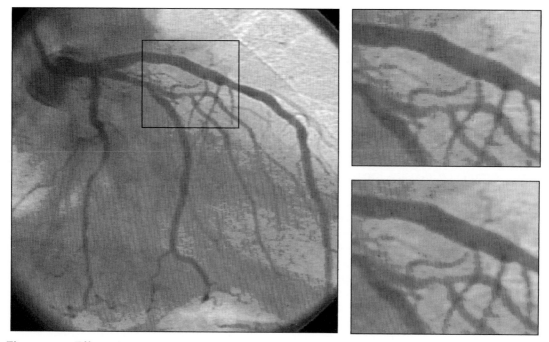

Figure 12.9. Effect of two different algorithms for image magnification (zoom). **Left panel.** The black square indicates the magnified area. **Right upper panel.** Magnification is achieved by pixel replication. **Lower right panel.** Interpolated zoom.

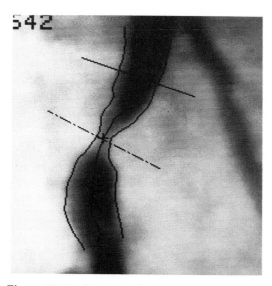

Figure 12.10. Automated tracking of vessel borders for stenosis quantification. *Dashed line,* Narrowest portion of the vessel. *Solid line,* A nearby reference segment used to determine stenosis.

ducibility for stenosis sizing with film-based quantitative angiography (5–7). However, film-derived quantitative measurements are available only off-line, a constraint that is acceptable for research but not for clinical decision making.

Because digital angiography records images directly in a computer system, quantitative angiography can be readily performed without the added step of film digitization. Improvements in computer technology have enabled some newer digital systems to provide nearly instantaneous quantitative angiography, a capability that enables measurement of severity of stenosis during the procedure. The ability to measure coronary diameter during interventional catheterization may facilitate device sizing and enable serial evaluation of the improvement in luminal diameter between successive treatments. Although intuition shows it to be useful, no randomized studies document improvement in outcome when interventional procedures are guided by quantitative angiography. Furthermore, few if any laboratories perform quantitative coronary angiography for all coronary interventions.

Traditional quantitative angiography employs geometric calculations to determine severity of stenosis. An alternative method employs computer-derived density measurements obtained by analysis of digital angiographic images. This densitometric approach to stenosis sizing calculates percentage reduction in luminal area by measuring summated density for two regions of interest, one over the lesion and the other over the nearest adjacent normal site. Theoretically densitometric stenosis measurements should be independent of the radiographic projection. Although superficially attractive, the densitometric method is seriously flawed, primarily because of inability to image both the stenosis and reference sites in a single orthogonal projection. There is a weak correlation between densitometric stenosis measurements obtained from alternative radiographic projections. Accordingly, clinical decision making based upon densitometric stenosis sizing cannot be recommended.

Digital Subtraction Ventriculography

Although misregistration artifacts have prevented application of digital subtraction ventriculography (DSA) to routine coronary arteriography, subtraction is sometimes employed to assist ventriculography. (8, 9) Typically a reduced quantity, usually a third to half of the customary dose, of iodinated contrast is power-injected into the left ventricle (Fig. 12.11). Subsequently mask mode subtraction is employed to enhance image contrast, which often results in an acceptable image quality. Misregistration artifacts are common but do not impair the diagnostic value of the ventriculogram. The reduced-contrast dose may be useful in patients with renal insufficiency, diabetes mellitus, or hemodynamic instability. During the early 1980s several studies employed DSA to perform ventriculography following intravenous administration of contrast

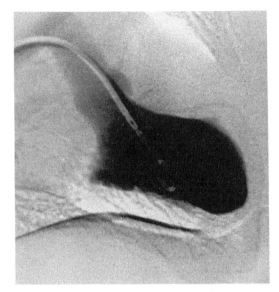

Figure 12.11. Digital subtraction left ventriculography performed by direct contrast administration. Only 15 mL of iodinated contrast generates this high quality of ventriculogram.

(8, 9). Although correlation with conventional ventriculography was close, intravenous DSA is no longer commonly applied, primarily because of the maturation of noninvasive imaging methods such as echocardiography.

In many laboratories digital ventriculograms obtained with or without subtraction are analyzed by computer. Most current digital imaging systems employ automated border detection to trace the ventricular silhouette and calculate ventricular volumes and ejection fraction using the area–length method. This technique can be more time efficient than the customary procedure, which requires projection of the cine film, tracing of ventricular borders, and planimetry of the end-diastolic and end-systolic silhouettes. Many digital imaging systems also provide computer-derived measurement of regional wall motion, often employing the well-validated method of Sheehan et al. (10). Computerized techniques for wall-motion analysis have become the standard for clinical studies evaluating and comparing interventions such as thrombolysis following acute myocardial infarction. Although comparable ventriculographic analyses are readily performed on film, digital angiography offers considerable advantages in speed and accessibility.

All film-based methods of evaluation of ventricular function rely on measurements of a silhouette of the left ventricle. Digital angiography with mask mode subtraction permits application of methods based upon the summated density of contrast within a ventricular region of interest (11–13). These video densitometric methods, which are analogous to nuclear techniques, have the potential to yield precise measures of ejection fraction that are independent of angle of view. Comparisons of densitometric ejection fraction to biplane area–length methods demonstrate a close correlation. Densitometric methods have also been applied to calculate right ventricle ejection fraction, a chamber difficult to analyze with conventional geometric methods (13). Despite considerable appeal, densitometric measurements are not widely applied, in part because of the disfavor of mask mode subtraction.

Coronary Flow Reserve by Digital Subtraction Angiography

Having recognized the limitations of stenosis sizing by angiography (14–19), more than 25 years ago investigators began to assess the functional significance of coronary lesions by analysis of density–time curves (20). A variety of computer analysis methods have been proposed for coronary reserve by digital angiography (21–25). Virtually all proposed algorithms rely upon precise measurement of density–time curves for regions of interest within the coronary or myocardial perfusion bed. Typically DSA has been employed to determine coronary flow reserve (CFR), defined as coronary blood flow (CBF) following pharmacologic vasodilation divided by CBF baseline (26, 27). Several alternative approaches for assessment of CFR have been introduced, although none has found major clinical acceptance.

FUTURE DIRECTIONS

Digital Archiving: Cineless Angiography

During the past decade advances in computer storage technology have made feasible the replacement of cine film by digital imaging for recording angiographic studies. To understand contemporary trends in filmless catheterization, it is essential to consider the various traditional roles played by 35-mm film over the past 3 decades. These roles include the functions of a **review** medium, an **archive** medium, and an **exchange** medium. A review medium is used locally to replay catheterization images for clinical decision making. An archive medium is used for semipermanent storage of angiographic studies for review during future work with the same patient. An exchange medium is used to convey images to other local or distant practitioners.

For the past 3 decades cine film has served all three functions. As laboratories make the transition to all-digital angiography, various technical approaches to digital image storage may or may not serve all three functions. For example, a laboratory may review digital images immediately after catheterization from a computer hard disk but eventually archive these images on a slower digital tape recorder for long-term storage. The computer technology enabling digital storage of images continues to evolve rapidly, which makes it difficult to predict the exact devices most suitable for transition to filmless archiving.

Despite significant uncertainties, it seems most likely that hospitals will adopt one of two systems for long-term digital storage of angiograms. One is a large digital storage device such as a tape jukebox, perhaps providing many terabytes (trillions of bytes) of capacity. An alternative may be to archive each angiographic study as a unit patient record on a single piece of medium such as a compact disk or CD. For jukebox-based systems the response time to retrieve a particular study may be several minutes. Therefore, most authorities envision a **hierarchic** structure in which a slower tape system complements a faster array of hard disks encompassing several hundred gigabytes. Ideally these systems would function automatically, so that admission of a patient or scheduling of an outpatient visit would trigger retrieval (prefetching) of relevant digital imaging studies from archival storage.

Advantages of Digital Archiving

Why the accelerating trend toward digital archiving of catheterization studies? Digital angiography offers many attractive features for long-term storage of cardiac catheterization studies. For coronary angiography the typical costs of film and development approach $100 per patient, not including long-term storage costs such as maintenance of film libraries. Digital image archiving allows substantial cost reduction with the potential to improve physicians' access to clinical studies. Digital technologies enable storage of a single angiographic procedure (approximately one gigabyte) for as little as $5 per patient, a twentieth of the cost of film.

Since 1970, every 18 months the computer industry has doubled storage density and halved cost of such storage, a trend known as Moore's Law. Given the continued improvements predicted by Moore's Law, computer storage technology will become more economical with each passing year, eventually overwhelming film storage by sheer economic advantages alone. Within the next decade technological developments may allow holographic storage of terabyte quantities of imaging data on a single small piece of medium. Such devices would enable virtually instantaneous access to a large bank of angiographic studies.

Many other important advantages are provided by digital archiving of catheterization images. Cine film is not easily copied; the original angiographic record must be physically conveyed to another physician who is seeing the patient. However, digital images can be readily duplicated, and the numeric nature of the digital image ensures that each copy is identical to the original. Thus several duplicates of an individual patient's angiograms can be stored concur-

rently in different places, such as the catheterization laboratory, cardiac surgery suite, and physician's office.

Evolution of Network Technology

Theoretically digital angiograms can be transmitted electronically over long distances for remote diagnosis and consultation. Although current transmission schemes are too slow to be practical, faster digital networks are planned for the late 1990s. To deliver digital images throughout a hospital will require evolution from the current Ethernet standard (10 megabits per second [Mbps]) to **Fast Ethernet** speeds (100 Mbps) or the even faster asynchronous transfer mode (ATM, 155 Mbps to more than 500 Mbps). Governments and private companies are making large investments to ensure that such high-speed links are widely available for commercial and medical applications. Development of the necessary software to track the thousands of examinations performed annually will be required for digital archiving in large hospitals.

The Transition to Digital Storage

Because of the economic and clinical advantages, most experts in radiographic imaging expect an accelerating transition from film to digital image storage during the coming few years (3, 4). A few laboratories have already abandoned cine film; some keep their archives on super VHS videocassette tape. Although transfer of digital images to analog videocassette tape is simple and inexpensive, the loss of image quality is clinically unacceptable. Under ideal circumstances super VHS videotape can record only about 50% of the spatial resolution available from modern digital angiographic acquisition systems. This visible reduction in image quality precludes use of videotape for critical applications, such as deciding the suitability of coronary anatomy for surgery or angioplasty. In addition, video tape steadily degrades over time, losing image quality. Thus use of analog video tape to replace cine film is clinically insupportable. Videotape may be useful to provide referring physicians with a copy of their patient's catheterization procedure but should not be used for primary decision making.

The DICOM Standard

Prior to 1993, in the zeal to replace cine film, some laboratories adopted a variety of nonstandard digital archiving media. Although image quality was much better than on analog videotape, the approach used by early adopters had significant disadvantages. Since there was no standard format, each device used a unique proprietary recording format. Accordingly, none of the early devices permitted playback of digital archives generated on competitors' products.

In the early 1990s existing archival devices lacked the one critical feature supplied by cine film: worldwide standardization. The result was that an angiogram performed and archived in one laboratory could not be reviewed in another, a phenomenon the ACC termed "the Tower of Babel in the catheterization laboratory" in a position paper (4). Under such conditions referral of the patient to an external institution for surgery, angioplasty, or a second opinion often required a repeat catheterization. The lack of an accepted standard also began to impair clinical investigations that require image analysis at a single core laboratory.

The obvious solution was development of an interchange standard to enable facile exchange of digital angiographic studies. Beginning in 1981 a radiology digital standards group began to develop an industrywide protocol for the image format and communication between devices. Initially the effort was jointly sponsored by the American College of Radiology (ACR) and the National Electrical Manufacturers Association (NEMA). In 1992 the ACC assembled interested parties to coordinate a cardiac angiographic standard. These working groups included representatives appointed by the ESC. Initial meetings led to an agreement by manufacturers through NEMA, and all three medical organizations (ACC, ASE and ESC) decided to work cooperatively toward the development of suitable standards. Eventually this effort was named the digital imaging and communication for medicine (DICOM) standard to reflect the broader composition of the committee.

Scope of the Angiographic Standard

Because of the many purposes served by cineangiographic film, the angiographic committee focused on solving the one critical problem facing digital cardiac catheterization: development of a format and medium for **interchange** of angiographic studies. The committee deliberately avoided any attempt to standardize the **acquisition, display,** or **archiving** of angiographic images. This approach allows vendors to develop a range of products to support the needs of hospitals and laboratories regardless of size. Since the interchange record is standardized, the only requirement for a laboratory to maintain compatibility is the ability to read and write images in a well-defined data format.

Emergence of the CD-R

Since 1992 the DICOM angiographic committee has met for 2 days each month in Washington to work out details of an interchange standard. After lengthy discussion and debate, the recordable 5.25-inch optical compact disk (CD–R) emerged as the optimal interchange medium for angiography. The medium, physically similar to the CD-ROM used in popular multimedia applications, has a capacity of approximately 680 MB. The exchange standard for cardiac angiography is nearly complete; it was first demonstrated in 1995 at the ACC scientific sessions and the annual meeting of the ESC. The DICOM format has been adopted by all major catheterization laboratory vendors and is appearing in many end-user products.

The CD-R storage capacity of 680 MB permits recording of approximately 2400 frames (512 × 512 × 8-bit gray scale) per disk. This capacity is insufficient to record on a single piece of medium all cardiovascular examinations, which can reach 4000 images or more. Accordingly, the Ad Hoc Standards Committee specified use of digital data compression to increase the storage capacity of the CD-R. The compression scheme adopted by the committee is the lossless Huffman method, which reduces by about two-thirds the amount of storage space required for each image frame. This increases the CD capacity to about 4800 angiographic frames, sufficient to store more than 98% of studies on a single piece of medium. The Ad Hoc Angiographic Committee did not include lossy compression for image exchange on CD-R because the clinical utility of a suitable compression scheme and acceptable compression ratio had not been determined.

Transfer Rates and Compression

Data transfer rates available in 1995, when the DICOM angiographic standard was introduced, limited the performance of the CD-R medium in the initial clinical applications. This technical limitation allowed display of angiographic images directly from the CD-R at no more than 7.5 frames per second. Thus full-motion display and review of DICOM images using available CD drives required uploading of images from the exchange medium to the computer workstation. Although future developments will gradually increase recording and playback performance of CD-R, drive speeds sufficient for viewing at 30 frames per second directly from the medium are unlikely in the immediate future. Because of the performance limits of CD-R, several equipment vendors have demonstrated an alternative approach to image exchange that uses lossy compression. Applying greater compression ratios on this proprietary CD increases the retrieval speed to 30 frames per second, but with some image degradation. This lossy approach to image compression is not yet a part of the official DICOM angiographic standard.

In evaluating appropriate methods of data compression, the Ad Hoc Angiographic Working Group did not rule out the use of lossy compression if clinical studies demonstrated no significant loss of diagnostic image quality. Therefore, as previously mentioned, the ACC, ESC, and industry have initiated a clinical study of lossy compression to determine whether this approach is suitable for inclusion in the DICOM standard. This complex study will examine the ability of observers to perform the subtle detection tasks required to interpret angiographic images. The results of this study should be available by late 1997 or early 1998.

Conversion Strategy: Conformance

In developing a conversion strategy practitioners must realize that DICOM standard is specialized for many modalities, and most equipment does not support all of them (e.g., a computed tomography scanner has little need to display echocardiograms). To specify precisely which aspects of DICOM are supported, vendors publish **conformance claims**, which should be studied carefully, most likely in consultation with a trusted adviser, to ensure that a given piece of equipment will meet the customer's need. Open architecture is critical to taking advantage of the ongoing computer revolution. One cannot expect any computer device to remain state-of-the-art for very long. Accordingly, an upgrade path—without being locked into a single vendor's proprietary hardware—will be important to ensure continuing cost competitiveness.

Barriers to Cineless Angiography

Despite the successful development of an exchange medium, there remain important obstacles to the development of a suitable replacement for cine film for long-term archiving. Ideally a cine replacement medium should permit rapid **random-access** review of any recorded digital angiographic injection sequence. Random-access archiving would permit review of imaging sequences in any order and viewing of individual injections in continuous cine loop. However, the density and speed of random-access computer storage technologies lag behind **sequential-access** devices, such as digital tape. Accordingly, the staggering quantities of digital imaging data cannot yet be stored economically in a random-access system. Nevertheless, the maturation of computer storage devices and the evolution of new storage technology will almost certainly overcome these limitations within the next few years.

Several additional issues must be resolved before development of an optimal strategy for replacement of cineangiography. Should the digital archive include non-imaging information, such as hemodynamic data and written reports? The standards committee has begun work on including these data in the interchange record, but some current systems may have difficulty with this. Is it clinically acceptable to employ any degree of lossy data compression, such as JPEG? Should the archiving of a particular hospital support nonradiographic images, such as echocardiography? Given the uncertainties, a prudent course of action requires close monitoring of DICOM standardization as the group further defines the format, devices, and media for digital archiving. Despite these obstacles, few expert observers doubt that digital angiography will constitute the dominant archiving method for cardiac catheterization images by the end of the decade.

SUMMARY

Digital technology is currently in widespread use in catheterization laboratories and its application will likely expand in the next decade. Digital imaging offers the potential for less radiation exposure, more accurate image quantitation, better image processing, more easily transmittable images, and less cost. As computer capabilities expand and data manipulation and storage

becomes more efficient and less costly, digital imaging should completely replace the hard film images in common use today. Development of a uniform standard through the DICOM effort underway will hasten this trend despite the technical obstacles still present.

References

1. Kruger RA, Mistretta CA, Houk TL, et al. Computer fluoroscopy in real time for noninvasive visualization of the cardiovascular system. Radiology 1979;130:49–57.
2. Gurley JC, Nissen SE, Booth DC, et al. Comparison of simultaneously performed digital and film-based angiography in the assessment of coronary artery disease. Circulation 1988;78:1411–1420.
3. Gurley JC, Nissen SE. Digital coronary angiography: is it ready to replace cine film? Cardiology 1991;8:82.
4. Nissen SE, Pepine CJ, Block PC, et al. Cardiac angiography without cine film: erecting a "Tower of Babel" in the catheterization laboratory. J Am Coll Cardiol 1994;24:834–837.
5. Brown BG, Bolson E, Frimer M, Dodge HT. Quantitative coronary arteriography: estimation of dimensions, hemodynamic resistance, and atheroma mass of coronary artery lesions using the arteriograms and digital computation. Circulation 1977;55:329–337.
6. Reiber JHC, Serruys PW, Kooijman CJ, et al. Assessment of short-, medium-, and long-term variations in arterial dimensions from computer-assisted quantitation of coronary cineangiograms. Circulation 1985;71:280–288.
7. Kirkeeide RL, Gould KL, Parsel L. Assessment of coronary stenoses by myocardial perfusion imaging during pharmacologic coronary vasodilation: 7. Validation of coronary flow reserve as a single integrated functional measure of stenosis severity reflecting all its geometric dimensions. J Am Coll Cardiol 1986;7:103–113.
8. Tobis J, Nalcioglu O, Johnston WD, et al. Left ventricular imaging with digital subtraction angiography using intravenous contrast injection and fluoroscopic exposure levels. Am Heart J 1982;104:20–27.
9. Nissen SE, Booth D, Waters J, et al. Evaluation of left ventricular contractile pattern by intravenous digital subtraction ventriculography: comparison with cineangiography and assessment of interobserver variability. Am J Cardiol 1983;52:1293–1298.
10. Sheehan FH, Schofer J, Mathey DG, et al. Measurement of regional wall motion from biplane contrast ventriculograms: a comparison of the 30 degree right anterior oblique and 60 degree left anterior oblique projections in patients with acute myocardial infarction. Circulation 1986;74:796–804.
11. Tobis J, Nalcioglu O, Seibert A, et al. Measurement of left ventricular ejection fraction by videodensito-

metric analysis of digital subtraction angiograms. Am J Cardiol 1983;52:871–875.

12. Nissen SE, Elion JL, Grayburn P, et al. Determination of left ventricular ejection fraction by computer densitometric analysis of digital subtraction angiography: experimental validation and correlation with area-length methods. Am J Cardiol 1987; 59:675–670.

13. Nissen SE, Elion JL, DeMaria AN. Value and limitations of densitometry in the calculation of right and left ventricular ejection fraction from digital angiography. In: Mancini GBJ, ed. Clinical applications of cardiac digital angiography. New York: Raven Press, 1988:115–130.

14. Zir LM, Miller SW, Dinsmore RE, et al. Interobserver variability in coronary angiography. Circulation 1976;53:627–632.

15. Galbraith JE, Murphy ML, Desoyza N. Coronary angiogram interpretation: interobserver variability. JAMA 1981;240:2053–2059.

16. Arnett EN, Isner JM, Redwood CR, et al. Coronary artery narrowing in coronary heart disease: comparison of cineangiographic and necropsy findings. Ann Intern Med 1979;91:350–356.

17. Grodin CM, Dyrda I, Pasternac A, et al. Discrepancies between cineangiographic and post-mortem findings in patients with coronary artery disease and recent myocardial revascularization. Circulation 1974;49:703–709.

18. Vlodaver Z, Frech R, van Tassel RA, Edwards JE. Correlation of the antemortem coronary angiogram and the postmortem specimen. Circulation 1973;47:162–168.

19. White CW, Wright CB, Doty DB, et al. Does visual interpretation of the coronary arteriogram predict the physiologic importance of a coronary stenosis? N Engl J Med 1984;310:819–824.

20. Smith HC, Frye RL, Donald DE, et al. Roentgen videodensitometric measure of coronary blood flow determination from simultaneous indicator-dilution curves at selected sites in the coronary circulation and in coronary artery saphenous vein grafts. Mayo Clin Proc 1971;46:800–806.

21. Vogel RA, LeFree MT, Bates ER, et al. Application of digital techniques to selective coronary arteriography: use of myocardial appearance time to measure coronary flow reserve. Am Heart J 1983;7: 153–164.

22. Nissen SE, Elion JL, Booth DC, et al. Value and limitations of computer analysis of digital subtraction angiography in the assessment of coronary flow reserve. Circulation 1986;73:562–571.

23. Whiting JS, Drury JK, Pfaff JM, et al. Digital angiographic measurement of radiographic contrast material kinetics for estimation of myocardial perfusion. Circulation 1986;73:789–798.

24. Cusma, JT, Toggart EJ, Folts JD, et al. Digital subtraction angiographic imaging of coronary flow reserve. Circulation 1987;74:461–472.

25. Pijls NHJ, Uijen GJH, Hoevelaken A, et al. Mean transit time for the assessment of myocardial perfusion by videodensitometry. Circulation 1990;81: 1331–1340.

26. Gould KL, Lipscomb K, Hamilton GW. Physiologic basis for assessing critical coronary stenosis: instantaneous flow response and regional distribution during coronary hyperemia as measures of coronary flow reserve. Am J Cardiol 1974;33:87–93.

27. Gould KL, Lipscomb K. Effects of coronary artery stenosis on coronary flow reserve and resistance. Am J Cardiol 1974;34:48–55.

13
Radiographic Contrast Agents

James A. Hill, MD, MS
Charles R. Lambert, MD, PhD
Carl J. Pepine, MD

INTRODUCTION

Radiographic examination of the cardiovascular system entails imaging structures of similar radiodensity, that is, blood and tissue. In general there is not enough difference between these densities to generate an image with conventional x-ray imaging techniques, so it is often necessary to enhance the minor degrees of contrast through use of a contrast agent. These agents absorb the beam of x-rays to a greater extent than surrounding tissue. Contrast agents are used in three basic ways in diagnostic imaging: direct injection into a vascular lumen to outline the lumen; intravenous administration to evaluate distribution in various compartments, as in contrast-enhanced computed tomography (CT); and intravenous or oral administration to show their excretion from the body, such as in diagnostic urography or biliary imaging. Except for occasional use with CT, at present direct visualization after intravascular injection is the principal way these agents are used.

As with any drug, **contrast agents should perform their function without causing untoward effects or altering physiologic function.** However, no contrast agent meets these criteria. This chapter provides an overview of intravascular radiographic contrast agents and their properties, discusses their adverse effects and how to manage them, and reviews agents now being used for cardiac angiography.

PHYSICAL PROPERTIES

All contrast agents today contain iodine, which in an appropriate concentration is an effective absorber of x-rays in the energy range of clinical imaging systems. While they differ structurally, contrast agents are all derivatives of tri-iodinated benzoic acids. Toxicology data suggest that all iodine-containing agents are relatively biologically inert, but they differ greatly in osmolality, viscosity, and other properties (Table 13.1). As the table shows, the amount of elemental iodine necessary to provide diagnostic imaging is often quite high, up to many times the body's average daily turnover of iodine. The molecular weights of the available agents range from 600 to 1700.

Agents used for vascular imaging may be divided into those that ionize in solution (ionic agents) and those that do not (nonionic agents). Conventional ionic contrast agents are all monomeric, generally with diatrizoate as the iodine carrier. This anion is combined with sodium and meglumine as cations. The ideal sodium–meglumine ratio, at least for coronary angiography, appears to be 1:6.6. The fact that these

Table 13.1.
Contrast Agents

Generic Name		Trade Name (Manufacturer)	Iodine (mg/mL)	Osmolality (mOsm/kg)	Viscosity 25°(cp)	Viscosity 37°	Sodium Content (mEq/L)	Additives
IONIC								
Diatrizoate		Renograffin-76	370	1940	13.80	8.40	190	Sodium citrate 0.32%
sodium	100 mg/mL	(E.R. Squibb)						Disodium EDTA 0.04%
meglumine	660 mg/mL							
Diatrizoate		Hypaque-76	370	2016	13.34	8.32	160	Calcium disodium
sodium	100 mg/mL	(Sanofi-						EDTA 0.01%
meglumine	660 mg/mL	Winthrop)						
Diatrizoate		Angiovist 370	370	2100	13.80	9.00	150	Calcium disodium EDT
sodium	100 mg/mL	(Berlex)						0.01%
meglumine	660 mg/mL							
Ioxaglate		Hexabrix	320	580	15.70	7.50	157	
sodium	19.6%	(Mallinckrodt)						
meglumine	39.3%							
NONIONIC								
Iohexol		Omnipaque	180	408	3.10[a]	2.00		
		(Sanofi-	240	520	5.80	3.40		Calcium disodium EDT
		Winthrop)	300	672	11.8	6.30		10 mg/dL
			350	844	20.4	10.4		Tromethamine 121 mg/dL
Iopamidol		Isovue 300	300	616	8.80[a]	4.70	200	Calcium disodium EDT
		Isovue 370	370	796	20.9	9.40	200	39 mg/dL (I-300)
		(E.R.Squibb)						48 mg/dL (I-370)
Ioversol		Optiray 320	320	702	9.90	5.80		EDTA 0.2 mg/mL
		Optiray 350	350	792	14.30	9.00		Tromethamine 3.6 mg/ mL (in both)
		(Mallinckrodt)						Tromethamine 100 mg/dL
Ioxilan		Oxilan 350	350	695	16.3	8.1	>1	Citric acid 0.576 mg/ mL
		(Cook Imaging)						Edetate calcium disodium 0.561 mg/ mL
Iodixanol		Visipaque 320	320	290	26.5[a]	11.8		Calcium chloride dihydrate 0.044 mg/ mL
								NaCl 1.11 mg/mL
								Tromethamine 1.2 mg/ mL
								Edetate calcium disodium 0.1 mg/mL

Reprinted with permission from Fischer HW. Catalog of intravascular contrast media. Radiology 1986;159:561–563.
[a] Measured at 20°.

agents ionize in solution is relevant to their effects on osmolality.

Osmolality is the number of particles in solution. The cations are radiologically inactive and serve only to increase the number of particles in solution. Thus osmolality can be reduced by providing a compound that does not ionize, thus increasing the number of particles in solution that contain iodine, or by providing more iodine molecules per particle in solution. The low-osmolality ionic agent sodium meglumine ioxaglate (Hexabrix) is a dimer, hence contains twice as much iodine per molecule compared to conventional ionic agents. This allows for much lower osmolality with equivalent io-dine concentrations than conventional high-osmolality ionic agents. Osmolality seems related to many physiologic and adverse effects caused by intravascular contrast agents. Considering that the osmolality of a widely used ionic contrast agent, meglumine sodium diatrizoate (Renografin-76), is approximately six times serum osmolality, the implications for adverse physiologic effects are obvious, and reducing osmolality is a desirable goal.

Nonionic contrast agents do not ionize in solution and so provide more particles that contain iodine in a given volume than do ionic agents. Therefore they can have an equivalent iodine content with a lower osmolality than conventional ionic agents. In addition, nonionic agents tend to associate in solution, further reducing the number of particles in solution and lowering the osmolality more than might be expected on a molecular basis alone. Iodixanol is a nonionic dimer providing six iodine molecules per osmotic particle. The osmolality of this compound is so low that addition of calcium and sodium is required to equal serum osmolality.

PHARMACOLOGY

Intravascular radiographic contrast agents have low lipid solubility and minimal plasma protein binding. They rapidly distribute in the body's extracellular space. Their molecular size and low lipid solubility prevent passage across cell membranes in any significant amount, and thus very little is absorbed. This size also allows them to be filtered by and almost entirely excreted by the kidneys.

The half-life for excretion in patients with normal renal function is 30 to 60 minutes. These agents are freely filtered by the kidney but are neither secreted nor absorbed. The amount of contrast agent entering tubules is determined by the glomerular filtration rate and plasma concentration. As water and sodium are reabsorbed, the contrast agent is concentrated to a level markedly higher than that entering the tubule. Although amounts of contrast present and the kinetics of distribution in various tissues differ widely, there seem to be few if any differences among the agents themselves (1). However, this generally has no consequence to standard cardiac imaging, as the images are made in real time immediately after injection. Even with signal-averaging imaging techniques, the imaging times are soon enough after injection that distribution kinetics do not significantly influence results.

Materials added to preserve or stabilize radiocontrast agents (e.g., ethylenediamine tetra-acetic acid [EDTA]) also vary among preparations. The major additives bind calcium, which contributes to adverse hemodynamic effects noted with intracoronary injection. Data suggest that the negative inotropic effects caused by calcium-binding actions of these agents can be reduced by adding calcium to the medium (2). Data from animal studies with Urografin-76, iopamidol, ioxaglate, and iohexol show that the agents with the lesser calcium-binding effect (i.e., iohexol, iopamidol, and ioxaglate) cause less of a decrease in coronary sinus calcium (3, 4). How calcium binding interacts with lower osmolality to produce fewer hemodynamic effects is not clear, but several studies have noted fewer hemodynamic alterations using non–calcium-binding nonionic agents (5, 6). In addition to adverse hemodynamic alterations, ventricular fibrillation associated with intracoronary injection is also increased with contrast agents that bind calcium (7–10). Repolarization is altered by calcium binding, contributing to ventricular fibrillation, and addition of calcium decreases the incidence. Although **serum calcium decreases transiently (11) when agents with these additives are administered,** this is unlikely to have important clinical implications.

Sodium content is likewise important. It was once assumed that the lower the sodium, the safer the intracoronary injection, because high-sodium agents were very toxic. Other data, however, suggest that no sodium in the medium is also toxic, and it appears that sodium content is optimal when it is near the physiologic level (12) except in the nonionic agents. Nonionic agents may change coronary venous sodium concentration less than conventional agents. How this contributes to the lower toxicity of these agents is not known.

ADVERSE EFFECTS

Adverse effects of contrast agents generally fall into two categories, anaphylactoid and toxic. Anaphylactoid reactions include urticaria, cardiovascular collapse, angioedema, and bronchospasm. Toxic reactions include hot flushing sensation, nausea, metallic taste, arrhythmias, vascular congestion, and renal failure. Anaphylactoid reactions generally are idiosyncratic, and toxic effects occur in most patients to some degree.

Anaphylactoid Reactions

Anaphylactoid reactions vary in severity. Often allergic, these include bronchospasm, urticaria, angioedema, and shock. While these reactions are related to neither dose nor injection rate, there are a number of hypotheses as to why they occur. Some appear to be immune (immunoglobulin E) mediated. There is some evidence that complement, alternate pathways, and kinin activation occur in these patients, but this does not occur consistently and may occur in the absence of an adverse reaction (13). Regardless of the mechanism involved, there appears to be at least some **increased risk of a repeat adverse reaction when one has occurred previously.** Skin testing for these reactions is generally not thought to be useful (14) and may be misleading. A repeat reaction may be lesser and may be obviated by various pretreatment regimens. However, an essential indication for the angiographic procedure should be clearly documented, and emergency equipment should be available in the event a repeat reaction is severe. Details of prevention are discussed subsequently.

Toxicity

As opposed to anaphylactoid reactions, toxic reactions are due to the inherent physical or chemical properties of contrast agents and the substances added to them. **Most toxic effects probably result from hyperosmolality, which causes major physiologic effects.** Locally, when exposed to contrast, erythrocytes lose cellular water very rapidly and increase internal viscosity. The cells are then unable to deform appropriately to cross the capillary beds, and acute capillary plugging can occur. This can be a problem in patients with pulmonary hypertension or sickle cell anemia when a high-osmolar agent is used. Endothelial damage can also result from the high osmolality of contrast injected near the endothelium, with resultant thrombophlebitis and thrombosis in the veins used. Hyperosmolality can cause a major increase in intravascular volume by drawing in extravascular water. Vasodilation also seems to be directly related to the osmolality, and neurotoxicity may be partially related to the capillary damage caused by the hyperosmolar contrast injection.

Hypotension

Hypotension and cardiovascular collapse that result from contrast agent administration may be anaphylactoid, directly toxic, or vasovagal. Recognition of the cause is essential if appropriate therapy is to be administered. Anaphylactoid reactions usually get worse quickly despite efforts to raise blood pressure. When this occurs, it is best to insert multiple large-bore intravenous lines and administer fluids, colloids, and vasopressors as rapidly as possible. The blood pressure decline is often very resistant to these measures, and it may take many liters of fluid and up to an hour or two of vasopressor support to raise and maintain the blood pressure. Direct toxic effects of the agent refer primarily to the hyperosmolality-induced drop in blood pressure. This is usually transient and generally does not require any treatment. If treatment is necessary, oxygen administration and leg elevation usually rapidly reverse the hypotension. If the hypotension persists or worsens despite these measures, other mechanisms should be considered. Vagal reactions should be considered, especially if there is also a decline in heart rate, although this is not universal, and a pure vasodepressor reaction can occur. These reactions are usually reversed promptly by atropine and fluids. Many cardiac patients poorly tolerate a fall in blood pressure. Hypotension may precipitate ischemia and left ventricular dysfunction, worsening the hypotension. For this reason every effort should be made to rapidly determine the cause of decreased blood pressure and correct it.

Nephrotoxicity

Contrast-associated nephrotoxicity is a well-known adverse effect. The mechanism for the development of this problem is controversial (15). Possible mechanisms include direct contrast toxicity, renal hemodynamic changes, tubular obstruction by protein or uric acid crystals, and immune reactions. While some data support all of these possible mechanisms, most agree that the injury is probably related to a combination of direct toxicity and changes in renal blood flow. Many patients with a minor degree of contrast-associated nephropathy do not have oliguria. However, some, particularly those with significant prior renal impairment, develop oliguria within the first 24 hours after contrast administration. This lasts for only 2 to 4 days, with the serum creatinine peaking at approximately 3 to 5 days and a gradual return to baseline levels in the large majority of cases. Occasionally hemodialysis is necessary, but this is unusual.

The exact incidence of contrast-associated nephropathy is unknown because of various definitions of renal toxicity, studies involving heterogeneous populations with differing risks, and the fact that changes in parameters of renal function are often clinically silent. In addition, serum creatinine, the most readily available measure of renal function, may not be as sensitive as is necessary to detect subtle changes in renal function. Some (16–18) have proposed the use of urinary enzymes, but these are neither generally available nor universally accepted.

Risk factors for the development of contrast-associated nephropathy include, among others, dehydration, congestive heart failure, diabetes mellitus, prior renal impairment, and repeated exposures to contrast (19). Advanced age has not been completely evaluated as an independent risk predictor but does not appear to contribute (20). Whether these risk factors are independent depends on the study, but many patients who develop nephrotoxicity have multiple risk factors, with one study finding 3.67 (mean) per patient (21). Parfrey et al. (22) reported data from 220 patients with some risk factor for renal damage (diabetes, pre-existing renal impairment, or both) undergoing either intravenous or intra-arterial contrast administration. The study was prospective but not randomized,

and 75% received high-osmolar contrast. They found an 8.8% chance of an increase in serum creatinine of more than 50% in the group with diabetes and pre-existing renal disease but did not find "clinically important" renal toxicity in the other patients. Manske et al. (23) likewise reported data from 59 azotemic diabetic patients (mean serum creatinine 5.9 mg/100 mL) undergoing coronary angiography but obtained different results. All had angiography with nonionic agents. They found that serum creatinine increased more than 25% in 50% of the patients studied, and 8 required dialysis. Moreover, doses of contrast higher than 30 mL were found to be an independent risk factor for development of renal impairment. Using iopamidol in a nonrandomized trial of cardiac angiography, Davidson et al. (24) found that pre-existing renal dysfunction was the only predictor of contrast-associated nephropathy.

Whether there are any differences between conventional and newer agents in the degree of renal dysfunction produced has not been completely resolved. Iopamidol may produce less protein aggregation in the tubules than diatrizoate, limiting any potential for nephrotoxicity from this mechanism (25). A number of clinical studies compare the incidence of contrast-associated nephropathy associated with nonionic and with ionic contrast media. Schwab et al. (26) randomly assigned patients to receive either iopamidol or diatrizoate during cardiac angiography. There were 283 considered at low risk and 160 at high risk (diabetes mellitus, heart failure, or pre-existing renal impairment). They were unable to demonstrate a difference between agents. Taliercio et al. (27) randomized a larger number of patients at high risk for renal impairment (diabetes mellitus or creatinine above 1.5 mg/100 mL) to receive either iopamidol or diatrizoate during cardiac angiography. In their 307 patients the mean change in creatinine at 24 hours was higher in the diatrizoate group than in the iopamidol group (0.22 versus 0.11 mg/100 mL), but there were no differences between the agents in the occurrence of severe renal impairment. In the largest randomized trial to date, 1196 patients, Rudnick et al. (28) reported that the risk of developing contrast-associated nephropathy was approximately 3.3 times as high with the use of diatrizoate as with iohexol. As with other smaller studies, this effect was found only in those with pre-existing renal insufficiency (creatinine at least 1.5 mg/100 mL).

Patients without pre-existing renal impairment do not seem to have a significant risk of nephrotoxicity irrespective of the agent used (28, 29), so no special precautions beyond standard care need be taken. However, for patients at higher risk several guidelines should be followed. All patients should receive adequate hydration before and after contrast exposure. Contrast load should be limited to the minimum amount necessary to perform the angiography needed, and the number of contrast studies within any 24- to 48-hour period should be limited in patients at high risk. All high-risk patients should be observed for urine output and serum creatinine for at least 24 hours after study. While it may be helpful, use of either mannitol or diuretics to maintain urine flow is controversial (30). One randomized study (31) showed that saline infusion alone was superior to saline plus furosemide or mannitol. Other measures such as theophylline (32, 33) and endothelin blockade are being investigated.

Volume Considerations

It is generally believed that contrast volume should be limited at any one time. The package inserts of contrast agents have various limits, but 250 mL is thought to be the upper limit for any one examination. There does not seem to be a sound scientific reason for this limitation. Available data seem to be related mainly to iodine concentration, which likely has minimal effect on cardiovascular toxicity. It is not clear that these limitations are still appropriate in view of the common practice of complex multivessel procedures and ad hoc percutaneous transluminal coronary angioplasty (PTCA), which commonly require high doses of contrast.

A number of factors influence the physiologic effects of a high volume of contrast: (*a*) hydration status, (*b*) left ventricular function, (*c*) ongoing myocardial ischemia, (*d*) blood pressure, and (*e*) pre-existing renal function. Because of the high osmolality of contrast media, considerable volume expansion can occur. This is less of a problem with the substantially lower osmolality of nonionic media. With the use of newer agents, such as iodixanol, which is equiosmolar to serum, there may be even less effect. Increased intravascular volume is poorly tolerated by many patients undergoing cardiac catheterization, especially those with severe left ventricular dysfunction.

Recent data from the Society for Cardiac Angiography and Interventions (SCA & I) Registry (34) reflecting data from 1991 show that the average dose of contrast used during diagnostic angiography was 132 mL, whereas with PTCA the average was 203 mL. This is likely to be higher today for the reasons previously stated. Kahn et al. (35) retrospectively identified 54 of 730 consecutive patients undergoing PTCA during a 6-month period who received more than 400 mL of ioxaglate during PTCA. The mean dose in this group was 496 plus or minus 76 mL (range 400 to 785), and 6 of the patients developed an increase in creatinine to 0.5 mg/dL or more after study. Of these, 5 had diabetes mellitus, elevated serum creatinine (more than 1.5 mg/dL), or both prior to PTCA. All serum creatinine levels were improving at the time of discharge. Patients with normal renal function did not have nephrotoxicity. No other adverse events resulted from contrast administration.

Many studies of the effect of contrast on renal function evaluate the effect of volume administered. The conclusions are mixed, largely because of the same limitations in these studies as for assessing contrast's effect on renal function in general. Higher volumes of contrast probably adversely affect the kidney, but exactly how much is safe and under what circumstances is unknown. High-dose contrast administration is likely to continue as more complex interventions are undertaken. The safety of such increased volumes should be addressed in a properly designed trial.

Thromboembolism

Data regarding thromboembolic complications of contrast agents must be interpreted in the context of the techniques used to perform the catheterization procedure and the type of patient studied. Use of systemic anticoagulation, the duration of time the catheters remain in the vascular system, and amount of catheter flushing all affect the incidence of thromboembolic problems. It appears that nonionic contrast agents do not have the same inhibitory effects on blood clotting and platelet aggregation (36) that conventional agents do. Several reports link nonionic contrast media to a higher incidence of adverse thrombotic outcomes, particularly with PTCA (37–41), but others refute this concept (42). This may be true particularly in those with unstable ischemic syndromes (43). Thrombotic problems generally result from breakdown in meticulous technique or inadequate anticoagulation or antiplatelet therapy during PTCA, but the contrast agent may play a role. When using any contrast agent, particularly the nonionic agents, the operator should consider systemic anticoagulation during cardiac angiographic procedures, avoid leaving blood and contrast mixtures in syringes for long periods, and maintain a meticulous routine of flushing catheters and cleaning guidewires. Adding heparin to the contrast medium has been advocated, but there is no evidence that it has any effect, and it cannot be recommended. As catheterization procedures, particularly interventional ones, continue to evolve, this is likely to remain controversial until more large-scale trials are done (44, 45).

CARDIAC EFFECTS

Electrocardiographic Changes and Arrhythmias

The major change in the electrocardiogram (ECG) as a result of intracoronary administration of contrast agents is sinus node slowing. This effect occurs 5 to 10 seconds after injection and persists for approximately 60 seconds. It occurs somewhat more frequently with right coronary than left coronary injection, probably because of direct effects on the sinus node and reflex vagal suppression. In addition, the QRS axis shifts, QRS is prolonged, the ST segment is depressed, the T wave inverts or peaks, and atrioventricular conduction, as manifested by P-R prolongation and occasionally development of higher degrees of heart block, increases. Some degree of ECG change is almost universal, especially with high osmolar ionic agents. It follows the same time course as the sinus slowing but may persist slightly longer. These ECG changes appear to be related to the osmolality and probably the electrolyte balance and are markedly attenuated with the newer nonionic agents (46).

Ventricular arrhythmias may also occur. They appear related to sodium and calcium content, as mentioned previously. These effects are irrespective of the coronary anatomy and do not seem any more frequent in patients with severe coronary artery disease than in normal patients, although they may not be as well tolerated by the more severely ill patients. The incidence and severity of both the ECG effects and the rhythm disturbances depend to a great extent on the contrast agent used. Among the agents in general use today, **diatrizoate seems to cause more severe effects** on these parameters than do the lower-osmolality agents.

Effects on Systemic Hemodynamic Parameters

Administration of a contrast medium generally causes some transient decrease in both systemic vascular resistance and blood pressure. This may be mild or marked, but the degree to which it occurs probably is related to the osmolality of the agent used, with the higher-osmolar agents having a greater effect. It occurs with systemic injection, suggesting peripheral vasodilation. Intracoronary administration also causes a decrease in systemic blood pressure, probably because of effects of the contrast agent on left ventricular function and various reflexes.

The effect of angiographic contrast media on ventricular function seems to be related to the method of administration.

When conventional agents are given directly into a coronary artery, there is a consistent rise in left ventricular end-diastolic pressure, but ejection fraction and ventricular volume are not affected to any major degree. Following left ventricular angiography, the left ventricular end-diastolic pressure generally rises, especially with the use of high-osmolality agents. Data comparing contrast agents and their effect on left ventricular hemodynamics conflict, but there appears to be less of an effect when lower-osmolality agents are used (47–49). Ejection fractions and ventricular volumes seem to exhibit only minor changes, at least in the early period after angiography (50). This may be more pronounced in patients with abnormal ventricular function. It may be related to a direct toxic effect (e.g., effect of calcium binding), an abnormality of the calcium–sodium relationship, enhanced myocardial ischemia causing compliance changes, an increase in intravascular volume secondary to the osmotic load, or some combination of these factors. Time after angiography is an important determinant in the responsible mechanism. There is evidence to support all of these ideas, and the mechanism probably differs from patient to patient.

Effects on Coronary Flow and Dilation

Injection of a conventional contrast agent into a coronary artery causes a transient increase in coronary flow and decrease in coronary resistance within seconds of injection (51). This appears similar in magnitude to the reactive hyperemia response to release of acute coronary occlusion and thus is probably related to coronary vascular reserve. This flow increase is at least in part due to hyperosmolality. However, in a recent study by Tatineni (52), there appeared to be little difference among agents regarding their effect on coronary flow velocity and vasodilator reserve. All agents studied, however, had a significantly higher osmolality than serum. This transient increase in coronary blood flow does seem to cause

only a small change in large coronary artery size. Using standard doses of Renografin-76, Hill et al. (53) have found only **minimal changes in epicardial coronary artery size.** It is unlikely that the minimal coronary dilating effects of contrast agents alter interpretation of angiograms for diagnostic purposes.

INCIDENCE OF ADVERSE EFFECTS

Prior to introduction of nonionic and low-osmolality agents, the most comprehensive data regarding adverse reactions with intravascular administration of contrast agents were collected by the Committee on Safety of Contrast Media of the International Society of Radiology (14, 54). **The overall incidence of adverse reactions is approximately 5%,** but with arterial injection it is only about half of that. In patients with a history of allergy the incidence is 10 to 12%, with the risk being highest in those with a shellfish or saltwater fish allergy, followed by various other food allergies, asthma, hay fever, and penicillin, in descending frequency. In those with a history of contrast reaction the frequency of adverse reaction is only 15 to 16%, with serious reactions rarely recurring. Mild adverse reactions for which no treatment is required and moderate ones for which treatment but not hospitalization is required constitute the overwhelming majority of adverse reactions. Occasionally hospitalization is necessary for a severe reaction (0.007%). The incidence of death following conventional contrast agent administration is estimated to be between 1 in 10,000 and 1 in 40,000. More recently the Royal Australasian Congress of Radiology (RACR) (55) and the Japanese Committee on the Safety of Contrast Media (56) surveys have reported safety data from large numbers of patients who received contrast media. Although these are registry data rather than clinical studies, the overall incidence of adverse reactions was reduced significantly with the use of nonionic media.

With cardiac angiography the incidence of adverse effects is probably different because of the relatively small numbers of patients in these radiologic surveys. Moreover, some specifically exclude such patients (57). A number of reports on the adverse reaction profiles of various contrast media used during cardiac angiography have recently become available. Hirshfeld et al. (58) collected data on the safety of high-osmolality contrast in 4630 cardiac angiographic procedures. They found 657 (14%) minor and 61 (1.3%) major reactions. Of the major reactions 51% were changes in arterial pressure requiring treatment and 34% were pulmonary vascular congestion. Ventricular fibrillation occurred in 8 patients and anaphylactoid reactions in 2, but there were no deaths. In addition, 5.4% of the procedures were abbreviated because of concern about an adverse reaction and 0.7% were abbreviated because of an actual reaction.

Data from a cohort of 8517 consecutive patients who received nonionic contrast, iopamidol or iohexol, for cardiac angiography was reported by Davidson et al. (38). They found a low incidence of cardiovascular complications. The incidence of ventricular tachycardia or fibrillation was 0.1%; severe bradycardia, 0.2%; prolonged angina, 0.3%; thrombotic events, 0.18% (coronary thromboembolus in 7, stroke or transient ischemic attack in 7, and a ventricular catheter thrombus in 1). There were 2 deaths, neither of which was thought to be related to contrast. Harding et al. (59) reported 41 patients who received both iopamidol and diatrizoate during different angiographic procedures. No patient had a major reaction with iopamidol, but 3 suffered a major reaction (prolonged angina in 2 and coronary occlusion in 1) with diatrizoate. In addition, there were 18 minor adverse cardiac events with diatrizoate but only 1 with iopamidol.

There also appear to be some differences in incidence of adverse reactions between nonionic agents and the ionic dimeric low-osmolality agent ioxaglate. Vacek et al. (60) found an 11% incidence of reaction with ioxaglate but only 3% with iohexol (p < .005) in 529 patients undergoing cardiac angiography or angioplasty. Other studies (61, 62) have shown similar or larger differences between nonionic and ionic low-osmolality contrast media.

In patients presumably at higher risk for cardiac adverse events, only limited data compare low-osmolality with high-osmolality contrast. Feldman et al. (63) randomized 82 patients with either heart failure or unstable ischemia to receive either ioxaglate or diatrizoate for their cardiac angiography. A higher incidence of severe adverse reactions was found with diatrizoate (16 versus 2%; p < .05).

Three large randomized studies comparing ionic with nonionic contrast in patients undergoing diagnostic cardiac angiography were reported by Barrett et al. (64), Steinberg et al. (65), and Matthai et al. (66). Barrett et al. randomized patients to receive either diatrizoate or nonionic contrast, mostly iopamidol. Of the 737 patients who received diatrizoate, 29% required treatment for adverse events, whereas only 9% of those receiving nonionic agent did. Likewise, severe reactions were more common with diatrizoate (2.9 compared to 0.8%; p = .035). Steinberg et al. randomized patients undergoing cardiac angiography to receive either iohexol or diatrizoate (Hypaque 76). In their group of 505 patients they found that use of high-osmolality contrast made patients three times as likely to suffer a moderate adverse reaction, but they found no difference in the incidence of severe reactions between the two agents. They also found that unstable angina, female gender, and age over 60 years seemed to place patients at higher risk. Matthai et al., in 2245 patients, found clinically important adverse events more frequently with diatrizoate, with an adjusted odds ratio of 1.59 (p = .07). They also found that a high-risk group could be identified and selective nonionic contrast use was feasible. **The criteria they identified (two were necessary to define high risk) were age at least 65, left ventricular pressure above 15 mm Hg, NYHA (New York Heart Association) class IV, and a history of contrast reaction.**

MANAGEMENT OF "CONTRAST-ALLERGIC" PATIENTS

Management of so-called contrast allergy has ranged from complete avoidance of contrast to skin testing and test dosing to various premedication regimens and finally to doing nothing at all because of the relatively low incidence of severe repeat reactions. None of these approaches is totally satisfactory, but premedication regimens appear to be the safest.

Greenberger et al. (67) reported a series of 857 contrast medium administrations to patients who had a history of anaphylactoid reactions to contrast media and who underwent repeat studies after various pretreatment regimens. In 695 cases prednisone and diphenhydramine were administered, and there was a 10.8% reaction rate with 0.7% developing transient hypotension. Subsequently 180 procedures were performed with ephedrine added to the regimen, and only a 5% rate was noted. Further addition of cimetidine did not change the rate significantly.

In another study reported by Ring et al. (68), various combinations of steroids and H_1 and H_2 receptor antagonists or normal saline were given prospectively to 800 patients undergoing intravenous contrast administration for renal study. In the normal saline group the incidence of adverse effects, excluding heat sensation, was 12.9%. In the combined H_1 and H_2 blocker group the incidence was 6.1% (p < .05). Nausea, urticaria, and angioedema were significantly less with this treatment. No other significant differences were noted. Only one type of contrast agent was used, so comparison among agents is not possible.

Lasser et al. (69) reported a series of 6763 patients with no history of reaction to contrast agents. These patients were given either two doses of methylprednisolone or placebo 12 and 2 hours prior or one dose of methylprednisolone or placebo 2 hours prior to contrast administration. They found that the incidence of contrast reactions was significantly less using the two-dose regimen than with the one-dose regimen (6.4 versus 9.4%). Moreover, the adverse reaction rate in the placebo groups was no different from that of the one-dose regimen (9.9 versus 9.4%). Comparing their data with uncontrolled data using nonionic contrast agents, they found no difference in the rate of reactions between the two-dose methylprednisolone group and the non-

ionic contrast group. They suggested that nonionic agents did not provide any benefit in routine use for preventing adverse effects to contrast agents.

From a practical standpoint, how should these data be applied to the patient undergoing cardiac angiography? A number of factors make available data somewhat less relevant to the average patient undergoing cardiac catheterization. Most studies report a broad group of patients receiving contrast material for a variety of procedures, not just those receiving arterial injection for angiography. Reaction rates with arterial as opposed to venous injection are probably different. Patients undergoing cardiac catheterization tend to be older than the population at large receiving contrast agents, making them somewhat less likely to have a reaction. However, the type of patient undergoing cardiac catheterization and angiography is not likely to tolerate a severe "allergic" reaction well.

For the population at large it is our practice not to premedicate with steroids but only with diphenhydramine orally 30 minutes before the procedure. We believe that premedication with steroids (60 mg of prednisone or the equivalent) the night before and immediately prior to the procedure is appropriate for the patient who has a history of severe reaction to contrast agents. Diphenhydramine (50 mg) and cimetidine (300 mg) should also be given because these agents are very well tolerated and may provide some additional protection. Sympathomimetic drugs, such as ephedrine, are dangerous in cardiac patients and should not be used routinely. While the data are not clear that this regimen is necessary or effective, it is imperative to take reasonable measures to avoid contrast reactions in such a patient. In any case all necessary emergency equipment and drugs for treating adverse reactions should be available for immediate use.

GUIDELINES FOR USE

A general principle of cardiac catheterization is that the procedure should be performed as safely and efficiently as possible

Table 13.2.
Guidelines for Use of Contrast Agents

Type of Angiography	Dose (mL)	Rate of Injection[a] (mL/sec)
Coronary		
Right	3–6	2–3
Left	4–7	2–3
Bypass grafts	4–7	2–3
Left ventricular	30–45	10–15
Aortic	30–60	15–30
Right ventricular	30–45	10–15
Pulmonary	30–60	15–30

[a] Both rate and volume of injection may be smaller with some digital imaging systems.

while obtaining the necessary diagnostic information. Use of contrast agents should be viewed in the same way. It is better to do one diagnostic angiogram than to have to repeat an angiogram because of inadequate visualization. Angiography views should also be obtained in order of decreasing clinical importance. The angiogram (site and projection) that will yield the most diagnostic information should be the first one obtained, especially if the patient has the potential to tolerate only a small volume of contrast. This way, if the procedure has to be aborted, useful information has been obtained.

The amount of contrast administered for any angiogram depends on a variety of factors, including the type of catheter used, the vessel or chamber to be visualized, rate of blood flow in the vessel, size of the patient, tissue density, total amount necessary for all of the angiograms to be performed, and type of contrast agent used. Likewise, rate of injection is related to many factors, the most important of which are the vessel or chamber to be visualized, the flow rate in the vessel, and the type of catheter. Guidelines are provided in Table 13.2. Digital imaging equipment may allow for less injection volume and a change in injection rate, particularly for ventricular or great vessel imaging. The capabilities of the imaging equipment used should be understood. However, these guidelines should be individualized to the patient undergoing study, and it is always better to have one good di-

agnostic angiogram than two of poor quality.

Choosing a Contrast Agent

A number of contrast agents suitable for cardiac angiography are available. Choosing among the different agents is to a certain extent a matter of personal preference. The major differences have been discussed, and this information can be used to guide choice. There has been considerable debate regarding the appropriate use of the newer nonionic, low-osmolality contrast agents (70–75) related to the fact that these agents are considerably more expensive than conventional agents. As competitive bidding and response of industry to pressures from buying consortia increased, however, the cost of these agents, particularly the nonionics, have come down to about half of what they were when first released. The policy statement of the American College of Cardiology (76) suggests that "nonionic contrast agents may be of use in selected patients at high risk for hemodynamic complications during cardiac catheterization and in patients with a history of allergic reaction to contrast material" but "there are no conclusive data to support the universal use of nonionic contrast agents in routine cardiac catheterization in view of the increased cost."

The guidelines listed in Table 13.3 provide a profile of indications for the routine use of nonionic low-osmolality contrast agents. However, many laboratories have

Table 13.3.
Indications for Use of Low Osmolar Contrast Agents

Unstable ischemic syndromes
Congestive heart failure
Diabetes mellitus
Renal insufficiency
Hypotension
Severe bradycardia
History of contrast allergy
Severe valvular heart disease
Need for internal mammary artery injection

chosen to use nonionic or low-osmolality contrast agents routinely in all patients undergoing cardiac angiography to avoid unpredictable so-called close calls (70). Administrative and cost concerns notwithstanding, it is the responsibility of the catheterizing physician to ensure the safety of the patient. As with any other component of catheterization equipment, this must be considered when choosing a contrast agent, and the choice must not be dictated by non-physicians.

SUMMARY

Contrast agents for intravascular administration have been refined so that they can provide diagnostic-quality angiography with minimal risk. Low-osmolality agents, many of which are nonionic, offer an excellent alternative to conventional high-osmolality agents, especially in unstable high-risk patients. In the current cost-conscious environment, however, their routine use is being increasingly scrutinized. The need is not for agents that will lower risk further while providing needed contrast but for a safer and more economical way to administer them.

References

1. Morris TW, Fischer HW. The pharmacology of intravascular radiocontrast media. Annu Rev Pharmacol Toxicol 1986;26:143–160.
2. Hanley PC, Holmes DR, Julsrud PR, Smith HC. Use of conventional and newer radiographic contrast agents in cardiac angiography. Prog Cardiovasc Dis 1986;28:435–448.
3. Thomson KR, Evill CA, Firzsche J, Benness G. Comparison of iopamidol, ioxaglate and diatrizoate during coronary arteriography in dogs. Invest Radiol 1980;115:234–241.
4. Bourdillon PD, Bettmann MD, McCracken S, et al. Effects of a new nonionic and a conventional ionic contrast agent on coronary sinus ionized calcium and left ventricular hemodynamics in dogs. J Am Coll Cardiol 1985;6:845–853.
5. Murdock DK, Walsh J, Euler DE, et al. Inotropic effects of ionic contrast media: the role of calcium binding additives. Cathet Cardiovasc Diagn 1984; 10:455–463.
6. Higgins CB, Gerber KH, Mattrey RF, Slutsky RA. Evaluation of the hemodynamic effects of intravenous administration of ionic and nonionic contrast materials. Radiology 1982;142:681–686.
7. Zukerman LS, Friehling TD, Wolf NM, et al. Effect of calcium binding additives on ventricular fibrillation and repolarization changes during coronary angiography. J Am Coll Cardiol 1987;10:1249–1253.
8. Murdock DK, Johnson SA, Loeb HS, Scanlon PJ. Ventricular fibrillation during coronary angiography: reduced incidence in man with contrast media lacking calcium binding additives. Cathet Cardiovasc Diagn 1985;59:153–159.
9. Murdock DK, Euler DE, Kozeny G, et al. Ventricular fibrillation during coronary angiography in dogs: the role of calcium binding additives. Am J Cardiol 1984;54:897–901.
10. Violante MR, Thomson KR, Fischer HW, Kenyon T. Ventricular fibrillation from diatrizoate with and without chelating agents. Radiology 1978;128:497–498.
11. Berger RE, Gomez LS, Mallette LE. Acute hypocalcemic effects of clinical contrast media injections. Am J Roentgenol 1982;138:282–288.
12. Paulin S, Adams DF. Increased ventricular fibrillation during coronary arteriography with a new contrast medium preparation. Radiology 1971;101:45–50.
13. Goldberg M. Systemic reactions to intravascular contrast media. Anesthesiology 1984;60:46–56.
14. Shehadi WH. Adverse reactions to intravascularly administered contrast media. Am J Roentgenol 1975;124:145–152.
15. Weisberg LS, Kurnik PB, Kurnik BRC. Radiocontrast-induced nephropathy in humans: role of renal vasoconstriction. Kidney Int 1992;41:1408–1415.
16. Hunter JV, Kind PR. Nonionic iodinated contrast media: potential renal damage assessed with enzymuria. Radiology 1992;183:101–104.
17. Thomsen HS. Contrast media- and pharmacologic-induced nephropathies: effects of diatrizoate and iohexol on urine profiles in rats. Invest Radiol 1990; 25:S129–S132.
18. Parvez Z, Ramamurthy S, Patel NB, Moncada R. Enzyme markers of contrast media-induced renal failure. Invest Radiol 1990;25:S133–S134.
19. Berns JS, Rudnick MR. Radiocontrast media associated nephrotoxicity. Kidney 1992;24:1–6.
20. Rich MW, Crecelius CA. Incidence, risk factors, and clinical course of acute renal insufficiency after cardiac catheterization in patients 70 years of age or older: a prospective study. Arch Intern Med 1990;150:1237–1242.
21. Byrd L, Sherman RL. Radiocontrast induced acute renal failure: a clinical and pathophysiologic review. Medicine 1979;58:270–278.
22. Parfrey PS, Griffiths SM, Barrett BJ, et al. Contrast material–induced renal failure in patients with diabetes mellitus, renal insufficiency or both. N Engl J Med 1989;320:143–149.
23. Manske CL, Sprafka JM, Strony JT, Wang Y. Contrast nephropathy in azotemic diabetic patients undergoing coronary angiography., Am J Med 1990;89:615–620.
24. Davidson CJ, Hlatky M, Morris KG, et al. Cardiovascular and renal toxicity of a nonionic radio-

graphic contrast agent after cardiac catheterization: a prospective trial. Ann Intern Med 1989;110: 119–124.

25. Humes HD, Cielinski DA, Messana JM. Effects of radiocontrast agents on renal tubule cell function: implications regarding the pathogenesis of contrast induced nephrotoxicity effects of contrast agents on renal function. Cardiology 1988;5:14–18.

26. Schwab SJ, Hlatky MA, Pieper KS, et al. Contrast nephrotoxicity: a randomized controlled trial of a nonionic and an ionic radiographic contrast agent. N Engl J Med 1989;320:149–153.

27. Taliercio CP, Vlietstra RE, Ilstrup DM, et al. A randomized comparison of the nephrotoxicity of iopamidol and diatrizoate in high risk patients undergoing cardiac angiography. J Am Coll Cardiol 1991;17:384–390.

28. Rudnick MR, Goldfarb S, Wexler L, et al. Nephrotoxicity of ionic and nonionic contrast media in 1196 patients: a randomized trial. Kidney Int 1995; 47:254–261.

29. Nunez BD, Allon M. Effect of cardiac catheterization on renal function. Clin Nephrol 1990;34: 263–266.

30. Taliercio CP, Burnett JC. Contrast nephropathy, cardiology and the newer radiocontrast agents. Int J Cardiol 1988;19:145–151.

31. Solomon R, Werner C, Mann D, et al. Effects of saline, mannitol, and furosemide on acute decreases in renal function induced by radiocontrast agents. N Engl J Med 1994;331:1416–1420.

32. Katholi RE, Taylor GJ, McCann WP, et al. Nephrotoxicity form contrast media: attenuation with theophylline. Radiology 1995;195:17–22.

33. Erley CM, Duda SH, Schlepckow S, et al. Adenosine antagonist theophylline prevents the reduction of glomerular filtration rate after contrast media application. Kidney Int 1994;45:1425–1431.

34. Johnson LW, Krone R. Cardiac catheterization 1991: a report of the registry of the Society for Cardiac Angiography and Interventions (SCA&I). Cathet Cardiovasc Diagn 1993;28:219–220.

35. Kahn JK, Rutherford BD, McConahay DR, et al. High-dose contrast agent administration during complex coronary angioplasty. Am Heart J 1990; 120:533–536.

36. Hardeman MR, Konijnenberg A, Sturk A, Reekers JA. Activation of platelets by low-osmolar contrast media: differential effects of ionic and nonionic agents. Radiology 1994;192:563–566.

37. Grollman JH, Liu CK, Astone RA, Lurie MD. Thromboembolic complications in coronary angiography associated with the use of nonionic contrast medium. Cathet Cardiovasc Diagn 1988;14: 159–164.

38. Davidson C, Mark D, Pieper K, et al. Thrombotic and cardiovascular complications related to nonionic contrast media during cardiac catheterization: analysis of 8,517 patients. Am J Cardiol 1990; 65:1481–1484.

39. Gasperetti CM, Feldman MD, Burwell LR, et al. Influence of contrast media on thrombus formation during coronary angioplasty. J Am Coll Cardiol 1991;18:443–450.

40. Piessens JH, Stammen F, Vrolix MC, et al. Effects of an ionic versus a nonionic low osmolar contrast

agent on the thrombotic complications of coronary angioplasty. Cathet Cardiovasc Diagn 1993;28: 99–105.

41. Esplugas E, Cequier A, Jara F, et al. Contrast media influence on thrombotic risk during coronary angioplasty. Semin Thromb Hemost 1993;19(Suppl 1):192–198.

42. Lembo NJ, King SB, Roubin GS, et al. Effects of nonionic versus ionic contrast media on complications of percutaneous transluminal coronary angioplasty. Am J Cardiol 1991;67:1046–1050.

43. Grines CL, Schrieber TL, Savas V, et al. A randomized trial of low osmolar ionic versus nonionic contrast media in patients with myocardial infarction or unstable angina undergoing percutaneous transluminal coronary angioplasty. J Am Coll Cardiol 1996;27:1381–1386.

44. Hill JA, Grabowski EF. Relationship of anticoagulation and radiographic contrast agents to thrombosis during coronary angiography and angioplasty: are there real concerns? Cathet Cardiovasc Diagn 1992;25:200–208.

45. Moliterno DJ, Topol EJ. Another step toward resolving the contrast controversy. J Am Coll Cardiol 1996;27:1387–1389.

46. Hill JA, Cohen MB, Kou WH, et al. Iodixanol, a new isosmotic nonionic contrast agent, compared with iohexol in cardiac angiography. Am J Cardiol 1994;74:57–63.

47. Gertz EW, Wisneski JA, Chiu D, et al. Clinical superiority of a new nonionic contrast agent (iopamidol) for cardiac angiography. J Am Coll Cardiol 1985;5:250–258.

48. Bettmann MA, Higgins CB. Comparison of an ionic with a nonionic contrast agent for cardiac angiography. Cardiac Angiogr 1985;29:S70–S74.

49. Mancini GBJ, Bloomquist JN, Bhargava V, et al. Hemodynamic and electrocardiographic effects in man of a new nonionic contrast agent (iohexol): advantages over standard ionic agents. Am J Cardiol 1983;51:1218–1222.

50. Stern L, Firth BG, Dehmer GJ, et al. Effect of selective coronary arteriography on left ventricular volumes and ejection fraction in man. Am J Cardiol 1980;46:827–831.

51. Kloster FE, Griesen WG, Green GS, Judkins MP. Effects of coronary arteriography on myocardial blood flow. Circulation 1972;46:438–444.

52. Tatineni S, Kern MJ, Deligonul U, Aguirre F. The effects of ionic and nonionic radiographic contrast media on coronary hyperemia in patients during coronary angiography. Am Heart J 1992;123:621.

53. Hill JA, Feldman RL, Conti CR, Pepine CJ. Effects of selective injection of contrast media on coronary artery diameter. Cathet Cardiovasc Diagn 1982;8: 547–552.

54. Shehadi WH. Contrast media adverse reactions: occurrence, recurrence and distribution patterns. Diagn Radiol 1982;143:11–17.

55. Palmer FJ. The R.A.C.R. survey of intravenous contrast media reactions: a preliminary report. Australas Radiol 1988;32:8–11.

56. Katayama H, Yamaguchi K, Kozuka T, et al. Adverse reactions to ionic and nonionic contrast media. Radiology 1990;175:621–628.

57. Caro JJ, Trindade E, McGregor M. The risks of

death and of severe nonfatal reactions with high- vs low-osmolality contrast media: a meta-analysis. AJR Am J Roentgenol 1991;156:825–832.

58. Hirshfeld JW, Kussmaul WG, DiBattiste PM. Safety of cardiac angiography with conventional ionic contrast agents. Am J Cardiol 1990;66:355–361.

59. Harding M, Davidson C, Pieper K, et al. Comparison of cardiovascular and renal toxicity after cardiac catheterization using a nonionic vs ionic radiographic contrast agent. Am J Cardiol 1991;68:1117–1119.

60. Vacek J, Gersema L, Woods M, et al. Frequencies of reactions to iohexol versus ioxaglate. Am J Cardiol 1990;66:1277–1278.

61. Wisneski JA, Gertz EW, Dahlgren M, Muslin A. Comparison of low osmolality ionic (ioxaglate) versus nonionic (iopamidol) contrast media in cardiac angiography. Am J Cardiol 1989;63:489–495.

62. Klinke WP, Grace M, Miller R, et al. A multicenter randomized trial of ionic (ioxaglate) and nonionic (iopamidol) low-osmolality contrast agents in cardiac angiography. Clin Cardiol 1989;12:689–696.

63. Feldman RL, Jalowiec DA, Hill JA, Lambert CR. Contrast media related complications during cardiac catheterization using Hexabrix or Renografin in high risk patients. Am J Cardiol 1988;61:1334–1337.

64. Barrett BJ, Parfrey PS, Vavasour HM, et al. A comparison of nonionic low-osmolality radiocontrast agents with ionic, high-osmolality agents during cardiac catheterization. N Engl J Med 1992;326:431–436.

65. Steinberg EP, Moore RD, Powe NR, et al. Safety and cost effectiveness of high-osmolality as compared with low-osmolality contrast material in patients undergoing cardiac catheterization. N Engl J Med 1992;326:425–430.

66. Matthai WH, Kussmaul WG, Krol J, et al. A comparison of low- with high-osmolality contrast agents in cardiac angiography: identification of criteria for selective use. Circulation 1994;89:291–301.

67. Greenberger WA, Patterson R, Tapio CM. Prophylaxis against repeated radiocontrast media reactions in 857 cases. Arch Intern Med 1985;145:2197–2200.

68. Ring J, Rothenberger KH, Clauss W. Prevention of anaphylactoid reactions after radiographic contrast media infusion by combined histamine H_1 and H_2 receptor antagonists: results of a prospective controlled trial. Int Arch Allergy Appl Immun 1985;78:9–14.

69. Lasser EC, Berry CC, Talner LB, et al. Pretreatment with corticosteroids to alleviate reactions to intravenous contrast material. N Engl J Med 1987;317:845–849.

70. Hirshfeld JW. Low-osmolality contrast agents: who needs them? N Engl J Med 1992;326:482–484.

71. Hlatky M, Morris K, Pieper K, et al. Randomized comparison of the cost and effectiveness of iopamidol and diatrizoate as contrast agents for cardiac angiography. J Am Coll Cardiol 1990;16:4:871–877.

72. Steinberg EP, Anderson GF, Powe NR, et al. Use of low-osmolality contrast media in a price-sensitive environment. AJR 1988;151:271–274.

73. Brinker JA. Low osmolal contrast: is it a luxury we can no longer afford? Cathet Cardiovasc Diagn 1994;33:20–21.

74. Powe NR, Davidoff AJ, Moore RD, et al. Net costs from three perspectives of using low versus high osmolality contrast medium in diagnostic angiocardiography. J Am Coll Cardiol 1993;21:1701–1709.

75. Hlatky MA. Economic evaluation of low osmolality contrast media. J Am Coll Cardiol 1993;21:1710–1711.

76. Statement of the use of nonionic or low-osmolar contrast agents in cardiovascular procedures. J Am Coll Cardiol 1993;21:269–273.

14
Recording Cardiovascular Variables

Wilmer W. Nichols, PhD
Charles R. Lambert, MD, PhD
Carl J. Pepine, MD

INTRODUCTION

Physiologic waveforms or cardiovascular variables recorded in the cardiac catheterization laboratory are usually time-varying periodic functions, such as the electrocardiogram, blood pressure (1–4), blood flow (1, 4–7), ventricular volume (8,9) and arterial diameter (10). Each variable has its own characteristic waveform, which changes relatively little from one beat to the next in a constant physiologic state. Various transducers are used to convert these physiologic events to electrical signals that are amplified, monitored, recorded, processed, and stored (Fig. 14.1). A large amount of information can be obtained from simple inspection of the wave contours (1–3), but more specific quantified data are even more valuable; for example, the reduced rate of rise of aortic and left ventricular pressures in aortic stenosis and myocardial disease, respectively. Recording of cardiovascular variables at the time of cardiac catheterization is therefore only a first step, to be followed by quantitative analysis. The goal of the analysis is to put the observations in a numeric form for easy tabulation and understanding.

The objective of physiologic recording in the diagnostic catheterization laboratory is to obtain a faithful reproduction of the cardiovascular variable of interest. If this is not entirely achieved, a measuring error must exist (4, 11). **Measuring errors may arise in any part of the recording system—the transducer, catheter, amplifier, recorder, or any other component.** Therefore, when testing for accuracy, the entire recording system should be evaluated.

Transducers, the instruments used to convert force, motion, or other cardiovascular variables into an electrical signal, are discussed in Chapters 21 and 22. This chapter is concerned with amplifying, recording, displaying, processing, and storing these signals. Any system designed for faithful reproduction of an event or variable must meet the following criteria: (*a*) amplitude linearity, (*b*) adequate frequency response, and (*c*) phase linearity (11).

AMPLITUDE LINEARITY

Amplitude linearity is the ability of the transducer–processor–reproducer system to produce an output signal that is directly proportional in magnitude to the amplitude of the input signal. This condition must be satisfied for measurements both above and below the zero baseline and should include the entire range of measurement (Fig. 14.2). Thus before calibration and linearity testing the approximate range of the variable to be measured should be known. This can usu-

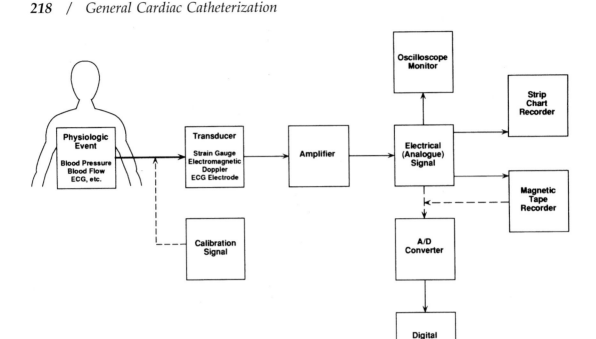

Figure 14.1. Data-handling schema for a cardiac catheterization laboratory. The physiologic event or cardiovascular variable being recorded may be blood pressure, blood flow, electrocardiogram, or other event that varies with time. The event detected by the sensor (transducer) is amplified and transmitted as an electrical signal to an oscilloscopic monitor, a strip chart recorder, and a magnetic tape recorder. If desired, the electrical analog signal may be converted to digital form and analyzed by a digital computer. The digitized signal may be stored on cards, tapes, or disks.

ally be obtained from the literature or a few preliminary measurements. In Figure 14.2 linearity of the electrical output of an electromagnetic flowmeter–catheter tip velocity transducer system was tested in a bidirectional hydraulic pump model (12). The velocity of the liquid (physiologic saline) detected by the electromagnetic velocity transducer, amplified by the flowmeter, and transmitted to the chart recorder, was linear (r = 0.996) over the range −103 to +110 cm/second, which covers the range of blood flow velocity measurements reported in the literature for normal humans (2, 13–15). Although the input–output characteristics of a system may be represented as a straight line, careful testing with accurate inputs usually reveals a small deviation from linearity (Fig. 14.2). Under these conditions regression analysis should be performed to obtain the line of best fit and this relation used in calibration.

Hysteresis

Another quality related to system linearity is hysteresis (i.e., lag), a measure of the ability of the system to produce an output that follows the input independent of the direction or change in magnitude of the input (16). When hysteresis is present in a system, an open curve (or Lissajou loop) results from linearity testing (Fig. 14.3). The amount of hysteresis is usually expressed in terms of the percentage of full-scale value. In the exaggerated example shown in Figure 14.3, the hysteresis error is approximately 20%. With most modern recording systems this error is less than 1%.

Noise

Another problem in recording systems is unwanted signals (noise) superimposed

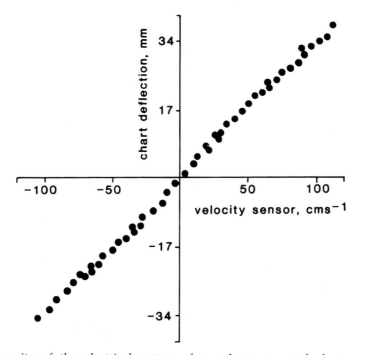

Figure 14.2. Linearity of the electrical output of a catheter-mounted electromagnetic velocity transducer–flowmeter system over the range of velocities recorded in normal humans. Linearity was determined in a bidirectional hydraulic pump model filled with physiologic saline. Reverse flow is indicated by a *minus sign*. The correlation coefficient was 0.996. (Reprinted with permission from Nichols WW, Paley DM, Thompson LV, Lambert CR. Experimental evaluation of a multisensor velocity-pressure catheter. Med Biol Eng Comput 1985;23:79–83.)

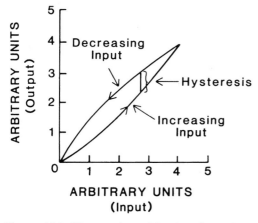

Figure 14.3. Hysteresis, or Lissajou, loop showing deviation from linearity during increases and decreases in system input and the corresponding variation in output.

on the cardiovascular variable of interest. The frequency of noise is usually much higher than that of the variable of interest. The **noise is part of the output of an instrument not related to the variable itself.** Sometimes it is generated within the instrument; at other times it is caused by external interference. In any recording system it is necessary to distinguish the signal from the noise. This can be done by measuring the signal-to-noise ratio and calculating the noise figure (17). The amount of noise in the output signal depends on the amount of noise amplified by the amplifier and presented to the output. The signal-to-noise ratio at the input divided by the signal-to-noise ratio at the output is the noise figure. Ideally it should equal unity.

Since the patient tends to act as an antenna, a spectral analysis of the noise (the amount of noise concentrated at each frequency) would show a rather large 60-Hz component. This is because most electrical instruments in the United States use 60-Hz current, and this 60-Hz noise is radiated from a variety of wires and devices.

The best way to manage noise is to identify its source and eliminate it. In most cases this can be accomplished by proper grounding. Every cardiac catheterization laboratory should be provided with a good reference ground. This means that electrostatic shields must be provided with an extremely low resistance path to the earth. In this way excess electrons can travel to and from the earth, which acts as an infinitely large source of electrons and an infinitely large sink into which electrons can flow (17). All electronic instruments in the laboratory should be grounded to this reference ground point, care being taken to avoid an excessive number of ground leads. In some cases it is necessary to ground the patient. However, the patient table and the particular instrument must not be grounded to the reference point and the table grounded to the instrument. If this is done, a ground loop is established, and the noise increases considerably (17). All ground wires should be arranged as symmetrically as possible and should be at least 12-gauge insulated wire.

High-frequency noise can also be eliminated or minimized by introducing a low-frequency bandpass electronic filter into the circuit. However, when adding electronic filters, it is important not to filter the cardiovascular variable itself (discussed later in this chapter). Another approach to removal of noise from periodic signals is digital signal averaging. Signal averaging is commonly used to derive the signal-averaged electrocardiogram. In this application efficient noise removal is crucial to record very low voltage afterpotentials. This degree of noise removal is not needed for routine clinical hemodynamic recording; however, it is useful in research applications.

Drift

The tendency of recording systems to drift or gradually change their output can complicate a catheterization. In most cases, in-

strumentation drift affects only the baseline calibration. If baseline drift does occur, the calibration, or linearity, curve (Fig. 14.2) moves up or down without a change in slope. If the calibration factor, or step, is affected, the slope of the calibration curve changes. Baseline drift in a fluid-filled pressure recording system can be detected and corrected by frequent checks of the zero baseline by opening a stopcock and exposing the pressure transducer to atmospheric pressure. When measuring blood flow velocity in the main pulmonary artery or ascending aorta, one assumes that the flat portion of the velocity curve in late diastole is zero baseline; electronic zero, especially of electromagnetic flowmeters, cannot always be trusted (4). Changes in the calibration factor can be detected only by recalibration. **No matter how carefully a system was calibrated initially, erroneous measurements are obtained if either the zero baseline or the calibration factor changes.** Fortunately, the recording systems used in modern cardiac catheterization laboratories are designed to minimize instrument drift and maintain constant calibration. However, it is still unwise to assume system stability, and catheterization procedures should allow for periodic checking and readjustment if necessary. Some transducers, especially those used to measure blood pressure, are particularly sensitive to environmental temperature; therefore, the recording system should be turned on well in advance of any measurement. In a busy laboratory it may be desirable to leave the recorder on all day.

Calibration

Calibration must be carried out over the range of input amplitudes to be measured (see earlier section). Calibration entails determination of the response of the entire system, including the recording apparatus and any other devices, such as strip chart recorders, oscilloscope monitors, and magnetic tape recorders. Fluid-filled catheter–manometer systems, those most commonly used in the cardiac catheterization laboratory for measuring blood pres-

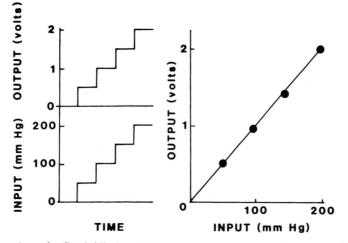

Figure 14.4. Calibration of a fluid-filled catheter–manometer system. Incremental increases in pressure are applied to the manometer and the resulting output voltage signal recorded (*left*). These input–output values are plotted as a linear relationship (*right*). (Reprinted with permission from Milnor WR. Hemodynamics. 2nd ed. Baltimore: Williams & Wilkins, 1989.)

sure, are usually calibrated against a column of mercury. **Calibration for every catheterization procedure is essential.** Incremental increases in mm Hg (input) are applied to the pressure transducer, and the resulting output signals are measured (Fig. 14.4). A plot of the input–output values results in a linear calibration relationship. Using the relationships of Figures 14.2 and 14.4, one obtains calibrated scales for the chart recording of ascending aortic blood pressure and blood flow velocity signals (Fig. 14.5). The velocity signal can be calibrated in volumetric flow units by multiplying by the cross-sectional area of the ascending aorta or main pulmonary artery or by comparison of the mean velocity signal with a simultaneous measurement of cardiac output (13).

ADEQUATE FREQUENCY RESPONSE AND PHASE LINEARITY

The dynamic frequency response and phase linearity are the ability of the recording system to provide a signal that is identical except in amplitude to the event presented to it. The dynamic frequency response of a re-

cording system must be great enough to detect the highest harmonic of the cardiovascular variable being recorded. Before the frequency response of such a system can be adequately discussed, it is necessary to establish the relationship between sine waves and waves of nonsinusoidal form. All periodic waves of nonsinusoidal form are designated complex waves (2, 4, 18, 19). It is possible to show with Fourier series analysis that any periodic complex wave can be dissected into a series of sine and cosine waves that when added, produce the original complex wave. Although this type of analysis was little used in cardiovascular physiology until it was introduced by Womersley (20) and McDonald (21), it was used theoretically by Otto Frank (22) many years earlier. Since Fourier series analysis is unfamiliar to most cardiologists, a general account of the nature and application of the series is given here. We make no attempt to be mathematically rigorous, especially in relation to the type of curves under concern, since they cannot be defined as a function of an algebraic variable on which the processes of integration can be performed. Instead these curves have to be dealt with as a finite sum of measured values.

A periodic function, $F(t)$, is defined as one that repeats itself after a given time, T.

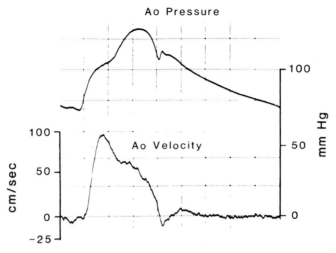

Figure 14.5. Calibrated high-fidelity ascending aortic (*Ao*) pressure and blood flow velocity waves recorded in a normal human subject using a Millar multisensor pressure–velocity catheter.

This may be expressed as $F(t) = F(t + T)$. This is familiar in the definition of a sinusoidal wave, which repeats after 2π radians so that $\sin x = \sin(x + n2\pi)$, as the frequency f is $1/T$, and then the angular frequency, ω, in radians per second, is given by $\omega = 2\pi/T = 2\pi f$. The Fourier theorem may be stated thus: if $y = F(t)$ is any continuous function of the variable t that repeats with a period T, then $F(t) = A_0 + A_1 \cos \omega t + A_2 \cos \omega t + A_3 \cos 3\omega t + \ldots + A_n \cos n\omega t + B_1 \sin \omega t + B_2 \sin 2\omega t + B_3 \sin 3\omega t + \ldots + B_n \sin n\omega t$, where n is an integer. A_0 is the mean value of the function over the period T, or from 0 to 2π. The sinusoidal components are called harmonics, with $n = 1$ being the first or fundamental harmonic. The frequency of the fundamental is that of a composite wave.

The Fourier coefficients A and B can be calculated from the following equations:

$$A_n = \frac{1}{\pi} \int_0^{2\pi} F(t) \cos n\omega t\,(dt)$$

and

$$B_n = \frac{1}{\pi} \int_0^{2\pi} F(t) \sin n\omega t\,(dt)$$

The Fourier coefficients can be converted to modulus (*M*) and phase (ω) by:

$$M_n = \sqrt{(A_n^2 + B_n^2)}$$

and

$$\tan \phi_n = \frac{B_n}{A_n}$$

This is the mathematical method for determining the Fourier series of a periodic function (4, 18, 19).

The actual calculation of the Fourier series of a curve (e.g., a cardiovascular variable) is performed by drawing a number, $2r$, of equally spaced ordinates, each of which has the value y_r. Then we may write

$$A_o = \frac{1}{2r} \sum_{r=1}^{2r-1} y_r,$$

$$A_n = \frac{1}{r} \sum_{r=1}^{2r-1} y_r \cos \left(\frac{n\pi}{r}\right)$$

and

$$B_n = \frac{1}{r} \sum_{r=1}^{2r-1} y_r \sin \left(\frac{n\pi}{r}\right)$$

The values of y_r are now given by the finite series.

$$y_r = A_o + \sum_{n=1}^{r} \left[A_n \cos \left(\frac{n\pi}{r}\right) + B_n \sin \left(\frac{n\pi}{r}\right)\right]$$

A digital computer program is used to carry out this operation (discussed later in this chapter).

The arterial blood pressure pulse is a good example of the application of Fourier series analysis to a periodic wave. Westerhof et al. (23), using a high-fidelity catheter tip pressure transducer, recorded the arterial pressure in the ascending aorta of a dog and subjected the wave to Fourier series analysis. Their results (Fig. 14.6) show the degree of fidelity obtainable by summing various harmonics. Individual harmonics are shown at the left, and the reconstructed, or resynthesized, curves are shown at the right. Reconstruction of the curve with the first six harmonics leads to a curve similar to the original arterial pressure wave; however, this is much improved by adding higher harmonics, up to 20 Hz.

Reproduction of the original curve from a given number of harmonic terms can by inspection give a qualitative check on the adequacy of the analysis. For a more quantitative measure the variance of the curve and of the Fourier series is compared (4, 18). The variance of a curve is the square of the standard deviation. Thus for a curve delineated by m ordinates with a mean value of y, we have

$$Variance = \frac{1}{m} \sum_{i=1}^{m} (y_i - \bar{y})^2$$

or more usually calculated as

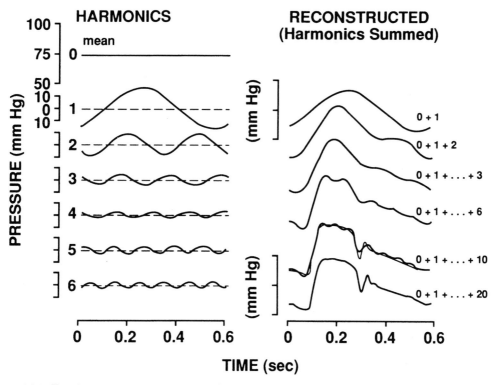

Figure 14.6. Fourier series representation of a periodic wave. *Left*, The mean term (or 0 harmonic) and harmonics 1 through 6 of a pressure wave, recorded in the ascending aorta of a dog. *Right*, individual harmonics are added to reconstruct or resynthesize the original measured wave. Agreement is relatively close with the first six harmonics (0 + 1 + ... + 6) summed and better with the first 10 harmonics (0 + 1 + ... + 10). The resynthesized wave is almost identical to the original wave (*thin line*) with the summation of the first 20 harmonics (0 + 1 + ... + 20). (Reprinted with permission from Westerhof N, Sipkema P, Elzinga G, et al. Arterial impedance. In: Hwang HC, Gross DR, Patel DJ, eds. Quantitative cardiovascular studies. Baltimore: University Park Press, 1979.)

$$Variance = \frac{1}{m}\sum_{i=1}^{m} y_i^2 - \left(\frac{1}{m}\sum_{i=1}^{m} y_i\right)^2$$

The variance of a Fourier series is given from the following equation resulting from Parseval's theorem:

$$Variance(series) = \frac{1}{2}\sum_{n=1}^{k} M_n^2$$

that is, half the sum of the squares of the moduli (M_n) of the harmonic terms used. The graphs shown in Figure 14.7 give the progressive sum of the variance of series rep-

resenting typical aortic and left ventricular pressure and aortic blood flow velocity waveforms as a percentage of the variance of the original curves. More than 99% of the variance of each curve is reached by the ninth or tenth harmonic. No appreciable improvement is achieved by going to 20 harmonics, and the residual loss appears to consist mostly of noise in the recording system and the low-energy content of cardiovascular sounds (4). It is evident from these results and those of others (24) that no significant propagated wave in relation to blood flow exists above 30 Hz (harmonic number × heart frequency) in humans, and those

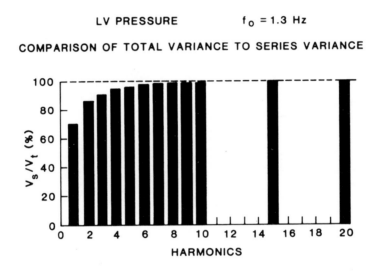

LV PRESSURE $f_o = 1.3$ Hz

COMPARISON OF TOTAL VARIANCE TO SERIES VARIANCE

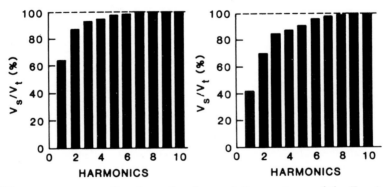

Ao PRESSURE $f_o = 1.3$ Hz   Ao VELOCITY $f_o = 1.3$ Hz

Figure 14.7. Histograms representing the ratio of cumulative variance of the Fourier series (V_s) to the total variance (V_t) of left ventricular (*LV*) pressure (*top*), ascending aortic (*Ao*) pressure (*bottom left*), and blood flow velocity (*bottom right*) waveforms. More than 99% of the variance of each waveform is in the first 10 harmonics.

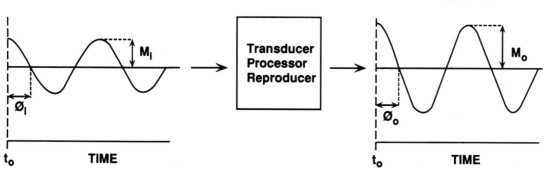

Figure 14.8. Sine wave input and output of a recording system. $\varnothing$ is the phase of the sine wave and M is the modulus or amplitude. Phase but not modulus of the output (o) should be identical to that of the input (i).

above 20 Hz are extremely small. Therefore the system used to record pressure and flow waves should have a dynamic frequency response that is flat plus or minus 5% to at least 20 Hz. A system capable of recording the pressure amplitude without distortion up to 60 Hz is mandatory for accurate peak left ventricular dP/dt determination (25). For electrocardiographic recordings the bandwidth of the system should be 0.05 to 100 Hz (11), and for electrophysiologic recordings the bandwidth should be 30 to 500 Hz.

The dynamic frequency characteristics of a recording system can be tested by using a sine wave forcing function as input and observing the output (Fig. 14.8). The output of the system should also be a sine wave of similar frequency and phase but not amplitude. If the phase of the output differs from that of the input, it must be linear with frequency (discussed later in this chapter) so that a correction factor can be introduced in analysis (4). The use of a sine wave generator to determine the frequency response of a fluid-filled catheter–manometer system is illustrated in Figure 14.9. The catheter–manometer system was used to measure left ventricular pressure, and this signal was compared with that measured with a high-fidelity catheter tip pressure manometer (26). It is evident that **blood pressure measured with the low–frequency response fluid-filled catheter–manometer system is much distorted in both phase and contour.** In this example the error is introduced in the fluid-filled catheter–manometer system

(see Chapter 22); however, the event or variable can be distorted by any component of the recording system. Therefore, before a cardiovascular variable is recorded, the entire recording system must be tested for amplitude linearity, adequate frequency response, and phase linearity. As mentioned previously, dynamic frequency response and phase linearity of a system can be tested by using a sine wave forcing function as input and recording the output. The frequency of the sine wave generator is increased in increments, and the relative amplitude (output divided by input) and phase lag (output minus input) are recorded and plotted against frequency (Fig. 14.10). Relative amplitude and phase lag are both influenced by the degree of damping in the system. With optimal damping, amplitude and phase distortion are minimal. In the example given in Figure 14.10, the frequency response of the system is almost flat to approximately 35 Hz, and the phase lag is relatively linear over this frequency range. Therefore, accurate recordings of pulsatile hemodynamic variables could be obtained with this system; however, recordings of the electrocardiogram would be in error.

Graphic Records

Recorders of cardiovascular variables in the cardiac catheterization laboratory are generally one of two types, direct thermal or

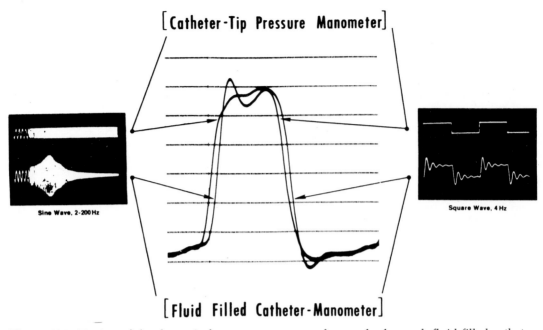

Figure 14.9. Testing of the dynamic frequency response of an underdamped, fluid-filled catheter–manometer system. Left ventricular blood pressure recorded with the low-frequency response, fluid-filled system is compared with the pressure recorded with a high-fidelity catheter tip pressure manometer. (Reprinted with permission from Nichols WW, Pepine CJ, Millar HD, et al. Percutaneous left ventricular catheterization with an ultraminiature catheter tip pressure transducer. Cardiovasc Res 1978;7:566–568.)

optical (18). The first type, the direct thermal recorder, is relatively new and is being used increasingly commonly in modern cardiac catheterization laboratories. Direct thermal recording is a technique similar to the one used in fax machines. It requires the following:

1. Temperature-sensitive paper
2. A thermal print head
3. A method for controlling the energy supplied to the print head

A thermal print head consists of a series of closely spaced resistive elements mounted on nonconductive material. The assembly is coated with a protective glaze and mounted on a heat sink. A drive roller or platen holds the thermal paper against the glaze. The platen is made of a soft rubber that ensures uniform contact between the print head and thermal paper. When voltage is applied to the resistive elements of the print head, current flows and generates heat. The heat is conducted through the

protective glaze to the paper. Heat is also conducted to the heat sink on which the print head is mounted. Thermal paper darkens with the application of sufficient heat. Thermal paper usually marks clearly when exposed to about 80° C. These recorders have a dynamic frequency response from DC to the kilohertz range. The second type, the optical recorder, uses photographic methods to record a beam of light reflected from a mirror galvanometer or the spot on a cathode ray tube. Optical recorders, especially the commonly used oscillographic type, also offer ultrahigh dynamic frequency characteristics. The frequency characteristics of any recording system are no better than their weakest link, which may be amplifier, recorder, transducer, or any other component. The frequency characteristics needed for faithful reproduction of physiologic events depends on the variable being recorded (see earlier discussion).

Amplifiers of many graphic recorders

have a filter control knob that allows the operator to filter out unwanted noise at the output. Noisy records can be made to look better in this way, but one must make certain that the cardiovascular variable itself is not being distorted at the same time. The frequency contents of several variables are given earlier. The so-called normal frequencies indicated on an instrument dial or in the manufacturer's operational manual are not always defined in the same way. Therefore, it is always wise to test the dynamic frequency response of a system under the experimental conditions in which it is to be used, plotting a frequency response curve like that in Figure 14.10. Usually the nominal frequency is the one at which the relative amplitude is reduced by approximately 30%.

The quantitative analysis of data in a finished graphic record begins with translation of selected points on the tracings into numbers or digits, a form of analog-to-digital (A-D) conversion. Measurement with a good millimeter scale and small calculator is the simplest method, but a higher degree of accuracy can be obtained with manually operated instruments designed for that purpose. The accuracy to be sought depends on the precision of the record itself, and it is rarely possible to resolve the measurements into units any smaller than a distance of 0.3 mm on the recording paper (18). The measurements obtained with the millimeter scale are calibrated by comparison with the recorded response to a known signal (Figs. 14.2 and 14.4).

Magnetic Records

Two types of magnetic data storage, analog and digital, are available. The analog form

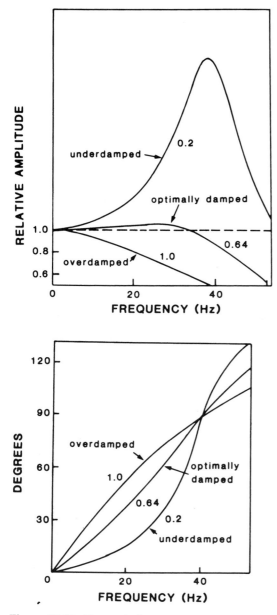

Figure 14.10. Dynamic frequency response of a recording system with different degrees of damping when driven by a sine wave forcing function. *Top,* Relative amplitude (output–input) versus frequency of the sine wave. When the system is underdamped, the amplitude tends to be augmented as the frequency approaches the resonant frequency of the system. With optimal damping the relative amplitude remains almost flat to a certain frequency and then declines. Overdamping limits the response to lower frequencies. *Bottom,* Phase lag (output–input) versus frequency of the sine wave. When the system is optimally damped, the phase lag is relatively linear with frequency; however, with overdamping and underdamping the relation deviates from linearity.

is essentially a continuous magnetic tape record of input voltage, its intensity varying with time in the same way as the original physiologic signal (Fig. 14.1). Reel-to-reel or cassette tape recorders used for this purpose are similar in design to those for recording and reproduction of sound. Because it is technically difficult to transform the DC components of the physiologic signal directly into magnetic code, the signal on the magnetic tape is usually a frequency-modulated version of the input voltage (18). The upper limit of the dynamic frequency response in such recordings depends on the tape speed; the faster the speed, the higher the frequency response. Relatively slow speeds are accurate for magnetic tape recording of most cardiovascular variables. Many magnetic tape recorders give a flat frequency response from 0 to 200 Hz at a tape speed of fifteen-sixteenths of an inch per second. A faster speed is necessary for electrophysiologic recordings.

In digital systems the analog voltage input is sampled at specified intervals, and each sample is converted into a number proportional to that voltage. The sampling rate is controlled by an internal clock, and a wide choice of intervals is usually available to the programer. Magnetic patterns represent digits in this method, and a series of coded numbers is stored on the recording medium (magnetic card, tape, or disk). Although the continuously changing input voltage is converted into a series of discrete readings, this list of numbers can represent almost any waveform adequately if the sampling interval is made sufficiently small. **The highest frequencies that can be recorded are related to the sampling interval;** a sampling interval of 5 or 10 milliseconds is adequate for most hemodynamic variables (4, 18). Calibration signals are recorded and used to translate the digital data into the proper units later.

DIGITAL COMPUTERS

The last step in the processing of cardiovascular variables or events obtained during cardiac catheterization is the calculation of desired variables (e.g., impedance spectra, ventricular work, ventricular wall stress). The amplified variable or electrical analog signal from the patient can be recorded on magnetic tape in analog form and analyzed later, after A-D conversion with a digital computer, or the signal can be converted to digital form and analyzed on line during the catheterization procedure (Fig. 14.1).

Before a calculation can be performed by the computer, the analog signal must be converted into a set of numbers, or digits. Mathematical operations and other manipulations are performed by the computer by means of a step-by-step sequence of instructions, the program. In recent years computer programing has become relatively simple, and commercial application packages to process routine clinical hemodynamic variables are available from several sources. Despite the apparent simplicity of such programs, it behooves the invasive cardiologist to use such applications critically to ensure quality control and measurement accuracy. **As digital applications for the cardiac catheterization laboratory continue to expand, computer literacy on the part of the cardiologist will become a necessity.**

SUMMARY

Cardiac catheterization laboratory recording systems are moving toward less analog and more digital technology. This applies to image (see Chapter 12) as well as hemodynamic, electrocardiographic, and electrophysiologic data. The laboratory of the not-too-distant future will be an all-digital operation with an option for final selective output of image and hemodynamic data to a digital transport medium and a digital archival medium. These data will be downloaded as part of the patient's unit record to a digital medium, probably a card or compact disk. The paperless laboratory will be the norm. Despite this inevitable evolution into all-digital black-box data acquisition, processing, and storage, the principles described in this chapter will still apply and must be understood by the operator to obtain accurate and precise data.

References

1. Murgo JP, Westerhof N, Giolma JP, Altobelli SA. Aortic input impedance in normal man: relationship to pressure wave shape. Circulation 1980;62:105–116.
2. O'Rourke MF. Arterial function in health and disease. London: Churchill Livingstone, 1982.
3. Wiggers CJ. The pressure pulses in the cardiovascular system. London: Longmans, 1928.
4. Nichols WW, O'Rourke MF. McDonald's blood flow in arteries. 4th ed. London: Edward Arnold, 1997.
5. Kern MJ, Anderson HV. The clinical applications of the intracoronary Doppler guidewire flow velocity in patients: understanding blood flow beyond the coronary stenosis. Am J Cardiol 1993;71:1D–86D.
6. Bertolet BD, Belardinelli L, Franco EA, et al. Selective attenuation by N-0861 (N^6-endonorboran-2-yl-9-methyladenine) of cardiac A_1 receptor-mediated effects in humans. Circulation 1996;93:1871–1976.
7. Nichols WW, Pepine CJ, Conti CR, Christie LG. Evaluation of a new catheter-mounted electromagnetic velocity sensor during cardiac catheterization. Cathet Cardiovasc Diagn 1980;6:1–11.
8. Schreuder JJ, van der Veen FH, van der Velde ET, et al. Beat-to-beat analysis of left ventricular pressure-volume relation and stroke volume by conductance catheter and aortic Modelflow in cardiomyoplasty patients. Circulation 1995;91:2010–2017.
9. Odake M, Takeuchi M, Takaoka H, et al. Determination of left ventricular volume using a conductance catheter in the diseased human heart. Eur Heart J 1992;13 (Suppl E):22–27.
10. Stefanadis C, Tsiamis E, Vlachopoulas C, et al. Unfavorable effect of smoking on the elastic properties of the human aorta. Circulation 1997;95:31–38.
11. Geddes LA, Baker LE. Principles of applied biomedical instrumentation. 2nd ed. New York: John Wiley & Sons, 1975.
12. Nichols WW, Paley DM, Thompson LV, Lambert CR. Experimental evaluation of a multisensor velocity-pressure catheter. Med Biol Eng Comput 1985;23:79–83.
13. Nichols WW, Conti CR, Walker WE, Milnor WR. Input impedance of the systemic circulation in man. Circ Res 1977;40:451–458.
14. Laskey WK, Kussmaul WG, Martin JL, et al. Characteristics of vascular hydraulic load in patients with heart failure. Circulation 1985;72:61–71.
15. Nichols WW, O'Rourke MF, Avolio AP, et al. Effects of age on ventricular-vascular coupling. Am J Cardiol 1985;55:1179–1184.
16. Cobbold RSC. Transducers for biomedical measurements: principles and applications. New York: John Wiley & Sons, 1974.
17. Yanof HM. Biomedical electronics. 2nd ed. Philadelphia: FA Davis, 1972.
18. Milnor WR. Hemodynamics. 2nd ed. Baltimore: Williams & Wilkins, 1989.
19. Geddes, LA. Handbook of blood pressure measurement. Clifton, NJ: Humana Press, 1991.
20. Womersley JR. Method for the calculation of velocity, rate of flow and viscous drag in arteries when the pressure gradient is known. J Physiol (Lond) 1955;127:553–563.
21. McDonald DA. The relation of pulsatile pressure to flow in arteries. J Physiol (Lond) 1955;127:533–552.
22. Frank O. Die Theorie der Pulswellen. zeitschriff für Biologie 1927;85:91–130.
23. Westerhof N, Sipkema P, Elzinga G, et al. Arterial impedance. In: Hwang HC, Gross DR, Patel DJ, eds. Quantitative cardiovascular studies. Baltimore: University Park Press, 1979.
24. Patel DJ, Mason DT, Ross J, Braunwald E. Harmonic analysis of pressure pulses obtained from the heart and great vessels in man. Am Heart J 1965;69:785–794.
25. Gersh BJ, Hahn CEW, Prys-Roberts C. Physical criteria for measurement of left ventricular pressure and its first derivative. Cardiovasc Res 1971;5:32–40.
26. Nichols WW, Pepine CJ, Millar HD, et al. Percutaneous left ventricular catheterization with an ultraminiature catheter tip pressure transducer. Cardiovasc Res 1978;7:566–568.

Section
4

DIAGNOSTIC CARDIAC CATHETERIZATION TECHNIQUES

15

Indications and Contraindications for Cardiac Catheterization

Charles R. Lambert, MD, PhD
James A. Hill, MD, MS
Carl J. Pepine, MD

INTRODUCTION

Since the previous edition of this text was published, diagnostic cardiac catheterization has continued to grow in volume. Trends in diagnostic and therapeutic cardiac catheterization are toward more outpatient procedures, fewer combined right and left heart studies, less use of ionic contrast material, and an increasing number of diagnostic procedures, largely coronary angiography, that lead to interventional procedures (1). It can be assumed that as therapeutic techniques such as coronary stent implantation continue to advance, the volume of diagnostic procedures will also continue to grow. However, growth in diagnostic and therapeutic modalities is raising costs, which may become prohibitive, especially in some managed care settings. The increasing cost of invasive cardiac diagnosis and treatment is being scrutinized with a need to improve intermediate- to long-term outcomes rather than acute procedural or short-term results. Therefore, it is more important than ever to be careful in development and revision of indications for procedures. Whereas in the past indication guidelines have been used primarily to guide patient care, more and more frequently the same guidelines are being used to justify performance of procedures a priori or to approve payment for them. Both **the cardiologist and primary care physician need to understand guidelines for cardiology to deal with payors and with use review agencies, as well as to provide optimal care for patients.**

The first American College of Cardiology–American Heart Association (ACC/AHA) Task Force guidelines for coronary angiography were published in 1987 (2). A large portion of the explosion in transcatheter therapeutics that is now fueling an increasing number of diagnostic coronary angiograms took place in the ensuing 10 years. It is therefore appropriate that these guidelines have recently been revised (3). This chapter reviews the new ACC/AHA guidelines for coronary angiography, angioscopy, intracoronary ultrasound, and Doppler velocimetry. In addition, comments illustrate differences between the 1987 and 1998 recommendations. A complementary document is the ACC/AHA Task Force Guidelines for cardiac catheterization and cardiac catheterization laboratories, which was published in 1991 (4).

The indication for cardiac catheterization still generally is **suspicion of structural heart disease or known heart disease that requires additional evaluation** and directions for therapy. Most commonly suspicion of coronary artery disease prompts cardiac catheterization in the United States. Valvular, congenital, myocardial, pericardial, great vessel, or other pathology may also necessitate an invasive study. The most widely performed invasive cardiac procedure in the United States and in most developed countries remains coronary angiography.

CLASSIFICATION GUIDELINES

A standard classification nomenclature from the ACC/AHA Task Force subcommittees is generally used in formulation of guidelines for cardiac procedures, tests, and therapies. For coronary angiography this has been modified in the newer guidelines as follows:

Class I describes conditions for which there is evidence or general agreement that coronary angiography is useful and effective. A Class I indication should not be taken to mean that coronary angiography is the only acceptable diagnostic procedure. Likewise, failure to elect coronary angiography for patients with Class I conditions is not necessarily medically or legally incorrect.

Class II describes conditions for which there is a divergence of opinion about usefulness and efficacy of performing the procedure. In the revised coronary angiography guidelines this class was subdivided. **In Class IIa the weight of evidence or opinion is in favor of performance of the procedure.** In Class IIb usefulness or efficacy is less well established by evidence and opinion. **Class III describes conditions for which there is evidence or general agreement that coronary angiography is not useful and effective and in some patients may be harmful** (e.g., risks outweigh benefits).

In addition, the weight of evidence in support of the recommendation for each listed indication is presented as follows in the 1998 revision:

A: Multiple randomized clinical trials
B: A single randomized clinical trial

C: Expert consensus

PATIENTS WITH KNOWN OR SUSPECTED CORONARY ARTERY DISEASE

The most common need for coronary angiography is to evaluate patients with known or suspected symptomatic ischemic heart disease. Asymptomatic patients are those with no symptoms to suggest cardiac ischemia in the previous 6 weeks. **Known coronary artery disease** (CAD) is CAD documented by either angiography or prior confirmed myocardial infarction according to World Health Organization criteria. **Suspect CAD** is taken to mean clinical characteristics or test results that suggest high risk of CAD and its related adverse outcomes in patients who are asymptomatic.

ASYMPTOMATIC PATIENTS

Class I

1. High risk for adverse outcome based on noninvasive testing (Table 15.1) (level of evidence C).
2. Successful resuscitation from cardiac arrest or sustained ventricular tachycardia without obvious precipitating cause (level of evidence B).

Class IIa

1. Periodic evaluation after cardiac transplantation (level of evidence C).
2. Abnormal but not high-risk stress testing result or multiple clinical features suggesting high risk in individuals whose occupation involves safety of others (e.g., pilots, bus drivers) (level of evidence C).

Class IIb

1. At least 1 but less than 2 mm of ischemic type of ST segment depression during exercise with concordant abnormalities on independent noninvasive stress test (i.e., stress thal-

Table 15.1.
Noninvasive Test Results Predicting High Risk[a] for Adverse Outcome

Exercise ECG
> Abnormal horizontal or down-sloping ST segment depression in patients with an interpretable[b] stress ECG who have any of these:
>> Onset at heart rate <120/min (off β-blockers) or ≤6.5 METS[c]
>> Magnitude ≥2.0 mm of depression
>> Postexercise duration ≥6 minutes
>> Depression in multiple leads reflecting multiple coronary artery regions
> Abnormal systolic blood pressure response during progressive exercise[d]:
>> With sustained decrease of >10 mm Hg or flat blood pressure response (≤130 mm Hg), associated with ECG evidence of ischemia
> Other potentially important determinants
> Exercise-induced ST segment elevation in leads other than aVR and without significant Q waves
> Exercise-induced ventricular tachycardia

Stress radionuclide myocardial perfusion imaging
> Abnormal myocardial tracer distribution in more than one coronary artery region at rest or with stress or a large single anterior defect that reperfuses
> With thallium, abnormal myocardial distribution associated with increased lung uptake during exercise in absence of severely depressed LV function at rest
> Cardiac enlargement with exercise

Stress radionuclide ventriculography
> Fall in left ventricular ejection fraction of ≥0.10 during exercise
> Exercise LV ejection fraction of <0.50 suspected due to coronary artery disease
> Rest EF ≤35% suspected due to coronary artery disease

Stress echocardiography
> Rest EF ≤35% suspected due to coronary artery disease
> Increased segmental wall motion score >1.0
> New early diastolic wall motion abnormalities

[a] High-risk patients generally are those with reduced event-free survival due to left main coronary artery obstruction to severe multivessel obstruction with impaired left ventricular function.

[b] At rest, no ST segment depression ≥1 mm, intraventricular conduction defects, electrolyte abnormalities, or drugs like digoxin.

[c] Energy expenditure at rest equivalent to an oxygen uptake of approximately 3.5 mL O_2/kg body weight per minute.

[d] A decline in systolic blood pressure may also occur in some patients without heart disease during sustained maximal exercise or if certain medications are in use at time of exercise.

EF, ejection fraction.

---

lium, radionuclide ventriculography, or stress echocardiography) but without criteria for high risk as listed in Class I or IIa (level of evidence C).

2. At least two clinical risk factors (e.g., male gender, hypertension, hypercholesterolemia) and abnormal but not high risk criteria on noninvasive testing in a man or postmenopausal woman without known coronary heart disease (level of evidence C).

3. Prior myocardial infarction (MI) with normal resting left ventricular function and ischemia on noninvasive testing but without high-risk criteria (level of evidence C).

4. After coronary artery bypass graft (CABG) or angioplasty when there is ischemia on noninvasive testing but without high risk criteria (level of evidence C).

5. Candidacy for liver, lung, or renal transplant in a patient at least 40 years old as part of evaluation for transplantation (level of evidence C).

Class III

1. As a screening test for CAD in asymptomatic patient without abnormalities on noninvasive testing (level of evidence C).

2. After CABG or angioplasty when there is no evidence of ischemia on noninvasive testing except when there is informed consent for research purposes (level of evidence C).

3. Abnormal electrocardiographic (ECG) exer-

cise test alone, excluding categories listed earlier (level of evidence C).

4. Coronary calcification on fluoroscopy, fast computed tomography (CT), or other screening tests without criteria for high risk listed earlier (level of evidence C).

STABLE ANGINA

Class I

1. Canadian Cardiovascular Society (CCS) Class III and IV with medical treatment (level of evidence B).
2. Regardless of severity of angina, high-risk criteria on noninvasive testing (Table 15.1) (level of evidence A).
3. Angina and survival of sudden cardiac death, sustained (longer than 30 seconds) monomorphic ventricular tachycardia, or nonsustained (less than 30 seconds) polymorphic ventricular tachycardia (level of evidence B).

Class IIa

1. CCS Class III and IV angina that with medical therapy improves to Class I or II (level of evidence C).
2. Serial noninvasive testing using identical protocols at the same level of medical therapy with increasing abnormalities (level of evidence C).
3. Because of disability, illness, or physical challenge, inadequate evaluation and risk stratification by other means (level of evidence C).
4. Need to know in persons who by occupation or strenuous activity constitute a risk to themselves or others (level of evidence C).
5. CCS Class I or II angina with intolerance to medical therapy, with failure to respond adequately, or with recurrence during adequate medical therapy consisting of at least two antianginal medications (level of evidence C).

Class IIb

1. CCS Class I and II with demonstrable ischemia but less than high-risk criteria on noninvasive testing (level of evidence C).
2. CCS Class I and II with a family history of premature coronary events in direct relatives or other serious risk factors accompanied by ischemia of less than high risk on noninvasive testing (level of evidence C).
3. CCS Class I and II angina with no evidence of high risk criteria on noninvasive testing and no adverse clinical risk markers (level of evidence B).
4. CCS Class I and II angina that responds to medical therapy with no evidence of silent ischemia on appropriate testing (level of evidence B).

Class III

1. Angina in a patient who refuses to consider revascularization even though it may be medically appropriate (level of evidence C).
2. Angina in a patient who is not a candidate for coronary revascularization or whose quality or duration of life cannot be improved by revascularization (level of evidence C). These are patients whose quality of life is limited by comorbid illness.

UNSTABLE CORONARY SYNDROMES

Class I

1. High- or intermediate-risk unstable angina (Table 15.2) refractory to aggressive medical therapy or recurrent symptoms after initial stabilization. Emergency catheterization is recommended (level of evidence B).
2. High-risk unstable angina for adverse outcome (Table 15.2). Urgent catheterization is recommended (level of evidence B).
3. High- or intermediate-risk unstable angina that stabilizes after initial treatment (level of evidence A).
4. Initially low-short-term risk unstable angina (Table 15.2) found to be high risk on noninvasive testing (Table 15.1) (level of evidence B).
5. Suspected Prinzmetal's variant angina (level of evidence C).

Class IIa

None.

Class IIb

Low short-term risk for adverse outcome (i.e., without high-risk criteria on noninvasive testing) (level of evidence C).

Table 15.2.
Short-Term Risk of Death or Nonfatal Myocardial Infarction in Patients with Unstable Angina

High Risk	Intermediate Risk	Low Risk
At least one of these features	No high-risk feature but any of the following:	No high or intermediate risk feature but may have any of the following:
Prolonged ongoing (>20 min) rest pain within previous 24 hrs	Prolonged (>20 min) rest angina, now resolved, with moderate or high likelihood of CAD	Increased angina frequency, severity, or duration
Pulmonary edema most likely related to ischemia	Rest angina (>20 min or relieved with rest or sublingual nitroglycerin)	Angina provoked at a lower threshold
Angina at rest with dynamic ST changes ≥1 mm	Nocturnal angina	New onset angina with onset 2 weeks to 2 months prior to presentation
Angina with new or worsening MR murmur	Angina with dynamic T-wave changes	Normal or unchanged ECG
Angina with S3 or new or worsening rales	New onset CCSC III or IV angina in the past 2 weeks with moderate or high likelihood of CAD	
Angina with hypotension	Pathologic Q waves or resting ST depression ≤1 mm in multiple lead groups (anterior, Inferior, lateral) Age >65 years	

CCSC, Canadian Cardiovascular Society classification.
Estimation of the short-term risks of death and nonfatal MI in unstable angina is a complex multivariable problem that cannot be fully specified in a table such as this. Therefore, the table is meant to offer general guidance and illustration rather than rigid algorithms.
MR, mitral regurgitation; *S3*, third beat sound.

Class III

1. Recurrent chest discomfort with a normal coronary angiogram during the past 5 years (level of evidence C).
2. Unstable angina in a noncandidate for coronary revascularization or in a patient for whom coronary revascularization will not improve the quality or duration of life (level of evidence C).

ISCHEMIA FOLLOWING REVASCULARIZATION

Class I

1. Suspect abrupt closure or subacute stent thrombosis after percutaneous revascularization (level of evidence B).

2. Recurrent angina or high-risk criteria by non-invasive evaluation (Table 15.1) within 9 months of percutaneous revascularization (level of evidence C).
3. Recurrent ischemia within 18 months of CABG (level of evidence B).

Class IIa

1. Late postoperative period with noninvasive test evidence of high-risk criteria (level of evidence B).
2. Postoperative recurrent angina inadequately controlled by medical means (level of evidence C).

Class IIb

1. Asymptomatic patient who has had percutaneous transluminal coronary angioplasty

(PTCA) and who is suspected of having restenosis but without high-risk criteria on noninvasive testing (level of evidence B).
2. Postoperative recurrent angina without high-risk criteria on noninvasive testing (level of evidence C).
3. Asymptomatic postoperative patient in whom a deterioration in serial noninvasive testing has been documented but who is not at high risk on noninvasive testing (level of evidence C).

Class III

Any postoperative patient who is not a candidate for repeat revascularization (level of evidence C).

ACUTE TREATMENT PHASE OF MYOCARDIAL INFARCTION SUSPECTED BY NEW ST SEGMENT ELEVATION OR LEFT BUNDLE BRANCH BLOCK

With Intention to Perform Primary Percutaneous Transluminal Coronary Angioplasty

Class I

Candidates for thrombolytic therapy in whom primary PTCA can be performed within 90 minutes of diagnosis by an experienced operator (more than 75 cases per year) in a high-volume laboratory (more than 200 cases per year) at a hospital with on-site cardiac surgical backup facilities or proven rapid transport to a nearby surgical center (level of evidence A).

Class IIa

1. Candidates for thrombolytic therapy who have a bleeding precaution; primary PTCA can be performed within 90 minutes from diagnosis by an experienced operator (more

than 75 cases per year) in a high-volume laboratory (more than 200 cases per year) at a hospital with on-site surgical backup facilities or proven rapid transport to a nearby surgical center (level of evidence C).
2. Cardiogenic shock, refractory to fluids and correction of rhythm disturbance, at presentation (level of evidence B).

Class IIb

Thrombolysis contraindicated for reasons other than bleeding; primary PTCA can be performed within 90 minutes of diagnosis by an experienced operator (more than 75 cases per year) in a high-volume laboratory (more than 200 cases per year) at a hospital with on-site surgical backup facilities or proven rapid transport to a nearby surgical center (level of evidence C).

Class III

None.

ACUTE MYOCARDIAL INFARCTION

In a Patient Who Has Not Had Primary PTCA

Class I

None.

Class IIa

Cardiogenic shock or persistent hemodynamic instability (level of evidence B).

Class IIb

1. Evolving large or anterior MI after thrombolytic treatment when it is believed that reperfusion has not occurred and rescue PTCA is planned (level of evidence B).

2. Marginal hemodynamic status but not actual cardiogenic shock when standard management (optimizing filling pressures and so on) does not result in improvement (level of evidence C).

Class III

Routine use of angiography and PTCA within 24 hours of the administration of thrombolytic agents (level of evidence A).

During the Acute Treatment Phase (Acute MI Suspected but no ST-Segment Elevation)

Class I

1. Recurrent (stuttering) episodes of ischemia with confirmatory ECG changes or evidence of shock, pulmonary congestion, or severe left ventricular dysfunction (level of evidence A).
2. Persistent ischemic type of chest discomfort despite medical therapy, with an abnormal ECG, a wall motion abnormality by echocardiography, or at least two coronary risk factors (level of evidence B).

Class IIa

The patient has chest discomfort, not necessarily ischemic in description, with hemodynamic instability and abnormal ECG (level of evidence B).

Class IIb

1. Persistent chest discomfort unresolved by therapy with an unchanged ECG (level of evidence C).
2. Persistent ischemic type of chest discomfort, a normal ECG, and more than two CAD risk factors (level of evidence C).

Class III

Prior normal coronary angiogram within the past 5 years without significant new ECG abnormality (level of evidence C).

During Hospital Management Phase for Patients with Q-Wave and Non–Q-Wave Infarction

Class I

1. Spontaneous myocardial ischemia or myocardial ischemia provoked by minimal exertion during recovery from infarction (level of evidence C).
2. Preparation for definitive therapy for a mechanical complication of infarction such as acute mitral regurgitation, ventricular septal defect, pseudoaneurysm, or left ventricular aneurysm (level of evidence C).
3. Persistent hemodynamic instability (level of evidence B).

Class IIa

1. Suspicion of MI occurring by a mechanism other than thrombotic occlusion at an atherosclerotic plaque (e.g., coronary embolism, arteritis, trauma, certain metabolic or hematologic diseases or coronary spasm) (level of evidence C).
2. Survival of acute MI with left ventricular ejection fraction no more than 40, congestive heart failure, prior revascularization, or malignant ventricular arrhythmias (level of evidence C).
3. Clinical heart failure during the acute episode but subsequent demonstration of preserved left ventricular function (left ventricular ejection fraction more than 40%) (level of evidence C).

Class IIb

1. Coronary angiography to find a persistently occluded infarct-related artery in an attempt to revascularize that artery (open artery hypothesis) (level of evidence C).
2. Coronary angiography performed without

other risk stratification to identify left main or three-vessel disease (level of evidence C).

3. Follow-up of all non–Q wave MI (level of evidence C).

4. Recurrent ventricular tachycardia and/or ventricular fibrillation despite antiarrhythmic therapy without evidence of ongoing myocardial ischemia (level of evidence C).

Class III

1. Routine use of coronary angiography and subsequent PTCA of infarct-related artery within 48 to 72 hours after thrombolytic therapy without evidence of spontaneous or provocable ischemia (level of evidence A).

2. Noncandidacy for or refusal of coronary revascularization (level of evidence C).

Risk Stratification Phase After Myocardial Infarction

Class I

Ischemia at low levels of exercise with ECG changes (at least 1 mm ST segment depression) and/or imaging abnormalities (generally accepted definitions of low-level exercise include exercise heart rates not more than 120 beats/minute, not more than 70% of the age-predicted heart rat or not more than 4 METS) (level of evidence B).

Class IIa

1. Clinically significant congestive heart failure during the hospital stay (level of evidence C).

2. Inability to perform exercise test with left ventricular ejection fraction below 45 (level of evidence C).

Class IIb

1. Ischemia at high levels of exercise (level of evidence C).

2. Non–Q wave MI in a patient who is an appropriate candidate for a revascularization procedure (level of evidence C).

3. Need to return to unusually active form of employment (level of evidence C).

4. Remote history of MI without evidence of congestive heart failure during the current event and without evidence of inducible ischemia (level of evidence C).

5. Recurrent ventricular tachycardia, fibrillation, or both despite antiarrhythmic therapy without ongoing myocardial ischemia (level of evidence C).

Class III

The patient is not a candidate for or refuses coronary revascularization (level of evidence C).

CHEST PAIN OF UNDETERMINED ORIGIN

Class I

1. Noninvasive testing indicates high risk for adverse outcome (Table 15.1) (level of evidence A).

2. Coronary artery spasm is suspected and provocative testing is planned (level of evidence C).

Class IIa

1. There is evidence of ischemia on noninvasive testing but no criteria of high risk (level of evidence C).

2. Noninvasive testing cannot be performed or is inconclusive for ischemia (level of evidence C).

3. The patient has a cardiac condition known to cause chest pain with equivocal noninvasive studies for ischemia (level of evidence C).

Class IIb

The patient has no evidence of myocardial ischemia by noninvasive testing but does have disabling recurrent symptoms (level of evidence C).

Class III

The patient has no objective signs of ischemia; an earlier technically satisfactory coronary angiogram for the same type of chest pain is normal (level of evidence C).

EVALUATION BEFORE OR AFTER NONCARDIAC SURGERY (TABLE 15.3)

Class I

1. Evidence of high risk of adverse outcome based on noninvasive test results (Table 15.1) (level of evidence C).
2. Angina unresponsive to adequate medical therapy (level of evidence C).
3. Unstable angina when planning intermediate- or high-risk noncardiac surgery (level of evidence C).

Table 15.3.
Definitions of Perioperative Risk

Low-risk surgical procedures
   Endoscopic procedures, superficial procedures, cataract, breast
Intermediate-risk surgical procedures
   Carotid endarterectomy, major head and neck, intraperitoneal and/or intrathoracic, orthopedic, prostate
High-risk surgical procedures
   Emergency major operations, aortic and major vascular, peripheral vascular, anticipated prolonged surgical procedure associated with large fluid shifts and/or blood loss
Characteristics of Patients at High Clinical Risk
   Unstable angina; recent MI and evidence of important residual ischemic risk; decompensated congestive heart failure; high-degree AV block; symptomatic ventricular arrhythmias with known structural heart disease; severe symptomatic valvular heart disease; multiple intermediate risk markers, such as prior MI, congestive heart failure, and diabetes
Characteristics of Patients at Intermediate Clinical Risk
   CCS Class I or II angina, prior MI by history or ECG, compensated or prior congestive heart failure, diabetes mellitus

4. Equivocal noninvasive test result in patient with high clinical risk and planned high-risk surgery (level of evidence C).

Class IIa

1. Multiple intermediate clinical risk markers and planned vascular surgery (level of evidence B).
2. Ischemia on noninvasive testing but without high-risk criteria (Table 15.1) (level of evidence B).
3. Equivocal noninvasive test result in a patient at intermediate clinical risk undergoing high-risk noncardiac surgery (level of evidence C).
4. Urgent noncardiac surgery while convalescing from acute MI (level of evidence C).

Class IIb

1. Perioperative MI (level of evidence B).
2. Evaluation for transplantation in a candidate for liver, lung, or renal transplant aged 40 years or older (level of evidence C).
3. Class III or IV angina and planned low-risk or minor surgery (level of evidence C).

Class III

1. Low-risk noncardiac surgery with known CAD and no high risk criteria on noninvasive testing (level of evidence B).
2. No symptoms after coronary revascularization with excellent exercise capacity (at least 7 METS) (level of evidence C).
3. Mild stable angina with good left ventricular function and no high-risk noninvasive test results (level of evidence B).
4. Unsuitable for coronary revascularization because of concomitant medical illness, severe left ventricular dysfunction (e.g., left ventricular ejection fraction less than 20%) or refusal to consider coronary revascularization.

VALVULAR HEART DISEASE

Class I

1. Preparation for valve surgery or balloon valvotomy in an adult with chest discomfort, is-

chemia by noninvasive testing, or both (level of evidence B).
2. Preparation for valve surgery in an adult free of chest pain but with multiple risk factors for coronary artery disease (level of evidence C).
3. Infective endocarditis with evidence for coronary embolization (level of evidence C).

Class IIa

None.

Class IIb

Left heart catheterization is being performed for hemodynamic evaluation prior to aortic or mitral valve surgery in patient without pre-existing evidence of CAD, advanced age, or multiple CAD risk factors (level of evidence C).

Class III

1. Before cardiac surgery for infective endocarditis when there are no risk factors for coronary disease or evidence for coronary embolization (level of evidence C).
2. No symptoms and cardiac surgery not being considered (level of evidence C).
3. Before cardiac surgery when preoperative hemodynamic assessment by catheterization is unnecessary and without pre-existing evidence of coronary disease (level of evidence C).

CONGENITAL HEART DISEASE

Class I

1. Before surgical correction of congenital heart disease when chest discomfort or noninvasive evidence suggests associated coronary artery disease (level of evidence C).
2. Before surgical correction of suspected congenital coronary anomalies such as congenital coronary artery stenosis, coronary arteriovenous fistula, and anomalous origin of the left coronary artery (level of evidence C).
3. Congenital heart disease frequently associated with coronary artery anomalies that may complicate surgical management (level of evidence C).
4. Unexplained sudden death in a young patient (level of evidence B).

Class IIa

Before corrective open heart surgery for congenital heart disease in an adult whose risk profile increases the likelihood of coexisting coronary disease (level of evidence C).

Class IIb

Coronary angiography may be performed during left heart catheterization for hemodynamic assessment of congenital heart disease in an adult whose risk of coronary disease is not high (level of evidence C).

Class III

An asymptomatic patient for whom heart surgery is not planned is being routinely evaluated for congenital heart disease (level of evidence C).

CONGESTIVE HEART FAILURE

Class I

1. Congestive heart failure due to systolic dysfunction with angina or regional wall motion abnormalities and/or scintigraphic evidence of reversible myocardial ischemia when revascularization is being considered (level of evidence B).
2. Preparation for cardiac transplantation (level of evidence C).
3. Normal systolic function but episodic heart failure raising suspicion of ischemically mediated left ventricular dysfunction (level of evidence C).
4. Congestive heart failure secondary to post-MI ventricular aneurysm or other mechanical complications of MI (level of evidence C).

Class IIa

The patient has systolic dysfunction with unexplained cause despite noninvasive testing (level of evidence C).

Class III

The patient has congestive heart failure with previous coronary angiograms showing normal coronary arteries but with no new evidence to suggest ischemic heart disease (level of evidence C).

OTHER CONDITIONS

Class I

1. Diseases affecting the aorta when knowledge of the presence or extent of coronary artery involvement is necessary for management (e.g., aortic dissection or aneurysm with known CAD) (level of evidence B).
2. Hypertrophic cardiomyopathy with angina despite medical therapy when knowledge of coronary anatomy might affect therapy (level of evidence C).
3. Hypertrophic cardiomyopathy with angina when heart surgery is planned (level of evidence B).

Class IIa

1. High risk for CAD when other cardiac surgery is planned (e.g., pericardiectomy or removal of chronic pulmonary emboli) (level of evidence C).
2. Prospective immediate cardiac transplant donor whose risk profile increases the likelihood of coronary artery disease (level of evidence B).
3. Asymptomatic patient with Kawasaki's disease who have coronary aneurysms on echocardiography (level of evidence B).
4. Patient awaiting surgery for aortic aneurysm or dissection without known coronary disease (level of evidence C).
5. Recent blunt chest trauma and suspicion of acute MI without evidence of pre-existing coronary artery disease (level of evidence C).

RECOMMENDATIONS FOR CORONARY INTRAVASCULAR ULTRASOUND

Class I

The patient has a positive functional study and a suspected flow-limiting stenosis and is considered a candidate for revascularization; it is desirable to evaluate lesion severity at a location difficult to image by angiography (level of evidence C).

Class IIa

1. Assessment of a suboptimal angiographic result following coronary intervention (level of evidence C).
2. Diagnosis and management of coronary disease following cardiac transplantation (level of evidence C).
3. Determination of plaque location and circumferential distribution for guidance of directional coronary atherectomy (level of evidence C).
4. Assessment of the adequacy of deployment of the Palmaz-Schatz coronary stent, including the extent of stent apposition and determination of the minimum luminal diameter within the stent (level of evidence B).
5. Further evaluation of patient with characteristic anginal symptoms and a positive functional study with no focal stenoses or mild CAD on angiography (level of evidence C).

Class IIb

1. Determination of the mechanism of stent restenosis (inadequate expansion versus neointimal proliferation) and selection of appropriate therapy (plaque ablation versus repeat balloon expansion) (level of evidence C).
2. Assessment of a lesion's characteristics as a means to select an optimal revascularization device (level of evidence C).

RECOMMENDATIONS FOR INTRACORONARY DOPPLER ULTRASOUND

Class I

None.

Class IIa

Assessment of the physiologic effects of intermediate coronary stenoses (30 to 70% luminal narrowing) in patient with symptoms of angina. Doppler velocimetry may also be useful as an alternative to performing a noninvasive functional study to determine whether an intervention is warranted for intermediate lesions or when the functional study is ambiguous (level of evidence C).

Class IIb

1. Evaluation of the success of percutaneous coronary revascularization in restoring flow reserve and prediction of the risk of restenosis (level of evidence C).
2. Following cardiac transplantation, diagnosis of impaired coronary flow reserve in patient with symptoms of angina but no apparent angiographic culprit lesion (level of evidence C).
3. Assessment of the severity of coronary flow abnormalities in patient with symptoms of angina and a positive noninvasive functional study but no apparent angiographic lesion (level of evidence C).

Class III

Routine assessment of the severity of angiographic disease is desirable for a patient with a positive noninvasive functional study.

RECOMMENDATIONS FOR CORONARY ANGIOSCOPY

Classes I and II

None.

Class III

Coronary angioscopy is a research tool for which there are no established clinical indications (level of evidence C).

RECOMMENDATIONS FOR PHARMACOLOGIC ASSESSMENT OF CORONARY DISEASE 48 HOURS AFTER WITHDRAWAL OF CORONARY VASODILATORS

Class I

None.

Class IIa

The patient has recurrent episodes of apparent ischemic cardiac pain at rest and is found to have a normal or mildly abnormal coronary angiogram, and no clinical observations substantiate the diagnosis of variant angina, that is, ST segment elevation during pain (level of evidence C).

Class IIb

The patient has recurrent episodes of ischemic cardiac pain at rest with associated transient ST segment elevation and is found to have a normal or mildly abnormal coronary angiogram (level of evidence C).

Class III

1. Any absolute contraindication to pharmacologic challenge, including possible pregnancy, severe hypertension, severe left ventricular dysfunction, moderate to severe aortic stenosis, and high-grade left main stenosis (level of evidence C).
2. Any relative contraindication to pharmacologic testing, including uncontrolled or unstable angina, uncontrolled ventricular arrhythmia, recent MI or severe three-vessel coronary disease (level of evidence C).

DIFFERENCES IN THE GUIDELINES BETWEEN 1987 AND 1998

During this decade much has transpired in invasive and interventional cardiology, and the guidelines for coronary angiography have been significantly revised. We outline some of the important differences here; however, possibly most important are the new class IIa and IIb categories with their structure of indications and weights of evidence to support recommendations. These changes make the new guidelines more relevant and much easier to relate to clinical practice. Other major differences are the inclusion of criteria for intracoronary ultrasound, Doppler velocimetry, and angioscopy. All of these techniques will undoubtedly continue to evolve as new applications are discovered and indications are re-evaluated through further study. Class I indications for angiography in asymptomatic patients are similar, except that a high-risk occupation alone is now coupled with an abnormal but not necessarily high-risk stress test or other features to make a class IIa indication. Class II indications have been expanded to include postmenopausal women and candidates in the process of liver, lung, or renal transplantation. Class III indications have been clarified and extended to use of some imaging modalities designed to pick up coronary calcification as a screen.

Indications for symptomatic patients have been reclassified in a more useful clinical format based upon clinical syndromes of no symptoms, stable angina, unstable coronary syndromes, previous revascularization, and MI. The basic premise according to which treatment of symptomatic patients warrants a class I indication for coronary angiography is uncontrolled symptoms, a high-risk clinical profile, or recurrent objective evidence of ischemia. Ischemia class I indications after revascularization include subacute stent thrombosis and any early recurrent ischemia after revascularization. Perhaps the most dramatic change in the indications is the class I status for acute MI when primary angioplasty is planned; in 1987 there was no class I indication in that setting. Although indications for performing angiography on patients after MI with high risk stress testing or recurrent ischemia are similar in the new guidelines, a new group of class II indications has evolved. These include low ejection fraction, generally whether routine angiography should be pursued after infarct, and whether non–Q-wave infarct patients should also be routinely studied. These areas are in evolution, and sufficient data to warrant class I indications are not available. Guidelines for evaluation of atypical chest pain are similar. However, indications for patients undergoing noncardiac surgery are much better defined, although a large number of patients fall into Class 2 indications. Congenital heart disease indications are similar; however, a class I indication is now included for sudden death. More defined criteria for investigation of congestive heart failure are also included in the current guidelines. Although this is the first appearance of two new testing modalities that are not significantly reimbursed, it is likely that indications for intracoronary ultrasound for both imaging and velocimetry will continue to evolve through further research and clinical use.

CONTRAINDICATIONS TO CARDIAC CATHETERIZATION

Perhaps the only absolute contraindications to cardiac catheterization are (*a*) lack of access to the heart and/or great vessels, (*b*) absence of a cardiologist or cardiovascular radiologist with appropriate training or skills, and (*c*) inadequate catheterization laboratory, support staff, or facilities.

Relative contraindications to catheterization irrespective of type of laboratory include the following:

1. Recent stroke (within 1 month)
2. Progressive renal insufficiency
3. Active gastrointestinal bleeding
4. Fever that may be due to infection
5. Active infection
6. Short life expectancy because of another illness, such as cancer or severe pulmonary, hepatic, or renal disease
7. Severe anemia
8. Severe uncontrolled systemic hypertension
9. Severe electrolyte imbalance
10. Severe systemic or psychological illness in which prognosis is doubtful or behavior is unpredictable, producing undue risk associated with cardiac catheterization
11. Very advanced physiologic (not chronologic) age
12. The patient's refusal to consider definitive treatment such as angioplasty, coronary artery bypass surgery, or valve replacement
13. In an unstable patient, lack of a cardiac surgical team in the hospital (such a patient refractory to maximal medical therapy should generally be transferred to a center where surgical backup is immediately available); under special circumstances, when the condition of a hospitalized patient can be readily stabilized, such as by use of balloon counterpulsation, catheterization may be undertaken in the hospital in the absence of a cardiac surgical team, provided that well-defined mechanisms are in place for rapid referral and acceptance of such patient by a hospital in which emergency surgery or angioplasty can be carried out with minimal delay
14. Digitalis intoxication
15. Documented anaphylaxis during previous exposure to angiographic contrast material; in most patients with a history of an immediate generalized anaphylactoid reaction to contrast material the reactions do not constitute anaphylaxis, and these individuals can safely undergo coronary angiography after medication with corticosteroids and antihistamines
16. Pregnancy

SUMMARY

Indications for expensive invasive cardiac procedures are important for patient care as well as for quality improvement, utilization review, and economic reasons. There is little doubt that after a careful history and physical examination the single test that can offer the most diagnostic, prognostic, and therapeutic information concerning cardiac disease is a thorough and careful cardiac hemodynamic and angiographic study performed by a skilled operator in a high-quality laboratory. Although catheterization carries risks associated with its invasive nature, the era of active aggressive acute cardiac intervention has taught us that the potential for lifesaving in catheterization and associated therapeutic procedures may far outweigh such risks.

The indications for cardiac catheterization and coronary angiography outlined in this chapter, as compared with the 1987 guidelines, have evolved as the result of important developments in interventional and medical therapies. With the current rate of clinical research in this area we anticipate the need for more frequent revisions of guidelines in the future.

References

1. Krone RJ, Johnson L, Noto, T. Five year trends in cardiac catheterization: a report from the Registry of the Society for Cardiac Angiography and Interventions. Cathet Cardiovasc Diagn 1996;31–35.
2. Ross J, Brandenburg RO, Dinsmore RE, et al. Guidelines for coronary angiography: a report of the American College of Cardiology/American Heart Association Task Force on Assessment of Diagnostic and Therapeutic Cardiovascular Procedures. J Am Coll Cardiol 1987;935–950.
3. Guidelines for coronary angiography. A report of the American College of Cardiology/American Heart Association Task Force on Assessment of Diagnostic and Therapeutic Cardiovascular Procedures. J Am Coll Cardiol 1998. In press.
4. ACC/AHA Guidelines for cardiac catheterization and cardiac catheterization laboratories. J Am Coll Cardiol 1991;1149–1182.

16
Ventriculography

Florence H. Sheehan, MD
J. Ward Kennedy, MD

INTRODUCTION

As the emphasis in adult cardiology drifted away from congenital heart disease and considerable experience was gained in the catheterization of patients with valvular heart disease, interest in more detailed assessment of ventricular function through the use of angiography increased. In the late 1950s Dodge et al. in this country and Ardvisson, working in Sweden, began to develop methods to measure cardiac chamber volumes using 6 and later 12 frames per second, biplane cut, or roll film contrast angiograms (1, 2). Sandler and Dodge (3), Rackley et al. (4), and Sauter et al. (5) established methods to determine left ventricular stroke volume, left ventricular muscle mass, and left atrial volume. Determining end-diastolic and end-systolic volume made it possible to calculate stroke volume and minute output of the left ventricle. Comparing left ventricular output with forward cardiac output as measured by standard dye dilution or Fick techniques allowed left ventricular regurgitant stroke volume and minute output to be calculated. It also became possible to integrate pressure and volume information during the cardiac cycle to clarify pressure–volume relationships. With knowledge of the ventricular pressure, chamber dimensions, and left ventricular wall thickness it was possible to measure left ventricular wall stress (6). With development of catheter tip pressure manometers and rapid biplane cine filming techniques, precise simultaneous pressure and volume information became available, and the mechanics of left ventricular performance could be determined in various types of heart disease in humans.

This type of information gradually became available in relatively large numbers of patients, as well as in a number of individuals in whom careful study revealed no anatomic or physiologic evidence of heart disease. The data from these normal persons accumulated and eventually provided reference standards for normal chamber size and function, in addition to the mass of the left ventricular myocardium for both men and women (7).

With further experience in evaluating left ventricular size and performance in patients with heart disease, various investigators began to appreciate the importance of the relationship between left ventricular stroke volume and end-diastolic volume. It became clear that the ratio of stroke volume to end-diastolic volume, that is, left ventricular ejection fraction, had great value for assessment of left ventricular pump function (8, 9). Now, nearly 2 decades later, the **ejection fraction is still the most frequently used method of assessing global left ventricular function.** This measurement is most useful in evaluation of left ventricular function in patients with valvular heart disease and cardiomyopathy, but it is also useful in assessing patients with ischemic heart disease (10).

247

In the mid and late 1960s, with widespread use of selective coronary angiography and development of coronary artery bypass surgery, evaluation of left ventricular function became essential. This was because it became apparent that ventricular performance was a major independent predictor of surgical risk and long-term survival in patients with ischemic heart disease. With simple visual assessment of ventricular size and distribution of regional contraction abnormalities, it was possible to divide patients into low-, medium-, and high-risk categories (11). Angiographers also noted several types of abnormalities in regional wall motion, both in the sequence of regional contraction and in the extent of wall movement. Herman et al. (12) defined **abnormalities of extent of contraction** as **hypokinesis** for reduced movement, **akinesis** for loss of contraction, and **dyskinesis** for paradoxic outward motion during systole. These terms have become the reference standards for describing abnormalities of contraction.

TECHNIQUE OF LEFT VENTRICULAR ANGIOGRAPHY

The left ventricle can be evaluated angiographically by injection of contrast material into the right side of the heart and filming the contrast material as it enters the left ventricle, and by injection of contrast material into the left atrium, the left ventricular chamber, or even the ascending aorta in patients with aortic valvular regurgitation. In most instances optimal examination is obtained when contrast material is injected directly into the left ventricular chamber. The techniques for catheterization of the left ventricle are detailed in Chapter 9. Briefly, a pigtail catheter is usually placed in the left ventricle retrograde through the aortic valve. Other multiple-hole catheters, such as multipurpose, Sones, and NIH, may be used.

CONTRAST INJECTION TECHNIQUES

To obtain high-quality angiograms for analysis of wall motion and mitral insufficiency, ventricular ectopic rhythms must be avoided by placing the catheter in the area of the ventricular cavity that is least likely to cause ectopy during power injection. Injection at the apex produces good image quality but is associated with a very high incidence of ectopy (13). The best injection site is **often midway between the apex of the ventricle and the aortic valve,** with the loop directed back toward the mitral valve. In some patients it may be necessary to move the catheter tip to another location until a region free of ectopy is found during test injection. This is done by a forceful test injection of 5 to 10 mL of contrast material to see if ectopy occurs and to assess the contrast material distribution. This information is also used to determine how much contrast material should be injected. The type of catheter used also influences contrast quality as well as the risk of inducing artifactual mitral regurgitation (14).

When an appropriate injection site is selected, a power injection of 30 to 50 mL of contrast material is made into the ventricular chamber at 10 to 20 mL per second. The volume and rate of injection of contrast material vary with the size of the patient, size of the chamber, function of the ventricle, hemodynamic state of the patient, and other factors. Larger volume and faster injection are required in large, hyperdynamic ventricles, seen in patients with aortic or mitral regurgitation. Smaller volume and slower injections are appropriate in small or hypokinetic ventricles. In patients with very poor left ventricular function and dilated ventricles, contrast material mixes slowly in the chamber, so that a relatively small amount of contrast material injected rapidly and allowed to mix over three to five cardiac cycles often provides excellent ventriculograms. In patients with recent anterior or apical myocardial infarction and in those with ventricular aneurysms, the possibility that a mural thrombus in the ventricle may be dislodged during manipulation of the catheter must be considered. In these patients the experienced angiographer places the catheter so as to avoid the area of possible mural thrombus, which is likely to be attached to the area of the wall that is most akinetic or dyskinetic.

FILMING TECHNIQUES

During the early years of cardiac angiography direct x-ray exposure of large cut or roll filming at 6 or 12 frames per second was used. Since the development of high-quality image intensifiers, cine recording, and television monitoring systems adapted for angiocardiography, these cumbersome devices have been replaced by cine filming in either single or biplane projections at 30, 50, 60, or 90 frames per second. **For visual and most quantitative analysis of left ventricular angiograms 30 frames per second is adequate,** but many laboratories prefer to film at 60 frames per second to provide a more pleasing image of ventricular filling and ejection and more frames for analysis. For patients with tachycardia, 60 frames per second is a more desirable filming rate.

FILMING PROJECTION

The left ventricle traditionally has been viewed by single-plane angiography in the 30° right anterior oblique (RAO) projection. With biplane filming, anteroposterior and lateral or RAO and left anterior oblique (LAO) projections have been used. Although biplane filming is ideal, the greater expense of biplane cineradiographic equipment and increased radiation exposure of the patient and operators militate against routine use of biplane cineradiography for most examinations in adults. In patients with valvular and congenital heart disease and in most with nonischemic cardiomyopathies ventricular contraction is relatively symmetric and reasonably represented in the RAO view. In patients with ischemic heart disease who have a prior myocardial infarction or ongoing ischemia at the time of study, segmental wall motion defects

may not be adequately represented in a single view.

The location of coronary obstructions can guide the angiographer in selecting the best single view for left ventriculography (see Chapter 17). The RAO view is preferable in patients with major obstruction in the left anterior descending and/or right coronary arteries. The LAO view is best in patients whose circumflex artery is the major site of obstruction. In patients with diffuse three-vessel disease the RAO view usually provides adequate information for assessment of surgical risk, as well as acting as a guide for the surgeon for the placement of revascularization conduits. In a minority of patients it is necessary to perform either biplane or two serial contrast injections, with filming in both RAO and LAO views. In these circumstances the most important view should be done first, and the second injection should be omitted in patients who respond unfavorably to the first. Fortunately, there are many ways to evaluate regional ventricular contraction, such as echocardiography and radionuclide angiography, so that unstable patients almost never must be subjected to more than one left ventriculogram. Some may not need ventriculography at all if they are at extremely high risk and have been adequately evaluated by another technique.

Some investigators have proposed using **sagittal plane angulated views of the left ventricle to improve examination of certain portions of the wall** (15–17). The most common is the cranial LAO view, which provides better definition of the lateral wall, septum, and outflow tract than standard 60° LAO or 90° lateral projections. A disadvantage is that the apex is often obscured by the overlapping liver shadow. Although this view is sometimes desirable, we do not use it routinely for biplane cineangiography.

QUALITATIVE ASSESSMENT OF LEFT VENTRICULAR ANGIOGRAMS

Although we advocate quantitative assessment of left ventricular contraction and valvular regurgitation, a great deal of information can be derived from subjective visual evaluation of left ventricular contraction patterns in patients with all types of heart disease. The angiographer must appreciate the way the ventricle responds to acute and chronic changes in both pressure and volume. These differences are most notable in patients with acute rather than chronic volume overload. In chronic volume overload of the left ventricle, such as occurs in aortic or mitral regurgitation, ventricular septal defect, and patent ductus arteriosus, the ventricle responds by progressive increase in end-diastolic volume and stroke volume and maintains a normal cardiac output at rest. So the **ratio of stroke volume to end-diastolic volume (ejection fraction)** remains normal or only modestly decreased in the patient with normal left ventricular function. When symptoms of congestive heart failure develop, however, angiography usually demonstrates an increase in end-diastolic volume and a fall in ejection fraction. Thus in well-compensated patients the enlarged end-diastolic volume is an index of the severity of volume overload, not an indication of diminished left ventricular performance.

Because of these relationships, the ejection fraction has great value in assessing the patient with volume overload of the left ventricle. There is, however, a special situation in which care must be taken in the interpretation of the ejection fraction. In chronic severe mitral regurgitation the left ventricle ejects a large portion of its stroke volume into the low-pressure left atrium. Since this reduces ventricular afterload, the ejection fraction is often higher for a given degree of left ventricular dysfunction than it would be under other circumstances without mitral regurgitation. This finding may mislead the physician into believing that left ventricular function or functional reserve is better than it is. In one small series of patients whose ejection fraction was measured before and several months after mitral valve surgery for severe mitral insufficiency, the ejection fraction deteriorated in half of the patients in whom it was abnormal preoperatively and in all of those in whom it was below 50% prior to surgery (18). This suggests that only a normal or high ejection fraction (more than 65 to 75%) reliably indicates relatively normal left ventricular function in patients with severe mitral insufficiency. This topic is discussed in more detail in Chapter 40.

In patients with acute volume overload, as seen in mitral or aortic valve endocarditis or ruptured mitral valve chordae tendineae, many patients had normal left ventricular function prior to the acute illness. In this situation the ventricle is unprepared for the acute volume overload and responds by minimal dilation, increase in ejection fraction, and marked increase in filling pressure. Most of these patients in whom regurgitation is severe present with acute pulmonary edema. Under most circumstances the appropriate therapy is early surgical correction of the valvular lesion. In patients who survive without surgery, the ventricle gradually dilates, the myocardium hypertrophies, and the filling pressure decreases, so that after several months the patient acquires characteristics of chronic volume overload.

The response of the patient with chronic pressure overload of either the right or left ventricle, as occurs in either pulmonic or aortic stenosis, is progressive myocardial hypertrophy without chamber dilation. These patients who present prior to the development of congestive heart failure have normal-sized, heavily trabeculated chambers with relatively normal contractile function and thick walls. However, since significant hypertrophy usually causes decreased compliance, the left ventricular end-diastolic pressure is usually elevated despite normal end-diastolic volume. When these patients develop congestive heart failure, the end-diastolic and end-systolic volumes increase, and the stroke volume and ejection fraction fall. Fortunately, in patients with aortic stenosis the ejection fraction usually improves after successful valve replacement (8, 19).

Today idiopathic hypertrophic subaortic stenosis and other forms of hypertrophic cardiomyopathy are most often evaluated by echocardiography, but in the past left ventriculography was the standard method of evaluation. In these patients the end-diastolic volume is normal or small and the ventricle often has a thick free wall and an increased ejection fraction. This may obliterate the apical portions of the chamber. In a 60° LAO or lateral view during systole, the anterior leaflet of the mitral valve can often be seen moving forward, even touching the septum. While simultaneous injections of contrast material in the right and left ventricles are not necessary for clinical purposes, these **biventricular angiographic studies can identify the markedly thickened basal portion of the interventricular septum** that is characteristic of patients with outflow obstruction. If only a single-plane RAO view is available, idiopathic hypertrophic subaortic stenosis can be suggested by a high ejection fraction, apical cavity obliteration, and a reduction in the density of the contrast material as a band separating the upper third of the chamber from the apex. This angiographic appearance is caused by the anterior leaflet of the mitral valve abutting the septum during systole.

Another condition usually evaluated with echocardiography is **mitral valve prolapse.** This condition is well demonstrated angiographically in the RAO projection. The mitral valve plane is easily appreciated in this view, as nonopacified blood enters the contrast-filled ventricle during diastole. With the onset of systole the mitral valve moves posteriorly and closes along the plane of the annulus. In patients with mitral valve prolapse the valve leaflets outlined by contrast behind them prolapse backward beyond the annulus into the left atrium. In its most severe form this appears as a large ring of contrast material extending around the annulus. Severe prolapse is nearly always associated with significant mitral regurgitation, while minor degrees of prolapse are usually not.

LEFT VENTRICULAR CONTRACTION PATTERNS IN ISCHEMIC HEART DISEASE

The most characteristic angiographic feature of the left ventricle in ischemic heart disease is the segmental localization of contraction and even relaxation abnormalities. Although many patients with severe coronary artery stenosis have normal left ventricular contraction patterns when resting, most patients with totally obstructed vessels or a history of or electrocardiographic (ECG) evidence of myocardial infarction have clear and distinct segmental contraction abnormalities. A very useful method of locating these segments and quantifying the severity of contraction abnormality was developed for the Coronary Artery Surgery Study (CASS) (20) (Figure 16.1). This method requires that 10 segments of the left ventricle, five in the RAO and five in the LAO projection, be scored 1 through 6 as follows:

1. Normal
2. Mild hypokinesis
3. Severe hypokinesis
4. Akinesis
5. Dyskinesis
6. Aneurysm

The segment scores are added so that when the method is applied to a single-plane RAO ventriculogram, a normal score is 5 and the most abnormal score is 30. This semiquantitative method of evaluating left ventricular function is superior to use of ejection fraction in defining surgical risk in patients with coronary artery disease (21).

The location of wall motion abnormalities is related to the location of artery stenosis. As viewed from the RAO projection, occlusion of the left anterior descending coronary artery and development of Q-wave infarction result in abnormalities of the anterolateral and apical segments (Fig. 16.2). In very proximal left anterior descending obstruction, the apical portion of the anterobasal segment may be involved. If the anterior descending artery extends around the apex, the wall motion abnormality may extend to involve the inferior portion of the apex as well. The severity of wall motion abnormality may vary from hypokinesis to dyskinesis, which indicates ventricular aneurysm. In nearly all patients motion of the basal portion of the anterobasal segment is preserved.

In inferior myocardial infarction due to occlusion of either the right coronary artery or anatomically dominant left circumflex artery, the inferior basal and inferior apical segments show contraction abnormalities.

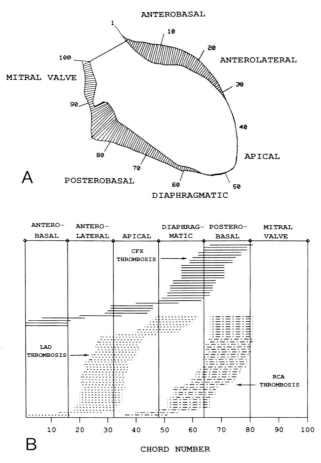

Figure 16.1. A. Left ventricular segments 1 to 5 analyzed from the RAO ventriculogram as defined in the CASS report (20). **B.** Quantitative analysis performed with the centerline method to locate the most hypokinetic fifth of the ventricle in patients with single-vessel coronary artery disease studied during acute myocardial infarction. The location of hypokinesis varies widely; as a result, attempts to measure wall motion in predefined segments underestimate abnormality (37). *CFX,* circumflex; *LAD,* left anterior descending; *RCA,* right coronary artery.

The extent of the abnormality depends on the distribution of the posterior descending. In some patients it extends to or around the apex, and in others it is short and does not reach the apex. Although akinesis frequently follows inferior infarction, dyskinesis is distinctly uncommon, and development of a large ventricular aneurysm is rare. This difference in severity of wall motion abnormalities between the inferior and anterior wall may also relate to splinting of the inferior wall by the diaphragm.

Wall motion abnormalities associated with myocardial infarctions resulting from circumflex coronary artery occlusion are often subtler in appearance from the RAO view than those associated with either left anterior descending or posterior descending occlusion. These wall motion abnormalities, which appear as a hypokinetic region at the junction between the anterolateral and anterior apical segments, are often associated with a similar abnormality in the inferoapical segment of the wall. In high-quality angiocardiograms a double density may be appreciated because of normal contraction of the anterior lateral segment with a hypokinetic or akinetic segment behind.

The LAO projection best reveals septal wall motion abnormalities resulting from

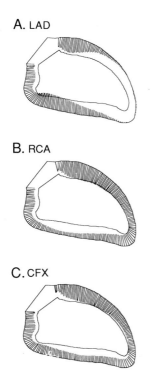

A. LAD

B. RCA

C. CFX

Figure 16.2. A–C. The location of hypokinesis due to isolated thrombosis of the left anterior descending (*LAD*, N at least 185), right coronary artery (*RCA*, N at least 132), and left circumflex coronary artery (*CFX*, N at least 57). In each panel the mean motion of the infarct is indicated by the length of the chords. For comparison the normal mean motion is presented by the solid end-diastolic contour.

anterior infarctions. This projection also provides an end-on view of inferior wall contraction abnormalities resulting from infarcts due to right coronary artery occlusions. The LAO projection best demonstrates the posterior wall motion abnormalities often seen in segments 9 and 10 in patients with posterior infarctions associated with left circumflex artery occlusion.

A **left ventricular aneurysm** may be defined as a region of the left ventricular wall that extends beyond the expected location of the wall during diastole and is akinetic or dyskinetic during systole. In other words, this abnormality distorts the diastolic contour of the chamber as well as having no contractile function. It most often follows Q-wave infarctions of the anterior free wall and apex, especially when the anterior

descending coronary artery is occluded proximal to the first diagonal branch of that vessel. Ventricular aneurysms frequently are attached to mural thrombus, which may be seen as a mass projecting into the chamber and occasionally is seen to move separately from the wall with each cardiac contraction. Mural thrombus is often seen more easily by echocardiography than by cardiac angiography. Older aneurysms may contain **calcified layers of thrombus** that are visible by fluoroscopy. This distortion of the left ventricular cavity by a large aneurysm often makes application of mode-dependent equations for calculation of ejection fraction difficult or impossible.

LEFT ATRIAL ANGIOGRAPHY

The left atrium is often visualized during left ventricular angiography because of mitral regurgitation. It may be selectively opacified by transseptal catheterization and retrograde mitral valve catheterization, or may be seen during right atrial angiography in patients with congenital heart disease and a right-to-left shunt. The left atrium may also be visualized by filming the levophase of a pulmonary artery injection. **The left atrium is normally a relatively small structure containing about half of the volume of the left ventricle in diastole.** In the absence of mitral regurgitation left atrial angiography may be useful for the identification of atrial mural thrombi and for the detection of left atrial myxomas, but both of these entities are usually best identified by echocardiography, and transseptal catheterization should not be done when either of these entities is suspected.

QUANTITATIVE VENTRICULAR ANGIOGRAPHY AND WALL MOTION ANALYSIS

Regional and global left ventricular function is commonly estimated by visual inspection of the contrast ventriculogram. However, quantitative analysis provides precise measurement of the severity of ventricular dysfunction, the ventricle's compensatory response, the effect of treatment in enhancing functional recovery, and a prognostic index. Furthermore, quantitative analysis permits objective comparisons between patients and between observers. The most commonly measured parameters are **left ventricular chamber volume** and **ejection fraction.** However, in patients with coronary artery stenosis, which causes local dysfunction, measurement of regional wall motion is more sensitive than the ejection fraction in defining the function of ischemic and nonischemic segments of myocardium. Although fewer studies have been performed on the right ventricle, its volume, ejection fraction, and wall motion can be measured with methods similar to those for the left ventricle.

DETERMINATION OF LEFT VENTRICULAR VOLUME

Because of its high degree of accuracy, measurement of left ventricular volume from contrast angiograms is the reference standard by which other imaging modalities are judged. This accuracy has repeatedly been verified by comparing the end-diastolic volumes calculated from angiograms of cadaver hearts with their directly measured volumes. In vivo validation has also been performed by comparing angiographic stroke volumes with volumes calculated with Fick or indicator–dilution techniques (1, 2, 20). Volumes calculated from ventriculograms with the area–length method agree closely with the known volumes ($r = 0.995$; standard error of the estimate = 8.2 mL) (1).

With the **area–length method** the projected image is likened to an ellipse and the ventricular chamber to an ellipsoid of revolution. The short-axis diameter of each ventricular image is calculated from the measured area and long axis length as $D = 4A/\pi L$, in which D is the diameter, A is the area of the projected image, and L is the length of the chamber. Volume (V) is then computed as $V = (\pi/6)(L)(D_a)(D_b)$, in which L is the longer measured length of two orthogonal projections and D_a and D_b are the calculated transverse diameters. Although volume can also be calculated with comparable accuracy with Simpson's rule, the area–length method has found greater acceptance because of its computational simplicity.

Calculated volumes are consistently larger than true volumes because of the volume of the papillary muscles, trabeculae carneae, and chordae tendineae. Therefore, regression equations are used to correct for this systematic error. Equations have been developed for each of the standard biplane projections (Table 16.1). Volume can also be

Table 16.1.
Regression Equations for Left Ventricular Volume Determination

Projection	Regression	Number of Observations	Standard Error of Estimate (mL)	Reference Standard	Reference
AP, lateral[a]	$V_O = 0.928\ V - 3.8$	54 (9)[b]	8.2	Casts	Dodge et al. (1)
AP	$V_O = 0.951\ V - 3.0$	1204 (55)	15.0	Biplane	Sandler and Dodge (3)
AP	$V_O = 1.00\ V + 9.6$	15[c]	24.0	Biplane	Kennedy et al. (23)
AP	$V_O = 0.788\ V + 8.4$	16[c]	28.8	Biplane	Kasser and Kennedy (24)
RAO 30°	$V_O = 0.81\ V + 1.9$	15	24.0	Biplane	Kennedy et al. (23)
RAO 30°	$V_O = 0.938\ V - 5.7$	11	5.5	Casts	Wynne et al. (15)
RAO 30°, LAO 60°	$V_O = 0.989\ V - 8.1$	11	8.0	Casts	Wynne et al. (15)

[a] AP, anteroposterior; V, volume computed from the cineimage using the area–length method; Vo, volume after correction by regression equation.
[b] Parentheses indicate the number of subjects if multiple images/subject were studied.
[c] These studies had 10 patients in common.

determined accurately from single-plane images in the anteroposterior or 30° RAO projections, because the transverse or short-axis diameter, calculated with the area–length method, is similar in orthogonal views (3, 15, 23, 24). The ventricle is usually foreshortened in the 60° LAO projection, which some investigators correct by adding 15 to 30° cranial angulation (16, 17).

Correction must also be made for **magnification** and **pincushion distortion** in the imaging system. This is usually accomplished by filming a calibration figure of known dimension, such as an aluminum sphere 7 cm in diameter, at the midchest level with the same imaging mode (intensifier magnification) and table-to-tube positions as during ventriculography. When the ventriculogram is projected for tracing, the image of the calibration figure is also examined. A correction factor is derived from the ratio of the number of the sphere diameter to its measured diameter (24). The correction factor can also be determined by measuring the distance between metallic bands on banded pigtail catheters (25); however, biplane imaging is required. Since the correction factor is applied to the diameters and long-axis length in the volume equation, errors as well as corrections are cubed.

In practice the **quality of the image and the care and confidence with which the ventricular endocardial contours are traced** are very important factors influencing the accuracy of volume determination. Reproducibility studies have shown that interobserver variation ranges from 6.6 to 20 mL for end-diastolic volume, from 5.7 to 10 mL for end-systolic volume, and from 4 to 5% units for ejection fraction (26–29). For patients who are in a regular rhythm, beat-to-beat variation is also low (26). The effect of contrast medium on volume and function is insignificant until seven beats after injection (30). Variation is greatest between serial studies, even in clinically stable patients (26). This is probably due to changes in the patient's hemodynamic condition between studies.

Calculation of left ventricular volume is the basis for the derivation of many other clinical parameters. Besides the end-diastolic volume, end-systolic volume, stroke volume, ejection fraction, cardiac output, and their indices (Fig. 16.3), the mass of the myocardium can be computed by adding a measurement of wall thickness (4). The area–length method has also been applied to calculation of right ventricular and left and right atrial volumes (5, 31, 32), but these measurements are rarely made for clinical purposes.

METHODS OF WALL MOTION ANALYSIS

The endocardial contours that were delineated for calculation of chamber volume can also be used to quantify regional wall motion. In patients with coronary artery disease (CAD) there may be dysfunction in nonischemic as well as ischemic regions (33). Regional hypokinesis has also been observed in patients with valvular heart disease and in those with nonischemic cardiomyopathy (34, 35). In addition to measuring the severity of such abnormalities in ventricular function for evaluation of disease progression or effect of therapy, regional wall motion analysis is useful for assessing prognosis (21, 35).

The **methodology used for analyzing regional wall motion is less widely accepted** than techniques used to determine ventricular volume and ejection fraction. This is due in part to the lack of a standard for testing the accuracy of wall motion measurements. As a result, a large number of methods have been developed and validated empirically, according to criteria such as accuracy in distinguishing the function of diseased patients from that of normal subjects or homogeneity of function in normal subjects. Although these methods have varying assumptions concerning the direction of regional motion, they fall into two categories according to whether or not the motion vectors derive from a coordinate system. The earliest methods were based on a rectangular coordinate system in which motion was measured along a hemiaxis perpendicular to the long axis (12). Another frequently used approach is motion measurement along radii from a central point in the ventricular chamber, such as the center of

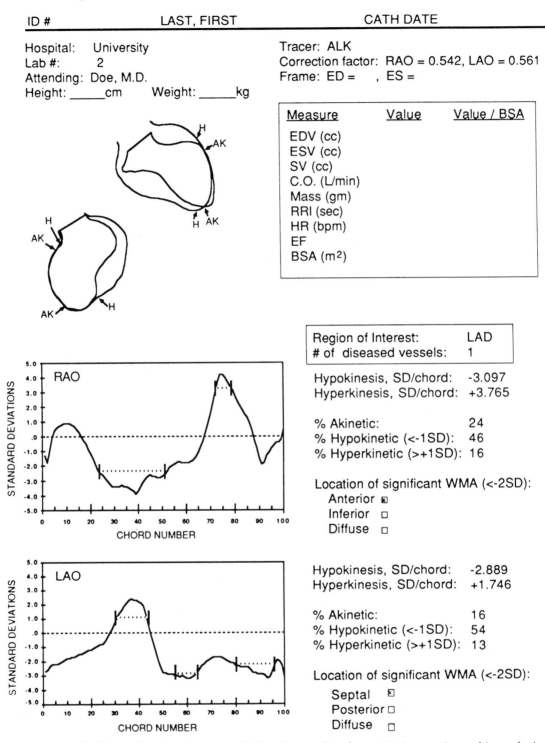

Figure 16.3. Cardiac catheterization report listing the results of quantitative angiographic analysis of the left ventricle. The volumes are shown in the upper box on the right: *EDV,* end-diastolic volume; *ESV,* end-systolic volume; *SV,* stroke volume; *CO,* cardiac output; *RRI,* R to R interval or cycle length; *HR,* heart rate; *EF,* ejection fraction; *BSA,* body surface area. *WMA,* wall motion abnormality.

mass or a point on the long axis. In these methods motion is usually expressed as a shortening fraction. Some investigators use the coordinate system to subdivide the ventricle into a number of regions and express wall motion in terms of an area or regional ejection fraction. This approach reduces variability in the measurement (36), but the severity of a regional abnormality may be underestimated if it spans more than one region (37).

Two coordinate system methods are based on observations in selected patient populations. Slager et al. analyzed the ventriculograms of normal subjects and used automated border recognition to track the motion of endocardial irregularities frame by frame throughout the cardiac cycle (38). After analyzing the trajectories of these landmarks, they defined 20 pathways in a rectangular coordinate system (38) along which they measured wall motion. Ingels et al. selected the origin of their radial coordinate system after analyzing the motion of metallic markers implanted in the midwall in patients undergoing coronary artery bypass graft surgery (39).

There are several problems associated with coordinate system methods. First, they constrain all motion to proceed toward a single origin or long axis, which is probably invalid (40, 41). Second, they use the apex as a landmark on which the coordinate system is constructed, which is unwise because the apical contour is often less well opacified and more difficult to identify with confidence (42–44). Also, since the ventricle is usually foreshortened in the LAO projection, methods that require identification of the apex cannot be accurately applied to this view. Because of the irregular shapes of projections of the right ventricle, which may be triangular or indented, neither radial nor rectangular coordinate system methods are applicable.

In view of these problems, more recently developed methods focus on alternative approaches to defining motion vectors. One approach is to divide the end-diastolic and end-systolic contours evenly into an equal number of points and measure motion as distance between corresponding points on the two contours. However, the implicit assumption that the ventricular contour short-ens homogeneously is invalid, since ischemia causes regional dysfunction.

Centerline Method of Wall Motion Analysis

The centerline method was developed to address many of these issues (Fig. 16.4) (37). Motion is measured along 100 chords constructed perpendicular to and evenly distributed along a centerline drawn midway between the end-diastolic and end-systolic contours. Thus the method makes no reference to any geometric figure, coordinate system, long axis, or apical landmark. Normalization for patient-to-patient differences in heart size is accomplished by dividing each chord's motion by the length of the end-diastolic perimeter to yield 100 **shortening fractions.**

The shortening fractions are converted into units of standard deviation from the mean motion of a normal reference population. This expresses the abnormality in terms of significance and allows comparison of function in different regions (36). Since the normal range for wall motion varies considerably from region to region around the ventricular contour (36, 45–47), any attempt to define a threshold for hypokinesis (e.g., shortening fraction less than 0.25) would erroneously include normally functioning myocardium at the apex and select only very severely dysfunctional myocardium at the anterobasal wall. This problem is avoided when the threshold is defined in standard deviations from normal, since all chords have comparable units for motion.

The standardization not only provides a uniform measure of motion around the contour but also allows calculation of an average motion value for chords lying within a region of interest (Figs. 16.3 and 16.4). The ability to measure function over a region is important, because it is more sensitive in detecting motion abnormalities than in measuring the function of discrete points on the ventricular contour (36). The greater sensitivity of area methods can be explained by their lesser variability, since averaging

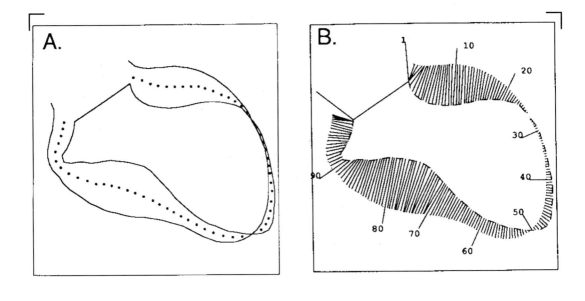

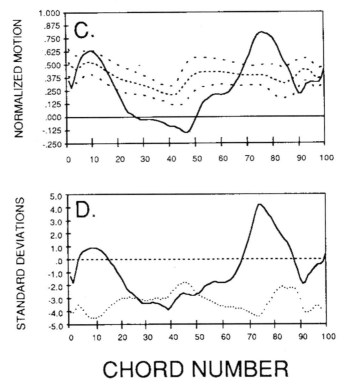

Figure 16.4. Centerline method of left ventricular wall motion analysis. **A.** A centerline is constructed midway between the end-diastolic and end-systolic endocardial contours. **B.** Motion is measured along 100 chords constructed perpendicular to the centerline. **C.** Motion at each chord is normalized by the end-diastolic perimeter length to yield a shortening fraction. The patient's motion (*solid line*) is compared with the mean plus or minus 1 standard deviation measured in a normal population (*dashed line*). **D.** The patient's wall motion is plotted in units of standard deviations from the normal mean (*dashed line*). Wall motion abnormality in the central infarct region, peripheral infarct region, and noninfarct region is calculated by averaging the motion of chords lying within these regions.

the motion of a sequence of chords significantly reduces point-to-point variation (43). For these reasons the centerline method calculates the severity of hypokinesis due to stenosis of a coronary artery by averaging the motion of chords lying in the most hypokinetic part of that artery's territory. This approach not only yields an area measurement but also focuses on the portion of the ventricle having the most abnormal function. Although coordinate system–based methods subdivide the ventricle into discrete regions, these predefined regions usually do not coincide with the part of the ventricle where motion is most depressed, and they often include either part of the border zone of intermediate dysfunction or a portion of normal ventricular wall (37).

Another advantage of the centerline method is its usefulness for calculating the circumferential extent of hypokinesis or hyperkinesis. That is, the number of chords having hypokinesis more severe than a given threshold can be easily determined and expressed as a percentage of the contour. **Commonly used thresholds of hypokinesis are one standard deviation and two standard deviations below normal akinesis.** Another way of viewing regional function is to measure the percent of the contour having normokinesis (48).

A three-dimensional representation of the location, extent, and severity of wall motion abnormality can be obtained by analyzing biplane ventriculograms (Fig. 16.5). This type of representation is useful for relating ventricular function to myocardial perfusion or metabolism studies using single photon emission computed tomography or positron emission tomography.

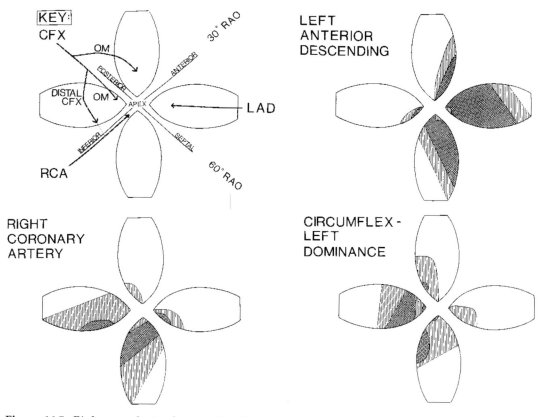

Figure 16.5. Biplane analysis of regional wall motion. The display presents the location, extent, and severity of regional dysfunction. This example shows the patterns of dysfunction observed in acute myocardial infarction resulting from isolated stenosis of the left anterior descending, circumflex, and right coronary arteries. The key is at the upper left of the figure.

Validation studies have demonstrated the sensitivity and specificity of the centerline method for identifying both hypokinesis and hyperkinesis (37, 49, 50) and its reproducibility (43). None of the methods of wall motion analysis, including the centerline method, can distinguish the motion of the ventricular walls from the motion of the heart within the chest. Methods of realigning the end-diastolic and end-systolic endocardial contours have been developed with empiric criteria, but they have no theoretic validity and may introduce systematic error and exacerbate variability (43).

Application of the Centerline Method in Ischemic Heart Disease

Because ischemic heart disease is inherently a regional disorder, analysis of wall motion is a very useful adjunct to calculating the global ejection fraction. The severity of hypokinesis measured by the centerline method has been correlated significantly with the minimum cross-sectional area of the stenosed coronary artery in question, and with infarct size measured from creatine phosphokinase release (37), intracoronary thallium scintigraphy (51), antimyosin antibody uptake (52), and magnetic resonance imaging (MRI) (53) in patients studied after acute myocardial infarction (AMI). Several studies have demonstrated the importance of measuring wall motion in ischemic and nonischemic regions. In patients with AMI the noninfarct region may be hypokinetic because of previous infarction or multivessel disease and may contribute to lowering the ejection fraction. In other patients hyperkinesis in the noninfarct region may be an acute compensatory mechanism to maintain the ejection fraction at a normal level (54, 55). Later on, chronic hyperkinesis may develop, particularly in those with single-vessel disease (56, 57). Since the ejection fraction integrates the effect of wall motion abnormalities in all regions, this parameter of global function may not sensitively reflect the severity of hypokinesis in either the infarcted or noninfarcted region. Likewise, the ejection

fraction may not reflect the effects of therapeutic interventions in salvaging myocardium or the time course of recovery (58–61). For these reasons the measurement of regional, as well as global, left ventricular function is particularly useful in evaluating response to treatment in patients with AMI and other ischemic syndromes (48).

Regional wall motion analysis is also being applied as a reference standard for evaluating tests of myocardial viability. The rationale is that viable myocardium will recover function if successfully reperfused; hence accurate prediction of functional recovery by metabolism and/or perfusion imaging techniques may be useful in planning reperfusion therapy for patients with resting dysfunction (62).

Newer Approaches to Imaging the Left Ventricle

Digital subtraction techniques are being used increasingly to facilitate the tedious task of delineating the endocardial contour of the left ventricle (see Chapter 12). The use of this and other image-processing techniques offers distinct advantages over the use of routine contrast cineventriculography. If injected into the left ventricle, the volume of contrast required is much smaller, as little as 7 to 10 mL (63–65). This reduces arrhythmias during injection and depression of myocardial function caused by the contrast material. Because of the lower contrast volume load, it is safe to perform repeated injections and serial studies to evaluate the effect of acute interventions on left ventricular performance. The addition of digital processing to a full-volume contrast injection yields excellent images, suitable for frame-by-frame analysis of function throughout the cardiac cycle. It is also possible to image the left ventricle after an intravenous injection of contrast material, but some patients are unable to suspend respiration until the end of the levophase, which is required to prevent motion artifact (63, 66).

Regardless of the quality of the image obtainable from contrast angiography, the accuracy of the volume, or the resolution of the wall motion analysis, the inescapable restriction is the invasiveness of the procedure. Two-dimensional echocardiography, radionuclide angiography, MRI, and cine computed tomography all can be used to obtain images of the cardiac chambers and evaluate ventricular function. All have their limitations and advantages. As nonangiographic methods are developed for the evaluation of cardiac performance, the standard by which these new techniques are evaluated will be cardiac angiography for some years to come.

The many investigators who helped develop quantitative methods to assess cardiac functions have laid the groundwork from which less invasive methods have been developed. As the invasive angiographic methods reviewed in this chapter are gradually replaced, it will be a credit to the investigators who developed our basic knowledge of cardiac function using invasive and at times difficult and complex procedures.

References

1. Dodge HT, Sandler H, Ballew DW, Lord JD. The use of biplane angiocardiography for the measurement of left ventricular volume in man. Am Heart J 1960;60:762–776.
2. Arvidsson H. Angiocardiographic determination of left ventricular volume. Acta Radiol 1961;56:321–339.
3. Sandler H, Dodge HT. The use of single plane angiocardiograms for the calculation of left ventricular volume in man. Am Heart J 1968;75:325–334.
4. Rackley CE, Dodge HT, Coble YD Jr, Hay RE. A method for determining left ventricular mass in man. Circulation 1964;29:666–679.
5. Sauter HJ, Dodge HT, Johnston RR, Graham TP. The relationship of left atrial pressure and volume in patients with heart disease. Am Heart J 1964;67:635–642.
6. Gault JH, Ross J, Braunwald E. Contractile state of the left ventricle in man: instantaneous tension-velocity-length relations in patients with and without disease of the left ventricular myocardium. Circ Res 1968;22:451–463.
7. Kennedy JW, Baxley WA, Figley MM, et al. Quantitative angiocardiography: 1. The normal left ventricle in man. Circulation 1966;34:272–278.
8. Kennedy JW, Twiss RD, Blackmon JR, Dodge HT. Quantitative angiocardiography: 3. Relationships of left ventricular pressure, volume and mass in aortic valve disease. Circulation 1968;38:838–845.
9. Kennedy JW, Yarnall SR, Murray JA, Figley MM. Quantitative angiocardiography: 4. Relationships of left atrial and ventricular pressure and volume in mitral valve disease. Circulation 1970;41:817–824.
10. Hamilton GW, Murray JA, Kennedy JW. Quantitative angiocardiography in ischemic heart disease: the spectrum of abnormal left ventricular function and the role of abnormally contracting segments. Circulation 1972;45:1065–1080.
11. Kennedy JW, Kaiser GC, Fisher LD, et al. Clinical and angiographic predictors of operative mortality from the Collaborative Study in Coronary Artery Surgery (CASS). Circulation 1981;63:793–802.
12. Herman MV, Heinle RA, Klein MD, Gorlin R. Localized disorders in myocardial contraction: asynergy and its role in congestive heart failure. N Engl J Med 1967;277:222–232.
13. Hildner FJ, Furst A, Krieger R, et al. New principles for optimum left ventriculography. Cathet Cardiovasc Diagn 1986;12:266–273.
14. Lehmann KG, Yang JC, Doria RJ, et al. Catheter optimization during contrast ventriculography: a prospective randomized trial. Am Heart J 1992;123:1273–1278.
15. Wynne J, Green LH, Mann T, et al. Estimation of left ventricular volumes in man from biplane cineangiograms filmed in oblique projections. Am J Cardiol 1978;41:726–732.
16. Als AV, Paulin S, Aroesty JM. Biplane angiographic volumetry using the right anterior oblique and half-axial left anterior oblique technique. Radiology 1978;126:511–514.
17. Rogers WJ, Smith LR, Bream PR, et al. Quantitative axial oblique contrast left ventriculography: validation of the method by demonstrating improved visualization of regional wall motion and mitral valve function with accurate volume determinations. Am Heart J 1982;103:185–193.
18. Kennedy JW, Doces JG, Stewart DK. Left ventricular function before and following surgical treatment of mitral valve disease. Am Heart J 1979;97:592–598.
19. Kennedy JW, Doces JG, Stewart DK. Left ventricular function before and following aortic valve replacement. Circulation 1977;56:944–950.
20. Principal Investigators of CASS and their Associates. The National Heart, Lung, and Blood Institute Coronary Artery Surgery Study: a multicenter comparison of the effects of randomized medical and surgical treatment of mildly symptomatic patients with coronary artery disease, and a registry of consecutive patients undergoing coronary angiography. Circulation 1981;63:I1–I81.
21. Kennedy JW, Kaiser GC, Fisher LD, et al. Multivariate discriminant analysis of the clinical and angiographic predictors of operative mortality from the collaborative study in coronary artery surgery (CASS). J Thorac Cardiovasc Surg 1980;80:876–887.
22. Hugenholtz PG, Wagner HR, Sandler H. The in vivo determination of left ventricular volume: comparison of the fiberoptic-indicator dilution and the angiocardiographic methods. Circulation 1968;37:489–508.
23. Kennedy JW, Trenholme SE, Kasser IS. Left ventricular volume and mass from single-plane ci-

neangiocardiogram: a comparison of anteroposterior and right anterior oblique methods. Am Heart J 1970;80:343–352.

24. Kasser IS, Kennedy JW. Measurement of left ventricular volumes in man by single-plane cineangiocardiography. Invest Radiol 1969;4:83–90.

25. Cha SD, Incarvito J, Maranhao V. Calculation of magnification factor from an intracardiac marker. Cathet Cardiovasc Diagn 1983;9:79–87.

26. Cohn PF, Levine JA, Bergeron GA, Gorlin R. Reproducibility of the angiographic left ventricular ejection fraction in patients with coronary artery disease. Am Heart J 1974;88:713–720.

27. Rogers WJ, Smith LR, Hood WP Jr, et al. Effect of filming projection and interobserver variability on angiographic biplane left ventricular volume determination. Circulation 1979;59:96–104.

28. Dodge HT, Sheehan FH, Stewart DK. Estimation of ventricular volume, fractional ejected volumes, stroke volume, and quantitation of regurgitant flow. In: Just H, Heintzen PH, eds. Angiocardiography: current status and future developments. Berlin: Springer-Verlag, 1986:99–108.

29. Chaitman BR, DeMots H, Bristow JD, et al. Objective and subjective analysis of left ventricular angiograms. Circulation 1975;52:420–425.

30. Vine DL, Hegg TD, Dodge HT, et al. Immediate effect of contrast medium injection on left ventricular volumes and ejection fraction: a study using metallic epicardial markers. Circulation 1977;56:379–384.

31. Lange PE, Onnasch D, Farr FL, Heintzen PH. Angiocardiographic right ventricular volume determination: accuracy, as determined from human casts, and clinical application. Eur J Cardiol 1978;8:477–501.

32. Graham TP Jr, Atwood GF, Faulkner SL, Nelson JH. Right atrial volume measurements from biplane cineangiocardiography. Circulation 1974;49:709–716.

33. Lang TW, Corday E, Gold H, et al. Consequences of reperfusion after coronary occlusion: effects on hemodynamic and regional myocardial metabolic function. Am J Cardiol 1974;33:69–81.

34. Thompson R, Ahmed M, Seabra-Gomes R, et al. Influence of preoperative left ventricular function on results of homograft replacement of the aortic valve for aortic regurgitation. J Thorac Cardiovasc Surg 1979;77:411–421.

35. Wallis DE, O'Connell JB, Henkin RE, et al. Segmental wall motion abnormalities in dilated cardiomyopathy: a common finding and good prognostic sign. J Am Coll Cardiol 1984;4:674–679.

36. Gelberg HJ, Brundage BH, Glantz S, Parmley WW. Quantitative left ventricular wall motion analysis: a comparison of area, chord and radial methods. Circulation 1979;59:991–1000.

37. Sheehan FH, Bolson EL, Dodge HT, et al. Advantages and applications of the centerline method for characterizing regional ventricular function. Circulation 1986;74:293–305.

38. Slager CJ, Hooghoudt TEH, Serruys PW, et al. Quantitative assessment of regional left ventricular motion using endocardial landmarks. J Am Coll Cardiol 1986;7:317–327.

39. Ingels NB Jr, Daughters GT II, Stinson EB, Alderman EL. Evaluation of methods for quantitating left ventricular segmental wall motion in man using myocardial markers as a standard. Circulation 1980;61:966–972.

40. Goodyer AVN, Langou RA. The multicentric character of normal left ventricular wall motion: implications for the evaluation of regional wall motion abnormalities by contrast angiography. Cathet Cardiovasc Diagn 1982;8:225–232.

41. McDonald IG. The shape and movements of the human left ventricle during systole. Am J Cardiol 1970;26:221–230.

42. Sandor T, Paulin S, Hanlon WB. Left ventricular wall motion analysis using operator-independent contour positioning. Comput Biomed Res 1984;17:129–142.

43. Sheehan FH, Stewart DK, Dodge HT, et al. Variability in the measurement of regional ventricular wall motion from contrast angiograms. Circulation 1983;68:550–559.

44. Brower RW. Evaluation of pattern recognition rules for the apex of the heart. Cathet Cardiovasc Diagn 1980;6:145–157.

45. Harris LD, Clayton PD, Marshall HW, Warner HR. A technique for the detection of asynergic motion in the left ventricle. Comput Biomed Res 1974;7:380–394.

46. Stewart DK, Dodge HT, Frimer M. Quantitative analysis of regional myocardial performance in coronary artery disease. Cardiovasc Imaging Image Processing 1975;72:217–224.

47. Ingles NB Jr, Daughters GT II, Stinson EB, Alderman EL. Measurement of midwall myocardial dynamics in intact man by radiography of surgically implanted markers. Circulation 1975;52:859–867.

48. The GUSTO Angiographic Investigators. The effects of tissue plasminogen activator, streptokinase, or both on coronary-artery patency, ventricular function, and survival after acute myocardial infarction. N Engl J Med 1993;329:1615–1622.

49. Sheehan FH, Bolson EL, Dodge HT, Mitten S. Centerline method: comparison with other methods for measuring regional left ventricular motion. In: Sigwart U, Heintzen PH, eds. Ventricular wall motion. Stuttgart: Georg Thieme Verlag, 1984:139–149.

50. Ginzton LE, Berntzen R, Lobodzinski S, et al. Computerized quantitative segmental wall motion analysis during exercise: radial vs. centerline left ventricular segmentation. In: Computers in Cardiology. Long Beach, CA: IEEE Computer Society, 1985:157–160.

51. Schofer J, Sheehan FH, Spielmann R, et al. Recovery of left ventricular function after myocardial infarction can be predicted immediately after thrombolysis by semiquantitative intracoronary thallium and technetium pyrophosphate scintigraphy. Eur Heart J 1988;9:1088–1097.

52. Khaw BA, Gold HK, Yasuda T, et al. Scintigraphic quantification of myocardial necrosis in patients after intravenous injection of myosin-specific antibody. Circulation 1986;74:501–508.

53. Johns JA, Leavitt MB, Newell JB, et al. Quantification of acute myocardial infarct size by nuclear magnetic resonance imaging. J Am Coll Cardiol 1990;15:143–149.

54. Stamm RB, Gibson RS, Bishop HL, et al. Echocardiographic detection of infarct-localized asynergy and remote asynergy during acute myocardial infarction: correlation with the extent of angiographic coronary disease. Circulation 1983;67:233–244.

55. Sheehan FH, Szente A, Mathey DG, Dodge HT. Assessment of left ventricular function in acute myocardial infarction: the relationship between global ejection fraction and regional wall motion. Eur Heart J 1985;6:E117–E125.

56. Martin GV, Sheehan FH, Stadius M, et al. Intravenous streptokinase: effects on global and regional systolic function. Circulation 1988;78:258–266.

57. Serruys PW, Simoons ML, Suryapranata H, et al. Preservation of global and regional left ventricular function after early thrombolysis in acute myocardial infarction. J Am Coll Cardiol 1986;7:729–742.

58. Stack RS, Phillips HR III, Grierson DS, et al. Functional improvement of jeopardized myocardium following intracoronary streptokinase infusion in acute myocardial infarction. J Clin Invest 1983;72:84–95.

59. Sheehan FH, Mathey DG, Schofer J, et al. Effect of interventions in salvaging left ventricular function in acute myocardial infarction: a study of intracoronary streptokinase. Am J Cardiol 1983;52:431–438.

60. Sheehan FH, Mathey DG, Schofer J, et al. Factors determining recovery of left ventricular function following thrombolysis in acute myocardial infarction. Circulation 1985;71:1121–1128.

61. Schmidt WG, Sheehan FH, von Essen R, et al. Evolution of left ventricular function after intracoronary thrombolysis for acute myocardial infarction. Am J Cardiol 1989;63:497–502.

62. Vom Dahl J, Altehoefer C, Sheehan FH, et al. Recovery of regional left ventricular dysfunction following coronary revascularization: impact of myocardial viability assessed by nuclear imaging and of vessel patency at follow-up. J Am Coll Cardiol (in press).

63. Tobis JM, Nalcioglu O, Johnston WD, et al. Correlation of 10-milliliter digital subtraction ventriculograms compared with standard cineangiograms. Am Heart J 1983;105:946–951.

64. Nichols AB, Martin EC, Fles TP, et al. Validation of the angiographic accuracy of digital left ventriculography. Am J Cardiol 1983;51:224–230.

65. Mancini GBJ, Hodgson JM, Legrand V, et al. Quantitative assessment of global and regional left ventricular function with low-contrast dose digital subtraction ventriculography. Chest 1985;87:598–602.

66. Nissen SE, Booth D, Waters J, et al. Evaluation of left ventricular contractile pattern by intravenous digital subtraction ventriculography: comparison with cineangiography and assessment of interobserver variability. Am J Cardiol 1983;52:1293–1298.

17
Coronary Angiography

Carl J. Pepine, MD
Charles R. Lambert, MD, PhD
James A. Hill, MD

INTRODUCTION

Coronary angiography is frequently performed to examine the coronary circulation selectively via contrast radiographic imaging techniques. The angiographic details of the lumen of both native coronary vessels and surgically constructed bypass grafts are examined. These details include the anatomic pattern of the vessel distribution, pathoanatomic and some pathophysiologic abnormalities as they influence the vessel lumen, collateral circulation, and congenital coronary anomalies. Coronary angiography is often performed in conjunction with a number of ancillary diagnostic and therapeutic procedures. Despite considerable limitations and dependence on noninvasive functional testing, selective coronary angiography remains the reference standard for clinical evaluation of patients with known or suspected coronary artery disease (CAD).

HISTORICAL PERSPECTIVE

The development of high-quality magnification cineradiography and the advent of coronary revascularization procedures led to incredible growth in the use of coronary angiography. This procedure is a benchmark in cardiovascular medicine for diagnosis, treatment, and research. Before addressing the details of this procedure, it seems appropriate to review its history and growth.

During the late 1940s investigators began working to develop **nonselective techniques** to visualize the coronary arteries (1). These indirect methods included flooding the aortic root with a large quantity of radiographic contrast material during maneuvers designed to enhance coronary filling (2, 3). Brief cardiac arrest by means of a bolus of acetylcholine (4, 5), a stimulated Valsalva-like maneuver, balloon occlusion of the ascending aorta, and a loop catheter to direct the injected contrast material toward the coronary ostia were all employed (6, 7).

Some of the techniques to enhance coronary artery and myocardial perfusion imaging by noninvasive methods have recently been reintroduced. In 1958 Mason Sones began to develop **selective coronary angiography** in animals. He used electronic image amplification, optical magnification, and high-speed cine filming. In 1959 he and his colleagues accidentally injected radiographic contrast material into the right coronary artery (RCA) of a patient during a planned aortogram (8). Although asystole occurred, the patient was resuscitated via coughs and had an uneventful recovery. Sones then developed a special catheter that selectively entered and opacified the coronary arteries when introduced from a brachial artery via a **surgical cutdown** (9). After he and his colleagues demonstrated that their procedure was safe, selective coronary angiography became the reference standard to assess the coronary arteries for both research and diagnostic purposes. By 1967 **percutaneous catheterization** was modified for selective coronary angiography by Judkins (10) and Amplatz et al. (11). These techniques used various preformed catheters designed to seek each coronary ostium after percutaneous introduction from a femoral artery. With the introduction of safe and effective coronary artery bypass surgery (CABG) in 1968 by Favalaro (12), selective coronary angiography also became the reference standard to select patients for revascularization therapy.

Growth of the procedure was initially slow, but it began to accelerate in the 1970s, fueled by the success of CABG. Although there are no data available specifically for coronary angiography, we estimate that catheterization procedures in 80% or more of adult patients include coronary angiography. This suggests that by the mid 1970s approximately 160,000 coronary angiographies were performed yearly (13). Development of percutaneous coronary revascularization in the late 1970s by Andreas and Gruentzig further accelerated growth of coronary angiography. According to catheterization volume data in hospitalized patients (14), we estimate that about 500,000 coronary angiograms were done yearly by the mid 1980s and at least a million per year by the early 1990s (15). Adding patients who underwent catheterization as outpatients suggests that by the early 1990s more than 1.5 million coronary angiographies were performed yearly, and the growth continues.

RADIOGRAPHIC ANATOMY

Normal Anatomic Distribution

Knowledge of the anatomic distribution of the coronary arteries is important for the physician participating in the care of patients undergoing cardiac catheterization.

For the physician planning to perform coronary angiography, the **radiographic anatomy must be committed to memory** before the first patient is approached. This brief summary is an introduction for physicians participating in the practice of coronary angiography. Each operator must be familiar with normal as well as abnormal radiographic anatomy of the coronary arteries. He or she should develop a personal protocol for radiographic projections that is modified to improve visualization of specific areas of a given patient's coronary vascular system as the need arises (Fig. 17.1). Prerequisites for better understanding this area include a review of some of the commonly used terminology: **coronary angiography** is a procedure performed during cardiac catheterization to visualize the lumen of the large and medium-sized (larger than 200 microns) coronary arteries.

Standard Radiographic Projections for Coronary Angiography

Left anterior oblique (LAO) projections are transverse-plane radiographic views obtained with the x-ray beam entering posteriorly on an oblique angle to exit anteriorly and to the patient's left at the location of the image acquisition device, usually the image intensifier. **Right anterior oblique** (RAO) projections are transverse-plane radiographic views obtained with the x-ray beam entering posteriorly on an oblique angle to exit anteriorly and to the patient's right (Fig. 17.2, *Top*). These oblique views are described by polar coordinates as viewed from the patient's feet and looking toward the patient's head, with 0° at the vertical position through 90° to either the left or right.

Cranial angulation refers to sagittal-plane views obtained with the x-ray beam entering posteriorly and exiting anteriorly and superiorly at the location of the image acquisition device (Fig. 17.2, *Bottom*). **Caudal angulation** refers to sagittal-plane views with the x-ray beam entering posteriorly and exiting anteriorly and inferiorly.

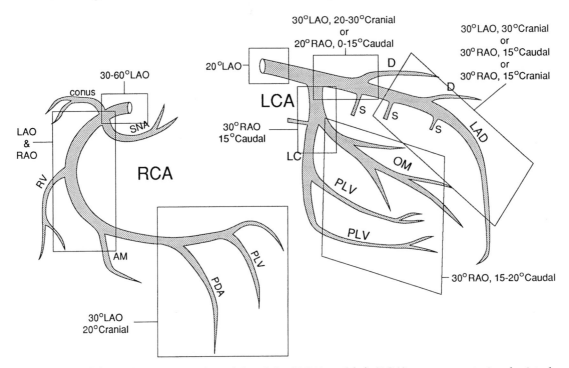

Figure 17.1. Schematic representation of the right (*RCA*) and left (*LCA*) coronary arteries depicted in the left anterior oblique (*LAO*) and right anterior oblique (*RAO*) projections, respectively. Approximate frontal and sagittal-plane projections and angulations for visualization of various portions of the coronary arteries are indicated. The LCA branches are noted as *SNA*, sinus node artery; *RV*, right ventricular; *AM*, acute marginal; *PDA*, posterior descending artery; *PLV*, posterior left ventricular; *LC*, left circumflex; *OM*, obtuse marginal; *S*, septal; *D*, diagonal; *LAD*, left anterior descending artery.

Coronary luminology is study of the radiographic shadows produced by the contrast-filled lumen of coronary arteries and bypass grafts. This type of study is only an approximation of the coronary lumen and provides little information about the state of the arterial wall.

Minimal or **intermediate lesions** are lesions that reduce the coronary lumen diameter not more than 50%; while they may not significantly limit blood flow at rest or stress, they may contribute to acute coronary events because they are vulnerable to rupture and result in acute worsening of the lumen obstruction so that blood flow is reduced.

Complex lesions are coronary narrowings with hazy borders on coronary angiography. They often have overhanging edges and are thought to be a result of recent plaque ulceration or disruption with associated thrombus formation.

Left Coronary Artery

The ostium of the left coronary artery (LCA) usually arises from the superior portion of the left coronary sinus, somewhat anterior to the coronal plane, from a position between the pulmonary artery and left atrial appendage (Figs. 17.3 and 17.4). The proximal portion of the left main coronary artery continues for a variable distance before it divides into its anterior descending and circumflex branches. The left main coronary artery may terminate in a trifurcation, with an intermediate branch bisecting the angle

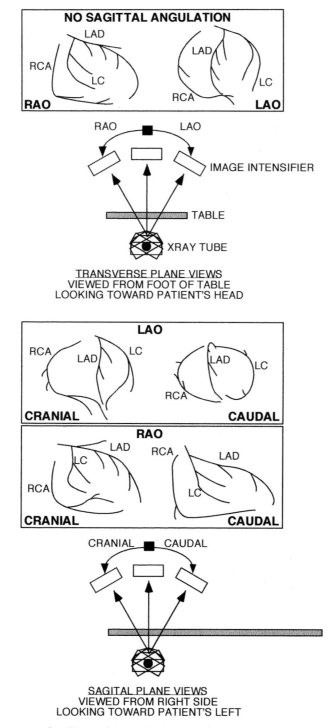

Figure 17.2. Diagrams of radiographic projections in the transverse (**top**) and sagittal (**bottom**) planes.

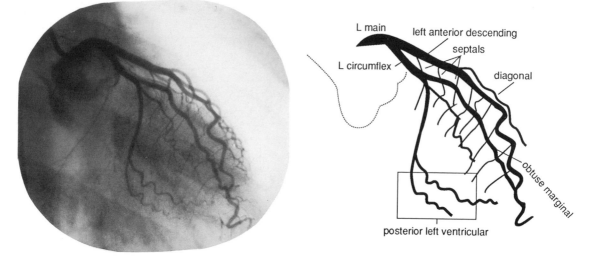

Figure 17.3. Normal radiographic anatomy of the LCA and its branches, as seen in the RAO projection with slight (15°) caudal angulation.

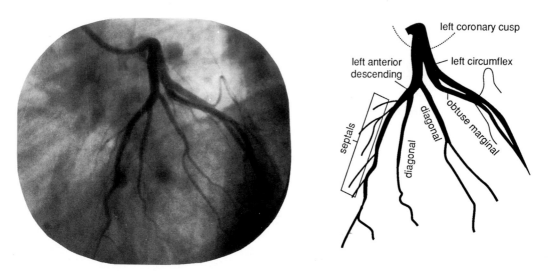

Figure 17.4. Normal radiographic anatomy of the LCA and its branches as seen in the LAO projection with cranial (20°) angulation.

between the anterior descending and circumflex branches. The left main artery usually does not supply secondary branches, and its ostium and proximal portions are often best visualized in the shallow (20 to 30°) left anterior oblique (LAO) projection (Fig. 17.1). Minimal (10 to 15%) cranial angulation in the sagittal plane may be help-

ful. The distal portion of the left main artery and bifurcation are best viewed in the shallow (20°) right anterior oblique (RAO) projection with minimal (0 to 15°) caudal or moderate (20 to 30°) cranial angulation. A secondary view for the distal left main and bifurcation is the 30 to 45° LAO with about 25° of caudal angulation.

Left Anterior Descending Artery

The left anterior descending (LAD) artery originates at an obtuse angle from the left main artery and courses anteriorly, inferiorly, and toward the patient's right to emerge from behind the pulmonary artery and descend in the anterior interventricular groove (Figs. 17.3 and 17.4). In most patients this vessel continues to the apex, and in some it also supplies the inferior apical region. Occasionally the LAD takes an intramyocardial route. Sometimes systolic compression from **muscular bridges** over the artery can be observed obstructing flow of contrast in systole (Fig. 17.5). In a few such cases obstruction over several centimeters during diastole is also present. Systolic compression caused by muscular bridges is usually accentuated after nitroglycerin. Recognition of these features helps to distinguish the bridge from other forms of obstruction, such as that caused by a pericardial band or CAD.

The proximal LAD is best visualized in LAO projections (30 to 60°) with cranial angulation (20 to 30°) (Figs. 17.3 and 17.4). The mid and distal portions are better seen in LAO projections without cranial angulation and in RAO projections (Fig. 17.3). In the RAO projections some caudal or cranial angulation (15 to 30°) may be used to minimize overlap of the mid LAD with diagonal branches. A useful secondary projection for the proximal mid LAD and its diagonal branches' origins is the shallow RAO (5 to 10°) with cranial angulation (30 to 60°).

Septal Perforating and Diagonal Branches

Septal branches arise at right angles from the LAD and course deep into the interventricular septum. They vary in number, and the first branch is sometimes large enough for angioplasty or bypass considerations.

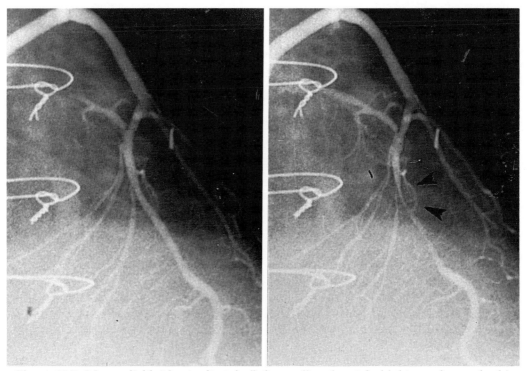

Figure 17.5. Myocardial bridge in diastole (**left panel**) and systole (**right panel,** *arrowheads*) involving the mid LAD, which is filled by a saphenous vein bypass graft.

Sometimes a large septal perforating trunk arises from the first or second septal branch position and supplies multiple secondary branches. Septal LAD branches supply the anterior two-thirds of the septum and form potential for anastomosis with septal perforating branches derived from the posterior descending branch of the right or left circumflex arteries. The proximal septal perforators are often large (1 to 1.5 mm in diameter), and their proximal portions are best visualized in the shallow (30°) LAO projection with cranial angulation (30°) and shallow (30°) RAO projection with caudal angulation (Fig. 17.3).

Diagonal Branches

The diagonal branches arise at oblique angles to the LAD and continue on the epicardial surface to descend diagonally toward the obtuse margin of the heart. Diagonal branches vary in number and size, but usually the first two or three are large enough for angioplasty or bypass consideration. On rare occasions a diagonal branch is quite large and even supplies septal perforating branches. Proximal parts of the diagonal branches are usually best viewed in the 30 to 45° LAO projection with 30° cranial angulation (Fig. 17.3). The 30° RAO projections with caudal (15°) or cranial (30°) angulation minimize overlap of the diagonal branches.

Left Circumflex Artery

The left circumflex (LC) artery often continues in the same general direction as the left main coronary artery, under the left atrial appendage to enter the left atrioventricular groove. The LC then continues to the patient's left and posteriorly at an oblique angle. After providing several posterior lateral ventricular branches, which parallel the LAD diagonal branches in their direction toward the obtuse margin, the LC supplies an obtuse marginal branch that continues along the obtuse margin of the heart. The continuation of the LC coronary in the atrioventricular groove is highly variable. In some patients with anatomically dominant LC artery circulation the LC continues to supply a large posterior descending branch. In the more common configuration the LC continues as a small terminal posterior left ventricular branch or branches and does not reach the posterior interventricular groove.

The proximal portion of the LC is best visualized in the RAO projection (30°) with about 15° caudal angulation (Fig. 17.3). A secondary view is the steep LAO projection (30 to 45°) with cranial angulation (15 to 20°). The obtuse marginal branch is best viewed in the RAO projections (30°) with 15 to 20° of caudal angulation.

Right Coronary Artery

The ostium of the right coronary artery (RCA) usually arises from an anterior position at approximately the middle portion of the right coronary sinus (Figs. 17.6 and 17.7). It is usually somewhat lower than the left coronary ostium. The RCA ostium is always more anterior than the left coronary ostium. From this position the RCA descends to the patient's right in the anterior right atrioventricular groove. The conus branch to the proximal pulmonary conus and right ventricular outflow region is its first branch. Alternatively the conus artery may originate from a separate ostium and not be visualized when the RCA ostium is selectively engaged, as in Figures 17.6 and 17.7. Ordinarily there are also two or three large right ventricular branches that arise anteriorly and course diagonally over the right ventricle. A sinus node branch usually originates posteriorly and courses toward the cranium to encircle the superior vena cava. A major branch at the acute margin usually supplies only right ventricular myocardium. On occasion this branch may continue to supply the apex. In most individuals the RCA continues along the diaphragmatic surface of the heart in the atrioventricular groove to reach the crux. In 90% of cases the RCA continues to supply a branch to the atrio-

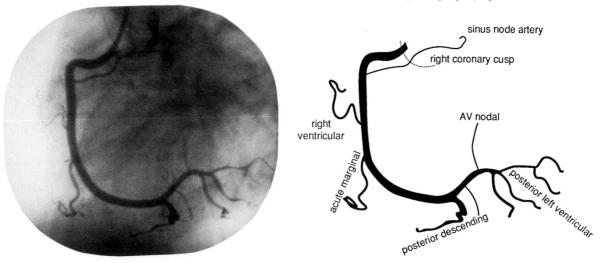

Figure 17.6. Normal radiographic anatomy of the RCA and its branches as seen in the left anterior oblique projection.

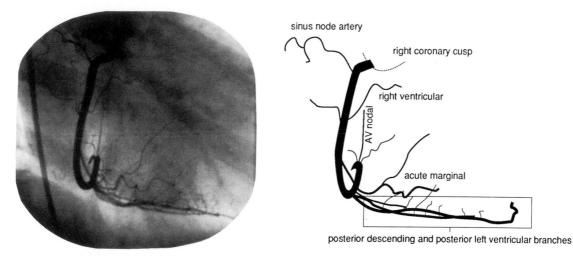

Figure 17.7. Normal radiographic anatomy of the RCA and its branches as seen in the right anterior oblique projection.

ventricular node and then descends in the interventricular groove to provide the posterior descending artery (PDA) branch. This PDA branch varies in size but in most individuals remains quite large. It courses anteriorly in the inferior interventricular groove to supply septal perforating branches. These ascend at right angles to supply the inferior third of the septum. These branches can provide a rich collateral pathway to the LAD via septal perforating arteries.

The right ostium and most proximal RCA are best viewed in the relatively steep (45 to 60°) LAO projections (Fig. 17.6). The midportion of the RCA is well seen in most LAO and RAO projections. The part of the RCA continuing along the diaphragmatic surface is best seen in the LAO projections. The RCA at the crux and PDA are best seen in the 30° LAO projection with cranial (20 to 30°) angulation (Fig. 17.6). A secondary view is the 20° RAO projection with cranial angulation.

Congenital Variations

Congenital anomalies of the coronary arteries are important considerations requiring accurate recognition in the approach to coronary angiography. Major anomalies occur in approximately 1 to 2% of patients undergoing coronary angiography, and most are considered benign. However, some forms may be associated with serious sequelae (e.g., angina, infarction, syncope, heart failure, arrhythmias, sudden death) (16, 17). They have a frequent association with other forms of congenital heart disease, and in these situations their identification and course are important in the surgical approach to correction of the congenital heart disease. Coronary anomalies may make selective opacification with preformed catheters, particularly the Judkins series, difficult.

The most common coronary artery anomaly observed in the angiographic laboratory is either an LCA or RCA branch arising from a **separate ostium.** As many as 50% of patients have a separate origin for the right coronary conus artery. This ostium is often located to the left (more anterior) of the right coronary ostium. This branch may be an important source of collaterals to visualize an occluded LAD artery. A separate ostium for the origin of the LAD and LC arteries occurs in about 1% of the cases. **High origin** of the coronary arteries may occur, with the LCA arising above the junction of the left coronary sinus and the aorta. It must be selectively entered to avoid erroneous interpretations with serious implications (Fig. 17.8). In a small proportion of cases the right coronary arises above the right coronary sinus–aorta junction. Both coronary arteries may even arise from the base of the ascending aorta rather than the coronary sinuses. If the high left ostium cannot be entered with a standard-sized left Judkins catheter, a catheter one size smaller may work. If not, either a left Amplatz or multipurpose catheter is usually successful. For a high right coronary ostium the standard sizes are usually adequate. The optimal projections noted previously for the course of these arteries are useful. While these high origins are benign, the cardiac surgeon should avoid accidental cross-clamping or transecting the vessel during surgery.

A **single coronary artery,** which is rare, may have any of various patterns. The single coronary artery may follow the course of one normal (e.g., either the RCA or LCA) coronary artery and then continue around the heart to supply the distribution of the second coronary artery. In another variation the ostium of the single coronary artery is in the position of one normal ostium, but branches originate proximally and cross the base of the heart to supply the artery to the other coronary territory. In a third type an irregular coronary distribution occurs as the LAD and LC arise separately from the proximal part of normal RCA. In any of these single-coronary variations the cross-sectional area of the single coronary artery may be less than that of the normal LCA plus the RCA, and/or various branches may be small or absent. In addition, the course of the anomalous artery relative to the aorta and pulmonary artery may be important because of possible compression. Accordingly, it has been suggested that this anomaly may have physiologic significance. Accelerated atherosclerosis may also be due to the irregular course, bending, high velocity of blood flow, and so on.

Origin of the LCA from the pulmonary artery is rare. Most patients with this condition demonstrate severe myocardial ischemia early in infancy or early childhood, with a syndrome of failure to thrive, tachypnea, wheezing, angina, and/or death. Origin of the LCA from the pulmonary artery results in low perfusion pressure and low oxygen content in blood perfusing the left ventricular wall. The few who survive to adulthood have mitral regurgitation, angina, congestive heart failure, and a high incidence of sudden death. Also, either the LAD or the RCA may arise separately from the pulmonary artery. Survival depends on development of collaterals from the other coronary arteries. However, a steal syndrome in which blood flows from the normal coronary system to the aberrant system or even into the pulmonary artery can develop. Treatment consists of occlusion by catheter-delivered balloon of the aberrant coronary artery at its origin from the pulmo-

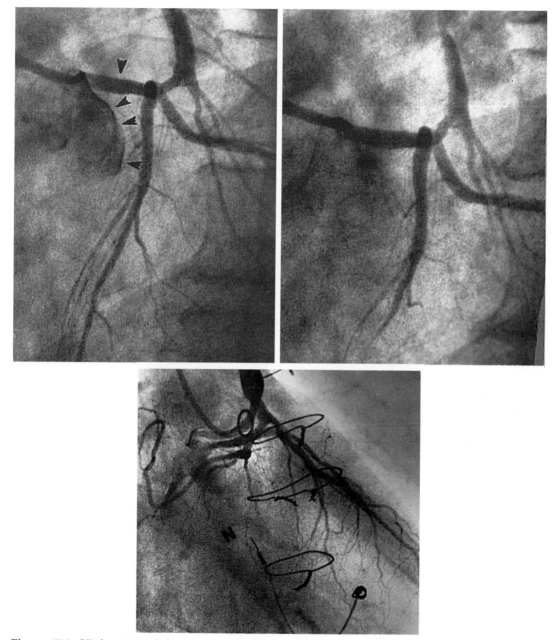

Figure 17.8. High origin of the LCA (*arrow*) above the left aortic sinus (*multiple arrowheads*) during nonselective opacification (**left panel**) which suggests possible narrowing in proximal part of LCA. This interpretation led to bypass surgery (note patent saphenous vein bypass graft). When the LCA is selectively opacified (**right panel**) or opacified in retrograde fashion by injection of SVBG (**lower panel**), no important obstruction is seen.

nary artery, if viable myocardium is not identified. If viable myocardium is present, occlusion and coronary artery bypass grafting or reimplantation of the coronary artery into the aorta is possible. **Congenital stenosis** or **atresia** of the proximal part of a coronary artery is relatively rare and usually accompanies other congenital heart disease.

Origin of either the LCA or RCA from the opposite coronary sinus is an important finding. The course of the anomalous vessel should be identified at coronary angiography. Some cases of this anomaly have been associated with sudden death, perhaps related to compression of the aberrant coronary artery because of a tethering effect of the great vessels. Five anatomic subtypes have been classified according to the relationship of the anomalous coronary artery with the aorta and pulmonary artery. The course of the anomalous vessel may be (*a*) **anterior,** (*b*) **interarterial,** (*c*) **septal,** (*d*) **posterior,** or **retroaortic,** or (*e*) **combined** (6). The septal subtype is most common and the interarterial (between) subtype rarest. Sometimes the portion of the artery between the great vessels appears ovoid and narrowed in an angiogram viewed in cross-section. This type of anomaly is first suggested from the left ventriculogram viewed in the right or oblique projection showing the location of the aberrant coronary artery at the base of the aorta. The course of the abnormal artery is confirmed by selective injection with filming in the steep (45 to 60°) left or oblique projection with steep (30 to 40°) cranial angulation and the RAO projection. The most common form of this anomaly seen during coronary angiography is **origin of the LC artery from the right coronary sinus or the RCA** (16, 17) (Figs. 17.9–17.13). Four of the five types are shown in detail in cross-section and the RAO projection. Selective opacification of an aberrant LCA or LC branch is important to identify obstruction for diagnostic purposes or for possible revascularization. When the anomalous artery arises from the right sinus, it is best cannulated selectively with a right Amplatz, multipurpose, or Sones catheter. When the anomalous artery arises from the left coronary sinus, it is best entered with a left Amplatz, multipurpose, or Sones catheter. It is essential to determine the vessel's course when the LCA arises from the right sinus or RCA and when the LAD arises from either the RCA or right coronary sinus.

Finally, **congenital coronary artery fistulas** with intracardiac shunts may be identified (Fig. 17.14). Fistulas may drain into a right heart chamber to function as right-to-left shunts, causing a volume overload syndrome that may be surgically or nonsurgically (catheter balloon occlusion) corrected.

TECHNIQUES FOR SELECTIVE CORONARY ARTERY OPACIFICATION

Current visualization techniques provide excellent resolution of large and medium-sized coronary vessels and even vessels as small as 100 mm in diameter. Repeated injections in multiple projections are needed for most diagnostic studies. Because of the potential for thromboembolism or thrombus formation at or distal to the site of catheter insertion, anticoagulation is often used routinely in many laboratories in patients undergoing coronary angiography. Heparin is administered intra-arterially or intravenously shortly after the first catheter enters a peripheral artery. The dose usually ranges from 3000 to 5000 units. This is based on the principle that bleeding can readily be controlled during or after catheterization but that thromboembolism cannot, and it has devastating consequences. For very brief procedures (< 10 min), the authors often omit heparin. The nonionic contrast agents have neither the anticoagulant nor antiplatelet aggregation properties of the ionic agents, nor do the nonionic agents potentiate the anticoagulant effects of heparin as do the ionic agents. Thus, in our opinion, when nonionic contrast agents are used for coronary angiography, heparin should almost always be used. Furthermore, use of these newer contrast agents demands even more meticulous attention to the safety details of coronary angiography. Blood in connecting tubes, manifolds, or syringes must not be left in contact with these agents. Manifolds with a port for heparinized flush solution are essential. Contrast agents and their use are discussed in more detail in Chapter 13.

There are two general approaches to selective coronary angiography. These are the

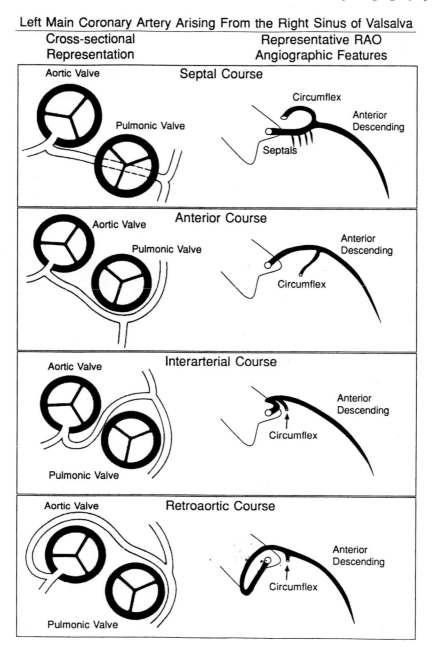

Figure 17.9. Diagram of possible anatomic paths taken with origin of the LCA from the right sinus of Valsalva (or the RCA). Representative RAO (30°) angiograms (**right panel**) illustrate characteristics of the LCA and its proximal branches, diagramed in cross-section (**left panel**) to define their relationship to the great vessels. With the septal course (**top panel**) the circumflex forms a cranial loop with respect to the left main and the proximal left main gives rise to one or more septal vessels. In the anterior course (*second from top*), with no cranial angulation, the circumflex is inferior to the left main and proximal anterior descending segments. The left main may be seen on end (*dot*) with the interarterial course (*third from top*) as it courses around the aorta anteriorly. The circumflex arises with a caudal orientation. The retroaortic course (**bottom**) is readily identified in this projection by the caudal and posterior initial course. The mixed course (not shown) is very rare and has various combinations of these four.

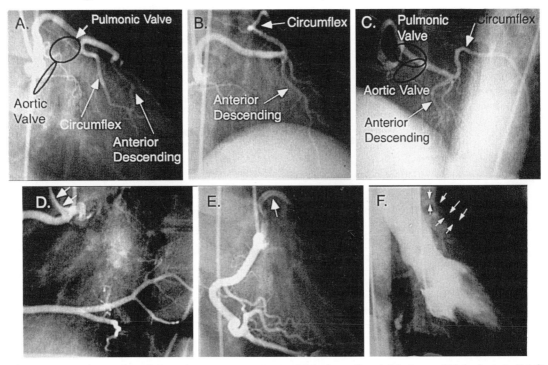

Figure 17.10. Anomalous left main coronary artery arising from the right sinus of Valsalva. **A.** RAO (no sagittal-plane angulation) angiogram illustrating the anterior course of the LCA as diagramed in Figure 17.8 (*second from top*). **B.** Addition of cranial angulation projects the circumflex branch superiorly. **C.** LAO projection illustrates left anterior descending and circumflex branches. **D.** An LAO projection of the right coronary artery (*arrows*), which arises from a common ostium in the right sinus of the Valsalva. **E.** An RAO projection of the right coronary artery illustrating the proximal portion of the left coronary artery (*arrow*). **F.** Left ventriculogram (RAO) revealing the proximal portion of the left main coronary artery.

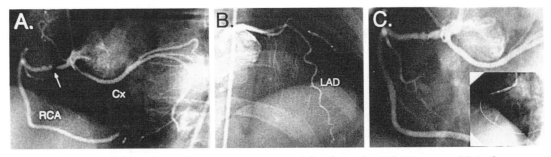

Figure 17.11. Anomalous circumflex coronary artery arising from the right coronary. Note the course of the anomalous circumflex posterior to the aorta and severe stenosis in the RCA distal to the circumflex origin (LAO projection) **A.** The left main segment arises from the left sinus and fills the anterior descending branch **B.** The stenosis was treated with angioplasty **C.** *Cx, ; RCA,* right coronary artery; *LAD,* left anterior descending artery.

femoral artery approach and the **brachial artery approach.** On very rare occasions another approach may be used because of lack of vascular access. Each approach may be used with any of several techniques, and each has its proponents. Many angiographers routinely use several techniques very capably. It is our belief, however, that an angiographer should attempt to achieve expertise with one technique and use it routinely, while reserving alternative techniques problems that preclude use of the primary technique. If the frequency of need for an alternative technique is not sufficient to maintain skills for its use in a safe and time-effective manner, patients requiring that technique should be referred to colleagues who use it regularly.

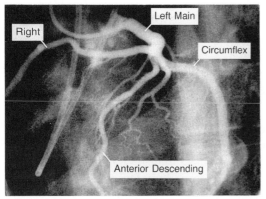

Figure 17.12. Anomalous RCA arising from the proximal LCA. (Adapted from Yamanaka O, Hobbs RE. Coronary artery anomalies in 126,595 patients undergoing coronary arteriography. Cathet Cardiovasc Diagn 1990;21:28–40).

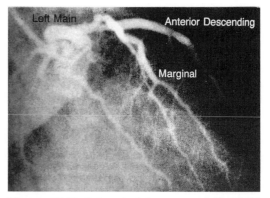

Figure 17.13. Interarterial course of the LCA arising from the proximal RCA. (Adapted from Yamanaka O, Hobbs RE. Coronary artery anomalies in 126,595 patients undergoing coronary angiography. Cathet Cardiovasc Diagn 1990;21: 28–40).

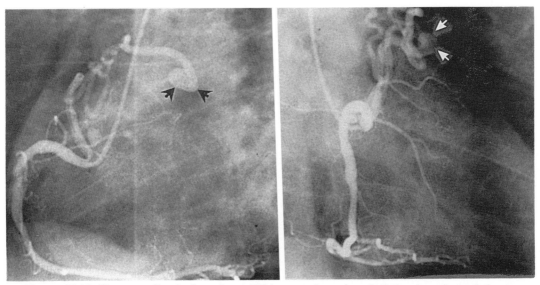

Figure 17.14. Coronary fistula from large RCA conus branches draining into the pulmonary artery.

Femoral Artery Approach

The femoral artery approach is the most widely used. It requires complete familiarity with the anatomy of the peripheral circulation and expertise in a technique for percutaneous vascular catheterization (10). The percutaneous technique is used to introduce the femoral artery catheter in almost all cases except in small children and other very special cases in which femoral artery cutdown may be needed.

The technique for percutaneous catheter insertion and the needles and wires used for this part of the procedure are described in detail in Chapters 9 and 10. Because it is essential that this technique be mastered to do coronary angiography rapidly, safely, and efficiently, it is reviewed in brief here. A special needle with a **blunt bevel** and appropriate obturator is introduced through the femoral artery. When adequate arterial pulsation is observed, the needle is advanced and the obturator or stylet is removed. Alternatively, a **sharp 18-gauge needle** without obturator or stylet is introduced through only the outer wall of the femoral artery. We prefer this technique for introduction of catheters for coronary angiography. We think the sharp needle without obturator has less potential to damage diseased, calcified femoral arteries. Furthermore, the sharp needle permits puncture through only the front of the arterial wall to minimize bleeding in anticoagulated patients. This is especially important in the setting of thrombolytic therapy. The sharp-needle technique is also faster.

When good pulsatile flow is observed, a guidewire, usually 0.035 inches in diameter, is introduced through the needle and advanced into the arterial system. After a fluoroscopic check to ensure that the guidewire has advanced retrograde into the iliac artery and aorta, pressure is maintained on the artery proximal to the insertion site with the left middle and fourth fingers, and the needle is removed with the right hand as the guidewire is wiped with a heparinized saline sponge held by the right thumb and forefinger. The guidewire is coiled as it is wiped, and the coil is secured by the left forefinger and thumb. Alternatively, an assistant may control the guidewire. A preselected coronary angiographic catheter is threaded over the guidewire and advanced to the appropriate artery. We prefer to modify the procedure by introduction of an appropriate arterial dilator and **valved catheter sheath** (see Chapter 10). The latter, although somewhat more costly, facilitates catheter exchanges, minimizes damage to the artery, and permits the catheter to be removed while the patient is transferred to a holding area before the sheath is removed and pressure is applied to effect tamponade.

Selective coronary angiography is done with special catheters (10, 11) and techniques described later in this chapter. There has been a tendency to use smaller catheters and sheaths in recent years compared with the 7-F catheters that have traditionally been used. The newer materials have improved torque control and increased lumen size so that adequate contrast flow rates can be delivered by hand injections in most cases. While these smaller-diameter catheters permit earlier ambulation and fewer peripheral vascular complications, concern has been raised about possible higher risk of coronary dissection. However, until large randomized trials are done, it is difficult to determine the relative benefit of routinely using catheters smaller than 7 F.

Judkins Catheters and Technique

These right and left coronary catheters (see Figs. 10.32 and 10.33) are usually 100 cm long and 5 to 8 F in diameter; they taper to approximately 5 F diameter at the tip. They have only an end hole and are preformed in various shapes. The preformed curves are designed on the principle that the proximal and transverse portions of the aortic arch, ascending aorta, and left coronary ostium lie in approximately the same plane. The body of a catheter advanced to the aortic root from below tends to lie against the lateral wall of the aorta opposite the direction of its tip (Fig. 17.15). Thus the operator should select the appropriately sized catheter prior to attempted engagement. This is

A.   B.   C.

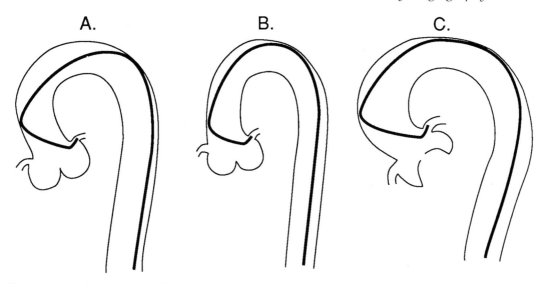

Figure 17.15. Approach to the LCA with Judkins catheters. Catheter positions in various types of aortic roots are shown in the LAO projection. When the catheter is advanced into the ascending aorta, the catheter tip moves along the left wall of the aorta to drop into the left coronary ostium. The secondary bend of the catheter touches the right lateral aortic wall. In the normal-sized aortic root (**A**), this is accomplished with a No. 4 left series catheter. In the small aortic root (**B**) a No. 3.5 catheter may be used. In the dilated aortic root (**C**) a No. 5 or 6 catheter is used as shown. Particular attention must be paid to the position of the catheter within the left coronary ostium. The catheter size should be appropriate so that withdrawal of the catheter allows the angle between the distal segment of the catheter and the main LCA to be minimal, preventing the tip from touching the coronary artery wall.

done by evaluating the patient's gender, body habitus, associated clinical findings (i.e., aortic stenosis), and aortic root size and shape from either chest film or fluoroscopic examination. Information about root size is also obtained from the behavior of the pigtail catheter, which may have been advanced to the left ventricle prior to coronary angiography.

The ascending aorta is assessed for size, coiling, and dilation or marked dilation. **Left coronary Judkins catheters** have primary (90°), secondary (180°), and tertiary curves (10) (Fig. 17.15). The radius of curvature for the tertiary curve is about 10 cm. The distance between primary and secondary curves varies from approximately 3.5 to 6 cm depending on the size. The size of the left coronary catheter is determined by the appropriate distance between primary and secondary curves (e.g., 4, 5, or 6 cm), and this also determines the angle that the distal segment forms with the coronary artery. For example, the longer the distance (e.g., 5 versus 4 cm), the greater the angle that the dis-

tal segment forms with the left coronary ostium. A No. 4 left Judkins has approximately 4 cm between the secondary and primary curves. This catheter size is applicable for most normal aortas and can be used in the large majority of patients. The distance between primary and secondary curves for the No. 5 Judkins is approximately 5 cm. This size is useful for the uncoiled or slightly enlarged aortas of hypertensive male patients. The No. 6 catheter's primary and secondary curves are approximately 6 cm apart; it is useful for the large poststenotic dilated aorta of the patient with aortic valve stenosis or aortic root disease (e.g., patients with Marfan's syndrome or syphilis). Occasionally catheters as large as No. 7 are needed. They may be shaped in the laboratory by heat gun. A No. 3 or 3.5 catheter is used in children and/or smaller adults, particularly young women. The **RCA Judkins catheter** has a secondary curve of 135° with a radius of 5 to 6 cm for the small and medium sizes and about 11 cm for the large size (Fig. 17.16). Chapter 10 has more details about these catheters.

The left Judkins catheter is usually used first (following ventriculography). As the catheter is advanced in the aortic arch, pressure is monitored. With the patient in a shallow LAO projection the catheter is advanced, and the tip moves down the left wall of the ascending aorta until it drops into the sinus of Valsalva and left coronary ostia (Fig 17.15). The pressure wave is inspected for alterations or damping. When these are absent, a test injection (1 to 2 mL) is observed on fluoroscopy. During this test the operator must pay particular attention to the position of catheter in LCA. The angle that the Judkins catheter tip makes with the direction of the proximal coronary artery must be minimal to ensure that the tip does not touch the artery wall. This is very important to avoid dissection of the coronary artery, should the catheter move unexpectedly to a deeper position within the artery, for example when the patient exhales. If there is any suspicion of left main coronary artery obstruction (e.g., calcification, unstable angina, marked electrocardiographic [ECG] changes during ischemia, or damp-

ing of systolic pressure on engagement), a cusp flush is essential before selective opacification.

After multiple injections are made with filming in different views, the left catheter is exchanged for the right coronary catheter (Fig. 17.16). This catheter is usually advanced so that its tip lies in the upper portion of the left sinus. Clockwise rotation is used to move the tip anteriorly until it enters the right ostium. This maneuver is best done in the 20° LAO projection.

If the operator has difficulty engaging either coronary artery ostium with the preselected catheter, it is important not to waste time attempting to manipulate an improperly sized catheter into a coronary orifice. A test injection should be done near the coronary ostium to help assess its position and size as well as the desired catheter size and shape. The catheter should then be replaced with one of a different size or shape. Selective engagement of the coronary arteries is generally easy and can be performed rapidly (within 1 minute) even by relatively inexperienced operators using Judkins catheters.

The major advantage of the Judkins

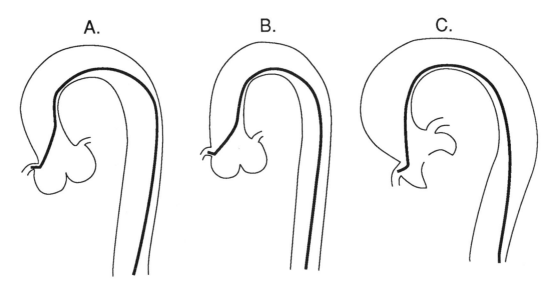

Figure 17.16. Approach to the RCA with Judkins catheters. The catheter is advanced to a point approximately 2 cm above the left coronary ostium and pointed toward the left ostium. From this position it is rotated clockwise until it enters the right coronary orifice. The figures illustrate the importance of catheter size relative to the aortic root in the LAO projection. In the normal-sized aortic root (**A**) a medium right catheter is used; in smaller aortas a smaller catheter may be needed (**B**); and in the larger poststenotic dilated aortas (**C**) a larger or longer configuration is required.

technique is its simplicity. It requires less dexterity and training than other techniques. Since the catheters have only an end hole, obstruction at the tip produces alteration of the pressure waveform. Recognition of pressure wave change may prevent the operator from injecting or embolizing a clot or damaging the intima of the coronary artery.

A disadvantage is that for practical purposes the technique is applicable only from the femoral arteries, although we have used it from the **left brachial artery** as well as **radial artery** (see Chapter 9). Thus, obstructive disease of the descending aorta, iliac, or femoral vessels can make catheterization impossible or difficult and/or create high risk for arterial damage, thrombosis, and cholesterol (athero) embolization. Multiple catheters must be used, increasing the chance of arterial damage and/or embolization. If one must re-examine both coronary arteries, for example after nitroglycerin and ergonovine or during chest pain, catheters must be exchanged. This limitation is minimized in our laboratories by use of a valved sheath. In some cases, when it is important to repeat either right or left coronary angiography several times rapidly during the procedure, we use the contralateral groin to introduce the other coronary artery catheter. One catheter is kept in the ascending aorta while the other is being used. Deliberate left ventricular catheterization between coronary injections to examine left ventricular end-diastolic pressure or perform a ventriculogram cannot be done easily with the left coronary catheter. Usually a guidewire is needed. The right coronary catheter can usually be guided into the left ventricle on clockwise rotation from the left cusp, but a guidewire may also be needed on occasion. In either case the Judkins coronary catheter must then be exchanged for another catheter for ventriculography. Finally, if one suspects an aberrant coronary artery origin, either congenital or secondary to disease of the aortic root, Judkins catheters may have to be abandoned.

Amplatz Catheters and Technique

This preformed catheter series is available in four left coronary tip sizes and the right

catheters in three sizes (Figs. 10.34 and 10.35). These catheters have hook shapes, which are very pronounced for the LCA and less pronounced for the RCA (11). The right coronary catheter has an additional curve to conform to the aortic arch. Again, as with Judkins catheters, selection of proper size is essential; it depends on the size and shape of the ascending aorta and aortic sinuses. Size 1 is for the smallest aortic root, 2 for normal, and 3 for large roots. Attempts to force engagement of a preformed catheter that does not conform to a particular aorta, aortic root, or aortic sinus only wastes time and increases risk of complication.

The left Amplatz catheter is advanced to the noncoronary cusp. The bottom of the hook is braced in this cusp in the LAO projection (Fig. 17.17A). The tip is rotated until

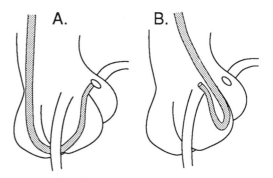

Figure 17.17. A. Approach to the LCA with Amplatz catheters. The LCA is approached by pointing the tip of the large hook-shaped left coronary catheter toward the patient's left and advancing until the catheter lies on the posterior or noncoronary cusp. From this position, if the catheter is appropriately sized for the aortic root, the tip will be easily engaged in the left coronary ostium with only slight withdrawal. If the tip lies below the left coronary ostium, the catheter is too small. If the hook cannot be opened, the catheter is too large. **B.** A similar approach can be used for the RCA if the right ostium is high and the root is moderately large, as shown. As the left catheter is advanced to touch the noncoronary cusp, the catheter is rotated until it is engaged into a high RCA. For arteries that lie in the midportion of the right sinus or lower, a right coronary catheter with a much smaller hook (not shown) must be used. The tip of the small hook is pointed leftward. This catheter generally is braced against the left aortic cusp and therefore lies directly opposite the RCA orifice.

it enters the left ostium, and displacement is prevented by slight withdrawal of the catheter body. If the tip does not reach the ostium (i.e., lies below it), the catheter is too small and should be replaced with the next larger size. If the tip lies above the ostium, the catheter is too large. After filming the LCA, the catheter is exchanged for the right coronary catheter. In the LAO projection the right catheter is braced in the left coronary cusp as it is rotated slightly to secure the tip in the right coronary ostium (Fig. 17.17B). When the right coronary ostium is very high, the left Amplatz catheter may be used to engage the right ostium.

Some advantages of Amplatz catheters are as follows: (*a*) They can be used percutaneously from either the femoral or the brachial artery. The brachial No. 2 and 3 catheters are variations of the left Amplatz design. (*b*) Attempts to seek a coronary ostium require less operator training, and for some operators less time, than with nonpreformed catheters. (*c*) They have only an end hole; thus, immediate dampening of the pressure waveform is produced when the tip is obstructed.

A disadvantage of the Amplatz technique is that multiple catheters must be used. Also, the LCA may be difficult to engage with the left catheter, particularly in smaller aortic roots and patients with short left main stem or low ostium. Subselective catheterization of either the LAD or LC may be unavoidable in some cases. If the coronaries must be re-examined after pharmacologic interventions, physiologic maneuvers, or pain, the operator may find that multiple catheter exchanges become an important inconvenience.

Multipurpose Catheter and Technique

This single-catheter technique usually uses a 7- or 8-F, 100-cm polyurethane or woven Dacron catheter with stainless steel wire incorporated (Fig. 10.36) that resembles Gensini and some Sones catheters (18). The tip is more flexible than that of the Gensini or even some Sones catheters. The different manufacturers have developed tips with different characteristics.

Torque control is very good, and the catheter tip usually can be manipulated into either coronary ostium or the left ventricle by maneuvers that are somewhat similar to those employed with the Sones (see next

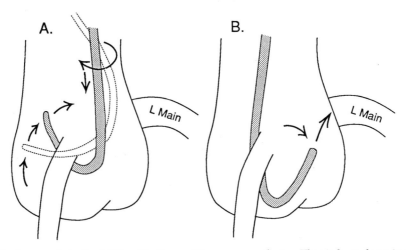

Figure 17.18. Approach to the LCA with the multipurpose catheter. This is best done in the 30° RAO projection with the tip pointed posteriorly. Advancement of the catheter allows a loop to be formed in the noncoronary or posterior sinus (**A**). From this position the catheter is rotated clockwise until the tip points toward the left coronary ostium (**B**). The catheter is advanced; the ostium is engaged; and then, as the patient inspires, the catheter is withdrawn slightly to secure the tip in the ostium of the LCA.

section) technique (Figs. 17.18 and 17.19). Most operators advocate starting from the posterior sinus or noncoronary cusp in the 30° RAO position (Fig. 17.18*A*). The catheter is advanced with the tip pointed toward the spine. When a loop has formed, slight clockwise rotation flips the tip to the left cusp

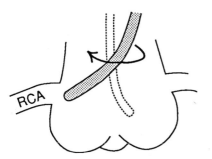

Figure 17.19. Approach to the RCA with the multipurpose technique. Best done in the LAO projection, this begins similarly to the approach to LCA; however, once the catheter tip points toward the LCA, continued clockwise rotation is used until the tip is oriented anteriorly toward the right coronary orifice. From this position the catheter is advanced and withdrawn until the tip is secured in the ostium.

and points it toward the ostium (Fig. 17.18*B*). The tip is then maneuvered into the left ostium by slight withdrawal or advancement of the catheter. Breathing maneuvers may also be helpful. The catheter is then withdrawn slightly to secure the tip and injections are made. The RCA is approached in the 45° LAO position. From the left cusp the catheter is rotated clockwise (Fig. 17.19). The tip is directed anteriorly and to the patient's right. The catheter is then slightly withdrawn to engage the right coronary ostium.

The multipurpose catheter technique requires more operator training than the other percutaneous techniques that use preformed catheters. The multipurpose catheter technique has the major advantage of using the same catheter for both right and left coronary arteries and left ventricular angiography. In routine practice, however, our experience is that only about 80% of procedures can be completed optimally with the single catheter and that ectopy during left ventriculography is common. The LCA may require a preformed catheter for good selective visualization in the remainder of cases.

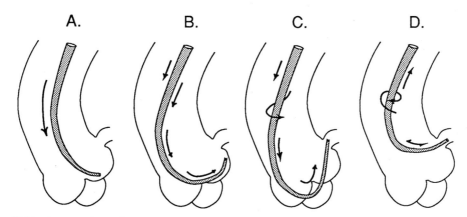

Figure 17.20. Approach to the LCA with Sones technique. This is best done in the LAO projection. The key to success with this technique is to advance the Sones catheter to the ascending aorta and position the tip in the left coronary cusp without major distortions of the primary angle (**A**). From this position gentle advancement (**B**) allows formation of a loop using the floor of the left cusp. When the loop begins to climb the left sinus and point upward, gradual additional advance and withdrawal plus counterclockwise torque produce posterior movement of the tip. From this position (**C**) advance and withdrawal to transmit the torque helps transmit movement of the tip to the left coronary ostium. When the catheter reaches this point and further advancement simply enlarges the loop, the tip can be firmly engaged in the left ostium by adding clockwise torque and withdrawing the catheter while the patient inspires. This secures the catheter tip in the ostium of the LCA (**D**).

Brachial Approach

Sones Catheter and Technique

Through a small antecubital cutdown the brachial artery is isolated by blunt dissection (19). The right brachial artery is preferred, but on occasion (e.g., prior scarring, brachial, or axillary–subclavian artery obstruction) the left arm can be used. One of several varieties of catheters ranging in diameter from about 6 to 8 F and in length from 80 to 125 cm is employed (see Fig. 10.31; see Chapter 10 for details about the construction of these catheters). The advantage of these catheters is that their shafts are relatively rigid at body temperature. This provides excellent torque control for maneuvering the tip through the subclavian artery and maintaining tip control in the high-velocity blood flow immediately above the aortic valve to cannulate the coronary ostia.

The tip of each Sones catheter tapers to about 5.5 F diameter over the distal 1 to 2 cm, depending on the type used, with type 1 longer than type 2. The two types have tapered sections of different lengths. This tapering makes the distal portion much more flexible and favors directing the catheter tip toward the coronary ostium by enabling this portion to be formed in a J shape. Each Sones catheter has an end hole and either two or four side holes that help stabilize the tip during injections. The tapered section of the catheter is generally maintained in an angled bend by a rigid wire before the catheter is used so that the distal section maintains an obtuse angle with the main catheter body. The tapered tip is more flexible than the main body of the catheter, allowing manipulation of the catheter from the subclavian artery into the ascending aorta and formation of a loop in the left aortic sinus. It is usually helpful to flex the catheter about 3 inches from its tip several times prior to insertion to facilitate building a loop on the left cusp.

For time-efficient use of the catheter it must be advanced to the ascending aorta without introducing major distortions in the tip or in the plane of the angle that the tip makes with the body of the catheter. We recommend use of a guidewire when difficulty is encountered at the subclavian brachiocephalic trunk. In addition, it is important to master the technique of building a loop in the left coronary cusp. This is accomplished by directing the tip of the catheter to the patient's left toward the left sinus as it enters the ascending aorta. When the tip touches the left cusp, the catheter is advanced to form a loop with its tip in the left sinus (Fig. 17.20). The catheter is advanced and withdrawn with short, sometimes rapid movements. Advancement and counterclockwise rotation of the catheter usually permit the tip to move superiorly and somewhat posteriorly to point toward and then enter the left ostium. Slight withdrawal and clockwise rotation of the catheter usually secure the tip in the left main coronary artery. This movement of the catheter tip is often enhanced if it is done as the patient is directed to inspire deeply.

After the LCA angiogram is recorded, the tip is withdrawn. The most reliable ap-

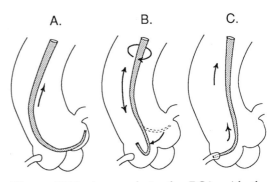

Figure 17.21. Approach to the RCA with the Sones catheter. Again the RCA is most readily approached from the initial configuration used for the LCA (i.e., the catheter tip is positioned in the left cusp (**A**) with the patient in the LAO projection). From the left cusp a small loop is formed, and when the tip begins to climb the left sinus but is relatively horizontal, the catheter is rotated clockwise. Slow advance and withdrawal again transmit this torque to the tip and allow the tip to traverse the commissure between the left and right aortic cusps. When this occurs, it is often necessary to provide counterclockwise torque to check the movement of the tip (**B**). From this position slightly withdrawing the catheter usually engages the tip in the ostium of the RCA (**C**). Again, inspiration is helpful to secure the tip.

proach to the RCA is again to build a loop in the left cusp (Fig. 17.21). While the tip is still nearly horizontal and anterior to the left ostium, the catheter is rotated clockwise. Again, short advance and withdrawal motions transmit this torque to the tip, so that the tip rotates anteriorly to cross the commissure between the left and right aortic cusps and enter the right ostium.

When the procedure is complete, the catheter is removed and the arteriotomy repaired when good antegrade and retrograde backflow are observed. Usually a purse-string or some form of everting mattress suture is employed with vascular suture (6–0 or 7–0 Tevdec or Proline).

Modified Brachial Technique

The brachial artery approach may be modified so that **percutaneous technique** is used with or without a sheath. We prefer a short 7-F valved sheath with modified catheters (19), but 6-F and 5.2-F catheters and sheaths are acceptable. This entry technique is particularly useful for patients with large muscular arms or previous scarring and for outpatient procedures. The sheath is secured to the arm, and maneuvers similar to those noted earlier with the Sones technique are followed. However, because the percutaneous modification restricts catheter movement and the feel obtained with the cutdown technique, modified catheters are sometimes helpful. A brachial 2 catheter may be used for the LCA, but it must be exchanged for either a pigtail or NIH type to obtain an acceptable left ventriculogram.

The brachial approach with Sones type of catheters has some advantages. A single catheter can be used in most cases for catheterization of both coronary arteries, left ventriculography, and selective CABG angiography. Obstructive disease of the abdominal aorta or iliofemoral arteries poses no problem. There is usually sufficient collateral circulation around the elbow to prevent tissue loss if brachial artery occlusion occurs. Any ischemic symptoms rarely persist after a few months. If they do persist, the artery can be repaired with simple local surgical techniques, often on an outpatient basis. If

bleeding occurs, for example after thrombolytic therapy or during anticoagulation, the arm is easier to tamponade than the groin. This feature makes the technique attractive for outpatient catheterization.

There are also disadvantages. Because of the multiple side holes, a clot can form at the tip of a Sones type of catheter or in one of the side holes without altering the pressure waveform. With subsequent injection the clot can dislodge and embolize. An aberrant or tortuous subclavian artery or distortion of the aortic root can make the technique difficult or impossible. But most important, the cutdown, arteriotomy, manipulation of a nonpreformed catheter, and arterial repair require considerable dexterity if the technique is to be employed in a time-efficient manner at minimum risk to the patient.

Other Approaches

Techniques for translumbar coronary angiography have been described for the rare patient with vascular access limited by obstruction of both axillary or subclavian arteries and both iliac or femoral arteries (20, 21). A small catheter exchange sheath, 5 or 6 F, modified to 20 cm long, may be used. An Amplatz or Judkins coronary catheter is used for selective coronary opacification. Bleeding from the periaortic area at the time of wire exchange may be a significant problem. We strongly recommend collaboration with a physician experienced in peripheral vascular angiographic techniques when this type of approach is necessary. The **radial artery** approach has received increased attention in recent years, and this requires a normal Allen test (22).

OTHER ANGIOGRAPHIC PROCEDURES FOR THE CORONARY CIRCULATION

Saphenous Vein Bypass Graft Angiography

The increasing numbers of patients returning for evaluation following coronary revascularization has made saphenous vein bypass graft angiography an essential procedure for the coronary angiographer. The techniques are essentially the same as those for selective coronary angiography, except that different catheters may be required. Saphenous vein grafts are usually attached to the anterior portion of the aorta well above the coronary sinuses. Generally we use the right Judkins catheter to enter these grafts selectively. If the aortic anastomosis can be localized from a radiopaque marker used at surgery or an aortic root angiogram, the catheter is positioned at this level or slightly above it. Rotating the catheter clockwise usually engages the tip in the bypass orifice. The LAO view is most helpful for catheterization of these grafts. If the right Judkins is unsuccessful (usually because the graft is very high, the root is dilated, or the graft exits the aorta at a very obtuse angle), a right or left saphenous vein bypass graft catheter may be used.

If the Sones or multipurpose catheter technique is used, these grafts are often accessible with the same catheter used for selective coronary angiography. A larger, longer loop is formed. Again the tip is positioned at or slightly above and to the left of the aortic anastomosis. Rotating the catheter clockwise engages the tip.

Internal Mammary Artery Graft Angiography

Internal mammary artery (IMA) grafts are used with increasing frequency, and this has made techniques to visualize the IMA a necessity for coronary angiographers. In our experience the IMA is best approached with a special preformed catheter (see Chapter 10, especially Fig. 10.36) made for this purpose. From either groin either mammary artery is approached with a guidewire advanced ahead of the catheter tip. The wire is first directed to the innominate and then to the subclavian artery. The internal mammary catheter is advanced over the wire, and when the tip reaches the subclavian artery, the wire is removed. The catheter tip then returns to its preshaped right-angle configuration, and the tip is directed inferi-

orly as the catheter is slowly withdrawn and rotated to engage the orifice of the internal mammary artery. A nonionic contrast agent should be used for test injection and selective angiography to minimize the intense burning chest pain perceived by patients with intact chest wall branches. Nitroglycerin should also be given into this arterial graft if its full potential size is to be evaluated.

In patients with severe iliofemoral atherosclerosis and for those using the brachial artery approach, alternative techniques are required. Either the right or left IMA can be rapidly cannulated from its respective brachial artery with the preshaped IMA catheter described for the femoral approach. The catheter is introduced, either percutaneously or via cutdown, into the brachial artery. If cutdown or sheath technique is used for the brachial approach, the IMA catheter must be preloaded with an 0.035-inch J-wire to protect the brachial, axillary, and subclavian arteries, because of the sharply angled tip. When the proximal subclavian is entered, the wire is removed and the catheter is withdrawn and rotated to engage the IMA. This is a very simple and rapid procedure for the ipsilateral IMA. The contralateral IMA can be approached by reintroduction of the catheter on that side. Alternatively, techniques to maneuver a guidewire and catheter into the aortic arch and to the contralateral IMA may be used. One technique is to advance a sidewinder catheter to the aortic root over a preloaded guidewire. When the wire is removed, the catheter assumes its preformed large hooklike shape. Selection of the size of the Simmons catheter depends on the size and configuration of the aortic root. Usually the medium or large size is used. The tip is rotated toward the contralateral shoulder and advanced into the subclavian artery. When it is introduced from the right brachial artery, it lies in the left subclavian artery, and this position should be confirmed by a small-volume contrast injection. An exchange guidewire (0.035-inch diameter, 260 cm length) is advanced through the catheter into the left subclavian artery. The Simmons catheter is then exchanged for a preshaped IMA bypass catheter. When the tip of this catheter is inserted into the contralateral subclavian artery beyond the origin of the IMA, the guidewire is removed. The catheter is slowly withdrawn and rotated until the IMA is engaged. After left IMA angiography the catheter is withdrawn to the ipsilateral subclavian artery, and the ipsilateral IMA (in this case right) is visualized.

Ventricular Angiography

Ventriculography (discussed in detail in Chapter 16) provides information that complements the coronary angiogram and assists in patient evaluation. Wall motion, aneurysm, septal perforation, and mitral insufficiency can be documented and quantified. Also, consider a patient in whom transient ischemic depression of the ST segment (spontaneously or during stress) develops in electrocardiographic leads I, aVL, V_5 and V_6. These changes may result from ischemic myocardium perfused by a diseased anterior descending, diagonal, or circumflex marginal branch of the LCA branch. In many instances an RAO ventriculogram may reveal a local area of hypokinesis in the anterior lateral region. Thus the relationship of the ischemia, regional wall motion abnormality, and coronary occlusive disease, viewed by coronary angiography, is helpful in deciding which coronary narrowing is responsible for production of ischemia.

Motion of hypokinetic myocardial regions can be improved by nitroglycerin or during postextrasystolic beats. It is possible to detect functionally jeopardized reversible ischemic or hibernating myocardium. Many laboratories, including ours, perform ventricular angiography before and after administration of sublingual nitroglycerin to patients with motion abnormalities. Since radiographic contrast material injected into the coronary circulation may alter left ventricular performance, many perform the left ventriculogram before coronary angiography. However, if one wishes to evoke areas of potential motion abnormality, induced perhaps by marginal areas of perfusion, it may be wise to consider performing coronary angiography before left ventriculography as a form of "stress." Abnormalities in

wall motion that may be reversed can then be assessed on postextrasystolic beats or after nitroglycerin administration. Very sick patients tolerate coronary angiography much better than left ventriculography. Therefore, it is sometimes clinically useful to perform coronary angiography early in the course of the procedure, attempting to obtain maximal information before performing the higher-risk ventriculographic procedure.

PRINCIPLES APPLICABLE TO ALL TECHNIQUES

The operator must know the radiographic anatomy of the heart and coronary circulation to choose the appropriate view. This includes not only the normal situations but also the not infrequent congenital variations. In general views should be chosen to minimize overlap of major vessels while avoiding the vertebrae and lungs. Appropriate shutter and collimator position should frame the area of interest. This minimizes radiation exposure and reduces scatter to improve the quality of the images. All filming should be done during inspiration with the diaphragm in its most inferior position. This may require a slow inspiration with initiation of injection just before maximum inspiration is reached, as some patients perform a Valsalva maneuver when told to inspire maximally. The Valsalva maneuver defeats the purpose by causing the diaphragm to move superiorly while reducing coronary perfusion pressure. The pressure from the catheter tip must be evaluated immediately before each injection of contrast. If damping of pressure is observed, before any contrast material is injected, the catheter should be withdrawn slowly until a normal pressure waveform is observed. A small-volume (1 to 2 mL) **test injection** should be made to determine the position of the tip and the status of the coronary artery. If attenuation of the pressure waveform is due to ostial obstruction or catheter-related dissection, an injection made when pressure is damped may enlarge the tear and create an occlusive dissection. In an extremely small coronary artery in which repeated damping is observed on entry, injection of 100 to 200 mg of nitroglycerin near the ostium often produces sufficient dilation to permit entry without pressure damping. If damping is still observed, a different-shaped catheter should be used.

Before any injection into the coronary arteries, the system (syringe, manifold, and catheter) must be free of air and blood. We recommend a closed manifold system filled with heparinized saline flush. This step helps to prevent air or blood from entering the system and to provide adequate transmission of pressure to permit recognition of waveform attenuations that may arise from catheter tip impaction in the artery wall or obstruction of the coronary orifice. Once these steps are mastered, they require only a few seconds and help avoid serious morbidity. After these measures are complete, contrast injection of sufficient volume and flow rate to opacify the artery under study is made. Inadequately opacified vessels generally result in overestimation of stenosis severity because of contrast streaming as it forms a layer with unopacified blood. When the heart rate is high and the coronary arteries are large, a higher-contrast flow rate is needed than for slow heart rate and small coronary arteries. Generally we use 3 to 4 mL injected over approximately two cardiac cycles for the RCA and 4 to 6 mL for the left. Occasionally larger volumes are needed. Cine filming should be started before contrast leaves the catheter tip and continued until most of the arterial phase of opacification is complete. In patients with obstruction, at least one filming run for each artery should be continued well after the arterial phase to look for collateral filling. Repeat filming after intracoronary nitroglycerin is always helpful in the evaluation of stenosis, coronary spasm, and collaterals.

With the use of an image intensifier field of 4.5 to 6 inches to provide optimal magnification of the coronary arteries and a collimator to minimize spine, lung, and diaphragm, the field of view may be considerably smaller than the myocardial distribution covered by the branches of either coronary artery. Accordingly, the tabletop or image intensifier tube must be moved to follow the distribution of a coronary artery and its branches filled with contrast medium. This movement, called panning, is a learned procedure that follows a specific pattern for each coronary artery in each projection. The initial field of view should permit optimal visualization of the ostium and proximal part of the coronary artery under study. From this position the field should follow the distribution of the artery and its major branches. Since most of the coronary artery obstructions of interest (e.g., for revascularization) are in the proximal and midportions of the artery under study, the time spent with these proximal portions in the field of view should occupy most of the duration of a cine film run. The remaining portion of the film run should be reserved to include the distal segments of the artery and possible collateral channels that may fill to supply segments of other arteries or branches. But the field of view should return to include the catheter tip at the end of each filming run. This permits identification of contrast staining at sites of intimal flaps, thrombus, or even catheter-related dissection.

PATHOPHYSIOLOGIC CONSIDERATIONS

Coronary angiography has made significant advances over the past 4 decades and is the reference standard by which severity of coronary artery obstruction is assessed. But a thorough understanding of some of the pathophysiologic processes that relate to ischemic heart disease is necessary to understand the uses and limits of the information provided by coronary angiography.

Revised Concepts of Ischemic Heart Disease

Ischemic heart disease is usually but not always the result of severe coronary atherosclerotic obstruction. Recent progress indicates a more complex origin than our previous static notion of only fixed athero-sclerotic obstructions rigid in passive conduits. Documentation of compensatory enlargement of stenotic coronary segments in a process called remodeling has replaced the rigid notion. Epicardial arteries, which may appear to be angiographically normal or to have only minor obstruction, as well as the nonvisualized microvasculature, have been documented to respond to certain influences with detrimental constriction. This process has been termed flow-mediated dysfunction. Central to our progress is understanding the expanded role of endothelium vascular smooth muscle and other components of the arterial wall in these processes. The endothelium generates vasoactive, anticoagulant, antiproliferative, and antiadhesive factors. It is likely that abnormal interaction between components of the arterial wall, circulating blood elements, and hemodynamic state leads to alterations in homeostatic equilibrium, resulting in constriction, thrombosis, smooth muscle growth, leukocyte recruitment, and other potentially deleterious processes in the broad context of ischemic heart disease. It should be apparent that the angiogram provides only a limited view of some of these processes. CAD becomes clinically manifest when it limits blood flow to result in cardiac ischemia. Ischemia is a functional disturbance of normal physiologic mechanisms that results from a variety of acute and chronic pathophysiologic processes involving the blood, coronary circulation, and myocardium.

Epicardial Coronary Stenosis and Angiography

Radiographic contrast angiography done under ideal circumstances provides only a shadow of the patent lumen of the large and medium-sized (more than 200 μm) coronary arteries, which carry only a fraction of the total coronary circulation. This shadow has been termed a **luminogram.** The misconceptions associated with preoccupation with luminology have been reviewed elsewhere (23). The size of the lumen and location of lumen narrowing can be relatively well assessed from an interpretation of this shadow. The actual magnitude of lumen narrowing, however, is less well assessed, and inferences of potential for ischemia-related adverse outcomes are even less reliable. There are a number of reasons for these limitations. One of them relates to the subjective method used in everyday clinical practice to assess severity of obstruction. Here substantial intraobserver and interobserver variability significantly limit the interpretation. The variability is reduced by use of quantitative methods, but even under these circumstances the information provided by quantifying the luminogram underestimates the severity judged by postmortem histology (24–29) and has not been shown to predict clinical outcome (30). Thus the luminogram is an **imperfect assessment** of the overall state of the coronary circulation's ability to deliver blood flow in an amount appropriate for myocardial oxygen demand. Thus cardiac ischemia and its potential for adverse outcome cannot be simply inferred or defined by angiographic narrowing, even when the narrowing is analyzed by quantitative methods.

Remodeling and Minimal, or Intermediate, Lesions

The development of luminal narrowing of a coronary artery by atherosclerosis is a complex process that is only partially understood. Review of the remodeling that occurs with the development of vascular disease clarifies the information provided by the angiogram. During atherogenesis raised plaque lesions develop from a damaged endothelial surface in an eccentric rather than concentric region along the surface of the lumen. These plaques, however, do not necessarily shrink the coronary lumen because of compensatory enlargement of the coronary lumen (e.g., remodeling). Some remodeling is related to thinning of the media adjacent to a plaque so the eccentric plaque shifts outward rather than bulging inward to encroach upon the lumen (31). As a result of this outward shift of plaque (e.g., so that the border lies outside of the original lumen position), large plaques are often not recognized on the luminogram because there is no apparent loss of lumen. Plaques that are detected as a small loss of diameter on the luminogram (e.g., appear as only minimal narrowings) are likely to be quite large. Because of re-modeling, the capacity to preserve lumen size is not overcome by plaque growth until the plaque area exceeds 40% of the original cross-sectional area of the vessel lumen (defined by the internal elastic lamina) (32, 33). So terms like **normal coronary arteries, mild disease,** and even **new lesions,** often used to describe changes noted on an angiogram or serial angiograms, are misnomers because the threshold for plaque detection as a result of lumen narrowing is not reached until the plaque is quite large (33). Lesions reaching the threshold for identification on the luminogram may have a hemodynamic effect that is difficult to quantify, and these lesions are often termed minimal or intermediate. Considerable evidence indicates that such minimal or intermediate lesions are associated with the majority of acute ischemic events, perhaps because they are more vulnerable to rupture than the better-established severely stenotic lesions (34, 35). These minimal or intermediate lesions, however, most frequently occur in patients with the better-established severe lesions. So the number of vessels containing severe stenoses, particularly when they are proximal, has evolved as an overall estimate of the severity of CAD. In studies completed in past decades these estimates have been found to predict intermediate- and long-term clinical outcome. However, with the changes observed over the past several decades in the mortality and incidence of the disease, the changing characteristics of our population (more elderly people), and the use of therapies that influence adverse outcome (e.g., aspirin, β-blockers, thrombolytics, HmG CoA reductase inhibitors and angiotensin-converting enzyme (ACE) inhibitors), it is unknown whether these angiographic estimates are useful as predictors of adverse outcome in patients seen today.

Complex Lumen Geometry and Distortion

Irregularities in the plaque surface, mural thrombus, and minor plaque fissuring complicate the geometry of many lesions. These lesions often appear with hazy borders on the luminogram, and it is difficult to assess the limits of the lumen even from multiple views. Even when the lesion is not complex and its borders are not hazy, the atherosclerotic artery's lumen is often crescent-shaped, so the severity of the obstruction is difficult to estimate from its appearance in two or even more orthogonal views (Fig. 17.6). The irregular lumen shape may have some of its dimensions distorted by foreshortening, but by convention the angiographer uses the view showing the most severe reduction in the lumen. Therefore there is considerable risk that foreshortening of some stenosis dimensions, but not the more circular reference lumen, limits the assessment of actual lumen size. In an attempt to circumvent limitations associated with haziness and geometric distortion of stenosis dimensions, some have advocated use of video densitometry, rather than edge detection, to quantify the coronary lumen size.

The usual method of analyzing angiograms in clinical practice is to detect areas of relative narrowing and to quantify the narrowing by comparing the minimal diameter of the narrowed coronary segment with the diameter of an adjacent "normal-appearing" reference segment. Since the atherosclerotic process is often not local, the reference coronary segment is likely also to be diseased. Therefore the degree of narrowing assessed in this manner is an underestimation of the severity of the atherosclerotic process in the narrowed segment (32, 36). To circumvent this reference segment problem, some have advocated measurement of minimal lumen diameter or area in absolute terms. While this approach has merit to study deterioration of the lumen over time or with intervention, it would require indexing for coronary artery, segment location, body size, state of myocardium, and so on.

Dynamic Coronary Obstruction

In certain cases, differences in coronary artery smooth muscle tone may lead to severe obstruction with little atherosclerotic mass. Indeed, most interventional cardiologists have planned percutaneous intervention on what appears to be a severe proximal narrowing only to find that the narrowing disappears or is much less severe after intracoronary nitroglycerin. Also coronary vessels may have abnormal flow-mediated vasodilation (37) and may undergo prominent circadian changes in their lumen size (38). Thus the consideration of coronary vasomotor tone is important in the angiographic assessment of any patient. In any patient in whom the clinical findings suggest coronary spasm or ischemia is documented but the degree of coronary narrowing fails to explain the ischemia findings, abnormal vasomotor tone must be considered.

Need for Physiologic and Pharmacologic Testing

These concerns justify a function assessment directed at providing cardiac ischemia, high-quality angiograms, multiple views, and absolute lumen dimension assessment rather than relative stenosis assessed by simple subjective inspection and frequent use of adjunctive procedures. The physiologic assessment that is clinically most useful usually comes from a noninvasive functional (stress) test for ischemia. The lumen measurement in all cases should be done with images recorded after administration of an endothelial-independent (direct-acting) vasodilator such as nitroglycerin. In many cases adjunctive non-angiographic procedures (see later section) to assess lumen size after pharmacologic agents, dimensions from intracoronary ultrasound, endothelial vasodilator function studies, flow reserve (Doppler evaluation), and exclusion of coronary spasm are essential to obtain a useful picture of the processes responsible for ischemia and related adverse outcome.

Despite these considerations, coronary angiography provides important information useful for the management of patients with a wide variety of diseases. This information includes an estimate of the anatomic severity of CAD that can complement the clinical and other findings derived from functional assessments. To make optimal use of the information provided by coronary angiography, it is most important to understand that the potential for cardiac ischemia and long-term adverse clinical outcome in any patient with CAD are results of complex interaction of multiple processes and not simply the incomplete picture provided by the coronary angiogram.

COGNITIVE AND TECHNICAL SKILLS

The cognitive and technical considerations required for coronary angiography may be grouped into those related to the evaluation, preparation, and care of the patient during and after the angiographic procedure and interpretation of the findings. This includes introduction of catheters into the arterial system and selective catheterization and opacification of coronary arteries or their CABG. These elements require considerable cognitive expertise on the part of the patient's primary care, hospital attending, and cardiac catheterization physicians. The last must have cognitive achievements that are difficult to separate from technical skills. The summaries to follow are intended as an introduction for physicians participating in the care of patients undergoing coronary angiography. Physicians actually practicing coronary angiography and those in need of more details should consult recent texts on this subject, including the other chapters of this book.

Training and Credentialing

Considerable formal training is required to acquire and maintain the cognitive and technical skills needed to perform coronary angiography competently. These skills, summarized in Tables 17.1 and 17.2, are often included in the local requirements for credentialing to perform coronary angiography.

Table 17.1.
Cognitive Skills Needed to Perform Coronary Angiography

Knowledge of
  Current indications, including reasons for selecting coronary angiography
  Risks (contraindications) and benefits of procedure and ability to communicate these to patient
  Preprocedural evaluation
  Anatomy, physiology, and pathology of systemic and coronary circulations and left ventricle
  Avoidance and management of complications
Ability to
  Identify situations that may lead to complications of cardiac catheterization and coronary angiography
  Recognize actual complications
  Understand and use x-ray and other laboratory equipment
  Interpret angiographic findings and integrate these with clinical findings
  Communicate risks, benefits, and results to patient, medical record, and others involved in care

Table 17.2.
Technical Skills Needed to Perform Coronary Angiography

Sufficient manual dexterity to perform procedure in time-efficient manner at acceptable risk
Operational skills in use of x-ray and other required equipment
Experience with general cardiac catheterization procedures and radiation safety
Additional demonstrated competence in coronary angiography
Technical aspects of recognition and management of complications
Demonstration of continued technical competence over time

Evaluation Before the Procedure

Evaluation before the procedure is critically important. It includes a review of the patient's records and clinical findings focusing on the indication for coronary angiography. Should the patient's primary physician also be the coronary angiographer, a second opinion about the need for the procedure is clearly advisable. In addition to a complete clinical examination, several laboratory studies are required. These include a recent chest x-ray film, complete blood count, blood urea nitrogen, creatinine, and ECG. Clotting function is assessed if there is a history suggesting that the patient either has a bleeding disorder or is taking an anticoagulant. Likewise, blood typing and cross-matching are not routinely needed unless the patient is either immediately going to surgery or actively bleeding.

While all **contraindications to coronary angiography** are relative, except in the rare patient with lack of vascular access to the coronary arteries, many patients have an increased risk related to other illness. Because such patients often benefit from correction of the other illness and related debility prior to coronary angiography, these illnesses must be recognized so that the coronary angiography can be properly timed. These patients include those with a **recent cerebrovascular accident, progressive renal insufficiency, active gastrointestinal bleeding, severe electrolyte imbalance, severe anemia, fever** that may be due to infection, **digitalis intoxication, severe hypertension,** and other diseases such as **cancer** and **severe respiratory or hepatic failure** that limit the patient's life span or quality of life more than does the suspected cardiac illness for which coronary angiography is contemplated. The patient who intends to **refuse therapeutic procedures** to which the coronary angiogram may lead, such as CABG and percutaneous coronary interventions, is best not subjected to the procedure. Patients with a **documented anaphylactic reaction** during a previous exposure to radiographic contrast agents require special consideration. In most instances history of an immediate, general anaphylactoid reaction to contrast does not constitute actual anaphylaxis, and these individuals can safely undergo coronary angiography after medication with corticosteroids and antihistamines. Finally, if the facility has no emergency cardiac surgery support, very unstable patients from the hemodynamic or clinical standpoint are often better served by transfer to a center where emergency surgery is available before their coronary angiography. This, for example, might be a patient in cardiogenic shock during the course of an acute myocardial infarction (MI) with mitral insufficiency due to suspected capillary muscle rupture. Such a patient would be better served by stabilization with an intra-aortic balloon pump plus nitroprusside infusion and transfer to a center where emergency cardiac surgery is available immediately following angiography.

Also important in this evaluation is determination of whether the patient can safely undergo an ambulatory catheterization (defined as no overnight stay in the hospital) or would be better served by hospitalization either before or after the procedure. A number of conditions are associated with an increase in risk for catheterization or angiography-related morbidity and mortality. These conditions must be sought and recognized so that the appropriate cardiac catheterization setting can be planned to minimize risks. Conditions that should specifically exclude coronary angiography in an ambulatory setting are summarized in Table 17.3. In general patients who are at relatively high risk for mortality or morbidity are those with severe ischemia on noninvasive testing (Table 17.4) that might be due

Table 17.3.
Characteristics of Patients Requiring Supervision After Angiography Who Would not be Candidates for Coronary Angiography in an Ambulatory Setting

High risk for vascular complications (e.g., severe obesity or severe peripheral vascular disease)
Mechanical prosthetic valve
General debility or cachexia
Ejection fraction ≤35%
Anticoagulation or bleeding diathesis
Uncontrolled systemic hypertension
Home more than a 2-hour drive from laboratory
Difficult-to-control diabetes mellitus
Chronic corticosteroid use
History of allergy to radiographic contrast material
Severe chronic obstructive lung disease
Youth (<21 years) or complex congenital heart disease
Recent (≤1 month) stroke
Severe ischemic response during noninvasive stress testing
Suspected moderate or severe pulmonary hypertension
Arterial oxygen desaturation

Table 17.4.
Criteria for Identifying High Risk for Adverse Outcomes in Patients with Angina Pectoris or Other Ischemic Syndromes

ETT criteria
  Failure to complete 6.5 METs or attain heart rate ≥120 beats/min
  ≥2 mm ST depression
  Postexercise ischemic ST depression >6 min
  Ischemic ST depression in multiple ECG leads
  Systolic blood pressure response flat or depressed >10 mm Hg
  ST elevation in leads without Q wave
  Exercise-induced ventricular tachycardia
Stress echocardiography or MUGA criteria
  Resting ejection fraction ≤35%
  Exercise decrease in ejection fraction ≥5%
  Increased segmental wall motion score during stress
  New defects at low workload
Radionuclide perfusion criteria
  New defect at low workload
  Multiple defects
  Increase in cardiac size with exercise
  Increase in lung uptake of thallium with exercise
Ambulatory ECG monitoring criteria
  Any ischemic ST shift lasting ≥1 minute in patients with ETT ischemia, unstable angina, or recent MI
  Other criteria still evolving

Adapted from Pepine CJ, Cohn PF, Ellenbogen KA. Advisory group reports on silent myocardial ischemia, coronary atherogenesis, and cardiac emergencies. Am J Cardiol 1994;73:39B–44B.
ETT, exercise treadmill test; MET, metabolic equivalent task; MUGA, multiple gated image acquisition analysis; MI, myocardial infarction.

to left main or severe multivessel stenosis, those with severe left ventricular dysfunction (ejection fraction below 30%), and those with Class IV heart failure or angina.

Another consideration is selection of adjunctive procedures that may be needed. Decisions about need for left ventricular angiography, right heart catheterization, other intracoronary procedures, and pharmacologic testing to assess coronary reactivity can often be made before the procedure. If the patient has a high-quality echocardiogram, left ventriculography may not be necessary. However, if the patient has valvular heart disease, signs and symptoms suggesting heart failure, or findings suggesting pulmonary hypertension, right heart catheterization is indicated. The general principle is that adjunctive procedures thought to be needed should be planned before coronary angiography because that way they are more likely to be done in an expedient fashion. Finally, written informed consent should be obtained by the physician who will perform the angiographic study.

Selection of Technique, Vascular Site, and Contrast Agent

Premedication should be tailored to the patient's needs, as sedation and analgesia are helpful in apprehensive patients. It is our practice to reduce premedications to a minimum, particularly when coronary spasm is suspected or the procedure is done in an ambulatory setting. During the preoperative evaluation the site for vascular cannulation is selected. In general the femoral artery approach is preferred in most laboratories using percutaneous technique, except when specific anatomic or pathologic problems limit access. In these cases the brachial artery approach is selected. Selection of the contrast agent is important because of the large difference in cost between the low-osmolality agents (high cost) and high-osmolality agents (very low cost). In the clinical conditions listed in Table 17.5 our choice is a low-osmolality agent. These issues are addressed in detail in Chapter 13.

Complications: Prevention and Management

In general coronary angiography can be performed very safely, so that the benefit to the patient far outweighs the risks and costs of the procedure. The frequency of a serious complication (e.g., death, nonfatal MI, or cerebrovascular accident) is approximately 1 in 1000 patients examined using data from several very large databases totaling more than 400,000 patients (Table 17.6 and Chapter 8). Briefly, the most frequent events are related to peripheral vascular complications, which occur in about 5 in 1000 patients. These events, which are related to vascular injury at the arterial access site, consist of hematoma, pseudoaneurysm, arteriovenous fistula, occlusion, bleeding requiring transfusion, limb ischemia, or atheroembolization. Multiple procedures in the same artery, inability to comply with bed rest and limb immobilization, age, female gender, and heparization after the proce-

Table 17.5.
Considerations for Use of Low-Osmolality Contrast Agent for Coronary Angiography

Unstable ischemic syndromes
Congestive heart failure ejection fraction ≤35%
Insulin-dependent diabetes
Renal insufficiency
Hypotension
Severe bradycardia
History of contrast agent allergy
Severe valvular heart disease
Internal mammary artery injection

Table 17.6.
Expected Rate of Complications of Coronary Angiography from Multiple Reports

Complication	%
Death	0.10
Myocardial infarction	0.08
Cerebrovascular accident	0.08
Arrhythmia	0.50
Vascular	0.50
Any other	0.50

dure are associated with these vascular complications. Factors associated with increased risk of death are increased severity of CAD and left ventricular dysfunction. About 2 or 3 patients in 1000 have an adverse reaction to the contrast agent. In patients with a history of reaction to contrast agent the frequency is about 15 in 1000 cases, and although the frequency of minor reactions (nausea, vomiting, bradycardia, hypotension) is reduced with the low-osmolality agents, it is uncertain whether serious reactions are diminished. Patients with clinical characteristics that necessitate an inpatient procedure require very close supervision after angiography because they are at increased risk for problems whose adverse consequences may be limited by early identification and treatment (Table 17.3).

Some complications of coronary angiography produce permanent damage; thus only supportive measures can be used. Complications such as stroke due to thromboembolism may result in dense loss of function. When this circumstance is suspected, prompt neurological consultation and computed tomography (CT) may suggest that thrombolysis can be helpful. Close monitoring of the puncture site is required. Occasionally occipital blindness occurs, probably because of hyperosmolarity of contrast material, but it usually disappears within a few hours after hydration and maintenance of blood pressure. Air embolus to the central nervous system can produce an agitated, confused, or comatose state, but in general it does not cause permanent damage. The hyperbaric oxygen chamber may be used to treat air embolism. MI occurring during coronary angiography may be the result of embolism (air or thrombus), arterial damage by the catheter (e.g., dissection), or toxic effects of the contrast material in patients with severe stenosis. In any patient developing signs and symptoms of severe ischemic injury during or shortly after a coronary angiographic procedure, both coronary arteries should be rapidly visualized to identify the location and severity of any new obstruction. In most of these instances the arterial problem causing the acute ischemic injury can be identified. Whenever possible myocardial oxygen demands should be reduced with intravenous

β-blockers and nitrates and anticoagulation considered. Reperfusion should be attempted if a new severe obstruction is identified. Intracoronary nitroglycerin should be given to determine whether a component of obstruction is due to coronary spasm. Thrombolytic agents may be given into the artery involved when the obstruction is thought to be due to thrombotic material. In cases of extensive occlusive dissection of an artery supplying a large amount of functional myocardium, prompt balloon reperfusion should be attempted. Intracoronary stenting may be helpful to treat the dissection. Circulatory support with the intra-aortic balloon pump may be advisable in some cases, and emergency CABG should be considered if a pharmacologic and/or percutaneous approach offers limited benefit. Ventricular fibrillation must be treated immediately with electrical defibrillation. Heart block or asystole, which is relatively infrequent, may require a temporary pacing electrode or external cardiac pacing. If asystole is persistent, intravenous epinephrine may help. In these situations cardiopulmonary resuscitation must be carried out until a stable rhythm and circulation are established. Rapid supraventricular tachycardia often requires rate-slowing drugs, overdrive pacing conversion, or sometimes electrical conversion. Vasovagal attacks can produce bradycardia and hypotension; they are treated with rapid administration of a bolus of atropine and with leg elevation. More profound hypotension secondary to vasovagal reactions, nitroglycerin, or contrast medium usually responds to fluid administration. If unresponsive, hypotension may require a vasoconstrictor (e.g., phenylephrine, dopamine) and should prompt evaluation for retroperitoneal bleeding. Allergic reactions to contrast material may be limited to rash, fever, and chills and may include hypotension. Antihistamines, antipyretics and/or corticosteroids are helpful. When hypotension is profound, H_2 receptor blockers with large volumes of fluid are added. Arterial complications must be recognized promptly and vascular surgical consultation sought. Loss of a distal pulse may be due to thrombosis, dissection, or hematoma. Flow usually can be restored by appropriate surgical procedures. Vascular perforation must be promptly treated. Local pressure and reversal of anticoagulant are usually adequate, but some patients need surgery.

Interpretation and Communication of Results

Standardization of Nomenclature and Description of Procedure

Proper communication of results and documentation for the permanent record, are essential parts of the procedure. To facilitate communication standard nomenclature must be used to describe the coronary arteries. Several systems have been widely accepted, including those advanced by the Coronary Artery Surgery Study (CASS) (39) and BARI (40) investigators. While the actual style varies among laboratories and angiographers, the report should include the reason for the procedure, preoperative medications, adjunctive procedures, site of vascular approach, and local anesthetic, contrast agent, and volume, as well as what arteries or grafts were visualized. Hemodynamic measurements from the ascending aorta and left ventricle and those done during any adjunctive procedures should be listed. Intraoperative medications or pharmacologic stimulation should be documented.

Angiographic Interpretation

In general angiographic interpretation should include an artery-by-artery analysis, for example beginning with the LCA and its branches and ending with the RCA. The artery size and location and extent of any lesions should be described. The specific arterial segments that have irregularities and stenoses should be noted along with any other findings, such as thrombus, aneurysms, complex stenoses, and collaterals. These same findings should be noted for any CABG along with the origin and distal anastomotic sites.

Approximations of coronary artery lumen diameters at given locations are important considerations for revascularization and also in development of a quantitative estimate of the severity of CAD. Measurement techniques for making these approximations are readily available for diagnostic clinical and research studies. A simple hand-held electronic caliper works well for cine films, and semiautomated calipers are a part of most digital imaging systems. Recent data suggest that the normal LCA measures 4.5 plus or minus 0.6 mm in diameter, and its size depends on whether the RCA or LCA is dominant. The size of the RCA is 3.9 plus or minus 0.6 mm and 2.8 plus or minus 0.5 mm, again depending on dominance. With disease these lumen diameters usually decrease, but the size depends on remodeling. The minimal lumen diameter of any stenoses detected in the proximal and mid segments should be noted. Computer-based digital image techniques provide an automated assessment of reference segments and narrowings by obtaining multiple diameters averaged across normal-appearing segments and narrowings. The digital recording techniques are supplanting conventional film-based image recording techniques for coronary angiography now that a standard transfer format and media (American College of Cardiology, American College of Radiology, European Society of Cardiology, and National Engineering Manufacturers Association digital image communication in medicine [DICOM] standard) have been adopted (see Chapter 12).

The exact amount of narrowing that defines hemodynamic significance varies from 50 to 70%, depending on the operator, but these data must be quantified. More accurate characterization of each coronary artery obstruction is highly desirable to minimize erroneous observations and to evaluate possible interventions and/or the course of the disease process.

The location of the coronary artery narrowings, proximal, mid, or distal, are noted. Narrowings in the RCA before the acute marginal branch, the LCA, the LAD branch before the first septal perforator, and the LC branch before the obtuse marginal branch are considered proximal. In addition to lo-

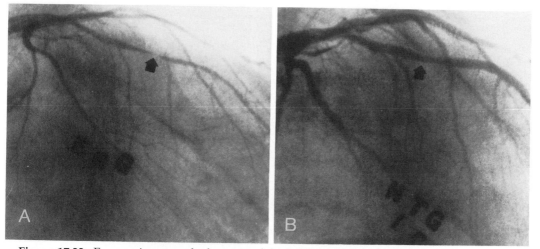

Figure 17.22. Ergonovine-provoked spasm of the LAD coronary artery (*arrow*) (**A**) promptly relieved by intracoronary nitroglycerin (*arrow*) (**B**).

cation and magnitude of any coronary narrowing, it is important to indicate estimated length. Other findings (e.g., areas of spasm, major diameter changes reversed by nitroglycerin, thrombus, myocardial bridges, anomalous coronary origins) must be noted (Figs. 17.22–17.24).

The angiographic anatomy of coronary spasm is characterized by dynamic lumen obstruction that may change from minute to minute. The process is usually limited to larger artery segments, and the RCA is most frequently involved. The LAD is next most frequently involved. Rarely, saphenous vein and internal mammary CABGs may be involved. In some cases spasm appears focal or limited to only a small segment of one artery. In others it may be multifocal, with several local sites in either the same or different arteries. In still others a much more diffuse process is manifested by general narrowing of one or more coronary arteries. A few patients have focal or multifocal spasm in one branch with diffuse spasm in another. Finally, some show a migratory process on repeated angiograms. As a general rule, however, spasm involves segments with atherosclerotic type of lumen irregularities, rather than the very smooth segments. However, spasm does not necessarily localize at sites of severe atherosclerotic type of obstruction. When spasm is relieved, either spontaneously or by

nitroglycerin, the lumen–endothelial border often appears hazy, suggesting that this layer of the vessel wall may be thickened or edematous or contain mural thrombus. Occasionally nonocclusive intraluminal thrombus is found at or just distal to a site of coronary spasm. Collaterals may appear during spasm and disappear when spasm is relieved.

It is also helpful for the coronary angiogram reader to diagram and report the location and extent of individual coronary narrowings. The degree of narrowing can be recorded, and vessel diameter at the narrowing and the length of narrowing can be noted. Although determining the exact location, degree, and length of narrowing is important, it is only part of the evaluation of the coronary circulation. Distal vessel anatomy must be considered, as must the function of the ventricular region perfused by that vessel. This is assessed by comparing the coronary angiography with the left ventricular angiography.

Quantitative assessment is made by measuring the diameter of the artery at its narrowest point and the diameter of the adjacent proximal segment where it is relatively wide. Objective techniques (e.g., electronic calipers or computer-assisted measurement) substantially reduce the wide observer variability regularly associated with only simple visual estimates. By

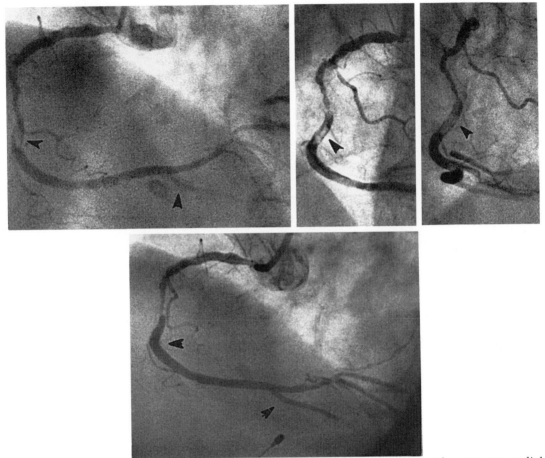

Figure 17.23. Large mid-RCA thrombus with distal embolization from patient with acute myocardial infarction. (**Top left**) LAO projection with filling defect (*arrow*) just distal to severe narrowing. Proximal part of posterior descending branch is occluded, probably as a result of embolization. Same filling defect is shown in shallow LAO (**center**) and RAO (**right**) projections. After 24 hours of only intravenous heparin, the filling defect is no longer visualized (**bottom**) and the posterior descending branch fills.

convention percent stenosis is assessed in a view demonstrating the most severe degree of narrowing, and the segment of vessel just proximal to the beginning of the stenosis is taken as the reference segment. Another assessment, flow, is estimated according to the thrombolysis in myocardial infarction (TIMI) method (42) (see Chapter 37). TIMI Grade 3 flow is considered normal; vessels with slow flow, Grade 2 or 1; and no contrast flow, Grade 0. Recently it has been shown that frame counts of the contrast–blood interface movement are needed to reduce variation in this estimate, particularly when trying to separate Grade 2 from

Grade 3 flow. Other findings (e.g., myocardial bridges, anomalous coronary arteries) must be noted and differentiated from atherosclerotic lesions. Intracoronary thrombus may appear as a discrete filling defect surrounded by contrast material. If complex plaque is present, it is likely to be responsible for an acute coronary syndrome. These lesions often appear eccentric, with overhanging edges, irregularities, ulceration, or abrupt shoulders. Grading systems are also available for thrombus and complex plaque (43).

A number of jeopardy scores have been used to assess the significance of multiple

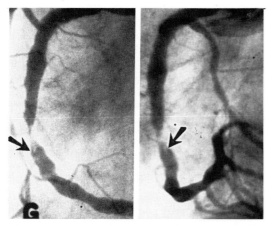

Figure 17.24. Small mid-RAC thrombus (*arrow*) in patient with unstable angina. Note filling defect just distal to subtotal occlusion (**left panel** LAO projection, **right panel** RAO projection).

Left Ventricular Pressure Recording and Angiography

Left ventricular hemodynamic evaluation provides information that complements the coronary angiogram. The left ventricular end diastolic pressure, wall motion, aneurysm, septal perforation, and mitral insufficiency can be documented. The anatomic relationship between any regional wall motion abnormality and coronary occlusive disease viewed by coronary angiography may be assessed. Abnormalities in wall motion that may be reversible can also be assessed on postextrasystolic beats or after nitroglycerin administration.

Right Heart Catheterization

Right heart catheterization is indicated in patients with suspected pulmonary hypertension, valvular or congenital lesions, and heart failure. It measures pulmonary artery and right heart filling pressures and cardiac output in addition to oxygen saturations if needed. It is usually done with a balloon flotation catheter at the time of coronary angiography. Routine right heart catheterization in all patients undergoing coronary angiography cannot be justified in our opinion.

Tests for Coronary Vasomotor and/or Endothelial Dysfunction

Visualization of **coronary spasm** during coronary angiography is the reference standard for this diagnosis. Catheter-related spasm occurs at or within 1 cm of the catheter tip and does not cause transient ischemia. In the ideal situation, when spontaneous ischemia (i.e., pain, changes in ST segment) occurs in the catheterization laboratory, the angiographer should attempt to visualize each coronary artery. If any coronary obstruction resolves with intracoronary nitroglycerin, the diagnosis of spasm as the basis for ischemia is established. Pro-

angiographic findings by one term. Yet conclusive evidence supporting their independent prognostic value is lacking. When eight indices were compared, "typically 80% of the prognostic information in one index was also contained in another" (39). When applied to 6-year outcome data from CASS, **number of vessels diseased, number of proximal segments diseased,** and **left wall motion** contained 80% of the prognostic information. Comprehensive reviews conclude that although such summary scores are useful for studies of the relation of atherosclerosis risk factors or treatments to extent or progression of disease, by definition they obscure the influence of individual severely stenotic lesions and thus are less useful for relating obstructive disease to clinical outcome (44).

SPECIAL TESTS AS ADJUNCTS TO CORONARY ANGIOGRAPHY

A number of procedures are helpful during coronary angiography. The frequently used adjunctive procedures are summarized next.

vocative tests may be required in patients without a spontaneous ischemic episode in the laboratory. Clinical situations in which provocative testing for coronary spasm may be helpful are outlined in Table 17.7. Situations in which provocative testing for spasm is contraindicated are summarized in Table 17.8.

A number of **provocative tests** have been used, but only those employing an **ergonovine derivative,** ergonovine maleate (Ergotrate) and methylergonovine maleate (Methergin) are in widespread use. These are nonspecific, direct-acting vasoconstrictors with structural similarities to several neurotransmitters. The response to an intravenous ergonovine derivative in patients without coronary spasm is minimal generalized vasoconstriction manifested by coronary diameter reduction of approximately 15% associated with a small increase in both systemic systolic and left ventricular end-diastolic pressures. Coronary diameter reduction after a low dose of ergonovine or methylergonovine (less than 0.3 mg), accompanied by objective evidence for ischemia without important increases in heart rate or blood pressure that can be reversed by intracoronary nitroglycerin, fulfills criteria for coronary spasm. Also, an ergonovine compound may be given directly into each coronary artery (5 to 10 mg, total cumulative dose of 50 mg) as a test for spasm. This eliminates systemic vasoconstriction and esophageal smooth muscle stimulation and separates right and left coronary responses. This route may be used in patients with moderate or severe hypertension when systemic administration is contraindicated.

Low doses (10 to 100 mg) of **acetylcholine** given directly into each coronary artery may test for spasm. This causes dilation in normal arteries and no changes or constriction where endothelial dysfunction is present. The response seen with this agent reverses spontaneously within 20 to 30 seconds. This agent may be used when intravenous ergonovine is contraindicated because of severe hypertension. The cold pressor test (i.e., hand immersion in ice water), hyperventilation, histamine, and exercise may be useful in selected patients to provoke coronary spasm, but use of these tests is recommended only when a patient's history suggests that these conditions are likely to be associated with either signs or symptoms of ischemia.

Recent clinical interest in coronary vasomotor changes as an index of coronary **endothelial dysfunction** has prompted increasing use of intracoronary **acetylcholine** for this evaluation. While this agent is very safe and sites of very severe constriction are often identified, its use for this purpose has been limited to research.

Table 17.7.
Clinical Situations Where Provocative Testing for Coronary Spasm May be Helpful

Rest pain associated with the following:
 No preceding heart rate and/or blood pressure rise
 Preserved effort tolerance
 Cyclic recurrence often in early morning
 Transient ST segment elevation or ventricular dysrhythmia
 Nonspecific or no ECG change
 ECG pattern prohibiting interpretation of ST segment (e.g., pacer, left bundle branch block)
Angina associated with the following:
 Variable threshold onset
 ST segment elevation during stress testing
 Syncope and/or ventricular dysrhythmia
 Patent coronary bypass grafts
 A ≤50% coronary stenosis and history of smoking

Table 17.8.
Contraindications to Provocative Testing for Coronary Spasm

Relative
 Myocardial infarction within 5 days
 Uncontrolled angina or ischemia
 Uncontrolled ventricular dysrhythmia
Absolute
 Amenorrhea in premenopausal women[a]
 Severe hypertension[b]
 Severe left ventricular dysfunction
 Severe aortic stenosis
 Significant left main coronary stenosis

[a] May use intracoronary acetylcholine.
[b] May use either intracoronary ergonovine derivative or acetylcholine.

Other Useful Procedures

Intraluminal ultrasound is used to provide a cross-sectional image of the wall of the larger coronary artery segments from a small catheter-mounted ultraminiature transducer (45). Plaque and dissections that are not well seen on the contrast angiogram can be visualized, and coronary artery wall thickness and plaque characteristics can be quantified. Intraluminal ultrasound also permits accurate measurements of coronary artery lumen size that are model independent. Intracoronary ultrasound is particularly useful for evaluation of dissection, tubular or diffuse types of coronary atherosclerosis in which focal obstruction may be absent, and branch stenosis, all of which may be difficult to visualize on angiography. **Coronary angioscopy** uses a miniature fiberoptic catheter to visualize the endothelial surface of the coronary artery lumen. New (red) and old (gray) mural thrombus and flaplike dissections can be detected. Angioscopy is superior to angiography for identification of mural thrombus. Coronary blood flow reserve can be assessed from an ultraminiature **Doppler blood flow velocity transducer** mounted on a guidewire suitable for intracoronary use. These newer catheter-based techniques provide additional information not available from coronary angiography alone and are useful in selected cases to clarify the presence and severity of disease and reasons for cardiac ischemia.

CONTROVERSIAL AREAS

Overuse

The most important controversy about coronary angiography in our opinion is the proper level of use. This question is generating considerable concern because of the suggestion that perhaps coronary angiography is being overused (46). This controversy is fueled by data showing widely varying use rates among geographic regions within the United States and between the United States and Canada (47–56). Use rates have been strongly linked to physicians' financial incentives, availability of a catheterization laboratory, and geographic area. Some reports suggest that a substantial proportion of procedures are done for inappropriate or equivocal indications (57, 58). Data on the relation between higher rates of angiography and clinical outcome are limited and difficult to interpret. Some observational reports suggest that there is no beneficial relationship (47, 59–61). Others suggest that there may be an early beneficial relationship (62). One problem with these latter data is that one would not expect angiography and revascularization to improve survival after only 30 days. Older randomized trials noted survival benefit with revascularization, but benefit did not become apparent until 3 to 7 years after CABG (63). Furthermore, a similar proportion of patients with either left main or three-vessel obstruction was found in the recent observational reports and the older randomized trials. Since no difference in benefit from revascularization between these two conditions was found, it is difficult to understand how increased angiography and revascularization can contribute to an early mortality benefit, particularly among the older patients, who are more likely to have high surgical risk, in these recent reports.

Whether higher levels of testing represent better or worse health care is very important; nonetheless, we believe that it is difficult, if not impossible, to address it without well-designed randomized trials that compare various strategies for coronary angiography and clinical outcome. Findings are muddied by changing statistics for atherosclerotic disease (e.g., reduced incidence and death rates for MI), our changing population demographics (more elderly and minority patients), our rapidly changing health care environment (more care by primary care physicians and nonphysicians), and more and more treatments that benefit outcome (e.g., aspirin, β-blockers, thrombolytics, statins, ACE inhibitors). Unfortunately, just as epidemiologic data are limited and only generate hypotheses for the design of randomized trials, the administrative data on use tell little about the most appropriate level of use for coronary angiography. They provide little guidance for the practicing physician who must decide whether or not to refer a specific patient for coronary angiography. Lower rates of coronary angiography do not necessarily mean better care. But if more coronary angiography is not necessarily better, at least we should know what level is best. When coronary angiography and revascularization use go up or down, we need to know in whom use rates have changed and what such change means in terms of health outcomes and cost-effective care (64).

We observe two general strategies for use of coronary angiography in common practice in the United States. One is as an **unrestricted** or routine procedure early in the clinical presentation of a patient with known or suspected coronary artery disease, followed by angiography-directed care along the steps summarized in Table 17.9. The other is as a **restricted** procedure whose use is delayed and based upon either risk stratification by noninvasive testing or unacceptable symptoms during medical management.

The important question that we think ought to be addressed is this: does a management strategy for a particular CAD syndrome (e.g., chronic stable angina or acute ischemic syndrome) that is guided by **early unrestricted use** of coronary angiography improve the clinical outcome (e.g., reduce death, nonfatal MI, and need for costly hospitalization) to a greater or lesser extent than a strategy centered on the **restricted use** of coronary angiography? **Restricted use** may be based on noninvasive test findings that predict high risk of adverse outcome. Alternatively, restricted use may be very conservative care based on unacceptable symptoms or lifestyle during an attempt at maximal medical therapy. While it would be very attractive to believe that early unrestricted use of coronary angiography is efficient and cost effective, no objective evidence supports this case. This is unlikely in our opinion, at least for patients in the chronic stable stage of CAD, whose risk of adverse outcome as a group is already very low and decreasing over time. An attempt at use of a noninvasive technique to identify the subgroup of patients within this low-risk group who are most at risk seems to be a logical approach. Whether this should be done with or without an attempt at maximal medical treatment is also a subject of debate.

Table 17.9.
Common Strategies for Use of Coronary Angiography

Unrestricted
  Early (initial) coronary angiography followed by angiography-directed management
    Left main or 3-vessel disease with reduced ejection fraction N CABG
    Multivessel disease N CABG or PTCA
    Single-vessel disease N PTCA
    Not revascularizable or no severe stenoses N medication
Restricted
  Early risk stratification (based on clinical and noninvasive test findings) followed by angiography-directed management only in those with findings suggesting high risk for adverse outcome
  Medical therapy followed by angiography-directed management only for those with unacceptable lifestyle during adequate medical therapy

PTCA, percutaneous transluminal coronary angioplasty.

Testing–Interventional Procedure–Testing Cycle

Another controversial area that has recently emerged is the increasingly strong link between testing and procedures. Data derived from a private insurance company's database on patients who have had MI suggest that fewer than 10% of patients undergoing coronary angiography is the late 1980s had had a stress test. More recent data, however, suggest that use of stress testing has increased dramatically, so that approximately 4% of the Medicare population undergo stress tests annually, and 56% of the time an imaging procedure is used (65). Moreover, there is a very strong link between the performance of the stress test and subsequent coronary angiography as well as revascularization. That the relationship between total stress tests and angiography is so robust suggests that it is the **performance of**

TEST - PROCEDURE - TEST CYCLE

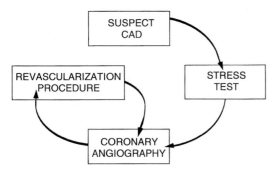

Figure 17.25. Test-procedure retest cycle.

the test rather than the **result of the test** that is driving the angiographic procedure and likewise the performance of angiography that drives revascularization (Fig. 17.25).

An even more difficult situation is what we call the **cycle** linking percutaneous revascularization and coronary angiography (Fig. 17.25). One of the best historical predictors of coronary angiography in many hospitals is a prior percutaneous revascularization. Once a patient enters such a cycle, it is not clear that variables drive the decision to perform the diagnostic procedure and the revascularization. It is even less clear whether these cycles have any relation to improvement in patient care or outcome, but they clearly increase the cost of care.

It is certain that while we do not know the "right" rate of testing, the decision to do a test, whether it be a stress test or a coronary angiogram, is very close to being a decision to treat with revascularization. Just how we deal with these issues in the future will have an extremely important influence on cardiovascular disease specialty care and training as well as physicians' responsibilities (66). It seems to us that in many patients coronary angiography is now used as a basis for suspicion of disease (e.g., case finding), and when an obstruction is identified, its presence is used as a reason for percutaneous intervention. But the potential reservoir of CAD is extraordinarily large, with about half of our general population having two or more CAD risk factors and a quarter of our elderly population

complaining of chest pain (67). Given the size of this pool of potential patients, the specific strategies used for their evaluation and treatment become extremely important, not only to those patients but also to our specialty.

FUTURE DIRECTIONS

Although the basic practice of coronary angiography is most likely to continue to be founded upon the methods and procedures outlined in this chapter, our changing population, disease characteristics, and new technology will no doubt alter certain aspects of angiography. We will be facing questions about whether to evaluate older patients and dealing less with acute MI. Instead our future patients will be more likely to have chronic stable ischemic disease, and many will have heart failure.

New catheter design, construction, and materials will allow use of smaller and less traumatic systems. Less-toxic contrast agents will continue to emerge as well as perhaps a method to allow contrast to persist for several minutes after injection. Use of smaller catheter systems and less-toxic contrast media with persistence in the coronary lumen will translate to fewer injections or even nonselective injection. These advances should facilitate more studies in ambulatory elderly patients with chronic ischemic syndromes and make studies in critically ill hospitalized patients safer.

Advances in both analog and digital components of radiographic imaging chains should enable remarkable change in technique and the appearance of laboratories. We should see replacement of conventional high-level radiation and bulky x-ray equipment and image intensifiers with low-level, less bulky radiation equipment and small solid-state image detectors.

Coronary angiograms recorded from pairs of images obtained from several radiographic views will be reconstructed as viewed from any desired projection. The entirety of coronary angiographic laboratory data collection and processing will be done from a computer workstation to generate a paperless and filmless unit record subject to transmission to distant sites for storage or exchange with other institutions. This digital record will combine the coronary angiography images with other imaging data (e.g., echocardiography, CT, magnetic resonance imaging) as well as clinical data. These innovations will obviate many paper-based and film-based procedures and personnel now required in day-to-day catheterization laboratory operations. Coronary angiography will continue to be closely allied with newer and evolving revascularization techniques. Optical coherence tomography (67) appears to be one of several attractive new technologies for intracoronary diagnostics. This technique has the potential to provide tomographic imaging of the wall and internal microstructure of coronary blood vessels. Knowledge of the coronary anatomy and principles of coronary angiography will continue to be important for physicians. More-rigorous training and credentialing will be required to maintain an acceptable standard of care as this field continues to evolve in the future.

References

1. Radner S. An attempt at the roentgenologic visualization of coronary blood vessels in man. Acta Radiol 1945;26:497–502.
2. Gensini GG, Di Giorgi S, Black A. New approaches to coronary arteriography. Angiology 1961;12:223–238.
3. Richards LS, Thal AP. Phasic dye injection control system for coronary arteriography in the human. Surg Gynecol Obstet 1958;107:739–743.
4. Arnulf G, Chacornac R. L'artériographie méthodique des artères coronaires grâace a l'utilisation de l'acetylcholine. Données expérimentales et cliniques. Bull Acad Natl Med (Paris) 1958;25, 26:661–673.
5. Lehman JS, Boyer RA, Winter FS. Coronary arteriography. Am J Roentgenol 1959;81:749–763.
6. Bellman S, Frank HA, Lambert PB, et al. Coronary arteriography: 1. Differential opacification of the aortic stream by catheters of special design–experimental development. N Engl J Med 1960;262:325–328.
7. Williams JA, Littmann D, Hall JH, et al. Coronary arteriography: 2. Clinical experiences with the loop-end catheter. N Engl J Med 1960;262:328–332.
8. Sones MF, Shirey EK, Proudfit WL, Westcott RN. Cine coronary arteriography. Circulation 1959;20:773 (abstract).
9. Sones FM, Shirey EK. Cine coronary arteriography. Mod Concepts Cardiovasc Dis 1962;31:735–738.
10. Judkins MP. Selective coronary arteriography: 1. A percutaneous transfemoral technic. Radiology 1967;89:815–824.
11. Amplatz K, Formanek G, Stanger P, Wilson W. Mechanics of selective coronary artery catheterization via femoral approach. Radiology 1967;89:1040–1047.
12. Favalaro RG. Saphenous vein autograft replacement of severe segmental coronary artery occlusion: operative technique. Ann Thorac Surg 1968;5:334–339.
13. Bernstein SJ, Laorui M, Hilborne LH, et al. A literature review and ratings of appropriateness and necessity. Coronary Angiography. Santa Monica: RAND, 1992.
14. Vital & Health Statistics. National Center for Health Statistics. National hospital discharge summary: detailed diagnoses and procedures. U.S. Department of Health and Human Services (DHHS PHS-88–1756), 1988.
15. Heart and stroke facts: 1996 statistical supplement. American Heart Association 1996:22.
16. Yamanaka O, Hobbs RE. Coronary artery anomalies in 126,595 patients undergoing coronary arteriography. Cathet Cardiovasc Diagn 1990;21:28–40.
17. Roberts WC, Siegel RJ, Zipes DP. Origin of the RCA from the left sinus of Valsalva and its functional consequences: analysis of 10 necropsy patients. Am J Cardiol 1982;49:863–868.
18. Schoonmaker FW, King SB. Coronary arteriography by the single catheter percutaneous femoral technique. Experience in 6800 cases. Circulation 1974;50:735–740.
19. Pepine CJ, von Gunten C, Hill JA, et al. Percutaneous brachial catheterization using a modified sheath and new catheter system. Cathet Cardiovasc Diagn 1984;10:637–642.
20. Argrenal AD, Baker MS. Selective coronary arteriography via translumbar catheterization. Am Heart J 1991;121:198–199.
21. Marcus R, Grollman JH Jr. Translumbar coronary and brachiocephalic arteriography using a modified Desilets-Hoffman sheath. Cathet Cardiovasc Diagn 1987;13:288–290.
22. Campeau L. Percutaneous radial artery approach for coronary angiography. Cathet Cardiovasc Diagn 1989;16:3–7.
23. Topol EJ, Nissen SE. Our preoccupation with coronary luminology: the dissociation between clinical and angiographic findings in ischemic heart disease. Circulation 1995;92:2333–2342.
24. Arnett EN, Isner JM, Redwood CR, et al. Coronary artery narrowing in coronary heart disease: comparison of cineangiographic and necropsy findings. Ann Intern Med 1979;91:350–356.
25. Grodin CM, Dyrda I, Pasternac A, et al. Discrepancies between cineangiographic and post-mortem findings in patients with coronary artery disease and recent myocardial revascularization. Circulation 1974;49:703–709.
26. Blankenhorn DH, Curry PJ. The accuracy of arteriography and ultrasound imaging for atherosclerosis measurement: a review. Arch Pathol Lab Med 1982;106:483–490.

27. Isner JM, Kishel J, Kent KM. Accuracy of angiographic determination of left main coronary arterial narrowing. Circulation 1981;63:1056–1061.

28. Roberts WC, Jones AA. Quantitation of coronary arterial narrowing at necropsy in sudden coronary death. Am J Cardiol 1979;44:39–44.

29. Vlaodaver Z, French R, van Tassel RA, Edwards JE. Correlation of the antemortem coronary angiogram and the postmortem specimen. Circulation 1973;47:162–168.

30. Folland ED, Vogel RA, Hartigan P, et al. Relation between coronary artery stenosis assessed by visual caliper, and computer methods and exercise capacity in patients with single-vessel coronary artery disease. Circulation 1994;89:2005–2014.

31. Crawford T, Levine CI. Medical thinning in atheroma. J Pathol Bacteriol 1953;66:19–23.

32. Stiel GM, Stiel LS, Schofer J, et al. Impact of compensatory enlargement of atherosclerotic coronary arteries on angiographic assessment of coronary artery disease. Circulation 1989;80:1603–1609.

33. Glagov S, Weisenberg E, Zarins CK, et al. Compensatory enlargement of human atherosclerotic coronary arteries. N Engl J Med 1987;316:1371–1375.

34. Little WC, Constantinescu M, Applegate RJ, et al. Can arteriography predict the site of a subsequent myocardial infarction inpatients with mild-to-moderate coronary artery disease? Circulation 1988;78:1157–1166.

35. Fuster V, Lewis A. Conner Memorial Lecture: Mechanisms leading to myocardial infarction: insights from studies of vascular biology. Conner Memorial Lecture. Circulation 1994;90:2126–2146.

36. Thomas AC, Davies MJ, Dilly S, et al. Potential errors in the estimation of coronary araterial stenosis from clinical arteriography with reference to the shape of the coronary arterial lumen. Br Heart J 1986;55:129–139.

37. El-Tamimi H, Mansour M, Wargovich T, et al. Constrictor and dilator responses in adjacent segments of the same coronary artery to intracoronary acetylcholine in patients with coronary artery disease: the endothelial function revisited. Circulation 1994;89:45–51.

38. El-Tamimi H, Mansour M, Pepine CJ, et al. Circadian variation in coronary tone in patients with stable angina: protective role of the endothelium. Circulation 1995;92:3201–3205.

39. Ringqvist I, Fisher LD, Mock M, et al. Prognostic value of angiographic indices of coronary artery disease from the Coronary Artery Surgery Study (CASS). J Clin Invest 1983;71:1854–1866.

40. Alderman EL, Stadius M. The angiographic definitions of the bypass angioplasty revascularization investigation (BARI). Coron Artery Dis 1992;3:1189–1207.

41. Detre KM, Takaro T, Hultgren H, Peduzzi P. Long-term mortality and morbidity results of the Veterans Administration randomized trial of coronary artery bypass surgery. Circulation 1985;72:V84–V89.

42. The TIMI Study Group. The thrombolysis in myocardial infarction (TIMI) trial: Phase I findings. N Engl J Med 1985;312:932–936.

43. Sharaf BL, Williams DO, Miele NJ, et al. A detailed angiographic analysis of patients with ambulatory electrocardiographic ischemia: results from the asymptomatic cardiac ischemia pilot (ACIP) study Angiographic Core Laboratory. J Am Coll Cardiol 1997;29:78–84.

44. Crouse JR III, Thompson CJ. An evaluation of methods for imaging and quantifying coronary and carotid lumen stenosis and atherosclerosis. Circulation 1993;87:II17–II33.

45. Scanlon PJ, Faxon DP, Audet AM, et al. ACC/AHA guidelines for coronary angiography. a report of the American College of Cardiology/American Heart Association Task Force on Practice Guidelines (Committee on Coronary Angiography). J Am Coll Cardiol 1998, in press.

46. Graboys TB, Biegelsen B, Lampert S, et al. Results of a second-opinion trial among patients recommended for coronary angiography. JAMA 1992;268:2537–2540.

47. Rouleau JL, Moye LA, Pfeffer MA, et al. A comparison of management patterns after acute myocardial infarction in Canada and the United States. N Engl J Med 1993;328:779–784.

48. Leape LL, Park RE, Solomon DH, et al. Does inappropriate use explain small-area variations in the use of health care services? JAMA 1990;263:669–672.

49. Gittelsohn Am, Halpern J, Sanchez Rl. Income, race, and surgery in Maryland. Am J Public Health 1991;81:1435–1441.

50. Ayanian JZ, Udvarhelyi IS, Gatsonis CA, et al. Racial differences in the use of revascularization procedures after coronary angiography. JAMA 1993;269:2642–2646.

51. Whittle J, Conigliaro J, Good CB, Lofgren RP. Racial differences in the use of cardiovascular procedures in the Department of Veternas Affairs medical system. N Engl J Med 1993;329:621–627.

52. Kostis JB, Wilson AC, O'Dowd K, et al. Sex differences in the management and long-term outcome of acute myocardial infarction: A statewide study: MIDAS Study Group. Circulation 1994;90:1715–1730.

53. Langa KM, Sussman EJ. The effect of cost-containment policies on the rates of coronary revascularization in California. N Engl J Med 1993;329:1784–1789.

54. Every NR, Larson EB, Litwin PE, et al. The association between on-site cardiac catheterization facilities and the use of coronary angiography after acute myocardial infarction. N Engl J Med 1993;329:546–551.

55. McClellan M, McNeil BJ, Newhouse JP. Does more intensive treatment of acute myocardial infarction in the elderly reduce the mortality? JAMA 1994;272:859–866.

56. Maynard C, Litwin PE, Martin JS, Weaver WD. Gender differences in the treatment and outcome of acute myocardial infarction: results from the Myocardial Infarction Triage and Intervention Registry. Arch Intern Med 1992;152:972–976.

57. McGlynn EA, Naylor CD, Anderson GM, et al. Comparison of the appropriateness of coronary angiography and coronary artery bypass graft

surgery between Canada and New York State. JAMA 1994;272:934–940.

58. Hilborne LH, Leape LL, Bernstein SJ, et al. The appropriateness of use of percutaneous transluminal angioplasty in New York State. JAMA 1993; 269:761–765.

59. Mark DB, Naylor CD, Hlatky MA, et al. Use of medical resources and quality of life after acute myocardial infarction in Canada and the United States. N Engl J Med 1994;331:1130–1135.

60. Pilote L, Califf Rm, Sapp S, et al. Regional variation across the United States in the management of aucte myocardial infarction. N Engl J Med 1995;333:565–572.

61. Guadagnoli E, Hauptman PJ, Ayanian JZ, et al. Variation in the use of cardiac procedures after acute myocardial infarction. N Engl J Med 1995; 3333:573–578.

62. Jollis JG, DeLong ER, Peterson ED, et al. Outcome of acute myocardial infarction according to the specialty of the admitting physician. N Engl J Med 1996;335:1880–1887.

63. Yusuf S, Zucker D, Peduzzi P, et al. Effect of coronary artery bypass graft surgery on survival: overview of 10-year results from randomized trials by the Coronary Artery Bypass Graft Surgery Trialists Collaboration. Lancet 1994;334: 563–570.

64. Epstein AM. Use of diagnostic tests and therapeutic procedures in a changing health care environment. JAMA 1996;275:1197–1198 (editorial).

65. Wennberg DE, Kellett MA, Dickins JD, et al. The association between local diagnostic testing intensity and invasive cardiac procedures. JAMA 1996; 275:1161–1164.

66. Goldman L. The value of cardiology. N Engl J Med 1996;335:1918–1919 (editorial).

67. Tearney GJ, Brezinski ME, Boppart SA, et al. Catheter-based optical imaging of a human coronary artery. Circulation 1996;94:3013.

18
Intravascular Ultrasound

Jay D. Schlaifer, MD
Steven E. Nissen, MD

INTRODUCTION

Coronary angiography is the standard for evaluating the presence and degree of coronary stenoses. However, angiography has a number of limitations, one of which is a rather **large degree of interobserver and intraobserver variation in interpretation** (1). Quantitative coronary angiographic techniques have improved this variation, but there are still significant differences between angiographic assessment of atherosclerotic disease and quantitative histologic postmortem findings (2, 3). Necropsy studies show that lesions are often inhomogeneous, complex, and eccentric, with varying degrees of fracturing and dissection within the lesion. Angiography outlines a two-dimensional planar silhouette of the contrast-filled vessel lumen that may not accurately delineate the three-dimensional complex cross-sectional anatomy of a diseased vessel. Furthermore, much of the plaque can lie within the vessel wall before encroaching upon the lumen and go undetected by angiography. Attempts to complement contrast angiography with alternative imaging modalities have been made with fluorescence spectroscopy and fiberoptic angioscopy. Although it provides excellent qualitative visualization of the intimal surface and detection of intraluminal thrombus, **angioscopy** is difficult to use and does not visualize the subintimal layers of the vessel. Intravascular ultrasound (IVUS) provides intraluminal real-time, two-dimensional, cross-sectional im-

ages of the vessel wall and plaque. IVUS used in conjunction with contrast angiography at the time of catheterization allows accurate assessment of disease severity and plaque composition in vivo. In its early years IVUS served mostly as a tool of research concentrating on tissue characterization. With further technological advances in miniaturization, downsizing of catheters (2.9 F), better image quality, and greater flexibility, IVUS has become more widely applicable clinically. Furthermore, improved insights into the pathophysiology of coronary artery disease and mechanisms of catheter-based interventional techniques have increased the clinical applicability of IVUS.

INTRAVASCULAR ULTRASOUND DEVICES

Today's IVUS imaging catheters use piezoelectric transducers that expand and contract in response to an electrical pulse. These changes in shape of the transducer result in compressions, rarefaction, or sound wave generation. The reverse is also true; when the transducer is struck by sound waves, it produces an electrical impulse. Tissues of different acoustic properties cause variations in the sound wave reflections that are represented on the video displayed monitor. The transducer must be optimized with regard to catheter size, field of view, and image resolution according to its clinical application (4, 5). Low-frequency devices (10 to 20 MHz) have been used to image intracardiac structures such as cardiac valves, intracardiac chambers, and larger vessels (i.e., aorta) with good penetration. However, there are several unique technical limitations on intracoronary ultrasound imaging devices. The catheter must have a low profile, and the catheter shaft must be flexible, especially if it is to be used in the tortuous coronary circulation without causing vessel injury. To increase the resolution of the microscopic vascular layers close to the transducer, the frequencies used in the intravascular catheters are usually 20 to 40 MHz. This increase in resolution is achieved at the expense of lower tissue penetration. Because of these higher frequencies, one can reduce the transducer aperture size and therefore catheter size without impairing lateral resolution. **Commercial imaging catheters come as small as 2.9 F** (0.96 mm diameter), and it is anticipated that an ultrasound-tipped guidewire will soon be available. One potential limitation of the higher-frequency (40 MHz) transducer is that the resolution is too good. Reflections from red blood cells produce a spontaneous echo contrast effect that may be difficult to distinguish from the intimal surface or thrombus. Therefore, 20- to 30-MHz catheters are most often used for intracoronary imaging.

The two classes of IVUS devices are mechanical and phased array. **Mechanical catheters** use a single ultrasound element, emitting and receiving echo beams while rotating the acoustic beam perpendicular to the catheter's axis. In this system one of two designs enables the ultrasound transducer either to rotate on a mechanical shaft through the catheter or to remain stationary while a mirror rotates around the transducer in the same housing. The mirror has a longer distance from the transducer to the tissue being interrogated, which minimizes some of the near-field or ring-down artifact that is seen immediately around the catheter. In either case the rotating mechanical force (up to 1,800 rpm) is generated through a flexible drive shaft connected to a proximal motor. The phased-array device uses a series of 64 fine ultrasound elements arranged circumferentially around the tip of the catheter. These elements are electronically fired sequentially so that each sends and receives its own signal from individual sectors perpendicular to the long axis of the catheter. These signals are summed, and computer reconstruction produces a single cross-sectional image of the vessel analogous to the technique used for computed tomography.

Both systems can be safely used in the peripheral and coronary circulation. There are advantages and disadvantages to both systems and considerable debate regarding the superiority of one device over the other. The phased-array catheter has a 3.5-F profile and a central lumen that accommodates an 0.014-inch (0.036 cm) guidewire for over-the-wire use. This coaxial design makes this catheter more flexible and easier to manipulate into distal or tortuous segments of the coronary circulation than mechanical catheters, which use a rounded tip or monorail design. The other advantages of the **phased-array catheter** are that they have no moving parts and that no special catheter preparation is required before inserting into the guide catheter. The mechanical catheters have a flexible drive shaft that runs down the center of the catheter, preventing an over-the-wire design. However, the more recent modifications include monorail systems using 0.014- to 0.018-inch guidewires, improving the flexibility and handling characteristics of the mechanical systems. The monorail guidewire can interfere with imaging in a full 360° arc by obscuring 10 to 30° of the vessel's circumference. More recently catheters have been designed with a transparent sheath that can be advanced distal to the stenosis or site of interest via a monorail system. The guidewire can then be pulled back, allowing advancement and withdrawal of the transducer freely within the sheath without interference from the guidewire or trauma to the vessel. Unlike the phased-array catheters, these must be flushed carefully before insertion into the guide catheter to remove all traces of air, which would otherwise interfere with acoustic transmission or perhaps result in coronary embolization.

Despite the better tracking of the

phased-array catheters, many investigators find that the mechanical catheters provide superior quality images. Artifacts are inherent in both types of catheter systems (6). During transmission and reception of ultrasound signals the mechanical imaging system uses the predetermined mechanical scan pattern to place the received acoustic data at the appropriate place on the video display. This requires a one-to-one rotational transmission from the motor to the scanning tip, even when the catheter follows a tortuous pathway. Otherwise constant drag and friction between the drive shaft and the catheter lumen cause the image as a whole to rotate on the screen, interfering with the orientation of anatomic structures. Bends or kinks in the catheter may cause nonuniform rotational distortion of the image because the shaft speeds up and slows down as it rotates around the bend. Because this occurs with each revolution, the image remains stationary but various image sectors are compressed or expanded. Intracoronary catheters also must have a high temporal resolution because of the rapid cardiac motion with systole and diastole. Most mechanical systems acquire images at 30 frames per second. The phased-array system acquires images at only 10 frames per second; it smooths the image visually by frame averaging. However, this still results in suboptimal image quality.

Ring-down artifact, which occurs in both mechanical and phased-array catheters, appears as a blurring or halo affect around the catheter that produces an image of the catheter that is slightly larger than its true size. This artifact arises from acoustic oscillations in the piezoelectric transducer material resulting in high-amplitude ultrasound signals that obscure the near-field image. The mechanical designs that use the rotating acoustical mirror have less ring-down artifact. By increasing the distance from the transducer to the vessel wall, the rotating mirror design confines the near-field distortion to the inside of the apparatus. The phased-array system is particularly prone to exhibit ring-down artifact, since the ultrasound elements are mounted on the surface of the catheter. To deal with this,

operators can digitally subtract the central portion of the image by collecting a reference image in a large vessel (i.e., aorta) before advancing the catheter into the target vessel. This procedure does not usually entirely eliminate the artifact.

ULTRASOUND APPEARANCE OF NORMAL VESSELS

To interpret abnormal coronary morphology accurately necessitates a good understanding of normal coronary structures as seen by ultrasound. However, there has been some degree of controversy regarding normal vessels' appearance on ultrasound. Early in vitro studies demonstrated a three-layer appearance in normal peripheral vessels with 20-MHz mechanical systems (7). Relatively bright intimal and adventitial signals were separated by a hypoechoic region corresponding histologically to the medial layer. Others have reported a monolayer appearance in normal arteries and medial thickening and subintimal plaque accumulation resulting in a three-layer appearance in abnormal arteries (8). Gussenhoven et al. compared in vitro ultrasound with histologic cross-sections from pressurized human necropsy specimens of both muscular and elastic arteries (9). The normal ultrasound pattern of the two types of arteries demonstrated a difference corresponding to the histologic differences of the medial layer. The media of a muscular artery composed of smooth muscle cells and practically devoid of elastin fibers was seen as a hypoechoic media with clear definition of the echogenic internal and external elastic lamina. The media of an elastic artery, in contrast, is largely composed of densely packed, concentrically arranged elastin fibers among smooth muscle cells. On ultrasound the regularly arranged elastin fibers produce significant acoustic backscatter comparable with that from the intima and adventitia, resulting in a monolayer appearance. Other investigators using 20- to 45-MHz devices confirmed that the normal ultrasound pattern depends on the relative content, density, and location of elastin and smooth muscle (10–12). Coronary arteries are generally muscular, with the exception of the proximal left main coronary artery, which is transitional.

Today's ultrasound catheters do not have the resolution to reveal the intima, which is only a few cell layers thick. Fitzgerald et al. (13) used a 30-MHz ultrasound catheter to image histologic sections of coronary arteries at autopsy of patients without a clinical history of coronary artery disease. Histologic analysis revealed significantly more intimal thickening in segments with three layers (243 plus or minus 105 mm) than in monolayer segments (112 plus or minus 55 mm). Young, nondiseased coronary vessels showed a monolayer appearance, and three layers were not observed in older, mildly diseased vessels until the intimal layer thickened sufficiently that the overall thickness became resolvable at 30 MHz (178 mm). Yet use of microsurgical and enzymatic dissection techniques demonstrated that the relatively broad echogenic intimal layer is predominantly caused by strong acoustical reflectance of the internal elastic lamina and does not correlate with the true width of the normal intima (12, 13). Angiographic studies of normal subjects aged 37 to 51 years demonstrated a discrete ultrasonic reflectance at the acoustic interface between the lumen and the intima averaging 180 plus or minus 60 mm wide at 25 of 33 sites; 8 sites showed a monolayer appearance (14). Much of the controversy surrounding the normal appearance of an artery stems from the use of different imaging systems with different degrees of resolution and variations between types of arteries and degree of disease. Most clinical investigators consider that there are two variants of "normal" ultrasound morphology: a monolayer appearance and a trilaminar structure with an intimal thickness less than 0.25 mm (Fig. 18.1).

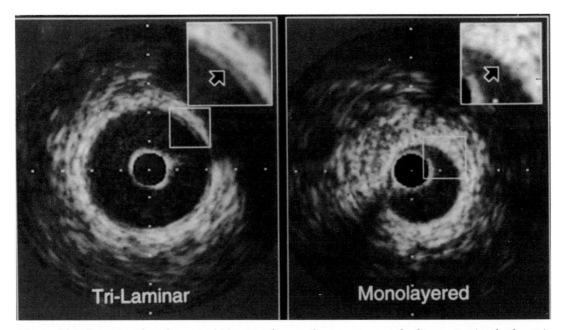

Figure 18.1. Intravascular ultrasound images of normal coronary vessels demonstrating both a trilaminar (**left panel**) and monolayered (**right panel**) appearances. Magnified **insets** show that the discrete intimal layer with subadjacent sonolucent zone seen in the trilaminar artery is absent in the monolayer artery. (Reprinted with permission from Nissen SE, Tuzcu EM, DeFranco AC, Moliterno DJ. Evaluating stenosis severity: quantitative angiography, coronary flow reserve, and IVUS. In: Ellis S, Holmes D Jr, eds. Strategic approaches in coronary intervention. Baltimore: Williams & Wilkins, 1996:207–234.)

ATHEROSCLEROTIC MORPHOLOGY

Validation of Morphologic Characterization

Appearance of atheromatous disease by IVUS depends on the extent of disease, tissue composition, eccentricity, and degree of fissuring or dissection. Most atherosclerotic plaques appear on ultrasound as varying degrees of intimal thickening separated from the adventitia by an echogenic internal elastic lamina and a sonolucent layer thought to represent remnants of the media. Because the **internal elastic lamina** is often disrupted and the media is destroyed at the base of large atherosclerotic plaques, the ultrasound image may not show a three-layer appearance (15, 16). Much of the early work with IVUS centered on the tissue characterization of plaque morphology as compared with histologic analysis. Although ultrasound does not record actual histologic images, it can often differentiate normal from fatty, fibrous, and calcified components within the vessel wall by detecting differences in acoustic properties of the tissues (9, 10, 15, 17). Areas within the intima that are hypoechoic correspond to deposits of lipids within the plaque on histologic section. A fibromuscular lesion, which contains smooth muscle cells and disorderly arranged elastin and collagen, is less echogenic then the more densely packed adventitia. These plaques on ultrasound are often termed **soft** (Fig. 18.2A). Dense fibrous or calcified tissue is seen as bright echogenic areas similar to the surrounding adventitia and is called **hard** plaque. However, unlike dense fibrous tissue, calcified tissue can be identified by characteristic acoustical **shadowing,** which obscures deeper structures such as the internal and external elastic lamina (Fig. 18.2B). Most plaques contain a variable amount of fibrous tissue and many have a mixed pattern, with an assortment of tissue components, including lipid or calcium deposits. A **dense fibrous cap** may sometimes be seen as a bright echoreflective layer overlying a fibromuscular plaque.

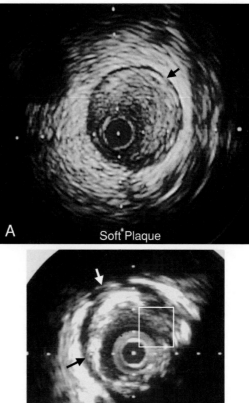

Figure 18.2. **A.** Soft plaque consistent with a fibromuscular lesion containing smooth muscle cells and disorderly arranged elastin and collagen. Note the inhomogeneous pattern which appears less echodense than the surrounding adventitia (*arrow*). **B.** Hard plaque with both dense fibrous (*black arrow*) and calcified (*white arrow*) components. Note the shadowing, or loss of echo reflectance deep to the calcified tissue compared with the dense fibrous tissue, where the underlying adventitia is still visible. This plaque also has a soft component adjacent to the calcium (*inside the box*).

Calcium deposits in atherosclerotic lesions occur in various forms, and IVUS is a sensitive technique to detect calcium in coronary arteries. Calcium deposits may be defined as either superficial or deep, depending on the location within the vessel wall relative to the lumen (Fig. 18.3). Compared with histologic sections, IVUS de-

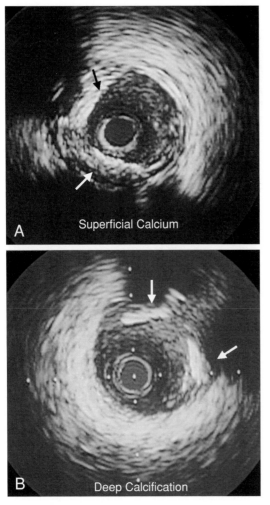

Figure 18.3. **A.** Superficial calcium adjacent to the vessel lumen with characteristic acoustic shadowing of the underlying structures (*arrows*). **B.** Calcium deeper within the atheromatous plaque. There is more superficial soft plaque adjacent to the lumen, as well as acoustical shadowing of underlying structures (*white arrows*).

tected dense calcification with a sensitivity of 90% and specificity of 100% (18). However, ultrasound has a much lower sensitivity for detecting microcalcification defined as small (less than 0.05 mm) calcium flecks. This is most likely because of the limited resolution of the 30-MHz catheter used in this study. Compared with electron beam computed tomography and histology, ultrasound also accurately quantitates cross-sectional area and volume of intralesional

calcium, especially if deep at the base of the plaque. Because of incomplete penetration of the ultrasound beam with subsequent signal drop-off, ultrasound is thought to underestimate the amount of calcium in lesions where the calcium is dense and superficial (19).

Unstable lesions are characterized histologically by intimal injury and fissuring with varying degrees of intraplaque and intraluminal thrombus formation (20). Pandian et al. (21) demonstrated the ability of IVUS to identify all intimal flaps created experimentally both in vitro and in vivo. In another study, in vitro ultrasound images accurately predicted the histologic presence or absence of tears in 11 of 13 arterial segments following balloon angioplasty (22). Two dissections were missed because the catheter tacked the flap against the vessel wall. Dissections appear as sonolucent communications between the lumen and adventitia with or without evidence of an intimal flap within the lumen (Fig. 18.4). In some cases the dissection plane can be difficult to differentiate from other hypoechoic structures beneath an atheromatous plaque. In this situation the smokelike appearance of moving blood within the sonolucent area can establish that this structure communicates with the vessel lumen. Intracoronary

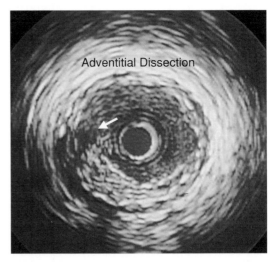

Figure 18.4. Adventitial dissection. *Arrow,* The sonolucent communication between the lumen and adventitia creating a small flap within the lumen.

injection of saline or iodinated contrast can increase the echogenicity of moving blood because of the microbubbles within the medium, and therefore such injection aids in the identification of a dissection. Siegel et al. (23) showed that IVUS had moderate sensitivity, 81%, for detecting intimal disruption by histology; the specificity, accuracy, and predictive values were greater than 90%.

IVUS was also accurate in detecting experimentally induced intraluminal thrombus in normal arteries without atheromatous disease (24). But when vessels with complex morphologic lesions were evaluated, IVUS had a lower sensitivity (57%) for detecting thrombus (23). One of the difficulties in interpreting the presence of thrombi by ultrasound is the varying echogenic patterns of thrombus. Intraluminal thrombus typically has a speckled echogenic pattern that is less dense than fibrous plaque but difficult to differentiate from adjacent fibromuscular plaque (25). IVUS demonstrated thrombus following myocardial infarction with a sensitivity of 84%, specificity of 71%, and predictive value of 89% when compared with atherectomy tissue samples (26). This compared favorably with angiography, which identified thrombus in only 27% of patients. In this study most thrombi were detected by ultrasound if studied less than 5 days after thrombolytic therapy. Thrombus had the characteristic speckled echogenic pattern often protruding into the lumen of the vessel but was rarely seen more than 5 days after thrombolytic therapy. Because of resorption into a fibrous structure, late thrombi appeared as linear structures close to the vessel wall and were difficult to differentiate from surrounding fibrous tissue.

Validation of Quantitative Measurements

IVUS can accurately quantitate normal and atherosclerotic vessel dimensions, including lesion and vessel wall thickness and plaque area, with minimal intraobserver and interobserver variability (r > 0.92) (17, 26, 27). Ultrasound measurements of luminal dimensions have been validated against phantom models and histologic measurements with correlation coefficients ranging from 0.85 to 0.98 for lumen cross-sectional area, diameter, and percent narrowing (9, 10, 17, 28, 29). Furthermore, necropsy studies have demonstrated a good correlation between ultrasound and direct histologic measurements of plaque thickness with less accuracy in measuring total wall thickness (9, 17, 28–31). Although the medial–adventitial border is frequently distinct, the penetration of current coronary ultrasound catheters is not high enough to image the true thickness of the adventitial layer except in the case of saphenous vein grafts, which do not have an extensive surrounding connective tissue. Furthermore, because of calcification-induced shadowing, plaque and total wall thickness cannot always be determined. Mallery et al. (30) found that the ultrasound measurements overestimated the mean intimal and mean total wall thickness by 0.3 and 0.7 mm, respectively, compared with histologic measurements. This is perhaps due to the strong echoreflectance of the internal elastic lamina and fibrous adventitia or artifactual shrinkage with histologic preparations. Measurement of plaque thickness requires the identification of a distinct medial layer that becomes thinner in association with atherosclerosis because of increased collagen content in the media (31, 32). Most investigators combine the inner echogenic and sonolucent layers in measuring plaque area. This correlates well with direct measurements (r > 0.96).

Clinical studies have demonstrated a close correlation between cineangiography and ultrasound measurements of lumen diameter (r = 0.98) and cross-sectional area (r = 0.96) in normal, nonatherosclerotic peripheral vessels. However, correlation between these two techniques decreased after balloon dilation (r = 0.86 and 0.81), reflecting an increase in measured vessel eccentricity (33–35). Clinical studies in patients with and without coronary artery disease demonstrate similar findings (14). In normal patients with circular coronary arteries on angiography, ultrasound measurement of luminal diameter closely correlates with angiographic diameter (r = 0.92). Correlation between angiographic and ultrasound assessment of lumen diameter was highest (r = 0.93) in patients with ultrasound evidence of concentric stenosis and was not as good in arteries with eccentric lesions (r = 0.77) . Similar findings are evident when comparing ultrasound with quantitative coronary angiography (34, 35). Angulation of the imaging catheter off the longitudinal axis of the vessel may cause an increase in ultrasound measurement of luminal area because of elliptical distortion of the image. However, the effect of eccentric catheter position on luminal measurements in small coronary vessels is probably not significant (35). The accuracy of IVUS in the assessment of luminal dimensions of saphenous vein grafts as large as 5 mm appears to be comparable with that for normal native coronary arteries (36).

DIAGNOSTIC APPLICATIONS

Detecting Angiographically Silent Disease

Necropsy studies demonstrate that coronary artery disease is frequently diffuse and underestimated by angiography (2, 3). Angiography produces longitudinal images of vessel lumens filled with contrast, and atherosclerosis is identified as defects in the planar silhouette. Diffuse concentric disease may be present without creating the typical peaks and valleys in the angiographic lumenogram. Eccentric stenoses may yield normal-appearing angiograms if the vessel is not imaged at the appropriate angle. However, vascular remodeling is perhaps the most important mechanism behind angiographically silent disease (37). Atherosclerosis develops within the vessel wall, and the artery compensates by enlarging. Because the circumference of the vessel wall expands within the external elastic lamina, the lumen area is conserved and appears normal angiographically as the atheroma accumulates. Encroachment of the plaque on the lumen occurs when arterial enlargement no longer keeps pace with increases in plaque size and is usually associated with more than 40% plaque burden (37).

IVUS confirms these findings in vivo, demonstrating more diffuse disease in coro-nary arteries than appreciated by angiography (38). Nissen et al. (14) reported that 81% of angiographically normal sites demonstrate vessel wall abnormalities by intracoronary ultrasound in patients brought to the catheterization laboratory for evaluation of chest pain. Patients studied before undergoing coronary intervention had ultrasound evidence of atheroma in 93% of angiographically "normal" reference sites. Compared with stenotic segments undergoing intervention, these angiographically silent lesions were more often eccentric, with soft, hypoechoic elements and less often had fibrotic or calcified components (39) (Fig. 18.5). Identification of angiographically silent disease with IVUS may have important implications for long-term prognosis, since cardiovascular morbidity and mortality correlate with total plaque burden and the eccentric, soft composition of these plaques may be associated with greater risk of rupture and thrombosis.

Nowhere is angiographically silent disease more evident than in the left main coronary artery. Measurements of the left main artery are the least accurate of any coronary segment analyzed by angiography. First of all, there is no reference segment. Second, foreshortening and superimposition on other branches often limit angiographic detection of left main stenoses on standard projections. IVUS has proved to be an excellent technique to evaluate left main disease. A very high percentage (89%) of patients with angiographically normal vessels have left main disease by ultrasound, including more than 40% area stenoses. This is despite a plaque burden that is comparable with that of angiographically abnormal left main coronary arteries (40, 41). The clinical implications of this are not yet well defined. Following 30 patients with angiographically silent or minimal coronary disease for a mean of 3 years, Burns et al. (42) identified an increased risk of cardiovascular events in patients with more than 20% area reduction of their left main artery by IVUS. As we have noted, this may just reflect more diffuse disease in the coronary arteries, and further studies are needed before revascularization recommendations can be based on ultrasound measurements of left main coronary disease. However, this information is im-

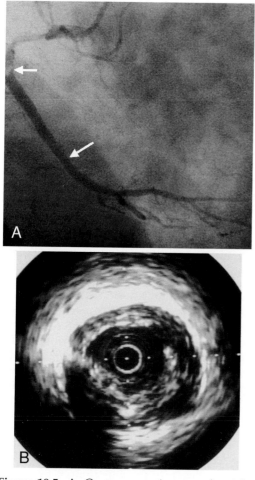

Figure 18.5. A. Coronary angiogram of a right coronary artery in the LAO projection demonstrating an ulcerated plaque with overhanging edges (*large arrow*). **B.** Ultrasound imaging before intervention demonstrates significant concentric soft plaque in the distal artery that was not apparent by angiography (*small arrow*).

Assessing Disease Severity

Decisions regarding revascularization are usually based on angiographic determination of percent luminal diameter reduction compared with a "normal" reference segment. The hemodynamic significance of a moderate angiographic stenosis ranging from 40 to 70% diameter narrowing is often not clear. Undetected diffuse disease in the reference segment can lead to an underestimation of lesion severity. Although IVUS does not directly assess hemodynamic significance of a stenosis, as does Doppler analysis or nuclear scintigraphy, it can help to determine the true anatomic severity of stenoses. In addition to preventing underestimation of stenosis by recognizing reference segment disease, **IVUS can also prevent overestimation of atherosclerotic disease** in aneurysmal arteries (43). Tomographic imaging is especially useful for evaluating the severity of ostial or bifurcating stenoses that are difficult to assess by angiography because of catheter tip location or vessel superimposition. Although IVUS appears useful for clinical decision making, including decisions about revascularization, no prospective data assess this use of IVUS. One retrospective analysis supports this approach, finding a low frequency (10%) of target lesion revascularization at 1 year when plans for interventions were abandoned as a result of ultrasound assessment of severity. The threshold for intervention in this study was a lumen area less than 3.5 mm^2 for native coronary lesions or less than 5 mm^2 for vein graft or left main lesions (44).

portant to the cardiologist planning percutaneous revascularization for an artery within the left coronary system. Guide catheter selection and techniques to avoid trauma to the diseased left main artery may be altered. On several occasions, we have elected to forgo percutaneous revascularization altogether for coronary artery bypass surgery when significant left main disease identified by ultrasound was thought to interfere with guide catheter or balloon placement.

Transplant Vasculopathy

Early stages of allograft vasculopathy are characterized histologically by diffuse homogeneous and concentric intimal proliferation of smooth muscle and collagen. Because of the diffuse and concentric nature of allograft vasculopathy, it often eludes early detection by angiographic lumenograms (45). IVUS, which provides detailed images of the vessel wall, can detect and quantitate transplant coronary disease early in its course (46). Vascular disease was classified by the Stanford group according to intimal thickness and degree of vessel circumference involved: Class 0, no measurable intimal layer; Class I (minimal), an initial thickness less than 0.3 mm involving less than 180°; Class II (mild), an intimal thickness less than 0.3 mm but extending more than 180°; Class III (moderate), an intimal layer 0.3 to 0.5 mm thick or an intimal layer more than 0.5 mm thick involving less than 180° of vessel circumference; and Class IV (severe), more than 0.5 mm involving less than 180° or more than 1 mm in any area of the vessel.

Although most patients have normal ultrasound appearance early (within a month) after transplant, up to 25% of donor hearts are transplanted with pre-existing coronary disease, and by 1 year, most patients demonstrate some degree of intimal thickening (47). Early studies, however, used large catheters with poor tractability, limiting examinations to the proximal segments of a single large epicardial vessel. Smaller catheters with better handling characteristics permit more extensive evaluations of the coronary tree. In contrast to histopathologic findings, recent IVUS studies have demonstrated a more heterogeneous pattern identifying a higher incidence of Class III or IV intimal thickening in proximal segments than in more distal segments (48). Thus analysis of a limited number of segments may misrepresent the degree of disease. Recently an observational study reported ultrasound data in 132 patients 1 to 9 years after transplantation. Again, the proximal segments had the highest prevalence of disease, and more than half the segments analyzed had focal rather than diffuse disease. This pattern of disease was irrespective of time from transplantation. In accordance with these results, it was proposed that transplant coronary disease has two causes; the diffuse and circumferential involvement seen in the mid and distal segments is consistent with immune-mediated allograft vasculopathy, and the focal disease seen proximally is consistent with pre-existing atherosclerosis (49). The early detection of vasculopathy in the transplant population using ultrasound imaging will assist in the assessment of treatment strategies.

INTERVENTIONAL APPLICATIONS

Preinterventional Lesion Assessment

Perhaps the greatest clinical benefit of IVUS is in interventional cardiology. IVUS is used to evaluate vessel morphology before and after intervention, to assist in device selection and sizing, and to guide interventional therapy. With the advent of newer catheter techniques designed to remove or ablate plaque, ultrasound assessment of plaque composition, distribution, and depth promises to have clinical utility in guiding such therapy.

Because of vascular remodeling, the plaque burden and true vessel diameter at the target site are much greater than suggested by the angiographic reference segment. Since operators size the catheter device according to the reference segment's diameter, coronary intervention using angiography alone may be too conservative. **IVUS accurately measures lumen, plaque thickness, and vessel wall size, enabling accurate sizing of interventional devices.** Other important IVUS findings that may affect the clinical success of an intervention include the location and degree of lesion calcification, degree of lesion eccentricity, intimal dissections, and thrombus. Certain devices may be better suited to treat lesions with particular plaque compositions and distributions than others. IVUS provides a unique opportunity to identify different mechanisms of lumen enlargement and clinical outcome amongst the different catheter techniques. Understanding the mechanisms of the available techniques allows interventionalists to tailor the therapy to the plaque's composition and character.

Balloon angioplasty is a nondirectional technique, and factors such as differences in plaque thickness and composition may cause an unequal transmission of forces to the vessel wall, resulting in a geometric distortion of that wall. Necropsy studies have indicated five possible mechanisms for balloon angioplasty: (*a*) plaque compression, (*b*) focal plaque **fracture** or **splitting,** (*c*) stretching of coronary segments without plaque damaging, (*d*) focal plaque rupture with localized dissection, and (*e*) stretching of the plaque-free wall in eccentric lesions (43, 50). Eccentric plaques with a disease-free wall are mainly dilated by local wall stretching, and concentric plaques are mainly dilated by compression or fracturing (43, 50). Ultrasound studies indicate that lumen enlargement with balloon dilation is a result of combined dissection, arterial expansion, and axial plaque redistribution (51, 52). Ultrasound data also confirm that disease-free wall has considerable effect on the mechanisms of lumen enlargement. Compared with stenoses without a disease-free wall, stenotic segments with a disease-free wall are associated with significantly lower lumen gains after balloon dilation, and this lumen enlargement is mainly obtained by wall stretch (52). This may increase restenosis because of **late relaxation,** and these lesions may be better treated with directional atherectomy and/or stenting. IVUS showed this phenomenon to be specifically related to the presence of a disease-free wall rather than to eccentricity alone, and there is a significant discordance between angiography and IVUS in assessing plaque distribution. One study of 1446 target lesions showed that while 55% of target lesions were eccentric by angiography, only 15% of target sites had an arc of normal arterial wall within the lesion by ultrasound (53).

Calcium is thought to increase shear forces during balloon inflation and increase the likelihood of dissection (54). IVUS studies indeed demonstrate that arterial dissection occurs more frequently at the site of angioplasty in calcified plaques, and arterial expansion occurs more frequently in noncalcified plaques (54–56). In more than 80% of cases dissections were adjacent to the calcific portion of the vessel wall (57). Moreover, the juxtaposition of soft plaque to calcified plaque is the most important independent predictor of angiographic dissection following balloon angioplasty (58). Angiography, however, detects less than 50% of the target lesion's calcification seen with IVUS (55, 56, 58–60). IVUS's greatest benefit is in assessing the precise location

and extent of target lesion calcification when there is angiographic evidence of calcium elsewhere in the coronary tree. In the absence of visible calcium anywhere in the coronary tree, there is a relatively low likelihood of a target lesion with more than 90° of superficial calcification (60).

Directional atherectomy has been particularly successful in the treatment of eccentric lesions as well as in lesions with intimal flaps, thrombus, or ulceration (61, 62). Unlike balloon angioplasty, most lumen enlargement with directional coronary atherectomy comes from a reduction in plaque, with a minor contribution of vessel expansion (63, 64). Both stretch and dissection are uncommon after atherectomy. However, the degree of plaque removal and final lumen area are limited by the extent of superficial calcification. Lesions with at least 90° arc of superficial calcification identified by IVUS had significantly greater residual plaque and smaller residual lumens than lesions with either less than 90° arc of calcium or no calcium (65). Rotational atherectomy, by contrast, preferentially removes atherosclerotic plaque composed of fibrous and calcific elements without extensive plaque disruption or arterial expansion (66, 67). Others have suggested that excimer laser coronary angioplasty may be effective treatment for long, calcified stenoses (68).

With the development of smaller ultrasound catheters and sheaths to protect the surface of the vessel, preoperative IVUS imaging is safe and feasible in most patients undergoing percutaneous revascularization. IVUS assessment of reference segment disease, lesion calcification, eccentricity, luminal flaps, and thrombus can aid the interventionalist in selecting and sizing the appropriate device for each individual target lesion (69). Lesions with significant superficial calcium may be better treated with rotational atherectomy or excimer laser angioplasty, and eccentric lesions free from significant superficial calcification may be better treated with directional atherectomy or stenting. Dissections and true aneurysms can be treated with stent placement even if calcified. Thrombus-containing lesions may require adjunctive treatment with thrombolytic or platelet-inhibiting agents. A lesion that appears hazy on angiogram may be su-

perimposed thrombus, dissection, or calcium and often cannot be differentiated by
angiography alone. The exact cause of the
hazy appearance can determine the success
or failure of a particular therapeutic approach. A number of lesion characteristics
that can affect the success of an intervention
cannot be determined by ultrasound, such
as side branch compromise, angulation, tortuosity, and collateral supply. Obviously,
IVUS imaging before intervention is useful
only in centers that have alternatives to balloon angioplasty. Finally, it is important to
realize that no prospective data look at early
and late outcome using this strategic approach, and crossing a stenosis with a catheter is not without risks.

Assessment of Results of Intervention

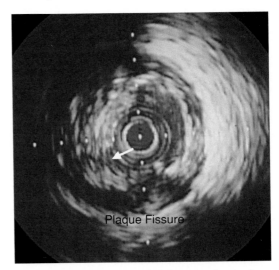

Figure 18.6. After successful angioplasty ultrasound demonstrates plaque fissuring that extends to but does not include the media (*arrow*).
Compare with Figure 18.4, which demonstrates
a type C pattern of dissection.

Plaque disruption, dissection, and residual
flaps were readily identified after angioplasty in vitro with tomographic ultrasound
imaging (20). Honye et al. (69) described six
morphologic patterns after angioplasty as
seen by ultrasound. Type A consists of a
linear partial tear of the plaque from the
lumen toward the media. Type B appears
as a split in the plaque that extends to the
media but does not include it (Fig. 18.6).
Type C demonstrates a dissection behind
the plaque that subtends an arc of up to 180°
around the circumference. Type D is a more
extensive dissection that encompasses an
arc of more than 180°. Type E is defined as
plaque without evidence of a fracture or dissection and may be either concentric (E_1) or
eccentric (E_2). Only 59% of type C or D dissections following angioplasty were identified by angiography. However, 23% of angiographic dissections were not apparent
by ultrasound, presumably because of a
stenting effect of the imaging catheter itself
in relatively small vessels. Also, severe calcium may interfere with identification of
dissections because of the poor penetration
of ultrasound signals. Thus IVUS has moderate sensitivity for detecting postangioplasty dissections, appearing to be more
sensitive than angiography alone (55, 70).

Although angiographic detection of dissection is considered a significant predictor of
ischemic outcome after percutaneous transluminal coronary angioplasty (PTCA), it remains to be determined whether ultrasound
detection will improve either acute or long-
term outcome. In some studies with small
numbers, ultrasound detection of major dissection is associated with restenosis but
minor dissections or fractures are not (71,
72). However, larger studies do not demonstrate such an association (70, 73–75).

In addition to evaluating morphologic
outcome following coronary intervention,
IVUS is particularly useful for quantitative
assessment of outcomes of interventions.
Although lumen dimensions measured by
ultrasound and angiography closely correlate in normal vessels, the correlation between these two techniques diverges as the
lumen becomes more irregular and eccentric (14, 33). The fractures and dissections
created with angioplasty can fill with contrast dye and "normalize" the angiographic
silhouette even on orthogonal views. Studies have shown that angiography commonly overestimates the residual lumen
size following balloon angioplasty (15, 22,
70). However, the comparison between an-

giographic and ultrasound lumen dimensions varies with the interventional device. Like conventional balloon angioplasty, atherectomy results in considerable angiographic overestimation of postprocedural lumen size, while rotational atherectomy results in less overestimation (76). This is not due to improved plaque removal with rotablation but probably due to the creation of a more nearly circular lumen than with balloon angioplasty or directional atherectomy. Since ultrasound measurements correlate with direct measurements from histologic cross-sections and angiography does not, IVUS most likely provides a more accurate assessment of lumen size post intervention.

Interestingly, despite results showing residual diameter stenoses 15 to 25% by angiography following coronary intervention, plaque burden is often more than 50% of the vessel's area by IVUS assessment (23, 52) (Fig. 18.7). This is true not only with conventional balloon angioplasty but also with plaque-removing devices such as directional or rotational atherectomy (63–67). Perhaps the underestimation of residual plaque burden by angiography explains the inability to predict clinical outcome from angiographic results. Thus far, only a few

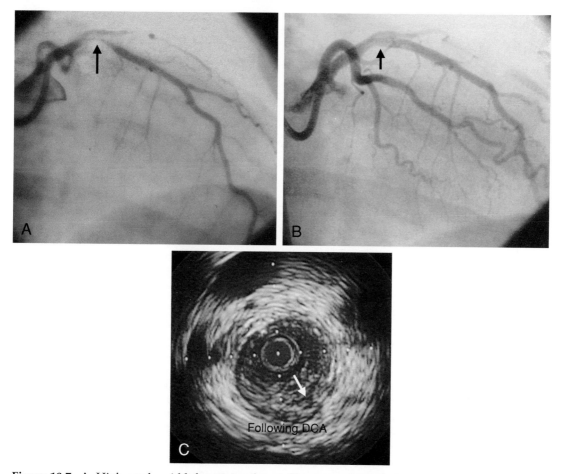

Figure 18.7. **A.** High-grade mid left anterior descending artery stenosis (*arrow*) in an RAO projection with cranial angulation. **B.** After directional coronary atherectomy a 10% residual narrowing was observed in its most severe projection (*arrow*). **C.** However, ultrasound imaging after the intervention reveals significant plaque burden encroaching upon the lumen. The small divot (*arrow*) created by the atherectomy cutter was enough to account for the improvement seen in the angiographic silhouette.

retrospective studies of small numbers of patients have looked at ultrasound predictors of clinical outcome. In an observational study by Jain et al. (72) the absence of plaque fracture, the existence of a major dissection, and residual plaque burden more than 40% of vessel area were associated with restenosis. More recently a large retrospective analysis was reported for 360 patients with 91% angiographic follow-up data. In this study the most consistent and powerful predictor of restenosis was the postintervention IVUS assessment of percent cross-sectional area narrowing, an index of plaque burden (73). Interim analysis from the Guidance by Ultrasound Imaging for Decision Endpoints (GUIDE) Trial, a prospective multicenter study designed to identify morphologic predictors of restenosis via IVUS, agrees that residual plaque burden is the most significant predictor and that angiographic predictors are not significant (74). Nevertheless, prospective studies are needed to determine whether additional intervention to maximize ultrasound end points will lead to a decrease in frequency of restenosis. An overaggressive approach may result in excessive vessel trauma and actually increase the incidence of restenosis or acute procedural complications. Several trials now under way are to determine whether ultrasound-guided therapy will improve clinical outcome in angioplasty, DCA, and rotational atherectomy.

Stent Deployment

It has been hypothesized that underdeployment of stents is responsible for the high rate of stent thrombosis. Studies show that stents were not adequately deployed with standard techniques (77–79). IVUS revealed that stents were asymmetrically and incompletely deployed, with nonuniform apposition of stent struts against the vessel wall (Fig. 18.8). Also, the average residual lumen area was 51% compared with the reference segment despite good angiographic results. Because of the nature of the coil or tubular slotted designs of today's stents, radiographic contrast material can surround the stent, producing an angiographic appear-

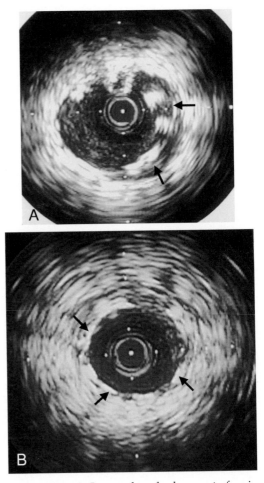

Figure 18.8. A. Incomplete deployment of an intracoronary Palmaz-Schatz stent demonstrating inadequate apposition of stent struts against the vessel wall, leaving a visible space between wall and struts (*arrows*). **B.** Optimal stent deployment of an intracoronary Palmaz-Schatz stent. *Arrows,* Flattened appearance of stent struts against the vessel wall.

ance of a large lumen although the struts do not make contact with the vessel wall. One large observational study has shown that ultrasound-guided high-pressure inflation using noncompliant balloons is associated with a lower thrombosis rate (0.3%) despite use of antiplatelet therapy only with no systematic anticoagulation (79). A number of other anecdotal studies have produced similar findings, prompting interventionalists to use high-pressure inflation following stent deployment with less anti-coagulation.

Ultrasound criteria commonly employed for optimal stent deployment include (*a*) minimal lumen cross-sectional area more than 80% the average reference segment area (proximal reference area minus distal reference area, or more than 100% distal reference area) (*b*) good apposition of struts against the vessel wall so that no space separates the stent and vessel (*c*) no dissection at the stent margins, and (*d*) circular or symmetric stent expansion. This last criterion has been abandoned by many operators, since it is difficult to change with current optimization techniques. Whether or not IVUS guidance is required to achieve optimal results with use of high-pressure inflation is extremely controversial. High-pressure inflation following stent deployment under angiographic guidance alone does not achieve optimal stent expansion in more than 50% cases, and further ultrasound-guided high-pressure dilations can improve expansion (80–81). However, it is not apparent that further stent expansion based on ultrasound findings will improve clinical outcome. Two prospective multicenter trials evaluating the usefulness of ultrasound in optimizing stent deployment are now under way. Interim analysis from the AVID trial, a prospective randomized multicenter trial comparing IVUS-directed stent placement with angiography-directed placement, shows no significant difference in the 30-day clinical event rate between the two treatments (82). Long-term outcome data on restenosis rates are still pending.

SAFETY

IVUS can be performed safely in the hands of cardiologists trained in interventions. In the setting of a severe stenosis the catheter can obstruct flow and cause myocardial ischemia, but this is usually relieved promptly upon withdrawal of the catheter into the guide. In a multicenter survey of 2207 IVUS studies, ultrasound was associated with minimal acute complications (83). The most common complication, transient spasm relieved with nitroglycerin, occurred in 2.9% of the patients. There was less than 1% major complication rate, including acute occlusion, embolism, dissection, thrombus, and myocardial infarction possibly related to ultrasound imaging. These major complications usually occurred in patients with acute coronary syndromes undergoing therapeutic intervention. Most operators administer systemic heparin (5000 to 10,000 IU) prior to coronary instrumentation. Despite the low complication rate, it is our opinion that only practitioners trained in interventional cardiology should perform intracoronary ultrasound imaging. In the event of a complication from intimal disruption, an interventional cardiologist can manage the problem effectively. Because of the possibility of endothelial denudation with the catheter, there has been some concern regarding the possibility of accelerating atherosclerosis, especially in patients in whom ultrasound is used for diagnostic purposes only. To date only one retrospective study has looked at the long-term safety of ultrasound imaging. Serial quantitative angiographic analysis of 49 vessels imaged with a 5-F device were compared with 61 matched vessels not previously imaged. A year after ultrasound imaging there was no difference in diameter change between the imaged and nonimaged vessels, suggesting that atherosclerosis is not accelerated by the device (84).

FUTURE OF INTRAVASCULAR ULTRASOUND

Advancements in catheter designs are being made. A combined phased-array imaging transducer and balloon catheter has already been approved by the Food and Drug Administration and is being studied in a multicenter trial (85). This design would reduce the number of catheter exchanges needed. Further modifications may allow for controlled pressure inflations as the operator watches the plaque crack. An atherectomy device has a single transducer in the body of the cutter so as to directly image the area of plaque being cut. Experimental studies have shown encouraging potential for aggressive debulking without significant subintimal injury (86). On the horizon is an imaging guidewire analogous to the Doppler-tipped guidewire now on the market. If the technical issues, such as miniaturizing the transducer without impairing the resolution, are solved, this will be a great advancement. Very few lesions would be unsuitable for imaging, and there would be less potential for intimal injury at a tight stenosis. Forward-viewing catheters in early development would enable visualization of total occlusions and avoid crossing the lesion with a catheter altogether (87).

Three-dimensional imaging is another advance in technology (88). With the aid of a motorized device that slowly pulls back the ultrasound transducer at a constant speed, two-dimensional slices can be reconstructed into three-dimensional images with special computer software. This would reveal the plaque composition throughout the length of the target lesion, evaluate stent expansion, or accurately calculate plaque volume. One of the major limitations at present is that the three-dimensional image is reconstructed as a straight vessel even if the actual vessel is tortuous. Other future directions include automated border detection and improved vessel wall boundary detection using sonicated contrast agents. Investigators are developing software to process radiofrequency backscatter sounds for tissue characterization and in vivo bioassay of plaque. In experimental studies this technique has improved the ability of ultrasound to differentiate soft plaque from thrombus (89). This could have a tremendous influence on our understanding of the pathophysiology of atherosclerosis and response to therapy.

The ability to predict clinical outcome and which lesions are prone to rupture will be the most important advancement in ultrasound imaging. There is a significantly greater frequency of soft plaque in patients with unstable angina, and hard plaque was more frequently seen in patients with stable angina (90). This correlates with pathologic studies showing that rupture-prone atherosclerotic lesions tend to be cholesterol rich with a thin overlying fibrous cap (20). This type of plaque may be best treated with lipid lowering or other plaque regression therapy, while the harder plaques may be better suited for revascularization. However, prospective data are needed to determine the usefulness of IVUS in predicting unstable lesions.

SUMMARY

While IVUS has been well validated in both experimental and research settings, its clinical usefulness is still emerging. Prospective clinical trials are needed to improve our knowledge of coronary atherosclerosis and define how IVUS will improve the success of coronary interventions and clinical outcome.

References

1. Zir L, Miller S, Dinsmore R, et al. Interobserver variability in coronary angiography. Circulation 1976;53:627–632.
2. Arnett EN, Isner JM, Redwood CR, et al. Coronary artery narrowing in coronary heart disease: comparison of cineangiographic and necropsy findings. Ann Intern Med 1979;91:350–356.
3. Grodin CM, Dydra I, Pastgernac A, et al. Discrepancies between cineangiographic and post-mortem findings in patients with coronary artery disease and recent myocardial revascularization. Circulation 1974;49:703–709.
4. Crowley RJ, von Behren PL, Couvillon LA, et al. Optimized ultrasound imaging catheters for use in the vascular system. Int J Cardiac Imag 1989;4:145–151.
5. Martin RW, Johnson CC. Design characteristics for intravascular ultrasound catheters. Int J Cardiac Imag 1989;4:201–216.
6. TenHoff H, Korbijn A, Smit THH, et al. Image artifacts in mechanically driven ultrasound catheters. Int J Cardiac Imag 1989;4:195–199.
7. Yock PG, Linker DT, Angelsen BAJ, Tech D. Two-dimensional intravascular ultrasound: technical development and initial clinical experience. J Am Soc Echo 1989;2:296–304.
8. Graham SP, Brands D, Savakus A, Hodgson JMcB. Utility of an intravascular ultrasound imaging device for arterial wall definition and atherectomy guidance. J Am Coll Cardiol 1989;13:222A (abstract).
9. Gussenhoven EJ, Essed CE, Lancee CT, et al. Arterial wall characteristics determined by intravascular ultrasound imaging: an in vitro study. J Am Coll Cardiol 1989;14:947–952.

10. Nishimura RA, Edwards WD, Warnes CA, et al. Intravascular ultrasound imaging: in-vitro validation and pathologic correlation. J Am Coll Cardiol 1990;16:145–154.

11. Lockwood GR, Ryan LK, Gotleb AI, et al. In vitro high resolution intravascular imaging in muscular and elastic arteries. J Am Coll Cardiol 1992; 20:153–160.

12. Siegel RJ, Chae JS, Maurer G, et al. Histopathologic correlation of the three-layered intravascular ultrasound appearance of normal adult human muscular arteries. Am Heart J 1993;126:872–878.

13. Fitzgerald PJ, St. Goar FG, Connolly AJ, et al. Intravascular ultrasound imaging of coronary arteries: is three layers the norm? Circulation 1992; 86:154–158.

14. Nissen SE, Gurley JC, Grines CL, et al. Intravascular ultrasound assessment of lumen size and wall morphology in normal subjects and patients with coronary disease. Circulation 1991;84:1087–1099.

15. Tobis JM, Mallery J, Mahon D, et al. Intravascular ultrasound imaging of human coronary arteries in vivo: analysis of tissue characterizations with comparison to in vitro histological specimens. Circulation 1991;83:913–926.

16. Maheswaran B, Leung CY, Gutfinger DE, et al. Intravascular ultrasound appearance of normal and mildly diseased coronary arteries: correlation with histologic specimens. Am Heart J 1995;130: 76–986.

17. Potkin BN, Bartorelli AL, Gessert JM, et al. Coronary artery imaging with intravascular high-frequency ultrasound. Circulation 1990; 81:1575–1585.

18. Friedrich GJ, Moes NY, Mühlberger, et al. Detection of intralesional calcium by intracoronary ultrasound depends on the histologic pattern. Am Heart J 1994;128:435–441.

19. Gutfinger DE, Leung CY, Hiro T, et al. In vitro atherosclerotic plaque and calcium quantitation by intravascular ultrasound and electron-beam computed tomography. Am Heart J 1996;131:899–906.

20. Davies MJ. A macro and micro view of coronary vascular insult in ischemic heart disease. Circulation 1990;82 (suppl II):II38–II46.

21. Pandian NG, Kreis A, Brockway B, et al. Intravascular high frequency two-dimensional ultrasound detection of arterial dissection and intimal flaps. Am J Cardiol 1990;65:1278–1280.

22. Tobis JM, Mallery JA, Gessert J, et al. Intravascular ultrasound cross-sectional arterial imaging before and after balloon angioplasty in vitro. Circulation 1989;80:873–882.

23. Siegel RJ, Ariani M, Fishbein MC, et al. Histopathologic validation of angioscopy and intravascular ultrasound. Circulation 1991;84:109–117.

24. Pandian NG, Kreis A, Brockway B. Detection of intraarterial thrombus by intravascular high frequency two-dimensional ultrasound imaging in vitro and in vivo studies. Am J Cardiol 1990; 65:1280–1283.

25. Frimerman A, Miller H, Hallman M, et al. Intravascular ultrasound characterization of thrombi of different composition. Am J Cardiol 1994;73: 1053–1057.

26. Chemarin-Alibelli MJ, Pieraggi MT, Elbaz M, et al. Identification of coronary thrombus after myocardial infarction by intracoronary ultrasound compared with histology of tissues sampled by atherectomy. Am J Cardiol 1996;77:344–349.

27. Hausmann D, Lundkuist AJS, Friedrich GJ, et al. Intracoronary ultrasound imaging: intraobserver and interobserver variability of morphometric measurements. Am Heart J 1994;128:674–680.

28. Pandian NG, Kreis A, Brockway B, et al. Ultrasound angioscopy: real-time, two-dimensional, intraluminal ultrasound imaging of blood vessels. Am J Cardiol 1988;62:493–494.

29. Hodgson JMcB, Graham SP, Savakus AD, et al. Clinical percutaneous imaging of coronary anatomy using an over-the-wire ultrasound catheter system. Int J Cardiac Imag 1989;4:187–193.

30. Mallery JA, Tobis JM, Griffith J, et al. Assessment of normal and atherosclerotic arterial wall thickness with an intravascular ultrasound imaging catheter. Am Heart J 1990;119:1392–1400.

31. Gussenhoven EJ, Frietman PAV, The SHK, et al. Assessment of medial thinning in atherosclerosis by intravascular ultrasound. Am J Cardiol 1991; 68:1625–1632.

32. Porter TR, Radio SJ, Anderson JA, et al. Composition of coronary atherosclerotic plaque in the intima and media affects intravascular ultrasound measurements of intimal thickness. J Am Coll Cardiol 1994;23:1079–1084.

33. Nissen SE, Grines CL, Gurley JC, et al. Application of a new phased-array ultrasound imaging catheter in assessment of vascular dimensions: in vivo comparison to cineangiography. Circulation 1990; 81:660–666.

34. DeScheereder I, DeMan F, Herregods MC, et al. Intravascular ultrasound versus angiography for measurement of luminal diameters in normal and diseased coronary arteries. Am Heart J 1994; 127:243–251.

35. St. Goar FG, Pinto FJ, Alderman EL, et al. Intravascular ultrasound imaging of angiographically normal coronary arteries: an in vivo comparison with quantitative angiography. J Am Coll Cardiol 1991; 18:952–958.

36. Jain SP, Roubin GS, Nanda NC, et al. Intravascular ultrasound imaging of saphenous vein graft stenosis. Am J Cardiol 1992;69:133–136.

37. Glagov S, Wisenberg E, Zarins CK, et al. Compensatory enlargement of human atherosclerotic coronary arteries. N Engl J Med 1987;316:1371–1375.

38. Hermiller JB, Tenaglia A, Kisslo KB, et al. In vivo validation of compensatory enlargement of atherosclerotic coronary arteries. Am J Cardiol 1993; 71:665–668.

39. Mintz GS, Painter JA, Pichard AD, et al. Atherosclerosis in angiographically "normal" coronary artery reference segments: an intravascular ultrasound study with clinical correlations. J Am Coll Cardiol 1995;25:1479–1485.

40. Hermiller JB, Buller CE, Tenaglia AN, et al. Unrecognized left main coronary artery disease in patients undergoing interventional procedures. Am J Cardiol 1993;71:173–176.

41. Gerber TC, Erbel R, Görge G, et al. Extent of atherosclerosis and remodeling of the left main coronary

artery determined by intravascular ultrasound. Am J Cardiol 1994;73:666–671.

42. Burns WB, Hermiller JB, Kisslo K, et al. Prognostic significance of left main coronary artery disease detected by intravascular ultrasound. J Invest Cardiol 1995;7:119–121.

43. Waller BF. The eccentric coronary atherosclerotic plaque: morphologic observations and clinical relevance. Clin Cardiol 1989;12:14–20.

44. Mintz GS, Bucher TA, Kent KM, et al. Clinical outcomes of patients not undergoing coronary artery revascularization as a result of intravascular ultrasound imaging. J Am Coll Cardiol 1995;25:61A (abstract).

45. Johnson DE, Alderman EL, Schroeder JS, et al. Transplant coronary artery disease: histopathologic correlations with angiographic morphology. J Am Coll Cardiol 1991;17:449–457.

46. St. Goar FG, Pinto FJ, Alderman EL, et al. Intracoronary ultrasound in cardiac transplant recipients: in vivo evidence of "angiographically silent" intimal thickening. Circulation 1992;85:979–987.

47. St. Goar FG, Pinto FJ, Alderman EL, et al. Detection of coronary atherosclerosis in young adult hearts using intravascular ultrasound. Circulation 1992; 86:756–763.

48. Klauss V, Mudra H, U;aUberfuhr P, Theisen K. Intraindividual variability of cardiac allograft vasculopathy as assessed by intravascular ultrasound. Am J Cardiol 1995;76:463–466.

49. Tuzcu EM, DeFranco AC, Goormastic M, et al. Dichotomous pattern of coronary atherosclerosis 1 to 9 years after transplantation: insights from systematic intravascular ultrasound imaging. J Am Coll Cardiol 1996;27:839–846.

50. Waller BF. "Crackers, breakers, stretchers, drillers, scrapers, shavers, burners, welders and melters": the future treatment of atherosclerotic coronary artery disease? A clinical–morphologic assessment. J Am Coll Cardiol 1989;13:969–987.

51. Mintz GS, Pichard AD, Dent KM, et al. Axial plaque redistribution as a mechanism of percutaneous transluminal coronary angioplasty. Am J Cardiol 1996;77:427–430.

52. Baptista J, di Mario C, Ozaki Y, et al. Impact of plaque morphology and composition on the mechanisms of lumen enlargement using intracoronary ultrasound and quantitative angiography after balloon angioplasty. Am J Cardiol 1996;77:115–121.

53. Mintz GS, Popma JJ, Pichard AD, et al. Limitations of angiography in the assessment of plaque distribution in coronary artery disease: a systematic study of target lesion eccentricity in 1446 lesions. Circulation 1996;93:924–931.

54. Demer LL. Effect of calcification on in vivo mechanical response of rabbit arteries to balloon dilation. Circulation 1991;83:2083–2093.

55. Potkin BN, Keren G, Mintz GS, et al. Arterial responses to balloon coronary angioplasty: an intravascular ultrasound study. J Am Coll Cardiol 1992; 20:942–951.

56. Fitzgerald PJ, Ports TA, Yock PG. Contribution of localized calcium deposits to dissection after angioplasty: an observational study using intravascular ultrasound. Circulation 1992;86:64–70.

57. De Franco AC, Nissen SE, Tuzcu EM, et al. Ultrasound plaque morphology predicts major dissections following stand-alone and adjunctive balloon angioplasty. Circulation 1994;90 (suppl 2):I-59 (abstract).

58. Mintz GS, Popma JJ, Pichard AD, et al. Patterns of calcification in coronary artery disease: a statistical analysis of intravascular ultrasound and coronary angiography in 1155 lesions. Circulation 1995; 91:1959–1965.

59. Mintz GS, Kouek P, Pichard AD, et al. Target lesion calcification in coronary artery disease: an intravascular ultrasound study. J Am Coll Cardiol 1992; 20:1149–1155.

60. Tuzcu EM, Berkalp B, De Franco AC, et al. The dilemma of diagnosing coronary calcification: angiography versus intravascular ultrasound. J Am Coll Cardiol 1996;27:832–838.

61. Hinohara T, Rowe MH, Robertson GC, et al. Effect of lesion characteristics on outcome of directional coronary atherectomy. J Am Coll Cardiol 1991; 17:112–1120.

62. Ellis SG, De Cesare NB, Pinkerton CA, et al. Relation of stenosis morphology and clinical presentation to the procedural results of directional coronary atherectomy. Circulation 1991;84:644–653.

63. Braden GA, Herrington DM, Downes TR, et al. Qualitative and quantitative contrasts in the mechanisms of lumen enlargement by coronary balloon angioplasty and directional coronary atherectomy. J Am Coll Cardiol 1994;23:40–48.

64. Tenaglia AN, Buller CE, Kisslo DB, et al. Mechanisms of balloon angioplasty and directional coronary atherectomy as assessed by intracoronary ultrasound. J Am Coll Cardiol 1992;20:685–691.

65. Popma JJ, Mintz GS, Satler LF, et al. Clinical and angiographic outcome after directional coronary atherectomy: a qualitative and quantitative analysis using coronary arteriography and intravascular ultrasound. Am J Cardiol 1993;72:55E–64E.

66. Mintz GS, Potkin BN, Keren G, et al. Intravascular ultrasound evaluation of the effect of rotational atherectomy in obstructive atherosclerotic coronary artery disease. Circulation 1992;86: 1383–1393.

67. Kovach JA, Mintz GS, Pichard AD, et al. Sequential intravascular ultrasound characterization of the mechanisms of rotational atherectomy and adjunct balloon angioplasty. J Am Coll Cardiol 1993; 22:1024–1032.

68. Cook SL, Eigler NL, Shefer A, et al. Percutaneous excimer laser coronary angioplasty of lesions not ideal for balloon angioplasty. Circulation 1991; 84:632–643.

69. Mintz GS, Pichard AD, Kovach JA, et al. Impact of preintervention intravascular ultrasound imaging on transcatheter treatment strategies in coronary artery disease. Am J Cardiol 1994;73:423–430.

70. Honye J, Mahon DJ, Jain A, et al. Morphological effects of coronary balloon angioplasty in vivo assessed by intravascular ultrasound imaging. Circulation 1992;85:1012–1025.

71. Tenaglia AN, Buller CE, Kisslo KB, et al. Intracoronary ultrasound predictors of adverse outcomes after coronary artery interventions. J Am Coll Cardiol 1992;20:1385–1390.

72. Jain SP, Jain A, Collins TJ, et al. Predictors of reste-

nosis: a morphometric and quantitative evaluation by intravascular ultrasound. Am Heart J 1994; 128:664–673.

73. Mintz GS, Popma JJ, Pichard AD, et al. Intravascular ultrasound predictors of restenosis after percutaneous transcatheter coronary revascularization. J Am Coll Cardiol 1996;27:1678–1687.

74. The Guide Trial Investigators. IVUS-determined predictors of restenosis in PTCA and DCA: an interim report from the GUIDE Trial, phase II. Circulation 1994;90:I-23.

75. Feld S, Ganim M, Carell ES. Comparison of angioscopy, intravascular ultrasound imaging and quantitative coronary angiography in predicting clinical outcome after coronary intervention in high risk patients. J Am Coll Cardiol 1996; 28:97–105.

76. De Franco AC, Nissen SE, Tuzcu EM, Witlow PL. Incremental value of intravascular ultrasound during rotational coronary atherectomy. Cathet Cardiovasc Diagn 1996;3(suppl):23–33.

77. Nakamura S, Colombo A, Galglione S, et al. Intracoronary ultrasound observations during stent implantation. Circulation 1994;89:2026–2034.

78. Goldberg SL, Colombo A, Nakamura S, et al. Benefit of intracoronary ultrasound in the deployment of Plamaz-Schatz stents. J Am Coll Cardiol 1994; 24(4):996–1003.

79. Colombo A, Hall P, Nakamura S, et al. Intracoronary stenting without anticoagulation accomplished with intravascular ultrasound guidance. Circulation 1995;91:1676–1688.

80. Görge G, Haude M, Ge J, et al. Intravascular ultrasound after low and high inflation pressure coronary artery stent implantation. J Am Coll Cardiol 1995;26:725–730.

81. Goldberg SL, Hall P, Nakamura S, et al. Is there a benefit from intravascular ultrasound when high-pressure stent expansion is routinely performed prior to ultrasound imaging? J Am Coll Cardiol 1996;27(suppl):306A (abstract).

82. Russo RJ, Teirstein PS. Angiography versus intravascular ultrasound-directed stent placement. J Am Coll Cardiol 1996;27(suppl):306A (abstract).

83. Hausmann D, Erbel R, Alibelli-Chemarin MJ, et al. The safety of intracoronary ultrasound: a multicenter survey of 2207 examinations. Circulation 1995; 91:623–630.

84. Pinto FJ, St. Goar FG, Gao SZ, et al. Immediate and one-year safety of intracoronary ultrasonic imaging: evaluation with serial quantitative angiography. Circulation 1993;88(part 1):1709–1714.

85. Stone GW, St. Goar FG, Klette MA, et al. Clinical experience with a novel low-profile integrated coronary ultrasound–angioplasty catheter: implications for routine use. J Am Coll Cardiol 1993; 21(suppl):134A (abstract).

86. Fitzgerald PJ, Belef M, Connolly AJ, et al. Design and initial testing of an ultrasound-guided directional atherectomy device. Am Heart J 1995; 129:593–598.

87. Evans JL, Ng KH, Vonesh MJ, et al. Arterial imaging with a new forward-viewing intravascular ultrasound catheter: phase I initial studies. Circulation 1994;89:712–717.

88. Rossenfield K, Losordo DW, Ramaswamy K, et al. Three-dimensional reconstruction of human coronary and peripheral arteries from images recorded during two-dimensional intravascular ultrasound examination. Circulation 1991;84:1938–1956.

89. Metz JA, Preuss P, Komiyama N, et al. Discrimination between soft plaque and thrombus based on radiofrequency analysis of intravascular ultrasound. J Am Coll Cardiol 1996;27(suppl):200A (abstract).

90. Rasheed Q, Nair R, Sheehan H, Hodgson J McB. Correlation of intracoronary ultrasound plaque characteristics in atherosclerotic coronary artery disease patients with clinical variables. Am J Cardiol 1994;73:753–758.

19
Angioscopy for Interventional Cardiovascular Diagnosis

Joel D. Eisenberg, MD
Sergio Waxman, MD
George S. Abela, MSc, MD

INTRODUCTION

Angioscopy may be defined as the visualization of the inner surfaces of blood vessels by use of an optical instrument. Although it was first introduced over 80 years ago, its clinical application was limited until recently by use of large ridged instruments (1, 2). Technical improvements in the scope and the explosive growth of interventional cardiology have led to renewed interest in coronary angioscopy (3–7).

Miniaturization of angioscopes has been made possible by the availability of small flexible fiberoptic bundles. The flexible angioscope as a part of a catheter system provides a means of clearing the visual field from blood with a clear crystalloid solution. Also, the multichannel angioscope allows incorporation of a soft balloon occluder to maintain a clear field of view for long periods (about 1 minute). Most systems include several of these features to make percutaneous angioscopy feasible.

Angioscopy is a reliable method of the **direct visualization of gross intravascular pathomorphology** by a three-dimensional color image. Angioscopic images are magnified, greatly enhancing anatomic detail. This yields a large amount of information that at present is underused. Thus the dilemma for angioscopy has been how to use the information from the impressive images obtained. In addressing this issue, one must recognize that angioscopy has been perceived as a qualitative rather than a quantitative technique. This is unfortunate, since angioscopic images have a great abundance of data that can be used quantitatively and as a means to predict lesion behavior. This chapter describes angioscopic techniques that provide new insights into coronary pathophysiology and that may serve as an adjunct to the interventional cardiologist while still acknowledging angioscopy's limitations.

EQUIPMENT NEEDED TO PERFORM ANGIOSCOPY

The basic items required to perform angioscopy include an angioscope, a light source, a color video camera, a monitor, and a video recorder (Fig. 19.1). Other related materials are those used for routine angioplasty (8).

326

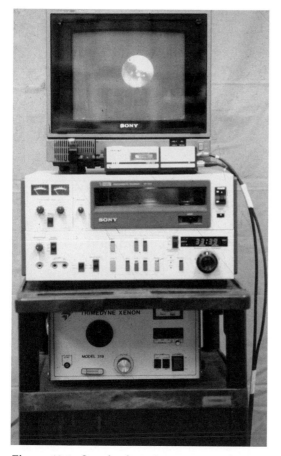

Figure 19.1. Standard angioscopy console. **Top to bottom.** A high-resolution monitor, a 0.75-inch video recorder, a color camera on top of the recorder, and a xenon light source below the top shelf. This system can be transported as a unit on a cart.

The Angioscope

The basic components of an angioscope are a fiberoptic imaging bundle composed of 3000 optical fibers, usually packed in a hexagonal pattern, and an illumination bundle. A **microlens** is placed at the tip of the imaging bundle to focus the light reflected from an object. The angle of view of these lenses is typically 55° in air and 45° in water. The depth of field, which is the ability of the lens to focus on two objects at different distances, is approximately 5 to 8 mm. The image bundle is 0.2 mm in diameter, and the final image on a 13-inch video monitor

screen is 75 mm, which is over 300× magnification. The focal length of the system is fixed and cannot be changed by the coupler adjustments.

The catheter that houses the fiberoptic elements is built specifically for the angioscope in the coronary circulation. This includes a relatively small (4 to 5 F) catheter and an occluder balloon and flush port to interrupt the blood flow and displace the blood column in the arterial lumen with an optically clear solution. The coronary guidewire provides not only the track for catheter advancement but also the coaxial position that aligns the lens to view the intraluminal area. This configuration allows visualization of a long segment (10 cm) of artery.

Various angioscopes and methods have been used to establish the three-dimensional video of the arterial lumen. Early studies were performed in the operating room, often during arterial bypass surgery (4, 6). Under these controlled and optimized conditions there is no blood flow, and residual blood requires minimal flushing and often causes no occlusion. Many of these angioscopes were large and bulky. Percutaneous methods required a balloon occluder proximal to the arterial segment being visualized, allowing for interruption and flushing of the blood to clear the field of view. In one system the angioscope ran over the wire and had a proximally occluding pressure-dependent balloon made of a percutaneous transluminal coronary angioplasty (PTCA) balloon material (9). This limited both the size of the artery examined (3-, 3.5-, and 4-mm balloons) and required several balloon inflations and deflations as the catheter was advanced down the artery. Moreover, it was time-consuming because it required an exchange over 300 cm of coronary wire. Subsequent advances (American Edwards) resolved this stepwise approach by allowing the optic bundle to track over the guidewire up to 5 to 10 cm beyond the catheter tip (10). And with the use of a single Silastic volume-dependent balloon occlusion, a column of saline solution can allow visualization of up to 10 cm of artery. Lastly, a monorail system allows for quicker exchanges (Fig. 19.2).

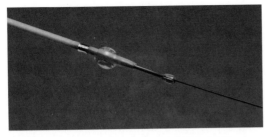

Figure 19.2. The distal part of the angioscope demonstrating a catheter shaft with a metallic marker proximal to a soft Silastic rubber balloon. There is an irrigation port at the tip of the catheter. Extending from the catheter tip are the imaging and illumination bundles, shown to be tracking a 0.014-inch guidewire that guides the optical system for viewing over several centimeters of artery.

Illumination Source, Coupler, Camera, and Video System

Most systems use a xenon cold lamp. The early systems employed a Karl Storz 487 with various color filters that improved image definition by reducing the halo generated by reflection of white light. The Baxter system, which is the most widely employed, uses an OPTX 300 xenon light. A fiberoptic cable is used to transmit the light from the source to the illumination bundle in the angioscope. A miniature color video camera (11.5 × 8.75 × 2.5 inches high) is used to generate the images with a focusing coupler. A high-resolution Sony video monitor and a 0.75-inch high-resolution video cassette recorder system complete the system. It is all mounted on a cart for mobility between catheterization suites.

The coupler takes the first step in the transfer of the image from the fiber to the monitor. It magnifies the image (7.5×) and focuses it on the camera's sensor surface. The image size is limited by the size of the charged couple device (CCD) and the brightness of the picture on the surface of the image bundle. The camera has a half-inch CCD format and an electronic shutter to eliminate the reflection of the white light that emanates from the very near filed tip of the angioscope. The camera resolution is specified as at least 300 horizontal and at least 300 vertical TV lines with a 5-lux sensitivity. Shutter speed is automatic (1/60; 1/100; 1/1000 of a second). The camera mount is a standard C-mount, and video connections are BNC.

PERCUTANEOUS CORONARY ANGIOSCOPY

Preparation of the Angioscope

The camera and light source are attached to the image fiber hub and light post, respectively. The angioscope is removed from the dispenser tube and the lens pointed at a white surface (i.e. a white 4 × 4) and the white balance button on the camera pressed. The power injector (Medrad) is set at a minimum of 0.5 mL per second, and the tube set is attached to the infusion port of the angioscope catheter. The flush fluid is typically either heparinized normal saline or lactated Ringer's solution warmed to 98°F by the Medrad warmer pad.

Insertion of Angioscope into the Patient

The insertion procedure, which is very similar to that of monorail balloon angioplasty, should be performed only by a physician competent in coronary angioplasty. The patient should be premedicated with soluble aspirin (325 mg) and systemically heparinized prior to advancement of the system. Before insertion a vacuum should be drawn at the balloon inflation port with a 3-mL syringe and the gate valve closed. Then a 1-mL syringe is filled with contrast agent, attached to the gate valve, and opened. The guidewire lumen is flushed with heparinized saline. The irrigating lumen is connected to the Medrad via tubing and a Y-connector and is also flushed with heparinized saline. The system should be devoid of air bubbles. An 8-F thin-walled catheter appropriate for the target vessel is advanced and the vessel engaged as in angioplasty. Nitroglycerin (50 to 200 μg) is injected into the coronary artery. A radiopaque 0.014-inch floppy tip coronary wire is advanced and positioned in the distal vessel. (The fully radiopaque wire allows for visualization of any buckling of the tip of the angioscope during its advancement.) The angioscope is then loaded onto the back of the coronary wire and advanced as a typical monorail balloon catheter. The inflation cuff on the angioscope is monitored by volume, not pressure, and overinflation must be avoided, with just enough fluid injected to prevent forward injection of contrast medium to be visualized beyond the inflated balloon (approximately 0.1 mL).

Imaging with the Angioscope

Imaging with the angioscope requires the tip to be in a coaxial position with the arterial lumen. Otherwise a whiteout on the screen will occur. This indicates that the angioscope tip is facing or is buried in the arterial wall. The angioscope is then pulled back and repositioned by manipulating the wire and catheter system. Thus the preferred quality of angioscopic images is often obtained on a pull-back viewing. The optimal time to limit the duration of ischemia during individual viewing is about 30 seconds. The average time added to the whole event by angioscopy is about 12 to 15 minutes.

INDICATIONS FOR ANGIOSCOPY

Assessment of Therapeutic Intervention

The accepted clinical indications for angioscopy include imaging of the target vessel both before and after intervention, including balloon and laser angioplasty (5, 9, 11) (Fig. 19.3), stent deployment (12) (Fig. 19.4), and lytic therapy (13) (Fig. 19.5). Characterization of the vascular obstruction may help in the selection of the appropriate interventional device. Angioscopy more clearly defines the nature of the luminal obstruction than does angiography. This is true especially for the detection and characterization of any thrombus, ulceration, and calcification within the lesion. Thrombus in the lesion is a relative contraindication to both stent deployment and rotational atherectomy. Expensive therapies such as intravenous administration of the monoclonal antiplatelet antibody agent abciximab (Reo-

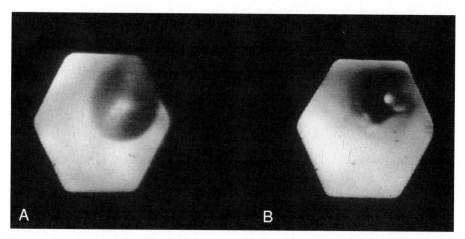

Figure 19.3. A. The 2-mm hybrid laser probe engaged in the center of a totally occluded femoral artery. The fiber tip is at the 5-o'clock position. The picture was taken at the initiation of laser activation. **B.** After laser recanalization a new vascular lumen appearing as a dark tunnel in the upper quadrant. The charred edges are due to the laser. (Reprinted with permission from Uchida Y. Percutaneous cardiovascular angioscopy. In: Abela GS, ed. Lasers in cardiovascular medicine and surgery. Norwell, MA: Kluwer Academic, 1990:399–410.)

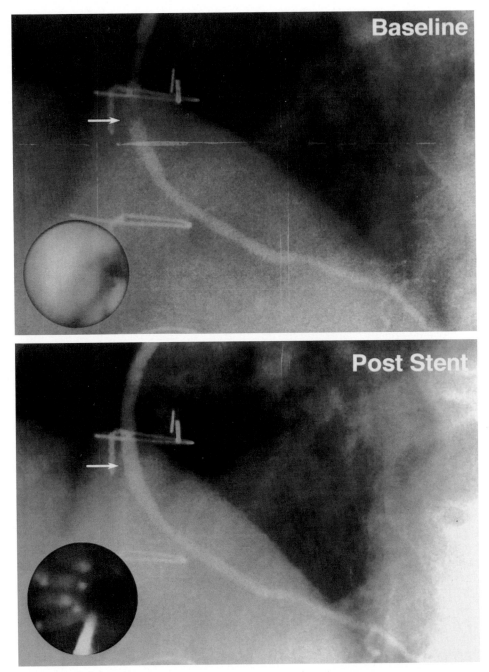

Figure 19.4. High-grade stenosis of saphenous vein graft to the right coronary. **Top.** Angiogram showing graft stenosis (*white arrow*) above the sternal wire. Angioscope insert demonstrates ruptured white plaque protruding into the lumen. **Bottom.** Angiogram showing widely patent graft (*white arrow*) following Palmaz (154 Biliary) stent deployment to 4 mm after 12 atmospheres. Angioscope insert shows typical scaffolding of the lumen, which is highlighted by the reflected light. (Courtesy of Dr. Christopher White, Dept of Invasive Cardiology, HCI International Medical Center, Clydebank, Scotland, UK.)

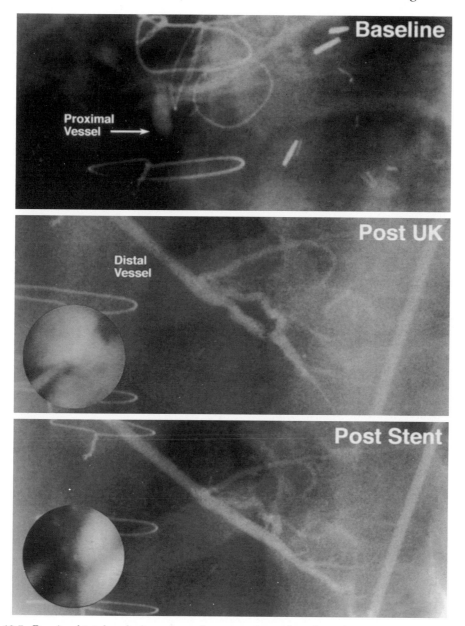

Figure 19.5. Proximal total occlusion of a saphenous vein graft to the right coronary. **Top.** Angiogram with proximal total cutoff of the contrast column. **Middle.** After 18 hours of urokinase infusion at 2000 units/minute an underlying lesion is seen in the native vessel. Angioscopy insert demonstrates a high-grade stenosis totally engulfing the guidewire. **Bottom.** After a Wiktor stent (3 mm) a widely patent vessel is seen by angiography and typical scaffolding noted by angioscopy. (Courtesy of Dr. Christopher White, Dept of Invasive Cardiology, HCI International Medical Center, Clydebank, Scotland, UK.)

Pro) may be more judiciously employed. The eccentricity and composition of the plaque may contribute to the decision to use directional and rotational atherectomy.

Angioscopy after intervention can identify **dissections, intraluminal flap dissections, the adequacy of stent deployment, and residual thrombus.**

Characterization of Lesions by Angiography Versus Angioscopy

The ability of angioscopy and angiography to evaluate the morphology of coronary lesions has been compared (14, 15). Manzo et al. tested it in 36 patients undergoing interventional procedures with the 4.5-F extendable coronary angioscope (15). Lesions were interpreted either angiographically or angioscopically by readers masked to the results of the other method. Angiographically lesions were categorized as a filling defect, a hazy lesion, or a smooth stenosis. The last two were considered thrombotic. According to these criteria 9 of 36 lesions were labeled as thrombotic by angiography. Lesions on angioscopy were characterized by both plaque morphology and the presence and type of thrombus identified. Thrombus was characterized as either red, when a gelatinous red material protruded into the lumen, or white, often billowing into the lumen from a disrupted intima. Plaque morphology was defined as either flat or elevated and further characterized by a pearly white or yellow color. By angioscopy 12 patients had thrombus. With angioscopy as the reference standard, angiography had a sensitivity of 67% and a specificity of 96% (Table 19.1). Teirstein et al. (16) in their series of 75 patients found an even lower sensitivity, 21%, but with a high specificity, 94%, for detection of thrombus by angiography as compared with angioscopy. Uretsky et al. (17) in a study of 40 patients found a sensitivity of 37% and a specificity of 100% for the angiographic detection of thrombus compared with an-

gioscopy. These three studies point to the relatively poor sensitivity of angiography for detection of thrombus. The importance of thrombus as a risk factor for both adverse outcome and restenosis has been stressed in recent studies (18, 19). Future trials with angioscopy should therefore focus on the influence of this technology on the acute management of thrombus and on long-term outcome with coronary intervention.

More recently Thieme et al. (20) validated angioscopic findings by histomorphologic analyses from specimens obtained by directional atherectomy. Gray-white plaque contained more fibrous tissue. Gray-yellow plaque was mixed and often degenerative. Deep yellow was soft degenerative atheroma. **Red and pink correlated well with the presence of thrombus.** The researchers also confirmed the tendency of yellow plaque (89% of specimens) to predominate in unstable angina, while stable patients had a more even distribution of white and yellow plaque.

Predictions of Procedural Outcomes

Since clinical and angiographic criteria have limited ability to predict adverse outcomes in patients with unstable angina, angioscopic characterization may provide some indicators. This was demonstrated in a study by Waxman et al. (21) in which angioscopy of the culprit lesion was performed in a high-risk group of 32 patients with unstable angina and 10 with non–Q-wave myocardial infarction. Plaque was

Table 19.1
Sensitivity and Specificity of Lesions By Angiography Versus Angioscopy

	Angioscopy Findings			
	Red Thrombus	White Thrombus	Plaque Only	Total
Angiography				
Filling defect	4	0	0	4
Hazy lesions	0	4	1	5
Smooth stenosis	0	4	23	27
Total	4	8	24	36

Adapted from Manzo K, Nesto R, Sassower M, et al. Coronary lesion morphology by angioscopy vs angiography: the ability of angiography to detect thrombi. J Am Coll Cardiol 1994;406A.

characterized as yellow (n = 18) or white (n = 24). An adverse outcome with balloon angioplasty, defined as an event within 24 hours of the procedure, included myocardial infarction, urgent bypass surgery, and repeat angioplasty. Of the patients with yellow plaque 6 had an event compared with only 1 with white plaque (p = .04). Confounding the issue of plaque color, however, was the tendency of those with events also to have disrupted plaque (n = 20 with 6 events) and thrombus. While yellow plaque may be the substrate for unstable lesions, White et al. (18) confirmed that it was thrombus that predicted an adverse outcome. This multicenter trial studied 122 patients undergoing angioplasty, the vast majority of whom had unstable angina. Some 61% of lesions were noted to have thrombus by angioscopy compared with only 20% by angiography. Major in-hospital complications (death, myocardial infarction, or emergency bypass surgery) occurred in 14% of those with thrombus on angioscopy versus only 2% in those without thrombus. Less dramatic recurrent ischemia was also more frequent in the patients with thrombus (26% versus 10%).

Angioscopic findings may also predict trends in restenosis. Itoh et al. (22) implicated angioscopically detected white plaque as a risk for restenosis in a series of 47 patients. The restenosis rate was 58% in patients identified as having white plaque versus only 17% in those with yellow plaque. Only 22% of all patients had identified thrombus, which was not surprising given that this was a cohort of patients with stable angina. Bauters et al. (23), however, found no correlation between plaque color and restenosis in a larger series of 117 consecutive patients. They did, however, implicate thrombus, particularly protruding thrombus, as a risk for restenosis. The binary (more than 50% diameter narrowing) restenosis rate was 38% in those without thrombus on angioscopy, 47% in those with thrombus lining the lesion by angioscopy, and 65% (13 of 20 patients) in those with thrombus protruding into the arterial lumen during angioscopy. The majority of them either had recently sustained a myocardial infarction or were classified as having unstable angina. Thrombus detected an-

giographically has been implicated as a risk factor for restenosis as well (19).

Evaluating Abrupt Closure

Abrupt closure after PTCA is a significant complication with an incidence ranging between 2 and 11% (24–26). The cause is usually dissection; other causes include thrombosis and spasm. Angioscopy can better define these factors than angiography. White et al. (27) confirmed the cause of abrupt vessel closure following PTCA in 17 patients. In 14 cases the primary cause was dissection. In 3 patients it was thrombus (Fig. 19.6). Many of these dissections (10 of 14) were unrecognized on angiography, and only one thrombotic cause was correctly identified by angiography. Larger-scale studies are necessary to assess the potential for angioscopy to influence therapy in this unstable patient group. In another study Sassower et al. (10) demonstrated that herniated plaque was the underlying cause in two cases of abrupt closure.

Evaluating Stent Deployment

Teirstein et al. (11) confirmed stent deployment in 48 of 50 patients undergoing implantation of the Johnson & Johnson coronary stent. Angioscopy influenced therapy in 18 of these patients, determining the need for lytic therapy of thrombus in 11 patients and further stent deployment or higher balloon pressures for prolapsing tissue in 9 patients.

Complications and Limitations of Coronary Angioscopy

As with most interventions, the complications of angioscopy must be balanced with its potential benefits. In some of these small series ventricular arrhythmia requiring defibrillation occurred (23, 28). One investigator noted this with flushing of saline follow-

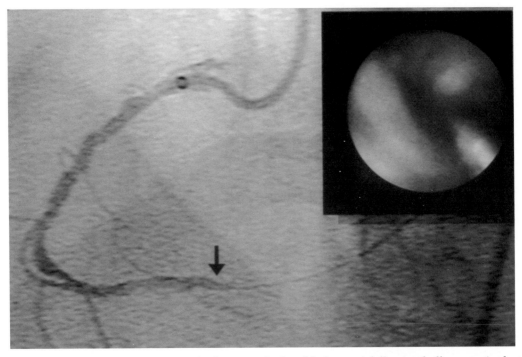

Figure 19.6. Right coronary artery with abrupt occlusion (*black arrow*) following balloon angioplasty. Angioscopy insert demonstrates that the lumen is occluded with a protuberant red thrombus (between 11 and 5 o'clock) and dense yellow plaque (between 5 and 11 o'clock). (Courtesy of Dr. Christopher White, Dept of Invasive Cardiology, HCI International Medical Center, Clydebank, Scotland, UK.)

ing balloon occlusion (22). This may be minimized by careful attention that the flush solution is warmed to body temperature. The relatively large size of the device compared with modern balloon catheters and other interventional systems may result in ischemia on preimaging of interventional lesions and the development of dissection, acute closure, and/or thrombus on postimaging. The latter was documented by Alfonso et al. (29) in 3 of 35 consecutive cases. The potential for barotrauma to the vessel by the occluding balloon also is a concern, although at least one series failed to reveal any progression of disease at these sites (30).

In addition to these concerns, today's device, although improved in size and flexibility from earlier angioscopes, remains large (4.5 F). It therefore cannot be advanced into vessels much under 2.5 mm in diameter, and it tracks poorly around tortuous bends. The requirement of a bloodless field for imaging precludes imaging of the left main coronary and the ostia of the right cor-onary, left anterior descending, and circumflex arteries, as the vessel can be imaged only beyond the balloon occlusion. Thus only the proximal to mid segments of relatively straight and large epicardial coronaries can be imaged.

ANGIOSCOPY COMPARED WITH INTRAVASCULAR ULTRASOUND

Although angioscopy and intravascular ultrasound should ideally be viewed as complementary, in an era of cost containment the options may be limited by cost effectiveness, safety, and ease of use. The overall safety of intracoronary ultrasound has been well demonstrated (31, 32), with transient coronary spasm being the most frequent sequela. The latest updates in ultrasound offer catheters ranging from 2.9 to 3.5 F, some of which are quite tractable over 0.014-inch coronary wires. At present angioscopy is limited to larger vessels. However, angioscopy is forward-viewing and shows surface morphology. Intravascular ultrasound provides primarily a cross-sectional view of the arterial wall and possibly some data on plaque composition (33). Feld et al. (34) recently published a small nonrandomized study comparing angioscopy, intracoronary ultrasound, and quantitative angiography on multivariate predictors of recurrent ischemia following interventional procedures. The only two predictors were angioscopic: plaque rupture on views taken before the procedure and thrombus identified on imaging after the procedure. Thus, although recent improvements may increase its diagnostic yield, the inability to image thrombus reproducibly remains the weakness of ultrasound (Fig. 19.7). If the identification of thrombus and its treatment are keys to decreasing acute complications and restenosis in interventional cardiology, the technology that ultimately addresses this issue will become paramount. Future issues, such as quantification and determining plaque vulnerability, will also play a major role in the use of these and other technologies.

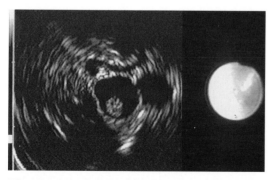

Figure 19.7. Comparison of imaging by intravascular ultrasound and angioscopy was performed in the aorta of a rabbit following balloon endothelial debridement. Intravascular ultrasound demonstrates a round filling defect without an exact definition. However, it suggests a pedunculated spherical thrombus. Angioscopy of the same lesion demonstrates an intimal flap that was confirmed at autopsy. This example illustrates the potential value of high-definition angioscopy that allows an exact identification of intraluminal pathology. (Courtesy of Dr. George Abela, Dept of Medicine, Division of Cardiology, Michigan State University, East Lansing, MI.)

FUTURE DIRECTIONS AND DEVELOPMENTS

Detection of Vulnerable Lesions

Plaques that are vulnerable to disruption and thrombosis have been described to have a thin collagenous cap overlying a lipid-rich pool (35, 36). Also, angioscopy of acute cardiovascular syndromes has demonstrated that disrupted plaques are predominantly yellow (37–39) (Fig. 19.8 and 19.9). A study was conducted by Miyamoto et al. (40) to evaluate the hypothesis that the yellow color of vulnerable lesions is due to the reflection of the lipid core seen through a thin cap. A software package was developed to quantify yellow color saturation of digitized angioscopic images. This was tested in a model consisting of lipid β-carotene emulsion injected subintimally at various depths in bovine aorta. The surface was viewed by an angioscope and the images captured and digitized. Normal aorta and the pure β-carotene–lipid emulsion were used as white and yellow standards respectively. On the chromaticity diagram white was represented as (0.33, 0.33). Also, each color was represented by a vector determined by its coordinates using white color as the site of origin. Yellow saturation was derived from the vector magnitude ratio of the difference between normal aorta (0% saturation) and the plaque sample over the difference between the normal aorta and the lipid emulsion (100%). Yellow saturation of 37 model plaques was evaluated by computed colorimetry, which uses the tristimulus color system. Results were compared with yellow color perception scored by 5 human observers as white, yellow, or intermediate. Initial medical cap thickness was calculated by computed planimetry of cross-sectional digitized images of the aortic plaque models.

Cap thickness less than 300 mm was highly correlated with yellow color (r = 0.86). Plaques with yellow saturation greater than 60% had a cap thickness of less than 75 mm (Fig. 19.8). Yellow score by visual perception and computerized colorimetery were highly correlated (r^2 = 0.91). Yel-

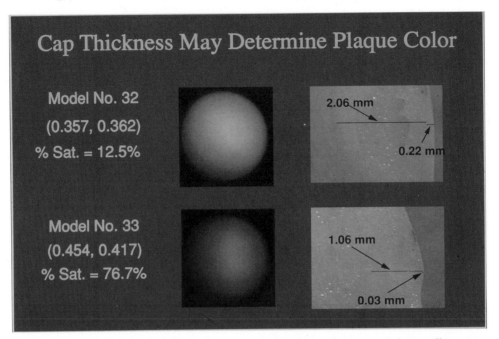

Figure 19.8. Angioscopic images of plaque models. **Top left.** Plaque with low yellow saturation (12.5%). **Top right.** Corresponding plaque cap thickness is 0.22 mm. **Bottom left.** Plaque with high yellow saturation (76.7%). **Bottom right.** Corresponding plaque cap is 0.03 mm thick. Thus higher yellow color saturation is associated with a thinner plaque cap. (Courtesy of Dr. George Abela, Dept of Medicine, Division of Cardiology, Michigan State University, East Lansing, MI, and Dr. Akira Myiamoto.)

low saturation was lower at smaller angles of view. However, the decrease was linear, which may allow for corrections. Overall these data indicated that cap thickness less than 300 mm was highly correlated with yellow color determined by either computer or visual perception. Thus **angioscopic colorimetry may provide an index of plaque thickness and hence its vulnerability to disruption and thrombosis.**

Quantitative Angioscopy

Current angioscopic systems are hampered by the inability to extract absolute dimensional measurements from the collected images. However, quantitative data can be useful in making decisions for various interventional procedures. The equipment required includes an angioscope, a light source, a color video camera, a monitor, and a personal computer with a numeric coprocessor. The image processing subsys-

tem is composed of an image processing card and customized software package. This technique has been reported by Friedl et al. (41).

Two separate sequences are required to make a measurement: first, calibration of the angioscope and second, the actual measurement. The calibration process produces a set of coefficients, stored permanently in a computer file and unique to the angioscope being used. Since the magnification of objects seen is nonlinear with respect to the distance of the angioscope tip to the object plane, the change in magnification of a calibrated angioscope can be used to determine exact image size (41).

Two in vitro experiments used this system to evaluate the accuracy of the quantification system. The first experiment entailed measuring circles with known dimensions and unknown distances to the circle surface. These measurements yielded a correlation coefficient r = 0.99. The percent error of the system was found to be 7.5%. The second

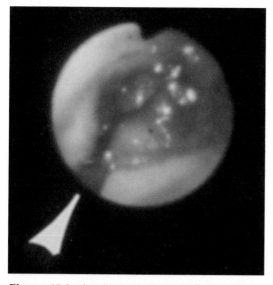

Figure 19.9. Angioscopic image of artery with ruptured plaque in a patient with an acute thrombotic event in a peripheral artery. There is yellow plaque at 6 and 8 o'clock with protruding lipomatous material in the lumen overlying a possible fissure at 7 o'clock (*arrowhead*). The remaining lumen is totally occluded with bulging red thrombus. (Courtesy of Dr. George Abela, and reprinted with permission from Uchida Y. Percutaneous cardiovascular angioscopy. In: Abela GS, ed. Lasers in cardiovascular medicine and surgery. Norwell, MA: Kluwer Academic, 1990:399–410.)

experiment was performed on cadaveric arteries with artificially induced stenoses of various severity. The results indicated a high correlation between the angioscopic measurements and those produced by planimetry of the arterial segment (r = 0.94). The angioscopic measurements had an average error of 15%.

A newer method uses a binocular system in which two fiberoptic bundles are used to view an image. Since the distance between the two bundles is known, triangulation of the image in the field allows exact measurement and dimension analysis (42).

SUMMARY

Angioscopy is an invasive diagnostic technique that provides detailed data on the intraluminal pathology of vessels, hence on the pathophysiology of intravascular occlu-

sive disease (i.e., thrombosis, herniated plaque). Also, it provides information to help in the selection of interventional devices and assessment of procedure outcomes (i.e., PTCA, laser, stents, and rotablation). The most promising aspect of angioscopy may be its ability to detect plaque that is vulnerable to disruption and thrombosis. As interventional techniques improve, the potential for angioscopy can be expected to evolve concomitantly.

References

1. Rhea L, Walker IC. Cited by Culver et al. Arch Surg 1913;9:689.
2. Gamble WJ, Irris RE. Experimental intracardiac visualization. N Engl J Med 1967;276:1397–1403.
3. Spears JR, Marais HJ, Serur J, et al. In vivo coronary angioscopy. J Am Coll Cardiol 1983;1:1311–1314.
4. Seeger JM, Abela GS. Angioscopy as an adjunct to arterial reconstructive surgery. J Vasc Surg 1986;4:315–320.
5. Abela GS, Seeger JM, Barbeiri E, et al. Laser angioplasty with angioscopic guidance in humans. J Am Coll Cardiol 1986;8:184–192.
6. Sherman TC, Litvack F, Grundfest W, et al. Coronary angioscopy in patients with unstable angina pectoris. N Engl J Med 1986;315:913–919.
7. Uchida Y, Tomaru T, Nakamura F, et al. Percutaneous coronary angioscopy in patients with ischemic heart disease. Am Heart J 1987;114:1216–1222.
8. Giacomino P, Abela GS, Baerbeau GR, et al. Angioscopy: current techniques. Dyn Cardiovasc Imaging 1989;2:178–187.
9. Ramee SR, White CJ, Collins TJ, et al. Percutaneous angioscopy during coronary angioplasty using a steerable microangioscope. J Am Coll Cardiol 1991;17:100–105.
10. Sassower MA, Abela GS, Koch JM, et al. Angioscopic evaluation of periprocedural and postprocedural abrupt closure after percutaneous coronary angioplasty. Am Heart J 1993;126:444–450.
11. Uchida Y. Percutaneous cardiovascular angioscopy. In: Abela GS, ed. Lasers in cardiovascular medicine and surgery. Norwell, MA: Kluwer Academic, 1990:399–410.
12. Teirstein PS, Schatz RA, Wong SC, Rocha-Singh KJ. Coronary stenting with angioscopic guidance. Am J Cardiol 1995;75:344–347.
13. Uchida Y, Masuo M, Tomaru T, et al. Fiberoptic observation of thrombosis and thrombolytic in isolated human coronary arteries. Am Heart J 1986;4:691–696.
14. Den Heifer P, Foley DP, Escaped J, et al. Angioscopic versus angiographic detection of intimal dissection and intracoronary thrombus. J Am Coll Cardiol 1994;24:649–54.
15. Manzo K, Nesto R, Sassower M, et al. Coronary lesion morphology by angioscopy vs angiography:

the ability of angiography to detect thrombi. J Am Coll Cardiol 1994;406A.

16. Teirstein PS, Schatz RA, DeNardo SJ, et al. Angioscopic versus angiographic detection of thrombus during coronary interventional procedures. Am J Cardol 1995;75:1083–1087.

17. Urestsky BF, Denys BG, Counihan PC, Ragosta M. Angioscopic evaluation of incompletely obstructing coronary intraluminal filling defects: comparison to angiography. Cathet Cardiovasc Diagn 1994; 33:323–329.

18. White CJ, Ramee SR, Collins TJ, et al. Coronary thrombi increase PTCA risk: angioscopy as a clinical tool. Circulation 1996;93:253–258.

19. Violaris AG, Melkert R, Herman JP, Serruys PW. Role of angiographically identifiable thrombus on long-term luminal renarrowing after coronary angioplasty: a quantitative angiographic analysis. Circulation 1996;93:889–897.

20. Thieme T, Wernecke KD, Meyer R, et al. Angioscopic evaluation of atherosclerotic plaque: validation by histomorphologic analysis and association with stable and unstable coronary syndromes. J Am Coll Cardiol 1996;28:1–6.

21. Waxman S, Sassower MA, Mittleman M, et al. Angioscopic predictors of early adverse outcome after coronary angioplasty in patients with unstable angina and non-Q wave myocardial infarction. Circulation 1996;93:2106–2113.

22. Itoh A, Miyazaki S, Nonogi H, et al. Angioscopic prediction of successful dilatation and of restenosis in precutaneous transluminal coronary angioplasty: significance of yellow plaque. Circulation 1995;91:1389–1396.

23. Bauters C, Lablanche JM, McFadden EP, et al. Relation of coronary angioscopic findings at coronary angioplasty to angiographic restenosis. Circulation 1995;92:2473–2479.

24. Detre KM, Holmes DR, Holubkov R, et al. Incidence and consequences of periprocedural occlusion. The 1985–1986 NHLBI PTCA Registry. Circulation 1990;92:739–750.

25. de Feyter PJ, van den Brand M, Jaarman G, et al. Acute coronary artery occlusion during and after percutaneous transluminal coronary angioplasty: frequency, prediction, clinical course, management, and follow-up. Circulation 1991;93:927–936.

26. Holmes DR, Holubkov R, Vlietstra RE, et al. Comparison of complications during percutaneous transluminal coronary angioplasty from 1977 to 1981 and from 1985 to 1986: the National Heart, Lung, and Blood Institute Percutaneous Transluminal Coronary Angioplasty Registry. J Am Coll Cardiol 1988;12:1149–1155.

27. White CJ, Ramee SR, Collins TJ, et al. Coronary angioscopy of abrupt occlusion after angioplasty. J Am Coll Cardiol 1995;25:1681–1684.

28. White C, Ramee SR, Collins TJ, et al. Percutaneous coronary angioscopy: applications in interventional cardiology. J Interven Cardiol 1993;6:61–67.

29. Alfonso F, Hernandez R, Goicolea J, et al. Angiographic deterioration of the previously dilated coronary segment induced by angioscopic examination. Am J Cardiol 1994;74:604–606.

30. Hamon M, Lablanche JM, Bauters C, et al. Effect of balloon inflation in angiographically normal coronary segments during coronary angioscopy: a quantitative angiographic study. Cathet Cardiovasc Diagn 1994;31:116–121.

31. Pinto FJ, St. Goar FG, Gao SZ, et al. Immediate and one-year safety of intracoronary ultrasound imaging: evaluation with serial qualitative angiography. Circulation 1993;88:1709–1714.

32. Hausmann D, Erbel R, Allibelli-Chemarin MJ, et al. The safety of intracoronary ultrasound: a multicenter survey of 2207 examinations. Circulation 1995;91:623–630.

33. Suarez De Lezo, J, Romero M, Medina A, et al. Intracoronary ultrasound assessment of directional coronary atherectomy: immediate and follow-up findings. J Am Coll Cardiol 1993;21:298–307.

34. Feld S, Mazen G, Carell ES, et al. Comparision of angioscopy, intravascular ultrasound and quantitative coronary angiography in predicting clinical outcome after coronary intervention in high risk patients. J Am Coll Cardiol 1996;28:97–105.

35. Richardson PD, Davies MJ, Born GV. Influence of plaque configuration and stress distribution on fissuring of coronary atherosclerotic plaques. Lancet 1989;2:941–944.

36. Loree HM, Kamm RD, Stringfellow RG, Lee RT. Effects of fibrous cap thickness on peak circumferential stress in model atherosclerotic vessels. Circ Res 1992;71:850–858.

37. Mizuno K, Miyamoto A, Satomura K. Angioscopic coronary macromorphology in patients with acute coronary disorders. Lancet 1991;337:809–812.

38. Nesto RW, Sassower M, Manzo KS, et al. Angioscopic differentiation of culprit lesions in unstable versus stable coronary artery disease. J Am Coll Cardiol 1993;21:195A (abstract).

39. Ueda, Y, Asakur M, Hirayama A, et al. Intracoronary morphology of culprit lesions after reperfusion in acute myocardial infarction: serial angioscopic observations. J Am Coll Cardiol 1996;27:606–610.

40. Miyamoto A, Friedl SE, Lin FC, et al. Plaque cap thickness can be detected by quantitative color analysis of angioscopic images in a plaque model. In: Anderson R, ed. Lasers in surgery: advanced characterization, therapeutics, and systems V. Bellingham, WA: Proceedings of the International Society for Optical Engineering, 1995:2395–429.

41. Friedl SE, Abela GS, Tomaru T, et al. Quantitative endovascular angioscopy: optical fibers in medicine IV. Bellingham, WA: International Society for Optical Engineering, 1989;1067:197–202.

42. Friedl SE, Abela GS. Stereoscopic angioscopy with quantitative image analysis. In: Diagnostic and therapeutic cardiovascular interventions III. Abela GS, ed. Proceedings of the Society of Photo-Optical Instrumentation Engineers, 1993;1878:224.

20
Noncardiac Angiography

Jeffrey Brinker, MD
Scott J. Savader, MD

INTRODUCTION

The cardiologist, although most concerned with imaging the heart and coronary arteries, frequently must visualize other vascular structures. Whether the result of necessity or opportunity, traditional procedural boundaries between the cardiologist and the vascular radiologist have become less distinct. A driving force for this has been the rapid evolution of interventional techniques by cardiologists. While innovations in other imaging modalities, such as ultrasound, magnetic resonance imaging (MRI), and computed tomography (CT), have lessened the need for more invasive diagnostic angiographic procedures in many instances, catheter intervention requires contrast visualization of the target vessel and occasionally the route to it. A growing number of invasive cardiologists are becoming specialists in angiographic intervention; their full-time activities center on a sophisticated angiographic suite equipped for many types of radiographic studies. Indeed many such individuals are routinely engaged in the diagnosis and catheter-based treatment of vascular disease throughout the body, including the renal, iliofemoral, and brachiocephalic arterial systems. Interventional cardiologists are among those pioneering new approaches to the treatment of noncardiac vascular disorders such as the stenting of carotid stenosis and the use of graft stents to address aneurysmal disease in the aorta and iliac arteries.

Rather than attempting to review every aspect of vascular radiology with which such individuals may be involved, this chapter is primarily concerned with the situations most commonly encountered in the practice of adult invasive cardiology. No text, of course, is an adequate substitute for experience. While the expertise of some cardiologists overlaps that of interventional radiologists in many areas, clearly sometimes collaboration between the disciplines is helpful. If the need arises for the extension of a procedure to an area not within the cardiac angiographer's expertise, appropriate radiology consultation must be obtained. This is true especially when combined procedures are to include areas with which the cardiologist has limited experience. For many angiographers this may be exemplified by the inclusion of a digital carotid examination after a diagnostic cardiac catheterization in a patient with a coronary disease and ultrasound evidence of carotid stenosis.

While one may sympathize with attempts to avoid a second invasive procedure for the patient, a poorly performed study may be worse than no study at all. Furthermore, interpretation of the angiography is often more demanding than its performance, and it is unjustifiable for this to rest with a physician who is unable to name the vessels in the study.

The extracardiac structures most often requiring angiographic definition by the cardiologist are the pulmonary arteries, the

339

great veins, and the aorta and its major branches. Contrast injection at these sites may be necessary in a number of clinical scenarios:

1. **Evaluation of cardiac disease.** Ascending aortography or pulmonary angiography may be necessary or desirable for visualization of the heart itself. The levophase of a pulmonary artery injection may be used to assess the left atrium and ventricle. Ascending aortography may be necessary to evaluate the aortic valve and in the presence of aortic regurgitation, the left ventricle and mitral valve; or to locate bypass grafts.
2. **Assessment of noncardiac pathology in a patient with cardiac symptoms.** Extension of the catheterization may be necessary to document unsuspected disease such as aortic dissection (Fig 20.1), coarctation (Fig 20.2), or pulmonary embolism (Fig 20.3) in a patient with chest pain.

3. **Anatomic assessment because of difficulty or anomaly encountered during an otherwise routine cardiac investigation.** Angiography may be helpful when there is trouble negotiating tortuous and stenotic vessels in the periphery. Aortography may be indicated for the evaluation of the distal aorta and iliofemoral arteries prior to a contemplated procedure such as intra-aortic balloon placement, balloon catheter valvuloplasty, or the use of the peripheral cardiopulmonary bypass system. Venography may be helpful in delineating anomalous persistent left superior vena cava entering the coronary sinus or the left atrium (Fig 20.4) or thoracic outlet obstruction complicating pacemaker implantation.
4. **Assessment of a possible complication encountered on this or a previous catheterization.** Peripheral arterial injection may reveal a dissection, pseudoaneurysm (Fig 20.5), or

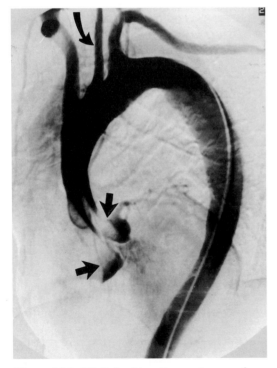

Figure 20.1. Digital subtraction aortogram demonstrating a type A aortic dissection beginning at the level of the aortic valve (*arrows*). This dissection extends to the level of the iliac arteries. The right coronary artery arises from the false lumen and the left coronary artery from the true lumen. The dissection involves the proximal portion of the left common carotid artery (*curved arrow*).

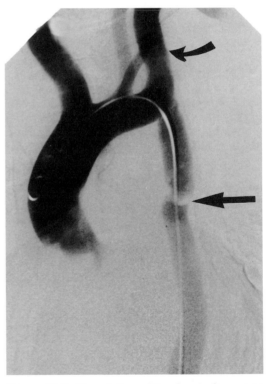

Figure 20.2. Coarctation of the descending aorta (*arrow*). Note the relative dilation of the left subclavian artery (*curved arrow*) and the rather hypoplastic appearance of the descending thoracic aorta. Angioplasty of this stenosis with double 8-mm × 4-cm balloons reduced the gradient from 120 mm Hg before dilation to 18 mm Hg afterward.

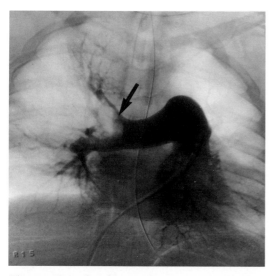

Figure 20.3. Cut-film pulmonary arteriogram demonstrating a massive saddle embolus (*arrow*) of the right pulmonary artery. Note the significant wedge-shaped areas of hypoperfusion in the right lung.

arteriovenous fistula (Fig 20.6). Venography can be used to document subclavian or superior vena caval obstruction secondary to prior or currently indwelling catheters, pacing leads (Fig 20.7), or spinal fluid shunts.

5. **Screening noncardiac anatomy.** Having an intravascular catheter in place for a cardiac study may be an opportunity to obtain a relatively low risk study of a noncardiac structure, provided a clear indication exists. For example, in selected patients with a neck bruit digital carotid angiography may be useful. In certain hypertensive patients a descending aortogram or selective renal arteriogram may identify or exclude renal artery stenosis.

6. **Combining procedures to avoid a second study.** Patients with known or highly suspected vascular abnormalities may benefit from extension of the cardiac study. An example is descending aortography to evaluate an abdominal aortic aneurysm. Certainly there is sometimes an economy of scale relative to both cost and discomfort for the patient.

7. **Evaluation of postoperative anatomy.** One may wish to visualize the site of previous catheter intervention or vascular surgery as an addendum to a cardiac procedure, such as aortography, to view a coarctation repair in a patient who now has aortic stenosis.

8. **Angiography primarily directed at noncardiac disease.** Finally, at some centers cardiologists may have or share responsibility for an-

giographic evaluation of pulmonary embolic disease or dissecting aortic aneurysm. Many cardiac interventionists have expanded their interests beyond the heart and great vessels. The properly credentialed individual may be involved in all aspects of vascular angiography and intervention.

GENERAL GUIDELINES

Since no angiography is entirely without risk, careful consideration should be given to each proposed procedure. No matter how routine the study appears, each patient brings unique circumstances that may require a customization of the procedure. It is helpful to adopt a systematic approach similar to that outlined in Table 20.1 for every study. While the best views, injection rates, and imaging modality vary with the area of interest, and the individual situation, some common principles are applicable to most angiographic procedures (Table 20.2).

PULMONARY ANGIOGRAPHY

Contrast in the pulmonary artery provides important information concerning the pulmonary arterial and venous system. It may also allow for visualization of the left atrium, left ventricle, and ascending aorta when more direct injection is difficult or risky. Pulmonary angiography is indicated for the evaluation of a variety of congenital and acquired diseases, including **pulmonary arterial branch stenosis, pulmonary arteriovenous malformations, anomalous pulmonary venous connections, and obstructive venous disease.** It is, however, most frequently performed in the setting of **suspected pulmonary embolic disease**. The general approach to this procedure, although applicable to the other disorders, is discussed in the context of embolic disease.

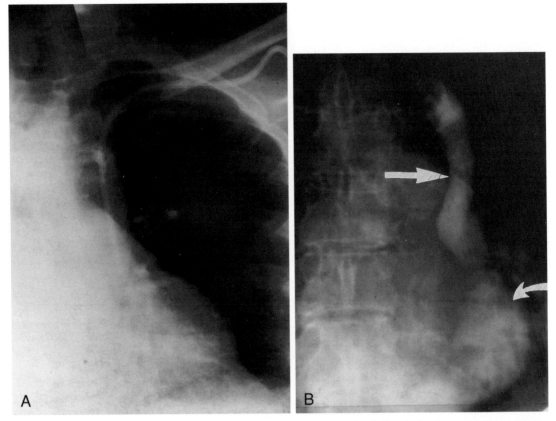

Figure 20.4. A. Double lumen Hickman catheter placed from the left subclavian vein lies with its distal tip to the left of the mediastinum. This portion of the catheter is in a persistent left superior vena cava. **B.** Injection of the Hickman catheter shows emptying of the persistent left superior vena cava (*arrow*) into the coronary sinus (*curved arrow*).

PULMONARY ANGIONGRAPHY FOR SUSPECTED EMBOLIC DISEASE

Physiologic Monitoring

Performance of pulmonary angiography entails a catheter manipulated through the right heart chambers and positioned in the pulmonary arterial tree. Adherence to proper cardiac catheterization technique, including attention to hemodynamic recordings and monitoring the electrocardiogram, is essential. In some situations an oxygen saturation run should be performed. Determination of the overall hemodynamic profile of the patient may add information important to performance of

angiography and ultimately to patient care (1, 2). The data may suggest alternative diagnoses, such as left ventricular failure, pulmonary venous disease, mitral valve disorder, pulmonary artery hypertension, intracardiac communications, or pericardial disease. In patients without pre-existent cardiopulmonary disease, mean pulmonary artery pressure correlates well with the degree of embolic obstruction (3, 4). Right ventricular failure, especially if the right ventricular end diastolic pressure is above 20 mm Hg, indicates a poor prognosis (5). The risk of pulmonary angiography is increased in patients with **pulmonary hypertension**, especially if the right heart is failing (6). These findings should alert the physician to take special precautions (reduced amounts of contrast material, low-osmolality con-

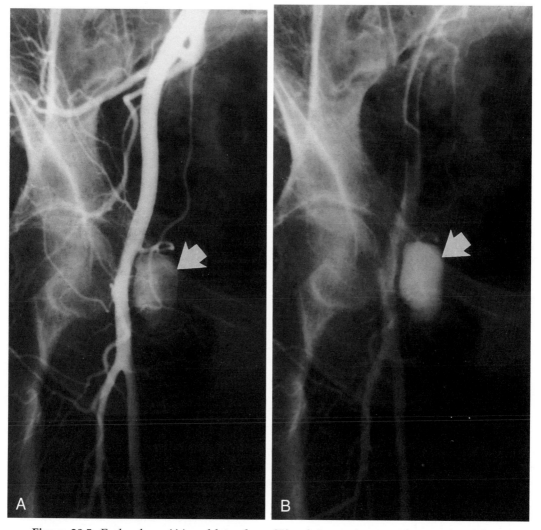

Figure 20.5. Early-phase (**A**) and late-phase (**B**) pelvic arteriograms demonstrate a large post–cardiac catheterization pseudoaneurysm (*arrow*) of the common femoral artery.

trast, superselective injections) when angiography is necessary.

Pressure monitoring is helpful to verify catheter location during manipulation. Fluoroscopy in the anteroposterior (AP) view is not always adequate to define catheter position. For example, the coronary sinus, which is not uncommonly entered when either the brachial or subclavian technique is used, may be indistinguishable from the right ventricular outflow tract in the AP view. Recognition of a right atrial pressure waveform from a catheter so placed makes this differentiation before any contrast material is injected and provides a measure of safety as one advances the catheter through the heart. This is most pertinent when using stiffer non–balloon directed catheters, which are capable of perforating the heart. Loss of an appropriate pressure waveform should caution the operator against advancing the catheter, especially when resistance is felt or the catheter tip appears to be hung up. **Electrocardiographic monitoring** is essential and should be initiated as soon as the patient arrives in the laboratory. Sinus

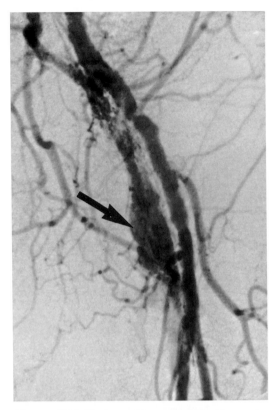

Figure 20.6. Post–cardiac catheterization arteriovenous fistula of the common femoral artery. Note the filling of the common femoral and external iliac vein (*arrow*) during the early arterial phase of the pelvic arteriogram.

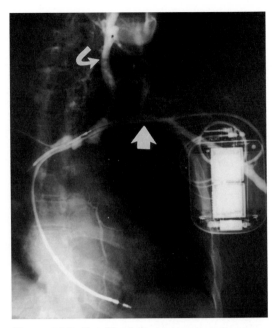

Figure 20.7. Cut-film left upper extremity venogram obtained prior to placement of a dialysis catheter demonstrates a high-grade subclavian artery stenosis (*arrow*) at the venous entrance site of the automated implanted cardiac defibrillator (AICD) lead. Note the significant retrograde filling of the right internal jugular vein (*curved arrow*).

bradycardia or heart block may occur as a vagal response while the cardiologist is gaining vascular access. Supraventricular as well as ventricular arrhythmias may be provoked during the procedure and may be poorly tolerated. Attention to the rhythm during catheter manipulation allows for the early detection of irritability and prevents sustained tachyarrhythmias. Particular care should be taken in the performance of the right heart catheterization necessary for placement of the pulmonary angiography catheter in patients with left bundle branch block. Catheter bruising of the right bundle may cause heart block resulting in profound symptoms. Some angiographers routinely place a temporary pacing catheter in such patients.

VASCULAR ACCESS

Although the brachiocephalic route often allows a balloon-directed catheter to take a natural course to the pulmonary artery, in most institutions the percutaneous femoral venous approach to pulmonary angiography has supplanted that from the neck or arm. The Seldinger method allows for quick and easy entry into the large femoral vein. One has the option of using a sheath or introducing the angiography catheter percutaneously over a wire. Venous spasm is not encountered, and no sutures are used to close the wound. Another advantage of this technique is the relative ease with which one may enter the branches of the pulmonary artery superselectively. Entry into the left pulmonary artery may be difficult from the arm, and catheter placement in specific segments may not be possible. The right femoral vein offers a more direct path to the

Table 20.1.
Systematic Approach to Angiography

1. What are the problems?
2. Is angiography necessary?
   A. Will treatment strategy be based on its results?
   B. Can other diagnostic modalities supply similar information at lower risk?
   C. Are there special risks (e.g., allergy, impaired renal function, peripheral vascular disease) that may influence the risk–benefit ratio?
3. What are the goals of angiography?
4. Is there a need for hemodynamic evaluation?
5. What are the optimal radiographic modalities (e.g., cine, serial cut film, digital subtraction, dynamic digital acquisition, single or biplane)?
6. What vascular access is optimal?
7. What is the specific sequence of contrast injections (sites, projections, filming modalities)?
8. Is intervention at this sitting contemplated?
9. What is a reasonable ceiling for the amount of contrast to be used?
10. Is help (e.g., radiology or surgery) needed in planning or carrying out the procedure?

heart and is preferred over the left, which may enter the inferior vena cava at an abrupt angle.

The principal drawback of femoral catheterization is the **potential for dislodging thrombi from iliac veins or vena cava** (7). This disadvantage is more theoretical than real (8), and we have yet to encounter a clinically evident complication of this type. However, when performing pulmonary angiography for suspected embolic disease, we routinely hand-inject about 10 mL of contrast material into the femoral vein and follow it fluoroscopically through the iliac vein and into the vena cava. If there is a suggestion of abnormality, an inferior vena cavogram is performed (discussed later in the chapter). If no thrombi are seen within the iliac vein or vena cava, the catheter is advanced over a guidewire to the heart.

A number of catheter types are available for pulmonary angiography. The Grollman pulmonary artery–seeking catheter (Cook Inc., Bloomington, IN) is used frequently at Johns Hopkins (9) (Fig. 20.8). This polyethylene pigtailed catheter has a gentle reverse

Table 20.2.
Principles Applicable to Most Angiography

1. The most important information (i.e., that unobtainable with other diagnostic modalities) should in most cases be acquired first.
2. Hemodynamics should be recorded prior to and after contrast administration when appropriate.
3. Test-inject under fluoroscopy with low pressure before power injection.
4. Ensure that the entire field of interest can be visualized with selected technique (e.g., cut filming encompasses desired area) or that adequate panning can be achieved during cineangiography given the projection chosen and the rate and volume of contrast material injected.
5. Consider multiple injections or biplane projections.
6. Optimal opacification is usually achieved by upstream injection as close to the area of interest as possible. However:
   A. Downstream injection with adequate force may be necessary if one cannot get past obstruction from below.
   B. High upstream injection may be necessary to delineate collateralization.
7. Limit contrast and radiation exposure to that compatible with a diagnostic study.
8. Coordinate injection rate and filming technique so that optimal opacification is recorded.
   A. High flow through a vascular bed requires injection of larger volumes of contrast material over shorter intervals and rapid filming.
   B. Delayed imaging may be necessary for collateral or venous phase visualization.
9. Motion caused by an uncooperative patient or by reaction to contrast material (e.g., pain, cough) reduces the quality of the study. Consider low-osmolality agents, the addition of lidocaine to contrast medium, and if necessary, sedation or anesthesia.
10. Catheters must be frequently flushed, especially when nonionic contrast is used or if anticoagulation is omitted.
11. Catheters must be adequate for desired injection rate. Excess pressure may rupture the catheter.
12. Consider the effects of recoil of the catheter during power injection.
13. Position the catheter to limit potential for migration into a smaller branch.
14. Radiographic images, including plain films, should be carefully studied to exclude unanticipated findings that might require further diagnosis or therapy (Fig. 20.1).

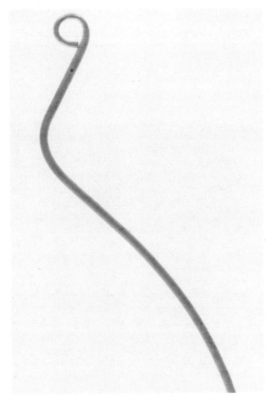

Figure 20.8. Standard Grollman pulmonary artery–seeking catheter.

per second), may be used. There is a 7-F Grollman polyurethane catheter with a single 90° curve 6 cm from its pigtail ring. This catheter has 12 side holes and good torque control, and it has been used with success (10), especially in patients with enlarged right heart chambers.

The technique of pulmonary artery catheterization with the Grollman catheter is shown in Figure 20.9. The anteromedial portion of the right atrium is probed with the tip of the catheter until the right ventricle is entered. This is marked by a change in pressure and perhaps the elicitation of ventricular ectopy. Counterclockwise rotation should direct the distal curve upward the ventricular outflow tract. From this point gently advancing the catheter causes it to enter the pulmonary artery. On occasion the catheter may get hung up in the outflow tract and buckle at the tricuspid valve when force is applied. Having the patient take a deep breath orients the heart more vertically, allowing the catheter to pass into the pulmonary artery. If this is unsuccessful, a soft-tipped guidewire such as the Benston (Cook Inc.) may be used to prevent buckling by stiffening the catheter. Care should be exercised when using a guidewire because one loses the opportunity to monitor pressure.

In patients with right atrial enlargement the distal tip of the catheter may be too short to enter the right ventricle directly. One may then bend the proximal end of a guidewire into a curve approximately 4 cm in diameter (11) and advance it into the catheter to a point just proximal to the pigtail. **It is imperative to ensure that this stiff end of the wire is never advanced beyond the tip of the catheter.** The guidewire generally adds enough additional curvature to allow the catheter to be directed through the tricuspid valve into the right ventricle. It may then be advanced into the pulmonary artery as described earlier (Fig. 20.10). A tip-deflecting guidewire system from Cook that offers an alternative to the stiff end of the guidewire may also be helpful in this situation.

A similar technique has been used to shape a 5- or 7-F high-flow pigtail catheter to access the pulmonary artery in patients with normal-sized hearts.

secondary curve proximal to the distal 3 cm that is angled 90° from the shaft. Its configuration facilitates passage through the heart and limits the likelihood of the tip getting caught in the trabeculated right ventricle. The soft material combined with the catheter's other attributes virtually eliminates the possibility of cardiac perforation.

This catheter may be introduced percutaneously over a guidewire or through a sheath. The ability to accept a guidewire facilitates its manipulation into virtually any pulmonary arterial segment. It is stable and exhibits minimal recoil during contrast injection. The standard catheter is available in 6.7- and 8.3-F diameters. The former, which is used more frequently, allows for a high enough flow rate (26 mL per second) for selective angiography. Injection to the main pulmonary artery is now rarely performed for assessment of embolic disease, but if it is required for other studies, the larger catheter, having a higher flow rate (up to 45 mL

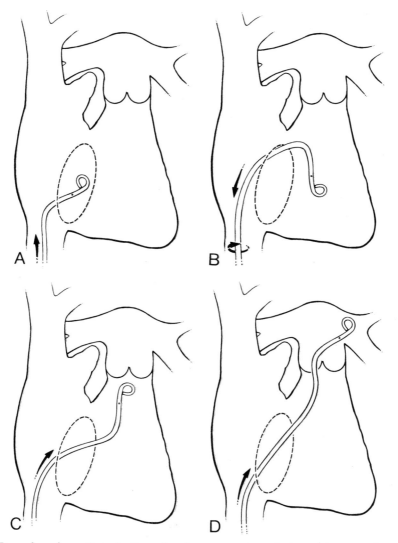

Figure 20.9. Procedure for catheterization of pulmonary artery via femoral approach with Grollman catheter. Once in the right atrium, the catheter is directed toward the tricuspid valve (**A**). With further advancement the right ventricle is entered. The catheter is then withdrawn slightly and rotated (**B**) so that the distal segment is directed toward the right ventricular outflow tract (**C**), from which it can be easily positioned in the pulmonary artery (**D**).

Catheters inserted from the femoral vein preferentially enter the left pulmonary artery. If superselective injection of the left lower lobe branches is necessary, further advancement of the catheter is usually all that is required. For selective right pulmonary artery angiography, withdrawal of the catheter into the main pulmonary artery, rotation of the tip toward the right side, and advancement will often be successful. If not,

a J-tipped guidewire may be directed into the right pulmonary artery and the catheter threaded over it. Torquable guidewires such as the TAD, the Wholley Hi-Torque Modified J (both from Peripheral Systems Group, Mountain View, CA), and the Magic Wire (Meditech, Watertown, MA) may also be helpful in these situations (see Chapter 9). Alternatively, the pigtail catheter may be exchanged over a long guidewire for a mul-

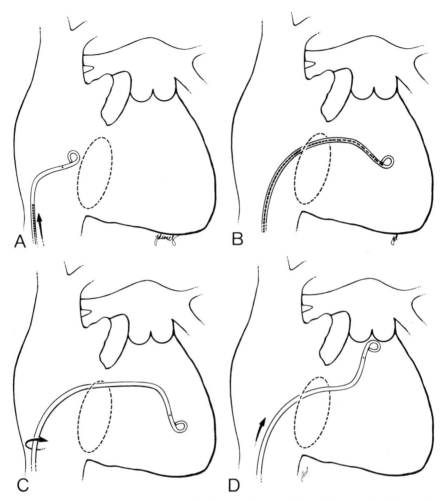

Figure 20.10. Pulmonary artery catheterization in a patient with cardiomegaly. Curved back end of guidewire is inserted to the pigtail (**A**) allowing the catheter to be advanced through the tricuspid valve and into the right ventricle (**B**). Guidewire is then removed and right ventricular pressure measured (**C**). Rotation of catheter directs it to the outflow tract and into pulmonary artery (**D**).

tipurpose catheter that can be directed toward the right pulmonary artery. Advancement of the exchange wire into the more distal vessel allows for replacement of the pigtail into the right pulmonary artery.

Balloon-tipped angiographic catheters may also be used from the femoral approach through an indwelling sheath. The Berman (Critikon Inc., Tampa, FL) catheter allows for flow direction while maintaining torque control. This device may facilitate catheterization of the pulmonary artery in some cases, although the balloon may be a hindrance in the presence of significant tri-

cuspid regurgitation. A 7-F catheter delivers flows of 20 mL per second and fits through a 7-F sheath. Since it has no end hole, it cannot be used with a guidewire. This catheter may be manipulated into the pulmonary artery in either of two ways: Once through the sheath, the balloon is inflated with room air or CO_2 (the latter if an abnormal communication between the right- and left-sided circulations is suspected) and advanced into the right atrium. The catheter may then be turned anteromedially, directed through the tricuspid valve, and rotated so as to point up toward the ventricular outflow tract. A deep breath at this time augments pulmonary flow, which is especially helpful with balloon catheters. Care should be taken not to advance the catheter too far into the ventricle before rotation and to avoid overtorque, which may kink the catheter. Once properly aligned, the catheter is usually easily advanced into the pulmonary artery with a preference to enter the left branch. If right pulmonary injection is required, one may take a second approach by looping the catheter around the lateral wall of the right atrium so that it crosses the tricuspid valve and enters the right ventricle pointing up. Advancement of this loop causes the tip of the catheter to enter the right pulmonary artery preferentially in much the same way as from the brachial approach (Fig. 20.11). This method may also help in the presence of tricuspid regurgitation by adding support and in effect stiffening the catheter. One should position the Berman catheter somewhat more distally to compensate for recoil during contrast injection.

A flow-directed pulmonary wedge catheter may also be used to enter the pulmonary circulation and provide a means for

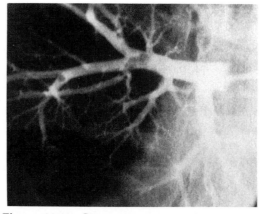

Figure 20.12. Cineangiographic frame demonstrating balloon occlusion pulmonary angiogram with emboli in right pulmonary artery.

selective balloon occlusion pulmonary angiography (Fig. 20.12). In addition, once in the pulmonary artery, it may be directed by flow or with a torquable wire to an area of interest and then provide a means for catheter exchange with a long guidewire. We have used this technique to introduce end hole catheters to deliver snares for retrieval of foreign body emboli from pulmonary arterial branches.

The pulmonary artery may also be catheterized from venous access in an upper extremity or via a percutaneous approach into a jugular or subclavian vein. These sites may be considered in cases of clinically recognized thrombosis of the iliofemoral veins or inferior vena cava, previous inferior vena cava ligation or caval filter placement, or an inaccessible groin (e.g., dermatitis, infection). A previously inserted central line may be used in seriously ill patients. A percutaneous technique may be employed from the arm if an antecubital vein of sufficient size is recognizable from the surface. The brachial approach requires a medially directed vein to enter the axillary and subclavian directly. **Laterally directed antecubital veins usually lead to the cephalic system,** which enters the axillary vein at an unfavorable angle for catheterization. In most cases an antecubital cutdown readily reveals a big enough vein. An intravascular sheath should be used even when access is via a venotomy to facilitate catheter exchange and lessen the incidence of venous spasm.

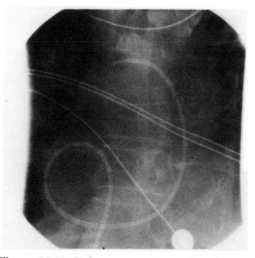

Figure 20.11. Pulmonary artery catheterization in the setting of tricuspid regurgitation. Balloon catheter was looped around lateral wall of the right atrium, allowing support for crossing tricuspid valve. When introduced in this fashion, the catheter commonly enters the right pulmonary artery.

A variety of catheters are available for pulmonary catheterization via the brachial approach. The traditional woven Dacron catheters have given way to balloon-tipped angiographic catheters at our institution because of the latter's lower likelihood of myocardial perforation and ease of use. While the incidence of clinically recognized perforation with stiffer catheters is low, the risk of tamponade increases if vigorous anticoagulation is employed. Pigtail catheters for use via the brachial approach include a modified Grollman catheter without the reverse curve (12) and a 5-F multiple-bend pigtail catheter (Cordis Corp., Miami, FL) available in three configurations. The last are said to have a maximum injection rate of 22 mL per second and have good torque control, especially when used with a guidewire (13).

The technique of catheterizing the pulmonary artery from a brachiocephalic vein is similar for most catheters. The catheter is directed into the right atrium and the tip advanced toward the lateral wall opposite the tricuspid valve so as to form a loop. Counterclockwise rotation is applied, and when the tricuspid valve is approached, gentle retraction allows the tip of the catheter to fall across the valve into the right ventricle, still pointing up toward the outflow tract. This position should be confirmed by pressure monitoring, because entry into the coronary sinus may not be discerned by AP fluoroscopy alone. When the catheter is properly positioned in the outflow tract, gentle advancement while the patient takes a deep breath usually results in entry into the pulmonary artery. Further advancement most often leads the catheter into the right lung. If the catheter loses its upward orientation after crossing the tricuspid valve, it is unlikely to enter the pulmonary artery, and the whole process must be repeated. Attempts to force the catheter into a more favorable position in the right ventricle are accompanied by ventricular ectopy and the possibility of perforation. This is true especially with the stiffer catheters and when the assistance of straight or stiffer guidewires is necessary. While monitoring pressure from the catheter will not guarantee safety, ignoring it invites complication.

Entry into the left pulmonary artery from the brachiocephalic approach may be difficult, as the natural course of a catheter delivered from this route is to the right pulmonary artery. If selective left pulmonary angiography is required and catheterization must be from above, one may try using a torquable guidewire through an end hole angiographic catheter. Alternatively, the proximal end of a guidewire may be formed into an "S-curve" and advanced carefully into a Berman catheter placed in the main pulmonary artery.

ANGIOGRAPHIC TECHNIQUE

Diagnosis of pulmonary embolic disease requires selective or superselective angiography. Injection of contrast material in the main pulmonary artery is less sensitive (14, 15) and is rarely indicated for the evaluation of either pulmonary emboli or arteriovenous malformations. Selective angiography is performed on the side of maximum abnormality revealed on the ventilation–perfusion lung scan (14, 16, 17). Superselective injections using oblique projections and/or magnification techniques (14, 17) are used when the scan defects are small or if the initial selective arteriogram is equivocal.

Contrast material is injected with a flow rate determined by the site of injection and the pulmonary artery pressure. If the latter is less than 40 mm Hg systolic, 20 mL per second for 2 seconds is used in the right or left pulmonary artery and 15 mL per second for 2 seconds if the catheter is placed more selectively. If pulmonary arterial systolic pressure is between 40 and 70 mm Hg, the injection rates are reduced to 15 mL per second and 10 mL per second over 2 seconds for the two sites respectively. Pulmonary angiography should be performed with caution if pulmonary arterial systolic pressure is greater than 70 mm Hg because contrast material may acutely elevate the pressure and produce right heart failure (6, 18). Superselective catheter position and small volumes of contrast material should be employed in this situation. Right heart failure, as evidenced by a right ventricular end-diastolic pressure of 20 mm Hg or more, is associated with an increased risk of death from pulmonary angiography (6), and this finding should cause the operator to reconsider the necessity of angiography. If angiography is still deemed essential, superselective techniques using very small doses of contrast material (5 to 10 mL) should be employed. Options include digital pulmonary angiography using dilute contrast (19) and wedged pulmonary angiography using balloon-tipped end hole catheters (20). Low-osmolality contrast, particularly a nonionic agent, should be used in patients with pulmonary hypertension or right heart failure as well as in those otherwise thought to be at increased risk for angiography. An additional advantage to the use of low-osmolality contrast for all pulmonary angiography is a reduction in discomfort and urge to cough, which may increase the quality of the angiogram.

Cineradiography, which has been advocated in selected situations (21), is logistically straightforward for catheterization laboratory personnel and allows for assessment of contrast flow. Serial cut films (14 × 14 inch), however, have greater spatial resolution, cover a larger area of the lung, and are generally recommended for pulmonary angiography. Filming is carried out at 3 films per second for 3 seconds and then 1 film per second for an additional 3 seconds for a total of 12 exposures. Exposure should be no longer than 20 milliseconds to minimize motion. For nonmagnification angiography 70 to 75 kilovolt peak (kVp) at 1000 milliamperes (mA) is used for maximum contrast resolution. A 1.2-mm x-ray tube focal spot is usually employed; however, magnification angiography requires a 0.3-mm focal spot. In the latter situation 90 to 95 kVp is used to compensate for the lower milliamperage (approximately 150 mA) necessitated by the small focal spot. Depending upon the x-ray tube's heat capacity and the size of the patient, magnification angiography may require a filming rate slower than 3 frames per second.

DIGITAL PULMONARY ANGIOGRAPHY

Digital subtraction angiography (DSA) has been advocated by some for pulmonary angiography (19, 22–24), especially in patients who are hemodynamically unstable, have pulmonary hypertension, or are suspected of having large emboli. While this technique does not mandate the placement of a catheter in the pulmonary artery, (avoiding the potential for complications in right heart catheterization), superior imaging is obtained with selective pulmonary artery catheterization. Subtraction techniques are used if the patient can hold his or her breath for the procedure; if not, digital spot filming is preferred.

Adequate studies may be obtained by injection into the superior vena cava or right atrium of 20 mL of contrast material per second, for a total of 30 to 40 mL. Digital arteriograms may also be obtained by injecting contrast medium (5 mL per second for 2 seconds) through the end hole of an indwelling balloon-tipped pulmonary arterial pressure monitoring catheter (19). The location of the catheter tip determines the lung imaged. The opposite lung may be visualized by injecting contrast medium (10 mL per second for 2 seconds) through the proximal port of the thermodilution catheter. Care should be taken in power-injecting low-osmolality contrast through such catheters because of the high viscosity of these agents.

The major disadvantage of DSA is the requirement for the patient to remain motionless; patients suspected of having acute pulmonary emboli may not be able to suspend respiration long enough to complete a digital subtraction study. Cardiac motion can make evaluation of the vessels adjacent to the heart difficult, although postprocessing techniques (i.e., mask shifting) can minimize this problem. Digital angiography has less spatial resolution than standard pulmonary angiography; however, the digitally acquired image can be diagnostically sharper than cut-film images, which poorly compensate for the density differences between the heart and lung (Fig. 20.13). While it has been suggested that digital techniques are most useful for detection of emboli in the larger branches (19, 22, 24), there is no convincing evidence that emboli in the smaller peripheral pulmonary arterial branches are better diagnosed by cut-film technique. Digital imaging of selective pulmonary arterial injections of dilute contrast

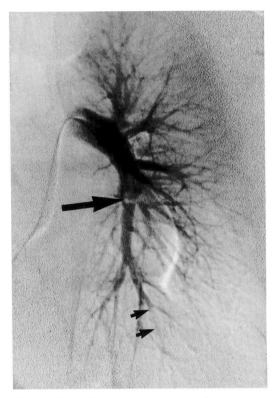

Figure 20.13. Digital subtraction pulmonary arteriogram of the right pulmonary artery clearly demonstrates a moderate-sized filling defect at the origin of the lower-lobe pulmonary artery (*large arrow*) and occlusion of a distal lower lobe branch (*small arrows*) secondary to thrombus.

material is advantageous in the evaluation of patients with pulmonary arteriovenous malformations and their treatment with embolization techniques (25). These patients can suspend respiration long enough for such procedures, and DSA has adequate resolution, can be performed quickly, and requires less contrast than conventional filming techniques.

BEDSIDE WEDGED PULMONARY ANGIOGRAPHY

Balloon occlusion pulmonary angiography with an indwelling flow-directed catheter has been suggested for the diagnosis of pulmonary emboli in patients thought too ill to

undergo conventional angiography (20, 24, 26, 27). The procedure may be performed at the bedside in unstable patients with a portable chest x-ray machine. The technique requires inflating the balloon and then advancing to a pulmonary wedge position. This is followed by a hand injection of 10 mL of a low-osmolality contrast material (or a mixture of 8.5 mL of standard contrast material and 1.5 mL of 2% lidocaine to suppress the cough response initiated by the injection). A single radiograph is taken at the conclusion of the injection, after which the balloon is deflated. This procedure is logistically easily accomplished with minimal risk but has low sensitivity (28). Although a positive study may be taken as indicative of pulmonary emboli, a negative examination has little meaning, since only a small area of the pulmonary circulation is seen with each injection and emboli in other areas cannot be excluded. Inasmuch as the balloon catheter cannot be easily directed to selected parts of the pulmonary circulation, its position proximal to an embolus would be fortuitous. While pulmonary emboli most often occur in the lower lobes and flow-directed catheters commonly are carried there (27), pulmonary blood flow is reduced in embolized beds, lessening the likelihood that the catheter will enter those segments. This method of establishing the diagnosis of embolic disease has limited value and little justification now that catheterization laboratories have the support staff and logistics to support the study of even the sickest patients.

COMPLICATIONS OF PULMONARY ANGIOGRAPHY

Although pulmonary angiography is relatively safe when performed by an experienced team, it is an invasive technique often used in compromised patients, and complications may occur. The overall incidence of significant morbidity ranges from 1 to 4%, with mortality 0.2 to 0.4% (1, 6, 29, 30). Complications may be classified as being due to the right heart catheterization or secondary to injection of contrast material. The former include atrial and ventricular extrasystoles, sustained tachycardia or fibrillation (supraventricular and ventricular), right bundle branch block (which may result in complete heart block with pre-existing left bundle branch block), and myocardial perforation with or without pericardial tamponade. Digitalis intoxication, recent myocardial infarction (1), and blood gas and electrolyte abnormalities may all predispose to malignant arrhythmia. Intense anticoagulation or thrombolytic therapy increases the risk of pericardial bleeding in case of perforation, as well as bleeding at the site of vascular access.

Injection of contrast material may be accompanied by allergic reaction, cardiac depression, or an acute increase in pulmonary vascular resistance. The last may be particularly risky in patients with marked pulmonary hypertension and/or right heart failure.

ROLE OF PULMONARY ANGIOGRAPHY IN SUSPECTED EMBOLIC DISEASE

Pulmonary embolism is a common disorder with a mortality as high as 30% in untreated patients (29, 31, 32). If it is diagnosed and properly treated, the risk of death is reduced to about 8% (29, 32). There are hazards associated with the overdiagnosis of this entity, since heparin therapy is a leading cause of drug-related complications, significant bleeding occurring in as many as 15% of those so treated (33). The iatrogenic risk may be increased if thrombolytic therapy or surgical embolectomy is considered.

Clinical recognition of pulmonary embolism may be difficult. Symptoms and common laboratory tests (systemic arterial oxygen saturation, electrocardiogram, chest x-ray) are often suggestive but are not specific. Ventilation–perfusion lung scanning and pulmonary angiography are the two primary imaging modalities used in the detection of embolism, although MRI and angiography, spiral CT, ultrasound, and angioscopy have also been used (34, 35). A normal perfusion scan virtually excludes the diagnosis (30, 33, 36, 37). Other disease states, however, may result in diminished

regional pulmonary arterial flow and limit the specificity of perfusion scanning. Combined ventilation–perfusion scanning is generally (38–42) although not universally (33) considered to improve specificity and should be performed whenever possible. A high-quality chest x-ray film is important in the interpretation of the scans and should always be available (43).

Characteristic findings of pulmonary embolism are perfusion defects in segmental areas of the lung that are normally ventilated and appear normal on chest radiograph (41, 42, 44). Publication of the Prospective Investigation of Pulmonary Embolism Diagnosis (PIOPED) trial established criteria for interpretation of abnormal lung scans in patients with suspected pulmonary embolism (45) (Table 20.3) A high-probability lung scan in a patient with strong clinical indications of pulmonary embolism has been shown to have a diagnostic accuracy of 96% compared with angiography. Thus such patients may be treated without pulmonary angiography (46). These cases, however, account for only a small percentage of patients in the PIOPED study (29 of 887).

It is often difficult to exclude pulmonary embolism in patients with severe chronic obstructive pulmonary disease having extensive ventilation defects (47). Lung scanning is usually indeterminate in such cases, as it is when perfusion–ventilation defects occur in areas of abnormality on the chest x-ray film (39, 40, 44, 48). Unfortunately, abnormal chest films are fairly common in patients with embolic disease (29, 43). Consolidation, pleural effusion, and atelectasis may accompany embolism but may also be due to other disorders that can result in defects on lung scans. Lung scans with corresponding ventilation–perfusion abnormalities and abnormalities in the chest roentgenogram cannot exclude the possibility of pulmonary embolism. Spiral volumetric CT may be a helpful noninvasive test in patients with nondiagnostic V/Q scans. A preliminary study demonstrated that spiral volumetric CT was associated with a sensitivity of 95% and a specificity of 97% compared with angiography in the diagnosis of pulmonary embolism (49).

In a patient clinically suspected of hav-

Table 20.3.
PIOPED Scan Interpretation Criteria

High probability

Two or more large segmental perfusion defects without corresponding ventilation or roentgenographic abnormalities or substantially larger than either matching ventilation or chest x-ray abnormalities

Two or more moderate segmental perfusion defects without matching ventilation or chest x-ray abnormalities and one large mismatched segmental defect

Four or more moderate segmental perfusion defects without ventilation or chest x-ray abnormalities

Intermediate probability (indeterminate)

Not falling into normal, very low, or high-probability categories

Borderline high or borderline low

Difficult to categorize as low or high

Low probability

Nonsegmental perfusion defects (e.g., very small effusion causing blunting of costophrenic angle, cardiomegaly, enlarged aorta, hila, mediastinum, elevated diaphragm)

Single moderate mismatched segmental perfusion defect with normal chest x-ray

Any perfusion defect with a substantially larger chest x-ray abnormality

Large or moderate segmental perfusion defects involving no more than four segments in one lung and no more than three segments in one lung region with matching ventilation defects either equal to or larger in size, and chest x-ray either normal or with abnormalities substantially smaller than perfusion defects

More than three small segmental perfusion defects with normal chest x-ray

Very low probability

Three or fewer small segmental perfusion defects with normal chest x-ray

Normal

No perfusion defects

Perfusion outlines exactly the shape of the lungs as seen on the chest x-ray (hilar and aortic impressions may be seen, chest x-ray and/or ventilation study may be abnormal)

Adapted from the PIOPED Investigators. Value of the ventilation–perfusion scan in acute pulmonary embolism. JAMA 1990;263:2753–2759.

ing pulmonary embolism, a ventilation–perfusion lung scan and a chest radiograph should be the initial screening procedures. Patients with a high-probability scan generally do not require pulmonary angiography unless there is a strong contraindication to heparin or thrombolytic therapy or invasive intervention is contemplated. Patients with low-probability scans may require angiography if the clinical impression of embolism is high. An indeterminate scan most often leads to angiography. Rarely is patient in extremis with a strong clinical suggestion of massive pulmonary emboli but too unstable for either scanning or emergency angiography. It has been suggested that an echocardiogram demonstrating right ventricular dysfunction, a compressed left ventricle, and tricuspid regurgitation justifies thrombolytic therapy if there are no specific contraindications to its use (46).

When required, pulmonary angiography should be performed within the first few days after the suggestive clinical episode. Resolution of the emboli may begin within a day and be complete by 1 to 2 weeks (29, 31, 50, 51). **Heparin** may be suspended for 2 to 4 hours prior to angiography, although this is not absolutely necessary if the procedure is done carefully.

Angiography should be directed by the lung scan. Selective right or left pulmonary angiography should be performed first in patients with large lobar defects. For smaller segmental or subsegmental defects, superselective angiography in the respective lobar or segmental branch may be necessary to diagnose small peripheral emboli (14, 17). Selective injections minimize dilution of contrast material and overlapping of vessels from adjacent portions of the lung. When initial views are equivocal, use of oblique projections may further aid in isolating the area of interest (15, 52). Magnification angiography may further improve detection of small emboli (14, 17). Once emboli are found, the procedure can be terminated. If angiography is negative in one area of scan defect, selective angiography must be performed in any other areas of scan abnormality. There is no need to image areas shown to be normal by scan.

Venography of the lower extremities is not an adequate substitute for pulmonary angiography in diagnosing pulmonary embolus. It may be negative in up to 30% of the patients with documented emboli (44), and venous thrombosis may occur in patients with abnormal lung scans not due to emboli. Bilateral leg venography has been recommended, however, to improve the detection of "thromboembolic disease" in patients with lung scan defects and negative angiography (44). Duplex ultrasound examination is considered an adequate substitute for contrast venography in detection of venous thrombosis in leg veins above the knee (53, 54).

INTERPRETATION OF THE PULMONARY ANGIOGRAM

Demonstration of an intraluminal filling defect within the pulmonary arteries establishes pulmonary embolism angiographically (Fig. 20.14) (52, 55, 56). If blood

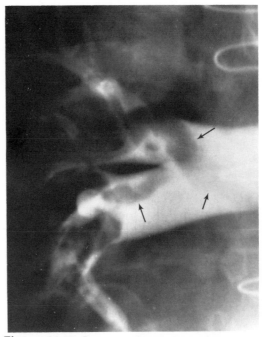

Figure 20.15. Large pulmonary embolus obstructing the right upper and lower lobe pulmonary arteries. Thrombus proximal to occlusion is seen within the arterial lumen (*arrows*).

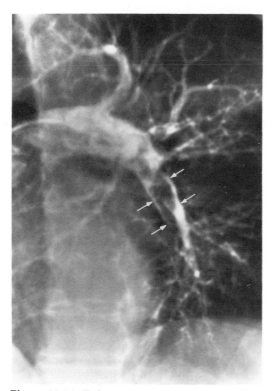

Figure 20.14. Pulmonary embolus: an intraluminal filling defect (*arrows*) within left lobe pulmonary artery.

flow is completely obstructed, the proximal end of the clot must be demonstrated to protrude into the lumen of the artery (Fig. 20.15). Vascular occlusion without evidence of a filling defect is nonspecific. Abrupt cutoff of pulmonary vessels has been seen with pulmonary abscess, neoplasm, and tuberculosis (21). Slow or diminished flow in a limited area is also nonspecific and may be seen in a multitude of other conditions. Selective angiography has diminished the incidence of equivocal angiography, which was common when injections were made only in the main pulmonary artery (1) (Fig. 20.16).

The syndrome of chronic pulmonary embolism (57) occurs when pulmonary emboli organize and become fibrotic. This may result from repeated bouts of emboli over years or from large emboli that fragment but do not completely lyse. These patients may have chronic dyspnea and suffer recurrent thrombophlebitis. Most have pulmonary hypertension. The angiographic manifestations include occluded vessels and those with stenoses and webs (Fig. 20.17).

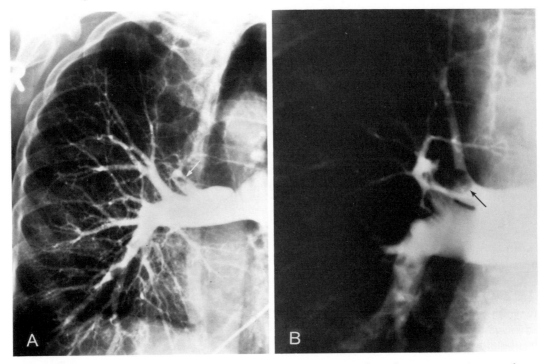

Figure 20.16. Embolus confirmed by superselective injection. **A.** Right pulmonary arteriogram shows possible defect in upper lobe branch. **B.** Superselective arteriography demonstrates an intraluminal filling defect (*arrow*) diagnostic of embolus.

Although these angiographic findings are not entirely specific, this syndrome should be considered in patients within the appropriate clinical setting.

PULMONARY ANGIOGRAPHY FOR NONEMBOLIC DISORDERS

Pulmonary Arteriovenous Malformation

Pulmonary arteriovenous malformation (PAVM) is a congenital abnormality that may be an isolated entity but is commonly associated with Osler-Weber-Rendu syndrome (58, 59). Clinical manifestations include dyspnea and cyanosis due to shunting of unoxygenated blood through the lung. This may be complicated by brain abscess, paradoxic embolization (including stroke),

or hemoptysis, and it carries with it a substantial risk of death. Pregnancy may be a predisposing factor for the development of acute hemothorax complicating PAVM. It has been suggested that women with hereditary telangiectasia be screened for PAVM before becoming pregnant (60). Transesophageal echocardiography may be helpful in the detection of PAVM (61). About 80% of PAVM consists of a single pulmonary arterial branch communicating directly with a draining vein through an aneurysmal vascular segment (Fig. 20.18) (25). The remaining cases are more complex, consisting of several arterial branches communicating with a septate aneurysmal segment and two or more draining veins (Fig. 20.19). Pulmonary angiography is diagnostic and a prerequisite for **transcatheter embolization,** the treatment of choice for PAVM (25, 62–65) because it eliminates the need for thoracotomy and preserves maximal lung function. It is indicated in all patients with symptoms and in those with lower-lobe PAVM greater than 3

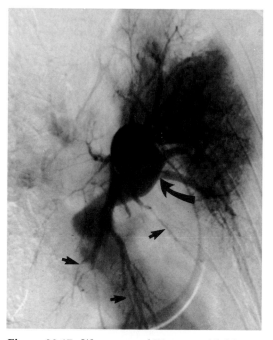

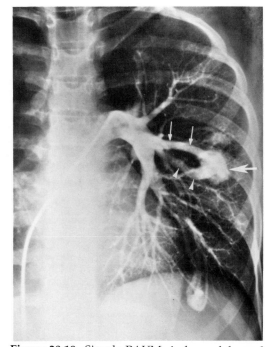

Figure 20.17. Woman aged 54 years with history of chronic pulmonary embolism and new exacerbation of shortness of breath. The lower-lobe pulmonary arteries show multiple irregularities and stenoses (*arrows*) consistent with chronic pulmonary embolism. A small rounded filling defect in the lingular artery (*curved arrow*) is consistent with acute pulmonary embolism. A larger acute embolism (not shown) was noted within the right pulmonary artery.

Figure 20.18. Simple PAVMs in lower lobe and lingula. Each malformation consists of a single feeding artery (*small arrows*), aneurysmal segment (*large arrow*), and a draining vein (*arrowheads*).

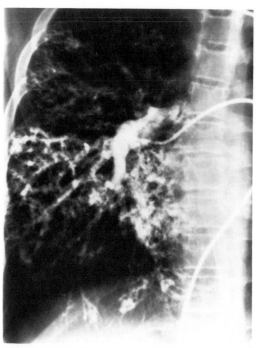

mm in diameter, regardless of symptoms, because of the risk of paradoxic embolization, brain abscess, and stroke.

Therapeutic embolization of PAVM has been performed with steel coils (Cook Inc.) (Fig 20.20) (64, 65) and detachable silicone balloons (Becton-Dickinson, Inc., Rutherford, NJ) (Fig. 20.21) (25, 62, 63). Silicone balloons are particularly advantageous because they can be positioned precisely within the feeding artery and repositioned if necessary prior to final detachment. However, the U.S. Food and Drug Administration (FDA) has approved no balloons for use in the pulmonary circulation. Thus coils are predominantly used for therapeutic embolization in this country. Diagnostic pulmonary angiography of both lungs is required before embolotherapy. Selective pulmonary arteriograms in several projec-

Figure 20.19. Complex PAVMs with multiple diffuse arteriovenous communications throughout the right lower lobe.

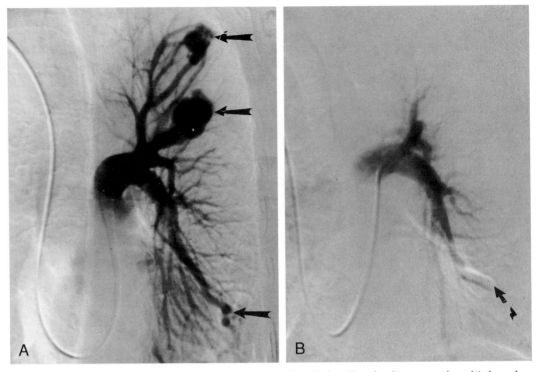

Figure 20.20. A. A 71-year-old patient with known Osler-Weber-Rendu disease and multiple pulmonary artery arteriovenous malformations (*arrows*) shown on this arteriogram. **B.** After embolization the arteriovenous malformations fail to fill. Coils were used for the two upper lobe malformations, and a balloon (*arrow*) was used for the lower-lobe malformation.

tions are necessary to localize the feeding vessels. This is usually performed at a separate session to limit the dose of contrast to the patient. In one early series (25) that included both simple and complex PAVMs, 91 arteriovenous fistulas were found in 17 patients. Therapeutic embolization with the detachable balloon technique was successful in 14 of 16 treated patients and was associated with an increase in arterial Po_2 from a mean of 44 mm Hg to a mean of 65 mm Hg. Recurrence due to collateral development has not been a problem, and complications (e.g., embolization to the systemic circulation, occlusion of normal arteries) have been infrequent and usually occur early in an operator's experience.

Rarely a bronchial arteriovenous malformation may cause hemoptysis. Pulmonary angiography in such cases may be normal, and the angiographic diagnosis depends on digital subtraction aortography (66).

Pulmonary Branch Stenosis

Congenital stenosis of the pulmonary artery may occur in either a diffuse or a focal pattern. Focal patterns consist of discrete obstructions with relatively normal-sized vessels before and beyond. Diffuse patterns manifest as abrupt tapering of the arteries, which remain small in their peripheral distribution. Pulmonary branch stenosis may also arise as a complication of surgery for congenital heart disease. Angiography plays an important role in the diagnosis and is necessary for the performance and evaluation of **balloon dilation** and stenting (67, 68). Pressure recordings are helpful in establishing the hemodynamic burden of the stenoses. Complete cardiac catheterization should be considered to exclude associated congenital defects. We have a patient with unilateral peripheral pulmonic stenosis as-

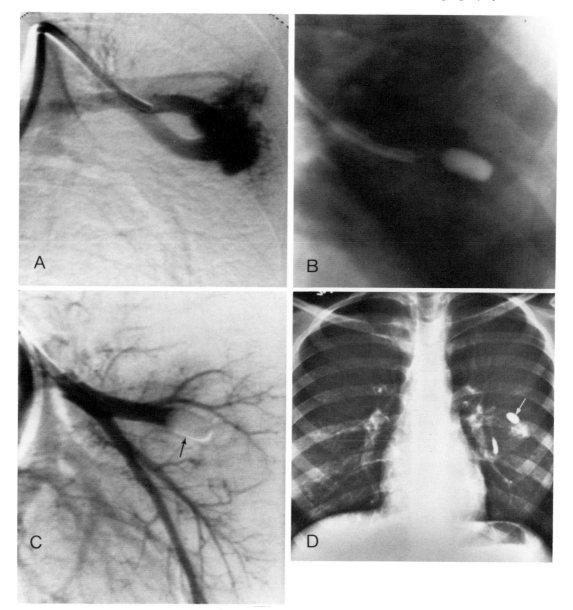

Figure 20.21. Balloon occlusion of PAVM. Selective DSA within feeding artery of malformation (**A**). Balloon is inflated within feeding artery (**B**) and is seen occluding malformation (*arrow*) (**C**). Follow-up chest film (**D**) shows balloon in place (*arrow*), as well as second balloon occluding feeding artery to lower-lobe PAVM.

sociated with the scimitar syndrome on the contralateral side (Fig. 20.22) (69). Pulmonary arterial stenosis may also be associated with Takayasu's arteritis (Fig 20.23). MRI may also contribute to diagnosis of pulmonary branch stenosis (Fig. 20.24).

Partial Anomalous Pulmonary Venous Return

Partial anomalous pulmonary venous return most frequently occurs in association

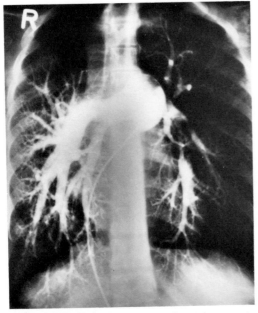

Figure 20.22. Pulmonary artery branch stenosis. Multiple discrete stenoses involving the left pulmonary artery. (Reprinted with permission from Platia EV, Brinker JA. Scimitar syndrome with peripheral left pulmonary artery branch stenoses. Am Heart J 1984;107:594–596.)

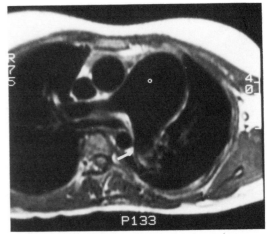

Figure 20.24. Diffuse pulmonary arterial stenoses demonstrated by MRI. Transition from dilated proximal pulmonary artery to hypoplastic branch vessel (*arrow*).

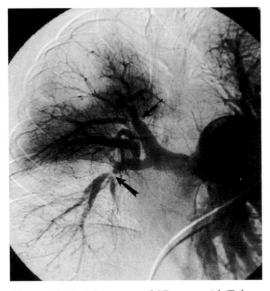

Figure 20.23. Woman aged 27 years with Takayasu arteritis involving the pulmonary arteries presents with multiple branch stenosis (*arrows*).

with atrial septal defect. On occasion, however, it is an isolated entity presenting as an abnormal finding on chest x-ray film or with the clinical picture of an atrial septal defect. A solitary left anomalous pulmonary venous connection is particularly unusual and may pose a diagnostic puzzle, being missed at catheterization unless blood from the high superior vena cava and left innominate vein is sampled for oxygen saturation (70). Analysis of dye dilution curves obtained by selective injection in both the right and left pulmonary arteries may also be helpful. Pulmonary angiography with delayed filming to include the venous phase is diagnostic (Fig. 20.25). CT and MRI are less invasive (71) but may offer little benefit if pulmonary arterial access is necessary for hemodynamic characterization and oximetry.

When associated with atrial septal defect, anomalous veins most often enter in or near the right atrium, and the condition is easily identified at surgery when both defects are corrected. Thus demonstration of an atrial septal defect at catheterization usually obviates angiographic definition of the pulmonary veins. Rarely an anomalous vein enters the systemic venous circulation remote from the atria and is not identified at the time of atrial septal defect repair. While this does not justify routine pulmo-

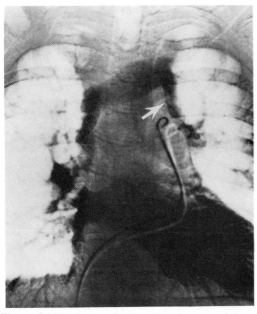

Figure 20.25. Anomalous pulmonary venous return. Venous phase of pulmonary angiogram demonstrating anomalous vein from left lung (*arrow*). This was an isolated finding in a patient thought to have an atrial septal defect. (Reprinted with permission from McGaughey MD, Traill TA, Brinker JA. Partial left anomalous pulmonary venous return: a diagnostic dilemma.)

nary angiography or selective dye curves for every patient with atrial septal defect, abnormalities on chest x-ray film or oximetry suggesting such a problem should be pursued at catheterization.

Pulmonary Varix

A perihilar or mediastinal mass on chest x-ray film may be the presenting feature of pulmonary varix. This is an aneurysmal enlargement of a segment of a pulmonary vein thought most often to be secondary to venous hypertension resulting from mitral valve disease. Three types of varix, saccular, tortuous, and confluent, have been described by Uyama, et al. (72). The varix may be demonstrated by pulmonary angiography, but less invasive studies, such as CT and MRI, are also diagnostic (73).

Neoplastic masses may compress the pulmonary veins and cause varying degrees of obstruction. Transesophageal echocardiography has been used to document this entity and follow its response to therapy (74).

Other Indications for Pulmonary Angiography

A number of other congenital and acquired abnormalities of the pulmonary vascular system may be revealed angiographically. While the need for angiography has been lessened by the availability of other imaging modalities, it is still considered the gold standard and is often required if surgical intervention is being considered. In many situations catheterization is performed to exclude other pathology and to get a physiologic assessment of the pulmonary abnormality. Pulmonary angiography in these situations is usually easily obtained with a minimum of risk. It may be used to demonstrate idiopathic dilation of the pulmonary artery, unilateral absence of a pulmonary artery (75, 76), pulmonary artery to atrial shunt (77), pulmonary artery sling (78), and pulmonary arterial aneurysm (Fig 20.26) (79–81). Sarcoma of the pulmonary artery may be visualized by contrast injection in the right ventricle or pulmonary artery (82). Pulmonary venous obstruction may be documented by wedge and subselective pulmonary angiography (83, 84). Rarely massive large thrombi may develop in the central pulmonary arteries of patients having primary pulmonary hypertension. These thrombi may not be associated with segmental or larger defects on V/Q scans, and the diagnosis is established by angiography (85).

On occasion it is necessary to visualize the pulmonary arterial system by other than routine techniques. In patients with a variety of congenital heart defects, pulmonary blood flow is maintained by surgical shunts or systemic-to-pulmonary collateralization. Not only may patency of a surgical shunt be assessed, but so may collateralization around it (Fig. 20.27). In some patients the opportunity for surgical intervention depends on the assessment of a confluence between the right and left pulmonary arteries, the size of the pulmonary vessels, the pressure in the circulation, and extent of any collateralization. Enlargement of small pulmo-

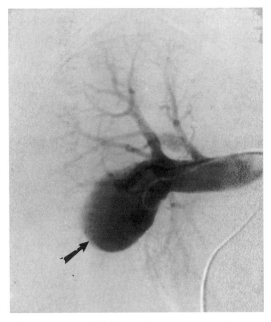

Figure 20.26. Right pulmonary arteriogram demonstrates a massive pulmonary artery aneurysm (*arrow*) in a 30-year-old woman with a history of chronic intravenous drug abuse.

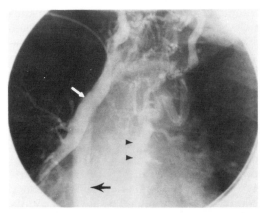

Figure 20.27. Superior vena cavagram in patient with Glenn shunt. Right pulmonary artery is opacified, as is a network of collaterals to azygos (*arrow*) and hemizygous (*arrowheads*) veins. *White arrow,* Superior vena cava.

nary arteries by a palliative procedure may be documented by angiography (86).

Access to the pulmonary arterial system may require catheterization of the shunt or a bronchial collateral. We have negotiated Blalock-Taussig shunts and bronchial collaterals with standard Judkins right coronary catheters. Pressure measurements and contrast injections can be performed through this catheter, or if necessary, an exchange guidewire enables other catheters to be positioned properly. Selective catheterization and angiography of the pulmonary artery in such cases enable one to obtain hemodynamic data and acquire angiography superior to aortography or right ventriculography (87). Biplane imaging (AP and lateral) is optimal, and relatively steep cranial angulation in the AP projection best reveals the pulmonary artery bifurcation.

A portion of the lung may receive its blood supply from a systemic artery. Frequently this is in association with bronchopulmonary sequestration, although rarely it may occur without sequestration. The anomalous systemic artery may be documented angiographically or by less invasive imaging techniques (88).

Pulmonary Angiography to Visualize the Left Heart

Contrast material injected into the pulmonary artery may be used to image the left atrium, left ventricle, and ascending aorta. We have used this technique to evaluate left ventricular function when direct injection was thought to be associated with increased risk, such as in the presence of left ventricular thrombus, aortic valvular endocarditis, and in some patients with aortic valve prosthesis. This technique has been suggested as a means of demonstrating cardiac thrombi in patients with cerebral infarction (89). Aortic dissection may also be visualized by cineangiography following pulmonary arterial injection.

Disadvantages of this approach include dilution of contrast as it passes through the pulmonary circulation, additional radiation dosage to patient and operator as one follows the contrast through the lungs, the chance of missing information by delaying imaging by an arbitrary time period (usually 3 to 5 seconds), direct exposure of the lungs to contrast, and inability to assess valvular regurgitation. Digital subtraction angiography may be an alternative to cineangiography, but it has other potential problems (e.g., motion artifact if injection of contrast material causes discomfort or stimulates cough and inability to image the full contraction sequence of left ventricle). Alternative imaging techniques, such as echocardiography with Doppler flow, gated blood pool scanning, MRI, and CT, can yield important information with less risk.

VENOGRAPHY

Intravenous injection of contrast material is used to document obstructive venous disease, as well as to document aberrant anatomy. Pertinent to the invasive cardiologist is venography of the brachiocephalic system. This is most often done when difficulties arise during the course of catheterization or pacemaker implantation. It may, however, also be part of a more thorough evaluation in a patient with symptoms of venous occlusion. Venography may be performed by advancing a catheter to the site in question and injecting selectively or by a bolus injection through a peripheral intravenous canula. Injection of 15 to 20 mL of contrast material through a vein in an upper extremity may be followed by a bolus of saline to arrive in the subclavian system relatively undiluted. We have used cineangiography and acquisition to document subclavian thrombosis (Fig. 20.28), thoracic outlet syndrome (Fig. 20.29), and superior vena cava obstruction (Fig. 20.30). Anomalous drainage of a left superior vena cava into the coronary sinus has been demonstrated by injecting in a left upper extremity vein or by passing a catheter from below through the coronary sinus (Fig. 20.31). Documentation of superior vena caval obstruction may lead to attempts at balloon angioplasty (90) with (91) or without stenting. While the prognosis for this entity is poor when associated with malignancy,

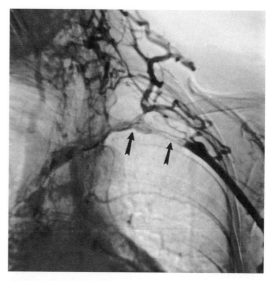

Figure 20.28. Digital subtraction left upper extremity venogram demonstrating occlusion of the left subclavian vein (*arrows*) with extensive collateralization via the superficial and deep veins of the neck. The patient had a history of a Hickman catheter on the left side.

long-term improvement may be achieved when obstruction results from a stenosing process, such as accompanies chronic catheter placement (91).

Venography of the lower extremity and intra-abdominal veins is performed less frequently now that noninvasive techniques are available. Ultrasound is considered by some to be the standard for diagnosing femoropopliteal deep venous thrombosis (53, 54, 92). On occasion, however, these modalities yield equivocal findings, and use of contrast is necessary (Fig. 20.32). The course of venous thrombosis has been characterized by acute (less than 1 week), subacute (1 to 4 weeks), and chronic stages. Angiographic findings similarly vary, and experience is necessary to avoid many pitfalls in interpretation of these studies (93).

Inferior vena cava angiography may be necessary for the placement and follow-up of a percutaneously introduced vena cava filter (94). It is used to detect anatomic variations, to size the inferior vena cava, to exclude thrombus, and to locate the renal veins. The inferior vena cava can be imaged well with digital techniques (2 frames per

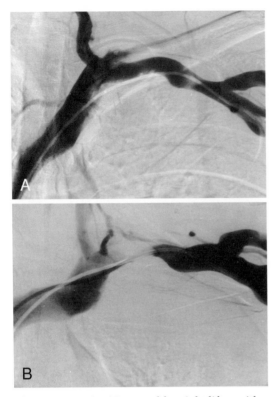

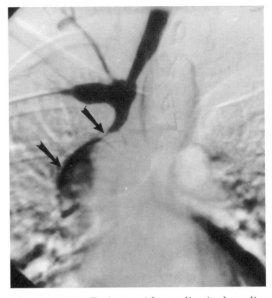

Figure 20.30. Patient with mediastinal malignancy resulting in superior vena cava obstruction (*arrows*) and superior vena cava syndrome.

Figure 20.29. An 18-year-old weight lifter with a prior episode of left subclavian vein thrombosis recanalized with thrombolytic therapy and having symptoms during exercise. **A**. In the neutral position the venogram is essentially normal, and no pressure gradient was recorded across the subclavian vein. **B**. On Adson's maneuver (ipsilateral hand behind head with head turned to contralateral side) essentially complete obstruction of the subclavian vein was noted and a 35-mm gradient was measured across the stenosis.

second) with an injection of 40 mL of contrast delivered at 20 mL per second.

VENA CAVAL FILTERS

Vena caval filters provide protection against recurrent pulmonary embolism. They are indicated to prevent recurrent pulmonary emboli in patients experiencing pulmonary embolism on adequate anticoagulation and in those who are not candidates for anticoagulation (i.e., recent history of gastrointestinal hemorrhage, hemor-

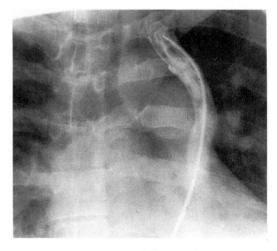

Figure 20.31. Persistent left superior vena cava shown by injection of catheter passing through coronary sinus.

rhagic stroke, noncompliant). Caval filters may also have a role in prophylaxis for high-risk patients. For example, patients with known lower-extremity deep venous thrombosis may experience pulmonary embolism in up to 25% of the time during lower extremity orthopedic surgery such as

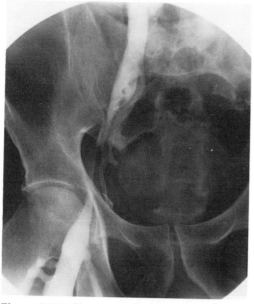

Figure 20.32. Venogram demonstrating femoral vein compression by a hematoma. No thrombosis is seen. Ultrasound examination was equivocal.

a knee or hip replacement. These individuals may benefit significantly from an inferior vena cava filter prior to surgery.

There are five FDA-approved caval filters on the market. These include the stainless steel and titanium Greenfield filters (Medi-Tech, Watertown, MA), the Bird's Nest filter (Cook Inc.) (Fig. 20.33), the Vena Tech filter (Braun, Evanston, IL) (Fig. 20.34), and the Simon Nitinol filter (Nitinol Medical Technologies, Woburn, MA). Each device has its own advantages and disadvantages. Some have a relatively small delivery system and can thus be inserted from a wide variety of access sites. Others are larger and can be used in patients with mega–inferior vena cavae (more than 28 mm in diameter). The manufacturers also claim superiority of prevention of recurrent embolism and/or a higher incidence of vena caval patency. With experience most physicians come to prefer one of the devices over the others.

Caval filters may be inserted by venous cut-down or percutaneously from the jugular, subclavian, or femoral approach with a high degree of success (95). They are typically performed from the right common

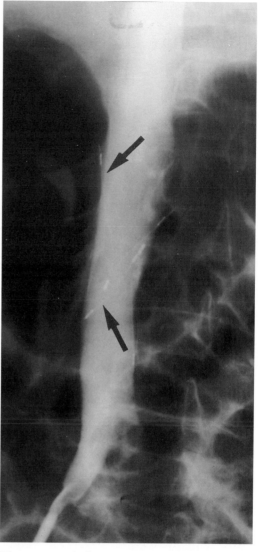

Figure 20.33. Inferior vena cavagram following placement of a Bird's Nest inferior vena cava filter. Note the two V-shaped struts (*arrows*). The small tangled wires forming the actual nest are not visible because of their small gauge.

femoral vein. Once access to this vessel is gained, a small amount of contrast is injected to establish the presence or absence of clot in the right iliac system. If no clot is present, filter placement can continue from this approach. However, it is suggested that if clot is documented, placement be attempted from the contralateral femoral vein or the right internal jugular vein to avoid

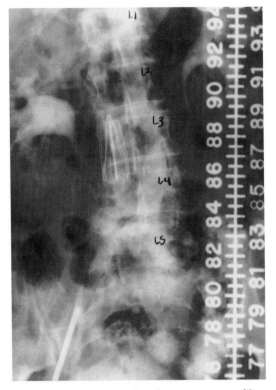

Figure 20.34. Vena Tech inferior vena cava filter in a patient with documented deep venous thrombosis and a recent gastrointestinal hemorrhage.

dislodgement of the clot and iatrogenic embolization. A vena cavogram should initially be performed with a 5-F pigtail to document the position of the renal veins and the transverse diameter of the inferior vena cava. While all of today's filters can be used in cavae that are 28 mm or less in diameter, only the Bird's Nest is approved for cavae up to 48 mm in diameter. After the vena cavogram is performed, the pigtail catheter is exchanged for a stiff guidewire, and the delivery system for the filter is gently advanced into the inferior vena cava and positioned below the level of the renal veins.

Each filter has a specific delivery release mechanism, so the operator should be thoroughly familiar with the particular device prior to implantation. Filters should be released so that the top of the filter cone is at the level of the renal veins. The inferior vena cava typically widens at the point of the renal veins, and positioning the filter at this point may result in failure to engage the caval wall. Should this occur, the filter could enter the renal vein and lodge at this location, tilt to a point that renders it ineffective, or migrate to the heart or pulmonary circulation. Once the filter has been released, a follow-up vena cavogram is recommended to document the position of the filter with respect to the walls of the cava and the renal veins.

Sometimes suprarenal placement of the inferior vena cava filter is desired. These include the following:

1. Clot within the inferior vena cava to the level of the renal veins
2. Renal vein thrombosis with recurrent pulmonary emboli
3. Female patient of child-bearing age
4. Tumor thrombus within the cava specifically from a renal vein or adrenal vein source

Patients with a documented upper-extremity source of recurrent pulmonary embolism can have a filter placed in the superior vena cava, although the clinical necessity of this approach has not been clearly established.

Upon completion of filter implantation, the catheters are removed from the groin and hemostasis obtained. In some cases the patient may be anticoagulated, which may help maintain inferior vena cava patency and prevent clot formation within the cone of the filter. While vena caval filters are relatively effective, their use has been complicated by caval occlusion; device migration, including embolization to the heart or pulmonary artery (96); tilting; and penetration of the venous wall. Their effectiveness may be compromised by the development of large collaterals. There is a relatively high short-term mortality of patients receiving vena cava filters, predominantly because of underlying disease. It is possible to stratify patients as to the likelihood of mortality based on analysis of their underlying disease (97).

AORTOGRAPHY

The aortogram is an important tool in the diagnosis and follow-up of a number of dis-

Table 20.4.
Indications for Aortography

1. Aortic valve integrity
2. Nonselective views of coronary arteries or grafts
3. Supravalvular aortic stenosis
4. Disease of the brachiocephalic and other branch vessels
5. Aortic aneurysm
6. Aortic dissection
7. Coarctation
8. Detection of systemic to pulmonary communications
9. Definition of pulmonary circulation by shunts or collaterals
10. Postvascular surgery
11. Trauma
12. Aortic neoplasia
13. Arterial thromboembolic disease
14. Atherosclerotic narrowing
15. Inflammatory arterial disease

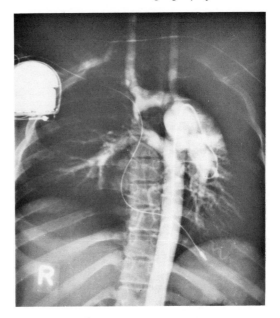

Figure 20.35. Aortography to delineate pulmonary circulation. Aortogram demonstrates pulmonary arterial system via functioning Blalock-Taussig shunt. Patient has a single ventricle with atretic pulmonary valve.

orders (Table 20.4). While the remarkable advances attained in noninvasive imaging have lessened the need for this procedure, aortography still plays an important role in the delineation of anatomy, is especially useful if surgery is contemplated, and is essential if catheter intervention is to be undertaken.

Contrast radiographs of the aorta and its branches may be recorded in a variety of ways, including cine, serial cut film, 105-mm photofluorography, and digital techniques (dynamic, subtraction, and serial spot acquisition). Each has advantages and disadvantages. Cineangiography is logistically simple, views structures in motion, and allows one to extend the area of visualization by panning along the path of contrast flow without motion artifact. It is ideal for the evaluation of aortic regurgitation and may be helpful in dissection by revealing the motion of an intimal flap. We have found it useful for visualizing the distal aorta and iliofemoral system as part of a cardiac catheterization. It lacks, however, the scope of coverage and resolution of serial cut filming. Cut filming may be the technique of choice when fine anatomic detail is required and when there is a large field of interest. It has been routinely employed in the study of aortic aneurysm and dissec-

tion and when the pulmonary arterial system is filled by systemic flow (Fig. 20.35)

Digital acquisition is being used with increasing frequency, especially for the evaluation of small discrete vascular areas. The mode of choice in the performance of interventional procedures, it offers advantages of postprocessing, facilitated storage of data, less contrast use, and possibly less radiation exposure. Subtraction techniques provide a relatively easy way to screen the carotid and vertebral vessels in patients coming to cardiac catheterization with signs or symptoms of cerebrovascular disease. It may be useful in locating a radiolucent intravascular foreign body (Fig. 20.36) (98).

While digital angiography has largely replaced 105-mm photofluorography in our laboratory, photofluorography can yield excellent studies, especially when selective injections of smaller vessels are necessary. It provides better resolution with less total radiation to the patient than cineangiography and may be available in laboratories that lack the ability to perform serial cut filming or digital acquisition.

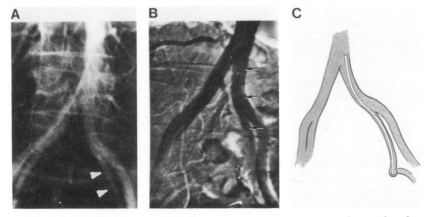

Figure 20.36. Detection of a radiolucent foreign body, an angioplasty catheter sheath, accidentally dislodged in the ascending aorta. It was searched for angiographically. Cineangiography in the descending aorta revealed a straightening of the left internal iliac vessel (**A**, *arrowheads*). Digital angiography revealed the sheath to extend proximally into the descending aorta (**B**). The foreign body was removed with a snare introduced from the right femoral artery (**C**). (Reprinted with permission from McIvor ME, Kaufman SL, Satre S, et al. Search and retrieval of an unidentifiable foreign object. Cathet Cardiovasc Diagn 1989;16:19–23.)

Ascending Aortography

Contrast material is injected into the ascending aorta to assess the anatomy of the aortic root, arch, and branch vessels, including aberrant coronary vessels. It may also be injected to locate coronary bypass grafts or determine their patency, to demonstrate abnormal vascular communication, or to quantitate aortic insufficiency. Since optimal opacification necessitates a relatively large amount of contrast material delivered over a short time, pigtail catheters capable of handling high flow rates are most often used. These have the advantage of accepting a guidewire, which allows for safe and easy placement, especially if the aortic wall is fragile (e.g., Marfan's syndrome or aortic dissection). The pigtail dissipates the pressure of the injection without a jet of contrast exiting the end hole. This reduces catheter recoil and the possibility of damage should the catheter migrate toward a small branch or a weakened area of the aorta. Since the aortogram is commonly only part of a diagnostic catheterization, one can use a pigtail catheter of the same outer diameter as the other arterial catheters employed during the procedure. There has been a growing tendency to use smaller catheters (5 to 6 F)

for these procedures; however, some of these devices do not provide very high flow rates, especially if the more viscous low-osmolality contrast agents are used at room temperature. It is essential that the pressure limit of the power injector be set appropriately and that the catheter accept the pressure and flow desired. Straight end hole or multi–side hole catheters should not be used for aortography in general because the high flow rates required cause considerable catheter recoil and possibly vascular damage.

The catheter should be positioned a few centimeters above the aortic valve for opacification of the entire aortic root. Too low a placement may interfere with the aortic valve, possibly inducing artifactual regurgitation. If the catheter dips into the ventricle, dilution of the contrast bolus may degrade visualization of the aorta. If the catheter is placed too high, opacification of the lower portion of root may be inadequate and aortic regurgitation underestimated.

While angiography can be safely performed in most patients, in rare instances even obtaining arterial access may pose a risk (e.g., Ehler Danlos syndrome, homocystinuria). In such cases intravenous DSA may be particularly helpful (Fig. 20.37) (99). Re-

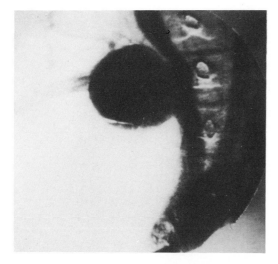

Figure 20.37. Aneurysm of innominate artery. Digital angiogram following intravenous contrast injection in a patient with Ehlers-Danlos syndrome IV in whom arterial access was thought too risky. (Reprinted with permission from Pyeritz RE, Stolle CA, Parfrey NA, Myers JC. Ehlers-Danlos syndrome IV due to a novel defect in type III procollagen. Am J Med Gen 1984;19:607–622.)

cently transesophageal echocardiography has been used to demonstrate protruding atheromas in the aortic arch at the time of cardiopulmonary bypass. Such disease can predict postoperative stroke (100). It is possible that such friable atheroma may be dislodged during aortography, accounting for the small but finite incidence of cerebral events accompanying this procedure.

The optimal positioning of the patient for aortography depends on the clinical objectives. In general the ascending aorta is best visualized in the steep left anterior oblique (LAO) projection (45 to 60°). This allows for assessment of aortic insufficiency and spreads out the ascending aorta and arch. Supravalvular stenosis, coarctation, and aortopulmonary communications are well seen. Aortocoronary grafts may also be detected in this view, although biplane filming (LAO and right anterior oblique, or RAO) is commonly used so that the origin and course of the grafts, especially grafts to the left anterior descending artery, which may be foreshortened and overlapped in the LAO projection, can be delineated. On

occasion, when there is significant aortic regurgitation, left ventricular function can be assessed from the aortogram. This may obviate crossing a prosthetic aortic valve and lessens the contrast load. RAO or biplane filming should be used.

Serial cut films are often used for aortic aneurysms, dissections, and evaluation of aortic-to-pulmonary communications, be they iatrogenic or congenital. Biplane aortograms in the AP and lateral projections are most often obtained. Biplane filming limits the total number and rate of images that can be recorded because of the need to expose the film alternately to avoid image degradation by x-ray scatter. If faster filming or a greater number of images are required, a single plane in either the steep LAO or AP projection may be substituted. The programing of serial films depends on the information desired. The ascending aorta is best visualized during the first 2 to 3 seconds of injection, and filming should be performed at 2 to 3 exposures per second over this time. The total number of images recorded and the programing of the remaining films in the run vary. Late filming is necessary to visualize the collaterals in coarctation (Fig. 20.38), a false lumen in cases of dissection, and the pulmonary anatomy in the presence of systemic-to-pulmonary communications. A total of 12 to 15 films in each projection, with an exposure rate of 1 film per second after the first 2 to 4 seconds, is usually obtained. The dedicated cardiac catheterization laboratory may not be able to perform cut-film angiography. Digital angiography or cineangiography may be an acceptable alternative. While biplane cineangiography is often available, biplane digital acquisition is less widespread.

The rate and amount of contrast material needed for aortography depends on the size of the patient, the cardiac output, and the specific anatomy. Usually 50 to 70 mL is delivered over 2 to 3 seconds. The larger amounts of contrast material are needed if flow is high or large aneurysms (such as occasionally encountered in Marfan's syndrome) require opacification. The use of nonionic contrast is recommended for patients who have precarious hemodynamics, who are otherwise at increased risk, or who

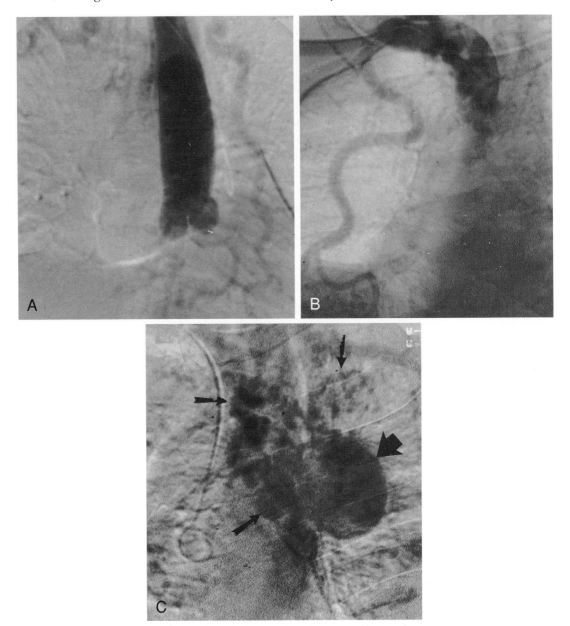

Figure 20.38. Woman aged 40 years with a 30-year history of hypertension and aortic stenosis. **A.** RAO view of the ascending aorta shows a bicuspid aortic valve. **B.** The aortic arch is obstructed distal to the left subclavian artery. Note the large internal mammary artery (*arrow*), which collateralizes to the internal iliac arteries and abdominal aorta. **C.** Late phase from the arch aortogram shows significant collaterals around the region of the obstruction (*small arrows*) and a large aneurysm (*large arrow*).

require a great deal of contrast medium to complete the study.

In general, less contrast material is needed and better pictures obtained if the injection is made as close to the area of inter-

est as possible. While the ascending aortogram gives information about the origins of the brachiocephalic vessels, digital subtraction techniques or selective injections provide better definition. Similarly, there may be little reason to inject dye into the ascending aorta if the object of the study is to evaluate a descending aortic aneurysm or to assess the pulmonary arterial system via bronchial collateralization. Proximal and distal injections may be necessary, however, to define the full extent of the disease process, to document other pathology, or to evaluate the nature and extent of collateralization.

Aortic Dissection

Aortic dissection may have a characteristic clinical picture; however, this is not always the case (101). It may be characterized as **one of the great masqueraders**, with fever, heart murmur, neurologic signs, and abnormal chest x-ray mimicking a variety of pathologic processes. Similarly, a variety of disorders can cause signs and symptoms compatible with acute dissection and be so mistaken (102). It is especially important to differentiate dissection from acute myocardial infarction so that thrombolytic and anticoagulant therapy are not inadvertently given (103, 104). The definitive diagnosis of dissecting aneurysm (actually a dissecting hematoma) has traditionally rested with aortography, and this is still the reference standard required by some surgeons before operation is considered. False-negative aortograms do occur, however, and other diagnostic modalities should be pursued as clinically indicated (105). The goals of aortography in patients with the clinical suspicion of dissection are to establish the diagnosis and to identify whether the process involves the ascending aorta or arch (proximal dissection; Fig. 20.39) or exists solely distal to the left subclavian artery (Fig. 20.40). Secondary objectives are to evaluate the integrity of the aortic valve and to determine patency of major branch vessels (Fig. 20.41). In older patients and those with a history of coronary disease it may be necessary to assess coronary anatomy for atherosclerotic obstruction so that a combined surgical procedure may be performed. Rarely rupture into a contiguous structure is documented (Fig. 20.42).

The angiographic diagnosis of dissec-

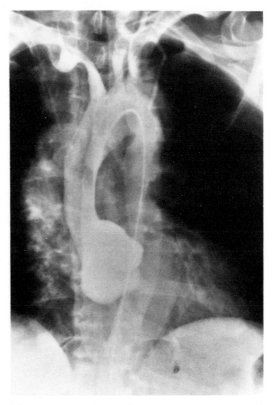

Figure 20.39. Ascending aortography reveals dissection involving proximal aorta and extending into brachycephalic vessels.

tion rests with the demonstration of a false lumen or intimal flap. Occlusion of branch vessels and compression of the contrast-filled aorta by intramural clot are highly suggestive. Traditionally, serial cut-film aortography in the steep LAO or AP–lateral biplane projections is performed. This allows for visualization of the ascending aorta, the arch, its major branch vessels, and the descending thoracic aorta. On occasion it is necessary to perform a second injection to evaluate the abdominal aorta and its branches. Cineangiography has the advantage of documenting the presence and degree of aortic regurgitation. It also images the aorta in motion, easily detecting any intimal flap (106); however, the field of view and resolution are less than are obtainable with serial cut filming. Noninvasive imaging techniques vary in their sensitivity and specificity compared with aortography, and each has some limitations. Transthoracic

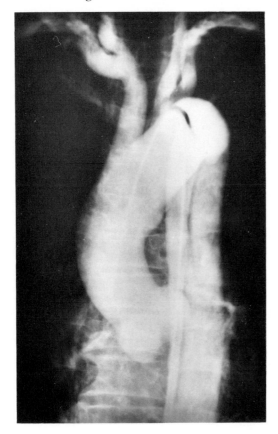

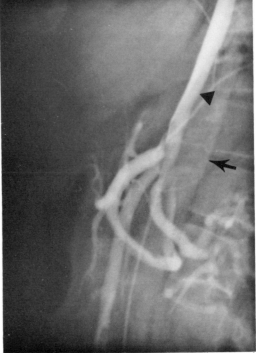

Figure 20.41. Aortic dissection. Lateral view of descending aortogram demonstrating true lumen compressed (*arrowhead*) and then occluded by false lumen (*arrow*).

Figure 20.40. Angiography demonstrates dissection limited to distal aorta.

echocardiography can be quickly obtained at the patient's bedside if necessary, but adequate studies cannot be recorded in every patient. Dissections limited to the descending thoracic aorta are rarely diagnosed by transthoracic sonography (107). While M-mode echocardiography lacks the sensitivity and specificity of CT or MRI (108), two-dimensional, transesophageal, and Doppler color flow echocardiography offer significant improvement and may reveal dissection missed by other techniques, including aortography (109–112). Rarely there remains some doubt as to whether a dissection is present. We have used intra-aortic ultrasound in these cases to assist in diagnosis.

Contrast-enhanced CT has proven value in the diagnosis of thoracic aortic disease and in expert hands appears to be as effica-

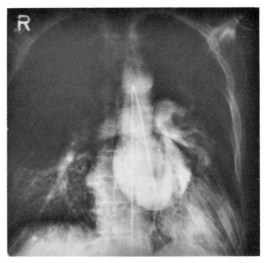

Figure 20.42. Ascending aortography revealing a rupture of dissecting aneurysm into pulmonary artery in patient with Marfan's syndrome.

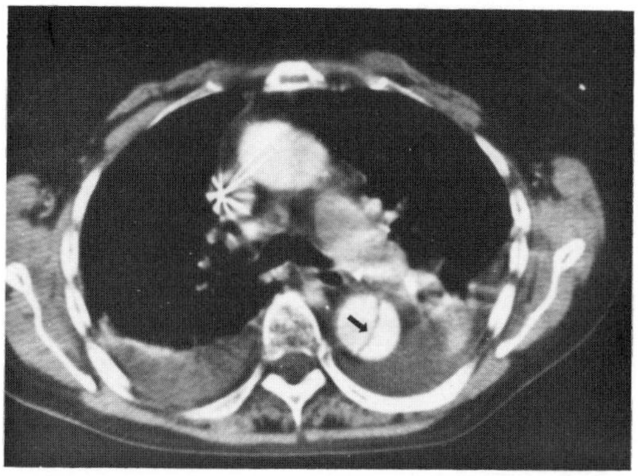

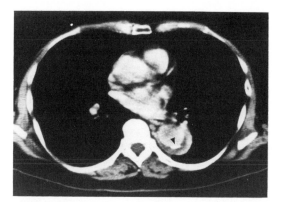

Figure 20.43. Aortic dissection. Contrast-enhanced CT demonstrates intimal flap (*arrow*) within aorta.

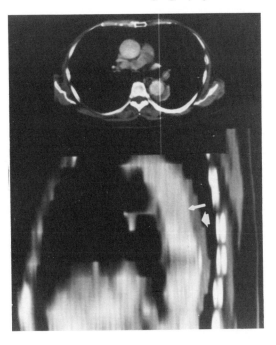

Figure 20.45. Aortic dissection. Reformatted CT demonstrating true (*arrow*) and false (*arrowhead*) lumens.

Figure 20.44. Aortic dissection. CT scan reveals medial displacement of intimal calcification (*arrowhead*).

cious as aortography in diagnosing dissection (113). The finding of a dual lumen with an intervening intimal flap is diagnostic (Fig. 20.43), and intimal calcification displaced by the false lumen (Fig. 20.44), a thickened aortic wall, disparity between the ascending and descending aorta, and compression of the true lumen are suggestive (114). Dynamic CT and reformatted images add to the study (Fig. 20.45) (115). There may be pitfalls in the diagnosis of dissection by CT (116, 117), including the differentiation of an intramural hematoma from mural thrombus in an aneurysm (118).

MRI can provide a diagnosis of dissection by demonstrating an intimal flap and double lumen (119) (Fig. 20.46). It does not require contrast injection or radiation expo-

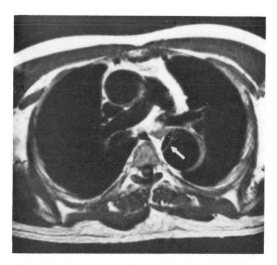

Figure 20.46. Aortic dissection. MRI revealing intimal flap (*arrow*) in descending aorta.

sure and may be superior to CT in assessment of aortic branches (120, 121). Since this method does not image calcium, it cannot detect its displacement. Other limitations of MRI include difficulty in imaging acutely ill patients and those with pacemakers or artificial ventilation. The introduction of advanced techniques allowing for three-dimensional reconstruction using multiple-intensity projection have increased the imaging capability of MRI.

The success of the less invasive procedures to screen for dissection has limited the use of angiography to cases in which there remains a high level of clinical suspicion despite negative or equivocal noninvasive studies and to patients in whom specific surgically relevant issues must be resolved. Despite the rigors of angiography the catheterization laboratory is often the best place for the acutely ill patient undergoing a diagnostic procedure because of the availability of physiologic monitoring and a staff experienced in handling such individuals. The use of nonionic contrast, soft torquable guidewires, and small pigtail catheters may further reduce the overall risk of angiography. Angiography is necessary if an interventional procedure is contemplated. There are reports of dilation of an obstructed aorta secondary to a healed dissection (122), as well as fenestration of the dissection flap and stenting (123).

Transesophageal echocardiography may be useful in following patients' postoperative repair of dissection. A persistent open false lumen is readily detected and may be related to later complications (124).

Aortic Aneurysm

Aneurysmal dilation of the aorta may be true (contain all three layers of the vessel wall) or false (encapsulated only by elements of the adventitia and reactive fibrosis). Causes of true aneurysm include atherosclerosis, inflammation, infection, and hereditary defects. False aneurysms are usually the result of trauma but may be secondary to infection, especially with *Mycobacterium tuberculosis.* While aneurysms of the ascending and descending aorta may remain clinically silent for long periods, those involving the arch tend to compress structures in the upper mediastinum and thus become evident at an earlier stage. Compression of the left recurrent laryngeal

nerve (Ortner's syndrome) may be the first indication of aortic aneurysm. The objective of angiography in the evaluation of aortic aneurysms is to demonstrate the extent of the process, the involvement of major branches, and any additional pathology (e.g., other aneurysms, stenoses, shunts). Thoracic aortic aneurysms are usually approached with an initial ascending aortic injection in the LAO projection. A second injection may be required for adequate visualization of the descending aorta (usually in the AP and lateral biplane or the LAO).

Atherosclerotic aneurysms are most common. They are usually fusiform but on occasion are saccular and are most often located in the arch or descending portions of the aorta (Fig. 20.47). The atherosclerotic process produces elongation, as well as dilation, of the aorta and may affect multiple locations along the entire course of this vessel (Fig. 20.48). Calcification in an ascending aortic aneurysm in the past suggested syphilitic involvement. At present, however, such a finding is most frequently the result of atherosclerosis. While not common, luetic aortitis may be suggested by a thin dep-

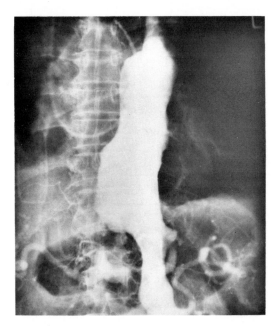

Figure 20.47. Atherosclerotic aneurysm of thoracic aorta.

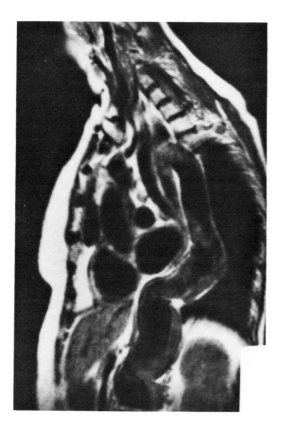

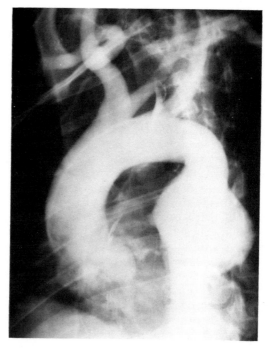

Figure 20.49. Mycotic aneurysm of descending aorta in young drug addict. Culture revealed *Staphylococcus.*

Figure 20.48. Atherosclerotic aneurysmal dilation of the thoracic and abdominal aorta demonstrated by MRI.

osition of calcium limited to the ascending aorta, by aortic regurgitation, and by serologic evidence of the disease. Narrowing of the aortocoronary ostia may also result from this disorder.

Aneurysms caused by infection (mycotic aneurysms; Fig. 20.49) may be classified as primary (not associated with an identifiable intravascular source) or secondary (having an intravascular or contiguous extravascular source of infection) (125). Mycotic aneurysms now most commonly are associated with arterial trauma or endocarditis and involve the abdominal aorta or femoral artery. If a causative agent is recoverable, most likely it is *Staphylococcus aureus* or *Salmonella* species (126).

Sinus of Valsalva aneurysms may be congenital or acquired via endocarditis. They usually involve the right or noncoro-

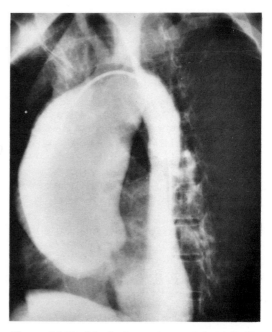

Figure 20.50. Marfan's syndrome. Massive dilation of ascending aorta associated with moderate aortic regurgitation.

nary aortic sinus and produce signs and symptoms when they rupture into a cardiac chamber. Rarely there is symptomatic obstruction of the right ventricular outflow tract. Echocardiography with color flow Doppler is valuable in the diagnosis of aneurysm and its rupture (126–129), differentiating the latter from aortic regurgitation, which it often mimics. Angiography is usually reserved for those with a complication such that surgery is being considered. On occasion an unsuspected and uncomplicated sinus of Valsalva aneurysm is found fortuitously during cardiac catheterization for other disease.

Blunt chest trauma may result in a fistulous communication between the right sinus of Valsalva and right atrium. Diagnosis may be suggested by physical examination and confirmed by noninvasive studies and catheterization (130).

Dilation of all three aortic sinuses and the ascending aorta may occur in **Marfan's syndrome** (Fig. 20.50). When such aortic dilation occurs in the absence of involvement of other organs, the term **idiopathic annuloaortic ectasia** may be used (131). The aortic dilation may be accompanied by regurgitation, dissection, or rupture, which account for the vast majority of deaths in these patients (132). This poor prognosis has prompted an aggressive approach to the management of the disorder, which includes the insertion of a composite prosthetic valve graft in selected patients (133). This implant as a unit replaces the aortic valve and the sinuses of Valsalva. Coronary flow is established by anastomosing the aortic origins of the coronary arteries to side holes created in the graft. If this not feasible, bypass grafts are constructed from the prosthesis to the coronaries. Patients with proximal aortic dissections, severe aortic regurgitation, or dilation of the aortic root in excess of 5.5 to 6 cm may be considered for this procedure. Echocardiography, MRI, or CT can be used to follow the extent of aortic dilation and to document any dissection. Aortography is reserved for patients thought to require surgery on the basis of the noninvasive work-up and is usually part of a complete catheterization, including coronary angiography. The presence and extent of mitral valve disease, the degree of dilation of the

sinuses of Valsalva, and the location of the origins of the coronary arteries with respect to this dilation have surgical importance. Angiography also plays a role in the evaluation of postoperative patients who are thought to have a complication (134) (Figs. 20.51 and 20.52).

A variety of other disorders may be associated with dilations and/or narrowing of the aorta or its major branches, including Takayasu's arteritis (Fig. 20.53), rheumatoid arthritis, ankylosing spondylitis, giant cell arteritis (Fig 20.54), relapsing polychondritis, Reiter's syndrome, polyarteritis nodosa, and Kawasaki's disease. Each of these entities has other features that afford distinction.

Traumatic aneurysms may be due to blunt or penetrating injuries. The locations most frequently affected by the former are those where the aorta undergoes transition from being relatively free to being fixed. These include the aortic isthmus (region just beyond the origin of the left subclavian artery) and the site of attachment of the aorta to the heart. Angiography plays a major role

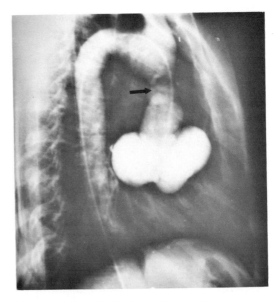

Figure 20.51. Marfan's syndrome. Previous surgery to replace portion of ascending aorta above aortic sinuses with subsequently dramatic enlargement of the sinuses. Distal anastomosis of graft with aorta (*arrow*) appears obstructive; however, no pressure gradient was detected.

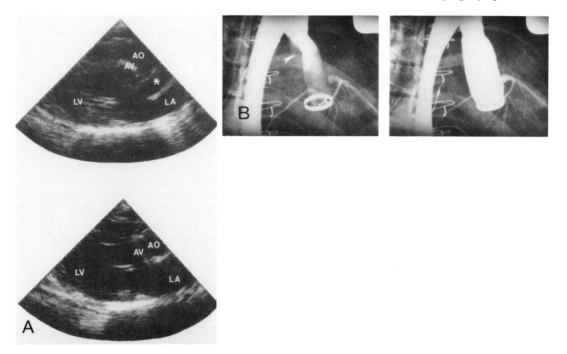

Figure 20.52. Dehiscence of valve prosthesis. Asymptomatic patient with Marfan's syndrome status after composite valve–graft insertion. Routine two-dimensional echocardiography reveals space between aorta and left atrium during ventricular systole (*asterisk*) that disappears in diastole (**A, top and bottom panels respectively**). Ascending aortography demonstrates systolic collapse of graft (**B**) because of partial dehiscence of valve prosthesis from annular insertion site. (Reprinted with permission from Josephson RA, Singer I, Levine JH, et al. Systolic expansion of the aortic root: an echocardiographic and angiographic sign of aortic composite graft dehiscence. Cathet Cardiovasc Diagn 1988; 14:105–107.)

in the evaluation of the patient thought to have a traumatic injury to the aorta; it may be accomplished by the techniques described previously. Penetrating trauma, including knife and bullet wounds, may require urgent angiography to document site of bleeding. It is advantageous in some cases to use digital acquisition with or without subtraction of intra-arterial injections, because it may be performed faster, with less contrast, and at a lower cost than conventional cut-film aortography (135). While aortography is considered the method of choice in the evaluation of aortic laceration and is relatively safe, fatal complications may occur. It has been suggested that attempts to pursue aortography by the retrograde approach be abandoned if difficulty is encountered in passage of the guidewire or catheter in cases of suspected aortic trauma (136). On occasion aortic trauma

may result from iatrogenic manipulations and be documented as part of the procedure (Fig. 20.55). Helical CT has been shown to be an alternative to aortography in some patients suspected of having traumatic aortic rupture (137).

Coarctation of the Aorta

The diagnosis of coarctation of the aorta in the adolescent and adult is usually made clinically, although on occasion it is discovered when the patient presents with an associated disorder. We have encountered two cases of unsuspected coarctation in patients with symptomatic aortic regurgitation undergoing catheterization. Angiography is used to assess the precise location and length of the coarct, the nature of collat-

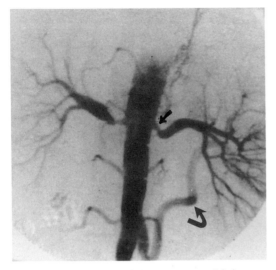

Figure 20.53. Young Asian woman with hypertension who underwent abdominal aortography. Bilateral renal artery stenoses (*arrow*) and filling of a large dilated inferior mesenteric artery (*curved arrow*) indicate critical stenosis or occlusion of the superior mesenteric artery and celiac axis.

eral vessels, and the presence and significance of other cardiovascular abnormalities. This procedure is necessary if percutaneous angioplasty of the defect is being considered and may be helpful in the assessment of restenosis or aneurysm formation following surgery or angioplasty (138) (Fig. 20.56). Hemodynamic characterization should be obtained, the translesional gradient being a function of the severity of the narrowing and the adequacy of collateralization.

The coarctation can often be negotiated from the retrograde approach using a soft torquable guidewire. In lieu of this, brachial arterial catheterization is relatively easy. The aortic narrowing is well visualized by ascending aortography in the steep LAO projection. Digital evaluation may be helpful. MRI has been shown to be useful in the diagnosis and appears superior to the echocardiogram in children with this defect (139, 140).

Balloon angioplasty of coarctation (Fig 20.2) has been performed with reasonable success and relatively low restenosis rates (141). Aneurysm formation at the site of balloon dilation has been reported with vary-

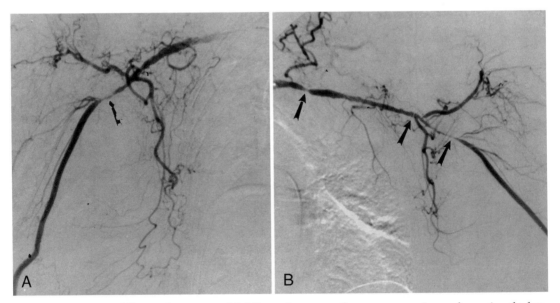

Figure 20.54. A middle-aged woman with bilateral arm weakness on exercise and spuriously low blood pressure readings bilaterally. Digital subtraction angiography of the (**A**) right and (**B**) left upper extremities shows multiple stenoses and irregularities bilaterally consistent with giant cell arteritis. Patient's erythrocyte sedimentation rate was more than 100.

ing frequency. In some cases it requires surgical correction. Changes in configuration following angioplasty may be secondary to alterations in flow (142).

Aortic aneurysm may arise in patients treated with patch aortoplasty for coarctation (143). This may be detected on routine chest radiography and confirmed by ascending aortic or DSA. Less invasive diagnostic techniques, such as CT and MRI, may also be used.

Systemic-to-Pulmonary Shunts

Communications from the systemic to pulmonary circulation may be congenital or acquired. **Patent ductus arteriosus**, the most common example of the former, is usually easily diagnosed on the basis of clinical and noninvasive study. The ductus is the fetal connection between the aortic arch and the left pulmonary artery (Fig. 20.57). Most adults with this disorder should probably undergo catheterization for hemodynamic and angiographic studies. It has been suggested that there is a significant incidence of additional cardiovascular anomalies in patients referred for transcatheter closure of a patent ductus and that all such patients should have a complete catheterization (144). Aortography may identify coexisting aortopulmonary communications and allow for catheter intervention (145). In many cases it is easy to pass through the ductus from either the pulmonary or the

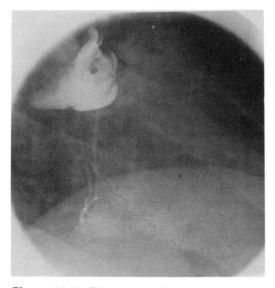

Figure 20.55. Dissection of aortic root subsequent to right coronary angiography. Contrast stains aorta at termination of coronary injection.

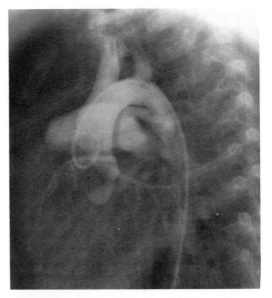

Figure 20.57. Aortogram in lateral projection demonstrating filling of pulmonary artery through a ductus arteriosus.

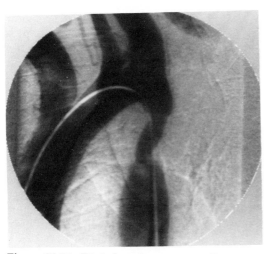

Figure 20.56. Digital angiogram revealing restenosis of coarctation. Gradient across stenosis was 60 mm Hg.

aortic side. Ascending aortography filmed in the steep LAO projection demonstrates the defect well and affords evaluation of the length and width of the connection, which is of some import to the surgeon and is necessary for a percutaneous closure (146).

ABDOMINAL AORTOGRAPHY

Angiography of the abdominal aorta may be considered in the evaluation of abdominal aortic aneurysms (Fig. 20.58), dissections, stenoses (Fig. 20.59), clots (Fig. 20.60), and branch integrity (Fig. 20.61). The cardiologist usually performs this procedure to evaluate the distal circulation because of a planned procedure (e.g., intra-aortic balloon placement, aortic valvuloplasty, peripheral cardiopulmonary bypass) in a patient having clinical evidence of disease, because of manifest difficulty negotiating the lower aorta during routine catheterization (Fig. 20.62), or as a screening test for renal artery stenosis.

The role of routine abdominal aortography in the evaluation of aneurysm is controversial (147–150). The diagnosis of this disorder and estimation of its size certainly do not rest with angiography; physical exami-

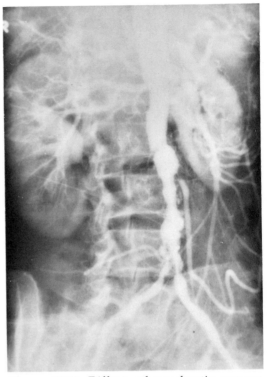

Figure 20.59. Diffuse atherosclerotic narrowings in the aorta of a patient with abdominal angina.

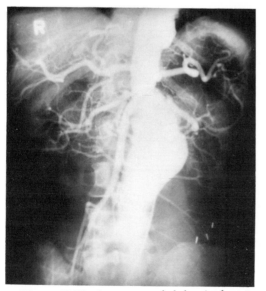

Figure 20.58. Aneurysm of abdominal aorta with involvement of renal arteries.

nation, plain films of the abdomen, and ultrasonography offer less risk. More recently CT (151), MRI (152), and DSA (153) have been shown to be advantageous in sizing and describing the aneurysm. The angiogram does give information concerning the extent of the aneurysm and the associated atherosclerotic process, including involvement of major branch vessels, such as the renal arteries, the superior mesenteric, and the iliofemoral system. The procedure, whose risk is relatively small, may be successfully performed via the femoral retrograde approach. A pigtail catheter advanced over a wire is typically positioned at the level of the twelfth thoracic vertebra. Alternatively, one of a number of catheters capable of providing aortic and more selective injections may be used (154, 155). Treatment of aortic aneurysms with an intraluminal stent–graft combination is an intriguing prospect (156).

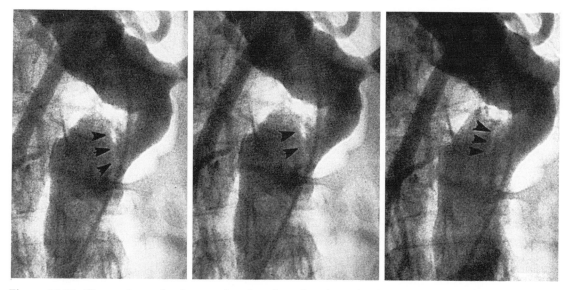

Figure 20.60. Cineangiography frames showing thrombus (*arrowheads*) attached to lower portion of narrowing within an aneurysm in the abdominal aorta. This aneurysm and the associated thrombus were first noted during an attempt to advance catheter for coronary angiography.

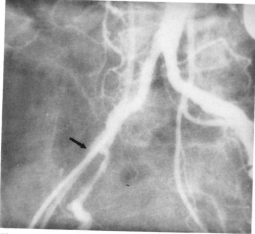

Figure 20.61. Cineangiographic frame revealing occlusion of right external iliac artery by indwelling arterial sheath (*arrow*) in a patient with right lower extremity pain following aortic valvuloplasty.

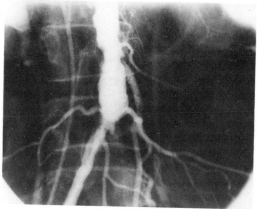

Figure 20.62. Occlusion of left iliac artery. Cineangiographic frame from distal aortogram obtained because of difficulty encountered during arterial entry in patient undergoing coronary angiography. Total occlusion of left iliac artery and atherosclerotic disease of distal aorta and right iliac artery are visible.

Injection of 40 to 50 mL of contrast material over 2 seconds is usually adequate, and filming is performed in the AP and lateral biplane views. On occasion filming in the right posterior oblique projection is necessary to evaluate the renal arteries properly (157). Serial cut filming has been thought superior to cineangiography. The exposure sequence should stress early acquisition, with a total of 12 films recorded in each plane. Cineangiography and digital studies may be considered in lieu of serial cut filming (158).

While the cardiologist has traditionally had little need to visualize any of the branches of the abdominal aorta, the use of the right gastroepiploic artery as a bypass graft may demand imaging of this vessel postoperatively. Black and Gibbons (159) have described a method for selective injection of the gastroepiploic artery with a coaxial catheter system. With an 8-F Judkins right coronary guide catheter used to enter the celiac axis, a torquable guidewire may be advanced through the hepatic, gastroduodenal, and then into the gastroepiploic artery. This procedure may be used to direct an angioplasty system to a site of stenosis in the graft or distal coronary vessel (160). Angiography of the gastroepiploic may more easily be accomplished with a 5-F Cobra or Simmons catheter (Cook Inc.).

RENAL ANGIOGRAPHY AND INTERVENTION

Patients with significant renal artery stenosis may require intervention to treat hypertension and/or renal failure. Both groups of patients can be relatively difficult to evaluate, and it is not always clear which patients will benefit from percutaneous treatment and which will not. Hypertension associated with a critical renal artery stenosis certainly calls for some attempt at revascularization; however, patients with renal failure and renal artery stenosis can be more difficult to evaluate. Since the latter often have a significant degree of intrarenal vascular disease, it may be impossible to determine whose renal function will stabilize or improve and who will fail to gain any benefit. The decision to revascularize should be based on the patient's entire clinical status. Hemodynamic measurements across a stenosis may be obtained with a small-caliber catheter. Gradients greater than 10 mm Hg may be considered significant. The utility of renal vein renins in helping one determine which lesions are critical is questionable, as up to 25% of patients with nonlateralizing renins correct their hypertension following percutaneous and/or surgical intervention. Routine screening angiography has not

been justified for all patients with hypertension undergoing cardiac catheterization. It may, however, be indicated in specific patients. The captopril renogram may be a good screen for patients with possible renal artery stenosis. Renal artery angioplasty may be considered in appropriate cases (Fig. 20.63) and may be facilitated by digital acquisition. Transvenous DSA may be useful for follow-up of patients having renal angioplasty (158).

Selective renal angiography may be accomplished with a 5-F cobra or shepherd's crook (Simmons, Cook Inc.). DSA is obtained at an injection rate of 5 mL per second for a total of 10 to 15 mL and is filmed at 2 frames per second through the venous phase. The arteries are imaged in the AP and the contralateral oblique planes (e.g., LAO for the right kidney).

After diagnostic angiography percutaneous intervention for critical stenosis can be pursued in a fashion analogous to angioplasty of other vessels. The renal artery is engaged with a 5-F diagnostic catheter through which a flexible soft-tipped torquable guidewire is advanced across the stenosis to secure access within the kidney. A hydrophilic guidewire is not recommended because of its potential to cause subintimal dissection. The catheter is then passed over the wire, and the wire is exchanged for a stiffer exchange guidewire such as a Rosen 3 mm J (Cook Inc.) that supports balloon angioplasty. Prior to balloon insertion the patient is heparinized; some operators elect to administer 10 mg of sublingual nifedipine to help prevent renal artery spasm. An angioplasty balloon is sized to the renal artery diameter obtained from the diagnostic angiogram. The balloon is advanced over the guidewire and when in place, inflated for 60 to 90 seconds. The balloon catheter is removed and the results are accessed angiographically via a 5-F pigtail catheter advanced from a contralateral femoral artery or a 4-F pigtail passed through the ipsilateral sheath adjacent to the guidewire. Hemodynamic results can also be ascertained using a small-lumen end hole catheter. If the results are not satisfactory, angioplasty can be repeated with the same size or larger balloon. If the result remains unsatisfactory, stenting should be considered.

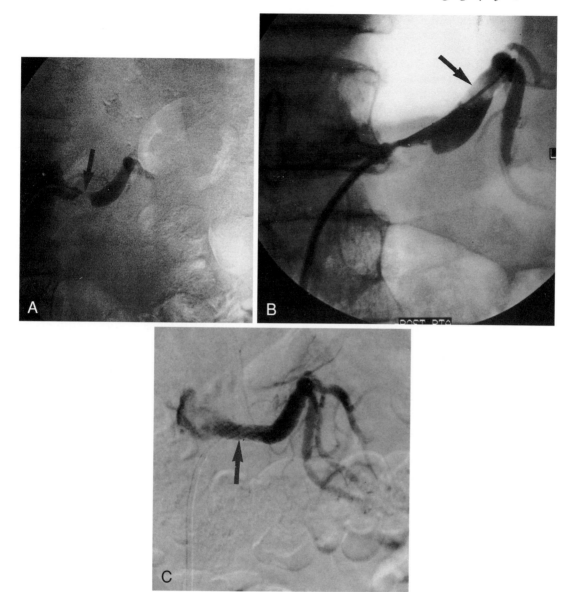

Figure 20.63. **A.** Selective left renal artery arteriogram demonstrates a very high grade stenosis (*arrow*) of the left renal artery. **B.** After PTA there is only minimal improvement in the angiographic appearance of the renal artery. **C.** After placement of a P294 Palmaz stent (*arrow*) the renal artery is widely patent. The thrombus noted in **B** was lysed with urokinase.

Renal arteries may be stented with a Palmaz stent (Johnson & Johnson, Warren, NJ) or the Wallstent (Schneider, Minneapolis MN). While the Palmaz stent can be placed more accurately, it must be used with a guiding catheter to avoid stripping the stent from the balloon. While the self-expanding Wallstent does not require the use of a guid-ing catheter, placement is more complicated because of the shortening of the device. A stent should be positioned so that it covers the region of the stenosis and extends a few millimeters into the aortic lumen. The aortic end should be flared to maximize inflow and prevent shifting of the device. The results are checked angiographically to confirm whether additional stenting is required. Since it is undesirable to have more than 5 mm of stent trailing into the aorta, the difficulty of predicting Wallstent shortening may present problems when this device is used. Some operators routinely heparinize renal stent patients overnight. Others treat with the antiplatelet regimen used for coronary stenting.

Renal artery stenting is associated with high procedural success and good long-term results that are not different for ostial as opposed to nonostial lesions (161). Preexisting renal dysfunction is an indicator of poor prognosis after stenting (162).

Iliofemoral Angiography and Intervention

Many patients with ischemic heart disease have concomitant atherosclerotic lesions in the lower abdominal aorta as well as arteries of the pelvis and lower extremity. Intervention for symptomatic disease requires accurate and thorough imaging of the arterial system from the infrarenal aorta to the feet so that appropriate decisions can be made concerning therapy. Overaggressive attempts at percutaneous revascularization without complete mapping of the pelvic and lower extremity vascular system typically result in poor long-term outcomes.

Diagnostic imaging is most commonly performed from a common femoral artery approach. A 5-F pigtail catheter is placed at the level of the renal arteries and an infrarenal aortogram and runoff arteriogram are obtained in one of a number of ways. The standard cut-film arteriogram, though widely available, can be difficult to perform because of the timing required between contrast injection and the actual filming of the runoff. New systems that allow for digital subtraction imaging of the lower extremities are much more efficient and provide highly detailed images with minimal contrast. Standard spot film DSA may be performed; however, some systems offer digital stepping, or Perivision (Siemens, Iselin, NJ), which provides for a continuously filmed digital subtraction runoff study with one contrast injection.

For a cut-film study contrast injection rates for the abdominal aorta are 20 mL per second for a total of 40 mL while filming at two frames per second. The runoff portion of the examination most often requires an injection of 7 to 10 mL per second for a total of 70 to 100 mL of contrast. The stepping sequence must be timed out initially, depending on the rate of flow of a test contrast bolus performed prior to the final filming. Digital subtraction allows for a somewhat reduced contrast load, but because of the significant hemodilution that commonly occurs in patients with complex peripheral vascular disease, injections rates of 7 to 8 mL per second for a total of 50 to 70 mL are still required. Once digital subtraction arteriography is performed, areas that were not well visualized are filled in with single-position DSA. The volume of contrast to be injected is adjusted to match the flow requirements of the specific area. Filming at one or two frames per second is usually sufficient.

For the cardiologist it is often adequate and logistically simpler to use cineangiography to evaluate the distal aorta and iliofemoral system. Imaging of the distal aorta can be accomplished by an injection of 8 to 15 mL per second for a total 20 to 40 mL depending on the size of the vessel and its runoff. The AP projection is used with a cine rate of 30 frames per second. It is often possible to pan down one iliofemoral system with this injection, but because of the limited field of view, a longer injection using more contrast is necessary if both iliofemoral systems are to be evaluated (Fig 20.64). Alternatively, two injections can be performed with imaging restricted for each to a single arterial system. Since these studies may be painful, the patient should be sedated and either lidocaine added to high-osmolality contrast or a low-osmolality agent should be used. The newer isosmotic contrast may be especially beneficial for these studies.

The cardiologist may be interested in visualizing the distal aorta and iliofemoral systems because of (*a*) difficulties in negotiating this pathway during attempted retrograde heart catheterization, (*b*) suspicion of a complication (e.g., dissection, pseudoaneurysm, arteriovenous fistula) of the cur-

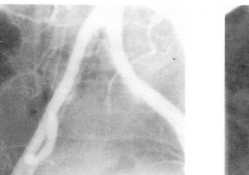

Figure 20.64. Distal aortogram performed after completion of cardiac catheterization to evaluate right iliac artery after it was dissected during attempts at access.

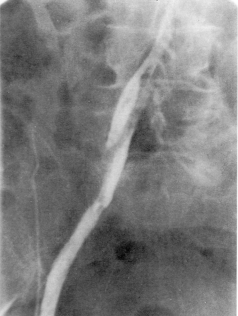

Figure 20.65. Injection through femoral artery sheath showing iatrogenic dissection of right iliac artery.

rent or a previous procedure (Fig 20.65), or (*c*) The desire to evaluate these vessels in a patient with signs or symptoms of claudication in anticipation of revascularization if necessary.

Contrast may be injected through an indwelling sheath or catheter to visualize the upstream pathway. Most catheterization laboratories have digital equipment that stores the image for review. Some even have the ability to roadmap, providing a mechanism for the properly selected guidewire to be directed through a tortuous and partially obstructed pathway. During injection through a sheath or partially advanced catheter, care should be taken to ensure that the tip of the sheath or catheter is intraluminal (i.e., having easily aspirated blood and a good pressure wave recording). One should always perform a test injection, which should reveal adequate washout of contrast and no staining prior to a power injection. The definitive imaging run must be performed with enough total contrast and enough force to visualize the upstream course well. Inadequate opacification of any

vessel may falsely suggest occlusion or disease of the vessel.

Access site complications such as pseudoaneurysm and arteriovenous fistula (Figs. 20.5 and 20.6) occur more frequently when vascular entry is low and into a branch of the femoral artery rather than the common trunk (163). The use of larger sheaths and more intensive anticoagulation increases the risk of peripheral vascular complication. Arteriovenous fistulas resulting from catheterization are usually small but may be large enough to cause heart failure (164). Until recently pseudoaneurysms, unless very small, have been considered best treated by surgery. The use of duplex ultrasonography, however, provides a mechanism for diagnosis and for directed compression that is highly successful in obliterating the aneurysm, especially if there is a narrow neck connecting it the artery (165, 166) (Fig 20.66). Angiography is rarely necessary for the diagnosis of pseudoaneurysm but may be requested if surgical repair is indicated. Similarly arteriovenous fistulas

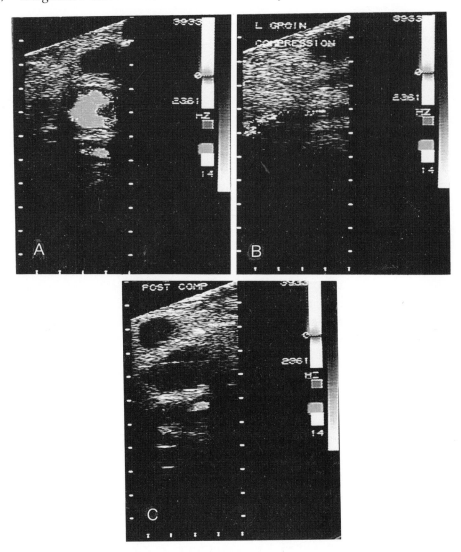

Figure 20.66. A. Color flow Doppler demonstrating large pseudoaneurysm above femoral artery with a clear space representing hematoma above pseudoaneurysm. **B.** Compression of groin by ultrasound probe obliterates pseudoaneurysm. **C.** Postcompression ultrasound demonstrating thrombosis of pseudoaneurysm. (Reprinted with permission from Resar JR, Trerotola SO, Osterman FA, et al. Ultrasound guided ablation of pseudoaneurysm following coronary artery stent placement: a preliminary report. Cathet Cardiovasc Diagn 1992;26:215–218.)

that require surgical repair should probably also be angiographically defined.

Peripheral vascular angioplasty, including that of the distal aorta (167, 168), is aggressively practiced by both radiologist and cardiologist. The periphery has long been a proving ground for new interventional devices prior to introduction into the coronary circulation. Stenoses in the symptomatic pa-

tient should be evaluated hemodynamically prior to intervention. Pressure gradients of more than 10 mm Hg (mean or systolic) are usually thought significant. Tolazoline (Priscolene, 25 mg diluted in 10 to 20 mL of normal saline) may be injected to provide a stress test to unmask gradients that are not detectable at rest but may become significant with exercise. Gradients across pelvic arteries may be measured by introducing a catheter from each femoral artery and positioning them above and below the stenosis. For lesions below the inguinal ligament the catheter is gently passed across the stenosis, a hemodynamic measurement made, and the catheter pulled back while recording the gradient. While the size of the catheter can impart some degree of error to the reading, particularly in the case of marked stenosis, it still provides a reference by which one can objectively measure the degree of improvement brought about by intervention.

Significant stenoses are addressed by angioplasty. All lesions should initially be crossed with a soft floppy-tipped guidewire and a 4- to 5-F diagnostic catheter. Hydrophilic guidewires should be used with care (if at all) because of the potential to dissect subintimally. Roadmapping capabilities are often helpful in crossing tight stenoses. Once across the obstruction, the floppy-tipped guide is exchanged for a more rigid exchange wire such as the Rosen (Cook Inc.). The "normal" vessel diameter is determined from the diagnostic angiogram and an appropriately sized balloon catheter chosen. The results of balloon angioplasty are assessed with angiography as well as by pressure gradient. The latter should be reduced to below 10 mm Hg. It the result is unsatisfactory, repeat inflations or use of a larger balloon is considered.

Lesions that do not respond appropriately to balloon angioplasty are usually stented (Fig 20.67). Both the Palmaz stent and Wallstent are available for use in the iliac artery. These stents are available in a wide variety of sizes matched to the vessel's diameter and lesion length. The Wallstent is preferred by some because it is premounted and relatively easy to deliver. This stent, however, undergoes considerable shortening during deployment, and it is not always easy to predict the final stent placement. The Palmaz device can be more accurately placed, but it requires mounting and must be delivered via a sheath or guide catheter to prevent inadvertent displacement and possible loss of it within the patient. Hemodynamic and angiographic assessment of the stenting procedure is performed after stent deployment. Further angioplasty and stenting may be necessary to optimize re-

sults. The long-term results of iliac stenting appear quite good. Because of the size of the vessel there is no need for aggressive anticoagulant therapy and only aspirin is given for at least 3 to 6 months. It is generally recommended that stents not be placed across the inguinal ligament. For lesions below this site the Wallstent is probably more suitable than the Palmaz stent, as it is flexible and more resistant to crush injury. The rigid Palmaz stent has been reported on occasion to be compressed by external forces, resulting in vessel occlusion.

Brachiocephalic System

Suspected disorders of the brachiocephalic and extracranial cerebrovascular system may be evaluated angiographically as part of cardiac catheterization. DSA with injections in the ascending aorta has been used to visualize these vessels in patients with symptomatic cerebrovascular disease, as well as those with asymptomatic neck bruits (169). While this technique does not achieve the resolution of a selective carotid angiography, it may suffice to reveal or exclude hemodynamically significant stenoses (Fig. 20.68). These studies are typically performed upon completion of the cardiac procedure. A pigtail catheter is placed in the ascending aorta and 30 to 40 mL of dilute contrast medium (60% contrast medium mixed with an equal volume of saline or 76% contrast medium diluted with twice its volume of saline) injected over 2 seconds for each injection. The aortic arch and origin of the great vessels are imaged first in the 45° LAO view. Suggested injections to view various segments of the brachiocephalic vessels are shown in Table 20.5 (169). To evaluate the carotid arteries it is necessary to visualize these vessels in two projections in which the vertebral arteries have been rotated so there is no overlap of the carotid bifurcations. The success of this technique depends on the ability of the patient to cooperate. The images may be severely degraded if the patient is unable to suspend respiration or refrain from swallowing during the examination.

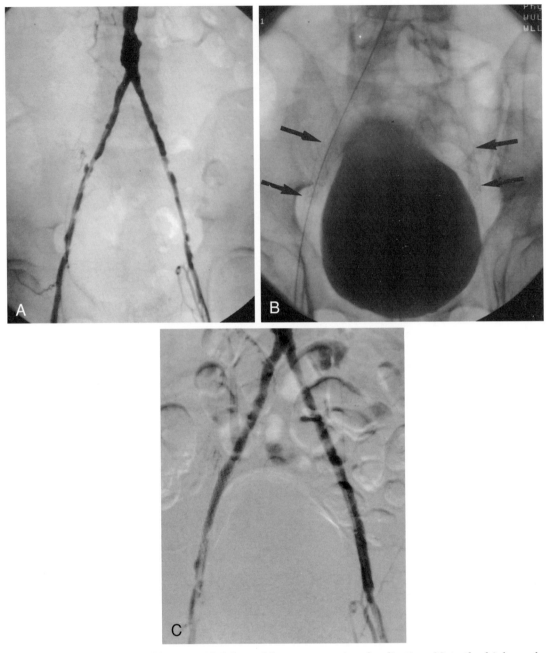

Figure 20.67. A. 57-year-old man with bilateral lower extremity claudication. Note the high-grade strictures throughout the external iliac arteries. Gradients of 50 mm Hg on the left and 15 mm Hg on the right were recorded across the iliac system. **B.** A series of four P294 Palmaz stents were placed (*arrows*) in the external iliac systems. **C.** Follow-up angiogram demonstrates marked improvement in the appearance of both iliacs. The gradient across the left system was reduced to zero and the gradient on the right was reduced to 1 mm Hg.

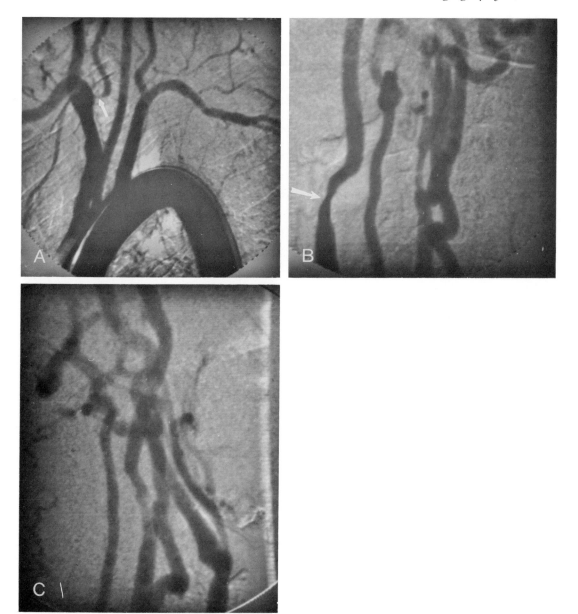

Figure 20.68. Sequence of intra-arterial digital carotid angiography. **A.** Aortic arch, imaged first, reveals stenosis of right vertebral artery (*arrow*). **B.** LAO view of carotids (second injection) reveals stenosis of right internal carotid (*arrow*) and flush occlusion of external carotid. **C.** Third injection filmed in the RAO unwraps left carotid system.

Selective catheterization of the carotid arterial systems is usually necessary when revascularization is considered. This should be performed only after the arch study is obtained so that the origins of the brachiocephalic and left carotid artery are imaged and the extent of disease, if present, is defined. Critical stenoses at these locations should be approached very gingerly with a soft guidewire and catheter. Selective catheterization of the brachiocephalic and left common carotid arteries can be performed

Table 20.5.
Digital Subtraction Angiography of Brachiocephalic Vessels

Objective	Patient Position	Image Intensifier Angle
AA and origin of its branches	Supine, head rotated about 45° to right	20–30° LAO
LCC bifurcation; posterior wall RCC	Supine, head rotated about 45° to right	20–30° LAO or change, depending on first view
RCC bifurcation; posterior wall LCC	Supine, head rotated about 45° to left	20–30° RAO
Both CC bifurcations if not well seen on oblique views	Supine, head AP, chin elevated	AP with caudal angulation to project lower margin of mandible over occipital rim
Intracranial; IC bifurcations, basilar artery	Supine, head AP	10–15° cranial to superimpose petrous ridge on superior orbital rim
Carotid siphons, basilar artery	Supine, head AP	70° oblique off lateral

Reprinted with permission from Cerebrovascular disease. In: van Breda A, Katzen BT. Angiography: practical aspects. Thorofare, NJ: Slack, Inc., 1986.
AA, aortic arch; AP, anteroposterior; CC, common carotid; IC, internal carotid; LCC, left common carotid; RCC, right common carotid.

with a Simmons or hockey stick type of catheter with a soft guidewire such as a Bentsen. The internal carotids are effectively imaged by injection into their respective common trunks. Care should be taken when catheterizing the common carotid to avoid extension of the guidewire into a diseased area, which may result in vessel dissection, occlusion, or embolus formation. Once the catheter is satisfactorily seated in the common carotid, DSA with filming rates of two frames per second is performed. In general, injection rates as low as 5 mL per second for a total of 7 to 10 mL are used. AP and lateral views of the common carotid bifurcation, a lateral intracranial view, and a Townes view are recommended.

Despite the lack of well-controlled studies comparing surgical carotid endarterectomy with percutaneous angioplasty and stenting, the enthusiasm for catheter intervention in the treatment of carotid stenosis is growing rapidly. Early registry studies (170) suggest that stenting of the carotid arteries is associated with a high procedural success rate and an acceptable 30-day complication rate (2.8% major stroke or death).

Carotid intervention at this time usually involves combined angioplasty and stenting (Fig 20.69). Patients are pretreated with aspirin and ticlopidine and are given relatively low dose heparin during the procedure to keep the activated clotting time at about 200 to 250 seconds. Some operators prefer to insert a temporary pacemaker prophylactically because carotid intervention may cause marked bradycardia. Blood pressure is constantly monitored and adjusted appropriately with vasodilators or constrictors. Stenting entails the use of a guide catheter to deliver the dilation balloon and stent system. Balloon dilation is carried out before stenting. Multilumen systems using an occlusion balloon to limit embolization have been used, but there is little evidence that such an approach is beneficial. After dilation the diameter of the target vessel is measured from the diagnostic angiogram and an appropriately sized stent selected. Rigid stents are subject to compression injury and probably should not be used in this portion of the circulation. Wallstents appear to be reasonable devices for this application and are commonly used. When possible, the stent should be positioned so that the ostium of the external carotid artery is not covered, but the first priority is to properly address the lesion. If necessary this may include extending the stent into the common carotid. Techniques using bifurcational stenting are being pioneered. High-pressure ballooning after the stent implant

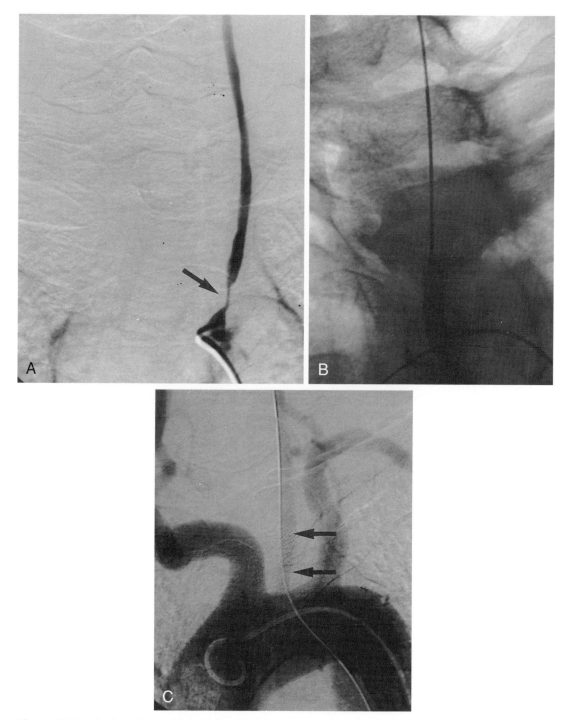

Figure 20.69. A. A patient with a right-sided transient ischemic episode was found to have a high-grade lesion (*arrow*) involving the origin of the left common carotid artery. **B.** Balloon angioplasty was performed. **C.** Placement of two 8 × 20 mm Wallstents (*arrows*).

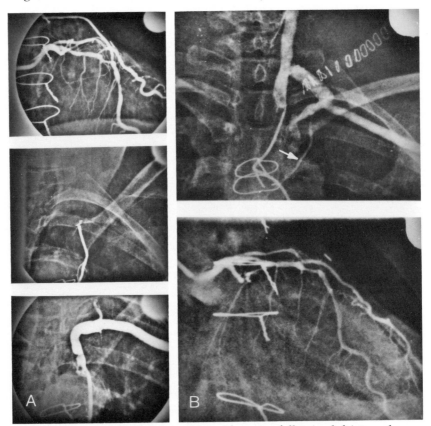

Figure 20.70. Subclavian artery stenosis in patient with angina following left internal mammary artery bypass to the left anterior descending artery. Injection of left coronary artery demonstrated retrograde filling of graft to subclavian artery. Selective injection of subclavian artery revealed stenosis with no antegrade flow through the left internal mammary artery. (**A**, top, middle, and lower panel respectively). Postcarotid-to-subclavian shunting, antegrade flow through the mammary artery (**B**, top, *arrow*) fails to opacify via injection of native coronary artery. (Reprinted with permission from McIvor ME, Williams GM, Brinker J. Subclavian–coronary steal through a LIMA-to-LAD bypass graft. Cathet Cardiovasc Diagn 1988;14:100–104.)

is often performed with care not to dilate to a diameter exceeding that of the self-expanding stent. Upon completion of the stenting procedure the results are assessed angiographically. The ipsilateral intracranial vessels should also be imaged to exclude guidewire damage or embolization.

The increased use of the internal mammary artery as a conduit for coronary bypass makes it essential that the cardiologist be able to perform selective angiography of this vessel in postoperative studies, as well as preoperatively if its integrity is suspect. Flow through the mammary may be compromised by disease proximal to its origin, and assessment of the subclavian artery

may be indicated during catheterization, especially if there is a significant blood pressure differential (171) (Fig. 20.70). Entrance into the internal mammary is not always easy, but it may be aided by use of the sharply angulated internal mammary–seeking catheter and on occasion by a torquable guidewire. The vessel arises from the inferior aspect of the proximal portion of the subclavian artery. It is close to the thyrocervical trunk and its branches (inferior thyroid, transverse scapular, and transverse cervical) and the vertebral artery. Rarely, tortuosity prevents selective engagement of the internal mammary artery, necessitating a retrograde approach from

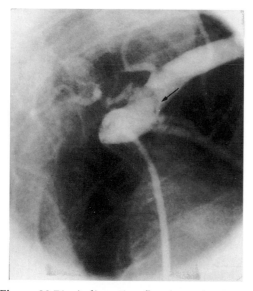

Figure 20.71. A dissection flap (*arrow*) was created in the left subclavian artery by a diagnostic angiography catheter attempting to engage the left internal mammary artery. This was asymptomatic and not associated with a pressure gradient. The patient was treated conservatively and is being followed by duplex ultrasonography.

the left brachial artery. A technique for catheterization of the internal mammary artery from the contralateral brachial artery has been described (172) (see Chapter 16). Care should be taken in the catheterization of the subclavian artery and internal mammary artery to limit the possibility of dissection. Iatrogenic injury to these vessels may cause acute coronary and/or upper extremity ischemia. When nonobstructive (no angiographic or hemodynamic evidence of impaired flow), the dissection may be treated conservatively (173, 174) (Fig 20.71). In the presence of clinical evidence of impaired blood flow however, catheter intervention (stenting) or surgical repair must be considered.

NEWER INVASIVE DIAGNOSTIC TECHNIQUES

Intravascular ultrasound imaging, flow velocity determinations, and angioscopy have been used in the diagnosis of coronary, pulmonary, and peripheral arterial disease. Ultrasound as a means of evaluating intraluminal dimensions correlates well with in vitro models (175) and in vivo angiography. Because of its ability to image the vessel wall, it may allow for the detection of atherosclerosis at an earlier stage than is possible with angiography (176). It may also be helpful in the diagnosis of aortic dissection and in the sizing of interventional devices. **Doppler flow velocity** is useful in the coronary circulation for the determination of flow reserve. Its utility in other vascular beds remains to be determined. The flexible angioscope produces elegant imaging of the vessel's lumen. It can detect clot and dissection but allows only an approximation of luminal diameter. While the pictures obtained are absorbing, the clinical utility of this device appears to be limited, and angioscopy is infrequently performed at present. All three of these techniques complement angiography but are more invasive and provide a limited view of the vessel and its branches. While they may be important for investigative purposes, their clinical role in the evaluation of vascular disease remains undefined at present.

References

1. Dalen JE, Brooks HL, Johnson LW, et al. Pulmonary angiography in acute pulmonary embolism: indications, techniques, and results in 367 patients. Am Heart J 1971;81:175–185.
2. Moser KM. Pulmonary embolism. Am Rev Resp Dis 1977;115:829–852.
3. McIntyre KM, Sasahara AA. Hemodynamic alterations related to extent of lung scan perfusion defect in pulmonary embolism. J Nucl Med 1971;12:166–170.
4. McIntyre KM, Sasahara AA. The hemodynamic response to pulmonary embolism in patients without prior cardiopulmonary disease. Am J Cardiol 1971;28:288–294.
5. Alpert JS, Smith R, Carlson J, et al. Mortality in patients treated for pulmonary embolism. JAMA 1976;236:1477–1480.
6. Mills SR, Jackson DC, Older RA, et al. The incidence, etiology, and avoidance of complications of pulmonary angiography in a large series. Radiology 1980;136:295–299.
7. Ferris EJ, Athanasoulis CA, Clapp PR. Inferior vena cavography correlated with pulmonary angiography. Chest 1971;59:651–653.
8. Stein MA, Winter J, Grollman JH Jr. The value of

the pulmonary artery-seeking catheter in percutaneous selective pulmonary arteriography. Radiology 1975;114:299–304.

9. Grollman JH Jr, Gyepes MT, Helmer E. Transfemoral selective bilateral pulmonary arteriography with a pulmonary artery–seeking catheter. Radiology 1978;96:202–204.

10. MILLS CS, Van Aman ME. Modified technique for percutaneous transfemoral pulmonary angiography. Cardiovasc Intervent Radiol 1986;9:52–53.

11. Courey WR, de Villasante JM, Waltman AC. A quick, simple method of percutaneous transfemoral pulmonary arteriography. Radiology 1975;113:475–477.

12. Grollman JH, Renner JW. Transfemoral pulmonary angiography: update on technique. Am J Roentgenol 1981;136:624–626.

13. Tempkin DL, Ladika JE. New catheter design and placement technique for pulmonary arteriography. Radiology 1987;163:275–276.

14. Bookstein JJ. Segmental arteriography in pulmonary embolism. Radiology 1969;93:1007–1013.

15. Johnson BA, James AE, White RI Jr. Oblique and selective pulmonary angiography in diagnosis of pulmonary embolism. Am J Roentgenol 1973;118:801–808.

16. Bookstein JJ, Feigin DS, Seo KW, Alazraki NP. Diagnosis of pulmonary embolism: experimental evaluation of the accuracy of scintigraphically guided pulmonary arteriography. Radiology 1980;136:15–23.

17. Novelline RA, Baltarowich QH, Athanasoulis CA, et al. The clinical course of patients with suspected pulmonary embolism and a negative pulmonary arteriogram. Radiology 1978;126:561–567.

18. Watson J. Severe pulmonary hypertensive episodes following angiocardiography with sodium metrizoate. Lancet 1964;2:732–733.

19. Goodman PC, Brant-Zawadzki M. Digital subtraction pulmonary angiography. Am J Roentgenol 1982;139:305–309.

20. Bynum LJ, Wilson JE, Christensen EE, Sorensen C. Radiographic techniques for balloon-occlusion pulmonary angiography. Radiology 1979;133:518–520.

21. Meister SG, Brooks HL, Szucs MM, et al. Pulmonary cineangiography in acute pulmonary embolism. Am Heart J 1972;84:33–37.

22. Pond GD, Ovitt TW, Capp MP. Comparison of conventional pulmonary angiography with intravenous digital subtraction angiography for pulmonary embolic disease. Radiology 1983;147:345–350.

23. Ludwig JW, Verhoeuen LA, Kersbergen JJ, Overtoom TT. Digital subtraction angiography of the pulmonary arteries for the diagnosis of pulmonary emboli. Radiology 1983;147:639–645.

24. Ferris EJ, Holder JC, Lim WM, et al. Angiography of pulmonary emboli: digital studies and balloon-occlusion cineangiography. Am J Roentgenol 1984;142:369–373.

25. White RI Jr, Mitchell SE, Barth KH, et al. Angioarchitecture of pulmonary arteriovenous malformations: an important consideration before embolotherapy. Am J Roentgenol 1983;140:681–686.

26. Greene R, Zapol WM, Snider MT, et al. Early bedside detection of pulmonary vascular occlusion during acute respiratory failure. Am Rev Respir Dis 1981;124:593–601.

27. Dougherty JE, LaSala AF, Fieldman A. Bedside pulmonary angiography utilizing an existing Swan-Ganz catheter. Chest 1980;77:43–46.

28. LePage JR, Garcia RM. The value of bedside wedge pulmonary angiography in the detection of pulmonary emboli: a predictive and prospective evaluation. Radiology 1982;144:67–73.

29. National Cooperative Study. The urokinase pulmonary embolism trial. Circulation 1973;47 (Suppl 2):1–108.

30. Bell WR, Simon TL. A comparative analysis of pulmonary perfusion scans with pulmonary angiograms. Am Heart J 1976;92:700–706.

31. Dalen JE, Alpert JS. Natural history of pulmonary embolism. Prog Cardiovasc Dis 1975;17:259–270.

32. Alpert JS, Smith R, Carlson J, et al. Mortality in patients treated for pulmonary embolism. JAMA 1976;236:1477–1480.

33. Robin ED. Overdiagnosis and overtreatment of pulmonary embolism: the emperor may have no clothes. Ann Intern Med 1977;87:775–781.

34. Gaither NS, Wortham DC, Brinker JB. Current recommendations for use of pulmonary angiography. Intern Med 1991;12:19.

35. Matsumoto AH, Tegtmeyer CJ. Contemporary diagnostic approaches to acute pulmonary emboli. Radiol Clin North Am 1995;33:167–183.

36. Stein PD, Willis PW III, Dalen JE. Importance of clinical assessment in selecting patients for pulmonary arteriography. Am J Cardiol 1979;43:669–671.

37. Kipper MS, Moser KM, Kortman KE, Ashbarn WL. Long-term follow-up of patients with suspected pulmonary embolism and a normal lung scan: perfusion scans in embolic suspects. Chest 1982;82:411–415.

38. Alderson PO, Doppman JL, Diamond SS, et al. Ventilation–perfusion lung imaging and selective pulmonary angiography in dogs with experimental pulmonary embolism. J Nucl Med 1978;19:164–171.

39. McNeil BJ. A diagnostic strategy using ventilation–perfusion studies in patients suspected for pulmonary embolism. J Nucl Med 1976;17:613–616.

40. Biello DR, Mattar AG, McKnight RC, Siegel BA. Ventilation–perfusion studies in suspected pulmonary embolism. Am J Roentgenol 1979;133:1033–1037.

41. Alderson PO, Rujanavech N, Sicker-Walker RH, McKnight RC. The role of 133Xe ventilation studies in the scintigraphic detection of pulmonary embolism. Radiology 1976;120:633–640.

42. Neumann RD, Sostman HD, Gottschalk A. Current status of ventilation–perfusion imaging. Semin Nucl Med 1980;10:198–217.

43. Moses DC, Silver TM, Bookstein JJ. The complementary role of chest radiography, lung scanning and selective pulmonary angiography in the diag-

nosis of pulmonary embolism. Circulation 1974; 49:179–188.

44. Hull RD, Hirsh J, Carter CJ, et al. Pulmonary angiography, ventilation lung scanning, and venography for clinically suspected pulmonary embolism with abnormal perfusion lung scan. Ann Intern Med 1983;98:891–899.

45. The PIOPED investigators. Value of the ventilation–perfusion scan in acute pulmonary embolism. JAMA 1990;263:2753–2759.

46. Goldhabe SZ. Evolving concepts in thrombolytic therapy for pulmonary embolism. Chest 1992;101 (Suppl):183S–185S.

47. Alderson PO, Biello DR, Khan AR, et al. Scintigraphic detection of pulmonary embolism in patients with obstructive lung disease. Radiology 1981;138:661–666.

48. Cavaluzzi JA, Alderson PO, White RI Jr. Pulmonary embolism with unilateral lung scan defects and matching infiltrates. J Can Assoc Radiol 1979; 30:162–164.

49. Van Rossum AB, Treurniet FE, Kieft GJ, et al. Role of spiral volumetric computed tomographic scanning in the assessment of patients with clinical suspicion of pulmonary embolism and an abnormal ventilation/perfusion lung scan. Thorax 1996;51:23–28.

50. Fred HL, Axelrad MA, Lewis JM, Alexander JK. Rapid resolution of pulmonary thromboemboli in man: an angiographic study. JAMA 1966;196: 1137–1139.

51. Murphy ML, Bullock H. Factors influencing the restoration of blood flow following pulmonary embolization as determined by angiography and scanning. Circulation 1968;38:1116–1126.

52. Weidner W, Swanson L, Wilson G. Roentgen techniques in the diagnosis of pulmonary thromboembolism. Am J Roentgenol 1967;100:397–407.

53. Dorfman GS, Cronan JJ. Sonographic diagnosis of thrombosis of the lower extremity veins. Semin Intervent Radiol 1990;7:9–19.

54. Comerota AJ, Katz ML, Greenwald LL, et al. Venous duplex imaging: should it replace hemodynamic tests for deep venous thrombosis? J Vasc Surg 1990;11:51–61.

55. Sagel SS, Greenspan RH. Nonuniform pulmonary artery perfusion. Radiology 1971;99:541–548.

56. Bookstein JJ, Silver TM. The angiographic differential diagnosis of pulmonary embolism. Radiology 1974;110:25–33.

57. Mills SR, Jackson DC, Sullivan DC, et al. Angiographic evaluation of chronic pulmonary embolism. Radiology 1980;136:301–308.

58. Dines DE, Arms RA, Bernatz PE, Gomes MR. Pulmonary arteriovenous fistulas. Mayo Clin Proc 1974;49:460–465.

59. Fox LS, Buntain WL, Brasfield D, et al. Pulmonary arteriovenous malformations in children. J Pediatr Surg 1979;14:53–57.

60. Larouche CM, Wells F, Shneerson J. Massive hemothorax due to enlarging arteriovenous fistula in pregnancy. Chest 1992;101:1452–1454.

61. Duch PM, Chandrasekaron K, Mulhern CB, et al. Transesophageal echocardiographic diagnosis of pulmonary arteriovenous malformation: role of

contrast and pulsed Doppler echocardiography. Chest 1994;105:1604–1605.

62. Terry PB, Barth KH, Kaufman SL, White RI Jr. Balloon embolization for treatment of pulmonary arteriovenous fistulas. N Engl J Med 1980;302: 1189–1190.

63. Barth KH, White RI Jr, Kaufman SL, et al. Embolotherapy of pulmonary arteriovenous malformations with detachable balloons. Radiology 1982; 142:599–606.

64. Taylor BG, Cockerill EM, Manfredi F, Klatte EC. Therapeutic embolization of the pulmonary artery in pulmonary arteriovenous fistula. Am J Med 1978;54:360–365.

65. Jonsson K, Hellekant C, Olsson O, Holen O. Percutaneous transcatheter occlusion of pulmonary arteriovenous malformation. Ann Radiol 1980;23: 335–337.

66. Sharif M, Messersmith R, Newman B, et al. Bronchial arteriovenous malformation in a child with hemoptysis: a case report. Angiology 1996;47: 203–209.

67. Rothman A, Perry SB, Keane JF, Lock JE. Early results and follow-up of balloon angioplasty for branch pulmonary stenosis. J Am Coll Cardiol 1990;15:1109–1117.

68. Gentles TL, Lock JE, Perry SB. High-pressure balloon angioplasty for branch pulmonary artery stenosis: early experience. J Am Coll Cardiol 1993; 22:867–872.

69. Platia EV, Brinker JA. Scimitar syndrome with peripheral left pulmonary artery branch stenoses. Am Heart J 1984;107:594–596.

70. McGaughey MD, Traill TA, Brinker JA. Partial left anomalous pulmonary venous return: a diagnostic dilemma. Cathet Cardiovasc Diagn 1986;12: 110–115.

71. Arlart IP, Bargon G, Sigel H. Anomalous intrapulmonal vein drainage and pulmonary vein connection in DSA. Eur J Radiol 1986;6:12–14.

72 Uyama T, Monden Y, Harada K, et al. Pulmonary varices: a case report and review of the literature. Jpn J Surg 1988;18:359–362.

73. Wildenhain PM, Bourekas EC. Pulmonary varix: magnetic resonance findings. Cathet Cardiovasc Diagn 1991;24:268–270.

74. Ren WD, Nicolosi GL, Lestuzzi C, et al. Role of transesophageal echocardiography in evaluation of pulmonary venous obstruction by paracardiac neoplastic masses. Am J Cardiol 1992;70: 1362–1366.

75. Kucera V, Fiser B, Tuma S, Hucin B. Unilateral absence of pulmonary artery: a report on 19 selected clinical cases. Thorac Cardiovasc Surg 1982; 30:152–158.

76. Kleinman, PK. Pleural telangiectasia and absence of a pulmonary artery. Radiology 1979;132: 281–284.

77. Lekuona I, Cabrera A, Inguanzo R, et al. Direct communication between the right pulmonary artery and left atrium. Thorax 1986;41:78–79.

78. Stone DN, Bein ME, Garris JB. Anomalous left pulmonary artery: two new adult cases. Am J Roentgenol 1980;135:1259–1263.

79. Davis SD, Neithamer CD, Schreiber TS, Sos TA. False pulmonary artery aneurysm induced by

Swan-Ganz catheter: diagnosis and embolotherapy. Radiology 1987;164:741–742.

80. Dillon WP, Taylor AT, Mineau DE, Datz FL. Traumatic pulmonary artery pseudoaneurysm simulating pulmonary embolism. Am J Roentgenol 1982;139:818–819.

81. Arom KV, Richardson JD, Grover FL, et al. Pulmonary artery aneurysm. Am Surg 1978;44: 688–692.

82. Hynes J, Smith HC, Holmes DR, et al. Preoperative angiographic diagnosis of primary sarcoma of the pulmonary artery. Circulation 1982;66: 672–674.

83. Bowen JS, Bookstein JJ, Johnson AD, et al. Wedge and subselective pulmonary angiography in pulmonary hypertension secondary to venous obstruction. Radiology 1985;155:599–603.

84. Tadavarthy SM, Klugman J, Castaneda-Zuniga WR, et al. Systemic-to-pulmonary collaterals in pathological states: a review. Radiology 1982;144: 55–59.

85. Moser KM, Fedullo PF, Finkbeiner WE, Golden J. Do patients with primary pulmonary hypertension develop extensive central thrombi. Circulation 1995;91:741–745.

86. Kirklin JW, Bargeron LM, Pacifico AD. The enlargement of small pulmonary arteries by preliminary palliative operations. Circulation 1977;56: 612–617.

87. White RI. Technique and preliminary results of selective catheterization of patients with Blalock-Taussig shunts. Radiology 1972;105:703–706.

88. Flisak ME, Chandrasekar AJ, Marsan RE, Ali MM. Systemic arterialization of lung without sequestration. Am J Roentgenol 1982;138:751–753.

89. Eriksson S, Osterman G, Asplund K, et al. Pulmonary-artery cineangiocardiography to demonstrate cardiac thrombi in patients with cerebral infarction. Acta Neurol Scand 1984;69:27–33.

90. Montgomery JH, D'Souza VJ, Dyer RB, et al. Nonsurgical treatment of the superior vena cava syndrome. Am J Cardiol 1985;56:829–830.

91. Solomon N, Wholey MH, Jarmolowski CR. Intravascular stents in the management of superior vena cava syndrome. Cathet Cardiovasc Diagn 1991;23:245–252.

92. Mitchell DC, Grasty MS, Stebbings WSL, et al. Comparison of duplex ultrasonography and venography in the diagnosis of deep venous thrombosis. Br J Surg 1991;78:611–613.

93. Kim D, Orron DE, Porter DH. Venographic anatomy, technique, and interpretation. In: Kim D, Orron DE, eds. Peripheral vascular imaging and intervention. St Louis: Mosby–Year Book, 1992: 269–349.

94. Rogoff PA, Hilgenberg AD, Miller SL, Stephan SM. Cephalic migration of the bird's nest inferior vena caval filter: report of two cases. Radiology 1992;184:819–822.

95. Ricco JB, Dubreuil F, Le Douarec P, et al. The LGM Veno Tech caval filter: results of a multicenter study. Ann Vasc Surg 1995;9 (Suppl):S89–S100.

96. Ritchie AJ, Mitchell L, Forty J. Migration of a vena caval filter to the pulmonary artery. Br J Surg 1995;207.

97. McLoughlin RF, Sirkis H, So CB, et al. Severity of disease score as a predictor of mortality after caval filter insertion. J Vasc Interv Radiol 1995;6: 715–719.

98. McIvor ME, Kaufman SL, Satre S, et al. Search and retrieval of an unidentifiable foreign object. Cathet Cardiovasc Diagn. 1989;16:19–23.

99. Pyeritz RE, Stolle CA, Parfrey NA, Myers JC. Ehlers-Danlos syndrome IV due to a novel defect in type III procollagen. Am J Med Gen 1984;19: 607–622.

100. Pernes JM, Grenier P, Desbleds MT, de Brux JL. MR evaluation of chronic aorta dissection. J Comput Assist Tomogr 1987;11:975–981.

101. White TJ, Pinstein ML, Scott RL, Gold RE. Aortic dissection manifested as leg ischemia. Am J Roentgenol 1980;135:353–356.

102. Eagle KA, Quertermous T, Kritzer GA, et al. Spectrum of conditions initially suggesting acute aortic dissection but with negative aortograms. Am J Cardiol 1986;57:322–326.

103. Satler LF, Levine S, Kent KM, et al. Aortic dissection masquerading as acute myocardial infarction: implication for thrombolytic therapy without cardiac catheterization. Am J Cardiol 1984;54: 1134–1135.

104. Blankenship JC, Almquist AK. Cardiovascular complications of thrombolytic therapy in patients with a mistaken diagnosis of acute myocardial infarction. J Am Coll Cardiol 1989;14:1579–1582.

105. Strouse PJ, Shea MJ, Guy GE, Santinga JT. Aortic dissection presenting as spinal cord ischemia with a false-negative aortogram. Cardiovasc Intervent Radiol 1990;13:77–82.

106. Arciniegas JG, Soto B, Little WC, Papapietro SE. Cineangiography in the diagnosis of aortic dissection. Am J Cardiol 1981;47:890–94.

107. Bondestam S, Hekali P, Landtman M. Sonographic diagnosis of dissection of the descending thoracic aorta. Ann Chir Gynaecol 1981;70: 210–212.

108. Matsumoto M, Matsuo H, O'Hara T, et al. A two-dimensional echoaortocardiographic approach to dissecting aneurysms of the aorta to prevent false-positive diagnoses. Radiology 1978;127:491–499.

109. Erbel R, Borner N, Steller D, et al. Detection of aortic dissection by transoesophageal echocardiography. Br Heart J 1987;58:45–51.

110. Goldman AP, Kotler MN, Scanlon MH, et al. The complementary role of magnetic resonance imaging, Doppler echocardiography, and computed tomography in the diagnosis of dissecting thoracic aneurysms. Am Heart J 1986;5:970–981.

111. Hitter H, Ranquin R, Mortelmans L, Parizel G. Diagnosis of aortic dissection: comparison of investigatory methods—case report. Angiology 1987;38:859–863.

112. Chia BL, Yan, PC, Ee BK, et al. Two-dimensional echocardiography and Doppler color flow abnormalities in aortic root dissection. Am Heart J 1988; 116:192–194.

113. White RD, Lipton MJ, Higgins CB, et al. Noninvasive evaluation of suspected thoracic aortic disease by contrast-enhanced computed tomography. Am J Cardiol 1986;57:282–290.

114. Heiberg E, Wolverson M, Sundaram M, et al. CT

findings in thoracic aortic dissections. Am J Roentgenol 1981;136:13–17.

115. Godwin JD, Herfkens RL, Skioldebrand CG, et al. Evaluation of dissections and aneurysms of the thoracic aorta by conventional and dynamic CT scanning. Radiology 1980;136:125–133.

116. Hekali P, Velt P, Gutierrez O, et al. Radiology of aortic dissection: pitfalls in diagnosis. Eur J Radiol 1986;6:314–318.

117. Goodwin JD, Breiman RS, Speckman JM. Problems and pitfalls in the evaluation of thoracic aortic dissection by computed tomography. J Comput Assist Tomogr 1982;6:750–756.

118. Egan TJ, Neiman HL, Herman RJ, et al. Computed tomography in the diagnosis of aortic aneurysm dissection or traumatic injury. Radiology 1980; 136:141–146.

119. Pernes JM, Grenier P, Desbleds MT, de Brux JL. MR evaluation of chronic aortic dissection. J Comput Assist Tomogr 1987;11:975–981.

120. Dinsmore RE, Wedeen VJ, Miller SW, et al. MRI of dissection of the aorta: recognition of the intimal tear and differential flow velocities. Am J Roentgenol 1986;146:1286–1288.

121. Amparo EG, Higgins CB, Hricak H, Sollitto R. Aortic dissection: magnetic resonance imaging. Radiology 1985;155:399–406.

122. Shimshak TM, Giorgi LV, Hartzler GO. Successful percutaneous transluminal angioplasty of an obstructed abdominal aorta secondary to a chronic dissection. Am J Cardiol 1988;61:486–487.

123. Trerotola SO. Use of a stone basket as a target during fenestration of aortic dissection. J Vasc Interv Radiol 1996;7:687–690.

124. Roudaut RP, Marcaggi XL, Deville C, et al. Value of transesophageal echocardiography combined with computed tomography for assessing repaired type A aortic dissection. Am J Cardiol 1992:1468–1476.

125. Crane AR. Primary multiocular mycotic aneurysms of the aorta. Arch Pathol 1937;24:634–641.

126. Brown SL, Busuttil RW, Baker JD, et al. Bacteriologic and surgical determinants of survival in patients with mycotic aneurysms. J Vasc Surg 1985; 1:541–548.

127. Desai AG, Sharma S, Kumar A, et al. Echocardiographic diagnosis of unruptured aneurysm of right sinus of Valsalva: an unusual cause of right ventricular outflow obstruction. Am Heart J 1985; 109:363–364.

128. Terdjman M, Bourdarias JP, Farcot HC, et al. Aneurysms of sinus of Valsalva: two-dimensional echocardiographic diagnosis and recognition of rupture into the right heart cavities. J Am Coll Cardiol 1984;3:1227–1235.

129. Sakakibara S, Donno S. Congenital aneurysm of sinus of Valsalva: a clinical study. Am Heart J 1962;63:708–719.

130. DeSa'Neto A, Padnick MB, Desser KB, Steinhoff NG. Right sinus of Valsalva: right atrial fistula secondary to nonpenetrating chest trauma. Circulation 1979;60:205–209.

131. Lemon DK, White C. Annuloaortic ectasia: angiographic, hemodynamic and clinical comparison with aortic valve insufficiency. Am J Cardiol 1978; 41:482–486.

132. Murdoch JL, Walker BA, Halpern BL, et al. Life expectancy and causes of death in the Marfan syndrome. N Engl J Med 1972;286:804–808.

133. Bentall H, Debono A. A technique for complete replacement of the ascending aorta. Thorax 1968; 23:338–339.

134. Nath PH, Zollikofer C, Castaneda-Zuniga WR, et al. Radiological evaluation of composite aortic grafts. Radiology 1979;131:43–51.

135. Josephson RA, Singer I, Levine JH, et al. Systolic expansion of the aortic root: an echocardiographic and angiographic sign of aortic composite graft dehiscence. Cathet Cardiovasc Diagn 1988; 14: 105–107.

136. Mirvis SE, Pais SO, Gens DR. Thoracic aortic rupture: advantages of intra-arterial digital subtraction angiography. Am J Roentgenol 1986;146: 987–991.

137. Schnyder P, Chapuis L, Mayor B, et al. Helical CT angiography for traumatic aortic rupture: correlation with aortography and surgery in five cases. J Thorac Imaging 1996;11:39–45.

138. LaBerge JM, Jeffrey RB. Aortic lacerations: fatal complications of thoracic aortography. Radiology 1987;165:367–369.

139. Clark RA, Colley DP, Siedlecki E. Late complications at repair site of operated coarctation of aorta. Am J Roentgenol 1979;133:1071–1075.

140. Fletcher BD, Jacobstein MD. MRI of congenital abnormalities of the great arteries. Am J Roentgenol 1984;146:941–948.

141. Rao PS, Thepar MK, Kutayli F, Carey P. Causes of recoarctation after balloon angioplasty of unoperated aortic coarctation. J Am Coll Cardiol 1989;13:109–115.

142. De Lezo JS, Sanch M, Pan M, et al. Angiographic follow-up after balloon angioplasty for coarctation of the aorta. J Am Coll Cardiol 1989;13: 689–695.

143. Rheuban KS, Carpenter MA, Jedeikin R, et al. Aortic aneurysm after patch aortoplasty for coarctation in childhood. Am J Cardiol 1985;55:612.

144. Gelb BD, O'Laughlin MP, Mullins CE. Prevalence of additional cardiovascular anomalies in patients referred for transcatheter closure of patent ductus arteriosus. J Am Coll Cardiol 1990;16:1680–1686.

145. Ing FF, Laskuri C, Bierman FZ. Additional aortopulmonary collaterals in patients referred for coil occlusion of a patent ductus arteriosus. Cathet Cardiovasc Diagn 1996;37:5–8.

146. Sievert H, Bussmann WD, Kaltenbach M, et al. Transfemoral catheter closure of persistent ductus arteriosus in patients over 60 years old. Z Kardiol 1991;80:330–332.

147. Bauer GM, Porter JM, Eidemiller LR, et al. The role of arteriography in abdominal aortic aneurysm. Am J Surg 1978;136:184–189.

148. Bell DD, Gaspar MR. Routine aortography before abdominal aortic aneurysmectomy: a prospective study. Am J Surg 1982;144:191–193.

149. Nuno IN, Collins GM, Bardin JA, Berstein EF. Should aortography be used routinely in the elective management of abdominal aortic aneurysm? Am J Surg 1982;144:53–57.

150. Eriksson I, Forsberg JO, Hemmingsson A, Lindgren PG. Preoperative evaluation of abdominal

aortic aneurysms: is there a need for aortography? Acta Chir Scand 1981;147:533–537.

151. Johnson WC, Paley RH, Castronuovo JJ, et al. Computed tomographic angiography. Am J Surg 1981;141:434–440. 152 Flak B, Li DKB, Ho BYB, et al. Magnetic resonance imaging of aneurysms of the abdominal aorta. Am J Roentgenol 1985;144: 991–996.

153. Passariello R, Simonetti G, Rossi P, et al. Angiographic characterization of aortic aneurysms by digital intravenous angiography. Ann Radiol 1983;26:599–600.

154. Hawkins IF, Haseman MK, Gelfand FN. Single mini-catheter technique for abdominal aortography and selective injection. Radiology 1979;132: 755–757.

155. Kogutt MS, Jander HP, Use of a curved multi-hole catheter for abdominal and femoral arteriography. Radiology 1978;128:817–818.

156. Laborde JC, Parodi JC, Clem MF, et al. Intraluminal bypass of abdominal aortic aneurysm: feasibility study. Radiology 1992;184:185–190.

157. Gerlock AJ, Goncharenko V, Sloan OM. Right posterior oblique: the projection of choice in aortography of hypertensive patients. Radiology 1978;127:45–48.

158. Arlart HIP, Dewitz GB. Transvenous digital subtraction angiography (DSA) for diagnostic control following percutaneous transluminal angioplasty (PTA) in patients with renovascular hypertension. Eur J Radiol 1985;5:115–119.

159. Black AJR, Gibbons F. Angiographic visualization of a right gastroepiploic artery–left circumflex coronary artery graft. Cathet Cardiovasc Diagn 1987;13:121–124.

160. Watson LE, Schoolar EJ. PTCA of gastroepiploic bypass. Cath Cardiovasc Diagn 1991;22:193–196.

161. Henry M, Amor M, Henry I, et al. Renal arterial stenting: a 6 year single center experience with a series of 151 stented arteries. J Am Coll Cardiol 1997;29:221A (abstract).

162. Dorros G, Jaff M, Dorros I, et al. Renal dysfunction is a poor prognosticator of patient survival after Palmaz stent revascularization for renal artery stenosis. J Am Coll Cardiol 1997;29:486A (abstract).

163. Kim D, Orron DE, Skillman JJ, et al. Role of superficial femoral artery puncture in the development of pseudoaneurysm and arteriovenous fistula complicating percutaneous transfemoral cardiac catheterization. Cathet Cardiovasc Diagn 1992;25: 91–97.

164. Sly AO, Plantholt S. Congestive heart failure secondary to an arteriovenous fistula from cardiac catheterization and angioplasty. Cathet Cardiovasc Diagn 1991;23:136–138.

165. Agrawal SK, Pinheiro L, Roubin GS, et al. Nonsurgical closure of femoral pseudoaneurysms complicating cardiac catheterization and percutaneous transluminal coronary angioplasty. J Am Coll Cardiol 1992;20:610–615.

166. Resar JR, Trerotola SO, Osterman FA, et al. Ultrasound guided ablation of pseudoaneurysm following coronary artery stent placement: a preliminary report. Cathet Cardiovasc Diagn 1992;26: 215–218.

167. Grollman JH, Del Vicario M, Mittal AK. Percutaneous transluminal abdominal aortic angioplasty. Am J Roentgenol 1980;134:1053–1054.

168. Khalilullah M, Tyagi S, Lochan R, et al. Percutaneous transluminal balloon angioplasty of the aorta in patients with aortitis. Circulation 1987;76: 597–600.

169. van Breda A, Katzen BT. Cerebrovascular disease. In: van Breda A, Katzen BT, eds. Digital subtraction angiography: practical aspects. Thorofare, NJ: Slack, 1986.

170. Yadav JS, Roubin GS, Iyer S, et al. Elective stenting of the extracranial carotid arteries. Circulation 1997;95:376–381.

171. McIvor ME, Williams GM, Brinker J. Subclavian-coronary steal through a LIMA-to-LAD bypass graft. Cathet Cardiovasc Diagn 1988;14:100–104.

172. Dorros G, Lewin RF. Angiography of the internal mammary artery via the contralateral brachial artery. Cathet Cardiovasc Diagn 1987;13:138–140.

173. Schmitter SP, Marx M, Bernstein R, et al. Angioplasty-induced subclavian artery dissection in a patient with internal mammary artery graft. Treatment with endovascular stent and stent-graft. Am J Roentgenol 1995;165:449–51.

174. Frohwein S, Ververis JJ, Marshall JJ. Subclavian artery dissection during diagnostic cardiac catheterization: the role conservative management. Cathet Cardiovasc Diagn 1995;34:313–317.

175. Nishimura RA, Edwards WD, Warnes CA, et al. Intravascular ultrasound imaging: in vitro validation and pathologic correlation. J Am Coll Cardiol 1990;16:145–154.

176. Davidson CJ, Sheikh KH, Harrison JK, et al. Intravascular ultrasonography versus DSA: a human in vivo comparison of vessel size and morphology. J Am Coll Cardiol 1990;16:633–636.

21
Blood Flow Measurement and Quantification of Vascular Stenoses

Michael D. Winniford, MD
Morton J. Kern, MD
Charles R. Lambert, MD, PhD

INTRODUCTION

The determination of blood flow complements that of pressure in formulating a rigorous description of cardiovascular hemodynamics in health and disease. Flow
measurements performed in the modern
cardiac catheterization laboratory vary
from standard thermodilution determination of cardiac output to subselective coronary blood flow velocity derived from
Doppler catheter studies. Although the
technology used to make such measurements has evolved greatly, the basic physiologic principles applied to measurement of
blood flow have been modified very little
since their original descriptions. Measurements of blood flow in the coronary circulation complement anatomic information
from the coronary angiogram in the assessment of the physiologic significance of coronary vascular stenoses. This chapter reviews the basic physiologic principles
involved in measurement of blood flow,
outlines the limitations of today's methods,
and describes the general application of
blood flow determination to description of
pathophysiologic states in the cardiac catheterization laboratory. In addition, methods
of quantifying the physiologic severity of
coronary vascular stenoses are reviewed.

CARDIAC OUTPUT

Cardiac output is the blood flow measurement most frequently performed in the cardiac catheterization laboratory. Cardiac
output, determined at rest and in some
cases during exercise, is an extremely useful
finding in the overall assessment of cardiovascular function and is essential for the calculation of **vascular resistance, valve orifice area, and regurgitant fraction**. The two
most common methods used clinically to
measure cardiac output are the Fick and indicator dilution techniques.

Fick Method

Theory

The Fick principle is based on the simple
concept of conservation of mass. It can be
applied to flow through any system in
which a substance (indicator) either enters
or leaves the flowing stream at a measurable
rate. The principle is illustrated by the
model in Figure 21.1. Fluid containing a
known concentration of an indicator (C_{in})
enters a chamber at a flow rate of Q. If additional indicator is added to the fluid in the

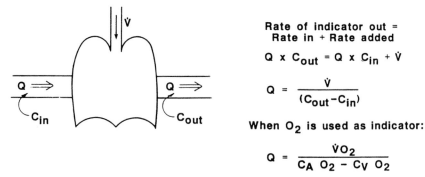

Figure 21.1. Flow measurement with the Fick principle. Fluid containing a known concentration of an indicator (C_{in}) enters a system at flow rate Q. As the fluid passes through the system, indicator is continuously added at rate $\dot{V}$, raising the concentration in the outflow to C_{out}. In a steady state the rate of indicator leaving the system (QC_{out}) must equal the rate at which it enters (QC_{in}) plus the rate at which it is added ($\dot{V}$). When O_2 is used as the indicator, cardiac output can be determined by measuring O_2 consumption ($\dot{V}_{O2}$), arterial O_2 content (C_{AO2}), and mixed venous O_2 content (C_{VO2}).

chamber at a constant rate ($\dot{V}$), the concentration of indicator at the outflow increases to C_{out}. The Fick principle states that the rate at which the indicator leaves the system (QC_{out}) must equal the rate at which it enters (QC_{in}) plus the rate at which it is added:

$$QC_{out} = QC_{in} + \dot{V} \qquad (1)$$

Solving Equation 1 for Q:

$$Q = \dot{V}/(C_{out} - C_{in}) \qquad (2)$$

When the Fick principle is applied to measurement of cardiac output, O_2 is an ideal indicator because both the rate of O_2 uptake by the lungs and the difference between arterial and mixed venous O_2 content can be accurately measured. The Fick principle is valid only in a steady state when both cardiac output and O_2 consumption are constant.

Oxygen Consumption

Accurate measurement of cardiac output with the Fick principle requires that both O_2 consumption and O_2 content in arterial and mixed venous blood be carefully determined. In many laboratories O_2 consumption is estimated from a formula, table, or nomogram (1, 2). There are major limita-

tions to this approach. Many factors that can influence O_2 consumption, such as level of sedation, medications, body temperature, and posture, are not accounted for in assumptions of an empiric value. In a study by Dehmer et al. (3), the average O_2 consumption in 108 patients undergoing cardiac catheterization was 126 mL/minute per square meter, but the standard deviation (plus or minus 26 mL/minute per square meter) and range (65 to 250 mL/minute per square meter) were wide. Kendrick et al. (1) examined the reliability of five methods of estimating O_2 consumption by comparing assumed and measured values in 80 adults during cardiac catheterization. For four of the five estimation methods the assumed O_2 consumption value differed from the actual value by more than 10% in 65% of subjects and by more than 25% in 35%. As shown in Figure 21.2, the "best" relationship, obtained when O_2 consumption was estimated from formulas developed by LaFarge and Miettinen (4), was still poor. Crocker et al. (5) developed estimates for O_2 consumption for adults undergoing cardiac catheterization but noted that only a portion of the variation in O_2 consumption could be accounted for by age, sex, and heart rate. More recently Bergstra et al. (6) developed a regression formula for estimating O_2 consumption that they found to be more reliable than that of LaFarge.

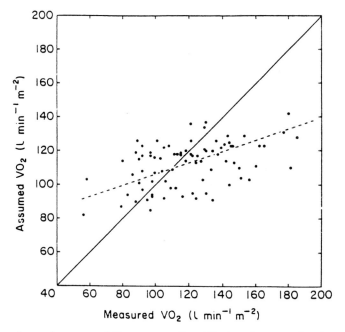

Figure 21.2. Comparison of measured O_2 consumption (V_{O2}) and assumed values from LaFarge and Miettinen in adults at the time of cardiac catheterization. There is a poor relation between measured and estimated O_2 consumption. (Reprinted with permission from Kendrick AH, West J, Papouchado M, Rozkovec A. Direct Fick cardiac output: are assumed values of O_2 consumption acceptable? Eur Heart J 1988;9:337–342.)

Methods

O_2 uptake by the lungs over a given period is the difference between the volume of O_2 inspired and expired. Determination of O_2 uptake requires knowledge of volume and O_2 concentration of both inspired and expired air. In practice inspired air volume is not measured but is inferred from the O_2 and CO_2 concentrations and volume of the expired air. When breathing room air, O_2 uptake ($\dot{V}_{O2}$) in milliliters of O_2 per minute is calculated according to this formula:

$$\dot{V}_{O_2} = \dot{V}_E\,[0.265(1 - F_ECO_2) - 1.265F_EO_2 \quad (3)$$

where $\dot{V}_E$ = minute volume of expired air, F_ECO_2 = fractional content of CO_2 in expired air, and F_EO_2 = fractional content of O_2 in expired air. The fractional amount of O_2 in inspired air is assumed to be 0.209. The derivation of Equation 3 is described in detail by Janicki et al. (7).

O_2 uptake can be measured in several ways, including Douglas bag collection, mixing chamber, and breath-by-breath techniques (7). In the mixing chamber technique expired air is directed from a mouthpiece or face mask into a large (5 to 10 L) chamber where expired gases are completely mixed. The fractional amounts of O_2 and CO_2 in the mixing chamber are measured continuously, and expired air volume is measured with a spirometer or other flow-sensing device. There are several commercial mixing chamber systems (e.g., SensorMedics Horizon System). The most recently developed O_2 uptake measurement technique uses rapidly responding O_2 and CO_2 analyzers to provide breath-by-breath measurement of O_2 uptake. Air flow and fractional content of O_2 and CO_2 from the expired air port of the mouthpiece or face mask are continuously measured. Data from each breath are integrated over time, and the system's computer provides a real-time continuous display of O_2 uptake. Commercial mobile cart breath-by-breath units are available (e.g., Medical Graphics Med-

Graphics System). Both the mixing chamber and breath-by-breath systems provide an on-line readout of O_2 uptake without manual analysis of expired air. This makes it easy to identify a steady state of O_2 uptake and allows Fick cardiac output to be determined immediately during the catheterization procedure. The breath-by-breath system responds most rapidly to changes in O_2 uptake and is well suited for use during exercise testing.

O_2 consumption can also be measured by a metabolic rate monitor (MRM-2, Waters Instruments, Rochester, MN) (8, 9). A clear plastic hood is placed over the subject's head and a blower in the MRM-2 draws room air through the hood fast enough to ensure that all of the patient's expired air is collected. A polarographic O_2 sensor is used to provide on-line time-averaged O_2 consumption values, assuming a respiratory quotient of 1. Lange et al. (10) found that Fick cardiac output with the MRM-2 was consistently lower than cardiac output obtained with either the standard Douglas bag method or thermodilution (Fig. 21.3). In 15 patients (38%), this differ-

ence was more than 25%. More compelling validation studies are needed before this device can be used with confidence to measure O_2 consumption in the cardiac catheterization laboratory.

Sources of Error

Determination of O_2 consumption is usually the least precise component of the Fick measurement of cardiac output. One of the most common sources of error is incomplete collection of expired air because of leakage around the mouthpiece or face mask. When CO_2 content is not measured, there is a small error (usually less than 5%) if the patient's respiratory quotient differs significantly from the assumed value. All of the methods described measure O_2 uptake by the lungs, which in a steady state is equal to O_2 consumption. However, O_2 uptake and consumption can differ widely over a short period (11). For example, **hyperventilation** or an increase in functional residual capacity results in a transient increase in the amount of O_2 entering the lungs with little change in the amount crossing the alveolar–pulmonary capillary membrane, causing an overestimation of O_2 consumption. O_2 uptake should be measured with the patient as relaxed and comfortable as possible, and a 1- to 2-minute equilibration period should follow placement of the mouthpiece, face mask, or hood.

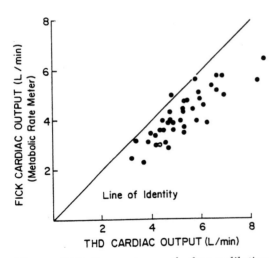

Figure 21.3. Comparison of thermodilution (*THD*) cardiac output and Fick cardiac output obtained with the metabolic rate meter (MRM-2). The Fick output using the MRM-2 is consistently lower than the simultaneous thermodilution output. (Reprinted with permission from Lange RA, Dehmer GJ, Wells PJ, et al. Limitations of the metabolic rate meter for measuring O_2 consumption and cardiac output. Am J Cardiol 1989; 64:783–786.)

Difference Between Arterial and Venous Oxygen Content

Methods

The second step in calculation of cardiac output by the Fick principle is determination of arterial and mixed venous O_2 contents. Systemic arterial and mixed venous blood samples are obtained simultaneously as O_2 consumption is determined. Because of **incomplete mixing** of inferior and superior vena cavae and coronary sinus drainage in the right atrium and right ventricle, the mixed venous blood sample should be obtained from the pulmonary artery. O_2 content is determined directly by means of an O_2-sensitive fuel cell (Lex-O_2-Con) or is calculated from a spectrophotometric measurement of O_2 saturation and hemoglobin concentration. Since the O_2-carrying capacity of fully saturated hemoglobin is 1.36 mL of O_2 per gram, O_2 content (percent by volume) equals O_2 saturation times 1.36 (mL of O_2 per gram) times hemoglobin (grams per 100 mL). (This ignores the small amount of O_2 dissolved in plasma.) For example, assume arterial and mixed venous O_2 saturations are 95 and 70%, respectively, and hemoglobin concentration is 14 g/100 mL:

$$C_{O_2art} = 0.95 \times 1.36 \ (mL \ of \ O_2/g)$$
$$\times \ 14 \ (g/100 \ mL)$$
$$= 18.1 \ mL \ of \ O_2/100 \ mL$$

$$C_{O_2MV} = 0.70 \times 1.36 \ (mL \ of \ O_2/g)$$
$$\times \ 14 \ (g/100 \ mL)$$
$$= 13.3 \ mL \ of \ O_2/100 \ mL$$

where C_{O2art} = arterial O_2 content and C_{O2MV} = mixed venous O_2 content. If O_2 consumption is 240 mL of O_2 per minute, cardiac output (Q) can be calculated with Equation 2:

$$Q = \dot{V}_{O_2}/(C_{O_2art} - C_{O_2MV})$$
$$= 240 \ (mL \ of \ O_2/min)/[(18.1 - 13.3)$$
$$(mL \ of \ O_2/100 \ mL) \times 10 \ (100 \ mL/L)]$$
$$= 5.0 \ (L/min)$$

Sources of Error

The difference between arterial and mixed venous O_2 content can usually be determined with greater accuracy than O_2 consumption, especially when an O_2-sensitive fuel cell is used. Errors can occur if blood samples are diluted with excess heparin, contain large air bubbles, or are allowed to sit at room temperature for several minutes before being analyzed. Indocyanine green dye has a maximum spectral absorbance at about 800 nm and can interfere with O_2 saturation measurements made with spectrophotometers operating at wavelengths near 800 nm. Green dye does not interfere with spectrophotometers that operate in the 530- to 630-nm range (e.g., IL-282 CO-Oximeter from Instrumentation Laboratory or OSM2

Hemoximeter from Radiometer) (12). Abnormal hemoglobins (methemoglobin, sulfhemoglobin), bilirubin, and markedly lipemic samples also interfere with spectrophotometric determination of O_2 saturation. Falsely elevated values for pulmonary arterial O_2 content may be obtained if the tip of the pulmonary artery catheter is being intermittently thrust into the wedge position by cardiac or respiratory motion. Finally, the Fick method assumes that the measured O_2 contents of the arterial and mixed venous blood samples are representative of average O_2 concentrations during the measurement period. An error can be caused by phasic changes in pulmonary or systemic arterial O_2 saturation during the cardiac or respiratory cycle. During steady-state normal respiration phasic changes in the difference between arterial and mixed venous O_2 content are negligible (13). In mechanically ventilated patients phasic changes in O_2 content may be more marked.

Errors in measurement of arterial or mixed venous O_2 content have a greater effect on the accuracy of Fick cardiac output when the difference between arterial and mixed venous O_2 content is very small. Therefore, the Fick method is generally regarded as being most accurate when cardiac output is low and difference between arterial and venous O_2 content is large (14). This should not imply that the Fick method is unreliable at high outputs, and several studies have demonstrated good correlation between Fick and thermodilution for cardiac outputs up to 15 L/minute (15).

Determination of the accuracy of a cardiac output method in humans is hindered by the lack of a direct way of measuring true output (e.g. timed blood collection). In animal studies the Fick cardiac output agrees well with direct measurements of flow. In humans the Fick output is often considered a gold standard for cardiac output measurements, and the accuracy of other techniques is determined by comparison with the Fick method. If all the assumptions on which the Fick technique is based were true and all the required analytical techniques were performed perfectly, the Fick method would be infallible. In fact, there is ample opportunity for error, and disagreement between Fick and an alternative method (e.g., thermodilution or green dye) is not a priori evidence that the alternative method is inaccurate. Reproducibility is the agreement between repeated measurements over a short period. It demonstrates not only variability in the measurement technique but also physiologic instability of cardiac output. Reproducibility is usually expressed as the percentage difference between two repeated measurements (the absolute difference divided by the average value) or the standard deviation of the difference between repeated measurements. For measurement of O_2 consumption the percentage difference between repeated measurements is 5 to 8%, and for measurement of the difference between arterial and mixed venous O_2 content, 5 to 7%. The median percentage difference for Fick cardiac output determinations is 6 to 10% (16).

Indicator Dilution

Like the Fick method, indicator dilution techniques are based on the conservation of mass principle (17). The two most common indicator dilution techniques used in the cardiac catheterization laboratory are the dye dilution and thermodilution methods. The indicator dilution principle can be ap-

plied when the indicator is infused continuously or given as a bolus. Since the continuous-infusion method is rarely used clinically, only the bolus technique is discussed here.

Theory

A schematic illustration of the indicator dilution principle is shown in Figure 21.4. When a known mass of indicator (M) is suddenly introduced as a bolus into the flowing stream entering a chamber, the concentration of indicator in the fluid exiting the chamber (C_{out}) increases in a curvilinear fashion. After reaching a peak, the concentration of indicator falls until all indicator has left the system. At any given moment the rate at which indicator leaves the system is the product of flow (Q) and the concentration of indicator at that time C(t). If there is no indicator present before the bolus ($C_{in} = 0$), the total amount of indicator that leaves the system is given by the formula:

$$\text{Amount of indicator out} = Q \int_0^\infty C_{out}(t)dt$$

The integral term $Q \int_0^\infty C_{out}(t)dt$ represents the area beneath the concentration–time curve. Assuming that all of the indicator

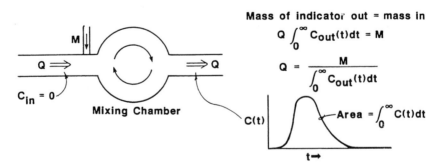

Figure 21.4. Bolus indicator dilution method of determining flow. A known quantity indicator (*M*) is added to blood entering a mixing chamber at flow rate *Q*. The concentration of indicator in blood leaving the mixing chamber is continuously recorded and plotted as a function of time, *C(t)*. The total amount of indicator leaving the system is the product of flow and the integrated area under the concentration–time curve. By the principle of conservation of mass, the total mass of indicator that leaves the chamber must equal the amount that enters. In this example the concentration of indicator entering the chamber (C_{in}) is assumed to be 0. C_{out} is the concentration of indicator at the outflow.

that was added to the system (M) eventually leaves:

$$M = Q \int_0^\infty C_{out}(t)dt$$

and

$$Q = M/[Q \int_0^\infty C_{out}(t)dt] \qquad (4)$$

To be valid the indicator dilution method described by Equation 4 requires (*a*) steady-state flow, (*b*) complete mixing of indicator and blood, (*c*) either no recirculation of indicator or elimination of the effect of recirculation on the concentration–time curve, and (*d*) no loss of indicator (e.g., by diffusion, metabolism, or warming) between the injection and sampling sites (17).

Dye Dilution

Methods

Of the numerous dyes used as indicators, the only one in common use today is indocyanine green. It is rapidly metabolized and excreted by the liver (half-life approximately 10 minutes) and easily measured by spectrophotometry. Allergic reactions to green dye are exceptionally rare (18). A precisely measured amount of green dye, usually 5 mg, is rapidly injected as a bolus through a catheter placed proximal to a mixing chamber. Blood from a site distal to the mixing chamber is withdrawn at a constant rate (15 to 40 mL/minute) through a densitometer, a simple photoelectric device that produces a voltage output proportional to the dye concentration. The concentration of dye is continuously recorded until recirculation is detected. If a sterile closed system has been used, withdrawn blood can be reinfused to the patient after each dye curve has been recorded. The injection site is as close to the sampling point as possible, as long as adequate mixing of the dye and blood can be ensured. In the cardiac catheterization laboratory the pulmonary artery is usually the injection site, mixing occurs in the left atrium and left ventricle, and the concentration of dye is sampled in the aorta

or femoral or brachial artery. Reliable dye outputs can also be obtained with injection to the right atrium or superior vena cava. Injecting to the left ventricle and sampling from the femoral or brachial artery allows dye dilution cardiac output to be determined without a right heart catheterization (19, 20).

According to Equation 4, cardiac output is equal to the amount of green dye injected divided by the area under the concentration–time curve (Fig. 21.4). In practice the area under the concentration curve cannot be measured directly because the dye recirculates before the concentration falls to zero. However, since the downslope of the curve before recirculation follows an exponential decline, the curve can be extrapolated to the baseline. There are several manual ways to eliminate the effect of recirculation and obtain the area under the concentration curve (21, 22). Analysis of dye dilution curves is simplified by the use of analog output computers (23, 24). Most of these units deal with the problem of recirculation by calculating an exponential decay constant from an early portion of the downslope of the dye curve that is normally well above the onset of recirculation. This decay constant is used to extrapolate the curve to baseline.

Calibration is necessary to convert the voltage output of the densitometer to dye concentration. Precisely measured amounts of green dye are mixed with aliquots of the patient's blood to prepare samples with known dye concentrations (usually in the range of 1 to 10 mg/L). These samples are withdrawn through the densitometer, and the voltage output is recorded on paper or used to calibrate the analog output computer. So-called dynamic calibration requires a smaller volume of blood and eliminates the need to prepare blood–dye samples (25, 26). Sullivan et al. (27) found that the voltage output of a densitometer for a given concentration of dye in blood was stable for up to 4 weeks. They described an electronic calibration method that requires only periodic blood calibration of the densitometer. Prior to each study the gain of the analog output computer is adjusted to the predetermined calibration factor for the densitometer being used. While this simplifies the green dye technique, there are few published data on the reliability of dye dilution outputs performed in this way.

Sources of Error

Errors in the green dye method occur if the amount of dye delivered to the blood is inaccurately measured, if there is incomplete mixing of dye and blood, if the concentration–time curve is distorted, if the densitometer is improperly calibrated, or if the area under the curve is imprecisely determined. Since indocyanine green dye deteriorates with **exposure to light**, it should be used within 2 hours of preparation. The rate of blood withdrawal through the densitometer must be constant, and the tubing between sampling site and densitometer should be kept as short as possible to avoid distorting the concentration curve (28). When an analog output computer is used, the first half of the downslope of the dye curve must be exponential so that an accurate decay constant can be determined. Inspection of the dye curve may reveal the cause of erroneous outputs, such as air leak, nonuniform or slow withdrawal rate, early recirculation, and baseline drift.

Numerous reports have demonstrated a good correlation between Fick and green dye measurements of cardiac output over a wide range of outputs (29–31). Several authors have found a greater disparity between Fick and dye outputs in patients with low cardiac output (less than 2 L/minute per square meter) and in those with significant mitral or aortic regurgitation (31, 32) (Fig. 21.5). In these individuals the downslope of the concentration curve is prolonged, and recirculation distorts the curve before an accurate area can be calculated, resulting in underestimation of cardiac output. This can sometimes be corrected by moving the injection and sampling sites closer together or by determining the area under the curve manually if an analog output computer was used. A **nonrecirculated indicator** (e.g., thermal) or Fick method is preferable in these patients. The downslope of the curve is also distorted by early recirculation of dye in patients with a left-to-right intracardiac shunt. The percentage difference between

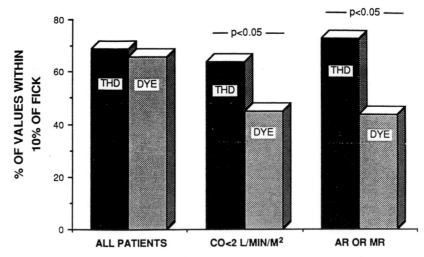

Figure 21.5. Comparison of thermodilution and dye dilution cardiac output determinations. Cardiac output *(CO)* was measured by Fick and either thermodilution *(THD)* (242 patients) or dye dilution (DYE) (556 patients). Overall the difference between the Fick and the THD or dye output was less than 10% in approximately 70% of patients. However, dye output was within 10% of the Fick output in only about 45% of patients with low cardiac output, aortic regurgitation *(AR)* or mitral regurgitation *(MR)*. (From data in Hillis LD, Firth BG, Winniford MD. Analysis of factors affecting the variation of Fick versus indicator dilution measurements of cardiac output. Am J Cardiol 1985;56:764–768.)

repeated green dye cardiac outputs at rest has been reported to be 6 to 9%.

Thermodilution

Methods

The thermodilution technique is based on the same principle as the dye dilution method described earlier (33, 34). In this case the indicator is "cold," and the "concentration" of indicator is temperature. A thermistor-tipped triple-lumen balloon catheter is positioned in the pulmonary artery. A carefully measured volume of iced or room temperature saline or 5% dextrose is injected as a bolus into the right atrium, and the temperature of the blood–injectate mixture in the pulmonary artery is continuously recorded. The cardiac output (Q), which is inversely proportional to the area under the temperature–time curve, can be calculated with the following formula:

$$Q = 60 V_I \, S_I \, C_I \, CF \, (T_B - T_I)/[S_B C_B \int_0^\infty \Delta T_B(t)dt],$$

$$= 60(V_I \, S_I \, C_I \, CF/S_B \, C_B)(T_B - T_I)/[\int_0^\infty \Delta T_B(t)dt]$$

$$(5)$$

where V_I = volume of injectate, S_I = specific gravity of injectate, C_I = specific heat of injectate, CF = correction factor accounting for warming of indicator during passage through the catheter, S_B = specific gravity of blood, C_B = specific heat of blood, T_B = blood temperature, T_I = injectate temperature, and $\int_0^\infty \Delta D T_B(t)dt$ = area under the temperature–time curve. The variables that must be measured are the temperature of blood and injectate and the area under the temperature–time curve. In practice analog cardiac output computers are routinely used to integrate the temperature–time curve and calculate cardiac output with Equation 5 (35, 36). The other factors in Equation 5 are entered into the computer as a single constant depending on the injectate volume and temperature and catheter model.

As injectate passes through the catheter in the body, it gains heat so that the temperature of injectate that enters the blood-stream is higher than that measured outside the body (37). The temperature gain (amount of indicator lost) varies with the injectate volume and temperature, injection rate, time between injections, and catheter construction. The correction factor CF in Equation 5 attempts to account for this unmeasured loss of indicator and is determined for each catheter model by the manufacturer under standardized conditions. Loss of indicator is greatest for the first injection of a series, since the catheter and the fluid it contains are closest to body temperature (38). Accordingly, the first cardiac output may be higher than subsequent outputs, especially when iced injectate is used (39). The correction factor supplied by the manufacturer assumes that (*a*) repeat injections are performed 1 to 2 minutes after the previous output is displayed by the computer, (*b*) injection rate is 10 mL within 4 seconds, (*c*) the first injection is disregarded when iced injectate is used, and (*d*) the catheter is not aspirated between injections.

The amount of indicator is determined by the volume and temperature of injectate. Although use of ice-cold indicator is frequently cited as having a greater signal-to-noise ratio, there is no clear difference in cardiac output measured with ice-cold (0 to 5°C) versus room temperature (20 to 25°C) injectate in most clinical settings (40–43). It is possible that the advantage of a greater signal-to-noise ratio is offset by increased uncertainty as to the amount of indicator (cold) lost during passage through the catheter. Some studies have found less variability between repeat measurements with ice-cold injectate (35, 44). Ice-cold injectate should be used in hypothermic patients and when room temperature exceeds 25°C. Ice-cold injectate may also be preferable when cardiac output is very high (e.g., during exercise), when the area under the temperature–time curve is small, when there are large fluctuations in pulmonary artery blood temperature, and when less than 10 mL of injectate is used. Regardless of injectate temperature, thermodilution cardiac output should always be determined from the average of three to five injections.

CO_2-powered injection devices can rapidly deliver injectate at a constant rate. However, there is little advantage to these devices over hand injection at a constant rate, provided injectate is delivered within about 4 seconds (45). Injections performed at an uneven rate result in distorted temperature–time curves and increase the variability of repeated measurements.

During normal respiration phasic changes in pulmonary artery blood temperature are negligible (46). Phasic temperature changes are more marked with deep breathing and hyperventilation (47), and this can lead to increased variability of output measurements. Mechanical ventilation causes exaggerated phasic changes in left ventricular stroke volume and cardiac output, with greater variation in thermodilution outputs. Reproducibility is improved in dyspneic or mechanically ventilated patients if injection is timed to begin at end expiration or peak inspiration (48). However, thermodilution outputs performed in this manner may not accurately reflect the average cardiac output throughout the respiratory cycle. Injection at regularly spaced intervals during the respiratory cycle has been suggested as a way to improve accuracy (49, 50) but may not be feasible in routine practice. Averaging three to five randomly timed injections of ice-cold injectate is probably adequate in most cases.

A newer thermodilution catheter system makes it possible to assess cardiac output continuously without fluid injection (51–53). A heating filament that can produce small changes in blood temperature at the site of the thermistor in the pulmonary artery is placed on the catheter in the right ventricle. The output computer cross-correlates the changes in blood temperature that occur in response to programed on–off cycling of the heating filament to calculate output according to the thermodilution principle described earlier. This system has been shown to correlate well with conventional bolus thermodilution and Fick cardiac output measurements (51, 52, 54, 55).

The thermodilution method has several advantages over Fick and dye dilution. It is the easiest and quickest of the three techniques. No arterial blood samples are required. Since there is negligible recirculation of indicator in the absence of an intracardiac shunt, calculation of the area under the temperature–time curve is sim-

plified. There is close agreement between the thermodilution and Fick methods over a wide range of cardiac outputs (15, 33, 56, 57). Unlike dye dilution techniques, accuracy of the thermodilution method is not reduced in patients with aortic or mitral regurgitation or moderately depressed cardiac output (31, 32). At extremely low outputs (less than 2.5 L/minute), the thermodilution method appears to overestimate cardiac output, presumably because of loss of thermal indicator between the injection site and pulmonary artery (58). The Fick method would be preferable to either of the indicator dilution techniques in these individuals.

Sources of Error

The thermodilution cardiac output method is used so frequently and seems so simple that it is easy to overlook the many technical factors that can lead to erroneous results. If ice-cold injectate is used, excessive handling of the syringe after removal from the ice bath warms the injectate (loss of indicator), resulting in overestimation of cardiac output. The temperature of iced injectate in a plastic syringe held in a gloved hand increases $1°C$ every 13 seconds (59). If it is held for 1 minute before injection, cardiac output is overestimated by about 12%. Theoretically this problem can be minimized if injectate temperature is measured by a thermistor placed in line between the injection syringe and the hub of the thermodilution catheter. A closed injection system with in-line thermistor probes is Model 93–510, CO-Set, American Edwards) (60, 61). The rapid administration of intravenous fluids during output measurements can lead to a significant underestimation of cardiac output (62). Other sources of error include fibrin or thrombus accumulation on the catheter tip (63) and migration of the catheter tip to a wedge position.

Tricuspid regurgitation has been reported to cause underestimation (64), overestimation (57, 65), and no effect (66) on cardiac output by thermodilution. In 17 patients with tricuspid regurgitation studied by Cigarroa et al. (64), thermodilution

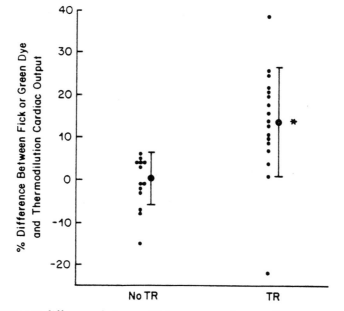

Figure 21.6. The percent difference between Fick or green dye cardiac output and thermodilution cardiac output in patients with and without tricuspid regurgitation (*TR*). There is a greater percent difference in those with tricuspid regurgitation. In nearly every case the thermodilution output was lower than the corresponding Fick or green dye value. (Reprinted with permission from Cigarroa RG, Lange RA, Williams RH, et al. Underestimation of cardiac output by thermodilution in patients with tricuspid regurgitation. Am J Med 1989;86:417–420.)

cardiac output was 15 plus or minus 14% (mean plus or minus one standard deviation) lower than Fick or green dye outputs (Fig. 21.6). This discrepancy was attributed to splaying and prolongation of the thermodilution temperature–time curve with a resultant overestimation of the curve area. In some patients with tricuspid regurgitation, unphysiologically high cardiac outputs can be recorded by thermodilution, presumably because of loss of indicator in the right heart (57). In patients with an intracardiac left-to-right shunt recirculation of indicator distorts the downslope of the temperature–time curve (67). This increases the measured area under the curve and leads to underestimation of pulmonary blood flow, especially when iced injectate is used. Accordingly, the **thermodilution technique should not be considered a reliable way to measure pulmonary blood flow in patients with a large left-to-right shunt**.

The reproducibility of the thermodilution method has been extensively examined (68). The standard deviation of the differ-

ence between repeated measurements is reported to be 4 to 9%. The 95% confidence limits for a thermodilution cardiac output determination is equal to twice the standard error of the mean (standard deviation divided by the square root of the number of injections). For example, if the standard deviation of the difference between repeated measurements is 7%, the reliability (95% confidence limits) of a cardiac output determination based on the average of 3 injections is plus or minus 8% (4.6 to 5.4 L/minute for a cardiac output of 5 L/minute) compared with plus or minus 14% (4.3 to 5.7 L/minute) when a single injection is used. When the average of three output measurements is used, reported 95% confidence limits range from plus or minus 4% to plus or minus 10%.

Other Techniques

Both Doppler (69–71) and electromagnetic (72–74) techniques have been adapted to catheter measurement of blood velocity in the pulmonary artery and aorta. When they are used in combination with high-fidelity catheter tip micromanometers, vascular impedance spectra and wave reflections can be studied (75, 76). Other uses include quantitation of valvular regurgitation (77). Effects of pharmacologic agents and oscillatory components of afterload can be quantified with these techniques (78, 79).

There are several practical problems with use of velocity catheters in the great vessels. First, as noted in the section on coronary velocity catheters, volumetric flow can be measured with these techniques only when vessel cross-sectional area is known or independent calibration is done. Vessel diameter can be estimated according to expected values for age, sex, and body size or measured by angiography or echocardiography, but each of these approaches has serious limitations. Alternatively, cardiac output measurement by thermodilution or other indicator dilution techniques can be used to calibrate the velocity catheter. Second, since blood flow velocity profiles in the great vessels in vivo are not flat, catheter sampling from one location may not represent an average of true blood velocity. Finally, instability of the catheter in the vessel limits the accuracy of these devices.

The noninvasive techniques for assessing cardiac output include impedance cardiography (80–82), Doppler echocardiography (83, 84), CO_2 rebreathing (85), nitrous oxide technique (86), and radionuclide imaging (87). These techniques are less reliable than the Fick and indicator dilution methods that we have described and cannot be recommended when accurate measurement of cardiac output is needed during cardiac catheterization.

Summary of Cardiac Output Determination

It should be evident from the preceding discussion that each of the most commonly used methods of measuring cardiac output has advantages and limitations. All require that the patient be in a steady state with a constant cardiac output during the measurement period. Traditionally, the Fick method has been used as the reference standard against which other techniques are compared. From a practical standpoint, there are many possible sources of error in measuring O_2 consumption and arterial and mixed venous O_2 contents. The thermodilution technique is easiest and quickest to perform but is subject to error in a patient with tricuspid regurgitation, intracardiac shunt, or extremely low cardiac output. The dye dilution method is the most cumbersome and time-consuming to perform, requires withdrawal of large amounts of blood and cleaning and resterilization of equipment, and is not well suited for patients with significant mitral or aortic regurgitation or low cardiac output. Use of this technique has declined sharply (88) in favor of thermodilution, which has become by far the most commonly used method of measuring cardiac output.

When a high level of precision is desired (e.g., calculation of a valve orifice area), **we routinely measure cardiac output by both Fick and thermodilution**. The Fick method is also employed in patients with low cardiac output, tricuspid regurgitation, or an intracardiac shunt. O_2 consumption is estimated only when it cannot be measured (e.g., ventilated, uncooperative, or acutely ill patients). The dye dilution technique is used mainly for patients with intracardiac shunts or tricuspid regurgitation and in the rare instance when the pulmonary artery cannot be cannulated.

CORONARY BLOOD FLOW

Several methods have been used to assess coronary blood flow or myocardial perfusion (flow per unit mass of tissue) in the cardiac catheterization laboratory (Table 21.1). Gas clearance and coronary sinus thermodilution techniques are important research tools, but these methods have limited ability to provide clinically useful information about the coronary circulation. Digital radiographic techniques can provide reliable information about regional coronary flow, and further technical advances

Table 21.1.
Invasive Methods of Assessing Coronary Blood Flow in Conscious Humans

Method	Advantages	Disadvantages
Inert gas clearance	Accurate at high flows	Poor spatial resolution
Nonradioactive	Flow per unit weight	Prolonged steady state required
	Safe	Complex chemical analysis
Radioactive	Assessment of regional flow	Inaccurate at high flows
(xenon-133)	Flow per unit weight	Requires intracoronary injection of tracer
		Limited number of flow measurements per study
Coronary venous thermodilution	Simple	Poor spatial resolution
	Volumetric flow measured	Affected by changes in catheter position, heart size
	Safe	
	Multiple flow measurements per study	Underestimates flow reserve
Contrast density; appearance time with digital subtraction angiography	Assessment of regional flow reserve	Requires specialized digital imaging equipment
	Accurate at high flows (some studies)	Requires intracoronary contrast injection
	Subselective coronary cannulation not required	Motion artifacts
Doppler probe	Simple	Requires intracoronary placement
	Assessment of regional flow reserve	Volumetric flow not measured
	Rapid time constant enabling assessment of phasic flow velocity pattern during cardiac cycle	Not feasible in some patients with severe proximal or diffuse coronary disease
	Well validated	
	Accurate at high flows	

should make these methods more feasible for clinical use. **Doppler flow probes have emerged as the most practical way of examining coronary flow** and are assuming an increasingly important role in the clinical evaluation of patients with known or suspected ischemic heart disease.

Gas Clearance

Theory and Methods

Gas clearance is used to measure the average left ventricular blood flow per unit weight. It is an adaptation of the Kety-Schmidt nitrous oxide technique originally applied to the quantitation of cerebral blood flow (89, 90). Gas clearance is based on the concept of conservation of mass described by the Fick principle (90, 91). A diffusible inert gas that is not metabolized by the myocardium is added to the systemic circula-

tion, usually by inhalation. The most commonly used nonradioactive inert gases are nitrous oxide, helium, hydrogen, and argon. As the gas saturates the myocardium, the coronary arterial and venous blood concentrations of gas are recorded periodically. According to the Fick principle, flow is equal to the myocardial gas uptake divided by the mean difference between arterial and venous gas content. That value is found by integrating the instantaneous differences over the period required to achieve saturation. Determination of myocardial gas uptake requires knowledge of the tissue–blood partition coefficient for the specific gas being used. See the review by Klocke (91) for a detailed discussion of this method.

The inert gas clearance technique can also be used to measure average left ventricular flow following the bolus intracoronary injection of a radioactive tracer such as xenon-133 (89, 92, 93). The xenon-133 washout curve is analyzed by precordial counting of radioactivity with a scintillation camera. When a multicrystal camera is used, washout from specific regions of the heart can be recorded and regional blood flow estimated.

Limitations of Gas Clearance

Several assumptions are made when the Kety-Schmidt approach is applied to measurement of coronary blood flow. First, there must be a steady state of coronary flow during the 5 to 20 minutes required to make the flow measurement. Thus rapid changes in flow cannot be assessed. Second, the accuracy of the technique is reduced when the coronary sinus blood sample contains venous drainage from structures other than the left ventricle or when venous drainage from certain regions of the left ventricle does not go into the coronary sinus. For example, drainage from regions of the left ventricle supplied by the posterior descending artery enters the coronary sinus near the ostium and is usually not represented in blood obtained from a catheter positioned 2 or 3 cm within the sinus (94). Third, the measured flow per unit weight represents the average flow in the entire myocardial region draining into the coronary sinus upstream from the sampling catheter. At best an attempt can be made to measure regional flow in the territory of the left anterior descending artery by sampling from the great cardiac vein. Finally, the technique tends to overestimate flow in patients with coronary artery disease (CAD) who have heterogeneous perfusion and in some cases myocardial scar (91, 95).

The xenon-133 precordial counting method is technically demanding and has several limitations (91, 93). Because xenon-133 is highly soluble in fat, adipose tissue contributes a large fraction of the total radioactivity detected by precordial counting during the later portion of the washout curve. The high fat solubility also limits the number of measurements that can be made during each study. The accuracy of xenon-133 measurements of average left ventricular blood flow, especially at high flow rates, is controversial.

The nonradioactive and radioactive inert gas clearance techniques are time-consuming, require special equipment for sample analysis, and may not be accurate at high coronary flow rates. While not practical for clinical use, they continue to be used in a small number of laboratories for research studies examining physiologic regulation of coronary flow and the effect of pathologic conditions or pharmacologic agents on myocardial perfusion.

Coronary Sinus Thermodilution

Theory and Methods

In 1971 Ganz et al. (96) described a method of measuring coronary sinus blood flow using the thermodilution technique. Room temperature injectate (5% dextrose solution or saline) is injected into the coronary sinus through a 7- or 8-F thermodilution catheter at 35 to 55 mL/minute. The injectate mixes with the coronary sinus blood, and the temperature of the injectate–blood mixture is recorded by a thermistor placed on the external surface of the catheter 10 to 45 mm proximal to the injectate orifice. Use of thermodilution principles allows coronary sinus flow to be determined from the temperature difference between blood and the blood–injectate mixture. If the catheter is advanced into the great cardiac vein, venous flow from the anterior region of the left ventricle can be recorded. Catheters with two external thermistors (Regional Pepine 2, Webster Laboratories, Baldwin Park, CA; Baim, Electro-Catheter Corp., Rahway, NJ) permit simultaneous measurement of great cardiac vein and coronary sinus flow (97, 98).

The validity of the thermodilution technique has been convincingly demonstrated in models of the coronary sinus and in animal studies with the catheter secured within the coronary sinus. A poorer relationship between flow measured by thermodilution and krypton-85 washout was found when the catheter was placed in intact dogs (99).

Coronary sinus thermodilution has several advantages. It is relatively simple to perform, and with experience adequate flow signals from both great cardiac vein and coronary sinus can be obtained in more than 90% of patients studied. There is no significant accumulation of indicator (cold), so multiple measurements can be made over a relatively short time. The time constant of the method is rapid enough to permit detection of flow changes over 5 to 10 seconds. The thermodilution method is safer than techniques that require cannulation of a coronary artery. Transient atrial arrhythmias may occur during manipulation of the catheter in the right atrium. Perforation of the atrium or coronary sinus is extremely rare. Finally, volumetric flow in milliliters per minute, rather than flow per unit weight or flow velocity, is measured.

Limitations of Coronary Sinus Thermodilution

In common with all methods of measuring coronary flow in humans, the thermodilution technique has several limitations. As with gas clearance, the portion of left ventricular flow measured depends on the precise position of the catheter within the coronary sinus and the origin of venous blood entering the sinus proximal to the catheter. In normal subjects there is some variation in the entry site of veins draining the lateral and inferior regions of the left ventricle. In addition, human hearts may have extensive venous intercommunications (100). In the presence of severe coronary disease the pattern of venous drainage may be further distorted. Therefore it may be difficult to attribute coronary sinus flow to any specific portion of the left ventricle.

This limitation can be partially overcome by measuring great cardiac vein flow, as noted earlier, since the majority of resting great cardiac vein flow arises from the anterior region and conversely, the majority of anterior region flow drains into the great cardiac vein. Some validation studies in animals have shown excellent regionalization of coronary flow signals from the great cardiac vein to the anterior descending coronary artery perfusion bed (101, 102). Others have noted a significant discrepancy between great cardiac vein and anterior descending flow (103, 104). Nakazawa et al. (103) demonstrated that 37% of canine left anterior descending artery flow drained through routes other than the great cardiac vein. Cohen et al. (104) found that peak great cardiac vein flow during reactive hyperemia underestimated peak left anterior descending flow by nearly 40% in dogs. In humans Pepine et al. (98) have validated the regionalization of thermodilution coronary blood flow determinations during open heart surgery. An electromagnetic flow probe in the operating room was used to demonstrate a close relationship between thermodilution great cardiac vein flow and left anterior descending bypass graft flow in patients with occluded or partially occluded left anterior descending arteries.

When used in conscious patients during cardiac catheterization, thermodilution great cardiac vein flow appears to underestimate changes in flow in the left anterior descending artery. With use of Doppler or videodensitometric techniques coronary flow in normal subjects increases fourfold to sixfold above resting flow during maximal pharmacologic vasodilation. With the thermodilution technique great cardiac vein and coronary sinus flow rarely rise above three times the resting value (105–107). Rossen et al. (108) compared thermodilution great cardiac vein flow with simultaneous Doppler measurements of changes in flow velocity of the left anterior descending artery after administration of several vasodilators. Submaximal and maximal flow increases measured with the thermodilution method were substantially smaller than Doppler-derived measurements (Fig. 21.7). Coronary flow reserve, the ratio of peak to resting blood flow, was 3.7 plus or minus 1.7 by Doppler and 2 plus or minus 0.7 by thermodilution.

Thermodilution flow measurements are affected by changes in catheter position within the coronary sinus (109). The location of the catheter should be frequently checked radiographically, but it may not be possible to detect small changes in position caused by catheter softening, patient movement, coughing, and so on. An unrecognized change in catheter position may also occur if an intervention, such as rapid atrial

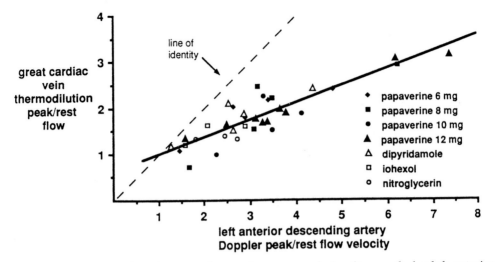

Figure 21.7. Comparison of peak-to-rest flow ratios measured simultaneously by left anterior descending Doppler and great cardiac vein thermodilution after a variety of vasodilator stimuli. Changes in great cardiac vein flow by thermodilution were consistently less than changes in left anterior descending Doppler flow velocity. (Reprinted with permission from Rossen JD, Oskarsson H, Stenberg RG, et al. Simultaneous measurement of coronary flow reserve by left anterior descending coronary artery Doppler and great cardiac vein thermodilution methods. J Am Coll Cardiol 1992;20:402–407.)

pacing, produces a change in heart size. Reflux of right atrial blood into the coronary sinus when right atrial pressure is increased may cause an overestimation of coronary sinus thermodilution flow (110). This can be detected by injecting room temperature saline into the low right atrium while recording from the coronary venous thermistors. There is limited experience with the coronary sinus thermodilution technique during exercise (111).

While coronary sinus thermodilution has not proved useful for clinical decision making in individual patients, it has provided valuable information about the pathophysiology of angina pectoris in patients with and without CAD, the mechanism of action of antianginal drugs, and the effect of myocardial revascularization on coronary blood flow. Like gas clearance, thermodilution is best suited for patients with homogeneous perfusion and normal coronary arteries. When used in patients with CAD, the measurement of great cardiac vein flow can be used to detect changes in left anterior descending flow, but the magnitude of flow changes may be underestimated. The use of coronary sinus thermodilution as a research tool has markedly

declined over the past 10 years in favor of intracoronary Doppler flow probes.

Doppler

Theory and Methods

The Doppler principle states that when sound waves are reflected from moving structures, such as red blood cells, the frequency of the reflected wave changes in proportion to the instantaneous flow velocity according to this formula:

$$v = (c\Delta f)/(2f_0 cos\tau) \qquad (6)$$

where v = flow velocity, c = speed of sound in blood, Δf = Doppler frequency shift, f_0 = frequency of the transmitted wave, and τ = angle between the sound wave vector and the bloodstream. For many years Doppler flow probes have been used to measure phasic coronary blood flow velocity in animals and have been applied to the surface of epicardial coronary arteries of patients undergoing coronary artery bypass surgery (112). Initial attempts to measure coronary flow velocity during cardiac catheterization were made with a Doppler crystal mounted on the tip of a Sones catheter (113). The development of small intracoronary Doppler catheters in the mid-1980s made it possible to record changes in phasic flow velocity in individual coronary arteries in awake humans during cardiac catheterization (114, 115). These 3-F catheters had a forward-facing Doppler crystal mounted on either the side (NuMED, Inc., Hopkinton, NY) or distal tip (DC-101, Millar Instruments, Houston, TX) of the catheter. The Doppler signal was analyzed with a zero-crossing detector velocimeter operating at 20 MHz.

More recently a Doppler crystal mounted on the end of an angioplasty guidewire has become available. As described and validated by Doucette et al. (116), the Doppler angioplasty guidewire (FloWire, Cardiometrics, Inc., Mountain View, CA) is a 175-cm-long, 0.018-inch-diameter flexible steerable guidewire with a piezoelectric ultrasound transducer in the tip. The forward-directed ultrasound beam diverges in a 27° arc from the long axis. The FloWire signal is coupled to a FloMap console with a real-time spectrum analyzer, videocassette recorder, and video page printer. The Doppler audio signals are processed by the spectrum analyzer and are available on a scrolling gray scale video display. The setup time of the Doppler guidewire system is usually less than 10 minutes. Intravenous heparin (5000 to 10,000 units) is administered before insertion of the Doppler guidewire. After diagnostic angiography or during angioplasty, the Doppler guidewire is passed through an angioplasty Y-connector attached to the diagnostic or guiding catheter. The guidewire is then advanced into the artery to the desired location of flow measurement. For measurement of flow velocity distal to a stenosis the wire tip is placed at least 5 to 10 artery diameter lengths (more than 2 cm) beyond the stenosis to avoid turbulence caused by the stenosis. Gentle manipulation of the wire is usually required to obtain a stable, high-quality velocity signal.

Doppler catheter and guidewire techniques have been extensively validated in animal studies (114, 116). Changes in velocity of coronary blood flow correlate closely with timed venous collection of coronary sinus blood over a wide range of coronary flows (114). In vitro and in vivo validation studies demonstrate that the Doppler guidewire system can accurately measure blood flow velocity over a wide range of flows (116).

There are several advantages to the intracoronary Doppler guidewire technique. A continuous record of flow velocity is provided over the entire range of flow velocities encountered in the coronary circulation. Maximal flow velocity is more accurately identified with spectral analysis than with Doppler catheters used with zero-crossing detectors because of the automatic edge detection, wide beam angle, and relative position insensitivity of the signal. The use of a guidewire rather than a catheter also allows safe interrogation of smaller, more diffusely diseased arteries and of artery segments distal to coronary stenoses. The rapid time constant permits measurement of instantaneous changes in blood flow velocity. The Doppler probe is easily incorporated into interventional procedures via angioplasty guidewires and can be used during diagnostic angiography without significant risk. Finally, the **Doppler probe technique of measuring flow velocity is relatively simple to perform**, making it by far the most clinically practical method of the assessment of coronary flow.

Limitations of Doppler Technique

Notwithstanding its advantages, the intracoronary Doppler method has significant limitations. Doppler techniques assess flow velocity; volumetric blood flow is not directly measured. Changes in flow velocity are proportional to changes in volumetric flow only when there is no change in vessel cross-sectional area at the site of the sample volume just distal to Doppler crystal. For example, if a potent vasodilator simultaneously produces both an increase in volumetric flow and epicardial vasodilation, the increase in flow is underestimated by the Doppler technique (117). Attempts to calcu-

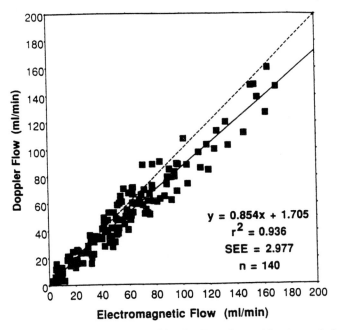

Figure 21.8. Correlation between flow measured by the Doppler guidewire and electromagnetic flow in the proximal left circumflex coronary artery in dogs. Volumetric flow by Doppler was determined from the average peak velocity from the spectral display and the vessel cross-sectional area. (Reprinted with permission from Doucette JW, Corl PD, Payne HM, et al. Validation of a Doppler guide wire for intravascular measurement of coronary artery flow velocity. Circulation 1992;85:1899–1911.)

late volumetric flow in milliliters per minute from the Doppler flow velocity in cm/sec and coronary cross-sectional area from quantitative angiography are limited by uncertainties about the angle of incidence (q), the nature of the flow profile, and the accuracy of zero-crossing detector velocity measurements (118). Using the Doppler guidewire in a tube model and an open chest dog preparation, Doucette et al. (116) found a good relationship between actual flow (by electromagnetic flow probe) and calculated flow using the time average of the fast Fourier transform peak spectral velocity (Fig. 21.8). Whether a similar relationship can be obtained in humans with tortuous, branching vessels and atherosclerosis is unknown.

The need for intracoronary placement means that there is always a risk associated with this technique. Careful patient selection, full systemic heparinization, and use by individuals skilled in coronary angioplasty minimize the risks of the procedure. Coronary artery dissection, thrombosis, and

spasm are obvious possible complications. The risk of vascular trauma with the flexible Doppler guidewire is extremely low, and extensive experience has proved that an experienced operator can safely place the device across coronary stenoses of intermediate severity. Worldwide, only 10 cases out of more than 40,000 uses have resulted in serious artery injury reported to the manufacturer or U.S. Food and Drug Administration. This incidence is lower than for diagnostic angiography alone. Even so, it should be used with caution in patients with severe, diffuse coronary disease.

The Doppler guidewire is durable, but it may be damaged by rough handling on insertion. Manipulation within the coronary system may bend the guidewire tip, but rarely is this severe enough to cause signal failure. Finally, damping or partial obstruction of the coronary ostium by the guiding catheter may restrict peak coronary flow; this may not be evident from the pressure waveform recorded from the tip of the guiding catheter. Use of the Doppler guidewire with a small (5 or 6 F) diagnostic catheter minimizes restriction of peak flow at the coronary ostium. The primary disadvantage of the Doppler guidewire system compared with the zero-crossing detector velocimeter and reusable Doppler catheters is the greater cost of the FloMap console and single-use guidewires.

Radiographic Techniques

Methods

The numerous radiographic methods to assess coronary blood flow and myocardial perfusion are extensively described in the review by Mancini (119). The first successful radiographic method to measure coronary blood flow was the transit time technique developed by Rutishauser et al. (120, 121) and Smith et al. (122). These investigators measured the density of injected contrast material at two locations in a proximal coronary vessel to determine the transit time of the contrast bolus between the two points. If the distance between the two points is known, the flow velocity can be calculated. Volumetric flow is obtained by multiplying the cross-sectional area of the vessel by the blood flow velocity. Limitations of this technique include the short distance between regions of interest, the pulsatile nature of coronary flow, and artifacts caused by cardiac and respiratory motion. Spiller et al. (123) used modern technology and reported a good correlation between flow measured by a videodensitometric technique and electromagnetic flow probes. These videodensitometric techniques work especially well in bypass grafts, which are long, straight, free of branches, and large in diameter (124). More recently Chappuis et al. (125) measured absolute coronary blood flow using a modification of the transit time method with arterial lengths and volumes calculated from a computerized three-dimensional reconstruction of the major coronary branches.

The indicator dilution principle described earlier for determination of cardiac output has also been applied to the measurement of coronary blood flow. Analyzing the contrast density–time curve created by a known amount of dye passing through a region of interest over a coronary artery at rest and during hyperemia lets coronary flow reserve be assessed (126, 127). These techniques do not require measurement of either coronary artery diameter or segment length. In a canine model Nissen et al. (128) demonstrated good agreement between coronary flow reserve measured by an indicator dilution videodensitometric approach and an electromagnetic flow probe. A simplified version of this approach not requiring power contrast injection or electrocardiographic gating has also been validated in an animal study (129).

Several methods of digital angiography based on an analysis of the contrast density–time curve from a myocardial region of interest have been used to assess myocardial perfusion and flow reserve (119). Ikeda et al. (130) used the Kety-Schmidt approach to analyze the disappearance of contrast from a region of interest over the myocardium. They showed that the disappearance half-life calculated from a contrast washout analysis of the density–time curve correlated well with the angiographic severity of coronary stenoses in patients studied during cardiac catheterization. Eigler et al. (131) used the entire wash-in and washout curve and transfer function analysis to calculate a mean transit time that correlated well with flowmeter measures of perfusion.

The most common radiographic approaches to assessing myocardial perfusion are modifications of the appearance time and density analysis developed by Vogel et al. (132) and Hodgson et al. (133). This approach is based on the principle that the ratio of contrast density to contrast appearance time over a region of myocardium is an index of myocardial perfusion. While there are major limitations to determining absolute myocardial perfusion from contrast density and appearance time, changes in perfusion can be assessed. For example, by measuring contrast density (D) and appearance time (AT) at rest and during maximal vasodilation, coronary flow reserve (CFR) can be determined thus:

$$CFR = \frac{maximal\ flow}{rest\ flow} = \frac{(D/AT)_{max}}{(D/AT)_{rest}} \quad (7)$$

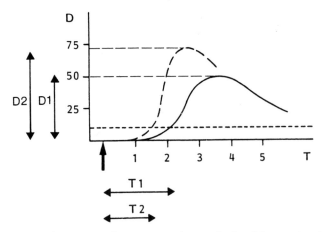

Figure 21.9. Measurement of coronary flow reserve by analysis of the contrast density–time curve. In the myocardial region of interest baseline (*solid line*) and hyperemic (*dashed line*) density–time curves are generated with the use of digital subtraction of end diastolic frames. The myocardial contrast appearance time (*T*) is the point at which the contrast density exceeds a fixed threshold and is measured at baseline (*T1*) and during maximal vasodilation (*T2*). The maximal contrast density is also measured at baseline (*D1*) and during vasodilation (*D2*). Coronary flow reserve is calculated according to Equation 10 in the text. (Reprinted with permission from Reiber JHC, Serruys PW. Quantitative coronary angiography. In: Marcus ML, Schelbert HR, Skorton DJ, Wolf GL, eds. Cardiac Imaging. Philadelphia: W.B. Saunders, 1991:211–280.)

where max = values during maximal coronary vasodilation (Fig. 21.9). Current versions of this approach use color- and intensity-coded parametric images to depict the appearance time and density of contrast (134, 135). In some studies regional flow reserve measured by this technique correlated well with measured flow reserve in animals (133, 134). In others only a modest correlation between flow reserve by parametric imaging and microspheres was found (135, 136). In human studies flow reserve by parametric imaging and intracoronary Doppler flow probe correlate reasonably well (137, 138). This approach has been used to assess the physiologic significance of coronary lesions (137, 139) and to examine the effect of coronary angioplasty on myocardial perfusion (140, 141).

Limitations of Radiographic Techniques

The invasive radiographic techniques have several limitations. First, most of these techniques only estimate flow reserve; absolute coronary blood flow or myocardial perfusion is not measured. Attempts to measure absolute coronary flow or perfusion are limited by many factors, including incomplete mixing of contrast with blood, inability to precisely measure vascular volume in the region of interest, the complex nonlinear relationship between contrast x-ray density and concentration, and the influence of the indicator (contrast) on flow. Second, the time constant of these techniques is slow; rapid changes in flow cannot be measured. Third, most of these techniques require the use of background subtraction, atrial pacing, and electrocardiographically triggered power injection of contrast into the coronary artery. This increases both the complexity of flow measurements and the opportunity for technical errors. Fourth, artifacts of patient motion and overlapping vessels or perfusion fields are common. Finally, most of these methods require specialized imaging and computer equipment not readily available in most catheterization laboratories. As further developments in digital imaging technology are made, these methods of measuring regional coronary blood flow and flow reserve will undoubtedly be refined. The success of the Doppler guidewire system for invasive assessment of coronary flow and flow reserve and the availability of accurate noninvasive methods of measuring regional myocardial perfusion (especially positron emission tomography) appear to have led to a decline in interest in the invasive radiographic techniques described earlier.

Noninvasive Imaging Techniques

The ability of four noninvasive imaging techniques, positron emission tomography, ultrafast computed tomography, magnetic resonance imaging (MRI), and contrast echocardiography, to quantitate regional myocardial perfusion is being actively investigated. Of these new modalities, positron emission tomography has proved most useful for perfusion imaging (142). A positron-emitting radionuclide suitable for perfusion imaging, such as rubidium-82, $[N^{13}]$ammonia, or $[O^{15}]$water, is injected intravenously and accumulates in the myocardium. As the isotope decays, the masses of a positron and an electron annihilate to form two 511-keV photons that are emitted 180° apart. These photons are detected by a circumferential array of external radiation detectors, and tomographic images are mathematically reconstructed. The resultant tomographic image represents the cross-sectional distribution of the tissue radioisotope concentration. Regional myocardial perfusion can then be quantitated by analyzing the kinetics of the tissue concentration of the isotope. By use of other positron-emitting tracers, such as $[C^{11}]$palmitate or $[F^{18}]$2-fluoro-2-deoxyglucose, regional myocardial metabolism can also be determined (143). Animal studies have confirmed the ability of positron emission tomography to measure myocardial perfusion, and human studies suggest that this technique can be clinically useful (144–148). Unfortunately, a positron emission tomography facility is tremendously expensive. An on-site cyclotron is necessary when imaging with tracers other than rubidium-82, which can be produced by an inexpensive generator. Other limitations of this technique include underestimation of high perfusion rates with some tracers, limited spatial resolution of positron cameras, and imaging motion artifacts. Ultrafast computed tomography (149, 150), MRI (151, 152), and contrast echocardiography (153–155) may also prove to be valuable methods to measure myocardial perfusion.

QUANTITATION OF VASCULAR STENOSIS

The development and widespread application of coronary angiography have revolutionized the evaluation and treatment of patients with coronary artery disease. Information regarding the extent, location, and severity of coronary atherosclerosis from angiography provides powerful information regarding prognosis and selection of appropriate therapy. However, when evaluating the physiologic significance of individual coronary stenoses, angiography has significant limitations. In routine clinical practice the physiologic significance of a stenosis is usually estimated by a visual assessment of the percent reduction in lumen diameter at the lesion site. A stenosis is considered significant if it reduces the lumen diameter by more than 50%, as this was the degree of narrowing required to restrict maximal coronary flow in experimental studies by Gould et al. (156) in the 1970s. There are major limitations to this approach. First, there is a large and well documented **intraobserver and interobserver variation** in coronary angiogram interpretation (157–159). Second, coronary atherosclerosis often produces **diffuse** as well as focal narrowing of the vessel lumen (160–162). Diffuse disease is not readily apparent on the coronary angiogram, which leads to an underestimation of the true degree of lumenal obstruction. Third, the **relationship between stenosis geometry and its effect on coronary flow is complex.** While minimum cross-sectional area is the most important determinant of the effect of a stenosis on coronary flow, lesion length, entrance angle, exit angle, and the presence of other stenoses in the vessel all contribute to energy loss across a coronary lesion (163–166). The contribution of these factors cannot be

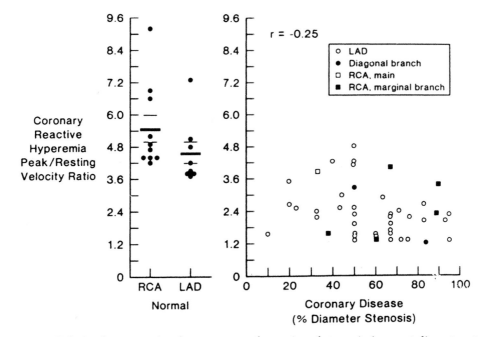

Figure 21.10. Relation between visual assessment of severity of stenosis (percent diameter stenosis) and coronary reactive hyperemia by epicardial Doppler flow probe. Values for reactive hyperemia, a measure of coronary vasodilator reserve, in angiographically normal vessels are shown in the left panel. The correlation between severity of stenosis as visually assessed and reactive hyperemia is poor. (Reprinted with permission from White CW, Wright CB, Doty DB, et al. Does visual interpretation of the coronary arteriogram predict the physiologic importance of a coronary stenosis? N Engl J Med 1984;310:819–824.)

accurately determined from visual inspection alone. Finally, abnormalities in the coronary **microvasculature** may be severe enough to cause myocardial ischemia even in the absence of angiographically apparent coronary disease (167, 168). Therefore the correlation between the severity of a stenosis as assessed by visual inspection of the coronary angiogram and its effect on coronary blood flow is poor (169) (Fig. 21.10). A more accurate assessment of the physiologic significance of a coronary stenosis can be provided by (*a*) precise measurement of stenosis geometry from quantitative analysis of the coronary angiogram and (*b*) direct determination of intracoronary flow and pressure.

Quantitative Angiography

There are two major reasons for the development of quantitative coronary angiogra-

phy. First, quantitative angiography markedly reduces the large intraobserver and interobserver variation inherent in visual coronary angiogram interpretation (170). Second, principles of fluid dynamics can more accurately predict the physiologic significance of a coronary stenosis when its geometry can be precisely defined (163, 170, 171).

Methods

The earliest form of quantitative coronary angiography involved the use of calipers to measure vessel diameter visually (172–174). By comparing the minimum diameter at the site of stenosis with the diameter of the normal-appearing adjacent vessel, percent diameter stenosis can be determined with much less variability than by visual inspection. Absolute vessel dimensions can be estimated by caliper measurement of a reference object of known diameter, such as the catheter tip. While superior to visual measurements, caliper techniques are less reproducible than computer-assisted quantitative angiographic techniques using automated edge detection (175).

The next generation of quantitative coronary angiography attempted a more complete three-dimensional reconstruction of artery lumen geometry. Brown et al. (170, 176) used a system in which optically magnified angiographic images from orthogonal views were manually traced on a digitizing tablet. After correcting for magnification and pincushion distortion, the two views were combined to construct a three-dimensional display of the vessel segment, assuming an elliptical lesion geometry. Use of hemodynamic principles and hypothetical blood flow values allowed estimates of stenosis resistance to be made. Although this approach has been validated by comparison with pressure-injected postmortem coronary arteries and was useful as a research technique, it is technically demanding and unsuitable for clinical use.

Several commercial film–based quantitative angiographic systems using computerized edge detection techniques have been developed (177–180). In addition, modern digital catheterization laboratory imaging systems routinely offer automated edge detection for measurement of vessel dimensions. Most automated edge detection methods require the operator to identify an approximate centerline or region of interest containing the opacified coronary vessel segment. The computer then analyzes pixel density along multiple scan lines perpendicular to the vessel's approximate centerline. The vessel edge is identified via a weighted first-second derivative function; the specific weighting algorithm varies from system to system. The coronary catheter image is usually used as a reference for dimensional scaling. Several automated edge detection systems have been well validated and proved to be accurate and reliable (178, 181–184). See recent reviews (180, 185, 186) for additional details.

An alternative approach to edge detection for lesion analysis is videodensitometry. According to the Beer-Lambert princi-

ple the background-subtracted attenuation profile of a coronary angiogram gives a value directly proportional to the cross-sectional area of the vessel if viewed perpendicular to its central axis. In theory application of this principle to cineangiographic images could obviate edge detection in assessing vessel dimensions. Automated videodensitometric techniques require the user to select a region of interest on a digitized cine frame. After background subtraction, density profiles are constructed along the vessel's centerline, and percent area reduction is calculated by application of the Beer-Lambert principles. Several investigators have demonstrated that careful attention to image acquisition and analysis permits the severity of stenosis to be accurately assessed (187, 188). However, the technique is technically demanding, requires meticulous angiographic procedure, and is not as useful for clinical stenosis assessment as automated edge detection in most settings (189–193).

Limitations and Clinical Utility of Quantitative Angiography

While computer-assisted quantitative angiographic methods significantly reduce the interobserver variability of vascular stenosis measurement, many technical factors can cause measurement errors (176, 180). Most modern systems rely on automated edge detection to identify the vessel borders. Overlap of the vascular segment of interest by adjacent vessels or radiopaque background structures may disrupt the automated edge detection algorithm, resulting in inaccurate identification of vessel borders. While computer-detected borders can be manually corrected, this is time-consuming and allows observer bias and variation. The accuracy of automated edge detection also depends on the concentration of contrast medium in the vessel; underfilling of the vessel because of poor catheter engagement, slow injection rate, or high coronary blood flow reduces the accuracy of border detection (194). Most automated edge detection algorithms cannot accurately find vessel borders in small coronary vessels (less than 1 mm diameter), so that the diameter of these vessels is usually overestimated (195). Other factors that can interfere with accurate vessel detection include blurring due to vessel motion, quantum mottle, beam hardening, and veiling glare.

The calibration factor required for dimensional scaling is usually derived from the angiographic catheter. Catheter borders are identified by either electronic caliper or automated edge detection, and a calibration factor (millimeters per pixel) is usually based on the catheter's outer diameter. Several investigators have shown that the x-ray intensity profile used to determine the catheter edges is influenced by catheter material and manufacturer and that the internal diameter may provide a more accurate calibration factor than the external diameter (196, 197). A more accurate calibration factor can be determined by use of a calibrated grid at approximately the same distance from the x-ray tube and image intensifier as the coronary artery segment. While pincushion distortion can also produce errors in accurate vessel sizing, the magnitude of error is small with modern x-ray equipment (198).

Measurement of **vessel cross-sectional area** requires information about the vessel's shape. When a coronary stenosis is imaged in orthogonal projections, calculation of the cross-sectional area can be based on the assumption that (*a*) the vessel is elliptical and (*b*) the location of the minimum diameter in one view matches the location of the minimum diameter in the orthogonal view (170). In practice it is often impossible to obtain true orthogonal views because of vessel overlap and foreshortening (176). In addition, the true shape of the vessel lumen at the site of a stenosis is often complex, with marked irregularity and eccentricity, so that even the use of true orthogonal views fails to eliminate significant errors (199). While some investigators have found a good correlation between measurements from orthogonal views and those from the single worst view (i.e., the view in which the lesion is most severe) (200), others have noted considerable variation in these measurements, especially after angioplasty (201).

In addition to the technical factors affecting the accuracy of quantitative angiography in assessing stenosis geometry, there are additional sources of error when quantitative coronary angiography is used to determine the functional significance of a coronary stenosis. In patients with limited coronary disease and no ventricular hypertrophy or prior infarction, there is a reasonably good correlation between severity of stenosis assessed by quantitative angiography and coronary flow reserve (202–204). In 50 patients with limited coronary disease, normal left ventricular function, and no left ventricular hypertrophy or prior myocardial infarction, Wilson et al. (203) found that lesions with a cross-sectional area larger than 2.5 mm^2 uniformly had a normal coronary flow reserve. However, 31 of 41 (76%) lesions with cross-sectional area less than 2.5 mm^2 had diminished flow reserve. Likewise, flow reserve was normal for all lesions with an area stenosis less than 70% and abnormal in the majority of those with more than 70% area stenosis. Uren et al. (202) examined the relationship between stenosis severity and myocardial blood flow by positron emission tomography in 35 patients with single-vessel disease and normal left ventricular function. Regional flow reserve was normal in patients with a diameter stenosis less than 40% and fell progressively as the severity of stenosis increased above 40%. Even in this select group of patients with limited coronary disease there was considerable variation in regional flow reserve in patients with angiographically intermediate stenoses (40 to 75% diameter narrowing); flow reserve was consistently abnormal only when the percent diameter stenosis was reduced by more than approximately 75% (Fig. 21.11). In patients with multivessel disease there is much greater variation in the relationship between stenosis dimensions and functional significance (163). This is due in part to angiographically inapparent diffuse atherosclerosis in the reference segment and the complex relationship between stenosis geometry and energy loss. Nevertheless, measurement of minimum stenosis dimension via quantitative angiography is superior to visual inspection in assessing functional significance of a lesion.

Quantitative coronary angiography has proved useful in studying (*a*) the effects of pharmacologic agents and neurohumoral

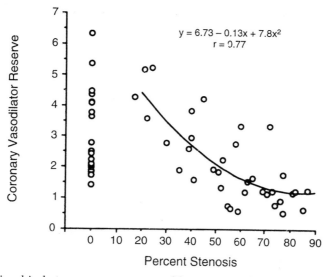

Figure 21.11. Relationship between coronary vasodilator reserve by positron emission tomography and percent diameter stenosis by quantitative angiography in patients with single-vessel coronary disease. There is a progressive decline in coronary reserve with increasing stenosis. While the relation between flow reserve and angiographic stenosis severity is better than that shown in Figure 21.10, there is considerable variation in flow reserve for stenoses of intermediate severity. (Reprinted with permission from Uren NG, Melin JA, De Bruyne B, et al. Relation between myocardial blood flow and the severity of coronary-artery stenosis. N Engl J Med 1994;330:1782–1788.)

factors on the coronary vasculature, (*b*) progression or regression of coronary atherosclerosis, and (*c*) geometric changes after coronary interventions. Quantitative angiography is routinely used to guide selection of appropriately sized interventional devices in many clinical laboratories. Despite improvements in the speed and accuracy of automated edge detection available on most modern digital imaging systems, quantitative angiography is still not being routinely used clinically in most laboratories to assess the functional significance of intermediate coronary lesions. This is likely due to both a recognition of the limitations described earlier and the availability of alternative methods of assessing stenosis significance, such as Doppler coronary flow reserve and translesional pressure gradient.

Coronary Flow and Pressure Techniques

Doppler Flow Velocity

The development of the **Doppler guidewire** (described earlier in this chapter) has greatly facilitated the clinical use of Doppler flow velocity indices of stenosis severity. With this device precise coronary flow velocity data can be measured in the distal or poststenotic region of a vessel, where coronary blood flow is most affected by a stenosis (205, 206). With the bulkier Doppler catheters flow could be measured only proximal to a stenosis, and it was difficult to acquire data during interventions. Since flow velocity measures of severity of stenosis can be affected by flow through unobstructed prelesional side branches, proximally measured coronary flow reserve may be nearly normal despite a severe stenosis or total occlusion of the distal vessel (207). Directly measured poststenotic coronary blood flow velocity has been used as an alternative to out-of-laboratory ischemic stress testing in some laboratories (204, 208–210), an approach with important clinical and economic implications for patients undergoing evaluation of coronary artery disease.

The use of flow velocity to assess hemodynamics of a coronary stenosis is based on the concept that the coronary circulation comprises two major components, a conduit (epicardial arteries) and a microcirculation (capillary and myocardial vascular bed). If poststenotic vasodilatory flow reserve is normal, both components can be assumed to be normal. If coronary vasodilatory reserve is abnormal, examination of lesion-specific indices separates conduit obstruction, which can be treated mechanically with angioplasty, from microcirculatory disturbances, which are treated medically. Lesion-specific indices of severity of stenosis include ratios of translesional coronary flow velocity and of diastolic-to-systolic velocity, translesional pressure gradient, and fractional flow reserve.

Coronary Flow Velocity Reserve

Coronary flow velocity reserve is computed as the quotient of hyperemic and basal mean flow velocity (Fig. 21.12). Coronary hyperemia is induced by intracoronary adenosine (6 to 8 μg in the right coronary artery and 12 to 18 μg in the left coronary artery) (211). There is no absolute contraindication to the use of intracoronary adenosine in the appropriate dosages for coronary vasodilatory reserve measurements. Some cardiac transplant patients are sensitive to standard doses of adenosine, which may cause heart block lasting 2 to 3 seconds. Unlike papaverine (212), intracoronary adenosine given for vasodilatory reserve measurements has not been reported to have any serious complications.

Although earlier studies report a coronary vasodilatory reserve ratio of 3.5 to 5 in normal patients (169, 213), lower values are more commonly observed in patients with chest pain and angiographically normal arteries (mean coronary vasodilatory reserve ratio, 2.7 plus or minus 0.6) (214). In transplanted hearts with angiographic normal arteries, coronary vasodilatory reserve ratios are usually higher (3.1 plus or minus 0.6).

Donohue et al. (205) measured coronary vasodilatory reserve with the Doppler guidewire in 17 normal patients and 29 patients with stenoses ranging from 50 to 85%

N.L., CFX

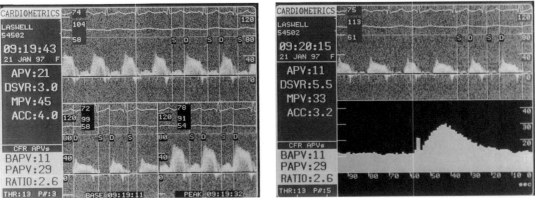

Figure 21.12. Left. Coronary flow velocity at baseline and peak hyperemia obtained from the Doppler velocimeter of the FloMap system. **Top left panel.** Continuous flow recording demonstrating electrocardiogram, aortic pressure, and spectral flow velocity signal. *S* and *D* identify the systolic and diastolic periods, respectively. The left side of the two lower panels is the basal flow velocity (*base*) and the right side is the peak hyperemic velocity. The time code indicates that peak hyperemic velocity was achieved 21 seconds after basal flow was recorded. *APV*, average peak velocity; *DSVR*, diastolic–systolic velocity ratio; *MPV*, maximal peak velocity; *BAPV*, basal average peak velocity; *PAPV*, peak average peak velocity (after adenosine administration); *ratio*, coronary flow reserve ratio of 2.6, normal in this case. **Right lower panel.** Trend plot of average peak velocity (*APV*) over 90 seconds showing the hyperemic response to intracoronary adenosine.

on angiography and translesional gradients from 0 to 85 mm Hg. In normal vessels coronary vasodilatory reserve was 2.5 plus or minus 0.7 proximally and 2.6 plus or minus 0.6 in the distal portion of the artery. In the diseased vessels the proximally measured coronary flow reserve was not significantly different for any translesional gradient and could not differentiate stenoses with gradients less than 20 mm Hg (2.1 plus or minus 0.7) from those above 20 mm Hg (1.7 plus or minus 0.6). The coronary flow reserve measured distal to the area of stenosis did differentiate between these two groups. Those with a gradient above 20 mm Hg had a distal flow reserve of 2.1 plus or minus 0.7, and those with a gradient below 20 mm Hg had a flow reserve of 1.4 plus or minus 0.6 (p < .01).

Strong correlations with myocardial perfusion imaging and poststenotic coronary flow reserve have been reported (204, 209, 215, 216). Miller et al. (204) correlated pharmacologic stress technetium-99m sestamibi tomographic myocardial perfusion imaging with poststenotic coronary flow reserve in 33 patients with angiographically intermediate (56 plus or minus 14%; range 20 to 84% diameter stenosis) coronary stenoses. Quantitative coronary stenosis of more than 50% diameter on angiography and poststenotic coronary flow velocity reserve of less than 2 were correlated in 20 of 27 patients (74%). The strongest correlation was noted between poststenotic flow velocity reserve and sestamibi perfusion imaging in 24 of 27 patients (89%). A similar correspondence between poststenotic coronary flow reserve and myocardial perfusion imaging has been described by Joye et al. (209).

Ratio of Proximal to Distal Translesional Coronary Flow Velocity

In a branching arterial system significant epicardial lesions increase resistance to blood flow, divert flow to side branches, and reduce flow velocity in the poststenotic region, with a resultant increase in the ratio of proximal to distal flow velocity (217). In 88 patients Donohue et al. (205) demonstrated a strong correlation between translesional pressure gradient and the ratio of the proximal to distal total flow velocity integrals. An integral ratio of more than 1.7 in the proximal to distal flow velocity was nearly always associated with a translesional pressure gradient of more than 30 mm Hg, and a ratio of less than 1.7 was associated with a gradient more than 30 mm Hg in 85% of patients. In angiographically intermediate stenoses (range 50 to 70%), angiography was a poor predictor of translesional gradient, but the flow velocity ratio continued to have a strong correlation. A subsequent study by these investigators found a poor correlation between the ratio of proximal to distal flow velocity and stress myocardial perfusion imaging (204), casting doubt on the reliability of this lesion-specific index of stenosis severity. In addition, this index cannot be used in nonbranching vascular segments, such as saphenous vein and internal mammary grafts, and in the right coronary artery, where there is no relationship between the proximal and distal flow velocity ratio and severity of stenosis. Given these limitations, this ratio has limited clinical utility as a measure of severity of stenosis.

Ratio of Phasic (Diastolic to Systolic) Velocity

For the unobstructed left anterior descending or circumflex, posterior descending, and proximal right coronary arteries, the expected ratios of phasic diastolic-to-systolic velocity are less than 1.8, 1.5, and 1.2, respectively (205, 206, 218, 219). A coronary stenosis reduces the normal diastolic predominance of the phasic pattern, and the ratio of diastolic to systolic velocity falls. This relationship requires a normally contracting myocardium in the region of the target stenosis. In patients with a significant coronary stenosis an abnormally low diastolic-to-systolic velocity ratio in the distal left anterior descending artery before angioplasty increased to the normal range after a successful procedure (218). A case example of the effect of a severe stenosis on coronary flow velocity is shown in Figure 21.13.

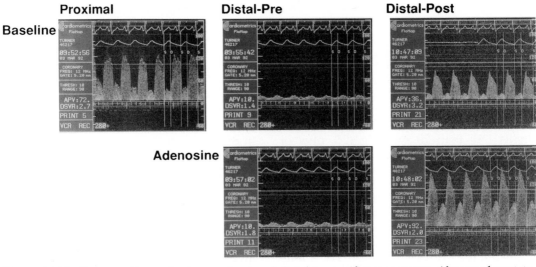

Figure 21.13. Coronary flow velocity proximal and distal to significant stenoses. Abnormal poststenotic flow (distal-preangioplasty, **middle panels**) is characterized by decreased phasic pattern, decreased absolute velocity, and inability to achieve hyperemia during adenosine infusion. After angioplasty (distal-postangioplasty, **right panels**), there is restoration of the phasic flow velocity pattern, increase in mean velocity, and return of coronary hyperemia with adenosine. Format as on Figure 21.12.

Continuity Equation for Stenosis Severity

The continuity equation can be used to define the luminal geometry of an angiographically indeterminate stenosis (118). The continuity equation is based on the conservation of mass, wherein the volume of flow proximal to a stenosis must equal the volume of flow within the stenosis. Since the volume of flow is equal to the product of cross-sectional area and velocity, the continuity equation can be written thus:

$$V_{prox} \times A_{prox} = V_{sten} \times A_{sten} \qquad (8)$$

where V_{prox} and A_{prox} = flow velocity and cross-sectional area proximal to the stenosis and V_{sten} and A_{sten} = flow velocity and area at the site of minimum lumenal narrowing. Solving Equation 8 for percent area stenosis yields this:

$$\text{Percent area stenosis} \qquad (9)$$
$$= (1 - V_{prox}/V_{sten}) \times 100$$

When high-quality Doppler flow velocity measurements can be obtained both proximal to and within a coronary stenosis, there is a good correlation between Doppler-derived and angiographic percent area stenoses (118, 220). However, in practical terms the use of the continuity equation requires no interference from side branch flow or turbulence in the poststenotic region, and precise determination of the high-velocity stenosis jet can be difficult or unobtainable in some cases (221).

Translesional Pressure Gradient and Fractional Flow Reserve

Coronary lesion resistance is best measured by use of both transstenotic pressure and flow, as demonstrated by Gould et al. (156). In some patients whose flow velocity measurements are indeterminate or unobtainable, a translesional pressure gradient measured during maximal hyperemia may help eliminate ambiguity. From guidewire pressure measurements during hyperemia, a new concept for the determination of coronary blood flow, the myocardial fractional flow reserve (FFR_{myo}), has emerged (222).

The FFR$_{myo}$, the ratio of maximal hyperemic flow in the stenotic artery to the theoretic maximal hyperemic flow in the same artery without a stenosis, is a specific index to describe the influence of the coronary stenosis on maximal perfusion of the subtended myocardium.

Theory and Methods

The transstenotic pressure gradient is highly dependent on transstenotic flow (167, 223). Under normal circumstances coronary flow varies over a wide range to meet changes in myocardial O$_2$ demand. Neither resting absolute coronary flow nor transstenotic pressure gradient can be related to stenosis severity unless the resistance is known or at least constant. During maximal pharmacologic vasodilation myocardial resistance is minimal and presumably constant. Flow traversing the stenosis under these circumstances theoretically represents maximal achievable flow and maximal achievable pressure gradient.

The concept of fractional flow reserve was developed from the relation between pressure gradient and myocardial blood flow during maximal arteriolar vasodilation (222). Fractional flow reserve is the maximal blood flow to the myocardium in the presence of a stenosis divided by the maximal flow that could be achieved if there were no obstruction. FFR$_{myo}$ can be calculated by this:

$$FFR_{myo} = (P_d - P_v)/(P_a - P_v) \qquad (10)$$

where P$_d$ = mean distal coronary (transstenotic) pressure, P$_v$ = mean central venous pressure, and P$_a$ = mean arterial pressure. P$_d$, P$_v$, and P$_a$ are all measured during maximal vasodilation, usually by intravenous or intracoronary adenosine. Since P$_v$ is usually much lower than P$_a$ or P$_d$, FFR$_{myo}$ can be estimated by the ratio of mean distal coronary pressure to mean arterial pressure:

$$FFR_{myo} = P_d/P_a \qquad (11)$$

In the absence of stenosis there is little difference between aortic and distal coronary

pressure, so that the "normal" value for FFR$_{myo}$ is 1. See Pijls et al. (222) for a detailed derivation of Equation 9.

Assessment of fractional flow reserve requires accurate measurement of pressure distal to the coronary stenosis. In the past transstenotic pressure was measured through angioplasty-sized catheters. Since the smallest available catheter is relatively large compared with the stenosed lumen, an unpredictable overestimation of the true pressure gradient occurs (224). To circumvent this, several pressure monitoring guidewires have recently been developed and validated. Commercially available only in Europe, the Pressure Guide (Radi Medical Systems, Uppsala, Sweden) is a 0.014-inch relatively stiff guidewire with a fiberoptic capability to detect changes in reflected light from a mirror source deformed by pressure changes (225). The high-fidelity signal produces phasic pressure waveforms equivalent to those of larger high-fidelity catheters. Another device, the Premo Wire (Schneider Corporation, Bulag, Switzerland), is a fluid-filled 0.014-inch diameter angioplasty guidewire (226). This wire has the same overall characteristics as a conventional angioplasty guidewire and can be connected to any pressure transducer, but it produces a damped phasic pressure because of its small inner lumen. The accuracy of the mean pressure signals recorded through fluid-filled guidewires has been validated (227). In contrast to pressure measurements through angioplasty balloon catheters, the Radi and fluid-filled pressure guidewires produce useful pressure signals without the artifact of a catheter shaft or balloon material in the artery lumen.

The guiding catheter is used to measure proximal coronary artery pressure, and the pressure wire measures artery pressure beyond the target lesion. After the pressure wire is positioned distal to the stenosis, the aortic and distal coronary pressures are simultaneously recorded at baseline and during hyperemia. The pressure sensor is then pulled back proximal to the stenosis. Any small difference between the aortic pressure and that measured proximal to the lesion is called the intrinsic gradient of the system and is subtracted from the transstenotic pressure gradient.

To determine threshold values of FFR_{myo} and ischemic exercise responses, De Bruyne et al. (228) studied 60 patients with an isolated epicardial coronary stenosis, normal left ventricular function, and no left ventricular hypertrophy. Anti-ischemic medications were withheld before a maximal exercise electrocardiogram was performed within 6 hours of cardiac catheterization. At catheterization baseline and hyperemic translesional pressure measurements were obtained with a pressure guidewire system. Both FFR_{myo} and hyperemic translesional pressure gradient correlated well with the magnitude of ST depression during exercise. No patient with a FFR_{myo} value above 0.72 showed an abnormal exercise electrocardiogram. Use of FFR_{myo} as an index of severity of stenosis has been well validated (227, 229, 230). Normal values (above 0.75) can reliably discriminate among stenoses responsible for a positive exercise stress test with excellent specificity and sensitivity and high diagnostic accuracy (227, 229).

Limitations

The Radi pressure guidewire and Tracker catheter produce excellent phasic signals. The Premo Wire (fluid-filled pressure monitoring guidewire) produces damped pressure tracings because of its small inner lumen. However, all three systems reliably reflect mean pressures. The evaluation of pressure gradients is useful only if a reliable pressure tracing can be obtained. The pressure gradient may be unreliable in vessels that are small (less than 2.5 mm diameter) or measured beyond acute artery bends or multiple lesions in a vessel. An artifactual pressure drop because of obstruction of the tip of the pressure catheter is unlikely when the catheter is aligned in a normal and relatively straight segment of a coronary artery. In contrast to angioplasty catheters, the pressure measurements made with guidewires and Tracker catheters are not generally affected by tortuosity of a proximal artery segment.

Utility of Doppler Flow and Pressure Measurements

The major clinical applications for coronary Doppler flow and pressure gradient measurements include assessment of the angiographically intermediate lesion (205, 206, 208), monitoring flow after angioplasty (231), and physiologic end point determination after balloon angioplasty.

Assessment of the "Intermediate Stenosis"

In the approximately 1 million coronary angiograms performed in the United States each year, an intermediate stenosis (40 to 70% diameter narrowing) may be encountered in nearly 50% of patients. Of these patients only 50% are estimated to have stress testing prior to an intervention (232). Doppler flow or pressure gradient measurements obtained at the time of diagnostic angiography, employing the criteria of lesion significance described earlier, can help identify important lesions and may save cost, hospital days, and catheterization laboratory resources.

Deferring angioplasty in clinically stable patients with "intermediate" (e.g., from 40 to 70% diameter reduction) lesions and normal translesional hemodynamics is safe and has an excellent clinical outcome (208). A prospective study determined the feasibility, safety, and outcome of deferring angioplasty according to normal translesional pressure and flow velocity data in 88 patients with 100 lesions (26 single vessel, 74 multivessel coronary artery stenoses) scheduled for angioplasty (208).

The percent lumen area reduction, percent diameter stenosis, and obstruction diameter in the deferred group were 77 plus or minus 8%, 54 plus or minus 7%, and 1.32 plus or minus 0.33 mm, respectively. Translesional pressure gradients were lower for the deferred group than for a reference angioplasty group (10 plus or minus 9 mm Hg versus 46 plus or minus 22 mm Hg; p < .01). Proximal-to-distal velocity ratios were similar for the normal and deferred groups and significantly lower than for the angioplasty group (1.1 plus or minus 0.35 normal, 1.3 plus or minus 0.55 deferred, and 2.3 plus or minus 1.2 angioplasty group). No patient had a complication related to translesional pressure or flow velocity measurements.

Clinical 6-month follow-up data for 84 of 88 patients were available. In the deferred group rehospitalization for either noncardiac or anginalike symptoms occurred in 18 patients, 12 of whom had cardiac events. No patient had a myocardial infarction. Also, 1 patient died of complications of angioplasty of a nontarget artery, and 1 with multivessel coronary artery disease and decreased left ventricular function died suddenly of ventricular fibrillation 12 months after lesion assessment. Some 7 patients had repeat coronary angiography without apparent change in the target lesion, and 10 patients required either coronary artery bypass grafting (n = 6) or coronary angioplasty (n = 4); only 6 involved revascularization of target arteries. Finally, 4 patients had new lesions not present at the initial evaluation. An example of the use of Doppler flow measurements to assess an intermediate coronary stenosis is shown in Figure 21.14.

This study demonstrated that in stable patients with angiographically intermediate lesions, translesional hemodynamic data can be acquired safely and can identify patients in whom angioplasty can be safely deferred. By visual angiographic and clinical criteria, a majority of these lesions would likely have been treated at the initial catheterization, many without any physiologic assessment of lesion significance, such as ischemic stress testing. While this approach may assist in selecting hemodynamically significant lesions in the routine practice of multivessel or multilesion angioplasty, further trials are needed to determine whether this reduces cost and improves outcome.

Use During Angioplasty and Stent Placement

One of the advantages of the Doppler flow wire is that it can be used as an angioplasty guidewire, enabling measurement of distal flow velocity continuously during the procedure. During coronary balloon occlusion flow velocity rapidly approaches zero. If persistent antegrade flow occurs, the balloon is undersized or there is collateral input distal to the balloon but proximal to the wire tip (233). If flow velocity initially falls to zero, then becomes visible below the baseline (negative), retrograde collateral flow is identified and can be quantitated. Retrograde collateral flow velocity during occlusion, which occurs in 10 to 15% of patients, may be a useful indicator of the patient's tolerance for prolonged balloon occlusions (234). After angioplasty a satisfactory result is demonstrated by normalization of coronary vasodilatory reserve, increase in the distal average flow, and return of diastolic predominant phasic flow velocity (206, 218) (Fig. 21.13).

Secondary lesions in multivessel coronary artery disease can be addressed at the time of angioplasty of the culprit vessel by means of flow velocity lesion assessment as described for the intermediate lesion. This approach has the potential to save the costs of additional hospital days, stress testing, angioplasty equipment, and complications.

Monitoring postprocedural coronary flow velocity for variations due to progressive dissection, thrombus, or vasospasm is easily performed with the mean velocity trend plot. Changes in the flow velocity trend often precede angiographic signs of vessel occlusion (235). Monitoring coronary flow can also reduce total radiographic contrast volume in assessing the stability of a borderline angioplasty result and can identify unstable flow associated with potential vessel closure.

To identify the predictive value of coronary flow velocity measurements after coronary angioplasty, the European multicenter prospective study DEBATE (Doppler Endpoint Balloon Angioplasty Trial Europe) examined the relation of immediate postangioplasty coronary vasodilatory reserve to early and late clinical events and angiographic restenosis (236). Preliminary data for 224 patients 6 months after single-vessel angioplasty indicated that 169 patients were free of ischemic events and 35 had either typical chest pain or a positive electrocardiographic exercise test. There was no dif-

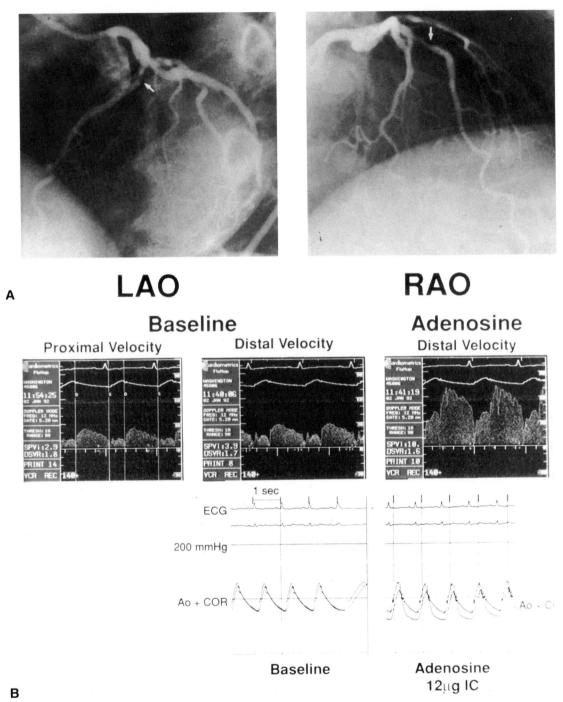

A

LAO   **RAO**

Baseline

Proximal Velocity   Distal Velocity   Adenosine
                                          Distal Velocity

B

Figure 21.14. A. Angiographic views of eccentric lesion in the left anterior descending coronary artery in a 59-year-old man with atypical chest pain. The lesion is severe (more than 70%) in the left anterior oblique (*LAO*) view. **B.** Flow velocity (**top panels**) and translesional gradients (**lower panels**) at rest and during maximal hyperemia with intracoronary (*IC*) adenosine (12μg). Proximal and distal flow velocity are nearly identical, with a ratio of 1.05. The rest gradient is zero. With adenosine distal flow increases 2.5 times baseline and the hyperemic gradient is 10 mm Hg. A thallium scintigraphic exercise study showed a minimal apical defect, and no angioplasty was performed. The patient's symptoms

ference in the angiographic minimal lumen diameter between the group with ischemic events and the asymptomatic patients. However, the poststenotic coronary vasodilatory reserve (2.73 plus or minus 0.93 versus 2.22 plus or minus 0.64; p < .05) and the diastolic-to-systolic velocity ratio in the left anterior descending (2.77 plus or minus 1.57 versus 2.14 plus or minus 0.69; p < .05) were higher in the asymptomatic than in the ischemic event patients. Because of overlap of values in the two groups, neither flow reserve nor diastolic-to-systolic velocity ratio alone could reliably predict outcome. However, in the 44 patients with both a postprocedural coronary flow reserve above 2.5 and a quantitative angiographic diameter stenosis below 35%, the rate of repeat angioplasty at 6 months was only 16%, a value similar to that found in stent trials. Additional prospective trials will determine whether physiologically guided decisions can improve the clinical outcome of coronary angioplasty.

Coronary flow velocity data were examined in 15 patients undergoing elective angioplasty followed by stent placement (237). Serial measurements of coronary flow velocity reserve and intravascular ultrasound imaging were obtained after balloon angioplasty and again after stent placement. The stenosis decreased from 71% plus or minus 10% of diameter to 37% plus or minus 11% after angioplasty and to 7% plus or minus 12% after stent placement. Coronary vasodilatory reserve increased from 1.3 plus or minus 0.6 to 1.6 plus or minus 0.6 after angioplasty and to 2.3 plus or minus 0.5 after stent placement, a value similar to that in a normal adjacent reference vessel. Intravascular ultrasound vessel cross-sectional area was significantly larger after stenting (4.5 mm^2 after angioplasty versus 7.6 mm^2 after stent; p < .01). A case example is shown in

Figure 21.15. The greater increase in coronary vasodilator reserve after stenting than after angioplasty suggests that a major mechanism of persistently impaired coronary vasodilatory reserve after balloon angioplasty is suboptimal lumen expansion that may not be identified by angiography. These preliminary data support a physiologically guided intervention to facilitate achieving an optimal lumen, which may lead to improved angioplasty results, as noted in the DEBATE study (236).

SUMMARY

Measurements of blood flow are an essential part of diagnostic cardiac catheterization. Cardiac output, or systemic blood flow, is one of the single most useful flow measurements. With attention to detail cardiac output can be accurately measured during cardiac catheterization of the great majority of patients. Advances in radiographic and Doppler technology, especially the development of the Doppler guidewire system, have greatly improved the feasibility of regional blood flow measurements in the coronary circulation for both research and clinical purposes. Despite well-described limitations, visual inspection of the coronary angiogram remains the most widely used method of assessing the functional significance of coronary vascular stenoses. Doppler flow and translesional pressure gradient measurements can improve the accuracy of this assessment and may also improve the results of coronary interventions, but additional clinical trials are needed to determine whether the routine use of these methods will reduce the cost and improve the quality of care.

Figure 21.14 *(continued)* abated spontaneously, and he was well at 8-month follow-up. *Ao,* aortic; *COR,* distal coronary artery pressure (mm Hg); *ECG,* electrocardiogram. (Reprinted with permission from Donohue TJ, Kern MJ, Aguirre FV, et al. Assessing the hemodynamic significance of coronary artery stenoses: analysis of translesional pressure–flow velocity relations in patients. J Am Coll Cardiol 1993;22:449–458.)

44 yr old Man

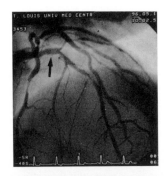

Proximal LAD, CFR=2.6

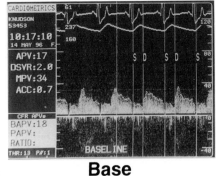

A **Base** **Adenosine**

Mid LAD

83% QCA

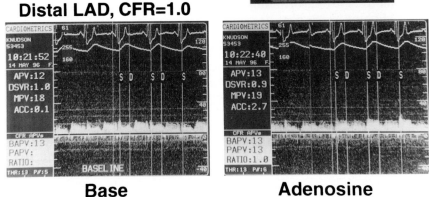

Distal LAD, CFR=1.0

B **Base** **Adenosine**

Figure 21.15. A. Angiogram and coronary flow velocity data before and after angioplasty and again after stent placement. Coronary flow reserve proximal to a severe left anterior descending stenosis is 2.6, indicating that flow through side branches can result in a normal flow reserve in the proximal vessel despite a critical stenosis further downstream in the vessel. **B.** Poststenotic flow velocity in the left anterior descending artery. Baseline average peak flow velocity is 13 cm/second and there is no increase after adenosine, so that flow reserve is 1.0 with no increase after adenosine in basal average peak velocity of 13 cm/second. Note the impaired phasic flow pattern.

432

Mid LAD
Post-PTCA
3.5 mm Balloon
28% QCA DS

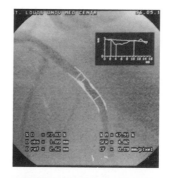

Distal LAD, CFR=2.0

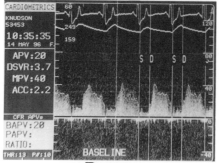

C   **Base**   **Adenosine**

Mid LAD
Post-Stent
3.5 P-S
0% QCA DS

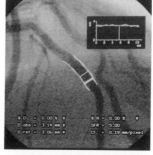

Distal LAD, CFR=2.7

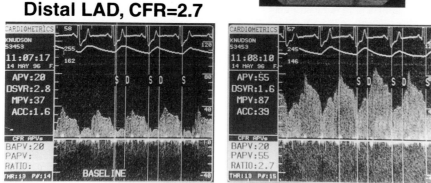

D   **Base**   **Adenosine**

Figure 21.15. *(continued)* **C.** After coronary angioplasty there is a residual 28% diameter stenosis and increase in coronary flow reserve to 2. **D.** After stent placement there is no residual stenosis, and coronary flow reserve has increased markedly to 2.7. There is also restoration of the normal phasic configuration of the distal flow velocity pattern. *APV,* average peak velocity; *DSVR,* diastolic–systolic velocity ratio; *MPV,* maximal peak velocity; *BAPV,* basal average peak velocity; *PAPV,* peak average peak velocity (after adenosine administration); *ratio,* coronary flow reserve ratio of 2.6, normal in this case.

Acknowledgment

We thank Dr. Richard G. Bach for his expert assistance with preparation of the sections describing the use of Doppler flow velocity measurements.

References

1. Kendrick AH, West J, Papouchado M, Rozkovec A. Direct Fick cardiac output: are assumed values of oxygen consumption acceptable? Eur Heart J 1988;9:337–342.
2. Dale J, Jespersen L. Determination of cardiac output with a modified Fick method using estimated instead of measured oxygen consumption. Scand J Clin Lab Invest 1987;47:759–763.
3. Dehmer GJ, Firth BG, Hillis LD. Oxygen consumption in adult patients during cardiac catheterization. Clin Cardiol 1982;5:436–440.
4. LaFarge CG, Miettinen OS. The estimation of oxygen consumption. Cardiovasc Res 1970;4:23–30.
5. Crocker RH, Ockene IS, Alpert JS, et al. Determinants of total body oxygen consumption in adults undergoing cardiac catheterization. Cathet Cardiovasc Diagn 1982;8:363–372.
6. Bergstra A, van Dijk RB, Hillege HL, et al. Assumed oxygen consumption based on calculation from dye dilution cardiac output: an improved formula. Eur Heart J 1995;16:698–703.
7. Janicki JS, Shroff SG, Weber KT. Instrumentation for monitoring respiratory gas exchange. In: Weber KT, Janicki JS, eds. Cardiopulmonary exercise testing: physiologic principles and clinical applications. Philadelphia: WB Saunders, 1986: 113–125.
8. Webb P, Troutman SJ Jr. An instrument for continuous measurement of oxygen consumption. J Appl Physiol 1970;28:867–871.
9. Grossman W. Blood flow measurement: the cardiac output. In: Grossman W, Baim DS, eds. Cardiac catheterization, angiography and intervention. 4th ed. Philadelphia: Lea & Febiger, 1991: 105–122.
10. Lange RA, Dehmer GJ, Wells PJ, et al. Limitations of the metabolic rate meter for measuring oxygen consumption and cardiac output. Am J Cardiol 1989;64:783–786.
11. Wessel HU, Stout RL, Bastanier CK, Paul MH. Breath-by-breath variation of FRC: effect on VO2 and VCO2 measured at the mouth. J Appl Physiol 1979;46:1122–1126.
12. Mook GA, Buursma A, Gerding A, et al. Spectrophotometric determination of oxygen saturation of blood independent of the presence of indocyanine green. Cardiovasc Res 1979;13:233–237.
13. Wood EH, Bowers D, Shephard JT, Fox IJ. O_2 content of mixed venous blood in man during various phases of the respiratory and cardiac cycles in relation to possible errors in measurement of cardiac output by conventional application of the Fick method. J Appl Physiol 1955;7:621–628.
14. Selzer A, Sudrann RB. Reliability of the determination of cardiac output in man by means of the Fick principle. Circ Res 1958;6:485–490.
15. Kubo SH, Burchenal JE, Cody RJ. Comparison of direct Fick and thermodilution cardiac output techniques at high flow rates. Am J Cardiol 1987; 59:384–386.
16. Fagard R, Conway J. Measurement of cardiac output: Fick principle using catheterization. Eur Heart J 1990;11(Suppl 1):1–5.
17. Zierler KL, Nichols RJ, Traber DL. Theoretical basis of indicator dilution methods for measuring flow and volume. Circ Res 1962;10:393–407.
18. Benya R, Quintana J, Brundage B. Adverse reactions to indocyanine green: a case report and a review of the literature. Cathet Cardiovasc Diagn 1989;17:231–233.
19. van den Berg E, Pacifico A, Lange RA, et al. Measurement of cardiac output without right heart catheterization: reliability, advantages, and limitations of a left-sided indicator dilution technique. Cathet Cardiovasc Diagn 1986;12:205–208.
20. Shepherd RL, Higgs LM, Glancy DL. Comparison of left ventricular and pulmonary arterial injection sites in determination of cardiac output by indicator dilution technique. Chest 1972;62: 175–178.
21. Kinsman JM, Moore JW, Hamilton WF. Studies on the circulation: 1. Injection method: physical and mathematical considerations. Am J Physiol 1929;89:322–330.
22. Guyton AC, Jones CE, Coleman TG. Indicator-dilution methods for determining cardiac output. In: Circulatory physiology: cardiac output and its regulation. 2nd ed. Philadelphia: WB Saunders, 1973:40–80.
23. Morkrid L, Lund Johansen P. Comparison of analog and numerical computation of cardiac output from dye dilution curves. Acta Med Scand Suppl 1977;603:15–21.
24. Leighton RF, Czekajewski J. Use of a new cardiac output computer for human hemodynamic studies. J Appl Physiol 1971;30:914–916.
25. Vollm KR, Rolett EL. Calibration of dye-dilution curves by a dynamic method. J Appl Physiol 1969; 26:147–150.
26. Shinebourne E, Fleming J, Hamer J. Calibration of indicator dilution curves in man by the dynamic method. Br Heart J 1967;29:920–925.
27. Sullivan FJ, Mroz EA, Miller RE. Electronic calibration for indocyanine dye-dilution curves. Am Heart J 1973;85:506–510.
28. Glassman E, Blesser W, Mitzner W. Correction of distortion in dye dilution curves due to sampling systems. Cardiovasc Res 1969;3:92–99.
29. Reddy PS, Curtiss EI, Bell B, et al. Determinants of variation between Fick and indicator dilution estimates of cardiac output during diagnostic catheterization. Fick vs. dye cardiac outputs. J Lab Clin Med 1976;87:568–576.
30. Nanas JN, Anastasiou Nana MI, Sutton RB, et al. Comparison of Fick and dye cardiac outputs during rest and exercise in 1,022 patients. Can J Cardiol 1986;2:195–199.

31. Hillis LD, Firth BG, Winniford MD. Analysis of factors affecting the variability of Fick versus indicator dilution measurements of cardiac output. Am J Cardiol 1985;56:764–768.

32. Hillis LD, Firth BG, Winniford MD. Comparison of thermodilution and indocyanine green dye in low cardiac output or left-sided regurgitation. Am J Cardiol 1986;57:1201–1202.

33. Branthwaite MA, Bradley RD. Measurement of cardiac output by thermal dilution in man. J Appl Physiol 1968;24:434–438.

34. Weisel RD, Berger RL, Hechtman HB. Current concepts measurement of cardiac output by thermodilution. N Engl J Med 1975;292:682–684.

35. Mackenzie JD, Haites NE, Rawles JM. Method of assessing the reproducibility of blood flow measurement: factors influencing the performance of thermodilution cardiac output computers. Br Heart J 1986;55:14–24.

36. Rubini A, Del Monte D, Catena V, et al. Cardiac output measurement by the thermodilution method: an in vitro test of accuracy of three commercial automatic cardiac output computers. Intensive Care Med 1995;21:154–158.

37. Meisner H, Glanert S, Steckmeier B, et al. Indicator loss during injection in the thermodilution system. Res Exp Med 1973;159:183–196.

38. Wong M, Skulsky A, Moon E. Loss of indicator in the thermodilution technique. Cathet Cardiovasc Diagn 1978;4:103–109.

39. Kadota LT. Reproducibility of thermodilution cardiac output measurements. Heart Lung 1986; 15:618–622.

40. Cross JA, Vargo RL. Cardiac output: iced versus room temperature solution. Dimens Crit Care Nurs 1988;7:146–149.

41. Elkayam U, Berkley R, Azen S, et al. Cardiac output by thermodilution technique: effect of injectate's volume and temperature on accuracy and reproducibility in the critically Ill patient. Chest 1983;84:418–422.

42. Shellock FG, Riedinger MS. Reproducibility and accuracy of using room-temperature vs. ice-temperature injectate for thermodilution cardiac output determination. Heart Lung 1983;12:175–176.

43. Lyons K, Dalbow M. Room temperature injectate and iced injectate for cardiac output: a comparative study. Crit Care Nurs 1986;6:48–50.

44. Bourdillon PD, Fineberg N. Comparison of iced and room temperature injectate for thermodilution cardiac output. Cathet Cardiovasc Diagn 1989;17:116–120.

45. Nelson LD, Houtchens BA. Automatic versus manual injections for thermodilution cardiac output determinations. Crit Care Med 1982;10: 190–192.

46. Wessel HU, James GW, Paul MH. Effects of respiration and circulation on central blood temperature of the dog. Am J Physiol 1966;211:1403–1412.

47. Afonso S, Rowe GG, Castillo CA, Crumpton CW. Intravascular and intracardiac blood temperatures in man. J Appl Physiol 1962;17:706–708.

48. Stevens JH, Raffin TA, Mihm FG, et al. Thermodilution cardiac output measurement: effects of the respiratory cycle on its reproducibility. JAMA 1985;253:2240–2242.

49. Thrush DN, Varlotta D. Thermodilution cardiac output: comparison between automated and manual injection of indicator. J Cardiothorac Vasc Anesth 1992;6:17–19.

50. Synder JV, Powner DJ. Effects of mechanical ventilation on the measurement of cardiac output by thermodilution. Crit Care Med 1982;10:677–682.

51. Bottiger BW, Soder M, Rauch H, et al. Semi-continuous versus injectate cardiac output measurement in intensive care patients after cardiac surgery. Intensive Care Med 1996;22:312–318.

52. Boldt J, Menges T, Wollbruck M, et al. Is continuous cardiac output measurement using thermodilution reliable in the critically ill patient? Crit Care Med 1994;22:1913–1918.

53. Mihaljevic T, von Segesser LK, Tonz M, et al. Continuous thermodilution measurement of cardiac output: in-vitro and in-vivo evaluation. Thorac Cardiovasc Surg 1994;42:32–35.

54. Lefrant JY, Bruelle P, Ripart J, et al. Cardiac output measurement in critically ill patients: comparison of continuous and conventional thermodilution techniques. Can J Anaesth 1995;42:972–976.

55. Thrush D, Downs JB, Smith RA. Continuous thermodilution cardiac output: agreement with Fick and bolus thermodilution methods. J Cardiothorac Vasc Anesth 1995;9:399–404.

56. Enghoff E, Michaelsson M, Pavek K, Sjogren S. A comparison between the thermal dilution method and the direct Fick and the dye dilution methods for cardiac output measurements in man. Acta Soc Med Ups 1970;75:157–170.

57. Lipkin DP, Poole Wilson PA. Measurement of cardiac output during exercise by the thermodilution and direct Fick techniques in patients with chronic congestive heart failure. Am J Cardiol 1985;56:321–324.

58. van Grondelle A, Ditchey RV, Groves BM, et al. Thermodilution method overestimates low cardiac output in humans. Am J Physiol 1983;245: H690–H692.

59. Powner JD. Thermodilution technique for cardiac output. N Engl J Med 1975;293:1210.

60. Gardner PE, Monat LA, Woods SL. Accuracy of the closed injectate delivery system in measuring thermodilution cardiac output. Heart Lung 1987; 16:552–561.

61. Barcelona M, Patague L, Bunoy M, et al. Cardiac output determination by the thermodilution method: comparison of ice-temperature injectate versus room-temperature injectate contained in prefilled syringes or a closed injectate delivery system. Heart Lung 1985;14:232–235.

62. Wetzel RC, Latson TW. Major errors in thermodilution cardiac output measurement during rapid volume infusion. Anesthesiology 1985;62: 684–687.

63. Bjoraker DG, Ketcham TR. Catheter thrombus artifactually decreases thermodilution cardiac output measurements. Anesth Analg 1983;62: 1031–1034.

64. Cigarroa RG, Lange RA, Williams RH, et al. Underestimation of cardiac output by thermodilution in patients with tricuspid regurgitation. Am J Med 1989;86:417–420.

65. Heerdt PM, Pond CG, Blessios GA, Rosenbloom

M. Inaccuracy of cardiac output by thermodilution during acute tricuspid regurgitation. Ann Thorac Surg 1992;53:706–708.

66. Hamilton MA, Stevenson LW, Woo M, et al. Effect of tricuspid regurgitation on the reliability of the thermodilution cardiac output technique in congestive heart failure. Am J Cardiol 1989;64: 945–948.

67. Morady F, Brundage BH, Gelberg HJ. Rapid method for determination of shunt ratio using a thermodilution technique. Am Heart J 1983;106: 369–373.

68. Stetz CW, Miller RG, Kelly GE, Raffin TA. Reliability of the thermodilution method in the determination of cardiac output in clinical practice. Am Rev Respir Dis 1982;126:1001–1004.

69. Segal J, Nassi M, Ford AJ Jr, Schuenemeyer TD. Instantaneous and continuous cardiac output in humans obtained with a Doppler pulmonary artery catheter. J Am Coll Cardiol 1990;16: 1398–1407.

70. Benchimol A, Desser KB, Gartlan JL Jr. Bidirectional blood flow velocity in the cardiac chambers and great vessels studied with the Doppler ultrasonic flowmeter. Am J Med 1972;52:467–473.

71. Segal J, Gaudiani V, Nishimura T. Continuous determination of cardiac output using a flow-directed Doppler pulmonary artery catheter. J Cardiothorac Vasc Anesth 1991;5:309–315.

72. Gabe IT, Gault JH, Ross J Jr, et al. Measurement of instantaneous blood flow velocity and pressure in conscious man with a catheter-tip velocity probe. Circulation 1969;40:603–614.

73. Uther JB, Peterson KL, Shabetai R, Braunwald E. Measurement of force–velocity–length relationships in man using an electromagnetic flowmeter catheter. Adv Cardiol 1974;12:198–209.

74. Nichols WW, Pepine CJ, Conti CR, et al. Evaluation of a new catheter-mounted electromagnetic velocity sensor during cardiac catheterization. Cathet Cardiovasc Diagn 1980;6:97–113.

75. Pepine CJ, Nichols WW. Aortic input impedance in cardiovascular disease. Prog Cardiovasc Dis 1982;24:307–318.

76. Nichols WW, Pepine CJ. Left ventricular afterload and aortic input impedance: implications of pulsatile blood flow. Prog Cardiovasc Dis 1982;24: 293–306.

77. Nichols WW, Pepine CJ, Conti CR, et al. Quantitation of aortic insufficiency using a catheter-tip velocity transducer. Circulation 1981;64:375–380.

78. Pepine CJ, Nichols WW, Curry RC Jr, Conti CR. Aortic input impedance during nitroprusside infusion: a reconsideration of afterload reduction and beneficial action. J Clin Invest 1979;64: 643–654.

79. Klinke WP, Christie LG, Nichols WW, et al. Use of catheter-tip velocity–pressure transducer to evaluate left ventricular function in man: effects of intravenous propranolol. Circulation 1980;61: 946–954.

80. White SW, Quail AW, de Leeuw PW, et al. Impedance cardiography for cardiac output measurement: an evaluation of accuracy and limitations. Eur Heart J 1990;11(Suppl 1):79–92.

81. Atallah MM, Demain AD. Cardiac output measurement: lack of agreement between thermodilution and thoracic electric bioimpedance in two clinical settings. J Clin Anesth 1995;7:182–185.

82. Yakimets J, Jensen L. Evaluation of impedance cardiography: comparison of NCCOM3-R7 with Fick and thermodilution methods. Heart Lung 1995;24:194–206.

83. Coats AJ. Doppler ultrasonic measurement of cardiac output: reproducibility and validation. Eur Heart J 1990;11(Suppl 1):49–61.

84. Kim WY, Poulsen JK, Terp K, Staalsen NH. A new Doppler method for quantification of volumetric flow: in vivo validation using color Doppler. J Am Coll Cardiol 1996;27:182–192.

85. Clausen JP, Larsen OA, Trap Jensen J. Cardiac output in middle-aged patients determined with CO_2 rebreathing method. J Appl Physiol 1970;28: 337–342.

86. Ayotte B, Seymour J, McIlroy MB. A new method for measurement of cardiac output with nitrous oxide. J Appl Physiol 1970;28:863–866.

87. Fouad Tarazi FM, MacIntyre WJ. Radionuclide methods for cardiac output determination. Eur Heart J 1990;11(Suppl 1):33–40.

88. Dehmer GJ, Rutala WA. Current use of green dye curves. Am J Cardiol 1995;75:170–171.

89. Cannon PJ, Weiss MB, Sciacca RR. Myocardial blood flow in coronary artery disease: studies at rest and during stress with inert gas washout techniques. Prog Cardiovasc Dis 1977;20:95–120.

90. Kety SS. The theory and applications of inert gas at the lungs and tissues. Pharmacol Rev 1951;3: 1–41.

91. Klocke FJ. Coronary blood flow in man. Prog Cardiovasc Dis 1976;19:117–166.

92. Cannon PJ, Dell RB, Dwyer EM Jr. Measurement of regional myocardial perfusion in man with 133 xenon and a scintillation camera. J Clin Invest 1972;51:964–977.

93. Cannon PJ, Sciacca RR, Fowler DL, et al. Measurement of regional myocardial blood flow in man: description and critique of the method using xenon-133 and a scintillation camera. Am J Cardiol 1975;36:783–792.

94. Gregg DE, Shipley RE. Studies of the venous drainage of the heart. Am J Physiol 1947;151: 13–25.

95. Klocke FJ, Bunnell IL, Greene DG, et al. Average coronary blood flow per unit weight of left ventricle in patients with and without coronary artery disease. Circulation 1974;50:547–559.

96. Ganz W, Tamura K, Marcus HS, et al. Measurement of coronary sinus blood flow by continuous thermodilution in man. Circulation 1971;44: 181–195.

97. Baim DS, Rothman MT, Harrison DC. Simultaneous measurement of coronary venous blood flow and oxygen saturation during transient alterations in myocardial oxygen supply and demand. Am J Cardiol 1982;49:743–752.

98. Pepine CJ, Mehta J, Webster WW, Nichols WW. In vivo validation of a thermodilution method to determine regional left ventricular blood flow in patients with coronary disease. Circulation 1978; 58:795–802.

99. Weisse AB, Regan TJ. A comparison of thermodi-

lution coronary sinus blood flows and krypton myocardial blood flows in the intact dog. Cardiovasc Res 1974;8:526–533.

100. Gensini GG, DiGeorge S, Coskum O, et al. Anatomy of the coronary circulation in living man: coronary venography. Circulation 1965;31:778–784.

101. Kurita A, Azorin J, Granier A, Bourassa MG. Estimation of coronary reserve in left anterior descending and circumflex coronary arteries by regional thermodilution technique. Jpn Circ J 1982; 46:964–973.

102. Roberts DL, Nakazawa HK, Klocke FJ. Origin of great cardiac vein and coronary sinus drainage within the left ventricle. Am J Physiol 1976;230: 486–492.

103. Nakazawa HK, Roberts DL, Klocke FJ. Quantitation of anterior descending vs. circumflex venous drainage in the canine great cardiac vein and coronary sinus. Am J Physiol 1978;234:H163–H166.

104. Cohen MV, Matsuki T, Downey JM. Pressure-flow characteristics and nutritional capacity of coronary veins in dogs. Am J Physiol 1988;255: H834–H846.

105. Cannon RO III, Schenke WH, Leon MB, et al. Limited coronary flow reserve after dipyridamole in patients with ergonovine-induced coronary vasoconstriction. Circulation 1987;75:163–174.

106. Picano E, Simonetti I, Masini M, et al. Transient myocardial dysfunction during pharmacologic vasodilation as an index of reduced coronary reserve: a coronary hemodynamic and echocardiographic study. J Am Coll Cardiol 1986;8:84–90.

107. Marchant E, Pichard A, Rodriguez JA, Casanegra P. Acute effect of systemic versus intracoronary dipyridamole on coronary circulation. Am J Cardiol 1986;57:1401–1404.

108. Rossen JD, Oskarsson H, Stenberg RG, et al. Simultaneous measurement of coronary flow reserve by left anterior descending coronary artery Doppler and great cardiac vein thermodilution methods. J Am Coll Cardiol 1992;20:402–407.

109. Bagger JP. Coronary sinus blood flow determination by the thermodilution technique: influence of catheter position and respiration. Cardiovasc Res 1985;19:27–31.

110. Mathey DG, Chatterjee K, Tyberg JV, et al. Coronary sinus reflux: a source of error in the measurement of thermodilution coronary sinus flow. Circulation 1978;57:778–786.

111. Magorien RD, Frederick J, Leier CV, Unverferth DV. Influence of exercise on coronary sinus blood flow determinations. Am J Cardiol 1987;59: 659–661.

112. Wright CB, Doty DB, Eastham CL, Marcus ML. Measurements of coronary reactive hyperemia with a Doppler probe: intraoperative guide to hemodynamically significant lesions. J Thorac Cardiovasc Surg 1980;80:888–897.

113. Cole JS, Hartley CJ. The pulsed Doppler coronary artery catheter preliminary report of a new technique for measuring rapid changes in coronary artery flow velocity in man. Circulation 1977;56: 18–25.

114. Wilson RF, Laughlin DE, Ackell PH, et al. Transluminal subselective measurement of coronary artery blood flow velocity and vasodilator reserve in man. Circulation 1985;72:82–92.

115. Sibley DH, Millar HD, Hartley CJ, Whitlow PL. Subselective measurement of coronary blood flow velocity using a steerable Doppler catheter. J Am Coll Cardiol 1986;8:1332–1340.

116. Doucette JW, Corl PD, Payne HM, et al. Validation of a Doppler guide wire for intravascular measurement of coronary artery flow velocity. Circulation 1992;85:1899–1911.

117. Zijlstra F, Reiber JH, Serruys PW. Does intracoronary papaverine dilate epicardial coronary arteries? Implications for the assessment of coronary flow reserve. Cathet Cardiovasc Diagn 1988;14: 1–6.

118. Johnson EL, Yock PG, Hargrave VK, et al. Assessment of severity of coronary stenoses using a Doppler catheter: validation of a method based on the continuity equation. Circulation 1989;80: 625–635.

119. Mancini GBJ. Digital angiography. In: Skorton DJ, Schelbert HR, Wolf GL, Brundage BH, eds. Marcus cardiac imaging. 2nd ed. Philadelphia: WB Saunders, 1996:257–271.

120. Rutishauser W, Noseda G, Bussmann WD, Preter B. Blood flow measurement through single coronary arteries by roentgen densitometry: right coronary artery flow in conscious man. Am J Roentgenol Rad Ther Nucl Med 1970;109:21–24.

121. Rutishauser W, Bussmann WD, Noseda G, et al. Blood flow measurement through single coronary arteries by roentgen densitometry: 1. A comparison of flow measured by a radiologic technique applicable in the intact organism and by electromagnetic flowmeter. Am J Roentgenol Rad Ther Nucl Med 1970;109:12–20.

122. Smith HC, Frye RL, Donald DE, et al. Roentgen videodensitometric measure of coronary blood flow: determination from simultaneous indicator–dilution curves at selected sites in the coronary circulation and in coronary artery–saphenous vein grafts. Mayo Clin Proc 1971;46:800–806.

123. Spiller P, Schmiel FK, Politz B, et al. Measurement of systolic and diastolic flow rates in the coronary artery system by x-ray densitometry. Circulation 1983;68:337–347.

124. Swanson DK, Kress DC, Pasaoglu I, et al. Quantitation of absolute flow in coronary artery bypass grafts using digital subtraction angiography. J Surg Res 1988;44:326–335.

125. Chappuis F, Guggenheim N, Suilen C, et al. Regional coronary flow in ml/min measured by conventional cineangiograms. Schweiz Med Wochenschr 1992;122:588–592.

126. Foerster JM, Link DP, Lantz BM, et al. Measurement of coronary reactive hyperemia during clinical angiography by video dilution technique. Acta Radiol (Diagn) 1981;22:209–216.

127. Foerster JM, Lantz BM, Holcroft JW, et al. Angiographic measurement of coronary blood flow by video dilution technique. Acta Radiol (Diagn) 1981;22:121–127.

128. Nissen SE, Elion JL, Booth DC, et al. Value and limitations of computer analysis of digital subtraction angiography in the assessment of coronary flow reserve. Circulation 1986;73:562–571.

129. Gurley JC, Nissen SE, Elion JL, et al. Determination of coronary flow reserve by digital angiography: validation of a practical method not requiring power injection or electrocardiographic gating. J Am Coll Cardiol 1990;16:190–197.

130. Ikeda H, Koga Y, Utsu F, Toshima H. Quantitative evaluation of regional myocardial blood flow by videodensitometric analysis of digital subtraction coronary arteriography in humans. J Am Coll Cardiol 1986;8:809–816.

131. Eigler NL, Schuhlen H, Whiting JS, et al. Digital angiographic impulse response analysis of regional myocardial perfusion: estimation of coronary flow, flow reserve, and distribution volume by compartmental transit time measurement in a canine model. Circ Res 1991;68:870–880.

132. Vogel R, LeFree M, Bates E, et al. Application of digital techniques to selective coronary arteriography: use of myocardial contrast appearance time to measure coronary flow reserve. Am Heart J 1984;107:153–164.

133. Hodgson JM, Legrand V, Bates ER, et al. Validation in dogs of a rapid digital angiographic technique to measure relative coronary blood flow during routine cardiac catheterization. Am J Cardiol 1985;55:188–193.

134. Cusma JT, Toggart EJ, Folts JD, et al. Digital subtraction angiographic imaging of coronary flow reserve. Circulation 1987;75:461–472.

135. Hess OM, McGillem MJ, DeBoe SF, et al. Determination of coronary flow reserve by parametric imaging. Circulation 1990;82:1438–1448.

136. Nishimura RA, Rogers PJ, Holmes DJR, et al. Assessment of myocardial perfusion by videodensitometry in the canine model. J Am Coll Cardiol 1987;9:891–897.

137. Serruys PW, Zijlstra F, Laarman GJ, et al. A comparison of two methods to measure coronary flow reserve in the setting of coronary angioplasty: intracoronary blood flow velocity measurements with a Doppler catheter, and digital subtraction cineangiography. Eur Heart J 1989;10:725–736.

138. Graham SP, Cohen MD, Hodgson JM. Estimation of coronary flow reserve by intracoronary Doppler flow probes and digital angiography. Cathet Cardiovasc Diagn 1990;19:214–221.

139. Legrand V, Mancini GB, Bates ER, et al. Comparative study of coronary flow reserve, coronary anatomy and results of radionuclide exercise tests in patients with coronary artery disease. J Am Coll Cardiol 1986;8:1022–1032.

140. Hodgson JM, Riley RS, Most AS, Williams DO. Assessment of coronary flow reserve using digital angiography before and after successful percutaneous transluminal coronary angioplasty. Am J Cardiol 1987;60:61–65.

141. Pijls NH, Aengevaeren WR, Uijen GJ, et al. Concept of maximal flow ratio for immediate evaluation of percutaneous transluminal coronary angioplasty result by videodensitometry. Circulation 1991;83:854–865.

142. Schelbert HR. Blood flow and metabolism by PET. Cardiol Clin 1994;12:303–315.

143. Grover McKay M. Positron emission tomography as an aid in understanding electrocardiographic changes of ischemia, infarction, and cardiomyopathy. Ann NY Acad Sci 1990;601:77–94.

144. Dayanikli F, Grambow D, Muzik O, et al. Early detection of abnormal coronary flow reserve in asymptomatic men at high risk for coronary artery disease using positron emission tomography. Circulation 1994;90:808–817.

145. Geltman EM, Henes CG, Senneff MJ, et al. Increased myocardial perfusion at rest and diminished perfusion reserve in patients with angina and angiographically normal coronary arteries. J Am Coll Cardiol 1994;16:586–595.

146. Gewirtz H, Fischman AJ, Abraham S, et al. Positron emission tomographic measurements of absolute regional myocardial blood flow permits identification of nonviable myocardium in patients with chronic myocardial infarction. J Am Coll Cardiol 1994;23:851–859.

147. Nitzsche EU, Choi Y, Czernin J, et al. Noninvasive quantification of myocardial blood flow in humans. A direct comparison of the [13N]ammonia and the [15O]water techniques. Circulation 1996;93:2000–2006.

148. Beanlands RS, Muzik O, Melon P, et al. Noninvasive quantification of regional myocardial flow reserve in patients with coronary atherosclerosis using nitrogen-13 ammonia positron emission tomography: determination of extent of altered vascular reactivity. J Am Coll Cardiol 1995;26:1465–1475.

149. Weiss RM, Otoadese EA, Noel MP, et al. Quantitation of absolute regional myocardial perfusion using cine computed tomography. J Am Coll Cardiol 1994;23:1186–1193.

150. Ludman PF, Coats AJ, Burger P, et al. Validation of measurement of regional myocardial perfusion in humans by ultrafast x-ray computed tomography. Am J Card Imaging 1993;7:267–279.

151. Clarke GD, Eckels R, Chaney C, et al. Measurement of absolute epicardial coronary artery flow and flow reserve with breath-hold cine phase-contrast magnetic resonance imaging. Circulation 1995;91:2627–2634.

152. Hundley WG, Lange RA, Clarke GD, et al. Assessment of coronary arterial flow and flow reserve in humans with magnetic resonance imaging. Circulation 1996;93:1502–1508.

153. Vandenberg BF, Kieso R, Fox Eastham K, et al. Quantitation of myocardial perfusion by contrast echocardiography: analysis of contrast gray level appearance variables and intracyclic variability. J Am Coll Cardiol 1989;13:200–206.

154. Mulvagh SL, Foley DA, Aeschbacher BC, et al. Second harmonic imaging of an intravenously administered echocardiographic contrast agent: visualization of coronary arteries and measurement of coronary blood flow. J Am Coll Cardiol 1996;27:1519–1525.

155. Meza M, Greener Y, Hunt R, et al. Myocardial contrast echocardiography: reliable, safe, and efficacious myocardial perfusion assessment after intravenous injections of a new echocardiographic contrast agent. Am Heart J 1996;132:871–881.

156. Gould KL, Lipscomb K, Hamilton GW. Physiologic basis for assessing critical coronary stenosis: instantaneous flow response and regional distri-

bution during coronary hyperemia as measures of coronary flow reserve. Am J Cardiol 1974;33: 87–94.

157. Detre KM, Wright E, Murphy ML, Takaro T. Observer agreement in evaluating coronary angiograms. Circulation 1975;52:979–986.

158. DeRouen TA, Murray JA, Owen W. Variability in the analysis of coronary arteriograms. Circulation 1977;55:324–328.

159. Zir LM, Miller SW, Dinsmore RE, et al. Interobserver variability in coronary angiography. Circulation 1976;53:627–632.

160. Arnett EN, Isner JM, Redwood DR, et al. Coronary artery narrowing in coronary heart disease: comparison of cineangiographic and necropsy findings. Ann Intern Med 1979;91:350–356.

161. Marcus ML, Harrison DG, White CW, et al. Assessing the physiologic significance of coronary obstructions in patients: importance of diffuse undetected atherosclerosis. Prog Cardiovasc Dis 1988;31:39–56.

162. Leung WH, Alderman EL, Lee TC, Stadius ML. Quantitative arteriography of apparently normal coronary segments with nearby or distant disease suggests presence of occult, nonvisualized atherosclerosis. J Am Coll Cardiol 1995;25:311–317.

163. Harrison DG, White CW, Hiratzka LF, et al. The value of lesion cross-sectional area determined by quantitative coronary angiography in assessing the physiologic significance of proximal left anterior descending coronary arterial stenoses. Circulation 1984;69:1111–1119.

164. Feldman RL, Nichols WW, Pepine CJ, Conti CR. Hemodynamic significance of the length of a coronary arterial narrowing. Am J Cardiol 1978;41: 865–871.

165. Young DF, Cholvin NR, Kirkeeide RL, Roth AC. Hemodynamics of arterial stenoses at elevated flow rates. Circ Res 1977;41:99–107.

166. Mates RE, Gupta RL, Bell AC, Klocke FJ. Fluid dynamics of coronary artery stenosis. Circ Res 1978;42:152–162.

167. Gould KL, Kirkeeide RL, Buchi M. Coronary flow reserve as a physiologic measure of stenosis severity. J Am Coll Cardiol 1990;15:459–474.

168. Sutsch G, Hess OM, Franzeck UK, et al. Cutaneous and coronary flow reserve in patients with microvascular angina. J Am Coll Cardiol 1992;20: 78–84.

169. White CW, Wright CB, Doty DB, et al. Does visual interpretation of the coronary arteriogram predict the physiologic importance of a coronary stenosis? N Engl J Med 1984;310:819–824.

170. Brown BG, Bolson E, Frimer M, Dodge HT. Quantitative coronary arteriography: estimation of dimensions, hemodynamic resistance, and atheroma mass of coronary artery lesions using the arteriogram and digital computation. Circulation 1977;55:329–337.

171. Demer L, Gould KL, Kirkeeide R. Assessing stenosis severity: coronary flow reserve, collateral function, quantitative coronary arteriography, positron imaging, and digital subtraction angiography: a review and analysis. Prog Cardiovasc Dis 1988;30:307–322.

172. Gensini GG, Kelly AE, Da Costa BC, Huntington

PP. Quantitative angiography: the measurement of coronary vasomobility in the intact animal and man. Chest 1971;60:522–530.

173. Scoblionko DP, Brown BG, Mitten S, et al. A new digital electronic caliper for measurement of coronary arterial stenosis: comparison with visual estimates and computer-assisted measurements. Am J Cardiol 1984;53:689–693.

174. Feldman RL, Pepine CJ, Curry RC, Conti CR. Quantitative coronary arteriography using 105-MM photospot angiography and an optical magnifying device. Cathet Cardiovasc Diagn 1979;5: 195–201.

175. Kalbfleisch SJ, McGillem MJ, Pinto IM, et al. Comparison of automated quantitative coronary angiography with caliper measurements of percent diameter stenosis. Am J Cardiol 1990;65:1181–1184.

176. Brown BG, Bolson EL, Dodge HT. Quantitative computer techniques for analyzing coronary arteriograms. Prog Cardiovasc Dis 1986;28:403–418.

177. Reiber JHC, Serruys PW, Kooijman CJ, et al. Assessment of short-, medium-, and long-term variations in arterial dimensions from computer-assisted quantitation of coronary cineangiograms. Circulation 1985;71:280–288.

178. Hausleiter J, Nolte CW, Jost S, et al. Comparison of different quantitative coronary analysis systems: ARTREK, CAAS, and CMS. Cathet Cardiovasc Diagn 1996;37:14–22; discussion 23.

179. Mancini GB. Quantitative coronary arteriographic methods in the interventional catheterization laboratory: an update and perspective. J Am Coll Cardiol 1991;17:23B–33B.

180. Hermiller JB, Cusma JT, Spero LA, et al. Quantitative and qualitative coronary angiographic analysis: review of methods, utility, and limitations. Cathet Cardiovasc Diagn 1992;25:110–131.

181. Cusma JT, Spero LA, van der Geest RJ, et al. Application of quantitative coronary angiography in a cineless environment: in vivo assessment of a fully automated system for clinical use. Am Heart J 1995;129:300–306.

182. Gronenschild E, Janssen J, Tijdens F. CAAS II: A second generation system for off-line and on-line quantitative coronary angiography. Cathet Cardiovasc Diagn 1994;33:61–75.

183. Keane D, Haase J, Slager CJ, et al. Comparative validation of quantitative coronary angiography systems: results and implications from a multicenter study using a standardized approach. Circulation 1995;91:2174–2183.

184. Bell MR, Britson PJ, Chu A, et al. Validation of a new UNIX-based quantitative coronary angiographic system for the measurement of coronary artery lesions. Cathet Cardiovasc Diagn 1997;40: 66–74.

185. Strauss BH, Escaned J, Foley DP, et al. Technologic considerations and practical limitations in the use of quantitative angiography during percutaneous coronary recanalization. Prog Cardiovasc Dis 1994;36:343–362.

186. Foley DP, Escaned J, Strauss BH, et al. Quantitative coronary angiography (QCA) in interventional cardiology: clinical application of QCA measurements. Prog Cardiovasc Dis 1994;36: 363–384.

187. Nichols AB, Gabrieli CF, Fenoglio JJ Jr, Esser PD. Quantification of relative coronary arterial stenosis by cinevideodensitometric analysis of coronary arteriograms. Circulation 1984;69:512–522.

188. Johnson MR, McPherson DD, Fleagle SR, et al. Videodensitometric analysis of human coronary stenoses: validation in vivo by intraoperative high-frequency epicardial echocardiography. Circulation 1988;77:328–336.

189. Haase J, Escaned J, van Swijndregt EM, et al. Experimental validation of geometric and densitometric coronary measurements on the new generation Cardiovascular Angiography Analysis System (CAAS II). Cathet Cardiovasc Diagn 1993; 30:104–114.

190. Doriot PA, Dorsaz PA, Dorsaz L, et al. The impact of vessel orientation in space on densitometric measurements of cross sectional areas of coronary arteries. Int J Card Imaging 1996;12:289–297.

191. Sugahara T, Kimura K, Yanagihara Y, et al. Limitation of detection and evaluation of coronary arterial stenosis by densitometry. Int J Card Imaging 1994;10:35–43.

192. Skelton TN, Kisslo KB, Bashore TM. Comparison of coronary stenosis quantitation results from on-line digital and digitized cine film images. Am J Cardiol 1988;62:381–386.

193. Sanz ML, Mancini J, LeFree MT, et al. Variability of quantitative digital subtraction coronary angiography before and after percutaneous transluminal coronary angioplasty. Am J Cardiol 1987;60: 55–60.

194. Spears JR, Sandor T, Als AV, et al. Computerized image analysis for quantitative measurement of vessel diameter from cineangiograms. Circulation 1983;68:453–461.

195. Sonka M, Reddy GK, Winniford MD, Collins SM. Adaptive approach to accurate analysis of small-diameter vessels in cineangiograms. IEEE Trans Med Imaging 1997;16:87–95.

196. Fortin DF, Spero LA, Cusma JT, et al. Pitfalls in the determination of absolute dimensions using angiographic catheters as calibration devices in quantitative angiography. Am J Cardiol 1991;68: 1176–1182.

197. Herrman JR, Keane D, Ozaki Y, et al. Radiological quality of coronary guiding catheters: a quantitative analysis. Cathet Cardiovasc Diagn 1994;33: 55–60.

198. van der Zwet PM, Meyer DJ, Reiber JH. Automated and accurate assessment of the distribution, magnitude, and direction of pincushion distortion in angiographic images. Invest Radiol 1995;30:204–213.

199. Spears JR, Sandor T, Baim DS, Paulin S. The minimum error in estimating coronary luminal cross-sectional area from cineangiographic diameter measurements. Cathet Cardiovasc Diagn 1983;9: 119–128.

200. Lesperance J, Hudon G, White CW, et al. Comparison by quantitative angiographic assessment of coronary stenoses of one view showing the severest narrowing to two orthogonal views. Am J Cardiol 1989;64:462–465.

201. Escaned J, Foley DP, Haase J, et al. Quantitative angiography during coronary angioplasty with a single angiographic view: a comparison of automated edge detection and videodensitometric techniques. Am Heart J 1993;126:1326–1333.

202. Uren NG, Melin JA, De Bruyne BW, et al. Relation between myocardial blood flow and the severity of coronary-artery stenosis. N Engl J Med 1994; 330:1782–1788.

203. Wilson RF, Marcus ML, White CW. Prediction of the physiologic significance of coronary arterial lesions by quantitative lesion geometry in patients with limited coronary artery disease. Circulation 1987;75:723–732.

204. Miller DD, Donohue TJ, Younis LT, et al. Correlation of pharmacological ^{99m}Tc-sestamibi myocardial perfusion imaging with poststenotic coronary flow reserve in patients with angiographically intermediate coronary artery stenoses. Circulation 1994;89:2150–2160.

205. Donohue TJ, Kern MJ, Aguirre FV, et al. Assessing the hemodynamic significance of coronary artery stenoses: analysis of translesional pressure-flow velocity relations in patients. J Am Coll Cardiol 1993;22:449–458.

206. Ofili EO, Kern MJ, Labovitz AJ, et al. Analysis of coronary blood flow velocity dynamics in angiographically normal and stenosed arteries before and after endolumen enlargement by angioplasty. J Am Coll Cardiol 1993;21:308–316.

207. Geschwind HJ, Dupouy P, Dubois-Rande JL, Zelinsky R. Restoration of coronary blood flow in severely narrowed and chronically occluded coronary arteries before and after angioplasty: implications regarding restenosis. Am Heart J 1994;127: 252–262.

208. Kern MJ, Donohue TJ, Aguirre FV, et al. Clinical outcome of deferring angioplasty in patients with normal translesional pressure-flow velocity measurements. J Am Coll Cardiol 1995;25:178–187.

209. Joye JD, Schulman DS, Lasorda D, et al. Intracoronary Doppler guide wire versus stress single-photon emission computed tomographic thallium-201 imaging in assessment of intermediate coronary stenoses. J Am Coll Cardiol 1994;24:940–947.

210. Di Mario C, Krams R, Gil R, Serruys PW. Slope of the instantaneous hyperemic diastolic coronary flow velocity-pressure relation: a new index for assessment of the physiological significance of coronary stenosis in humans. Circulation 1994;90: 1215–1224.

211. Wilson RF, Wyche K, Christensen BV, et al. Effects of adenosine on human coronary arterial circulation. Circulation 1990;82:1595–1606.

212. Talman CL, Winniford MD, Rossen JD, et al. Polymorphous ventricular tachycardia: a side effect of intracoronary papaverine. J Am Coll Cardiol 1990;15:275–278.

213. Wilson RF, White CW. Intracoronary papaverine: an ideal coronary vasodilator for studies of the coronary circulation in conscious humans. Circulation 1986;73:444–451.

214. Kern MJ, Bach RG, Mechem CJ, et al. Variations in normal coronary vasodilatory reserve stratified by artery, gender, heart transplantation and coronary artery disease. J Am Coll Cardiol 1996;28: 1154–1160.

215. Deychak YA, Segal J, Reiner JS, et al. Doppler

guide wire flow-velocity indexes measured distal to coronary stenoses associated with reversible thallium perfusion defects. Am Heart J 1995;129: 219–227.

216. Miller DD, Donohue TJ, Wolford TL, et al. Assessment of blood flow distal to coronary artery stenoses: correlations between myocardial positron emission tomography and poststenotic intracoronary doppler flow reserve. Circulation 1996;94: 2447–2454.

217. Kern MJ, Aguirre FV, Bach RG, et al. Fundamentals of translesional pressure-flow velocity measurements. Cathet Cardiovasc Diagn 1994;31: 137–143.

218. Segal J, Kern MJ, Scott NA, et al. Alterations of phasic coronary artery flow velocity in humans during percutaneous coronary angioplasty. J Am Coll Cardiol 1992;20:276–286.

219. Heller LI, Silver KH, Villegas BJ, et al. Blood flow velocity in the right coronary artery: assessment before and after angioplasty. J Am Coll Cardiol 1994;24:1012–1017.

220. Nakatani S, Yamagishi M, Tamai J, et al. Quantitative assessment of coronary artery stenosis by intravascular Doppler catheter technique: application of the continuity equation. Circulation 1992; 85:1786–1791.

221. Di Mario C, Meneveau N, Gil R, et al. Maximal blood flow velocity in severe coronary stenoses measured with a Doppler guidewire: limitations for the application of the continuity equation in the assessment of stenosis severity. Am J Cardiol 1993;71:54D–61D.

222. Pijls NH, van Son JA, Kirkeeide RL, et al. Experimental basis of determining maximum coronary, myocardial, and collateral blood flow by pressure measurements for assessing functional stenosis severity before and after percutaneous transluminal coronary angioplasty. Circulation 1993;87: 1354–1367.

223. Gould KL. Pressure-flow characteristics of coronary stenoses in unsedated dogs at rest and during coronary vasodilation. Circ Res 1978;43: 242–253.

224. De Bruyne B, Sys SU, Heyndrickx GR. Percutaneous transluminal coronary angioplasty catheters versus fluid-filled pressure monitoring guidewires for coronary pressure measurements and correlation with quantitative coronary angiography. Am J Cardiol 1993;72:1101–1106.

225. Emanuelsson H, Dohnal M, Lamm C, Tenerz L. Initial experiences with a miniaturized pressure transducer during coronary angioplasty. Cathet Cardiovasc Diagn 1991;24:137–143.

226. De Bruyne B, Pijls NH, Paulus WJ, et al. Transstenotic coronary pressure gradient measurement in humans: in vitro and in vivo evaluation of a new pressure monitoring angioplasty guide wire. J Am Coll Cardiol 1993;22:119–126.

227. De Bruyne B, Bartunek J, Sys SU, et al. Simultaneous coronary pressure and flow velocity measurements in humans: feasibility, reproducibility, and hemodynamic dependence of coronary flow velocity reserve, hyperemic flow versus pressure slope index, and fractional flow reserve. Circulation 1996;94:1842–1849.

228. De Bruyne B, Bartunek J, Sys SU, Heyndrickx GR. Relation between myocardial fractional flow reserve calculated from coronary pressure measurements and exercise-induced myocardial ischemia. Circulation 1995;92:39–46.

229. Pijls NH, De Bruyne B, Peels K, et al. Measurement of fractional flow reserve to assess the functional severity of coronary-artery stenoses. N Engl J Med 1996;334:1703–1708.

230. De Bruyne B, Baudhuin T, Melin JA, et al. Coronary flow reserve calculated from pressure measurements in humans: validation with positron emission tomography. Circulation 1994;89: 1013–1022.

231. Kern MJ, Donohue T, Bach R, et al. Monitoring cyclical coronary blood flow alterations after coronary angioplasty for stent restenosis with a Doppler guide wire. Am Heart J 1993;125: 1159–1161.

232. Topol EJ, Ellis SG, Cosgrove DM, et al. Analysis of coronary angioplasty practice in the United States with an insurance-claims data base. Circulation 1993;87:1489–1497.

233. Tron C, Donohue TJ, Bach RG, et al. Differential characterization of human coronary collateral blood flow velocity. Am Heart J 1996;132:508–515.

234. Donohue T, Kern MJ, Bach R, et al. Examination of the effects of hemodynamic and pharmacologic interventions on coronary collateral flow in a patient during cardiac catheterization. Cathet Cardiovasc Diagn 1993;28:155–161.

235. Kern MJ, Aguirre FV, Donohue TJ, et al. Continuous coronary flow velocity monitoring during coronary interventions: velocity trend patterns associated with adverse events. Am Heart J 1994; 128:426–434.

236. Serruys PW, Di Mario C. Prognostic value of coronary flow velocity and diameter stenosis in assessing the short and long term outcome of balloon angioplasty: the DEBATE study (Doppler Endpoints Balloon Angioplasty Trial Europe). Circulation 1996;94:317 (abstract).

237. Kern MJ, Dupouy P, Drury JH, et al. Role of coronary artery lumen enlargement in improving coronary blood flow after balloon angioplasty and stenting: a combined intravascular ultrasound Doppler flow and imaging study. J Am Coll Cardiol 1997;29:1520–1527.

22

Pressure Measurement and Determination of Vascular Resistance

Charles R. Lambert, MD, PhD
Carl J. Pepine, MD
Wilmer W. Nichols, PhD

INTRODUCTION

Ventricular systole produces systemic and pulmonary blood flow secondary to generation of pulsatile pressure that is transmitted throughout the vascular tree. It follows that measurement of pressure waveforms is a key element in evaluation of normal and abnormal cardiovascular physiology. Indeed, with current technology pressure should be the most accurate determination of all hemodynamic measurements made during cardiac catheterization. This chapter addresses the principles and application of pressure measurement in the cardiac catheterization laboratory.

THEORETICAL CONSIDERATIONS

By definition **pressure is force per unit of area**. The International System of Units defines the standard unit of pressure as the pascal (Pa). A pascal is the pressure, acting uniformly on an area of 1 m², to exert a vertical force of 1 newton. In cardiovascular physiology noncoherent technical units of pressure are used most commonly. Such units include the centimeter of water and millimeter of mercury (mm Hg). The millimeter of mercury is defined in accordance with the International Barometric Conventions of the World Meteorological Organization as the pressure exerted by a column of liquid 1 mm in height with a density of 13.5951 g/cm³ at 1 gravity. In practice this definition is realized by a column of mercury 1 mm in height at 0°C and standard atmospheric pressure. Conversions for some other commonly used units of pressure are given in Table 22.1. In clinical catheterization practice pressures are often measured in reference to a point at **midchest level** in the supine position and thus are relative, not absolute, values. Other choices include relating zero to the sternal angle or 10 cm above tabletop, but these levels have no reference to the patient's size. Some attempt to identify the center of the heart, using a lateral x-ray done with the patient standing, and relate zero to this point. This is very time-consuming and has no relation to the position of the heart when the patient is supine. In addition, pressures are usually measured without consideration to conversion of kinetic energy to pressure energy in flowing blood. This conversion may be

Table 22.1.
Pressure Conversions

1 mm Hg = 1.00000014 torr
1 mm Hg = 133.3 Pa
1 mm Hg = 1.36 cm H_2O
1 mm Hg = 1334 dyn/cm^2

measurable when using an end hole rather than a side hole fluid-filled system. The blood impinging on the end hole facing the stream loses some kinetic energy when the velocity of the blood near this point falls because of catheter obstruction. This gives rise to a small difference in **lateral versus end or impact pressure** in such systems. In vivo this difference is usually no more than 1 mm Hg, or so and thus has limited clinical importance.

PRESSURE TRANSDUCERS

Blood pressure has been measured with an enormous number of devices reviewed in an interesting monograph by Geddes (1). Perhaps the simplest direct-writing blood pressure transduction system was that described in 1872 by Landois, who used a needle in an artery to direct spraying blood onto a moving paper surface (2) (Fig. 22.1). This **"hemautogram"** yielded information of surprising accuracy regarding the amplitude and contour of the arterial pulse, including existence of the dicrotic notch. Many more recent transducers use various methods to convert pressure into electrical signals for recording and processing. Transduction devices used for pressure measurement include variable resistance, variable capacitance, variable inductance, and piezoelectric types. The most commonly used of these is the variable resistance transducer, which usually consists of a metal diaphragm upon which is applied a full or partial resistive bridge. This is connected to a pressure preamplifier or bridge amplifier in a configuration similar to that of a classical Wheatstone bridge. AC (alternating current) or DC (direct current) excitation voltage is applied to the bridge from the preamplifier through appropriate patient isolation transformers. A change in pressure of the fluid in the system causes a small move-

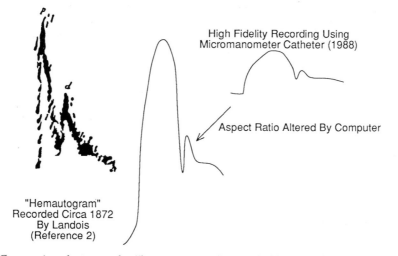

P

d

High Fidelity Recording Using Micromanometer Catheter (1988)

Aspect Ratio Altered By Computer

"Hemautogram" Recorded Circa 1872 By Landois (Reference 2)

Figure 22.1. Comparison between the "hemautogram" recorded in the 1800s by spraying blood from a dog artery onto a drum and a high-fidelity catheter tip micromanometer recording of arterial pressure. Altering the aspect ratio (vertical and horizontal gain) by computer shows that the records are strikingly similar in morphology. Thus it appears that Landois made the first high-fidelity pressure recordings in the nineteenth century (see Luciani L. Human physiology (Welby FA, trans). London: Macmillan, 1911;1:592).

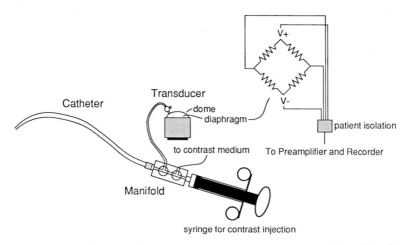

Figure 22.2. Components of a typical pressure measurement system used in clinical catheterization for a left heart study. A catheter is attached via Luer connectors to a manifold that in turn is connected to contrast medium and pressure transducer. The transducer may be attached directly to the manifold or via extension pressure tubing, as shown. The active element of the pressure transducer is a resistive bridge deposited on or attached to the diaphragm and connected via isolation amplifiers to the recording system.

ment of the diaphragm, which in turn changes the resistance of the bridge. This change is amplified, filtered, and recorded as a pressure waveform with respect to time. Components of such a system are illustrated in Figure 22.2. Details of pressure preamplifiers and recorders are given in Chapter 14.

The key to proper application of instruments to pressure recording is understanding the **dynamic frequency response** characteristics of the recording system and what factors modify these characteristics. For a given pressure measurement system the input signal is the true pressure being measured and the output signal is the analog signal, usually recorded on paper to be analyzed. For this discussion we assume that the recorder, or the portion of the system beyond the pressure transducer in Figure 22.2, has perfect response characteristics. Thus, our concerns are the catheter–connector–transducer (or manometer) apparatus and its response characteristics. If these components of a system were perfect, both the frequency and the amplitude of the input signal would be reproduced exactly at the output without distortion. In reality most commonly used catheterization laboratory pressure-measuring systems distort

the intravascular pressure waveform with respect to both amplitude and phase of the signal. The magnitude of this distortion generally depends on the frequency being considered; that is, the higher the frequency, the greater the distortion.

Neglecting phase shift distortion, which usually is too small to have clinical importance, a transducer system must be evaluated with regard to linearity and frequency characteristics of amplitude response. In this context linearity simply means that input plotted against output gives a straight line (Figure 22.3). For real systems, however, as the frequency of a given alternating signal increases, at some point the amplitude of the output signal is no longer equal to the amplitude of the input signal (Figure 22.3). This phenomenon, which defines the frequency response of the system with respect to signal amplitude, can be graphically demonstrated by plotting output amplitude against frequency (Figure 22.3). Real pressure-measuring systems usually exhibit a flat, or constant, frequency response curve to a certain level, at which point output either falls off toward zero or shows a second rise in amplitude at higher frequencies if the system is underdamped or resonates. The origin of these characteris-

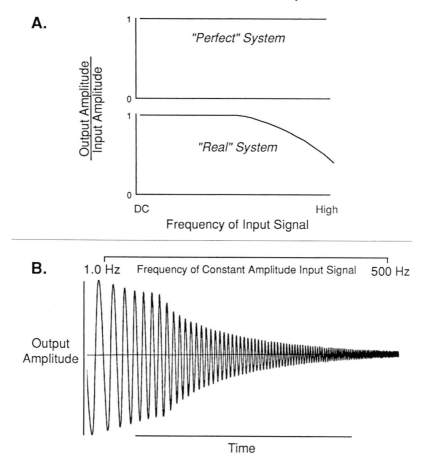

Figure 22.3. A. Ratio of output to input amplitude of a periodic signal for a theoretically perfect pressure measurement system would be 1 for all input frequencies. Real systems show a drop-off in output signal amplitude that may also be associated with a resonant effect at certain frequencies (not shown). The latter may cause the ratio of output to input to exceed 1 transiently, as described in the text. **B.** Output waveform from a real pressure measurement system as a constant amplitude sine wave input is applied and swept from low to high frequencies. As shown in the real system of **A,** as frequency increases, output signal amplitude decreases.

tics resides in mechanical properties, such as mass, inertia, and frictional resistance, and in electronic characteristics of the system. The dynamic behavior of most transducer systems can be described by a second-order differential equation as $F(t) = M (d^2y/dt^2) + R (dy/dt) + Sy$.

By this relation the response of the system (y) to the force exerted on the transducer by the pressure $(F(t))$ is governed by the mass of the moving liquid (M), frictional resistance (R), and stiffness, or elastance (S), of the system. The frequency response of such a system can be predicted if the damping constant (β_0) and undamped natural frequency (ω_0) are known. In terms of the physical properties of the system, these parameters are defined as follows:

$$\omega_0 = (S/M)^{1/2} = (\pi r^2 E/\rho L)^{1/2}$$

and

$$\beta_0 = R/(2M) = 4\mu/\rho r^2$$

$E = \Delta P/\Delta V$ is the volume elasticity, where P is pressure, V is volume, and L and r, respectively, are the length and internal radius of the catheters; ρ and μ are the density and viscosity of the liquid.

These equations can be applied to evaluate the frequency characteristics of a transducer system by the transient, or pop, method. Although the frequency response characteristics of modern measurement systems are most often determined by use of special pressure generators designed for this purpose, the transient method is still useful and is presented here to illustrate the principles involved (3, 4).

An apparatus consisting of a pressurized chamber closed with a thin rubber membrane (a surgical glove is satisfactory), is constructed and filled with degassed or boiled saline (Fig. 22.4). After all connections are tightened, the pressure in the chamber is increased to distend the membrane. The recording system is started at rapid speed, and the membrane is ruptured suddenly with a very sharp pointed instrument or lighted match. This drops the pressure essentially to 0 (atmospheric). A typical underdamped system undergoes several oscillations of decreasing amplitude before reaching a steady level (Fig. 22.4). After transient excitement such as this, the system oscillates at its damped natural frequency (ω_D) defined by $\omega_D = (\omega_0^2 - \beta_0^2)^{1/2}$.

The record is analyzed to determine the damped natural frequency (ω_D) by means of the following relationship, where T is the time interval (seconds) between the peaks of the oscillation, that is, $\omega_D = 2\pi f_D = 2\pi/T$.

The exponential rate at which the oscillations decrease in amplitude is defined by a logarithmic decrement Λ, defined as $\Lambda = \log_e(y_{n+1}/y_n)$, where y_1, y_2, and so on, represent successive peak-to-peak amplitudes of oscillation (Fig. 22.4).

It follows then that $\beta_0 = \Lambda/T$ and $\omega_0 = [SQR](4\pi^2 + \Lambda^2)^{1/2}/T$.

The damping coefficient (or factor) β is defined as $\beta = \beta_0/\omega_0 = \Lambda/[SQR](4\pi^2 + \Lambda^2) = (4\mu/r^3)(L/\rho\pi E)^{1/2}$.

In general an optimal damping coefficient is around 0.64, where there is minimal resonant peak, and the response of the system remains constant plus or minus 2% to about 67% of the undamped natural frequency (see Figure 13.10) (4–6). Phase lag is also relatively inert at a damping ratio of 0.64. The adequacy of a catheter–manometer system for recording certain events can be judged by determination of the frequency response and damping coefficient. These parameters can also be used to correct data retrospectively to those that would have been recorded with a system having perfect frequency characteristics (3). Examples of a step pressure response for an undamped, optimally damped, and overdamped system are shown in Figure 22.5.

In practice, if high-fidelity pressure data are critical in patient evaluation or for research purposes, catheter tip micromanometers are used (7). These catheters have a semiconductor strain gauge built into the catheter tip with frequency characteristics that enable not only precise measurements of pressure waveforms but also intravascular recording of sounds. Responses to a step

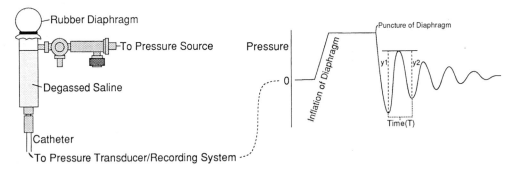

Figure 22.4. A system for the pop test to define the frequency response characteristics of a system, as described in the text. A closed chamber filled with degassed saline and capped with a rubber diaphragm is connected to a pressure source. The system is pressurized and the diaphragm is ruptured with a sharp instrument. The resulting pressure waveform is recorded at high speed for analysis of time (T) and pressure oscillations y_1 and y_2 for analysis, as given in the text.

change in pressure of a catheter tip micromanometer and a standard fluid-filled NIH catheter–transducer system are compared in Figure 22.6. Using a catheter tip micromanometer as a reference standard, it is useful to document the effects of altering frequency response characteristics with a typical clinical catheter–transducer system. Barring the presence of air or contrast medium in a system, errors in balancing or calibration, and inaccurate zero reference determination, the most common causes of pressure distortion clinically are addition of extensions and stopcocks between the catheter and transducer and catheter whip artifact. Such distortion is shown in Figure 22.7 for left ventricular pressure. Distortion is amplified with such a system when catheters are moved, such as during a pullback recording from left ventricle to aorta (Fig. 22.8).

The frequency response needed to record accurate pressure waveforms in man can be estimated by Fourier analysis, which breaks a complex periodic wave into a series of component sine waves of increasing frequency (see Chapter 14). When the harmonic contents of left ventricular and aortic pressure waves are examined in this manner, more than 99% of the signal content is contained in the first 10 harmonics (4, 8, 9) (Table 22.2). For a fundamental frequency or heart rate of 120 beats per minute the frequency of the tenth harmonic is 20 cycles/second (Hz). Experimental work has verified that a system with a frequency response range that is flat to 20 Hz is necessary for accurate pressure reproduction, although many systems routinely used in clinical catheterization studies have lower frequency response characteristics (Table 22.3). If recorded pressure data are to be used for further calculations, such as first- or second-time derivative computation, the transducer systems must have correspondingly better frequency characteristics (flat to 60 Hz) (10). Such applications usually employ catheter tip micromanometers.

NORMAL PRESSURE WAVEFORMS

Normal pressure waveforms for cardiac chambers and great vessels are illustrated

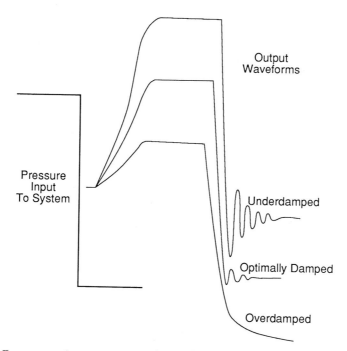

Figure 22.5. Representative output waveforms for underdamped, optimally damped, and overdamped pressure measurement systems to application of a stepped pressure change as input.

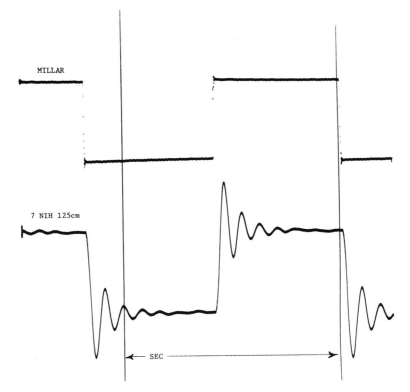

MILLAR

7 NIH 125cm

SEC

Figure 22.6. Simultaneously obtained pressure recordings in response to a step pressure input for a high-fidelity (Millar) catheter tip micromanometer and a standard fluid-filled NIH-Statham resistive bridge pressure measurement system. *SEC,* second.

in Figure 22.9 as recorded using a standard clinical fluid-filled system. Normal values for the phasic and mean components of these waveforms are listed in Table 22.4. To perform diagnostic cardiac catheterization properly, it is important to have a thorough knowledge of normal pressure waveform morphology. As a basis for understanding alterations of pressures in pathologic states, pertinent facts regarding normal pressures are addressed with reference to Figure 22.9.

A normal right atrial pressure waveform begins with the *a* wave, which follows the P wave of the electrocardiogram and has its origin from right atrial systole. Fall of pressure from this point proceeds along the *x* descent, to be interrupted by a small upward inflection, the *c* wave, which coincides with closure of the tricuspid valve. The *x* descent continues during atrial relaxation, to be followed by a slow rise in pressure because of atrial filling from the venous cir-

culation until inscription of the *v* wave, which coincides with right ventricular systole. The tricuspid valve then opens, and pressure falls as the atrium empties into the right ventricle along the *y* descent. Following the *y* descent, right atrial and right ventricular diastolic pressures equilibrate before the next cardiac cycle. Most reported data include mean right atrial pressure, as well as the peak value for the *a* and *v* waves. In the normal right atrium the *a* wave is usually the highest wave recorded.

A normal right ventricular pressure waveform consists of a small rapid-filling wave, a slow-filling wave, the *a* wave coincident with right atrial systole, and then systolic pressure generation. The shape is somewhat triangular with respect to the rise and fall of pressure during systole. Pressures usually reported include end-diastolic pressure, which is measured just after the *a* wave, and peak systolic pressure. With

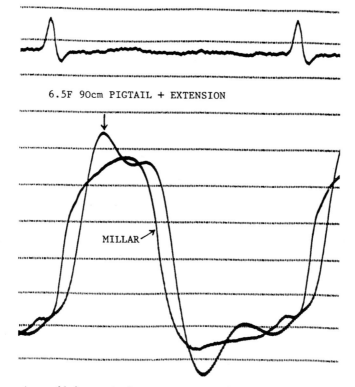

Figure 22.7. Comparison of left ventricular pressure recordings using a standard clinical fluid-filled catheter system and a high-fidelity catheter tip micromanometer (*Millar*) that were calibrated to respond in an equisensitive manner to the same static pressure using a mercury manometer. Note inaccuracy in peak systolic (overestimate) and early diastolic (underestimate) pressures recorded from the fluid-filled catheter (pigtail). Each horizontal line is 20 mm Hg.

atrial fibrillation, when no *a* wave is present, end-diastolic pressure is usually measured 0.04 seconds after the peak of the R wave on the electrocardiogram. There is no reason to measure the initial diastolic pressure when fluid-filled catheters are used.

A normal pulmonary artery pressure waveform consists of a systolic pulse coincident with right ventricular emptying. As right ventricular ejection ends, pulmonary pressure begins to fall, and the incisura occurs as right ventricular pressure falls below that in the pulmonary artery and the pulmonic valve closes. Pulmonary artery pressure continues to fall as blood runs off into the pulmonary venous circulation. The nadir of this phase is measured as pulmonary end-diastolic pressure and is usually reported along with peak systolic and mean pressures. The pulmonary capillary wedge pressure has a configuration similar to that

of left atrial pressure, with the added effects of delay with respect to time and damping of pressure waves because of transmission through the pulmonary capillary and venous beds. Similar to right atrial pressure discussed previously, *a* and *v* waves should be present and should correspond to left atrial systole and left atrial filling from the pulmonary venous system. In most cases distinct *x* and *y* descents are seen; however, a *c* wave is usually not apparent. Values reported should include mean pulmonary capillary wedge pressure, as well as peak values for the *a* and *v* waves. Normally pulmonary artery end-diastolic pressure is equal to mean pulmonary capillary wedge pressure, since the pulmonary circulation has low intrinsic resistance.

A normal left atrial pressure waveform is similar in morphology to that of the right atrium, with *a*, *c*, and *v* waves and corre-

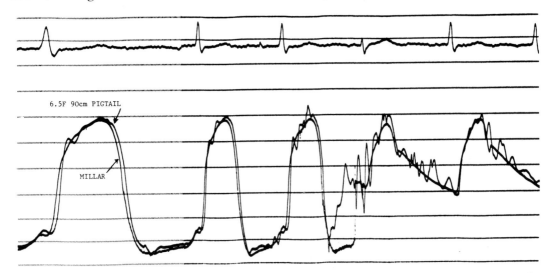

Figure 22.8. Artifact imposed during left ventricle to aorta pullback on recordings made with a standard fluid-filled catheter system (pigtail) compared with a high-fidelity catheter tip micromanometer (*Millar*).

Table 22.2.
Harmonic Content of Pressure Waves in Humans[a]

Harmonic No.	Left Ventricle		Aorta	
	mm Hg	Vs/Vt	mm Hg	Vs/Vt
1	59	73.0%	15	66.0%
2	37	86.0	6	89.0
3	17	91.0	2	93.0
4	10	94.0	1	95.0
5	7	95.0	1	96.0
6	6	97.0	1	97.0
7	5	97.0	1	98.0
8	4	98.0	0	99.0
9	3	99.0	0	99.6
10	2	99.3	0	99.7

From Nichols WW, Pepine CJ. Unpublished data.
[a] Heart rate, 76 beats/min (1.3 Hz).
Vs, series variance representing the component contribution of a given harmonic; Vt, total variance representing the relative proportion contributed to the total pressure signal by a given harmonic (expressed as a percentage).

sponding x and y descents. The v wave, however, is usually the highest wave in the normal left atrium. Unless transseptal catheterization is done, this pressure is not usually measured, and the pulmonary capillary wedge pressure is used as an estimate of left atrial pressure. In many cases this is adequate; however, error may be introduced unless care is taken to avoid overdamping and correct positioning is confirmed by flu-

oroscopy and if necessary, oxygen saturation in blood drawn from the catheter in wedge position is determined. The pulmonary capillary wedge pressure does not reflect left atrial pressure in the occasional patient with pulmonary venous obstruction or mechanically related anomalies such as an obstructive left atrial myxoma. Although the mean pulmonary wedge pressure correlates closely with left ventricular end-dia-

Table 22.3.
Frequency Response Characteristics of Some Catheter–Manometer Systems[a]

Catheter	Flat Frequency Cutoff (Hz)	Resonant Frequency (Hz)	Damping Coefficient
Sones 8 F			
80 cm	20	30	0.15
Dome with membrane	19	28	0.15
Renografin in system	19	22	0.31
NIH 7 F			
80 cm	13	20	0.19
NIH 8 F			
125 cm	14	22	0.19
NIH 8 F			
125 cm direct to transducer	30	39	0.17
NIH 8 F			
125 cm + 140 cm ext	2	7	0.24
Pigtail 6.5 F			
90 cm + 40 cm ext	5	11	0.21
Swan-Ganz 7 F	7	12	0.33
Cournand 7 F			
125 cm	11	17	0.20

From Nichols WW, Pepine CJ. Unpublished data.
[a] Values determined using Statham P23ID transducer, disposable dome, and three-way stopcock.
ext, extension tubing; NIH, National Institutes of Health.

stolic pressure in the absence of mitral valve obstruction, these two pressures may not necessarily be equivalent. The mean pulmonary wedge pressure relates most closely to the mean diastolic left ventricular pressure.

The normal left ventricular pressure waveform, however, is usually somewhat less triangular, with faster upstroke and descent than the right ventricular pressure pulse. The early filling wave is followed by late filling, the *a* wave of left atrial contraction, and systole. As ventricular pressure rises, the mitral valve closes, and isovolumic contraction continues until the aortic valve opens. The course of isovolumic pressure rise may be used as an index of left ventricular contractile state, and it is usually studied in this context as its first derivative or a function thereof. Following ventricular ejection, as ventricu-

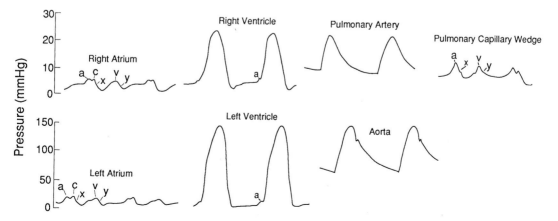

Figure 22.9. Supine right and left heart pressures recorded from standard fluid-filled catheter systems in humans.

Table 22.4.
Normal Supine Resting Pressure Values in Humans

	RA	RV	PA	PCW	LA	LV	Ao
Systolic		15–30	15–30			100–140	100–140
End-diastolic		0–8	3–12			3–12	60–90
Mean	0–8		9–16	1–10	1–10		70–105
α Wave	2–10			3–15	3–15		
ν Wave	2–10			3–12	3–12		

All values are in mm Hg.
Ao, aorta; LA, left atrium; LV, left ventricle; PA, pulmonary artery; PCW, pulmonary–capillary wedge; RA, right atrium; RV, right ventricle.

lar pressure falls below aortic pressure, the aortic valve closes. The period between aortic valve closure and mitral valve opening is **isovolumic relaxation.** The fall of pressure during this period has been shown to follow a monoexponential course, although other mathematical models have been used as well. The time constant describing the decay of left ventricular isovolumic pressure is sensitive to processes affecting myocardial relaxation and thus may be one of the earliest indicators of ischemia. Values reported include end-diastolic, which is measured at the end of the *a* wave or z point, and peak systolic left ventricular pressure. In atrial fibrillation it is customary to report end-diastolic pressure 0.04 seconds after peak of the *R* wave. There is little meaning in the initial diastolic pressure when fluid catheters are used, as this point is highly variable (Fig. 22.7).

Normal central aortic pressure is composed of a rapidly rising systolic pulse, an incisura, and a subsequent decay of pressure similar to that described previously for the pulmonary artery. Values usually reported include peak systolic, end-diastolic, and mean pressures. The composition of the central aortic pressure in man has been studied in detail, using harmonic analysis and related techniques useful in describing pulse transmission (11, 12). These studies have shown that the measured aortic pressure waveform is composed of both forward and antegrade pressure waves and reflected or retrograde pressure waves. The measured central aortic pressure wave is a conjugate of these **forward and reflected waves**. The component forward and re-

flected waves may vary with disease and with pharmacologic manipulation, as well as with the functional status of the left ventricle. These changes are reflected in the morphology of the central aortic pressure tracing (Fig. 22.10).

Peripheral arterial pressure waveforms, usually from the brachial or femoral arteries, are also commonly recorded in the catheterization laboratory. In general the contours of these waveforms are similar to those of the aortic pressure, with a slightly higher peak pressure and greater pulse pressure in the periphery. This phenomenon is due to a slight amplification resulting from wave reflection from the periphery, and it may be marked with the decreased arterial compliance and increased pulse wave velocity seen in older individuals. The mean peripheral and aortic pressures are usually equal, or there may be a slight decrease apparent in the periphery; however, this is rarely clinically important from a diagnostic standpoint (3, 4, 13)

ABNORMAL PRESSURE WAVEFORMS

Virtually every cardiovascular disease entity may be associated with abnormalities in systemic or pulmonary pressures. Many of these conditions and their associated pressure abnormalities are illustrated elsewhere in this volume. The following section discusses specific pathophysiologic entities that have characteristic pressure abnormalities and are common in the routine practice of diagnostic cardiac catheterization.

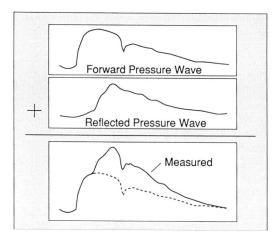

Figure 22.10. A representative high-fidelity recording of central aortic pressure in man and the component forward and reflected waves as described in the text. (Adapted from Murgo JP, Westerhof N, Giolma JP, Altobelli SA. Manipulation of ascending aortic pressure and flow wave reflections with the Valsalva maneuver: relationship to input impedance. Circulation 1981;63: 122–132.)

Atrioventricular Valve Insufficiency

Pressure waveform alterations are similar in morphology for both mitral and tricuspid insufficiency. The primary abnormality in recorded pressure waveforms is secondary to abnormal transmission of ventricular pressure to the corresponding atrial chamber via the incompetent valve. The right or left atrial pressure (pulmonary capillary wedge pressure) contains an accentuated *and early v* wave that may obscure other components of the normal waveform (Fig. 22.11). The magnitude of the *v* wave depends primarily on the degree of atrioventricular valve incompetence, the compliance of the receiving chamber, and ventricular function. Long-standing moderate mitral insufficiency and a dilated, compliant left atrium produces a less prominent *v* wave than in **acute mitral insufficiency** related to papillary muscle rupture, in which a similar volume of regurgitant blood ejected into a normal atrium produces a large *v* wave. In patients with large *v* waves in the pulmonary capillary wedge pressure recording, it

may be difficult to estimate left ventricular filling pressure in the intensive care unit with a balloon flotation catheter. It has recently been shown that the trough of the *x* descent is the best indicator of true left ventricular end-diastolic pressure in these cases (14). The absence of a large *v* wave does not exclude significant atrioventricular valve insufficiency. This may be the usual finding in patients with long-standing mitral insufficiency, dilated cardiomyopathy, and large left atrial volume. In general, angiographically severe mitral insufficiency is present when the height of the left atrial or pulmonary capillary wedge *v* wave is three to five times that of the mean left atrial or pulmonary capillary wedge pressure. Associated pressure abnormalities may include pulmonary or systemic venous hypertension and systemic hypotension with severe mitral insufficiency. In many cases, with large *v* waves in the pulmonary wedge pressure, the *v* waves are also seen in the pulmonary artery pressure waveform. In most patients with severe mitral insuffi-

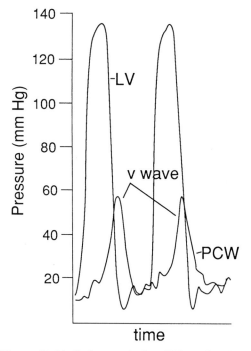

Figure 22.11. Left ventricular (*LV*) and pulmonary capillary wedge pressure (*PCW*) tracings in a patient with mitral insufficiency.

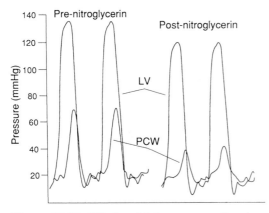

Figure 22.12. Effects of intravenous nitroglycerin on left ventricular (*LV*) and pulmonary capillary wedge (*PCW*) pressures in a patient with ischemia-related mitral insufficiency related to severe right coronary artery stenosis. With relief of angina pectoris by nitroglycerin (0.4 mg sl) the systolic LV pressure falls, the degree of mitral insufficiency improves with reduction in the &ygr, and wave of the PCW pressure and left ventricular end-diastolic pressure is reduced.

ciency, the magnitude of the regurgitant blood volume and corresponding *v* wave can be reduced with afterload reduction via sodium nitroprusside. If mitral insufficiency is due to myocardial ischemia affecting ventricular geometry, administration of nitroglycerin may produce dramatic relief (Fig. 22.12). Further discussion of hemodynamic abnormalities with atrioventricular valve incompetence may be found in Chapters 25 and 40.

Aortic Insufficiency

The principal pressure abnormality in isolated aortic insufficiency is directly related to regurgitant blood volume and systemic vascular impedance. This is manifested primarily by a widened systemic pulse pressure. This widening is due principally to decreased diastolic pressure with maintenance of systolic pressure unless cardiac failure intervenes. Associated with regurgitation of blood from the aorta into the left ventricle in diastole is rapid ventricular filling and premature closure of the mitral

valve as the rising ventricular diastolic pressure quickly exceeds that in the left atrium. This is particularly common with acute aortic insufficiency when compensatory ventricular enlargement has not taken place, as in chronic disease. An example of pressure tracings with acute aortic insufficiency is given in Figure 22.13. Again, other associated pressure abnormalities may include pulmonary hypertension and systemic hypotension.

Aortic Stenosis

In valvular aortic stenosis the left ventricular pressure is altered in keeping with the changes of chronic pressure overload and hypertrophy. These include primarily diastolic abnormalities because of diminished distensibility, such as elevated end-diastolic pressure, and an accentuated filling wave. The systolic ventricular pressure pulse depends on the state of left ventricular function but is generally normal in contour and increased in amplitude until cardiac failure intervenes. The stenotic aortic valve alters the characteristics of the aortic pressure contour by delaying the rate of pressure rise during systole and decreasing the absolute amplitude of peak systolic pressure (Fig. 22.14). Associated pressure abnormalities may include elevated pulmonary pressures and systemic hypotension. Simply having a catheter across the stenotic valve may increase the measured pressure gradient in patients with critical aortic stenosis. The hemodynamics of aortic stenosis are further discussed in Chapters 25 and 40.

Mitral Stenosis

As with any of the valvular abnormalities noted earlier, the pressure findings in mitral stenosis may vary with the state of the disease and compensation in the individual patient. This is true particularly of mitral stenosis, since the status of the pulmonary vasculature may undergo marked change in the course of this disease, as discussed in Chapters 25, 35 and 40. In general, **mitral**

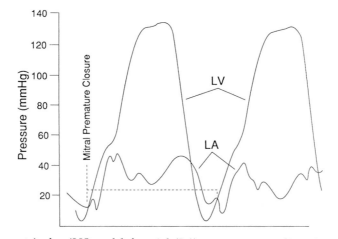

Figure 22.13. Left ventricular (*LV*) and left atrial (*LA*) pressure recordings in a patient with acute aortic insufficiency because of prosthetic valve dysfunction. LV end-diastolic pressure is markedly increased to approximately 50 mm Hg, causing early closure of the mitral valve, as indicated.

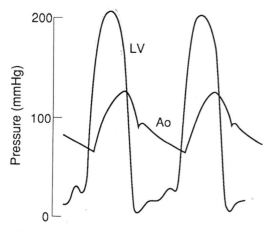

Figure 22.14. Left ventricular (*LV*) and aortic (*Ao*) pressure tracings in a patient with severe aortic stenosis.

As pulmonary vascular resistance increases with time, pulmonary hypertension becomes severe, and vasodilator administration may be necessary in the catheterization laboratory to determine how much of this increase is reversible. Concomitant mitral insufficiency or aortic insufficiency may further alter recorded pressure data in mitral stenosis. Recordings in a case of mitral stenosis are shown in Figure 22.15.

Obstructive Cardiomyopathy (Idiopathic Hypertrophic Subaortic Stenosis)

In this spectrum of disorders pressure measurements have been particularly interesting from a pathophysiologic and technical standpoint. The pressure finding of interest is a systolic left intraventricular gradient that may occur between the outflow tract and the apex or between other locations within the cavity. In some patients this gradient may be associated with asymmetric septal hypertrophy alone, and in others it appears to be primarily associated with obstruction of ventricular outflow by the mitral valve apparatus. The pathophysiology of this disorder has been addressed in several recent reviews (15–17). From a techni-

stenosis is evaluated by recording the diastolic pressure difference between the pulmonary capillary wedge catheter and a left ventricular catheter with simultaneously obtained cardiac output. Without intervening pulmonary venous disease or left atrial obstructive abnormalities this is generally valid; however, in some patients transseptal catheterization may be required to obtain accurate measurements (see Chapter 9). Significant mitral stenosis is accompanied by some degree of pulmonary hypertension and increases in right ventricular pressures.

cal standpoint this disorder presents several interesting problems with respect to pressure measurement. First, it is desirable, to measure continuously the intraventricular pressure gradient in such patients for documentation and also to assess the effects of interventions. We usually do this with a micromanometer catheter with two pressure sensors. The distance between the sensors may range from 2 to 4 cm or so. Extreme care must be exercised when making such measurements to ensure that the catheter is free-floating within the ventricular cavity. If this is not done, **entrapment** of the pressure sensors may occur within trabeculations, and a false gradient may be recorded. Entrapment can usually be detected with the combination of fluoroscopic visualization and observation of the diastolic pressure contour. The latter is altered when the catheter is entrapped, such that the two sensors read different pressures during diastasis. The contour of the usual diastolic filling wave is also usually distorted. In some patients it may be impossible to make such recordings because of ventricular irritability or geometric considerations. In such cases a pigtail catheter can be used to make a pullback recording from the ventricular apex to the outflow tract and across the aortic valve. It is very difficult to entrap a pigtail; however, localization of the gradient may be less precise, and measurements are not continuous with this method. A representative re-

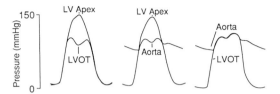

Figure 22.16. Pressure measurements in a patient with idiopathic hypertrophic subaortic stenosis at the left ventricular apex (*LV apex*), left ventricular outflow tract below the aortic valve (*LVOT*), and in the ascending aorta revealing an intracavitary gradient. (Adapted from Murgo JP, Alter BR, Dorethy JF, et al. Dynamics of left ventricular ejection in obstructive and nonobstructive hypertrophic cardiomyopathy. J Clin Invest 1980;66:1369–1382.)

cording from a patient with idiopathic hypertrophic subaortic stenosis is given in Figure 22.16.

DETERMINATION OF VASCULAR RESISTANCE

Vascular resistance, a derived function, is important in describing the interaction of cardiac pump function and the systemic and pulmonary circulations. Resistance has also been used to characterize valvular function as outlined in Chapter 25. Poiseuille's law states that the ratio of pressure gradient to flow is a function of tube dimension and viscosity moving through the tube. The ratio of mean pressure gradient to mean flow is thus a measure of the extent to which a system opposes or resists flow. In the context of the circulatory system this ratio is called vascular resistance (R) and is analogous to the definition of electrical resistance in Ohm's law. Stated mathematically, R equals mean pressure gradient divided by mean flow. Vascular resistance is commonly defined using either absolute resistance units or hybrid (Wood's) resistance units. Units for absolute resistance are dyne sec cm^{-5} and defined as R = [mean pressure gradient (dyne/cm^2)]/[mean flow (cm^3/sec)]. Hybrid or Wood's units are defined as R = [mean pressure gradient (mm

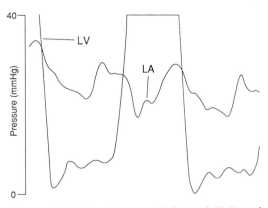

Figure 22.15. Simultaneous left atrial (*LA*) and left ventricular (*LV*) pressures in a patient with severe mitral stenosis.

Table 22.5.
Normal Values for Vascular Resistance

Measurement	Absolute Units (dyne sec cm^{-5})	Hybrid or Wood's Units (mm Hg min liter^1)
Systemic vascular resistance	$1130 + 178$	14.13 ± 2.23
Total pulmonary resistance	205 ± 51	2.56 ± 0.64
Pulmonary vascular resistance	67 ± 23	0.84 ± 0.29

From Barrett-Boyes BG, Wood EH. Cardiac output and related measurements and pressure values in the right heart and associated vessels together with an analysis of the hemodynamic response to the inhalation of high oxygen mixtures in healthy subjects. J Clin Lab Med 1958;51:72–82.
Values are mean ± standard deviation.

Hg)]/[mean flow (liter/min)]. Resistances using these two definitions are interchangeable as $[R$ (dyne sec cm^{-5})$] = [R$ (Wood's units) $\times 80]$ (4).

Vascular resistance is generally examined in clinical medicine for different cardiovascular segments. Thus pulmonary vascular resistance (*PVR*), total pulmonary vascular resistance (*TPR*), systemic vascular resistance (*SVR*) and total systemic resistance (*TSR*) are defined below (also see Appendix), where *PAM* is mean pulmonary artery pressure, *LAM* is mean left atrial pressure, *SAM* is mean systemic arterial pressure, *RAM* is mean right atrial pressure, and *CO* is cardiac output.

$$PVR = (PAM - LAM)/CO$$
$$TPR = PAM/CO$$
$$SVR = (SAM - RAM)/CO$$
$$TSR = SAM/CO$$

Normal values for vascular resistances are given in Table 22.5.

Vascular resistances as calculated by these formulas are based on and measure the opposition to mean blood flow only. They neglect the pulsatile components of cardiac loading, which may become very important in certain disease states. Rigorous description of total resistance to blood flow in a pulsatile system requires calculation of impedance, just as in electrical systems with alternating current. **Impedance** calculations can be made for both the pulmonary and systemic systems; however, they require calculations using high-fidelity pressure and velocity or flow recordings in the frequency domain, as described earlier in this chapter (3, 4). Such determinations are generally beyond the realm of routine clinical catheterization, although they are useful in hemodynamic research with particular regard to the intricacies of ventricular–vascular coupling.

Sources of error in calculation of vascular resistance arise from measurement of pressure and flow, usually cardiac output. Technical aspects of proper pressure measurement are outlined in this chapter, and similar considerations are applied to various techniques for determination of flow in Chapter 21. Standard methods for calculation of pulmonary vascular resistance have been criticized for possible influences from direct or indirect changes in critical closing pressure of pulmonary vessels. Such influences may be related to increased alveolar pressure such as may be seen with positive pressure ventilation or with pathophysiologic alterations in patients with chronic obstructive pulmonary disease (19). Despite these concerns, both pulmonary vascular resistance and total pulmonary resistance remain useful and valid expressions in the majority of cases.

SUMMARY

Of all hemodynamic measurements performed in the modern cardiac catheterization laboratory, pressure determination should be the most accurate and precise. This depends, however, on meticulous attention to detail and knowledge of catheters, transducers, recording systems, and the characteristics thereof. Accurate pressure measurement is extremely important in assessing the severity and functional significance of many pathophysiologic states, as discussed elsewhere in this volume. Invasive cardiologists should be especially aware of proper technique for pressure measurement and pitfalls involved therein. Combined with careful determination of blood flow, as outlined in Chapter 21, determination of vascular resistance adds another dimension to the hemodynamic description of a given pathophysiologic state only possible with accurate invasive measurement.

References

1. Geddes LA. The direct measurement of blood pressure. Chicago: Year Book Medical Publishers, 1970.
2. Luciani L. Human physiology (Welby FA, trans). London: Macmillan, 1911;1:592.
3. Milnor WR. Hemodynamics. Baltimore: Williams & Wilkins, 1982.
4. Nichols WW, O'Rourke MF. McDonald's blood flow in arteries. 3rd ed. Philadelphia: Lea & Febiger, 1990.
5. Geddes LE, Baker LE. Principles of applied biomedical instrumentation. New York: John Wiley & Sons, 1975.
6. Gabe IT. Pressure measurement in experimental physiology. In: Bergel DH, ed. Cardiovascular fluid dynamics. London: Academic Press, 1972;1:11–50.
7. Miller HD, Baker LE. A stable ultraminiature catheter tip pressure transducer. Med Biol Eng 1973;11:86–89.
8. Patel DJ, Mason OT, Ross J, Braunwald E. Harmonic analysis of pressure pulses obtained from the heart and great vessels of man. Am Heart J 1965;69:785–794.
9. Nichols WW, Pepine CJ, Conti CR. Catheter tip manometer system: pressure and velocity system. In: Ghista DN, ed. Advances in cardiovascular physics. New York: S. Karger, 1983;5:144–176.
10. Gersch BJ, Hahn CEW, Prys-Roberts C. Physical criteria for measurement of left ventricular pressure and its first derivative. Cardiovasc Res 1971; 5:32–40.
11. Murgo JP, Westerhof N, Giolma JP, Altobelli SA. Aortic input impedance in normal man: relationship to pressure waveforms. Circulation 1980;62:105–116.
12. Murgo JP, Westerhof N, Giolma JP, Altobelli SA. Manipulation of ascending aortic pressure and flow wave reflections with the Valsalva maneuver: relationship to input impedance. Circulation 1981; 63:122–132.
13. O'Rourke MF. Arterial function in health and disease. New York: Churchill Livingstone, 1982.
14. Haskell RJ, French WJ. Accuracy of left atrial and pulmonary artery wedge pressure in pure mitral regurgitation in predicting left ventricular end-diastolic pressure. Am J Cardiol 1988;61:136–141.
15. Maron BJ, Bonow RO, Cannon RO, et al. Hypertrophic cardiomyopathy: interrelations of clinical manifestations, pathophysiology, and therapy (Part 1). N Engl J Med 1987;316:780–789.
16. Maron BJ, Bonow RO, Cannon RO, et al. Hypertrophic cardiomyopathy: interrelations of clinical manifestations, pathophysiology, and therapy (Part 2). N Engl J Med 1987;316:844–852.
17. Murgo JP, Alter BR, Dorethy JF, et al. Dynamics of left ventricular ejection in obstructive and nonobstructive hypertrophic cardiomyopathy. J Clin Invest 1980;66:1369–1382.
18. Barratt-Boyes BG, Wood EH. Cardiac output and related measurements and pressure values in the right heart and associated vessels together with an analysis of the hemodynamic response to the inhalation of high oxygen mixtures in healthy subjects. J Clin Lab Med 1958;51:72–82.
19. McGregor M, Sniderman A. On pulmonary vascular resistance: the need for more precise definition. Am J Cardiol 1985;55:217–222.

23

Shunt Detection and Quantification

David C. Mayer, MD

INTRODUCTION

Because of echocardiography the cardiologist usually begins a cardiac catheterization in a child with a firm understanding of the intracardiac and great vessel anomalies, including central shunts. Transthoracic and transesophageal echocardiography together can reveal almost as much detail in the adult with congenital heart disease. The role of cardiac catheterization in adults with central shunts remains in the quantification of systemic and pulmonary blood flows and shunts. These data are vital to the timing and selection of catheter-based and surgical management.

This chapter focuses primarily on the use of oximetry (Fick method), as it is the major method used in most cardiac catheterization centers to detect and quantify central shunts. The major goal of this discussion is to provide practical information for the invasive cardiologist to use oximetric data to determine the systemic and pulmonary blood flows, the magnitude of the shunt or shunts, and the pulmonary-to-systemic flow ratio. A detailed explanation of **oximetric definitions** and normal blood O_2 values is presented as an introduction to these methods. This chapter also briefly discusses a much older method to detect and quantitate central shunts. This method, which uses indocyanine green (Cardiogreen) dye curves, is presented because it is still the reference standard with which other methods are usually compared. Finally, the noninvasive method of evaluating flows and flow ratios with two-dimensional and Doppler echocardiography is presented and integrated with the more commonly used Fick method.

OXYGEN IN BLOOD

Dissolved Oxygen, Oxygen Capacity, Oxygen Saturation, and Oxygen Content

When blood is exposed to gaseous O_2, O_2 is both dissolved in plasma and bound to hemoglobin. The amount of O_2 dissolved in plasma is determined by its solubility coefficient, temperature, and its partial pressure (pO_2). At 37°C, the solubility coefficient of O_2 in plasma is 0.03 mL/liter blood/mm Hg pO_2. Therefore, at a normal body temperature of 37°C, arterial blood with a pO_2 of 100 mm Hg has a **dissolved O_2** concentration of 3 mL/liter of blood. This amount of O_2 dissolved in plasma is relatively insignificant compared with the amount bound to hemoglobin. The maximal amount of O_2 that can be bound by hemoglobin is the **O_2 capacity.** Each gram of normal adult hemoglobin is capable of binding 1.36 mL of O_2. With a hemoglobin of 15 g/dL the calculated O_2 capacity is 204 mL/liter of blood (1.36 mL O_2/g × 15 g/dL × 10 dL/L).

In practice the most common way to evaluate blood O_2 uses **spectrophotometry** to measure the **O₂ saturation.** Spectrophotometry is based on Beer's law (1): "The absorption of light by a solution is a function of the concentration of its solute(s) and the depth of the solution." The absorption coefficients for light transmission of oxyhemoglobin and deoxyhemoglobin are measured at two different wavelengths, 600 nm for oxyhemoglobin, 506.5 nm for deoxyhemoglobin. The difference in the amount of light absorbed is proportional to the concentration of each form of hemoglobin. The concentrations of oxyhemoglobin and deoxyhemoglobin are determined from this difference in absorption. Thus the O₂ saturation is computed by the following:

$$percent\ O_2\ saturation =$$

$$\frac{oxyhemoglobin}{oxyhemoglobin + deoxyhemoglobin} \times 100$$

The spectrophotometric method of measuring O₂ saturation is relatively reliable, but a few sources of error are noteworthy (2). Clinical spectrophotometers cannot distinguish between carboxyhemoglobin and oxyhemoglobin, as they absorb light at virtually the same wavelength. This may be a major source of error in heavy smokers. Bilirubin also absorbs light at the same wavelength as oxyhemoglobin, so a marked elevation in serum bilirubin falsely increases the measured O₂ saturation. To circumvent these sources of error O₂ saturations should be calculated from the O₂–hemoglobin dissociation curve and the pO₂. In the absence of hyperbilirubinemia and elevated carboxyhemoglobin levels, the direct measurement of O₂ saturation has the advantage of being independent of factors that increase (alkalosis, hypothermia, fetal hemoglobin) or decrease (acidosis, fever) the affinity of hemoglobin for O₂ (Fig. 23.1).

O₂ content is the total quantity of O₂ in any blood sample, both combined with hemoglobin and dissolved in plasma. It is expressed as milliliters of O₂/100 mL blood (vol %) or as milliliters of O₂/liter of blood. The O₂ content can be directly measured by the manometric technique of Van Slyke and Neill (3), but this requires a large volume of blood and is time-consuming (20 to 30 minutes per sample). In most catheterization laboratories the O₂ content is calculated by multiplying the O₂ saturation by the O₂

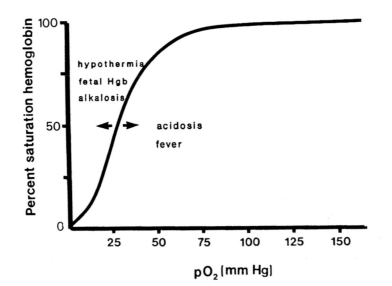

Figure 23.1. O₂–hemoglobin dissociation curve. This curve can be used to determine the percent O₂ saturation of hemoglobin at any given level of dissolved O₂ (pO₂) and vice versa. However, this curve can be shifted to the right or to the left (*arrows*) under the clinical situations indicated. Dissolved O₂ concentrations greater than 80 mm Hg are associated with very small increases in the percent O₂ saturation of hemoglobin.

capacity and adding the amount of dissolved O_2.

When the patient is breathing room air, adding the dissolved O_2 to determine the O_2 content is generally not necessary, since the relative amount of dissolved O_2 is negligible. For example, with a hemoglobin of 15 g/dL, the O_2 capacity is 1.36 mL O_2/g hemoglobin $\times$ 15 g/dL $\times$ 10 dL/L = 204 mL O_2/L blood. If the measured arterial O_2 saturation were 95%, the amount of O_2 bound to hemoglobin would be 0.95 $\times$ 204 mL O_2/L blood = 194 mL O_2/L blood. With a room air arterial pO_2 of 100 mm Hg, the dissolved O_2 would add only 3 mL O_2/liter blood (0.03 mL O_2/L blood/mm Hg pO_2 $\times$ 100 mm Hg). In this case the dissolved O_2 makes up only 1.5% of the total O_2 content.

$$\frac{3}{194 + 3} \times 100$$

However, if this same patient is breathing 100% O_2 and the arterial pO_2 increases to 600 mm Hg, 18 mL dissolved O_2/L blood (0.03 mL O_2/L blood/mm Hg pO_2 $\times$ 600 mm Hg) is added to the O_2 content. With the patient breathing 100% O_2, the O_2 saturation of the blood increases to 100%, and therefore the O_2 bound to hemoglobin increases to 204 mL O_2/liter blood (1 $\times$ 204 mL O_2/L blood). In this case the dissolved O_2 makes up 8% of the total O_2 content in the blood:

$$\frac{18}{204 + 18} \times 100$$

If this same patient, breathing 100% O_2, is anemic, with a hemoglobin of 8 g/100 mL, the O_2 capacity decreases to 109 mL O_2/liter blood (1.36 mL O_2/g hemoglobin $\times$ 8 g/dL $\times$ 10 dL/L). Dissolved O_2 makes up 14% of the total O_2 content.

$$\frac{18}{109 + 18} \times 100$$

This discussion shows that dissolved O_2 must be included in the O_2 content when shunts and flows are calculated in a patient breathing supplemental O_2, particularly if the subject is anemic. Therefore, a blood gas analyzer for the direct measurement of pO_2, a spectrophotometer for the direct measurement of O_2 saturation, and the capability to measure hemoglobin concentration are essential to a modern cardiac catheterization laboratory.

NORMAL BLOOD OXYGEN LEVELS

A major problem in using oximetry to detect and quantify central shunts involves determining the true **mixed venous O_2 saturation.** Even in the absence of a central shunt, blood samples in cardiac chambers proximal to the pulmonary artery yield unreliable measurements of mixed venous O_2 saturation because of streaming from the veins that enter the right heart. Blood enters the right atrium from three major sources. The superior vena cava (SVC) has an O_2 saturation of approximately 75%; the inferior vena cava (IVC) O_2 saturation is generally 5 to 7% higher because of highly saturated renal venous blood entering the IVC; and the coronary sinus saturation is in the range of 40 to 50%. **Complete mixing with a true average of the systemic venous return does not occur until blood enters the pulmonary artery.** Therefore, in the absence of a central shunt, the mixed venous O_2 saturation is most reliably obtained from the pulmonary artery.

When a central left-to-right shunt is present, the pulmonary artery saturation cannot be used because the pulmonary artery contains both mixed venous blood and well-oxygenated blood from the shunt. However, **studies of normal individuals without central shunts demonstrate that superior vena cava O_2 saturation very closely approximates the true mixed venous O_2 saturation found in the pulmonary artery.** Therefore, by convention, most catheterization laboratories use the SVC saturation as the mixed venous O_2 saturation in the detection and quantification of central shunts. The exception to this is left-to-right shunt proximal to or at the level of the SVC, such as anomalous pulmonary venous drainage into the SVC. In these patients the mixed venous O_2 saturation should be obtained

Table 23.1.
Normal Oxygen Saturations (Percent)

Site	Average	Range
Superior vena cava	74	67–83
Inferior vena cava	78	65–87
Right atrium	75	65–87
Right ventricle	75	67–84
Pulmonary artery	75	67–84
Left atrium	95	92–98
Left ventricle	95	93–98
Systemic artery	95	92–98

from the high SVC or innominate vein. Table 23.1 lists normal O_2 saturation data collected from various studies (1, 2, 4–6).

TECHNIQUES OF BLOOD SAMPLING

A common problem with using oximetry for the detection and quantification of central shunts occurs when blood samples in the various cardiac chambers and vessels are obtained over a relatively long time under changing conditions in the patient (e.g., changes in level of activity, respiration, heart rate). Ideally, samples should be obtained as quickly and accurately as possible. For this reason most operators prefer to begin the saturation run by sampling in the branch pulmonary arteries and withdrawing the catheter for sampling in the main pulmonary artery, right ventricle, and right atrium. Sampling in the superior and inferior vena cavae is then quickly performed. A femoral arterial (i.e., systemic arterial) sample is also obtained. If a patent foramen ovale or atrial septal defect (ASD) exists, the venous catheter can be advanced for sampling into the left atrium and left ventricle. Finally the catheter tip can be manipulated into one or two pulmonary veins to complete the saturation run. If the left heart chambers cannot be entered and a right-to-left intracardiac shunt is not suspected, the systemic arterial O_2 saturation obtained from the femoral artery may be substituted for the left atrial O_2 saturation in the calculation of flows and shunts.

It is important to record the time and

location of each sample to ascertain that sampling occurred over a relatively short time while the patient's condition remained unchanged. One must be careful when obtaining samples from angiographic catheters with multiple side holes (i.e., pigtail catheters). It is difficult to locate the sampling site accurately with these catheters. With any catheter it is important to flush the catheter well to obtain a true sample of blood from each site of interest.

SHUNT DETECTION BY OXIMETRY

Left-to-Right Shunts

Modern spectrophotometry equipment can measure blood O_2 saturations with an accuracy of approximately plus or minus 2%. The error is plus or minus 1% at O_2 saturations around 95% and plus or minus 2.5% at values around 70%. O_2 saturations measured by this method are relatively accurate to values of 40 to 50%. Spectrophotometry is not reliable at O_2 saturations lower than this (1). If necessary, saturations below 50% should be checked by the blood gas method (measuring the pO_2 and determining the O_2 saturation from the O_2–hemoglobin dissociation curve; Fig. 23.1).

Studies have been performed to determine the minimum change in the level of O_2 saturation required to demonstrate a left-to-right shunt (2). In adults chamber-to-chamber right heart O_2 saturation differences as small as 3% (right ventricle to pulmonary artery) or as large as 9% (SVC to pulmonary artery) reliably detect a left-to-right shunt. In practical terms an increase of 3% in O_2 saturation from the SVC to any downstream right heart chamber or vessel should raise the suspicion of a left-to-right shunt. An increase of 5% or more is considered to be definite evidence of a left-to-right shunt. **The ability to detect a left-to-right shunt reliably varies with the cardiac output.** If output is high and mixed venous blood is relatively well saturated, a shunt must be fairly large to be detected by oximetry. For example, if the mixed venous saturation measured in the SVC is 85% and pulmonary venous saturation is 95%, in the presence of a 2:1 left-to-right shunt (pulmonary flow twice systemic flow), the saturation in the pulmonary artery is 90%, or only 5% above the mixed venous saturation. Given a lower cardiac output with a mixed venous saturation of 75% and the same pulmonary venous saturation of 95%, the same 2:1 left-to-right shunt results in a pulmonary artery saturation of 85% (a 10% step up from the mixed venous saturation). Therefore, relatively small shunts (less than 2:1) can go undetected by oximetry in the presence of high cardiac output, low systemic O_2 extraction, and high mixed venous O_2 saturation.

Multiple sites of shunting can affect the ability to detect left-to-right shunting by oximetry. As an example, consider a patient with an ASD and a ventricular septal defect (VSD) with a systemic blood flow of 5 L/minute. At the atrial level 5 L/minute of pulmonary venous blood with an O_2 saturation of 95% crosses the ASD and mixes with 5 L/minute of systemic venous return with an O_2 saturation of 80%. The O_2 saturation of the 10 L/minute of blood entering the right ventricle is 87.5%, a significant increase, 7.5%, over the mixed venous saturation in the SVC. Then an additional 5 L/minute of blood with an O_2 saturation of 95% crosses the VSD to mix with the blood entering from the right atrium, resulting in a 15 L/minute flow of blood with an O_2 saturation of 90% entering the pulmonary artery. This increase of only 2.5% in the O_2 saturation from the right ventricle to pulmonary artery is not considered significant even though the shunt flow at the ventricular level is equal to that at the atrial level (Fig. 23.2).

Sampling errors can influence shunt de-

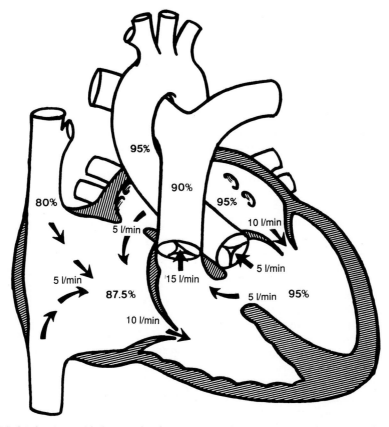

Figure 23.2. Multiple sites of left-to-right shunts affect the accuracy of detection of individual ones. As one moves downstream from right atrium to pulmonary artery, the ability to locate and quantify multiple left-to-right shunts decreases.

tection. Perimembranous or supracristal ventricular septal defects shunt saturated blood into the distal right ventricular outflow tract, resulting in streaming of saturated and desaturated blood within the main pulmonary artery. A left-to-right shunt may go undetected if only one sample is obtained from the desaturated stream in the main pulmonary artery. Sampling in the branch pulmonary arteries allows for specimen collection from blood that is better mixed downstream from the shunt. Falsely elevated mixed venous saturation from the SVC can occur with a VSD and tricuspid regurgitation or with a left ventricular to right atrial communication. In both instances well-saturated blood may regurgitate into the distal SVC. For this reason one should also measure the O_2 saturation of the blood in either the high SVC or the innominate vein.

Right-to-Left Shunts

Right-to-left shunts are detected by a decrease in O_2 saturation in left-sided cardiac chambers or vessels. For example, right-to-left shunting across the VSD in a patient with tetralogy of Fallot is detected by a decrease in O_2 saturation from the left atrium to the ascending aorta or femoral artery. For the purpose of precisely defining the level of right-to-left shunting with oximetry, a true measure of the mixed pulmonary venous O_2 saturation is sought. Ideally this measurement comes from a pulmonary venous sample. Many patients with congenital heart defects have an associated ASD or patent foramen ovale that readily allows the passage of a venous catheter into the left atrium and one or more pulmonary veins. However, O_2 saturations from the different pulmonary veins may vary widely. In normal individuals the lower (most dependent) portion of the lung has the lowest pulmonary venous O_2 saturation. Many children and adults with congenital heart lesions have atelectasis, as when left atrial enlargement causes compression of the left mainstem bronchus, and the pulmonary venous return from the atelectatic lung is desaturated.

For these reasons, in the absence of other indicators of right-to-left shunting at the atrial level, many cardiologists prefer to use the left atrial saturation as the mixed pulmonary venous O_2 saturation. As is the case for detection of left-to-right shunts, it is important to obtain blood samples as rapidly and as accurately as possible to avoid skewed results because of changes in the patient's condition.

No firm data as to how large a drop in O_2 saturation may be considered significant in detecting right-to-left shunts are available. A reasonable suspicion is justified when a decrease of at least 2 to 3% is detected (2). Decrements smaller than this may be explained by physiologic right-to-left shunting from thebesian and coronary veins draining into the left ventricle or left atrium or from bronchial veins draining into the left atrium or a pulmonary vein.

Detection of *small* right-to-left shunts is more easily accomplished via changes in the pO_2 rather than O_2 saturations. Pulmonary venous pO_2 in a normal young or middle-aged adult is approximately 100 mm Hg. A decrease to 70 mm Hg, measured in a downstream left-sided cardiac chamber or vessel, indicates a small right-to-left shunt that may not be detected by comparisons of the O_2 saturations. This is due to flattening of the O_2–hemoglobin dissociation curve at pO_2 levels at least 70 mm Hg, wherein large changes in pO_2 above 70 mm Hg do not result in large increases in O_2 saturation (Fig. 23.1).

If the left atrium cannot easily be entered because of an intact atrial septum, detection of a small right-to-left shunt by oximetry is extremely difficult. In the absence of pulmonary disease or hypoventilation because of heavy sedation, a systemic artery O_2 saturation of less than 95% strongly suggests an intracardiac right-to-left shunt. In equivocal cases one may measure systemic arterial pO_2 before and 10 minutes after 100% O_2 inhalation. If the systemic desaturation is due to a pulmonary ventilation–perfusion abnormality, the pO_2 usually rises above 300 mm Hg, but with a true right-to-left intracardiac shunt the pO_2 will not rise to these levels.

QUANTIFYING INTRACARDIAC SHUNTS AND BLOOD FLOW BY OXIMETRY

Fick Principle

All measurements of blood flow and shunt volumes are based on the indicator dilution method. This method is explained in detail in Chapter 18. Briefly, a known quantity of an indicator is added to fluid flowing through a pipe; thorough mixing of the indicator with the fluid is assumed. The concentration of indicator with respect to the time is measured downstream. Following the time course of indicator concentration from appearance to disappearance allows calculation of flow. Alternatively, instead of measuring the addition of an indicator to the fluid, one can measure removal of the indicator. This is the basis for measuring cardiac output by the Fick principle, which uses O_2 as the indicator. The formula:

$$Qs = CO = \frac{\dot{V}O_2}{A\dot{V}O_2 \ difference}$$

Qs (systemic blood flow) or CO (cardiac output) is the volume of blood delivered to the systemic circulation per unit time (liters/minute). $A\dot{V}O_2$ *difference* (arterial–venous O_2 difference) is the volume of O_2 extracted from the systemic circulation per volume of blood (mL O_2/L blood). $\dot{V}O_2$ (O_2 consumption) is the volume of O_2 consumed by the body per unit time (mL O_2/minute). The Fick principle also applies to the flow of blood across the pulmonary vascular bed (Qp), where:

$$Qp = \frac{\dot{V}O_2}{A\dot{V}O_2 \ difference \ across \ the \ lungs}$$

O$_2$ Consumption

In modern catheterization laboratories $\dot{V}O_2$ (O_2 consumption) is measured by a polarographic O_2 sensor (7). The device is zeroed by drawing room air through it. The patient's expired air is captured in a plastic hood placed over the head. All expired air mixed with room air is drawn across the O_2 sensor at a known constant rate. Since the volume of the air drawn through the hood is known and the initial O_2 concentration is known to be 20.93% (room air), the concentration of O_2 measured at the sensor can be used to calculate how much O_2 has been consumed by the patient. Modern $\dot{V}O_2$ instruments assume a respiratory exchange ratio of 0.85 between O_2 and CO_2. If O_2 consumption cannot be measured, one can use the tables of LaFarge and Miettinen (8) to estimate $\dot{V}O_2$ (Table 23.2). This $\dot{V}O_2$ table is based on calculations of average values from many normal sedated individuals and thus may not pertain to an individual patient's condition.

Quantification of Intracardiac Shunts

To calculate systemic blood flow (Qs), pulmonary blood flow (Qp), and the volumes of intracardiac shunts, one must know the $\dot{V}O_2$ and the O_2 saturations in the pulmonary artery (PA), the pulmonary veins or left atrium (PV or LA), a systemic artery (SA), and the mixed venous saturation (MV; commonly obtained from the SVC). It is important to collect these saturations as rapidly as possible to avoid any change in the patient's condition. **Accuracy depends on collecting truly representative samples** of the systemic and pulmonary venous returns (MV and PV), as well as thoroughly mixed samples distal to the shunt or shunts (SA and PA).

A left-to-right shunt is the amount of pulmonary venous (saturated) blood that bypasses the systemic vascular bed. A right-to-left shunt is the amount of systemic venous (desaturated) blood that bypasses the pulmonary vascular bed. The Qep (effective pulmonary blood flow) is the amount of systemic venous desaturated blood that is carried to the pulmonary vascular bed. The Qep is *equal* to the amount of pulmonary venous saturated blood that is delivered to the systemic capillaries. Qp/Qs is the ratio of pulmonary blood flow to systemic blood flow and is usually expressed with the denominator equal to 1. Table 23.3 gives the formulas required for quantitating intracardiac shunts and blood flow by oximetry.

Table 23.2.
Oxygen Consumption per Body Surface Area in Milliliters per Minute per Square Meter by Gender, Age, and Heart Rate

Age	Heart Rate (beats per minute)												
	50	60	70	80	90	100	110	120	130	140	150	160	170
Male patients													
3				155	159	163	167	171	175	178	182	186	190
4			149	152	156	160	163	168	171	175	179	182	186
6		141	144	148	151	155	159	162	167	171	174	178	181
8		136	141	145	148	152	156	159	163	167	171	175	178
10	130	134	139	142	146	149	153	157	160	165	169	172	176
12	128	132	136	140	144	147	151	155	158	162	167	170	174
14	127	130	134	137	142	146	149	153	157	160	165	169	172
16	125	129	132	136	141	144	148	152	155	159	162	167	
18	124	127	131	135	139	143	147	150	154	157	161	166	
20	123	126	130	134	137	142	145	149	153	156	160	165	
25	120	124	127	131	135	139	143	147	150	154	157		
30	118	122	125	129	133	136	141	145	148	152	155		
35	116	120	124	127	131	135	139	143	147	150			
40	115	119	122	126	130	133	137	141	145	149			
Female patients													
3				150	153	157	161	165	169	172	176	180	183
4			141	145	149	152	156	159	163	168	171	175	179
6		130	134	137	142	146	149	153	156	160	165	168	172
8		125	129	133	136	141	144	148	152	155	159	163	167
10	118	122	125	129	133	136	141	144	148	152	155	159	163
12	115	119	122	126	130	133	137	141	145	149	152	156	160
14	112	116	120	123	127	131	134	138	143	146	150	153	157
16	109	114	118	121	125	128	132	136	140	144	148	151	
18	107	111	116	119	123	127	130	134	137	142	146	149	
20	106	109	114	118	121	125	128	132	136	140	144	148	
25	102	106	109	114	118	121	125	128	132	136	140		
30	99	103	106	110	115	118	122	125	129	133	136		
35	97	100	104	107	111	116	119	123	127	130			
50	94	98	102	105	109	112	117	121	124	128			

Examples of Shunt Calculations

Example 1: Left-to-Right Shunt

This patient has a VSD. The hemoglobin is 15 g/dL, resulting in an O_2 capacity of 204 mL O_2/L blood ($15 \times 1.36 \times 10$). The O_2 consumption is measured to be 102 mL O_2/minute. The following O_2 saturations are obtained: systemic artery (SA), 95%; superior vena cava (MV), 75%; left atrium (PV), 95%; pulmonary artery (PA), 85%. Thus:

$$Qp = \frac{102}{(0.95 - 0.85)\,(204)} = 5 \text{ L/minute}$$

$$Qs = \frac{102}{(0.95 - 0.75)\,(204)} = 2.5 \text{ L/minute}$$

$$Qep = \frac{102}{(0.95 - 0.75)\,(204)} = 2.5 \text{ L/minute}$$

$$left\text{-}to\text{-}right\ shunt = Qp - Qep = 5 - 2.5 = 2.5 \text{ L/minute}$$

$$right\text{-}to\text{-}left\ shunt = Qs - Qep = 2.5 - 2.5 = 0$$

$$\frac{0.85 - 0.75}{0.95 - 0.75} \times 100 = 50\%$$

Figure 23.3 presents these data in the form of a box diagram. In this patient the left-to-right shunt equals the Qep. Thus total blood flow through the pulmonary circuit is twice that of the systemic circuit (Qp/Qs = 2/1). The magnitude of the shunt flow is often expressed as a percentage of the pulmonary blood flow. Thus 50% (2.5 L/minute) of the 5 L/minute total pulmonary blood flow is shunted blood. The patient has a 50% left-to-right shunt. The relation between Qp/Qs ratio and percent left-to-right shunt is expo-

Table 23.3.
Formulas for Quantifying Intracardiac Shunts and Blood Flows by Oximetry

	Room Air			Patient on Supplemental O_2
$QP =$	$\dfrac{VO_2}{PVO_2 \text{ content} - PAO_2 \text{ content}}$	$=$	$\dfrac{VO_2}{(Pv_{sat} - Pa_{sat})(O_2 \text{ capacity})}$	$= \dfrac{VO_2}{[Pv_{sat} \times O_2 \text{ capacity}) + PVO_2 \text{ diss}] - [(Pa_{sat} \times O_2 \text{ capacity}) + PAO_2 \text{ diss}]}$
$Qs =$	$\dfrac{VO_2}{SAO_2 \text{ content} - MVO_2 \text{ content}}$	$=$	$\dfrac{VO_2}{(Sa_{sat} - Mv_{sat})(O_2 \text{ capacity})}$	$= \dfrac{VO_2}{[(Sa_{sat} \times O_2 \text{ capacity}) + SAO_2 \text{ diss}] - [Mv_{sat} \times O_2 \text{ capacity}) + MVO_2 \text{ diss}]}$
$Qep =$	$\dfrac{VO_2}{PVO_2 \text{ content} - MVO_2 \text{ content}}$	$=$	$\dfrac{VO_2}{(Pv_{sat} - Mv_{sat})(O_2 \text{ capacity})}$	$= \dfrac{VO_2}{[(Pv_{sat} \times O_2 \text{ capacity}) + PVO_2 \text{ diss}] - [(Mv_{sat} \times O_2 \text{ capacity}) + MVO_2 \text{ diss}]}$
			$Qp/Qs = \dfrac{Sa_{sat} - Mv_{sat}}{Pv_{sat} - PA_{sat}}$	
	$L \rightarrow R \text{ shunt} = Qp - Qep$		$\%L \rightarrow R \text{ shunt} = \dfrac{Pa_{sat} - MV_{sat}}{Pv_{sat} - MV_{sat}} \times 100$	
	$R \rightarrow L \text{ shunt} = Qs - Qep$		$\%R \rightarrow L \text{ shunt} = \dfrac{PV_{sat} - SA_{sat}}{Pv_{sat} - Mv_{sat}} \times 100$	

O_2 content (mL/L), dissolved oxygen plus oxygen bound to hemoglobin; O_2 capacity (mL/L), $1.36 \times$ Hbg (gm/dl) $\times$ 10; O_2 diss (mL/L), dissolved $O_2 = pO_2 \times 0.03$ mL/L; Op (L/min), pulmonary blood flow; Qs (L/min), systemic blood flow; Qep (L/min), effective pulmonary blood flow; $L \rightarrow R$ shunt (L/min), amount of oxygenated blood that bypasses the systemic vascular bed; $R \rightarrow L$ shunt (L/min), amount of deoxygenated blood that bypasses the pulmonary vascular bed; PV_{sat}, pulmonary vein (or left atrium) oxygen saturation; PA_{sat}, pulmonary artery oxygen saturation; SA_{sat}, systemic artery oxygen saturation; MV_{sat}, mixed venous (usually superior vena cava) oxygen saturation; $\%L \rightarrow R$, $L \rightarrow R$ shunt expressed as percentage of pulmonary blood flow (Qp); $\%R \rightarrow L$, $R \rightarrow L$ shunt expressed as percentage of systemic blood flow (Qs).

nential. This is important to consider when estimating large shunts. For example, an increase in left-to-right shunt from 75 to 83% is associated with a change in Qp/Qs ratios from 4/1 to 6/1 (Fig. 23.4). Large shunts (above 80%) should probably just be expressed as a shunt greater than 80% and/or a Qp/Qs ratio greater than 5/1.

Example 2: Right-to-Left Shunt
This patient has tetralogy of Fallot (VSD with infundibular and valvular pulmonary stenosis). The hemoglobin is 16.9 g/dL with an O_2 capacity of 230 mL O_2/liter. $\dot{V}O_2$ is measured at 115 mL O_2/minute. The O_2 saturations are PV, 95%; SA, 85%; MVi, 70%; PA, 70%.

$$Qp = \frac{115}{(0.95 - 0.70)(230)} = 2.0 \; L/minute$$

$$Qs = \frac{115}{(0.85 - 0.70)(230)} = 3.3 \; L/minute$$

$$Qep = \frac{115}{(0.95 - 0.70)(230)} = 2.0 \; L/minute$$

left-to-right shunt

$$= Qp - Qep = 2 - 2 = 0$$

right-to-left shunt

$$= Qs - Qep = 3.3 - 2 = 1.3 \; L/minute$$

% right-to-left shunt

$$= \frac{0.95 - 0.85}{0.95 - 0.70} \times 100 = 40\%$$

In this example, as in all cases of pure right-to-left shunting, the pulmonary/systemic flow ratio (Qp/Qs) is less than 1.

$$Qp/Qs = \frac{0.85 - 0.70}{0.95 - 0.70} = 0.6 \; L/minute$$

Figure 23.5 is the box diagram of this patient's catheterization data. As in the first example, the amount of blood flow through either vascular bed (systemic or pulmonary) is Qep plus any volume shunted back to that vascular bed. In this example sys-

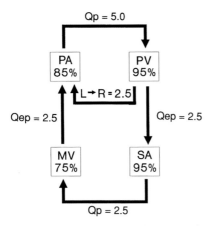

Figure 23.3. Example 1. Box diagram of a left-to-right shunt across a ventricular septal defect. Units for flow (Qp, Qs, Qep, and so on) and shunts (L → R, R → L) are in liters per minute. Numbers in boxes are percent O_2 saturation of hemoglobin measured from various cardiac chambers. *PV*, pulmonary vein; *SA*, systemic artery; *MV*, mixed venous (superior vena cava); PA, pulmonary artery. Arrows, blood flow or shunt from one cardiac chamber to another. See Table 23.3 for complete definitions of abbreviations.

temic blood flow is the Qep (all of the pulmonary venous return, or 2 L/minute), plus the right-to-left shunt (1.3 L/minute). The pulmonary blood flow is the Qep only; no left-to-right shunt is present.

Example 3: Bidirectional Shunt (Left-to-Right and Right-to-Left Shunts)
This patient had a palliative pulmonary artery banding to restrict pulmonary blood

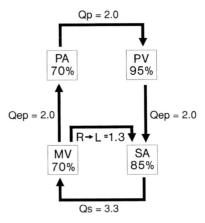

Figure 23.5. Example 2. Box diagram of right-to-left shunt in patient with tetralogy of Fallot. See Table 23.3 for definitions of abbreviations.

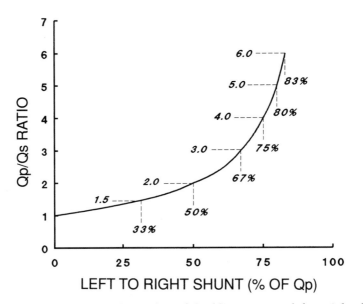

Figure 23.4. Exponential relationship of Qp/Qs to percent left-to-right shunt.

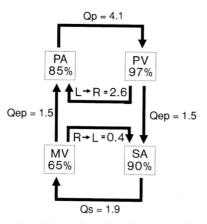

Figure 23.6. Example 3. Box diagram of bidirectional (right-to-left and left-to-right) shunts in patient with a ventricular septal defect and pulmonary artery band. See Table 23.3 for definitions of abbreviations.

flow because of a large left-to-right shunt across a VSD. The $\dot{V}O_2$ was 108 mL O_2/minute; hemoglobin was 16 g/dL; O_2 capacity was 218 mL O_2/minute. O_2 saturations were measured: PV, 97%; SA, 90%; MVi, 65%; PA, 85%.

$$Qp = \frac{108}{(0.97 - 0.85)(218)} = 4.1 \; L/minute$$

$$Qs = \frac{108}{(0.90 - 0.65)(218)} = 1.9 \; L/minute$$

$$Qep = \frac{108}{(0.97 - 0.65)(218)} = 1.5 \; L/minute$$

left-to-right shunt

$$= Qp - Qep = 4.1 - 1.5 = 2.6 \; L/minute$$

percent left-to-right shunt

$$= \frac{0.85 - 0.65}{0.97 - 0.65} \times 100 = 63\%$$

right-to-left shunt

$$= Qs - Qep = 1.9 - 1.5 = 0.4 \; L/minute$$

percent right-to-left shunt

$$= \frac{0.97 - 0.90}{0.97 - 0.65} \times 100 = 22\%$$

Figure 23.6 displays the data in the box diagram format. Although the patient has a bidirectional shunt, the magnitude of the left-

to-right shunt is approximately five times that of the right-to-left shunt, and pulmonary blood flow is twice systemic blood flow (Qp/Qs).

$$Qp/Qs = \frac{0.90 - 0.65}{0.97 - 0.85} = 2.1 \; L/minute$$

As before, the Qep is the same on both sides of the diagram because the volume of systemic venous blood going to the pulmonary circulation has to be equal to the volume of pulmonary venous blood that perfuses the systemic circulation.

Example 4: Left-to-Right Shunt During Oxygen Inhalation
In practice, including the dissolved O_2 in calculating pulmonary blood flow is important only in patients with left-to-right shunts who are breathing high concentrations of O_2. For example, a man has a large VSD and a measured $\dot{V}O_2$ of 160 mL O_2/minute. The hemoglobin is 12.5 g/dL. Therefore, the O_2 capacity is 170 mL O_2/L ($1.36 \times 12.5 \times 10 = 170$). The patient is breathing 100% O_2 and the following measurements are made: pulmonary vein O_2 saturation is 100% with a pO_2 of 500 mm Hg; pulmonary artery saturation is 95%, with a pO_2 equal to 80 mm Hg. The O_2 content of the pulmonary venous blood is 185 mL O_2/liter, consisting of 170 mL O_2/liter bound to hemoglobin ($1 \times 170 = 170$) plus 15 mL O_2/liter of dissolved O_2 (500 mm Hg $\times$ 0.03 mL O_2/L/mm Hg = 15 mL O_2/L). In the pulmonary artery the O_2 content is 163.9 mL O_2/liter (161.5 mL O_2/L bound to hemoglobin, plus 2.4 mL O_2/L O_2 dissolved in plasma). If one calculated the Qp using only the O_2 combined with hemoglobin, this would be the pulmonary blood flow:

$$Qp = \frac{160}{170 - 161.5} = 18.8 \; L/minute$$

However, if the dissolved O_2 values were included, the Qp would be calculated as follows:

$$Qp = \frac{160}{185 - 163.9} = 7.6 \; L/minute$$

As this example demonstrates, the dissolved O_2 must be included to determine the true O_2 contents of the pulmonary vein and artery whenever calculating the Qp in a patient breathing O_2 who has a left-to-right shunt. This is true especially if the patient is anemic, as the percentage of O_2 content that is made up of dissolved O_2 is even higher in patients with a low O_2 capacity.

Example 5: Multiple Left-to-Right Shunts
In practice the presence of multiple levels of shunting is important from an anatomic rather than a hemodynamic standpoint. The presence of multiple shunts is frequently known from precatheterization studies such as two-dimensional and Doppler echocardiography. In the usual situation one is interested primarily in quantitating the total amount of shunting. In fact, it is usually difficult to quantitate the relative contributions of shunting from each defect, primarily because complete mixing does not occur at each level.

Rather than using formulas for determining two left-to-right shunts, it is easier to determine the Qp, Qs, Qep, and left-to-right shunt as if only one shunt were present. Figure 23.7 diagrams the shunts, flows, and O_2 saturations in a patient with an ASD and a VSD. In this individual the $\dot{V}O_2$ is 135 mL O_2/minute, the hemoglobin is 13 g/dL,

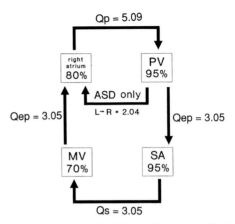

Figure 23.8. Example 5. Box diagram of left-to-right shunt from ASD alone in the patient from Figure 23.7 with an ASD and a VSD. See Table 23.3 for definitions of abbreviations.

and the O_2 capacity is 176.8 mL O_2/liter. The saturations are as shown in Figure 23.7.

The following calculations are made:

$$Qs = \frac{135}{(0.95 - 0.70)\,(176.8)} = 3.05\ L/minute$$

$$Qep = \frac{135}{(0.95 - 0.70)\,(176.8)} = 3.05\ L/minute$$

$$= 7.64\ L/minute$$

$$Qp = \frac{135}{(0.95 - 0.85)\,(176.8)} = 7.64\ L/minute$$

left-to-right shunt
$$= Qp - Qep = 7.64 - 3.05 = 4.59\ L/minute.$$

In this patient the total left-to-right shunt across the ASD and the VSD is 4.59 L/minute. How much of this shunt flows across the ASD alone can be calculated if one assumes complete mixing of saturated and desaturated blood in the right atrium. Figure 23.8 diagrams this situation if just the ASD is present. In this instance the Qs and Qep remain the same, but the Qp is recalculated as follows:

$$Qp = \frac{135}{(0.95 - 0.80)\,(176.8)} = 5.09\ L/minute$$

The left-to-right shunt from the ASD alone is calculated:

left-to-right shunt from ASD alone = Qp − Qep
$$= 5.09 - 3.05 = 2.04\ L/minute$$

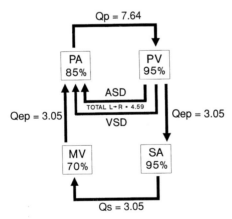

Figure 23.7. Example 4. Box diagram of two left-to-right shunts in patient with an atrial septal defect (ASD) and ventricular septal defect (VSD). Total left-to-right shunt resulting from both defects is shown (Total L → R shunt = 4. 59 L/minute). See Table 23.3 for definitions of abbreviations.

The contribution of the VSD left-to-right shunt to the total left-to-right shunt is obtained by subtracting 2.04 L/minute (ASD shunt alone) from 4.59 L/minute (ASD and VSD shunt total). The VSD contribution to the total left-to-right shunt equals 2.55 L/minute in this example.

INDICATOR DILUTION STUDIES

In years past dye dilution curves were used extensively for measuring cardiac output and to detect and quantify intracardiac shunts and valvular regurgitation (see Chapter 18). Many indicators or dyes have been used, but indocyanine green (Cardiogreen) became the standard in the 1960s. Indocyanine green is nontoxic, nonstaining, and soluble, and it absorbs light at a wavelength (805 nm) that is unaffected by the level of hemoglobin O_2 saturation. The light absorption of indocyanine green has a nearly linear relation to its concentration in the blood.

Although dye dilution curves are an accurate and reproducible method of evaluating cardiac physiology, their use has diminished in recent years because they are relatively cumbersome compared with newer techniques. Cardiac output can be accurately and more easily measured with thermodilution. Spectrophotometry for measuring blood O_2 saturation and polarography for measuring O_2 consumption have allowed accurate measurement of blood flows and accurate detection and quantitation of most intracardiac shunts. Echocardiography and angiography at 60 frames per second are the indicator dilution studies (e.g., bubbles and contrast medium) now used to define the anatomic details of almost all intracardiac shunts. Today dye dilution curves are rarely necessary.

Cardiac Output

To measure the cardiac output with indocyanine green, a calibration factor is deter-

mined, first by diluting a known amount of dye in a sample of the patient's blood so that the final concentration is 2.5 or 5 mg of indocyanine green per liter. This sample is drawn through a densitometer capable of measuring the concentration of green dye. The height that the calibration line is displaced from the baseline equals 2.5 or 5 mg/L (Fig. 23.9*A*). A known amount of green dye, usually 5 mg, is injected into the patient's venous system, usually into the pulmonary artery. Simultaneously, a constant flow of blood is withdrawn from the femoral artery into the densitometer, which measures the concentration of green dye with respect to time. A green dye curve is inscribed as illustrated in Figure 23.9*A*.

As stated in the section explaining the Fick principle, all catheterization methods of measuring cardiac output use an indicator dilution method. That is, one injects a known quantity of indicator and measures the concentration of the indicator downstream with respect to time. However, since the body is a closed system, recirculation of the indicator occurs before the initial bolus of indicator has completely passed downstream. **To determine cardiac output from a green dye curve, one must determine how much of the indicator concentration is due to the first pass and not to recycling.**

One method to assess recirculation is to plot the exponential disappearance of the green dye from the circulation on a three-cycle semilog graph (Figure 23.9*B*). If no recirculation occurred, the green dye would disappear in a linear fashion. However, in most patients the blood and dye recirculate about 10 seconds after the initial appearance of the dye. Where the straight line breaks is the beginning of recirculation. The straight line is extrapolated from the point where recirculation begins to 1% of the peak concentration of green dye (the point where the first pass is assumed to be complete). The average concentration of the green dye during the first pass is then calculated. To do this, one sums all of the first-pass deflections in millimeters per second and then divides this by the time in seconds required for the first pass to be complete. This average deflection during the first pass is multiplied by the calibration factor to give the average concentration during the first pass

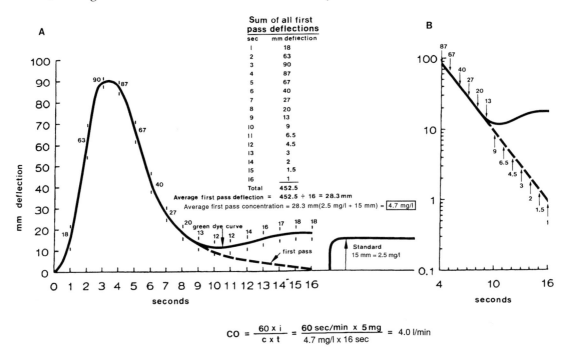

$$CO = \frac{60 \times i}{c \times t} = \frac{60 \text{ sec/min} \times 5 \text{mg}}{4.7 \text{ mg/l} \times 16 \text{ sec}} = 4.0 \text{ l/min}$$

Figure 23.9. Standard method of calculating cardiac output with indocyanine green. **A.** To calibrate the densitometer, a volume of the patient's arterial or venous blood is thoroughly mixed with a quantity of green dye to make a final concentration of 2.5 mg green dye per liter of blood. In this example, when specimen is drawn through the densitometer, it causes a deflection of 15 mm (as shown in lower right hand corner of **A**). Therefore, the standard calibration is 15 mm = 2.5 mg/ liter blood. Next 5 mg of green dye is injected into the patient's venous system (SVC or IVC) while a constant flow of blood is withdrawn from the femoral artery into the densitometer. As shown on the left side of **A**, by convention the green dye is first detected in the femoral artery at time 0. At 3 seconds the green dye curve is near its peak deflection at 90 mm. (Numbers shown along solid line curve give the height of deflection in mm for each second.) Beginning at 9 seconds the curve begins to rise a second time because of recirculation of dye. *Dashed line* labeled "first pass" indicates disappearance of dye if no recirculation occurred. **B.** To determine average first-pass concentration, disappearance of dye from the circulation is plotted on a three-cycle semilog graph (*solid line*). The straight line breaks at the beginning of recirculation. This straight line is extrapolated to 1% of the peak deflection (*dashed line*). First-pass deflections are summed and divided by the time in seconds of the first pass to give average first-pass deflection. Since the calibration standard of 2.5 mg/liter caused a 15-mm deflection, the average first-pass concentration in this example is 4.7 mg/liter (see earlier calculations). Cardiac output is then calculated from the equation shown at the bottom of this figure. *CO*, cardiac output; *60*, 60 seconds/minute; *i*, amount of green dye injected into the patient; *c*, average first pass concentration; and *t*, time of first pass deflection.

(Fig. 23.9*B*). The cardiac output is calculated by the following formula (9):

$$CO = \frac{60 \times i}{c \times t}$$

Where t = time of first pass (seconds), c = average concentration during first pass (milligrams per liter), i = amount green dye injected (mg), and 60 = 60 seconds/minute.

All formulas for calculating cardiac output from green dye curves entail determining the area under the curve inscribed by the first pass of dye. An easy and widely accepted alternative approach is the **forward triangle method,** which assumes that the area of the initial portion of the curve is proportional to the total area of the curve (Fig. 23.10). This method does not require plotting the disappearance of green dye

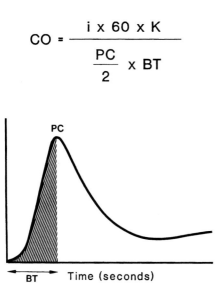

$$CO = \frac{i \times 60 \times K}{\frac{PC}{2} \times BT}$$

Figure 23.10. Forward triangle method of calculating cardiac output from a green dye curve (injection into the main pulmonary artery and withdrawal from the femoral artery). Peak concentration (PC) is determined by multiplying peak deflection (mm) by the calibration standard (milligrams per liter per millimeter). Calibration standard is not shown in this figure, but it is performed in the manner shown in Figure 23.9*A*. *CO*, cardiac output in liters per minute; *i*, amount injected in mg; *K*, constant of 0.37 or 0.35; *PC*, peak concentration in milligrams per liter; *BT*, buildup time to peak concentration.

from the circulation. If dye is injected into a peripheral vein, the initial portion of the curve represents 35% of the total area (37% if dye is injected centrally). The following formula was described by Hetzel et al. (10):

$$CO = \frac{i \times 60 \times K}{\frac{PC}{2} \times BT}$$

Where CO = cardiac output in L/minute, i = amount injected in mg, 60 = 60 seconds/minute, K = constant of 0.35 or 0.37, PC = peak concentration in milligrams per liter, and BT = buildup time in seconds to reach peak concentration.

Determining cardiac output from a green dye curve with the forward triangle method is especially useful in left-to-right shunts. In these situations recirculation of dye occurs earlier than usual in the downslope of the first-pass curve, which hampers

the ability to plot the disappearance of the dye from the bloodstream.

SHUNT DETECTION AND QUANTIFICATION BY INDICATOR DILUTION TECHNIQUES

Left-to-Right-Shunts

As stated previously, green dye curves are now rarely used for detecting intracardiac left-to-right shunts because improvements in oximetry, echocardiography, and angiography have made shunt detection easier. Figure 23.11 shows examples of detection of left-to-right shunts with green dye curves. Generally dye is injected into the main pulmonary artery and sampling is from the femoral artery. With modern angiography and echocardiography shunt localization by changing the injection and withdrawal sites is no longer required. Left-to-right shunts cause a lower peak concentration than normal curves because a percentage of the dye injected recirculates through the lungs rather than going directly to the sampling point in the arterial system. Left-to-right shunts decrease the slope of the downslope because the dye that recirculates through the lungs prolongs the appearance of the dye at the sampling point. Large left-to-right shunts depress the peak concentration and prolong the disappearance of the dye at the sampling site more than small left-to-right shunts.

Determining the amount of left-to-right shunting from a green dye curve with a smooth downstroke is best done with the Carter formula (11) (Fig. 23.12). This method determines the percentage of pulmonary blood flow that is due to left-to-right shunting based on the concentration of green dye at the arterial sampling site at twice and three times the time to peak concentration. The two values are averaged. If shunt recirculation is discrete, the formula of Victorica and Gessner (12) should be used. A dye curve of this type is illustrated in Figure 23.13. This method determines the percentage of pulmonary blood flow due to

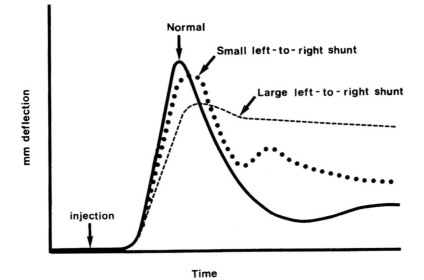

Figure 23.11. Detection of left-to-right shunts with green dye curves. For these examples dye is injected into the main pulmonary artery and sampling is from the femoral artery. The larger the left-to-right shunt, the lower the peak concentration and the more prolonged the disappearance of the dye at the sampling point.

left-to-right shunting from a simple ratio of the shunt peak concentration (P_2) to the primary peak due to pulmonary blood flow (P_1). Quantitating left-to-right shunts from the green dye curves using either of these methods can detect shunts greater than approximately 25 to 30%. Smaller shunts can be detected by inspection of the dye curves, but small left-to-right shunts cannot be accurately measured with these methods.

Right-to-Left Shunts

At present the major practical application of green dye curves is for detecting small right-to-left shunts that would not be measurable by oximetry. For example, a systemic arterial O_2 saturation of 93% and a left atrial O_2 saturation of 95% constitute equivocal evidence of a right-to-left shunt. Injecting green dye into the inferior vena cava and sampling in the femoral artery reveal an early appearance of the dye if a right-to-left shunt is present (Fig. 23.14). Green dye injected into the right heart that bypasses the pulmonary circulation arrives at a sampling site in a systemic artery much earlier than via normal

circulation through the lungs. The greater the magnitude of the early peak, the greater the percentage of right-to-left shunting. By changing the injection site and comparing the resulting curves, the site of right-to-left shunting can be determined. The most common situation entails localizing a right-to-left shunt to the atrial level. Injection into the right atrium with sampling from the femoral artery results in a curve with early appearance and subsequent recirculation of dye. The term **early appearance** is relative. It can be affected by hemodynamics, especially cardiac output, and technical aspects of performing and timing the injection. Therefore the injection site is moved to the right ventricle or main pulmonary (withdrawal continues from the femoral artery) and the resulting curve is compared with that obtained from the previous injection into the right atrium. As mentioned previously, shunt localization is readily performed with echocardiography and angiography. The major utility of green dye curves is to clarify the magnitude of the shunt.

The methods of quantifying right-to-left shunts are based on modifications of the forward triangle method, which determines the ratio of the magnitude of the early peak

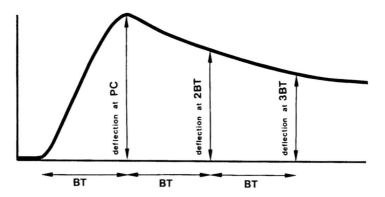

BT = buildup time (to peak concentration)

% Qp = percent of pulmonary blood flow
due to left-to-right shunt

$$\% \ Qp = 142 \left(\frac{\text{height of deflection at 2BT}}{\text{height of deflection at PC}} \right) - 42$$

$$\% \ Qp = 135 \left(\frac{\text{height of deflection at 3BT}}{\text{height of deflection at PC}} \right) - 14$$

Figure 23.12. Calculation of percent of pulmonary blood flow due to a left-to-right shunt using a green dye curve and the Carter formula (injection into the IVC with sampling from the femoral artery).

(right-to-left shunt) to the magnitude of the second peak (normal systemic flow). Figure 23.15 shows calculation of the percentage of systemic blood flow due to an atrial right-to-left shunt in which the dye is injected into the inferior vena cava and sampling is from the aorta. Right-to-left shunts as small as 2.5 to 5% of the systemic blood flow can be measured by this method (13).

QUANTIFYING FLOWS AND SHUNTS WITH TWO-DIMENSIONAL AND DOPPLER ECHOCARDIOGRAPHY

Pulmonary and systemic flow can be calculated from echocardiography data with the following formula (14):

Volumeric flow (L/minute)

$$= \frac{V \times CSA \times 60 \ seconds/minute}{100 \ cm_3/L}$$

Where V = mean velocity of flow (centimeters/second)

CSA = cross-sectional area (square centimeters)

Pulmonary blood flow (Qp) is usually measured by determining the mean velocity of flow from the Doppler spectral tracing distal to the pulmonary valve and measuring the cross-sectional area at the pulmonary annulus. Systemic blood flow (Qs) is usually measured by determining these same parameters in the ascending aorta and aortic annulus. However, other sites can be used depending on whether or not an intra-

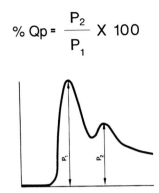

$$\% Qp = \frac{P_2}{P_1} \times 100$$

% Qp = percent of pulmonary blood flow
   due to left-to-right shunt

P_1 = height of first peak (mm)

P_2 = height of second peak (mm)

Figure 23.13. Calculation of percent of pulmonary blood flow due to a left-to-right shunt using the method of Victorica and Gessner (injection into the main pulmonary artery with sampling from the thoracic descending aorta). This method is useful if the green dye curve has a discrete recirculation peak (P_2).

$$\% Qs = \frac{(BT_1)(PC_1)}{(BT_1)(PC_1) + 0.44(T_2)(PC_2)} \times 100$$

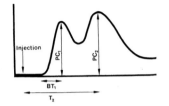

% Qs = percent of systemic blood flow
   due to right-to-left shunt

PC_1 = height of first peak (mm)

BT_1 = buildup time from appearance
   time to PC_1

PC_2 = height of second peak (mm)

T_2 = time from injection to PC_2

0.44 = constant

Figure 23.15. Calculation of percent of systemic blood flow due to a right-to-left shunt. For this example dye is injected to the inferior vena cava and sampling is from the abdominal aorta.

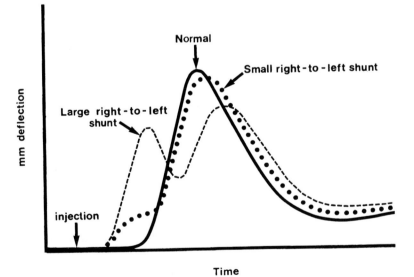

Figure 23.14. Detection of right-to-left shunts with green dye curves (injection into the inferior vena cava with sampling from the femoral artery). The larger the right-to-left shunt, the greater the magnitude of the early peak due to dye that bypasses the normal pulmonary circulation.

cardiac shunt is present and where it is. The magnitude of an intracardiac left-to-right shunt can be determined by calculating the pulmonary-to-systemic flow ratio (Qp/Qs).

Calculation of Mean Velocity

Mean velocity of flow is calculated from the Doppler spectral tracing. Most modern echocardiography machines have computer programs that allow calculation of the integrated area within the Doppler curve or the velocity time integral divided by the flow period of the traced beats. If a computer program is not available, the area under the curve can be calculated manually by drawing a straight line from the peak velocity to the baseline to divide the Doppler spectral tracing into two right triangles. The area of each triangle is one-half the base times the height. The areas of the two triangles are added, and this value is divided by the R-R interval in seconds to give the mean velocity of flow. Whichever method is used, the mean velocities of several Doppler spectral tracings should be measured and averaged.

There are two major sources of error in measuring mean velocity of flow with this technique. The first arises from the assumption that the velocity profile is uniform throughout the cross-sectional area of the vessel (15). For example, with a large left-to-right shunt or a left-to-right shunt close to the pulmonary artery, Doppler tracings from the pulmonary artery show spectral broadening, a sign of disturbed flow. In these cases a uniform velocity profile should not be assumed and another site should be chosen (mitral valve in a patient with a VSD) to calculate mean velocity of flow for the determination of pulmonary blood flow. The second source of error arises from the difficulty in recording the flow velocity in the center of the vessel with the Doppler beam parallel to the direction of flow so that no correction for intercept angle is required. Despite these two limitations, Gardin et al. (16) have shown good reproducibility in Doppler-derived measurements of mean velocity. In this study aortic mean velocity showed intraobserver variability of 3.2% plus or minus 2.9%, inter-observer variability of 5.4% plus or minus

3.4%, and day-to-day variability of 3.8% plus or minus 3.1%.

Calculation of Cross-Sectional Area

Vessel cross-sectional area is calculated by measuring the vessel diameter (usually annulus diameter) from the two-dimensional echocardiogram. The vessel is assumed to be circular and the formula for calculation of the area of the circle is CSA $= \pi(d^2)/4$, where d is the diameter.

The valve annulus is usually chosen as the site for measurement of vessel diameter because it is the smallest area, or flow-limiting point, in the vessel. The diameter is measured in early systole so the vessel is at or near its peak systolic dimension. Inaccurate measurement of the vessel or annulus diameter is the *major* source of error in determining flow and flow ratios by the two-dimensional and Doppler echo techniques. As can be seen from the equation for calculating the vessel cross-sectional area in which the value of the diameter is squared, a small change in the measured diameter results in a large change in the calculated area. Measuring the vessel diameter at the pulmonary annulus is particularly difficult. First, it is usually impossible to image the pulmonary artery in a view that allows axial resolution of the structures (i.e., the ultrasound beam cannot be aligned perpendicular to the walls of the vessel). Second, it is often impossible to visualize the left lateral border of the pulmonary artery or pulmonary artery annulus because of interference from adjacent lung tissue. Finally, with increasing flow the diameter of the pulmonary artery changes far more than that of the aorta. This reflects differences in the elasticity of the two vessels more than flow changes (17).

Clinical Applications

Studies (18–20) in patients with left-to-right shunts have shown that Doppler-derived values for Qp, Qs, and Qp/Qs correlated well with data obtained at cardiac catheterization using the Fick technique (oximetry). Correlation coefficients for systemic blood flow range from 0.78 to 0.91, with standard error of the estimate ranging from 0.6 to 0.81 L/minute. Similar correlation coefficients have been reported with pulmonary blood flow measurements but with a broader range in the standard error (range 1.1 to 2.4 L/minute). The Qp/Qs correlation coefficients have been reported at approximately 0.85 with a standard error of approximately 0.5.

SUMMARY

Central shunts today are routinely detected by the noninvasive methods of two-dimensional and Doppler transthoracic and transesophageal echocardiography. Although pulmonary and systemic blood flows and the pulmonary-to-systemic blood flow ratio can be estimated with echocardiography, the current standard of quantifying flows and shunts remains with analyzing oximetric data obtained during cardiac catheterization. This is true particularly in adults with limited echocardiographic windows, which may preclude accurate measurements of flow velocities or vessel diameters. Angiography is extremely useful for locating intracardiac or great vessel shunts. The older method, using indocyanine green dye injections and analyzing curves of concentration versus time, is comparatively cumbersome and therefore rarely used to locate or quantify central shunts. To quantify flows and shunts precisely using oximetric data, one must collect truly representative samples of the systemic and pulmonary venous returns and completely mixed samples distal to the shunt or shunts (systemic and pulmonary arteries). If these samples are collected at nearly the same time to avoid significant changes in the patient's condition and if dissolved O_2 is included in the measurements obtained from patients breathing supplemental O_2, calculations of flows and shunts using the Fick technique are extremely accurate.

References

1. Vargo TA. Cardiac catheterization: hemodynamic measurements. In: Garson A, Bricker JT, McNamara DG, eds. The science and practice of pediatric cardiology, vol 2. Philadelphia: Lea & Febiger, 1990:913–946.
2. Lock JE. Hemodynamic evaluation of congenital heart disease. In: Lock JE, Keane JF, Fellows KE, eds. Diagnostic and interventional catheterization in congenital heart disease. Boston: Martinus Nijhoff, 1987:33–62.
3. Van Slyke DD, Neill JM. Blood gases: 1. J Biol Chem 1924;61:523–573.
4. Pongpanich B, Ritter DG, Ougley PA. Hemodynamic findings in children without significant heart disease. Mayo Clin Proc 1969;44:13–24.
5. Freed MD. Invasive diagnostic and therapeutic techniques: 1. cardiac catheterization. In: Adams FH, Emmanouilides GC, Riemenschneider TA, eds. Moss' heart disease in infants, children, and adolescents. 4th ed. Baltimore: Williams & Wilkins, 1989:130–146.
6. Antman EM, Marsh JD, Green LH, Grossman W. Blood O_2 measurements in the assessment of intracardiac left to right shunts: a critical appraisal of methodology. Am J Cardiol 1980;46:265–271.
7. Lister G, Hoffman JIE, Rudolph AM. O_2 uptake in infants and children: a simple method for measurement. Pediatrics 1974;53:656–662.
8. LaFarge CG, Miettinen OS. The estimation of O_2 consumption. Cardiovasc Res 1970;4:23–30.
9. Hamilton WF, Moore JW, Kinsman JM, Spurling RG. Studies on the circulation: 4. Further analysis of the injection method and of changes in hemodynamics under physiological and pathological conditions. Am J Physiol 1932;99:534–551.
10. Hetzel PS, Swan HJC, Ramirez-DeArellano A, Wood EH. Estimation of cardiac output from first part of arterial dye dilution curves. J Appl Physiol 1958;13:92–96.
11. Carter SA, Bajec SF, Yannicelli E, Wood EH. Estimation of left to right shunts from arterial dilution curves. J Lab Clin Med 1960;55:77–88.
12. Victorica BE, Gessner IH. A simplified method for quantitating left-to-right shunts from arterial dilution curves. Circulation 1975;51:530–534.
13. Swan HJC, Zapata-Diaz J, Wood EH. Dye dilution curves in cyanotic congenital heart disease. Circulation 1953;8:70–81.
14. Nishimura RA, Callahan MJ, Schaff HV. Noninvasive measurement of cardiac output by continuous wave Doppler echocardiography: initial experience and review of the literature. Mayo Clin Proc 1984;59:484–489.
15. Snider AR, Serwer GA, eds. Echocardiography in pediatric heart disease. Chicago: Year Book, 1990.
16. Gardin JM, Tobis JM, Dabestani A. Superiority of two-dimensional measurement of aortic vessel diameter in Doppler echocardiographic estimates of left ventricular stroke volume. J Am Coll Cardiol 1985;6:66–74.
17. Stewart WJ, Jiang L, Mich R. Variable effects of changes in flow rate through the aortic, pulmonary, and mitral valves on valve area and flow ve-

locity: impact on quantitative Doppler flow calculations. J Am Coll Cardiol 1985;6:653–662.

18. Sanders SP, Yeager S, Williams RG. Measurements of systemic and pulmonary blood flow and Qp/Qs ratio using Doppler and two-dimensional echocardiography. Am J Cardiol 1983;51:952–956.

19. Barron JV, Sahn DJ, Valdes-Cruz LM. Clinical utility of two-dimensional Doppler echocardiographic techniques for estimating pulmonary to systemic blood flow ratios in children with left to right shunting atrial septal defect, ventricular septal defect, or patent ductus arteriosus. J Am Coll Cardiol 1984;3:169–178.

20. Goldberg SJ, Sahn DJ, Allen HD. Evaluation of pulmonary and systemic blood flow by 2-dimensional Doppler echocardiography using fast Fourier transform spectral analysis. Am J Cardiol 1982;50:1394–1400.

24
Assessment of Cardiovascular Function

Richard A. Lange, MD
L. David Hillis, MD

INTRODUCTION

A complete evaluation of the cardiovascular system entails an assessment of both anatomic and functional cardiac abnormalities. With physiologic testing, one may (*a*) assess the functional significance of an anatomic abnormality and (*b*) obtain prognostic and therapeutic information. Such a functional assessment may be performed during exercise (dynamic or isometric), rapid atrial pacing, a variety of hemodynamic maneuvers, and several pharmacologic interventions. The proper selection of each method and interpretation of the results require knowledge of the normal responses to each, as well as of the alterations produced by various kinds of cardiac disease.

PHYSIOLOGIC STRESS

Dynamic Exercise

Responses in Normal Subjects

In the cardiac catheterization laboratory, dynamic exercise is usually performed by bicycle ergometry with the subject in the supine position. In the exercise laboratory, it is performed by bicycle ergometry with the subject in the upright position or, more commonly, by having the subject walk or jog on a treadmill. During stepwise increases in the intensity of exertion, oxygen consumption, cardiac output, and intracardiac pressures can be measured, and the electrocardiogram (ECG) may be observed. From these variables, one may assess the cardiac response to exercise.

Dynamic exercise increases oxygen demand. The primary function of the cardiovascular system is to ensure that oxygen supply rises commensurately with the increase in oxygen demand. The relation between oxygen consumption and workload is linear until the maximal oxygen consumption is reached (Fig. 24.1) (1), at which time continued exercise is not accompanied by a further increase in oxygen consumption. As a result, **lactic acid** accumulates (2–4); minute ventilation increases disproportionately in comparison with cardiac output (the so-called ventilatory threshold); and exercise endurance declines (5). Although anaerobic metabolism may provide adequate energy for a brief period of exercise, it cannot sustain prolonged activity. Because anaerobic glycolysis may be present at rest in some individuals, and exercise-induced increases in lactate production may be caused by reduced lactate metabolism, some have suggested use of the term lactate

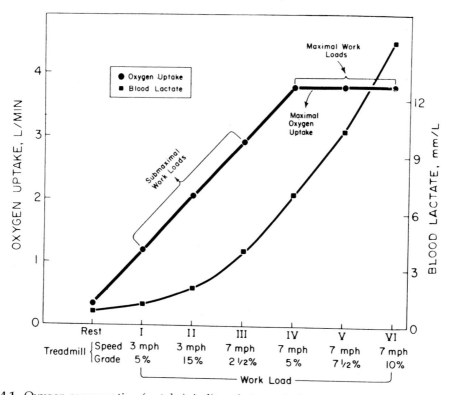

Figure 24.1. Oxygen consumption (uptake), in liters/minute (L/min), at increasing workloads. Note that this relation is linear until the maximal oxygen uptake is reached. Changes in blood lactate concentration are also shown. (Reprinted with permission from Mitchell JH, Blomqvist G. Maximal oxygen uptake. N Engl J Med 1971;284:1018–1022.)

threshold—rather than anaerobic threshold—to identify the maximal oxygen consumption at which the serum lactate concentration begins to increase dramatically.

Oxygen consumption is determined by cardiac output and the arteriovenous oxygen difference. Thus, if pulmonary function and the oxygen concentration of ambient air are normal, the maximal oxygen consumption is an index of maximal cardiovascular function. In patients with **coronary artery disease,** maximal oxygen consumption is usually 1 to 2 L/min; in normal sedentary individuals, it is approximately 3 L/min; and in endurance athletes, it may be as much as 6 L/min. Because the **maximal arteriovenous oxygen difference** is similar in these various individuals, the differences in maximal oxygen consumption are the result of differences in maximal cardiac output.

There is a linear relation between car-

diac output and oxygen consumption (Fig. 24.2). This relation, termed the exercise index, may be used to assess whether cardiac output during exercise is appropriate for a given oxygen consumption. A measured cardiac output less than 80% of that predicted (based on oxygen consumption) is considered abnormal. Similarly, cardiac output should increase by at least 600 mL/min for every 100 mL/min increase in O_2 consumption (the so-called exercise factor) (6). An exercise factor less than this indicates that the subject cannot respond to exercise by increasing cardiac output appropriately.

The hemodynamic responses to dynamic exercise are the result of a complex interplay of central and reflex neural mechanisms (7), local metabolic influences (8), and postural changes. In general, the response of the cardiovascular system is related to the intensity of physiologic stress. Heart rate increases early during exercise and rises linearly with increased exertion. During mild exercise, vagal withdrawal accounts for most of this chronotropic effect, whereas sympathetic activity predominates during intense exertion (9). Through complex humoral and neural interactions, blood flow is redistributed predominantly to working muscles, with a resultant decrease in systemic vascular resistance. Despite this fall in systemic vascular resistance, systolic and mean arterial pressures rise modestly because of a marked increase in cardiac output (10). Diastolic arterial pressure is usually unchanged or rises slightly, as do pulmonary arterial and pulmonary–capillary wedge pressures.

Hemodynamic responses to supine and upright exercise differ in certain respects. Resting left ventricular volumes are larger in the supine than in the standing position (11, 12), because venous return is diminished in the upright position. In comparison

with the supine position, the upright position at rest is accompanied by a higher heart rate and diastolic arterial pressure but a lower pulmonary–capillary wedge pressure, stroke volume, and cardiac output (10). With a comparable amount of exercise in the two positions, heart rate is higher in the upright position; pulmonary and intracardiac filling pressures are lower; and cardiac output is similar.

The increase in cardiac output that occurs with exercise is caused by an increase in both heart rate and stroke volume, but the contribution of each depends on the patient's position (13). Although stroke volume at maximal exercise is independent of position, the absolute and relative increases in stroke volume during exercise are greater in the upright position, because the initial stroke volume is lower in this position. Specifically, stroke volume increases by 20 to 50% with maximal exercise in the supine position (10, 14–16) and by approximately 100% in the upright position (13). Therefore, the increase

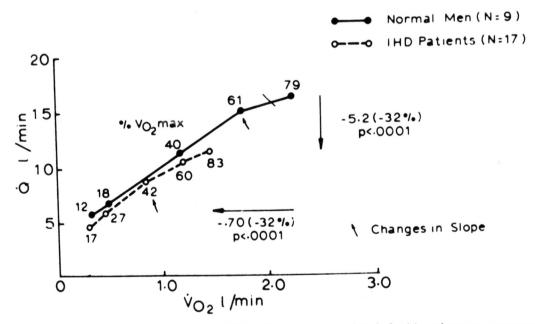

Figure 24.2. The relation of cardiac output (Q) in liters per minute (*vertical axis*), and oxygen consumption (*VO₂*) in liters/minute (*horizontal axis*), in normal men (*solid line*) and in patients with ischemic heart disease (IHD) (*dashed line*). Note that the normal subjects achieve a higher cardiac output and oxygen consumption than do those subjects with ischemic heart disease. (Reprinted with permission from Bruce RA, Petersen JL, Kusumi F. Hemodynamic responses to exercise in the upright posture in patients with ischemic heart disease. In: Dhalla HS, ed. Myocardial metabolism. Baltimore: University Park Press, 1973:849–865.)

in cardiac output in the supine position is primarily the result of an increased heart rate, whereas an increase in stroke volume contributes substantially to the increased cardiac output in the upright position.

The exercise-induced increase in stroke volume is caused by an increase in left ventricular contractility, which is caused by sympathetic nervous stimulation (17) and the Frank-Starling mechanism. The changes in left ventricular volumes that occur with mild to moderate exercise are shown in Figure 24.3. Both supine and upright exercise are accompanied by an increase in left ventricular end-diastolic volume and a decrease in end-systolic volume (14, 15, 18, 19); thus, ejection fraction increases. During intense exercise, left ventricular end-diastolic volume remains unchanged or decreases

slightly. However, increased myocardial contractility—as demonstrated by a decreased left ventricular end-systolic volume and increased ejection fraction—maintains stroke volume (Fig. 24.3). Hence, at low and moderate levels of exertion, the Frank-Starling mechanism predominates in increasing cardiac output; at peak exercise, enhanced contractility is the major mechanism for maintaining stroke volume (20, 21). In normals, left ventricular end-diastolic pressure is unchanged or falls slightly during exercise in young adults (22), whereas it usually rises modestly (by 6 to 8 mm Hg) in older adults (10, 23, 24). The diastolic pressure–volume relation is unchanged or shifted downward during exercise (Fig. 24.4) (25), indicating increased left ventricular compliance.

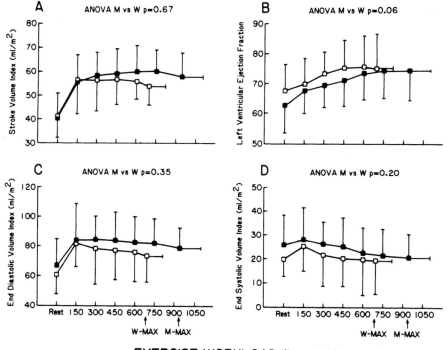

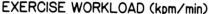

EXERCISE WORKLOAD (kpm/min)

Figure 24.3. Rest and exercise left ventricular stroke volume index (**A**), ejection fraction (**B**), end-diastolic volume index (**C**), and end-systolic volume index (**D**) in men (*M, closed squares*) and women (W, *open squares*). With intense exercise, left ventricular end-diastolic volume does not change or decreases slightly, but stroke volume is maintained because of a decrease in end-systolic volume. *MAX*, maximal. (Reprinted with permission from Sullivan MJ, Cobb FR, Higginbotham MB. Stroke volume increases by similar mechanisms during upright exercise in normal men and women. Am J Cardiol 1991;67:1405–1412.)

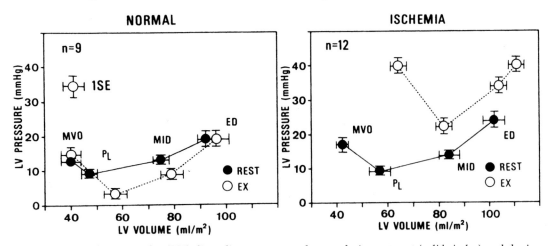

Figure 24.4. Left ventricular (*LV*) diastolic pressure–volume relations at rest (*solid circles*) and during exercise (*open circles*) in normal subjects (*normal*) and in patients with coronary artery disease (*ischemia*). With exercise, the pressure–volume curve shifts downward in the normal subjects (i.e., left ventricular compliance increases). In patients with exercise-induced ischemia, the pressure–volume curve shifts upward, indicating reduced left ventricular compliance. Coordinates of pressure and volume are shown for mitral valve opening (*MVO*), the lowest diastolic pressure (P_L), mid-diastole (*MID*), and end-diastole (*ED*). (Reprinted with permission from Nonogi H, Hess OM, Bortone AS, et al. Left ventricular pressure–length relation during exercise-induced ischemia. J Am Coll Cardiol 1989;13:1062–1070.)

Responses in Subjects with Cardiac Disease

Abnormalities in hemodynamic variables and in left ventricular function may be noted in patients with **coronary artery disease.** During submaximal exercise, these individuals often have normal oxygen consumption (26, 27) and maximal arteriovenous oxygen difference (i.e., a normal exercise index). During maximal exercise, however, cardiac output is reduced, owing primarily to a diminished stroke volume. Figure 24.5 displays the pathogenesis of this diminution in stroke volume. As in normal subjects, left ventricular end-diastolic volume increases with exercise, but end-systolic volume is unchanged or increases. Therefore, stroke volume is unchanged, and ejection fraction falls (15, 18, 25, 28–30). An increase in ejection fraction of less than 5 to 7% during exercise is considered abnormal, regardless of the subject's position (supine or upright) (18, 31). In patients with **coronary artery disease,** the changes in ejection fraction are often accompanied by segmen-

tal wall motion abnormalities (demonstrable by echocardiography (32), radionuclide ventriculography, or contrast ventriculography (14, 18, 29, 33–35).

Left ventricular diastolic function may be impaired in patients with **coronary artery disease** and may be manifested by impaired left ventricular filling (25, 29), an elevated left ventricular end-diastolic pressure (30), and an altered pressure–volume relation (15, 21, 25). In many patients, evidence of reduced left ventricular compliance precedes clinical and electrocardiographic evidence of ischemia. Figure 24.4 displays a diastolic pressure–volume relation at rest and during exercise-induced ischemia. During exercise, the curve is shifted upward so that a given end-diastolic volume is associated with an increased end-diastolic pressure. Consequently, pulmonary–capillary wedge and pulmonary arterial pressures may rise markedly during exercise in patients with exercise-induced ischemia (30, 36).

The specificity and sensitivity of routine exercise testing in identifying patients with **coronary artery disease** are improved if

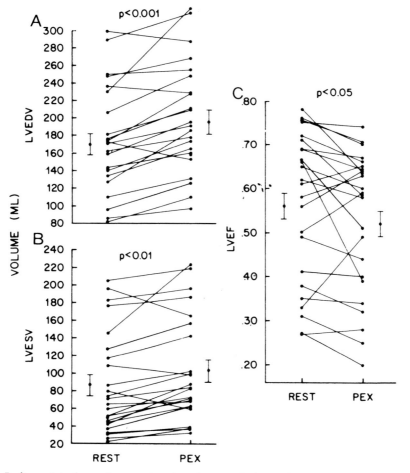

Figure 24.5. Left ventricular volumes at rest and at peak dynamic exercise (*PEX*) in patients with coronary artery disease. Each line represents the data from one patient, and the mean ± 1 SE is displayed on either side of each set of lines. At peak exercise, left ventricular end-diastolic volume (*LVEDV*, **A**) and left ventricular end-systolic volume (*LVESV*, **B**) increase, while ejection fraction (*LVEF*, **C**) declines. (Reprinted with permission from Dehmer GJ, Lewis SE, Hillis LD, et al. Exercise-induced alterations in left ventricular volumes and the pressure–volume relationship: a sensitive indicator of left ventricular dysfunction in patients with coronary artery disease. Circulation 1981; 63:1008–1018. By permission of the American Heart Association, Inc.)

these exercise-induced abnormalities of left ventricular systolic and diastolic function are added to standard clinical and electro-cardiographic variables (28, 37, 38). Although some authors report a sensitivity of 93 to 95% with such testing (33, 34), the specificity is lower because several kinds of cardiac disease other than **coronary artery disease** (i.e., dilated cardiomyopathy, hypertensive heart disease) may affect left ventricular performance during dynamic exercise (39–41).

The hemodynamic alterations that accompany physiologic stress in patients with **congestive heart failure** are well characterized. At rest, these patients usually have reduced right and left ventricular ejection fractions. The pulmonary–capillary wedge and pulmonary arterial pressures are elevated, as are the pulmonary and systemic vascular resistances. The severity of these resting hemodynamic derangements is reflective of the severity of heart failure (42, 43). With dynamic exercise, systemic vascular resistance falls, and pulmonary vascular resistance is unchanged (42, 44, 45). Oxygen consumption, systemic arterial pressure, cardiac output, heart rate, and stroke volume rise (42–45), but the magnitude of their increase is inadequate to meet oxygen demands, so that exercise tolerance and maximal oxygen consumption are diminished and anaerobic metabolism occurs at a low workload. In comparison with normal subjects, patients with **congestive heart failure** cannot manifest an appropriate increase in heart rate at an equivalent intensity of dynamic exercise (Fig. 24.6*A*) (46); in essence, they have "chronotropic incompetence" in response to stress. Similarly, these patients are unable to manifest an appropriate increase in systemic arterial pressure during exercise (Fig. 24.6*B*). The magnitude of the attenuated responses of heart rate and systemic arterial pressure to exercise is related to the severity of heart disease; it is caused by a blunted response of the sympathetic nervous system to exercise (46).

In subjects with heart failure, cardiac output rises during exercise, and the absolute change is determined by the severity of heart failure (Fig. 24.7) (43). As the magnitude of failure worsens, the exercise-induced increase in stroke volume declines because left ventricular end-diastolic and end-systolic volumes increase. In those with severe heart failure, the exercise-induced rise in cardiac output is almost entirely caused by an increase in heart rate (Fig. 24.7) (43). In these individuals, pulmonary–capillary wedge and pulmonary arterial pressures increase during exercise; so, at peak exercise, the wedge pressure may rise to 35 to 45 mm Hg, and the mean pulmonary arterial pressure may be 50 to 60 mm Hg (42–45, 47). Despite these marked exercise-induced increases in pulmonary–capillary wedge and pulmonary arterial pressures, the diminished exercise tolerance in patients with **congestive heart failure** is not the result of the ventilatory consequences of pulmonary congestion, because these patients do not manifest a decline in arterial oxygen tension or saturation or an increase in carbon dioxide tension with exercise (45). In addition, neither rest nor exercise pulmonary–capillary wedge pressures correlate with exercise tolerance.

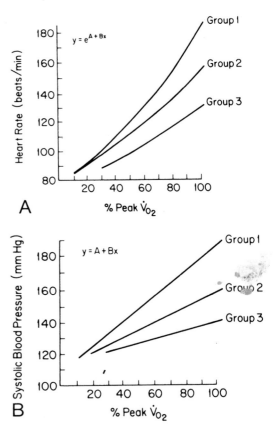

Figure 24.6. The relation of heart rate (**A**) and systolic blood pressure (**B**) (*vertical axes*) to the percent maximal oxygen consumption ($\dot{V}O_2$; *horizontal axes*) in normal subjects (group 1) and in patients with mild (group 2) or severe (group 3) congestive heart failure. Those with congestive heart failure cannot raise their heart rates or blood pressures to the same magnitude as normal subjects at similar relative work intensities. (Reprinted with permission from Francis GS, Goldsmith SR, Ziesche S, et al. Relative attenuation of sympathetic drive during exercise in patients with congestive heart failure. J Am Coll Cardiol 1985;5:832–839.)

Thus, in patients with **congestive heart failure,** exercise capacity is not limited by the pulmonary system, but rather by the inability of the cardiac system to increase cardiac output and oxygen delivery in response to increased demands (48).

Dynamic exercise testing may be used in patients with **congestive heart failure** to (*a*) grade the severity of heart failure objectively (49), (*b*) measure cardiac reserve (43),

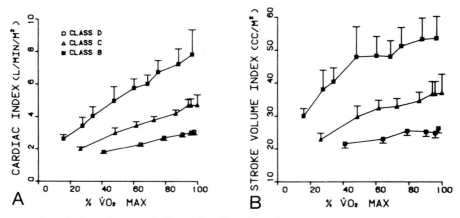

Figure 24.7. The relation of cardiac index (**A**) and stroke volume index (**B**) (*vertical axes*) to the percent maximal oxygen consumption ($\dot{V}O_2$; *horizontal axes*) in patients with mild (class B), moderate (class C), and severe (class D) congestive heart failure. With worsening heart failure, the increases in cardiac output and stroke volume that occur during dynamic exercise are attenuated. (Reprinted with permission from Weber KT, Kinasewitz GT, Janicki JS, et al. Oxygen utilization and ventilation during exercise in patients with chronic cardiac failure. Circulation 1982;65:1221–1223. By permission of the American Heart Association, Inc.)

Table 24.1.
Functional Classification Based on Maximal Oxygen Consumption

Class	Maximal Oxygen Consumption (mL/kg/min)
A	> 20
B	16–20
C	10–15
D	< 10

(*c*) quantitate the magnitude of improvement induced by a therapeutic intervention (50), and (*d*) provide information on prognosis (42). Historically, the severity of chronic **congestive heart failure** has been assessed subjectively, according to information provided by the patient (New York Heart Association [NYHA] classification). In contrast to this, a measurement of oxygen use during stress helps to provide a reproducible and objective assessment of the patient's cardiac status, and the quantitation of maximal oxygen consumption and anaerobic threshold provides an accurate reflection of functional capacity and cardiac reserve (Table 24.1). Such a functional classification offers valuable information concerning the severity of heart failure and the degree of cardiac reserve, and it is sub-

stantially more useful than resting hemodynamic variables (42, 43, 49).

Resting indices of left ventricular function correlate poorly with exercise capacity (49–55), and pharmacologic agents that improve resting left ventricular performance may not increase exercise capacity (56, 57). In contrast, maximal oxygen consumption and cardiac output during exercise correlate well with exercise capacity (42, 43, 58). Thus, functional classification of patients with **congestive heart failure** is best performed by dynamic exercise testing, rather than by assessment of resting hemodynamic variables.

Exercise capacity can provide information on prognosis, because short-term survival is improved in patients who achieve a high maximal oxygen consumption during exercise (Fig. 24.8). However, long-term survival cannot be predicted by exercise capacity (59). Although the efficacy of new pharmacologic agents for **congestive heart failure** is often assessed by measuring exercise capacity (60–64), the significance of this variable in assessing a drug response is not established.

In patients with **valvular heart disease,** dynamic exercise is used to help in assigning prognosis and to evaluate the efficacy of medical or surgical therapy. In addition,

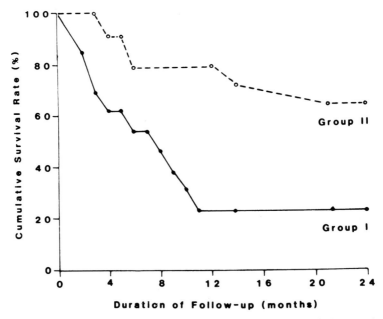

Figure 24.8. Cumulative survival rate for patients with congestive heart failure and severely (group I) or mildly (group II) impaired exercise tolerance over a 24-month period of observation. Those with severely impaired exercise tolerance (maximal oxygen consumption < 10 mL/kg/min) had a significantly higher mortality than those with only mildly impaired exercise tolerance (maximal oxygen consumption > 10 mL/kg/min). (Reprinted with permission from Szlachcic J, Massie BM, Kramer BL, et al. Correlates and prognostic implication of exercise capacity in chronic congestive heart failure. Am J Cardiol 1985;55:1037–1042.)

it may be used to evaluate the patient who has symptoms in the setting of normal resting hemodynamics. In the patient with mitral stenosis, exercise is usually accompanied by a slight increase in cardiac output and a substantial increase in left atrial and pulmonary arterial pressures (65, 66). In fact, the patient with elevated pressures at rest may develop pulmonary edema with only mild exercise. A transvalvular gradient that may be small at rest becomes larger with exercise, because of an increased cardiac output and a tachycardia-induced decrease in diastolic filling time (67, 68). In the patient with mitral stenosis whose cardiac output is low and whose transvalvular pressure gradient is small, exercise increases both variables, allowing a more reliable assessment of stenosis severity.

In most patients with aortic stenosis, an accurate measurement of the transvalvular gradient at rest allows one to calculate the valve area, even when the cardiac output is low; thus, dynamic exercise is rarely helpful

in these individuals. The risk of exercise-induced sudden death in these patients (because of peripheral vasodilation) provides a relative contraindication to dynamic exercise testing (40, 69). If the patient with aortic stenosis performs dynamic exercise, cardiac output increases, the transvalvular gradient increases, and both left atrial and pulmonary arterial pressures rise (70, 71). The calculated valve area may increase modestly with exercise, in all probability, because of improved leaflet movement with a higher flow across the valve (71).

Dynamic exercise may be helpful in assessing the cardiovascular status of patients with chronic mitral regurgitation, particularly in those whose symptoms are minimal and whose cardiac output, intracardiac filling pressures, and left ventricular function are relatively normal at rest (72). The patient with mitral regurgitation whose cardiac reserve is adequate responds to dynamic exercise with an appropriate increase in forward output, little change in intracardiac filling pressures, a fall in regurgitant fraction, and a modest decrease in left ventricular ejection fraction (73, 74). In contrast, the individual whose cardiac reserve is limited often demonstrates a blunted increase in forward cardiac output, a rise in intracardiac filling pressures, and a marked fall in left ventricular ejection fraction. In short, dynamic exercise in the patient with mitral regurgitation and minimal symptoms may help to identify the individual whose response to chronic volume overload is no longer normal, that is, whose cardiac reserve is limited.

Because of uncertainty as to when to proceed with valve replacement in patients with asymptomatic aortic regurgitation, several studies have investigated the response to dynamic exercise in patients with this valvular abnormality. Symptomatic patients consistently demonstrate a fall in left ventricular ejection fraction with exercise, whereas asymptomatic subjects demonstrate a heterogeneous response (i.e., ejection fraction may rise, fall, or be unchanged) (13, 75–78). Although a fall in left ventricular ejection fraction during exercise in the asymptomatic patient is thought to identify those who may require valve replacement in the near future, this finding alone is not an indication for surgery. In fact, only 25 to 30% of asymptomatic patients with aortic regurgitation and an abnormal exercise response require surgery for worsening symptoms over an average follow-up period of 4 years (79). Because operative and postoperative survival is not diminished if surgery is delayed until symptoms appear, valve replacement is generally delayed until the patient has symptoms or there is evidence of a progressive decline in left ventricular systolic function at rest on serial studies (79).

In short, dynamic exercise testing in the cardiac catheterization laboratory or the exercise laboratory may be used in patients with **valvular heart disease,** but its utility is substantially greater in those with valvular regurgitation than in those with predominant stenosis. In the patient with mitral or aortic stenosis, dynamic exercise provides the opportunity to calculate a valve area both at rest and during exercise, at a time when cardiac output and heart rate are aug-

mented. This may be especially important in the patient with mitral stenosis and a low cardiac output at rest, with a resultant small transvalvular gradient. In this individual, dynamic exercise may be used to increase the transvalvular gradient, thereby allowing a second calculation of the valve area. In the patient with mitral or aortic regurgitation who is asymptomatic or only minimally symptomatic, dynamic exercise provides the opportunity to assess cardiac reserve. The patient whose cardiac reserve is inadequate should be observed frequently and closely, because he or she may require valve replacement in the near future.

The alterations in cardiac function that occur during dynamic exercise with **aging** in the absence of cardiovascular disease should be recognized, so as not to confuse them with changes that are caused by cardiac disease. First, the elderly patient responds to sympathetic stimulation with only a modest increase in heart rate; similarly, in comparison with younger subjects, these individuals manifest a blunted increase in heart rate with vigorous exercise (80, 81). Because plasma catecholamine levels are markedly increased during exercise in the elderly, the mechanism of this diminished chronotropic response appears to be a diminished end-organ responsiveness to circulating catecholamines. Second, although cardiac output rises appropriately during exercise in elderly patients, it is the result of a greater reliance on the Frank-Starling mechanism—with a resultant increase in stroke volume—rather than to a marked increase in heart rate (82). Elderly patients often have a markedly increased end-diastolic and a modestly increased end-systolic volume. Third, aging is associated with an increased left ventricular mass and a reduced left ventricular compliance. Fourth, maximal oxygen consumption is known to decrease with age, but this may be caused by factors other than cardiovascular limitations, including sedentary lifestyle, motivation, orthopaedic considerations, and a decreased muscle mass. Thus, certain noncardiac factors may limit maximal oxygen consumption in the elderly population.

Isometric Exercise

Exercise in which skeletal muscle contraction causes primarily a change in tension with little change in length is termed isometric or static exercise. Isometric activities include lifting or pushing heavy objects and contracting muscles against immovable objects. In clinical practice, this is usually accomplished by having the subject perform handgrip, most often with a graded, hand dynamometer. The subject is asked to compress the dynamometer maximally several times, from which the maximal voluntary contraction is determined. Subsequently, hemodynamic variables and ventricular function are measured while the patient performs sustained handgrip at a percentage (usually 15 to 50%) of maximal contraction.

As with dynamic exercise, the effort magnitude expended during isometric exercise is an important determinant of the cardiovascular alterations that ensue. However, it is not the absolute tension developed during isometric exercise that is important, but rather the percentage of maximal voluntary contraction that is developed (83). Furthermore, the size of the involved muscle group is unimportant in determining the cardiovascular response. Thus, a 30% maximal voluntary contraction during handgrip requires an actual tension of 20 kg, whereas a 30% contraction of the leg requires a tension of 70 kg. Despite this difference in absolute tensions, muscle group masses, and energy expenditures, the same hemodynamic response is elicited in both situations (83) and, as a result, the same cardiovascular effects occur. The magnitude of the cardiovascular response to isometric exercise also depends on the duration of sustained tension (83). At 15% of maximal voluntary contraction, hemodynamic responses reach a steady state within 2 to 3 minutes. At tensions exceeding 15% maximal voluntary contraction, these hemodynamic variables do not reach a steady state but continue to increase until fatigue intervenes. Exercise duration varies with the tension exerted. At 50% maximal voluntary contraction, most subjects can sustain contraction for 2 to 3 minutes, whereas 3 to 5 minutes of sustained contraction are possible at 30% maximal voluntary contraction.

Because isometric exercise requires little equipment, it is simple and inexpensive. It is easily performed and easily repeated in the same subject. Handgrip does not involve body motion that may distort or interfere with the monitoring of hemodynamic variables or left ventricular function. Despite some concerns that isometric exercise might promote arrhythmias (84), numerous studies have been performed in normal subjects and in those with cardiac disease without serious arrhythmias (83, 85–100). As with any type of exercise, static exercise requires patient participation and cooperation that may limit its usefulness in some patients. In particular, one must ensure that isometric exercise is not confounded by the Valsalva maneuver, a frequent occurrence during unsupervised sustained static exertion. Careful respiration monitoring, as well as persistent coaxing and engagement of the subject in conversation during the procedure, minimizes the chance that this will occur.

Responses in Normal Subjects

Hemodynamic responses to isometric and dynamic exercise differ substantially from one another. With isometric exercise, systolic, diastolic, and mean arterial pressures rise markedly (by 25 to 50 mm Hg), whereas heart rate increases only modestly (by 20 to 30 beats per minute [bpm]) (85, 88, 89, 91). In contrast, dynamic exercise induces little change in diastolic arterial pressure, a modest rise in systolic and mean arterial pressures, and a considerable increase in heart rate. With isometric exercise, cardiac output increases modestly, and systemic vascular resistance is unchanged (83, 97). The increase in cardiac output is caused by an increase in heart rate, because stroke volume is unchanged (85, 87–89). There is no significant change in pulmonary arterial pressure or resistance during isometric exercise in normal subjects (88).

During dynamic exercise, stroke volume increases, and there is only a modest change in mean arterial pressure; thus, dynamic exercise causes primarily a volume load of the left ventricle. In contrast, isometric exercise induces no change in stroke volume and a substantial rise in systemic arterial pressure, resulting primarily in a pressure load of the left ventricle. Left ventricular end-diastolic volume decreases or is unchanged, and end-diastolic pressure is unchanged. Stroke volume against an increased aortic impedance is maintained by an increase in the inotropic state of the left ventricle; left ventricular preload is unchanged (11, 89, 95, 97, 100). In support of this, both invasively (92–94) and noninvasively measured (97, 99, 100) indices of left ventricular function (max dP/dt, dP/dt/P, V_{max}, fractional shortening, and shortening velocity) increase during isometric exercise.

Responses in Subjects with Cardiac Disease

In patients with **coronary artery disease,** isometric exercise rarely precipitates symptoms or electrocardiographic signs of ischemia (86, 89, 92, 101). Nevertheless, it may induce both left ventricular wall motion abnormalities (86, 90, 95, 101) and a fall in left ventricular ejection fraction. The latter is caused by an increase in end-systolic volume; end-diastolic volume is unchanged (89, 99). Stroke volume and cardiac output may decline during isometric exercise.

In patients with **congestive heart failure,** isometric exercise may be used to evaluate left ventricular function and cardiac reserve. During isometric exertion, those with heart failure cannot adequately increase left ventricular contractile function in response to the increased aortic impedance. Heart rate and systemic arterial pressure rise appropriately (102, 103), but cardiac output and stroke volume may fall, and left ventricular end-diastolic and pulmonary arterial pressures may rise. Aortic or mitral regurgitation, if present, increases in severity. Patients with mild heart failure often have normal hemodynamics at rest, but their response to isometric stress is abnormal in that an increased stroke work is accomplished at the expense of a high left

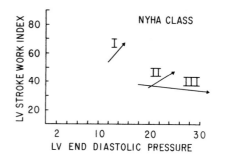

Figure 24.9. The relation between left ventricular stroke work index (*vertical axis*) and end-diastolic pressure (*horizontal axis*) in patients with congestive heart failure at rest and during isometric exercise (*arrow*). Patients with congestive heart failure at rest and during isometric exercise (*arrow*). Patients are segregated according to New York Heart Association (NYHA) classification. In class II and III patients, isometric exercise is associated with a marked rise in left ventricular end-diastolic pressure and little, if any, change in stroke work index. (Reprinted with permission from Kivowitz C, Parmley WW, Donoso R, et al. Effects of isometric exercise on cardiac performance. The grip test. Circulation 1971;44:994–1002. By permission of the American Heart Association, Inc.)

ventricular end-diastolic pressure (Fig. 24.9) (85, 89–93, 96).

Rapid Atrial Pacing

Although dynamic or isometric exercise can be performed in most individuals, alternative forms of stress are sometimes required. Exercise testing may be difficult in patients who are elderly, debilitated, poorly conditioned or motivated, or who have concomitant illnesses that preclude adequate exertion (i.e., chronic lung disease, peripheral vascular disease, arthritis, or neuromuscular disorders). In these subjects, rapid atrial pacing may serve as an alternative to exercise. Although atrial pacing may be useful in assessing left ventricular function, it is somewhat limited in identifying those with **coronary artery disease.**

Pacing is usually performed with the subject in the supine position. A pacing catheter is placed in the right atrium, coronary sinus, or esophagus (for transesophageal pacing of the left atrium). The heart rate is increased incrementally (by 10 to 20 bpm) every 2 to 3 minutes until (*a*) chest pain occurs, (*b*) a target heart rate is achieved (usually 140–160 bpm), or (*c*) atrioventricular block occurs. If 1:1 atrioventricular conduction does not occur at lower heart rates, 0.5 to 1.0 mg of atropine is given intravenously to enhance atrioventricular conduction.

Responses in Normal Subjects

Oxygen consumption increases slightly with rapid atrial pacing, but the magnitude of this increase is considerably less than that observed with exercise. Myocardial oxygen consumption increases because of the increase in heart rate and the augmented inotropic state that accompanies a tachycardia (termed the Treppe phenomenon or Bowditch effect) (104, 105). This increase in myocardial oxygen consumption is met by an appropriate increase in coronary blood flow, because the arteriovenous oxygen difference across the heart is unchanged (106–108). Although myocardial oxygen consumption rises during rapid atrial pacing, the magnitude of its rise is less than that observed with exercise. During rapid atrial pacing, systolic, diastolic, and mean arterial pressures are unchanged. Cardiac output is unchanged despite a marked increase in heart rate; thus, stroke volume declines incrementally as heart rate increases. Pulmonary arterial and right atrial pressures are unchanged (107–117).

During incremental atrial pacing, left ventricular end-diastolic volume falls precipitously, and end-systolic volume declines as well, although the magnitude of the fall in end-diastolic volume may be greater than that of end-systolic volume. As a result, the changes in ejection fraction caused by atrial pacing may vary from one individual to another, with some studies reporting an increase (118, 119) and others reporting no significant change in this variable (110, 111). This pacing-induced decline in left ventricular end-diastolic volume is accompanied by a decrease in left ventricular end-diastolic pressure; in normal subjects, end-diastolic pressure declines line-

arly as heart rate increases (115). Left ventricular contraction and relaxation, as reflected by positive and negative dP/dt (109, 111, 114, 120), peak diastolic filling rate (121), stroke volume to left ventricular end-diastolic pressure ratio (112, 115, 116), time constant of left ventricular pressure fall ([tau]) (122), and fiber shortening velocity (123) are enhanced during rapid atrial pacing (i.e., contractility and compliance are increased).

Responses in Subjects with Cardiac Disease

In early reports, angina induced by rapid atrial pacing was thought to be a sensitive and specific marker of **coronary artery disease** (124, 125). Accordingly, in some studies, symptoms served as the standard to which other markers of ischemia (i.e., lactate production, changes in left ventricular end-diastolic pressure, and electrocardiographic ST segment alterations) were compared. However, subsequent investigations have shown that chest pain is neither a sensitive nor a specific indicator of myocardial ischemia (118, 119, 126–131), because many patients cannot differentiate between ischemic chest pain and the palpitations associated with rapid atrial pacing. This may be particularly true at high pacing rates (> 140 bpm). On the one extreme, several studies of patients with angiographically normal coronary arteries reported angina-like chest pain in many of the subjects at high pacing rates (125, 126, 131). On the other extreme, patients with known **coronary artery disease** and metabolic evidence of pacing-induced ischemia (i.e., lactate production) may not have chest pain. In short, chest pain during rapid atrial pacing is unreliable in assessing the presence of **coronary artery disease.**

If angina occurs during atrial pacing in the setting of **coronary artery disease,** it usually resolves 30 seconds to 2 minutes after pacing is terminated (107), and it is reproducibly induced if pacing is performed again at the same rate. As a rule, angina that is induced by atrial pacing requires a higher heart rate (20 to 30 bpm) than that induced by dynamic exercise, because systemic arterial pressure is not affected substantially by pacing (107, 109, 115, 116, 124, 132). The heart rate at which angina occurs is unrelated to the severity of **coronary artery disease** (112, 124, 127).

The electrocardiographic changes that occur during pacing are difficult to interpret and are neither sensitive nor specific in identifying ischemia. A substantial frequency of false–negative and false–positive results are noted, especially at paced heart rates more than 160 bpm (125). Several factors may render the interpretation of electrocardiographic changes during pacing difficult (130). Alterations in the PR segment baseline may influence the assessment of ST segment changes (because the ST segment is compared with the PR segment), and placement of the pacing lead may influence the PR segment. Abnormal atrial repolarization may cause PR segment elevation, which may confuse the interpretation of ST segment depression. Prolongation of the PR interval occurs commonly at higher paced heart rates (>140 bpm), which may place the pacemaker spike on the T wave, ST segment, or J junction of the preceding QRS wave. Finally, a reentrant P wave induced by pacing is often located on the ST segment, making its interpretation difficult.

In an effort to improve the reliability of ECG alterations with pacing, some investigators have examined these changes immediately after pacing, and they have shown that ST segment alterations on a postpacing electrocardiogram offer excellent specificity and an acceptable sensitivity in the identification of subjects with **coronary artery disease** (118). In fact, if electrocardiographic alterations after pacing are used, the reliability of pacing in identifying patients with **coronary artery disease** approaches, but does not equal, that of standard exercise testing (133).

With rapid atrial pacing in patients with **coronary artery disease,** total oxygen consumption increases and is higher than in normal subjects at similarly paced heart rates (107). This has been attributed to the anxiety and increased ventilation associated with angina. Mean arterial pressure and cardiac output increase little, if any, and

stroke volume falls. Pulmonary arterial pressure is frequently elevated if there is evidence of ischemia with pacing.

The alterations in left ventricular volumes that occur during atrial pacing-induced ischemia are similar in many respects to those noted during dynamic exercise. With an incremental increase in heart rate, left ventricular end-diastolic volume decreases; at the same time, left ventricular end-systolic volume does not change or may even increase. As a result, ejection fraction remains the same or may actually fall during rapid atrial pacing (Fig. 24.10). Contrast left ventriculography at peak pacing may demonstrate a worsening of existing segmental wall motion abnormalities as well as the appearance of new wall motion alterations (110, 111, 118, 134–136).

The changes in left ventricular end-diastolic pressure that occur with rapid atrial pacing can be interpreted only in the context of the changes in left ventricular volumes described previously. During pacing, end-diastolic pressure usually falls (because end-diastolic volume falls), but in an occasional patient it may be unchanged from baseline. Although left ventricular end-diastolic pressure is not markedly elevated during pacing, a careful comparison with that of normal subjects shows that left ventricular end-diastolic pressure is higher at each level of pacing in subjects with ischemia than in normals (Fig. 24.11). When pacing is abruptly terminated in patients with pacing-induced ischemia, left ventricular end-diastolic volume returns to its prepacing level, and left ventricular end-diastolic pressure rises markedly and remains elevated for 30 seconds to 5 minutes (Fig. 24.12). In contrast, patients without **coronary artery disease,** as well as those with coronary disease but without ischemia, demonstrate no change or a minimal increase in end-diastolic pressure (in comparison with the prepacing values) after the abrupt termination of pacing. The cause of pacing-induced diastolic dysfunction has been investigated extensively. A pacing-induced reduction in peak negative dP/dt and an increase in the time constant of left ventricular pressure fall ([tau]) support the hypothesis that diastolic dysfunction is

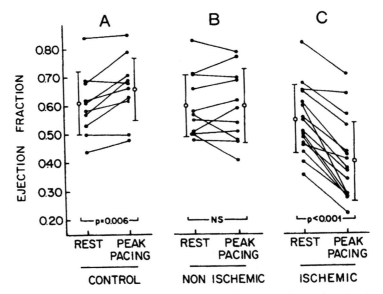

Figure 24.10. Left ventricular ejection fraction at rest and during peak atrial pacing in normal subjects (control, **A**) with coronary artery disease but without evidence of ischemia (nonischemic, **B**), and patients with coronary artery disease and pacing-induced ischemia (ischemic, **C**). With pacing, ejection fraction increases in the normal individuals, does not change in patients in the nonischemic group, and declines in those with ischemia. (Reprinted with permission from Dehmer GJ, Firth BG, Nicod P, et al. Alterations in left ventricular volumes and ejection fraction during atrial pacing in patients with coronary artery disease: assessment with radionuclide ventriculography. Am Heart J 1983;106:114–124.)

the result of a reduction in left ventricular compliance (122).

Hemodynamic Maneuvers

Valsalva Maneuver

With the Valsalva maneuver, the subject forcibly expires against a closed glottis. Its magnitude is quantitated by having the subject expire into a mouthpiece connected in parallel to a graduated manometer and pressure transducer. For most studies, a pressure of 30 to 50 mm Hg sustained for 10 to 15 seconds is sufficient to produce the characteristic hemodynamic changes. The Valsalva maneuver has been performed safely and without complications in numerous studies (137–144).

Responses in Normal Subjects

The hemodynamic alterations induced by the Valsalva maneuver, which are displayed in Figure 24.13 (145), are divided into four phases. Phase 1 begins with the onset of straining and is marked by a transient increase in intrathoracic pressure, which causes a transient increase in systemic arterial pressure. During phase 2, straining continues; venous return and cardiac output diminish; and peripheral vascular resistance increases. As a result of diminished cardiac output, systemic arterial pressure falls, and the pulse pressure narrows. Heart rate increases in response to the decline in arterial pressure. With the initial release of straining (phase 3), intrathoracic pressure decreases abruptly, and systemic arterial pressure transiently falls further as a result of blood pooling in the expanded pulmonary vascular bed. Phase 4 quickly follows, with an overshoot of the arterial

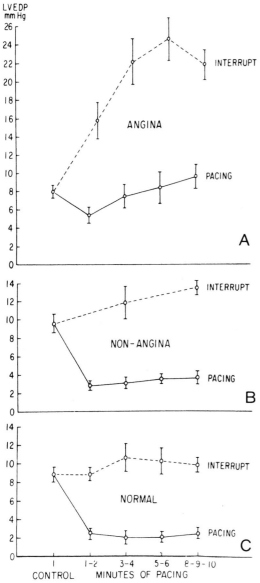

Figure 24.11. Left ventricular end-diastolic pressure (*LVEDP, vertical axes*) at rest (*control*), during rapid atrial pacing, and at points of interruption in normal subjects (**C**), and in patients with coronary artery disease with (**A**) or without (**B**) pacing-induced angina. In comparison with normals, LVEDP is elevated in the patients with pacing-induced ischemia (*angina group*) during pacing and with interruption of pacing. (Reprinted with permission from Parker JO, Ledwich JR, West RO, et al. Reversible cardiac failure during angina pectoris. Hemodynamic effects of atrial pacing in coronary artery disease. Circulation 1969;39:745–757. By permission of the American Heart Association, Inc.)

pressure caused by increased venous return and sympathetic activity. This overshoot of the pulse pressure and mean arterial pressure causes a reflex bradycardia, which is mediated by the parasympathetic nervous system.

During active straining, left ventricular end-diastolic and end-systolic volumes decrease by 45 to 50%, and stroke volume is diminished by 35 to 50%. Myocardial contractility is increased because of enhanced sympathetic stimulation, so that ejection fraction is increased. During recovery from straining, left ventricular end-diastolic volume returns to baseline, but end-systolic volume remains low because of increased sympathetic activity. As a result, stroke volume is increased in the recovery phase of the Valsalva maneuver.

During straining, right atrial, pulmonary arterial, and pulmonary–capillary wedge pressures rise markedly, but this is due primarily to the increased intrathoracic pressure generated by the maneuver. In fact, the transmural intracardiac pressures (intracavitary minus intrapleural) actually fall during the active straining phase of the Valsalva maneuver.

Responses in Subjects with Cardiac Disease

Rapid changes in intracardiac volumes induced by the Valsalva maneuver reflexly stimulate compensatory mechanisms via the autonomic nervous system, such that the changes in heart rate and arterial pressure that occur with this maneuver may provide insight into the integrity of the autonomic system. For example, the release of straining in phase 4, with its associated overshoot of arterial pressure, causes bradycardia by stimulating the carotid body receptor. The assessment of the heart rate response during phase 4 has been used as a noninvasive indicator of baroreceptor function (146). The magnitude of the change in heart rate during phase 4 diminishes with advanced age because of a depressed baroreceptor response (147), and patients with diabetes mellitus and autonomic dysfunction display a blunted heart rate response

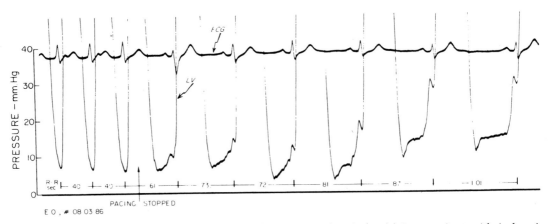

Figure 24.12. Left ventricular (*LV*) end-diastolic pressure (*vertical axis*) in a patient with ischemia induced by rapid atrial pacing. The LV end-diastolic pressure is normal during pacing but rapidly increases when pacing is terminated. (Reprinted with permission from O'Brien KP, Higgs LM, Glancy DL, et al. Hemodynamic accompaniments of angina. A comparison during angina induced by exercise and by atrial pacing. Circulation 1969;39:735–743. By permission of the American Heart Association, Inc.)

during phase 4 (148). In subjects with idiopathic orthostatic hypotension and in those on β-adrenergic blocking agents, the overshoot of arterial pressure in phase 4 may be absent (143, 149).

In patients with **congestive heart failure,** the heart rate behavior in all phases of the Valsalva maneuver is abnormal, in that it neither rises nor falls substantially (140, 142). During the straining phase (phase 2), arterial pressure does not fall as it does in normal subjects; rather, it remains the same or may even increase. When the release phase is reached, there is no arterial pressure overshoot. This is known as the "square wave response" and is shown in Figure 24.14 (138, 145, 150). This absence of marked changes in systemic arterial pressure and heart rate is believed to be caused by increased pulmonary blood volume in these patients, with continued left side heart filling for a sustained period of time, even during active straining. As a result, left ventricular volumes and stroke volume are not diminished (140). Hence, systemic arterial pressure does not fall, and heart rate does not reflexly change. Interestingly, one study has reported that effective therapy of heart failure resulted in normalization of the hemodynamic response to the Valsalva maneuver (138).

Some patients with **coronary artery disease** may manifest an abnormal hemody-

namic response to the Valsalva maneuver that is similar to that of subjects with **congestive heart failure.** These individuals have an attenuated response of heart rate and systolic arterial pressure during phases 2 and 4 of the Valsalva maneuver. This blunted hemodynamic response may be observed even in the absence of active ischemia (151).

In some patients with **coronary artery disease,** the Valsalva maneuver may help to alleviate episodes of myocardial ischemia (152). This occurs during the latter part of phase 2 (active straining) and is manifested as an abrupt reduction in left ventricular end-diastolic pressure, which is typically elevated during ischemia. Myocardial oxygen demand is decreased, as a result of diminished left ventricular volumes, and myocardial oxygen supply (coronary blood flow) is diminished during the Valsalva maneuver (153). The decrease in left ventricular volumes and pressures that occurs during the Valsalva maneuver may favorably affect the oxygen supply–demand relation in ischemic segments of the left ventricle, leading to augmentation of global and regional left ventricular function (139). No untoward effects are observed when a Valsalva maneuver is performed during an episode of ischemia (151, 152). The Valsalva maneuver has been used to recognize patients with **obstructive hypertrophic cardi-**

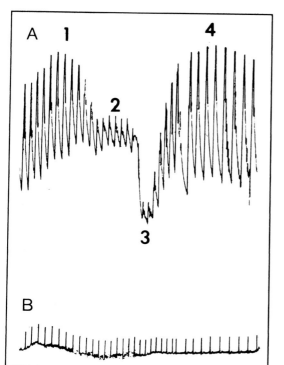

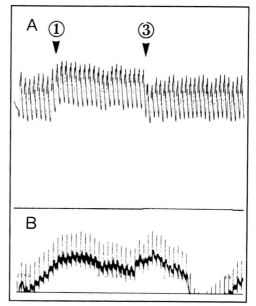

Figure 24.13. Systemic arterial pressure (**A**) and an electrocardiogram (**B**) during a Valsalva maneuver in a normal individual. With the onset of straining (*phase 1*), arterial pressure transiently increases. With continued straining (*phase 2*), systolic arterial pressure and pulse pressure decline, and heart rate increases reflexly. A further transient decrease in arterial pressure occurs in *phase 3* with release of straining and is followed by a characteristic pressure overshoot and bradycardia in *phase 4.* (Reprinted with permission from Nishimura RA, Tajik AJ. The Valsalva maneuver and response revisited. Mayo Clin Proc 1986;61:211–217.)

Figure 24.14. Systemic arterial pressure (**A**) and an electrocardiogram (**B**) during a Valsalva maneuver in a patient with congestive heart failure. *Phases 1* and *3* are marked as in Figure 24.13. Absence of a decreased arterial pressure in phase 2 and an overshoot of arterial pressure in phase 4 characterize the "square wave response" observed in these patients. Likewise, heart rate does not change during the Valsalva maneuver. (Reprinted with permission from Nishimura RA, Tajik AJ. The Valsalva maneuver and response revisited. Mayo Clin Proc 1986;61:211–217.)

omyopathy and to help in **differentiating right-** and **left-sided murmurs** (154). During forced expiration, the outflow tract gradient in patients with **obstructive hypertrophic cardiomyopathy** increases as peripheral pulse pressure and left ventricular volumes decline. As a result, the murmur increases in intensity (155, 156), whereas other systolic murmurs (i.e., aortic stenosis, mitral regurgitation) decrease in intensity or do not change with the Valsalva maneuver (157, 158). In an occasional patient with **obstructive hypertrophic cardio-**

myopathy, the murmur may paradoxically decrease in intensity during the Valsalva maneuver despite an increase in the gradient (159). This decrease is thought to be the result of a severe reduction in stroke volume and transaortic flow caused by the Valsalva maneuver. After release of the Valsalva maneuver, the intensity of a left-sided murmur usually returns to baseline in 4 to 11 cardiac cycles, whereas the intensity of a right-sided murmur returns to baseline in 1 to 2 cycles. This difference may be used to differentiate left- and right-sided murmurs (160).

In patients in whom a **patent foramen ovale** or **atrial septal defect** is suspected, the Valsalva maneuver may be performed to induce right-to-left intracardiac shunting of blood. With increased venous return that accompanies the release of straining, filling pressures in the right atrium transiently exceed those in the left atrium, and, if a defect in the interatrial septal is present, shunting of blood from the right to the left atrium can be detected by standard indication dilution techniques or echocardiography.

Mueller Maneuver

Responses in Normal Subjects

The Mueller maneuver involves inspiratory effort against a closed glottis; hence, it is the opposite of the Valsalva maneuver. It is usually performed by having the subject inhale with maximal effort against a closed one-way valve attached to a transducer, so that the subject begins at resting lung volume and generates -30 to -60 mm Hg for 20 to 30 seconds. The inspiratory pressure that is generated (161, 162), the time period (163), and the initial lung volume (162) influence the direction and magnitude of hemodynamic alterations. Thus, these variables must be standardized if one is to interpret the results meaningfully.

During the Mueller maneuver, several hemodynamic alterations occur. Right ventricular filling increases for 2 to 3 seconds (because of the negative intrathoracic pressure); this is followed by a prolonged period of diminished filling because of collapse of the superior and inferior vena cavae at the thoracic inlets (164, 165). Left ventricular afterload rises, causing an increase in left ventricular end-diastolic and end-systolic volumes, a diminished stroke volume, and a reduced ejection fraction in the upright patient (162, 163, 165–168). In the supine patient, left ventricular volumes may decline as a result of increased right ventricular volume (so-called ventricular interdependence) (168).

Responses in Subjects with Cardiac Disease

In patients with **coronary artery disease,** a decrease in left ventricular ejection fraction

is usually observed with the Mueller maneuver. However, a similar response often occurs in normal subjects. This maneuver may be helpful in distinguishing ischemic from infarcted myocardium. The regional wall motion of ischemic segments of myocardium is unaffected by the Mueller maneuver, but the appearance of new akinetic segments purportedly identifies areas of infarcted (scarred) myocardium (168).

The hemodynamic alterations induced by the Mueller maneuver may be useful in distinguishing **left-** and **right-sided heart murmurs** (169). The transient increase in right-sided filling may briefly increase the intensity of right-sided murmurs, such as tricuspid regurgitation or stenosis (68). Despite its wide clinical use, no studies document the usefulness of the Mueller maneuver in differentiating left- and right-sided heart murmurs (154).

In patients with **obstructive hypertrophic cardiomyopathy,** the Mueller maneuver causes a striking reduction in the left ventricular outflow gradient, the intensity of the systolic murmur, and the echocardiographically demonstrated systolic anterior movement of the anterior mitral valve leaflet (167, 170). These alterations are believed to be caused by the increase in left ventricular afterload caused by this maneuver.

Cold Pressor Testing

Responses in Normal Subjects

The cold pressor test is performed by placing the patient's hand in ice for 1 to 3 minutes. The exposure to cold stimulates α-adrenergic receptors (171), leading to a modest increase in heart rate (5 to 15 bpm), systolic and mean arterial pressures (15 to 30 mm Hg), and cardiac output. A maximal response occurs within 2 minutes. Left ventricular end-diastolic volume increases during exposure to cold, whereas the response of end-systolic volume, stroke volume, and ejection fraction is heterogeneous (172–179). In normal subjects, α-adrenergic activation increases coronary blood flow, and coronary vascular resistance is decreased or unchanged. Both an increase (180) and a small (6 to 8%) decrease in coronary artery diameter (181, 182) have been reported. Cold-induced, neurally mediated coronary vasoconstriction is offset by metabolically mediated vasodilation.

Responses in Subjects with Cardiac Disease

In patients with **coronary artery disease,** exposure to cold elicits similar modest elevations in heart rate and systemic arterial pressure (172, 173, 183–185), so that the heart rate-blood pressure product rises modestly (178, 179, 186). Precipitation of angina is caused by a concomitant reduction in oxygen supply, which, in turn, is caused by increased coronary vascular resistance and diminished coronary blood flow (Fig. 24.15) (172, 176, 181, 184). This cold-induced coronary vasoconstriction is mediated through stimulation of α-adrenergic receptors in diseased segments of coronary arteries (172, 174, 177); it is prevented with α-adrenergic blockade (181) and is potentiated by β-adrenergic blockade (184).

The usefulness of cold pressor testing in identifying patients with **coronary artery disease** is limited. Angina is precipitated uncommonly, even in the presence of documented ischemia; ECG changes are seldom observed (only in 25 to 30%) (177, 186). The cold pressor test is inferior to dynamic exercise testing in identifying patients with **coronary artery disease.** In direct comparisons of the two techniques, exercise offers a better sensitivity and specificity than does exposure to cold (173, 187–189). Systemic arterial hypertension impairs the vasodilator response of normal coronary arteries to cold pressor testing, and coronary vasoconstriction may be observed in hypertensive patients without angiographically evident **coronary artery disease** (180). Although stimulation of coronary α-adrenergic receptors has repeatedly been postulated as the cause of vasospastic (Prinzmetal's) angina, recent studies have shown that exposure to cold usually does not induce focal coronary vasospasm (171, 179, 186), although such

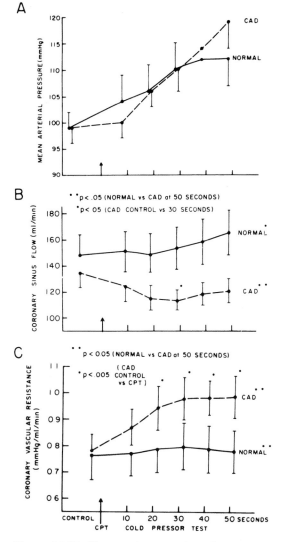

Figure 24.15. Changes in systemic and coronary vascular tone elicited by the cold pressor test (*CPT*) in normal subjects (*solid lines*) and in patients with CAD (*dashed lines*). Both groups demonstrate a systemic hypertensive response to cold (**A**). Unlike the normal subjects, however, patients with CAD have a cold-induced decrease in coronary blood flow (**B**) and an increase in coronary vascular resistance (**C**). (Reprinted with permission from Mudge GH Jr, Grossman W, Mills RM Jr, et al. Reflex increase in coronary vascular resistance in patients with ischemic heart disease. N Engl J Med 1976;295:1333–1337.)

spasm has occasionally been observed angiographically during cold provocation (182).

In patients with **congestive heart failure,** the increase in heart rate and systemic arterial pressure observed with cold pressor testing is blunted in comparison with normal subjects. This blunted response is likely caused by a diminished ability to increase cardiac output, impaired peripheral vasoconstriction, or both (189, 190). With exposure to cold, right atrial and pulmonary arterial pressures also rise in these patients.

Hyperventilation

Responses in Normal Subjects

Besides ergonovine and cold pressor, hyperventilation has been used as a maneuver to induce coronary arterial spasm. It is usually performed by having the patient take 30 deep respirations per minute for 5 minutes. If ischemia is precipitated, it may occur during hyperventilation; however, it more commonly develops within several minutes after the termination of hyperventilation (186). In response to hyperventilation, heart rate, oxygen consumption, the arteriovenous oxygen difference, and arterial pH increase, whereas mean arterial pressure, pulmonary arterial pressure, and arterial pCO_2 decline. Peripheral vascular resistance, cardiac output, and stroke volume are unchanged (190). In normal subjects, left ventricular ejection fraction increases (188).

Responses in Subjects with Cardiac Disease

Numerous reports have described ischemia induced by hyperventilation in patients with **stable** and **variant angina.** From 5 to 30% of patients with **coronary artery disease** develop angina and ischemic electrocardiographic alterations during vigorous hyperventilation (191–195). The ischemia is rapidly relieved by sublingual nitroglycerin, and it frequently responds chronically to calcium antagonists (196). In both normal subjects and those with **coronary artery disease,** coronary sinus blood flow falls during hyperventilation (191), and in those with atherosclerotic narrowings, hyperventilation may cause a significant reduction in coronary arterial diameter (by 25 to 100%) (194). Hyperventilation-induced ST segment depression changes that occur during rapid breathing are thought to be caused by increased myocardial oxygen demands, whereas those occurring during the recovery phase are attributed to reduced coronary blood flow. The sensitivity with which hyperventilation identifies patients with coronary vasospasm ranges from 70 to 80% (186, 188, 192, 195). It is thought that the hypocapnic alkalosis induced by hyperventilation decreases the concentration of hydrogen ions in vascular smooth muscle, thus allowing unbound calcium to induce smooth muscle contraction (197, 198). In support of this mechanism, hyperventilation that is performed with rebreathed air (so that arterial pH and pCO_2 do not change) does not induce coronary arterial spasm (195).

Mental Stress

In the laboratory setting, psychologic stress can be elicited passively (i.e., random bursts of noise) or actively, with assignment of a difficult or timed mental task (i.e., mental arithmetic). In normal subjects, such stress causes a modest increase in blood pressure, heart rate, and circulating catecholamines (199, 200). In some patients with **coronary artery disease,** the resultant increase in myocardial oxygen demands associated with mental stress may precipitate ischemia that is often clinically silent (201–209). In such patients, mental stress-induced ischemia may cause electrocardiographic changes (201–203), reversible myocardial perfusion defects (205, 208), or left ventricular dysfunction (203, 206, 208, 209). Although only a small percentage (10 to 15%) of asymptomatic ischemic episodes occur at a time when patients consider that their mental state is stressful, many more episodes may occur with routine mental activ-

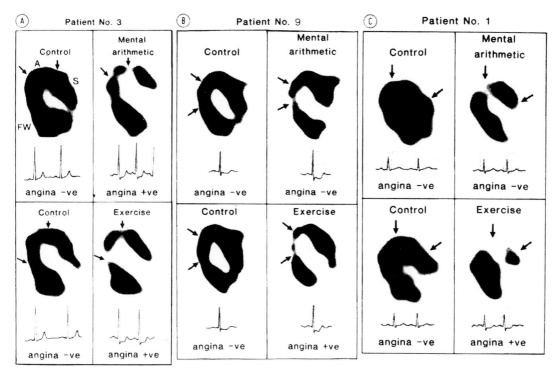

Figure 24.16. Changes in regional myocardial blood flow determined by rubidium-82 positron tomography before and after mental arithmetic in three patients with CAD. Resting (*control*) scans show homogenous uptake of cation. Mental arithmetic precipitates ischemic ECG changes and regional defects in rubidium uptake with angina, and similar changes with angina occur during exercise. −ve, absent; +ve, present. (Reprinted with permission from Deanfield JE, Shea M, Kensett M, et al. Silent myocardial ischemia due to mental stress. Lancet 1984;2:1001–1005.)

ity that is not perceived by the patient as stressful (202, 203, 207). In support of this, regional perfusion abnormalities may be demonstrated by positron tomography in a large percentage of patients with chronic stable angina during mental arithmetic that is not intended to upset or frustrate them (Fig. 24.16) (208).

In many patients with **coronary artery disease,** ischemia occurs with mental stress without a significant increase in myocardial oxygen demands (heart rate or blood pressure) (207). Although this is most likely the result of a primary reduction in coronary blood flow (200), quantitative coronary angiography of epicardial coronary arteries has not consistently demonstrated vasconstriction with mental stress (207). In these patients, vasoconstriction may occur at the microvascular level.

PHARMACOLOGIC STRESS

Nitroglycerin

Response in Normal Subjects

Nitrates cause smooth muscle relaxation in the venous capacitance vessels; as a result, venous pooling occurs, and venous return to the heart is diminished. Although nitrates act predominantly on veins rather than on arteries (210, 211), they acutely cause arterial vasodilation and decreased systemic vascular resistance at high doses. Thus, the hemodynamic responses that occur with nitrates depend on the dose administered.

At routine therapeutic doses, nitrates

cause a modest decrease in systolic and mean arterial pressures, as well as a slight fall in systemic vascular resistance. At the same time, they induce a more profound reduction in pulmonary arterial and left ventricular end-diastolic pressures (212, 213). Left ventricular volumes decline, because of reduced preload and diminished impedance to ejection, and stroke volume is reduced. Because there is usually little change in heart rate, cardiac output falls (214–216). Nitrates exert no demonstrable influence on left ventricular performance (217), unless a large dose causes a profound fall in systemic arterial pressure, with resultant reflex sympathetic stimulation.

Nitroglycerin is a powerful coronary vasodilator (218, 219) that decreases coronary vascular resistance and increases coronary blood flow (220–222), even in the absence of systemic hemodynamic effects. With exposure to nitroglycerin, the luminal area of normal epicardial coronary arteries increases by approximately 20%, and smaller coronary arteries dilate even more impressively (219, 220). As shown in Figure 24.17, diseased coronary arteries also retain the ability to dilate in response to nitroglycerin. Nitroglycerin prevents sympathetic coronary vasoconstriction (218), relieves focal coronary arterial spasm, augments blood flow through collaterals to ischemic myocardium (221), and (in animal studies) improves subendocardial perfusion.

Responses in Subjects with Cardiac Disease

The beneficial effects of nitroglycerin in patients with **coronary artery disease** result from its vasodilatory influence on various vascular beds. Similar to the changes noted in normal subjects, nitroglycerin in patients with **coronary artery disease** induces a fall in left ventricular volumes and pressures,

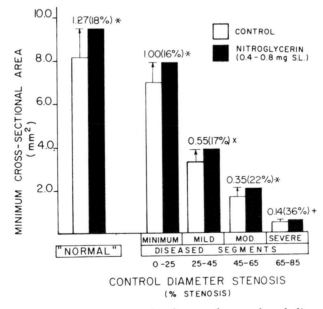

Figure 24.17. Changes in minimum cross-sectional area of normal and diseased coronary arteries after sublingual (*SL*) nitroglycerin. Coronary arteries are grouped according to severity of stenosis at baseline. All groups demonstrate significant increase in minimum cross-sectional area after nitroglycerin, regardless of severity of baseline stenosis. x, $P < 0.05$; *, $P < 0.01$; +, $P < 0.005$. *MOD*, moderate. (Reprinted with permission from Brown BG, Bolson E, Petersen RB, et al. The mechanisms of nitroglycerin action: stenosis vasodilation as a major component of the drug response. Circulation 1981;64:1089–1097. By permission of the American Heart Association, Inc.)

systemic vascular resistance, left ventricular wall tension, and myocardial oxygen demand. During dynamic exercise, patients with **coronary artery disease** who are pretreated with nitrates have an increased rate–pressure product at the onset of angina, a lower left ventricular end-diastolic volume and pressure, a lower pulmonary–capillary wedge pressure, and a higher ejection fraction at peak exercise than when these same patients are studied during exercise without nitrate pretreatment (213, 214, 216, 223). In addition to their favorable effects on oxygen demand, oxygen supply is increased because of nitrate-induced coronary vasodilation.

Because nitroglycerin may reverse the left ventricular asynergy associated with ischemia, it has been used to assess residual contractile function of ischemic myocardium. An improvement in global and regional left ventricular function has been noted in patients with **coronary artery disease** who are given nitroglycerin (224–226), and the regional ventricular response to nitroglycerin appears to be a reliable predictor of improvement in regional asynergy following successful coronary artery bypass surgery (227, 228). Asynergic areas that improve with nitroglycerin are thought to represent myocardium that is ischemic but not irreversibly injured.

When nitrates are given to subjects with **congestive heart failure,** they may induce a dramatic decrease in central venous and right atrial pressure, right ventricular end-systolic and end-diastolic pressures, and pulmonary arterial and left ventricular end-diastolic pressures. Heart rate is usually unchanged, whereas the response of stroke volume and cardiac output is variable. Those with a low cardiac output and a high left ventricular filling pressure before treatment are most likely to manifest an increase in stroke volume and cardiac output with nitrates (229, 230). In these individuals, cardiac output increases primarily because of a reduction in systemic vascular resistance. Subjects with elevated right atrial pressures often exhibit resistance to the hemodynamic effects of nitroglycerin; their response can be restored when right atrial pressures are lowered with diuresis (231).

Isoproterenol

Responses in Normal Subjects

Isoproterenol can be administered (as an intravenous infusion at 1 to 4 μg/min) as another means of provoking a stress response in the catheterization laboratory. Continuous hemodynamic and electrocardiographic monitoring is performed as the rate of infusion is increased until symptoms or electrocardiographic evidence of ischemia are observed. Its advantages are (*a*) it may be administered in situations where exercise is impossible; (*b*) as opposed to rapid atrial pacing, it can be given at the bedside without invasive monitoring; (*c*) the ECG is not obscured by motion or pacing artifact; and (*d*) it allows monitoring that may be technically difficult during active exercise. The hemodynamic changes that occur during an infusion of isoproterenol (232–239) are similar to those of dynamic exercise and are the consequence of β-adrenergic stimulation. Heart rate and cardiac output are increased. In young subjects, stroke volume increases substantially (236), whereas in older individuals the increased cardiac output is the result mainly of an increase in heart rate (237, 239, 240). The arterial pulse pressure widens as diastolic pressure falls and systolic pressure rises or is unchanged; mean arterial pressure declines. Systemic and pulmonary vascular resistances decline substantially, because of the vasodilating effects of β_2 stimulation. Pulmonary arterial pressure may decrease or be unchanged (233, 239).

During an isoproterenol infusion, left ventricular ejection fraction rises (241, 242). Increases in max dP/dt (234, 238), mean ejection rate (238, 240), and left ventricular work (in the setting of a decreased systemic vascular resistance) (233, 239, 243) provide evidence that ventricular contractility is enhanced. Left ventricular end-diastolic pressure is unchanged or falls (234, 238, 240). Myocardial oxygen consumption is increased, and coronary blood flow rises markedly; in fact, the increase in flow is out of proportion to the increase in demand, so that myocardial oxygen extraction declines.

Thus, isoproterenol causes direct coronary vasodilation (239, 244, 245).

Responses in Subjects with Cardiac Disease

The rate–pressure product that is achieved during an isoproterenol infusion is lower than that which occurs during dynamic exercise, primarily because isoproterenol does not cause a marked increase in systolic arterial pressure (236). Nevertheless, isoproterenol compares favorably with dynamic exercise in identifying patients with **coronary artery disease.** In these patients, an isoproterenol infusion has a sensitivity of 60 to 100% and a specificity of 70 to 80% in the identification of those with **coronary artery**

disease (237, 246–248). Despite the similar hemodynamic responses to exercise and isoproterenol in subjects with **coronary artery disease,** global and segmental left ventricular performance is affected differently by the two interventions. As Figure 24.18 shows, left ventricular ejection fraction falls with exercise in patients with ischemic heart disease, whereas it increases in response to the infusion of a β-agonist in the same patients (242). Dynamic exercise causes a worsening of regional wall motion abnormalities, whereas isoproterenol improves regional wall dyskinesia.

The infusion of isoproterenol may be associated with several adverse effects, including sweating, apprehension, facial flushing, tremor, headache, and ventricular premature beats. If used carefully, however,

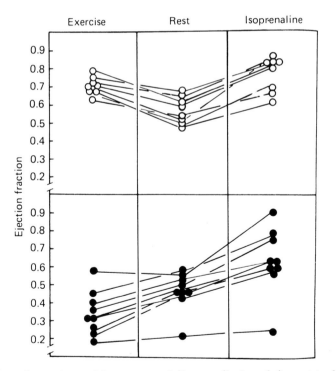

Figure 24.18. Effects of exercise and isoproterenol (*isoprenaline*) on left ventricular ejection fraction in normal subjects (*open circles*) and in patients with CAD (*closed circle*). Ejection fraction increases in normal subjects in response to both exercise and isoproterenol. In patients with CAD, left ventricular ejection fraction increases with isoproterenol but decreases with exercise. (Reprinted with permission from Sapru RP, Muir AL, Hannan WJ, et al. Effect of exercise and isoprenaline on left ventricular ejection fraction in patients with angina pectoris as assessed by radionuclide angiography. Cardiology 1982;69:91–97. With permission from S. Karger AG, Basel.)

it is safe, and its infusion rarely must be terminated because of intolerable side effects.

In patients with **congestive heart failure,** isoproterenol induces an increase in cardiac output, heart rate, stroke volume, and left and right ventricular stroke work, changes similar to those noted in normal subjects. Systemic and pulmonary vascular resistances fall. In those with heart failure, exercise causes pulmonary arterial pressure to rise, whereas isoproterenol is associated with a decrease in pulmonary arterial pressure (233, 243).

Ergonovine Maleate

Ergot alkaloids induce direct vasoconstriction by stimulating α-adrenergic and serotonin receptors in smooth muscle cells of veins and arteries. In 1949, Stein (249) introduced ergonovine as a provocative agent for coronary artery insufficiency, and in 1975, Heupler et al. (250) suggested that it was useful in provoking episodes of vasospastic angina. The reader is referred to the chapter on coronary arteriography for a description of its use in provoking coronary vasospasm.

Responses in Normal Subjects

The normal human subject responds to the administration of ergonovine with a small (10 to 15%) increase in systolic and mean arterial pressure and no change or a small (10%) increase in heart rate (251–255). Therefore, the rate–pressure product increases modestly (approximately 25%). Myocardial oxygen consumption usually increases (251, 255). Ergonovine causes an increase in left ventricular end-diastolic and end-systolic dimensions, in all probability because of increased venous return to the heart. Stroke volume and ejection fraction do not change significantly. Left ventricular end-diastolic pressure rises modestly (average, 3 mm Hg) with ergonovine (252). The epicardial coronary arteries demonstrate a 15 to 20% decrease in luminal diameter with

ergonovine (255–258), because of the drug's direct vasoconstricting effect (257).

Responses in Subjects with Cardiac Disease

Patients with **coronary artery disease** may exhibit symptoms or electrocardiographic changes of ischemia with ergonovine, despite the absence of demonstrable coronary arterial spasm (259). In all probability, this occurs because of an ergonovine-induced increase in myocardial oxygen demand and a concomitant fall in oxygen supply (because of direct vasoconstriction). Subjects with ergonovine-induced ischemia may manifest an increase in left ventricular dimensions and left ventricular end-diastolic pressure, as well as a profound decrease in stroke volume (20 to 30%) and left ventricular ejection fraction (16 to 20%) (252–254).

Amyl Nitrite

Responses in Normal Subjects

Amyl nitrite is a rapidly acting, direct vasodilator that is administered by inhalation. Its maximal hemodynamic effects are evident in 30 seconds and resolve in 2 to 5 minutes (153, 260, 261). Because of its pronounced hypotensive effects, it should be administered to patients in the recumbent position. Its quick onset of action and rapid resolution make it an ideal agent for bedside use.

Within seconds of the inhalation of amyl nitrite, systolic, diastolic, and mean arterial pressures fall dramatically (by 25 to 35%) (153, 260–265), and a reflex tachycardia occurs, with the heart rate increasing 50 to 80%. Cardiac output increases proportionately to the increase in heart rate because stroke volume does not change. Systemic and pulmonary vascular resistances decline. Left ventricular end-diastolic and end-systolic dimensions fall appreciably (18 and 57%, respectively) (261). Figure 24.19 demonstrates the time course of the changes in left ventricular volumes. Concomitant

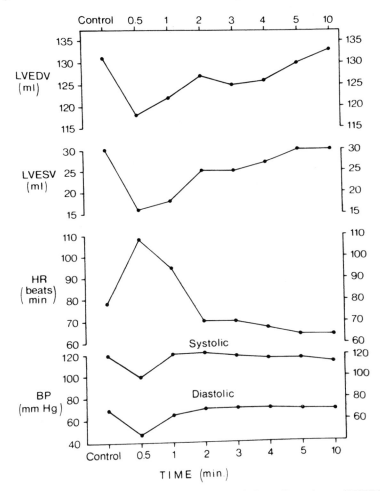

Figure 24.19. Time course of changes in left ventricular end-diastolic volume (*LVEDV*), end-systolic volume (*LVESV*), heart rate (*HR*), and blood pressure (*BP*) after the administration of amyl nitrite. Within 30 sec of amyl nitrite inhalation, there is a marked decline in left ventricular volumes and blood pressure, with a compensatory increase in heart rate. These variables return toward baseline 2 min after amyl nitrite administration. (From Burggraf GW, Parker JO. Left ventricular volume changes after amyl nitrite and nitroglycerin in man as measured by ultrasound. Circulation 1974;49: 136–143. By permission of the American Heart Association, Inc.)

with a decline in left ventricular end-diastolic volume, end-diastolic pressure falls (260, 261). Myocardial contractility increases because of the sympathetic overdrive that is precipitated by a marked fall in arterial pressure.

Responses in Subjects with Cardiac Disease

In response to amyl nitrite, patients with **coronary artery disease** exhibit the same alterations in hemodynamic variables and ventricular volumes as normal subjects. Although it decreases myocardial oxygen demand and acts as a direct coronary vasodilator (266), amyl nitrite may reduce coronary blood flow because of its profound influence on systemic arterial pressure (267). In fact, some reports have noted that amyl nitrite administration may induce ischemic ST-T wave alterations (268, 269), and others have suggested that it may be used to identify subjects with **coronary artery disease** (263).

SUMMARY

In summary, a complete understanding of cardiac hemodynamic function and its response to physiologic and pharmacologic maneuvers is essential for the cardiovascular specialist. In the cardiac catheterization laboratory these functional responses can be assessed directly and quantified in patients with a wide variety of disease states.

References

1. Mitchell JH, Blomqvist G. Maximal oxygen uptake. N Engl J Med 1971;284:1018–1022.
2. Douglas CG. Oliver-Sharpey lecture on the coordination of the respiration and circulation with variations in bodily activity. Lancet 1927;213:213–218.
3. Margaria R, Edwards HT, Dill DB. The possible mechanisms of contracting and paying the oxygen debt and the role of lactic acid in muscular contraction. Am J Physiol 1933;106:689–715.
4. Owles WH. Alterations in the lactic and acid content of the blood as a result of light exercise, and associated changes in the CO_2 combining power of the blood and in the alveolar CO_2 pressure. J Physiol (Lond) 1930;69:214–237.
5. Wasserman K. Determinants and detection of anaerobic threshold and consequences of exercise above it. Circulation 1987;76:V129–V139.
6. Lorell BH, Grossman W. Dynamic and isometric exercise during cardiac catheterization. In: Grossman W, ed. Cardiac catheterization and angiography. 3rd ed. Philadelphia: Lea & Febiger, 1986:251–266.
7. Mitchell JH. Cardiovascular control during exercise: central and reflex neural mechanisms. Am J Cardiol 1985;55:34D–41D.
8. Cohn JN. Quantitative testing for the cardiac patient: the value of monitoring gas exchange. Circulation 1987;76:VI1–VI2.
9. Robinson BF, Epstein SE, Beiser GD, et al. Control of heart rate by the autonomic nervous system. Studies in man on the interrelation between baroreceptor mechanisms and exercise. Circ Res 1966;19:400–411.
10. Thandani U, Parker JO. Hemodynamics at rest and during supine and sitting bicycle exercise in normal subjects. Am J Cardiol 1978;41:52–59.
11. Crawford MH, White DH, Amon KW. Echocardiographic evaluation of left ventricular size and performance during handgrip and supine and upright bicycle exercise. Circulation 1979;59:1188–1196.
12. Wilson M. Left ventricular diameter posture and exercise. Circ Res 1962;11:90–96.
13. Mitchell JH, Wildenthal K. Left ventricular function during exercise. In: Larsen OA, Malmborg RO, eds. Coronary heart disease and physical fitness. Copenhagen: Munksgaard, 1970:93–96.
14. Carroll JD, Hess OM, Studer NP, et al. Systolic function during exercise in patients with coronary artery disease. J Am Coll Cardiol 1983;2:206–216.
15. Dehmer GJ, Lewis SE, Hillis LD, et al. Exercise-induced alterations in left ventricular volumes and the pressure-volume relationship: a sensitive indicator of left ventricular dysfunction in patients with coronary artery disease. Circulation 1981;63:1008–1018.
16. Shen WF, Roubin GS, Hirasawa K, et al. Left ventricular volume and ejection fraction response to exercise in chronic congestive heart failure: difference between dilated cardiomyopathy and previous myocardial infarction. Am J Cardiol 1985;55:1027–1031.
17. Francis GS, Goldsmith SR, Ziesche SM, et al. Response of plasma norepinephrine and epinephrine to dynamic exercise in patients with congestive heart failure. Am J Cardiol 1982;49:1152–1156.
18. Freeman MR, Berman DS, Staniloff H, et al. Comparison of upright and supine bicycle exercise in the detection and evaluation of extent of coronary artery disease by equilibrium radionuclide ventriculography. Am Heart J 1981;102:182–189.
19. Poliner LR, Dehmer GJ, Lewis SE, et al. Left ventricular performance in normal subjects: a comparison of the responses to exercise in the upright and supine positions. Circulation 1980;62:528–534.
20. Sullivan MJ, Cobb FR, Higginbotham MB. Stroke volume increases by similar mechanisms during upright exercise in normal men and women. Am J Cardiol 1991;67:1405–1412.
21. Ginzton LE, Conant R, Brizendine M, et al. Effect of long-term high intensity aerobic training on left ventricular volume during maximal upright exercise. J Am Coll Cardiol 1989;14:364–371.
22. Gorlin R, Cohen LS, Elliott WC, et al. Effect of supine exercise on left ventricular volume and oxygen consumption in man. Circulation 1965;32:361–371.
23. Sharma B, Goodwin JF, Raphael MJ, et al. Left ventricular angiography on exercise. A new method of assessing left ventricular function in ischaemic heart disease. Br Heart J 1976;38:59–67.
24. Tebbe V, Hoffmeister N, Sauer G, et al. Changes in left ventricular diastolic function in coronary artery disease with and without angina pectoris assessed from exercise ventriculography. Clin Cardiol 1980;3:19–26.
25. Nonogi H, Hess OM, Bortone AS, et al. Left ventricular pressure-length relation during exercise-induced ischemia. J Am Coll Cardiol 1989;13:1062–1070.
26. Bruce RA, Petersen JL, Kusumi F. Hemodynamic responses to exercise in the upright posture in patients with ischemic heart disease. In: Dhalla HS, ed. Myocardial metabolism. Baltimore: University Park Press, 1973:849–865.
27. Forrester JS, Diamond GA, Swan HJC. Correlative classification of clinical and hemodynamic function after acute myocardial infarction. Am J Cardiol 1977;39:137–145.

28. Choi BW, Wasserman AG, Katz RJ, et al. Clinical and hemodynamic significance of left ventricular diastolic volume changes by exercise radionuclide ventricular in coronary artery disease. Am J Cardiol 1989;63:522–525.

29. Reduto LA, Wickemeyer WJ, Young JB, et al. Left ventricular diastolic performance at rest and during exercise in patients with coronary artery disease. Assessment with first-pass radionuclide angiography. Circulation 1981;63:1228–1237.

30. Wiener L, Dwyer EM Jr, Cox JW. Left ventricular hemodynamics in exercise-induced angina pectoris. Circulation 1968;38:240–249.

31. Iskandrian AS, Heo J, Askenase A, et al. Factors affecting exercise left ventricular performance in patients free of obstructive coronary artery disease. Am J Cardiol 1987;60:1173–1176.

32. Sugishita Y, Koseki S. Dynamic exercise echocardiography. Circulation 1979;60:743–752.

33. Borer JS, Bacharach SL, Green MV, et al. Real-time radionuclide cineangiography in the noninvasive evaluation of global and regional left ventricular function at rest and during exercise in patients with coronary artery disease. N Engl J Med 1977; 296:839–844.

34. Caldwell JH, Hamilton GW, Sorensen SG, et al. The detection of coronary artery disease with radionuclide techniques: a comparison of rest-exercise thallium imaging and ejection fraction response. Circulation 1980;61:610–619.

35. Kimchi A, Rozanski A, Fletcher C, et al. The clinical significance of exercise-induced left ventricular wall motion abnormality occurring at a low heart rate. Am Heart J 1987;114:724–730.

36. Thadani U, West RO, Mathew TM, et al. Hemodynamics at rest and during supine and sitting bicycle exercise in patients with coronary artery disease. Am J Cardiol 1977;39:776–783.

37. Clements IP, Gibbons RJ, Mankin HT, et al. Guidelines for the interpretation of the exercise radionuclide ventriculogram for diagnosing coronary artery disease. Am J Cardiol 1987;60: 1265–1268.

38. Rozanski A, Berman DS. The efficacy of cardiovascular nuclear medicine studies. Semin Nucl Med 1987;17:104–120.

39. Miller DD, Ruddy TD, Zusman RM, et al. Left ventricular ejection fraction response during exercise in asymptomatic systemic hypertension. Am J Cardiol 1987;59:409–413.

40. Ellestad MH. Stress testing: principles and practice. Philadelphia: FA Davis, 1986:113–126.

41. Sobue T, Yokota M, Iwase M, et al. Influence of left ventricular hypertrophy on left ventricular function during dynamic exercise in the presence or absence of coronary artery disease. J Am Coll Cardiol 1995;25:91–98.

42. Szlachcic J, Massie BM, Kramer BL, et al. Correlates and prognostic implication of exercise capacity in chronic congestive heart failure. Am J Cardiol 1985;55:1037–1042.

43. Weber KT, Kinasewitz GT, Janicki JS, et al. Oxygen utilization and ventilation during exercise in patients with chronic cardiac failure. Circulation 1982;65:1213–1223.

44. Walter M, Renard M, Dereppe H, et al. Influence of upright exercise on pulmonary hemodynamics in left heart failure. Acta Cardiol 1992;47:31–41.

45. Franciosa JA, Leddy CL, Wilen M, et al. Relation between hemodynamic and ventilatory responses in determining exercise capacity in severe congestive heart failure. Am J Cardiol 1984;53:127–134.

46. Francis GS, Goldsmith SR, Ziesche S, et al. Relative attenuation of sympathetic drive during exercise in patients with congestive heart failure. J Am Coll Cardiol 1985;5:832–839.

47. Gibbs JSR, Keegan J, Wright C, et al. Pulmonary artery pressure changes during exercise and daily activities in chronic heart failure. J Am Coll Cardiol 1990;15:52–61.

48. Clark A, Coats A. Mechanisms of exercise intolerance in cardiac failure: abnormalities of skeletal muscle and pulmonary function. Curr Opin Cardiol 1994;9:305–314.

49. Dunselman PHJM, Kuntze EE, van Bruggen A, et al. Value of New York Heart Association classification, radionuclide ventriculography, and cardiopulmonary exercise tests for selection of patients for congestive heart failure studies. Am Heart J 1988;116:1475–1482.

50. Franciosa JA, Ziesche S, Wilen M. Functional capacity of patients with chronic left ventricular failure. Relationship of bicycle exercise performance to clinical and hemodynamic characterization. Am J Med 1979;67:460–465.

51. Benge W, Litchfield RL, Marcus ML. Exercise capacity in patients with severe left ventricular dysfunction. Circulation 1980;61:955–959.

52. Franciosa JA, Park M, Levine TB. Lack of correlation between exercise capacity and indexes of resting left ventricular performance in heart failure. Am J Cardiol 1981;47:33–39.

53. Francis GS, Goldsmith SR, Cohn JN. Relationship of exercise capacity to resting left ventricular performance and basal plasma norepinephrine levels in patients with congestive heart failure. Am Heart J 1982;104:725–731.

54. Hakki AH, Weinreich DJ, Depace L, et al. Correlation between exercise capacity and left ventricular function in patients with severely depressed left ventricular function. J Cardiopulm Rehabil 1984; 4:38–43.

55. Higginbotham MB, Morris KG, Conn EH, et al. Determinants of variable exercise performance among patients with severe left ventricular dysfunction. Am J Cardiol 1983;51:52–60.

56. DiBianco R, Shabetai R, Silverman BD, et al., and the Amrinone Multicenter Study Investigators. Oral amrinone for the treatment of chronic congestive heart failure: results of a multicenter randomized double-blind and placebo-controlled withdrawal study. J Am Coll Cardiol 1984;4: 855–866.

57. Maskin CS, Forman R, Sonnenblick EH, et al. Failure of dobutamine to increase exercise capacity despite hemodynamic improvement in severe chronic heart failure. Am J Cardiol 1983;51: 177–182.

58. Sullivan MJ, Cobb FE. Central hemodynamic response to exercise in patients with chronic heart failure. Chest 1992;101(Suppl 5):340S–346S.

59. Wilson JR, Schwartz JS, St. John Sutton M, et al.

Prognosis in severe heart failure: relation to hemodynamic measurements and ventricular ectopy. J Am Coll Cardiol 1983;2:403–410.

60. Clausen JP. Circulatory adjustments to dynamic exercise and effect of physical training in normal subjects and in patients with coronary artery disease. Prog Cardiovasc Dis 1976;18:459–495.

61. Franciosa JA, Cohn JN. Effect of isosorbide dinitrate on response to submaximal and maximal exercise in patients with congestive heart failure. Am J Cardiol 1979;43:1009–1014.

62. Franciosa JA, Cohn JN. Immediate effects of hydralazine-isosorbide dinitrate combination on exercise capacity and exercise hemodynamics in patients with left ventricular failure. Circulation 1979;59:1085–1091.

63. Franciosa JA, Goldsmith SR, Cohn JN. Contrasting immediate and long term effects of isosorbide dinitrate on exercise capacity in congestive heart failure. Am J Med 1980;69:559–566.

64. Rubin SA, Chatterjee KJ, Parmley WW. Metabolic assessment of exercise in chronic heart failure patients treated with short-term vasodilators. Circulation 1980;61:543–548.

65. Gorlin R, Sawyer CG, Haynes FW, et al. Effects of exercise on circulatory dynamics in mitral stenosis. Am Heart J 1951;41:192–203.

66. Leavitt JI, Coats MH, Falk RH. Effects of exercise on transmittal gradient and pulmonary artery pressure in patients with mitral stenosis or a prosthetic valve: a Doppler echocardiographic study. J Am Coll Cardiol 1991;17:1520–1526.

67. Arandi DT, Carleton RA. The deleterious role of tachycardia in mitral stenosis. Circulation 1967;36:511–516.

68. Braunwald E. Heart disease: a textbook of cardiovascular medicine. 2nd ed. Philadelphia: WB Saunders, 1984;1064–1135.

69. Flamm MD, Braniff BA, Kimball R, et al. Mechanism of effort syncope in aortic stenosis [abstract]. Circulation 1967;35, 36:II109.

70. Bache RJ, Wang Y, Jorgensen CR. Hemodynamic effects of exercise in isolated valvular aortic stenosis. Circulation 1971;44:1003–1013.

71. Richardson JW, Anderson FL, Tsagaris TJ. Rest and exercise hemodynamic studies in patients with isolated aortic stenosis. Cardiology 1979;64:1–11.

72. Tischler MD, Battle RW, Saha M, et al. Observations suggesting a high incidence of exercise-induced severe mitral regurgitation in patients with mild rheumatic mitral valve disease at rest. J Am Coll Cardiol 1995;25:128–133.

73. Henze E, Schelbert HR, Wisenberg G, et al. Assessment of regurgitant fraction and right and left ventricular function at rest and during exercise: a new technique for determination of right ventricular stroke counts from gated equilibrium blood pool studies. Am Heart J 1982;104:953–962.

74. Tischler MD, Battle RW, Ashikaga T, et al. Effects of exercise on left ventricular performance determined by echocardiography in chronic, severe regurgitation secondary to mitral valve prolapse. Am J Cardiol 1996;77:397–402.

75. Borer JS, Bacharach SL, Green MV, et al. Exercise-induced left ventricular dysfunction in sympto-matic and asymptomatic patients with aortic regurgitation: assessment with radionuclide cine-angiography. Am J Cardiol 1978;42:351–357.

76. Huxley RL, Gaffney FA, Corbett JR, et al. Early detection of left ventricular dysfunction in chronic aortic regurgitation as assessed by contrast angiography, echocardiography, and rest and exercise scintigraphy. Am J Cardiol 1983;51:1542–1550.

77. Johnson LL, Powers ER, Tzall WR, et al. Left ventricular volume and ejection fraction response to exercise in aortic regurgitation. Am J Cardiol 1983;51:1379–1385.

78. Dehmer GJ, Firth BG, Hillis LD, et al. Alterations in left ventricular volumes and ejection fraction at rest and during exercise in patients with aortic regurgitation. Am J Cardiol 1981;48:17–27.

79. Bonow RO, Lakatos E, Maron BJ, et al. Serial long-term assessment of the natural history of asymptomatic patients with chronic aortic regurgitation and normal left ventricular systolic function. Circulation 1991;84:1625–1635.

80. Gerstenblith G, Lakatta EG, Wesifeldt ML. Age changes in myocardial function and exercise response. Prog Cardiovasc Dis 1976;19:1–21.

81. Raven PB, Mitchell J. The effect of aging on the cardiovascular response to dynamic and static exercise. Aging (Milano) 1980;12:269–296.

82. Rodeheffer RJ, Gerstenblith G, Becker LC, et al. Exercise cardiac output is maintained with advancing age in healthy human subjects: cardiac dilation and increased stroke volume compensate for a diminished heart rate. Circulation 1984;69:203–213.

83. Donald KW, Lind AR, McNicol GW, et al. Cardiovascular responses to sustained (static) contractions. Circ Res 1967;20, 21:115–130.

84. Atkins JM, Matthews OA, Blomqvist CG, et al. Incidence of arrhythmias induced by isometric and dynamic exercise. BR Heart J 1976;38(5):465–471.

85. Amende I, Krayenbuehl HP, Rutishauser W, et al. Left ventricular dynamics during handgrip. Br Heart J 1972;34:688–695.

86. Bodenheimer MM, Banka VS, Fooshee CM, et al. Detection of coronary heart disease using radionuclide determined regional ejection fraction at rest and during handgrip exercise: correlation with coronary arteriography. Circulation 1978;58:640–648.

87. Ewing DJ, Irving JB, Kerr F, et al. Static exercise in untreated systemic hypertension. Br Heart J 1973;35:413–421.

88. Fisher ML, Nutter DO, Jacobs W, et al. Haemodynamic responses to isometric exercise (handgrip) in patients with heart disease. Br Heart J 1973;35:422–432.

89. Flessas AP, Connelly GP, Handa S, et al. Effects of isometric exercise on the end-diastolic pressure, volumes, and function of the left ventricle in man. Circulation 1976;53:839–847.

90. Helfant RH, DeVilla MA, Banka VS. Evaluation of left ventricular performance in coronary heart disease: use of isometric handgrip stress test. Cathet Cardiovasc Diagn 1976;2:59–67.

91. Helfant RH, DeVilla MA, Meister SG. Effect of sustained isometric handgrip exercise on left ven-

tricular performance. Circulation 1971;44:982–993.

92. Kivowitz C, Parmley WW, Donoso R, et al. Effects of isometric exercise on cardiac performance. The grip test. Circulation 1971;44:994–1002.

93. Krayenbuehl HP, Rutishauser W, Schoenbeck M, et al. Evaluation of left ventricular function from isovolumic pressure measurements during isometric exercise. Am J Cardiol 1972;29:323–330.

94. Krayenbuehl HP, Rutishauser W, Wirz P, et al. High-fidelity left ventricular pressure measurements for the assessment of cardiac contractility in man. Am J Cardiol 1973;31:415–427.

95. Ludbrook P, Karliner JS, O'Rourke RA. Effects of submaximal isometric handgrip on left ventricular size and wall motion. Am J Cardiol 1974;33:30–36.

96. Payne RM, Horwitz LD, Mullins CB. Comparison of isometric exercise and angiotensin infusion as stress test for evaluation of left ventricular function. Am J Cardiol 1973;31:428–433.

97. Perez-Gonzales JF, Schiller NB, Parmley WW. Direct and noninvasive evaluation of the cardio-vascular response to isometric exercise. Circ Res 1981;48:I138–I148.

98. Savin WM, Alderman EL, Haskell WL, et al. Left ventricular response to isometric exercise in patients with denervated and innervated hearts. Circulation 1980;61:897–901.

99. Siegel W, Gilbert CA, Nutter DO, et al. Use of isometric handgrip for the indirect assessment of left ventricular function in patients with coronary atherosclerotic heart disease. Am J Cardiol 1972;30:48–54.

100. Sullivan J, Hanson P, Rahko PS, et al. Continuous measurement of left ventricular performance during and after maximal deadlift exercise. Circulation 1992;85:1406–1413.

101. Sagiv M, Hanson P, Besozzi M, et al. Left ventricular responses to upright isometric handgrip and deadlift in men with coronary artery disease. Am J Cardiol 1985;55:1298–1302.

102. Willenbrock R, Ozcelik C, Osterziel KJ, et al. Angiotensin-converting enzyme inhibition, autonomic activity and hemodynamics in patients with heart failure who perform isometric exercise. Am Heart J 1996;131:999–1006.

103. Elkayam U, Roth A, Weber L, et al. Isometric exercise in patients with chronic advanced heart failure: hemodynamic and neurohumoral evaluation. Circulation 1985;72:975–981.

104. Ricci DR, Orlick AE, Alderman EL, et al. Role of tachycardia as an inotropic stimulus in man. J Clin Invest 1979;63:695–703.

105. Sonnenblick EH, Morrow AG, Williams JF Jr. Effects of heart rate on the dynamics of force development in the intact human ventricle. Circulation 1966;33:945–951.

106. Forrester JS, Helfant RH, Pasternac A, et al. Atrial pacing in coronary heart disease. Effect on hemodynamics, metabolism, and coronary circulation. Am J Cardiol 1971;27:237–243.

107. Parker JO, Chiong MA, West RO, et al. Sequential alterations in myocardial lactate metabolism, S-T segments, and left ventricular function during angina induced by atrial pacing. Circulation 1969;40:113–131.

108. Kyriakides ZS, Antoniadis A, Iliodromitis E, et al. Short-term effects of right atrial, right ventricular apical, and atrioventricular sequential pacing on myocardial oxygen consumption and cardiac efficiency in patients with coronary artery disease. Br Heart J 1994;71:536–540 [published erratum appears in Br Heart J 1994;72:404].

109. Khaja F, Parker JO, Ledwich RJ, et al. Assessment of ventricular function in coronary artery disease by means of atrial pacing and exercise. Am J Cardiol 1970;26:107–116.

110. Krayenbuehl HP, Schoenbeck M, Rutishauser W, et al. Abnormal segmental contraction velocity in coronary artery disease produced by isometric exercise and atrial pacing. Am J Cardiol 1975;35:785–794.

111. Linhart JW. Pacing-induced changes in stroke volume in the evaluation of myocardial function. Circulation 1970;43:253–261.

112. Linhart JW. Myocardial function in coronary artery disease determined by atrial pacing. Circulation 1971;44:203–212.

113. Mann T, Brodie BR, Grossman W, et al. Effect of angina on the left ventricular diastolic pressure-volume relationship. Circulation 1977;55:761–766.

114. McLaurin LP, Rolett EL, Grossman W. Impaired left ventricular relaxation during pacing-induced ischemia. Am J Cardiol 1973;32:751–757.

115. Parker JO, Khaja F, Case RB. Analysis of left ventricular function by atrial pacing. Circulation 1971;43:241–252.

116. Parker JO, Ledwich JR, West RO, et al. Reversible cardiac failure during angina pectoris. Hemodynamic effects of atrial pacing in coronary artery disease. Circulation 1969;39:745–757.

117. Ross J Jr, Linhart JW, Braunwald E. Effects of changing heart rate in man by electrical stimulation of the right atrium. Studies at rest, during exercise, and with isoproterenol. Circulation 1965;32:549–558.

118. Dehmer GJ, Firth BG, Nicod P, et al. Alterations in left ventricular volumes and ejection fraction during atrial pacing in patients with coronary artery disease: assessment with radionuclide ventriculography. Am J Cardiol 1983;106:114–124.

119. Markham RV Jr, Winniford MD, Firth BG, et al. Symptomatic, electrocardiographic, metabolic, and hemodynamic alterations during pacing-induced myocardial ischemia. Am J Cardiol 1983;51:1589–1594.

120. Leighton RF, Zaron SJ, Robinson JL, et al. Effects of atrial pacing on left ventricular performance in patients with heart disease. Circulation 1969;40:615–622.

121. Aroesty JM, McKay RG, Heller GV, et al. Simultaneous assessment of left ventricular systolic and diastolic dysfunction during pacing-induced ischemia. Circulation 1985;71:889–900.

122. Mann T, Goldberg S, Mudge GH Jr, et al. Factors contributing to altered left ventricular diastolic properties during angina pectoris. Circulation 1979;59:14–20.

123. DeMaria AN, Neumann A, Schubart PJ, et al. Sys-

tematic correlation of cardiac chamber size and ventricular performance determined with echocardiography and alterations in heart rate in normal persons. Am J Cardiol 1979;43:1–9.

124. Bahler RC, Macleod CA. Atrial pacing and exercise in the evaluation of patients with angina pectoris. Circulation 1971;43:407–419.

125. Kelemen MH, Gillilan RE, Bouchard RJ, et al. Diagnosis of obstructive coronary disease by maximal exercise and atrial pacing. Circulation 1973; 48:1227–1233.

126. Boudoulas H, Cobb TC, Leighton RF, et al. Myocardial lactate production in patients with angina-like chest pain and angiographically normal coronary arteries and left ventricle. Am J Cardiol 1974; 34:501–505.

127. Helfant RH, Forrester JS, Hampton JR, et al. Coronary heart disease. Differential hemodynamic, metabolic, and electrocardiographic effects in subjects with and without angina pectoris during atrial pacing. Circulation 1970;42:601–610.

128. Linhart JW, Hildner FJ, Barold SS, et al. Left heart hemodynamics during angina pectoris induced by atrial pacing. Circulation 1969;40:483–492.

129. Mammohansingh P, Parker JO. Angina pectoris with normal coronary arteriograms: hemodynamic and metabolic response to atrial pacing. Am Heart J 1975;90:555–561.

130. Rios JC, Hurwitz LE. Electrocardiographic responses to atrial pacing and multistage treadmill exercise testing. Correlation with coronary arteriography. Am J Cardiol 1974;34:661–666.

131. Robson RH, Pridie R, Fluck DC. Evaluation of rapid atrial pacing in diagnosis of coronary artery disease. Evaluation of atrial pacing test. Br Heart J 1976;38:986–989.

132. O'Brien KP, Higgs LM, Glancy DL, et al. Hemodynamic accompaniments of angina. A comparison during angina induced by exercise and by atrial pacing. Circulation 1969;39:735–743.

133. Heller GV, Aroesty JM, McKay RG, et al. The pacing stress test: a reexamination of the relation between coronary artery disease and pacing-induced electrocardiographic changes. Am J Cardiol 1984;54:50–55.

134. Hecht HS, Chew CY, Burnam M, et al. Radionuclide ejection fraction and regional wall motion during atrial pacing in stable angina pectoris: comparison with metabolic and hemodynamic parameters. Am Heart J 1981;101:726–733.

135. Pasternac A, Gorlin R, Sonnenblick EH, et al. Abnormalities of ventricular motion induced by atrial pacing in coronary artery disease. Circulation 1972;45:1195–1205.

136. Stone D, Dymond D, Elliott AT, et al. Use of first-pass radionuclide ventriculography in assessment of wall motion abnormalities induced by incremental atrial pacing in patients with coronary artery disease. Br Heart J 1980;43:369–375.

137. Aebischer N, Malhotra R, Connors L, et al. Ventricular interdependence during the Valsalva maneuver as seen by two-dimensional echocardiography: new insights about an old method. J Am Soc Echocardiogr 1995;8:536–542.

138. Gorlin R, Knowles JH, Storey CF. The Valsalva maneuver as a test of cardiac function. Pathologic

physiology and clinical significance. Am J Med 1957;22:197–212.

139. Labovitz AJ, Dincer B, Mudd G, et al. The effects of Valsalva maneuver on global and segmental left ventricular function in presence and absence of coronary artery disease. Am Heart J 1985;109: 259–264.

140. Little WC, Barr WK, Crawford MH. Altered effect of the Valsalva maneuver on left ventricular volume in patients with cardiomyopathy. Circulation 1985;71:227–233.

141. Parisi AF, Harrington JJ, Askenazi J, et al. Echocardiographic evaluation of the Valsalva maneuver in healthy subjects and patients with and without heart failure. Circulation 1976;54: 921–927.

142. Robertson D, Stevens RM, Friesinger GC, et al. The effect of the Valsalva maneuver on echocardiographic dimensions in man. Circulation 1977; 55:596–602.

143. Hoshino PK, Blaustein AS, Gaasch WH. Effect of propranolol on the left ventricular response to the Valsalva maneuver in normal subjects. Am J Cardiol 1988;61:400–404.

144. Zema MJ, Restivo B, Sos T, et al. Left ventricular dysfunction—bedside Valsalva manoeuvre. Br Heart J 1980;44:560–569.

145. Nishimura RA, Tajik AJ. The Valsalva maneuver and response revisited. Mayo Clin Proc 1986;61: 211–217.

146. Palmero HA, Caeiro TF, Losa DJ, et al. Baroreceptor reflex sensitivity index derived from phase 4 of the Valsalva maneuver. Hypertension 1981;3: 134–137.

147. Kalbfleisch JH, Reinke JA, Porth CJ, et al. Effect of age on circulating response to postural and Valsalva tests. Proc Soc Exp Biol Med 1977;156: 100–103.

148. Ewing DJ, Campbell IW, Burt AA, et al. Vascular reflexes in diabetic autonomic neuropathy. Lancet 1973;2:1354–1356.

149. Ibrahim MM, Tarazi RC, Dustan HP. Orthostatic hypotension: mechanisms and management. Am Heart J 1975;90:513–520.

150. Ruskin J, Harley A, Greenfield JC Jr. Pressure flow studies in patients having a pressor response to the Valsalva maneuver. Circulation 1968;38: 277–281.

151. Pepine CJ, Wiener L. Effects of the Valsalva maneuver on myocardial ischemia in patients with coronary artery disease. Circulation 1979;59: 1304–1311.

152. Levine HJ, McIntyre KM, Glovsky MM. Relief of angina pectoris by Valsalva maneuver. N Engl J Med 1966;275:487–489.

153. Benchimol A, Wang TF, Desser KB, et al. The Valsalva maneuver and coronary arterial blood flow velocity. Studies in man. Ann Intern Med 1972; 77:357–360.

154. Rothman A, Goldberger AL. Aids to cardiac auscultation. Ann Intern Med 1983;99:346–353.

155. Moreyra E, Buteler B, Madoery R, Alday L. Drugs and maneuvers in the diagnosis of muscular subaortic stenosis. Am Heart J 1972;83:431–433.

156. Rosenblum R, Delman AJ. Valsalva's maneuver and the systolic murmur of hypertrophic subaor-

tic stenosis: a bedside diagnostic test. Am J Cardiol 1965;15:868–870.

157. Barlow JB, Pocock WA, Marchand P, et al. The significance of late systolic murmurs. Am Heart J 1963;66:443–452.

158. Erfan A, Abdel-Salam R. The effect of the Valsalva maneuver on cardiac vibrations: a phonocardiographic study. J Egypt Med Assoc 1966;49:1–23.

159. Stefadouros MA, Mucha E, Frank MJ. Paradoxic response of the murmur of idiopathic hypertrophic subaortic stenosis to the Valsalva maneuver. Am J Cardiol 1976;37:89–92.

160. Polis O, Cleempoel H, Hanson J, et al. Interet de l'epreuve de Valsalva en phonocardiographie. Acta Cardiol 1960;15:441–462.

161. Buda AJ, Pinsky MR, Ingels NB Jr, et al. Effect of intrathoracic pressure on left ventricular performance. N Engl J Med 1979;301:453–459.

162. Smucker ML, Cassidy SS, Nixon JV. Effect of the Mueller manoeuvre at different lung volumes on left ventricular performance in normal subjects. Clin Physiol 1983;3:411–421.

163. Scharf SM, Brown R, Tow DE, et al. Cardiac effects of increased lung volume and decreased pleural pressure in man. J Appl Physiol 1979;47:257–262.

164. Brinker JA, Weiss JL, Lappe DL, et al. Leftward septal displacement during right ventricular loading in man. Circulation 1980;61:626–633.

165. Condos WR Jr, Latham RD, Hoadley SD, et al. Hemodynamics of the Mueller maneuver in man: right and left heart micromanometry and Doppler echocardiography. Circulation 1987; 76:1020–1028.

166. Sharpey-Schafer EP. Effect of respiratory acts on the circulation. In: Hamilton WF, Dow P, eds. Handbook of physiology, section 2. Baltimore: Williams & Wilkins, 1965:1875–1886.

167. Buda AJ, MacKenzie GW, Wigle ED. Effect of negative intrathoracic pressure on left ventricular outflow tract obstruction in muscular subaortic stenosis. Circulation 1981;63:875–881.

168. Scharf SM, Woods BO, Brown R, et al. Effects of the Mueller maneuver on global and regional left ventricular function in angina pectoris with or without previous myocardial infarction. Am J Cardiol 1987;59:1305–1309.

169. Pennock RS, Kawai N, Segal BL. Physiologic and pharmacologic aids in cardiac auscultation. In: Fowler NO, ed. Diagnostic methods in cardiology. Philadelphia: FA Davis, 1975:29.

170. Bartall H, Amber S, Desser KB, et al. Normalization of the external carotid pulse tracing of hypertrophic subaortic stenosis during Muller's maneuver. Chest 1978;74:77–78.

171. Chierchia S, Davies G, Berkenboom G, et al. α-adrenergic receptors and coronary spasm: an elusive link. Circulation 1984;69:8–14.

172. Feldman RL, Whittle JL, Marx JD, et al. Regional coronary hemodynamic responses to cold stimulation in patients without variant angina. Am J Cardiol 1982;49:665–673.

173. Jordan LJ, Borer JS, Zullo M, et al. Exercise versus cold temperature stimulation during radionuclide cineangiography: diagnostic accuracy in coronary artery disease. Am J Cardiol 1983;51: 1091–1097.

174. Malacoff RF, Mudge GH Jr, Holman BL, et al. Effect of the cold pressor test on regional myocardial blood flow in patients with coronary artery disease. Am Heart J 1983;106:78–84.

175. Manyari DE, Nolewajka AJ, Purves P, et al. Comparative value of the cold-pressor test and supine bicycle exercise to detect subjects with coronary artery disease using radionuclide ventriculography. Circulation 1982;65:571–579.

176. Mudge GH Jr, Goldberg S, Gunther S, et al. Comparison of metabolic and vasoconstrictor stimuli on coronary vascular resistance in man. Circulation 1979;59:544–550.

177. Shea MJ, Deanfield JE, deLandsheere CM, et al. Asymptomatic myocardial ischemia following cold provocation. Am Heart J 1987;114:469–476.

178. Stratton JR, Halter JB, Hallstrom AP, et al. Comparative plasma catecholamine and hemodynamic responses to handgrip, cold pressor and supine bicycle exercise testing in normal subjects. J Am Coll Cardiol 1983;2:93–104.

179. Waters DD, Szlachcic J, Bonan R, et al. Comparative sensitivity of exercise, cold pressor and ergonovine testing in provoking attacks of variant angina in patients with active disease. Circulation 1983;67:310–315.

180. Nitenberg A, Antony I, Aptecar E, et al. Impairment of flow-dependent coronary dilation in hypertensive patients. Demonstration by cold pressor test induced low velocity increase. Am J Hypertens 1995;8:13S–18S.

181. Mudge GH Jr, Grossman W, Mills RM Jr, et al. Reflex increase in coronary vascular resistance in patients with ischemic heart disease. N Engl J Med 1976;295:1333–1337.

182. Raizner AE, Chahine RA, Ishimori T, et al. Provocation of coronary artery spasm by the cold pressor test. Hemodynamic, arteriographic and quantitative angiographic observations. Circulation 1980;62:925–932.

183. Gondi B, Nanda NC. Cold pressor test during two-dimensional echocardiography: usefulness in detection of patients with coronary disease. Am Heart J 1984;107:278–285.

184. Kern MJ, Ganz P, Horowitz JD, et al. Potentiation of coronary vasoconstriction by beta-adrenergic blockade in patients with coronary artery disease. Circulation 1983;67:1178–1185.

185. Mueller HS, Rao PS, Rao PB, et al. Enhanced transcardiac 1-norepinephrine response during cold pressor test in obstructive coronary artery disease. Am J Cardiol 1982;50:1223–1228.

186. Crea F, Davies G, Chierchia S, et al. Different susceptibility to myocardia ischemia provoked by hyperventilation and cold pressor test in exertional and variant angina pectoris. Am J Cardiol 1985;56:18–22.

187. Ahmad M, Dubiel JP, Haibach H. Cold pressor thallium-201 myocardial scintigraphy in the diagnosis of coronary artery disease. Am J Cardiol 1982;50:1253–1257.

188. Balino NAP, Liprandi AS, Masoli O, et al. Usefulness of radionuclide ventriculography in assessment of coronary artery spasm. Am J Cardiol 1987;59:552–558.

189. Oren RM, Roach PJ, Schobel HP, et al. Sympa-

thetic response of patients with congestive heart failure to cold pressor stimulus. Am J Cardiol 1991;67:67–77.

190. Westheim A, Os I, Thaulow E, et al. Hemodynamic and neurohumoral effects of cold pressor test in severe heart failure. Clin Physiol 1992;12: 95–106.

191. Rowe GG, Castillo CA, Crumpton CW. Effects of hyperventilation on systemic and coronary hemodynamics. Am Heart J 1962;63:67–77.

192. Girotti LA, Crosatto JR, Messuti H, et al. The hyperventilation test as a method for developing successful therapy in Prinzmetal's angina. Am J Cardiol 1982;49:834–841.

193. Ardissino D, DeServi S, Barberis P, et al. Significance of hyperventilation-induced ST segment depression in patients with coronary artery disease. J Am Coll Cardiol 1989;13:804–810.

194. Rasmussen K, Juul S, Bagger JP, et al. Usefulness of ST deviation induced by prolonged hyperventilation as a predictor of cardiac death in angina pectoris. Am J Cardiol 1987;59:763–768.

195. Ardissino D, De Servi S, Falcone C, et al. Role of hypocapnic alkalosis in hyperventilation-induced coronary artery spasm in variant angina. Am J Cardiol 1987;59:707–709.

196. Yasue H, Nagao M, Omote S, et al. Coronary arterial spasm and Prinzmetal's variant form of angina induced by hyperventilation and tris-buffer infusion. Circulation 1978;58:56–62.

197. Fleckenstein A, Nakayama K, Fleckenstein-Grun B, et al. Interaction of H ions, Ca antagonist drugs and cardiac glycosides with excitation contraction coupling of vascular smooth muscle. In: Betz E, ed. Ionic action on vascular smooth muscle. Berlin: Springer Verlag, 1976:117–125.

198. Mrwa U, Achtig I, Reugg JC. Influences of calcium concentration and pH on the tension development and ATPase activity of the arterial actomyosin contractile system. Blood Vessels 1974;11: 277–286.

199. Ushiyama K, Ogawa T, Ishii M, et al. Physiologic neuroendocrine arousal by mental arithmetic stress test in healthy subjects. Am J Cardiol 1991; 67:101–103.

200. Lacy CR, Contrada RJ, Robbins ML, et al. Coronary vasoconstriction induced by mental stress (simulated public speaking). Am J Cardiol 1995; 75:503–505.

201. Speechia G, Falcone C, Traversi C, et al. Mental stress as a provocative test in patients with various clinical syndromes of coronary artery disease. Circulation 1991;83 (Suppl II):II-108–II-114.

202. Barry J, Selwyn AP, Nabel EG, et al. Frequency of ST-segment depression produced by mental stress in stable angina pectoris from coronary artery disease. Am J Cardiol 1988;61:989–993.

203. Gottdiener JS, Krantz DS, Howell RH, et al. Induction of silent myocarial ischemia with mental stress testing: relation to the triggers of ischemia during daily life activities and to ischemic functional severity. J Am Coll Cardiol 1994;24: 1645–1651.

204. Rozanski A, Krantz DS, Bairey CN. Ventricular response to mental stress testing in patients with coronary artery disease; pathophysiological implications. Circulation 1991;83(Suppl II):II-137–II-144.

205. Giubbini R, Galli M, Campini R, et al. Effects of mental stress on myocardial perfusion in patients with ischemic heart disease. Circulation 1991; 83(Suppl II):II-100–II-107.

206. Jiang W, Babyak M, Krantz DS, et al. Mental stress-induced myocardial ischemia and cardiac events. JAMA 1996;275:1651–1656.

207. L'Abbate A, Simonetti I, Carpeggiani C, et al. Coronary dynamics and mental arithmetic stress in humans. Circulation 1991;83(Suppl II):II-94–II-99.

208. Deanfield JE, Shea M, Kensett M, et al. Silent myocardial ischemia due to mental stress. Lancet 1984; 2:1001–1005.

209. Jain D, Burg M, Soufer R, et al. Prognostic implications of mental stress-induced silent left ventricular dysfunction in patients with stable angina pectoris. Am J Cardiol 1995;76:31–35.

210. Miller RR, Vismara LA, Williams DO, et al. Pharmacologic mechanisms for left ventricular unloading in clinical congestive heart failure. Differential effects of nitroprusside, phentolamine and nitroglycerin on cardiac function and peripheral circulation. Circ Res 1976;39:127–133.

211. Opie LH. Nitrates. Lancet 1980;1:750–753.

212. Mookherjee S, Fuleihan D, Warner RA, et al. Effects of sublingual nitroglycerin on resting pulmonary gas exchange and hemodynamics in man. Circulation 1978;57:106–110.

213. Parker JO, di Giorgi S, West RO. A hemodynamic study of acute coronary insufficiency precipitated by exercise. With observations on the effects of nitroglycerin. Am J Cardiol 1966;17:470–483.

214. Choong CYP, Roubin GS, Bautovich GJ, et al. Antianginal effects of nitroglycerin during exercise-induced angina: hemodynamic and left ventricular function changes related to indexes of myocardial oxygen consumption. Am J Cardiol 1987;60:10H–14H.

215. De Coster PM, Chiechia S, Davies GJ, et al. Combined effects of nitrates on the coronary and peripheral circulation in exercise-induced ischemia. Circulation 1990;81:1881–1886.

216. Udhoji VN, Heng MK. Hemodynamic effects of high-dose sustained-action oral isosorbide dinitrate in stable angina. Am J Med 1984;76:234–240.

217. Kingma I, Smiseth OA, Belenkie I, et al. A mechanism for the nitroglycerin-induced downward shift of the left ventricular diastolic pressure-diameter relation. Am J Cardiol 1986;57:673–677.

218. Brown BG. Response of normal and diseased epicardial coronary arteries to vasoactive drugs: quantitative arteriographic studies. Am J Cardiol 1985;56:23E–29E.

219. Brown BG, Bolson E, Petersen RB, et al. The mechanisms of nitroglycerin action: stenosis vasodilation as a major component of the drug response. Circulation 1981;64:1089–1097.

220. Feldman RL, Marx JD, Pepine CJ, et al. Analysis of coronary responses to various doses of intracoronary nitroglycerin. Circulation 1982;66: 321–327.

221. Aoki M, Sakai K, Koyanagi S, et al. Effect of nitroglycerin on collateral function during exercise evaluated by quantitative analysis of thallium-201

single photon computed tomography. Am Heart J 1991;121:1361–1366.

222. May DC, Popma JJ, Black WH, et al. In vivo induction and reversal of nitroglycerin tolerance in human coronary arteries. N Engl J Med 1987;317:805–809.

223. Pepine CJ, Joyal M, Cremer KF, et al. Hemodynamic effects of nitroglycerin combined with diltiazem in patients with coronary artery disease. Am J Med 1984;76:47–51.

224. Dumesnil JG, Ritman EL, Davis GD, et al. Regional left ventricular wall dynamics before and after sublingual administration of nitroglycerin. Am J Cardiol 1975;36:419–425.

225. McAnulty JH, Hattenhauer MT, Rosch J, et al. Improvement in left ventricular wall motion following nitroglycerin. Circulation 1975;51:140–145.

226. Pepine CJ, Feldman RL, Ludbrook P, et al. Left ventricular dyskinesia reversed by intravenous nitroglycerin: a manifestation of silent myocardial ischemia. Am J Cardiol 1986;58:38B–42B.

227. Chesebro JH, Ritman EL, Frye RL, et al. Regional myocardial wall thickening response to nitroglycerin—a predictor of myocardial response to aortocoronary bypass surgery. Circulation 1978;57:952–957.

228. Helfant RH, Pine R, Meister SG, et al. Nitroglycerin to unmask reversible asynergy. Correlation with post coronary bypass ventriculography. Circulation 1974;50:108–113.

229. Franciosa JA, Blank RC, Cohn JN. Nitrate effects on cardiac output and left ventricular outflow resistance in chronic congestive heart failure. Am J Med 1978;64:207–213.

230. Gold HK, Leinbach RC, Sanders CA. Use of sublingual nitroglycerin in congestive heart failure following acute myocardial infarction. Circulation 1972;46:839–845.

231. Varriale P, David WJ, Chryssos BE. Hemodynamic resistance to intravenous nitroglycerin in severe congestive heart failure and restored response after diuresis. Am J Cardiol 1991;68:1400–1402.

232. Cokkinos DV, Tsartsalis GD, Heimonas ET, et al. Comparison of the inotropic action of digitalis and isoproterenol in younger and older individuals. Am Heart J 1980;100:802–806.

233. Dodge HT, Lord JD, Sandler H. Cardiovascular effects of isoproterenol in normal subjects and subjects with congestive heart failure. Am Heart J 1960;60:94–105.

234. Firth BG, Tan LB, Rajagopalan B, et al. Assessment of myocardial performance in ischaemic heart disease: from changes in left ventricular power output produced by graded-dose isoprenaline infusion. Cardiovasc Res 1981;15:351–364.

235. Fitzgerald DE, O'Shaughnessy AM. Cardiac and peripheral arterial responses to isoprenaline challenge. Cardiovasc Res 1984;18:414–418.

236. Kuramoto K, Matsushita S, Kuwajima I, et al. Comparison of hemodynamic effects of exercise and isoproterenol infusion in normal young and old men. Jpn Circ J 1979;43:71–76.

237. Kuramoto K, Matsushita S, Mifune J, et al. Electrocardiographic and hemodynamic evaluations of isoproterenol test in elderly ischemic heart disease. Jpn Circ J 1978;42:955–960.

238. Nathan D, Ongley PA, Rahimtoola SH. The dynamics of left ventricular ejection in "normal" man with infusion of isoproterenol. Chest 1977;71:746–752.

239. Stephens J, Ead H, Spurrell R. Haemodynamic effects of dobutamine with special reference to myocardial blood flow. A comparison with dopamine and isoprenaline. Br Heart J 1979;42:43–50.

240. Gundel W, Cherry G, Rajagopalan B, et al. Aortic input impedance in man: acute response to vasodilator drugs. Circulation 1981;63:1305–1314.

241. Sapru RP, Hannan WJ, Muir AL, et al. Effect of isoprenaline and propranolol on left ventricular function as determined by nuclear angiography. Br Heart J 1980;44:75–81.

242. Sapru RP, Muir AL, Hannan WJ, et al. Effect of exercise and isoprenaline on left ventricular ejection fraction in patients with angina pectoris as assessed by radionuclide angiography. Cardiology 1982;69:91–97.

243. Dodge HT, Murdaugh HV Jr. Cardiovascular-renal effects of isoproterenol in congestive heart failure [abstract]. Circulation 1957;16:873.

244. Horwitz LD, Curry GC, Parkey RW, et al. Differentiation of physiologically significant coronary artery lesions by coronary blood flow measurements during isoproterenol infusion. Circulation 1974;49:55–62.

245. Krasnow N, Rolett EL, Yurchak PM, et al. Isoproterenol and cardiovascular function. Am J Med 1964;37:514–525.

246. Combs DT, Martin CM. Evaluation of isoproterenol as a method of stress testing. Am Heart J 1974;87:711–715.

247. Kerber RE, Abboud FM, Marcus ML, et al. Effect of inotropic agents on the localized dyskinesis of acutely ischemic myocardium. An experimental ultrasound study. Circulation 1974;49:1038–1046.

248. Wexler H, Kuaity J, Simonson E. Electrocardiographic effects of isoprenaline in normal subjects and patients with coronary atherosclerosis. Br Heart J 1971;33:759–764.

249. Stein I. Observations on the action of ergonovine on the coronary circulation and its use in the diagnosis of coronary artery insufficiency. Am Heart J 1949;37:36–45.

250. Heupler F, Proudfit W, Siegel W, et al. The ergonovine maleate test for the diagnosis of coronary artery spasm [abstract]. Circulation 1975;52:II–11.

251. Schwartz AB, Donmichael TA, Botvinick EH, et al. Variability in coronary hemodynamics in response to ergonovine in patients with normal coronary arteries and atypical chest pain. J Am Coll Cardiol 1983;1:797–803.

252. Curry RC Jr, Pepine CJ, Sabom MB, et al. Hemodynamic and myocardial metabolic effects of ergonovine in patients with chest pain. Circulation 1978;58:648–654.

253. Feldman RL, Pepine CJ, Whittle JL, et al. Coronary hemodynamic findings during spontaneous angina in patients with variant angina. Circulation 1981;64:76–83.

254. Fragasso G, Davies GJ, Chierchia S, et al. Relative roles of preload increase and coronary constric-

tion in ergonovine-induced myocardial ischemia in stable angina pectoris. Am J Cardiol 1987;60: 238–243.

255. Orlick AE, Ricci DR, Cipriano PR, et al. Coronary hemodynamic effects of ergonovine maleate in human subjects. Am J Cardiol 1980;45:48–52.

256. Tousoulis D, Kaski JC, Bogaty P, et al. Reactivity of proximal and distal angiographically normal and stenotic coronary segments in chronic stable angina pectoris. Am J Cardiol 1991;67:1195–1200.

257. Cipriano PR, Guthaner DF, Orlick AE, et al. The effects of ergonovine maleate on coronary arterial size. Circulation 1979;59:82–89.

258. Tatineni S, Kern MJ, Aguirre F. The effect of ergonovine on coronary vasodilatory reserve in patients with angiographically normal coronary arteries. Am Heart J 1992;123:617–620.

259. Crea F, Davies G, Romeo F, et al. Myocardial ischemia during ergonovine testing: different susceptibility to coronary vasoconstriction in patients with exertional and variant angina. Circulation 1984;69:690–695.

260. Burggraf GW, Parker JO. Hemodynamic effects of amyl nitrite in coronary artery disease. Am J Cardiol 1973;32:772–778.

261. Burggraf GW, Parker JO. Left ventricular volume changes after amyl nitrite and nitroglycerin in man as measured by ultrasound. Circulation 1974;49:136–143.

262. de Leon AC, Perloff JK. The pulmonary hemodynamic effects of amyl nitrite in normal man. Am Heart J 1966;72:337–344.

263. Mitake H, Sawayama T, Nezuo S, et al. Significant coronary artery disease detected by amyl nitrite and systolic time intervals. Am J Cardiol 1984;54: 79–83.

264. Niarchos AP, Tahmooressi P, Tarazi RC. Comparison of heart rate and blood pressure response to amyl nitrite, isoproterenol, and standing before and during acute beta-adrenergic blockade with intravenous propranolol. Am Heart J 1978;96: 47–53.

265. Perloff JK, Calvin J, De Leon AC, et al. Systemic hemodynamic effects of amyl nitrite in normal man. Am Heart J 1963;66:460–469.

266. Miller H, Ostrzega E, Geva B, et al. Effect of amyl nitrite on coronary blood flow [abstract]. J Am Coll Cardiol 1983;1:695A.

267. Benchimol A, Desser KB, Raizada V. Effects of amyl nitrite on phasic aortocoronary bypass graft blood velocity in man. Am Heart J 1977;93: 592–595.

268. Contro S, Haring DM, Goldstein W. Paradoxic action of amyl nitrite in coronary patients. Circulation 1952;6:250–256.

269. Kerber RE, Harrison DC. Paradoxical electrocardiographic effects of amyl nitrite in coronary artery disease. Br Heart J 1972;34:851–857.

25
Valve Function: Stenosis and Insufficiency

Lawrence R. Blitz, MD
Daniel M. Kolansky, MD
John W. Hirshfeld Jr, MD

INTRODUCTION: GENERAL PRINCIPLES

Normal Valve Function

The heart is a pressure pump that propels blood through the circulatory system by raising chamber cavity pressure. When the pressure in one chamber exceeds the pressure in the next chamber downstream, blood flows to the downstream chamber. The proper operation of this system depends on the cardiac valves whose purpose is to allow unidirectional blood flow. A normal valve performs this function without obstructing forward flow or allowing any reverse flow. Any of the four cardiac valves can become either stenotic (obstructing the normal forward flow of blood) or regurgitant (allowing backward flow of blood), or both.

Objectives of Catheterization Assessment

Most valvular dysfunction can be recognized by physical examination and noninvasive diagnostic techniques. Accordingly, it should be unusual to discover previously unrecognized valve disease during a cardiac catheterization procedure. Instead, the assessment of abnormal valve function by cardiac catheterization has two general purposes: (*a*) to characterize and quantify the valvular dysfunction and (*b*) to characterize and quantify the response of the affected chamber(s) to the excessive hemodynamic burden caused by the valvular dysfunction.

VALVULAR STENOSIS

Functional Problems Caused by Cardiac Valve Stenosis

A stenotic cardiac valve predominantly affects the chamber immediately upstream from it. Although other cardiac chambers further upstream may also be burdened, these effects are indirect, resulting from the altered conditions in the chamber immediately upstream from the stenotic valve.

The reduced **orifice area** of a stenotic valve obstructs normal forward blood flow, requiring an abnormally increased pressure gradient across the valve. This, in turn, requires an increased cavity pressure in the

516

chamber upstream from the stenosed valve. Thus, the stenotic valve places a pressure load on the upstream chamber, which must adapt to the requirement to generate increased pressure.

Valvular stenosis, which can be either congenital or acquired, does not develop acutely. It is either present from birth or develops slowly over many years. Therefore, the affected cardiac chambers can adapt to the hemodynamic burden over time.

Determinants of Flow Velocity Across a Cardiac Valve

When considering flow across a cardiac valve, it is important to distinguish between flow rate (measured in volume per unit time such as milliliters per second) and flow velocity (measured in length per unit time such as centimeters per second). Each unit of measurement has its own physiologic significance. Flow rate is related to the cardiac output and measures the total volume of flow across the valve. Flow velocity, on the other hand, measures the speed at which blood moves and (as will be explained) is related to the pressure gradient across a valve orifice.

The flow velocity across any cardiac valve, stenotic or not, is determined by the interaction of two variables:

1. The total flow rate across the valve (generally the cardiac output divided by the fraction of time that flow actually occurs across the valve).
2. The area of the valve orifice through which flow must pass.

These variables are interrelated by the following mathematical expression:

$$Flow = Area \times Velocity \qquad (1)$$

This relationship, which is merely an expression of conservation of volume, has two pragmatic consequences:

1. At a given valve orifice area, an increase in flow rate requires a direct increase in flow velocity.
2. At a constant flow rate, a change in orifice area requires an inverse change in flow velocity.

Thus, either a decrease in orifice area or an increase in flow rate requires an increase in the flow velocity.

"Orifice Action": The Biophysics of Flow from One Cardiac Chamber to Another

The transfer of blood from a relatively stationary state within a cardiac chamber across an orifice to a downstream chamber or great vessel requires the addition of the kinetic energy associated with the increase in velocity of the blood as it moves across the orifice. In the heart, this kinetic energy is derived from the potential energy associated with the cavity pressure in the chamber immediately upstream from the orifice. As the velocity of the stationary blood within the chamber cavity is accelerated, some of its potential (or pressure) energy is transformed to kinetic (or velocity) energy. The Bernoulli principle (which is an expression of the conservation of energy) requires a decrease in pressure (pressure gradient) as the blood traverses the orifice (Fig. 25.1).

The hydraulic potential energy of a fluid is related to the volume of the fluid and its pressure:

$$E_p = P_g V \qquad (2)$$

where E_p = potential energy (ergs), P = pressure (cm H_2O), g = gravitational acceleration (cm/sec), and V = volume (cm^3). The hydraulic kinetic energy of a fluid is related to both its volume and its velocity.

$$E_k = \frac{1}{2} V v^2 \qquad (3)$$

where E_k = kinetic energy (ergs), V = volume (cm^3), and v = velocity (cm/sec).

The V term is actually mass ($E_k = \frac{1}{2} mv^2$). However, for simplicity of derivation, mass and volume are treated as being interchangeable. This assumption would be correct if the specific gravity of blood (which is 1.06) were 1.00.

If energy is conserved in the passage of blood across the orifice, there is no change

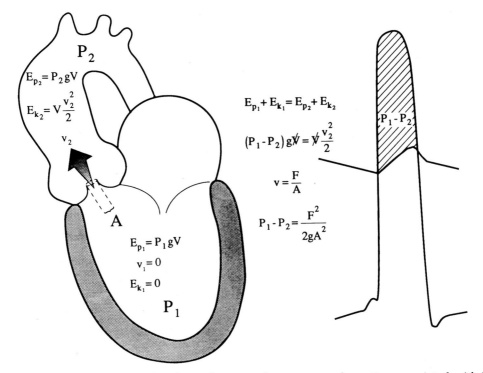

Figure 25.1. Diagram depicting biophysical events of energy transformation associated with blood flow across an orifice. In this example, a stenotic aortic valve with an orifice area A is depicted. Blood in the chamber upstream from the orifice (in this case the left ventricle) has potential energy E_{p1} (ergs) determined by its pressure (P) and volume (V). Because the blood is relatively stationary, its kinetic energy E_{k1} is considered to be zero. Blood in the chamber downstream from the orifice (in this case the aorta) has less potential energy E_{p2} and has acquired kinetic energy E_{k2}, which is determined by its velocity (v) and volume. Velocity (cm/sec) of blood flow across the orifice is determined by the volume flow rate F (mL/sec) and orifice area A (cm^2). As it passes through the orifice, the blood's loss of potential energy is equal to its gain of potential energy. Thus, the decrease in pressure ($P_1 - P_2$) as blood passes across the orifice is directly related to the square of the flow rate and inversely to the square of the orifice area. (See text for further details.)

in total energy content, and the decrease in potential energy is equal to the increase in kinetic energy.

$$Ep_1 + E_{k1} = E_{p2} + E_{k2} \qquad (4)$$

Assuming that the blood contained in the chamber upstream from the orifice has zero kinetic energy, and also assuming that no potential energy is transformed in other processes (not exactly correct, but an adequate approximation for this derivation), Equations 1 and 2 can be combined.

$$P_1gV = P_2gV + (Vv_2^2/2)$$
$$(P_1 - P_2)g = v_2^2/2 \qquad (5)$$
$$(P_1 - P_2) = v_2^2/2g$$

where $(P_1 - P_2)$ = the pressure gradient across the orifice (cm H_2O).

Because the potential energy content of blood is related linearly to pressure and the kinetic energy content of blood is related to the square of velocity, the decrement in pressure necessary to achieve a particular flow velocity is related directly to the square of the velocity. The flow velocity in Equation 5 can be derived by substituting measurements of flow rate into Equation 1.

$$P_1 - P_2 = F^2/2gA^2 \qquad (6)$$

where F = flow rate (cm^3/sec), and A = orifice area (cm^2).

Two consequences follow from Equa-

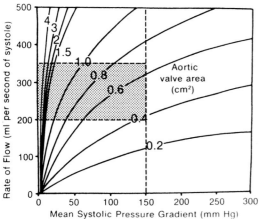

Figure 25.2. Hemodynamic characteristics of aortic stenosis. Graph of a family of curves illustrating the quadratic relationship between the aortic valve pressure gradient (*mm Hg*) and the transvalvular flow rate (*mL/sec*) for different aortic valve orifice areas. The two *horizontal dashed lines* represent the normal aortic valve flow rate at rest and the flow rate achieved during moderately intense exercise, respectively. The *vertical dashed line* represents the maximal aortic valve pressure gradient. The *stippled area* enclosed by these lines illustrates the boundaries within which the heart must operate. Note the parabolic shape of the curves and that the curves become increasingly horizontal as valve area decreases. This relationship demonstrates why an aortic valve area of 0.5 cm^2, which only enters the lower right corner of the operating range, represents critical aortic stenosis. (Modified from Wallace AG. Pathophysiology of cardiovascular disease. In: Smith LH, Thier SO, eds. Pathophysiology. The biological principles of disease. Philadelphia: WB Saunders, 1981:1200.)

tion 6: (*a*) at a particular flow rate, the pressure gradient across the orifice is related inversely to the square of the orifice area; (*b*) at a particular orifice area, the pressure gradient is related directly to the square of the flow rate. Thus, curves describing the relationship between pressure gradient and flow rate across an orifice are parabolic (Fig. 25.2).

The biophysical relationship derived above indicates that a pressure gradient should exist across a normal cardiac valve, which, in fact, is the case. Such a naturally occurring pressure gradient is termed "impulse gradient" to distinguish it from a gra-

dient across a stenosed valve (1, 2). It is caused by the energy loss needed to (*a*) overcome resistive forces, (*b*) achieve the velocity needed to cross the orifice, and (*c*) accomplish the acceleration to that velocity. The magnitude of a typical **impulse gradient** is too small to be detected with a conventional fluid-filled catheter system because the obligatory artifacts in recordings made with such systems (see Chapter 22) are large compared with the magnitude of the impulse gradient. Such gradients are recognizable, however, when pressure is recorded with precisely calibrated catheter-tip micromanometers (Fig. 25.3).

At rest, and probably during exercise, the "normal" pressure gradient that occurs across a normal cardiac valve does not contribute significantly to the hydraulic load faced by the cardiac chamber that generated it. This is because the orifice area of a normal cardiac valve is large enough to permit flow to occur at a relatively low velocity (3).

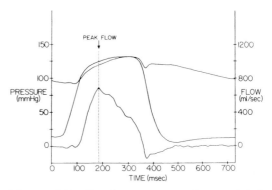

Figure 25.3. Simultaneous recordings of left ventricular (*LV*) pressure, ascending aortic (*Ao*) pressure, and ascending aortic flow velocity (*AoV*). Pressure recordings were made with catheter-mounted micromanometers and, accordingly, are free of the usual artifacts that distort recordings made with fluid-filled catheter systems. The velocity recording was made with a catheter-mounted velocity transducer. Flow velocity (*cm/sec*) has been multiplied by the cross-sectional area of the ascending aorta to yield the flow rate (*mL/sec*). Note the small systolic gradient between the left ventricle and aorta. As predicted by the Bernoulli theorem, peak magnitude of the pressure gradient coincides with peak magnitude of ascending aortic velocity.

Implications of Valve Orifice Area as a Quantification of the Severity of Valvular Stenosis

Ultimately, the most important determinant of valvular stenosis severity is the actual size of the valve orifice. It should be clear from the biophysics presented above that, in the setting of a stenosed cardiac valve, the absolute magnitude of the affected cardiac chamber's pressure and the pressure gradient across the valve change as hemodynamic conditions change. Thus, a particular valve orifice area is associated with a range of intracardiac pressures and pressure gradients. Consequently, the valve pressure gradient measurement alone is not adequate to define the stenosis severity.

Because the relationship between the flow across a valve orifice and the pressure gradient required to generate the flow is quadratic, **small changes in certain hemodynamic parameters, such as heart rate and cardiac output, can cause large changes in the pressure gradient.** For example, a small pressure gradient may exist across a severely stenotic valve if the cardiac output is low. Also, a change in heart rate may, because of its effect on the flow time, cause a substantial change in the pressure gradient across a valve even if the cardiac output does not change.

Application of the Bernoulli Principle to the Calculation of Valve Orifice Area

Theory of the Calculation of the Valve Orifice Area by the Gorlin Equation

The concept of calculation of valve orifice area from hemodynamic measurements was originally conceived by Gorlin and Gorlin as a means of explaining the wide range of variability of hemodynamic findings in valvular stenosis (4). Despite the fact that it was published more than 45 years ago, the validity of this concept has stood the test of time. The Gorlin equation applies the Bernoulli principle, as expressed in Equation 5, to the hemodynamic behavior of a stenotic cardiac valve. Equation 6 can be rearranged:

$$A^2 = F^2/2g(P_1 - P_2)$$
$$A = F/\sqrt{2g(P_1 - P_2)} \qquad (7)$$
$$since \ \sqrt{2g} = 44.3$$
$$A = F/C \ (44.3) \ \sqrt{P_1 - P_2}$$

where A = valve orifice area (cm^2), F = flow across the valve (cm^3/sec), $P_1 - P_2$ = pressure gradient (mm Hg), and C = an empiric constant to correct for the viscous properties of blood and the complexities of the geometry of the orifice, and to convert the pressure units from centimeters H$_2$O to the clinically used millimeters of mercury.

Equation for the Aortic Valve

In calculating the aortic valve orifice area, the average systolic pressure gradient between the left ventricle and the aorta is measured and substituted into the equation. Because aortic valve flow occurs during systole, the flow term (in mL/sec) is the cardiac output divided by the systolic ejection period in seconds of systole per minute. The systolic ejection period is calculated by multiplying the duration of systole in seconds per beat by the heart rate in beats per minute. The value of the constant was empirically determined by Gorlin and Gorlin to be 1.0 (4). Thus, for the aortic valve:

$$A = (CO/(sep \cdot HR))/44.3 \ \sqrt{P_1 - P_2} \quad (8)$$

where CO = cardiac output (mL/min), *sep* = systolic ejection period (seconds per beat), HR = heart rate (beats per minute), and $(P_1 - P_2)$ = mean (time averaged) systolic gradient, between the left ventricle and the aorta in millimeters of mercury.

Equation for the Mitral Valve

In calculating the mitral valve orifice area, the average diastolic pressure gradient between the left atrium and the left ventricle is measured and substituted into the equation. The flow term (mL/sec) in the equation is the cardiac output in milliliters per minute divided by the diastolic filling period in seconds of diastole per minute. The value of the constant (C) was originally determined by Gorlin and Gorlin to be 0.7. However, in the original determinations, left-sided heart catheterization was not done. Left atrial pressure was estimated from the pulmonary–capillary wedge pressure; left ventricular diastolic pressure was assumed to be 5 mm Hg; and the pressure gradient was calculated by subtracting 5 from the pulmonary–capillary wedge pressure. The diastolic filling period was estimated by subtracting the systolic ejection period (determined from a peripheral arterial recording) from 1 min. However, these approximations tend to overestimate the actual pressure gradient and diastolic flow period. Subsequent validation studies using direct measurement of left atrial and left ventricular pressures have recalculated the value of the constant to be 0.85 (5) or 0.90 (6). The value of 0.85 was determined using pulmonary–capillary wedge pressure recordings; the value of 0.90 was determined using direct left atrial pressure measurements. Thus, for the mitral valve when a direct left atrial pressure measurement is used:

$$A = (CO/dfp \cdot HR))/40.0 \sqrt{P_1 - P_2} \quad (9)$$

where CO = cardiac output (mL/min), dfp = diastolic filling period (seconds per beat), HR = heart rate (beats per minute), 40.0 = (44.3)(0.902), and $(P_1 - P_2)$ = mean (time averaged) diastolic pressure gradient between the left atrium and the left ventricle in millimeters of mercury. If the pulmonary–capillary wedge pressure is used, the constant 40.0 should be replaced by 37.6.

It is noteworthy to point out that the same principle (Bernoulli) on which the Gorlin equation is based is used to determine transvalvular pressure gradients from Doppler ultrasound measurements of flow velocity (7, 8). In this procedure, the principle is applied somewhat differently. The flow velocity is measured, and the estimated pressure gradient is calculated from it.

Alternative Equations for Calculation of Stenotic Valve Areas

Although the original Gorlin equation has stood up well over time, a simplification was proposed by Hakki and colleagues (9) that reduces the formula to:

$$A = CO/\sqrt{P_1 - P_2} \quad (10)$$

where CO = cardiac output (L/min) and $(P_1 - P_2)$ = mean (time averaged) pressure gradient across either the aortic or mitral valve in millimeters of mercury. They demonstrated that this formula correlated closely with the Gorlin formula over a wide range of valve areas. This simplification is possible because the product of (heart rate) × (systolic ejection period or diastolic filling period) × (the appropriate empiric constant) was close to 1000 for most patients, allowing these terms to drop out of the equation. Note that the cardiac output is expressed in liters per minute, in contrast to milliliters per minute as in the original formula. Subsequently, a modification of this simplified formula was proposed because of inaccuracies related to heart rate, because the heart rate has an influence on either systolic ejection period or diastolic filling period, and because these parameters are excluded in the Hakki simplification. This modification proposes that for a heart rate greater than 90 beats per minute in aortic stenosis, or less than 75 beats per minute in mitral stenosis, the valve area calculated by the simplified formula should be divided by 1.35 (10).

Requirements for Accurate Determination of Valve Area

Accurate determination of valve area requires a thorough understanding of the biophysical principles that underlie the Gorlin equation and acquisition of accurate valid hemodynamic data. Several basic principles apply:

1. Because cardiac output, pressure gradient, and flow time all appear in the equation, they

must be measured simultaneously. It is not correct to measure cardiac output at one point in the procedure, pressure gradient at another, and then to substitute the two values into the same equation. If the hemodynamic situation changes between the two determinations, the calculated valve area is not valid.

2. Because transvalvular flow enters the equation linearly and the pressure gradient enters the equation as a square root function, the valve area calculation is more strongly influenced by the cardiac output and the flow time measurements. Thus, it is particularly important that these measurements be precise. In a low cardiac output state, a deceptively small valve pressure gradient can exist across a valve with a very small orifice area.

3. Accurate determination of the transvalvular pressure gradient requires simultaneous, high-fidelity, properly damped pressure recordings from the chambers upstream and downstream from the valve in question. Pullback gradients are not accurate enough and should not be used. If the pulmonary–capillary wedge pressure is used to represent left atrial pressure, great care must be taken to obtain a recording with as high a frequency response as possible. This is generally best obtained using an end-hole catheter. Recordings from flow-directed balloon-tipped catheters can also be used, but such recordings may show attenuation of descent pressure rate from the peak of the V wave, resulting in a systematic overestimation of the pressure gradient. If balloon-tipped catheters are used, only large lumen catheters (e.g., *Arrow Wedge*) should be used. Recordings should be made at a paper speed of 100 mm/sec at a gain that produces a recorded image of the gradient large enough to measure accurately. Average gradients should be determined by planimetric methods. If the patient is in sinus rhythm, five consecutive cardiac cycles should be measured and averaged. If the patient is in atrial fibrillation, no less than 10 consecutive cardiac cycles should be measured and averaged. Failure to use consecutive cardiac cycles risks the selection of nonrepresentative beats.

Simplifications Inherent in the Gorlin Equation

The Gorlin equation is a simplified application of a physical principle to the circulation. Two approximations, which are not

exactly correct, are involved in the actual calculation:

1. The equation uses the average pressure gradient and average flow across the valve orifice. These variables change from one cardiac cycle to the next and, over time, within each cardiac cycle.
2. The equation assumes that the valve orifice is a so-called "ideal" orifice, which is known not to be the case.

In fact, the geometry of the orifices of stenotic cardiac valves is so complex as to defy precise measurement of orifice area. The equation attempts to deal with this problem by the insertion of a correction factor that was derived by comparing orifice areas calculated from the uncorrected equation with estimations of actual orifice area at the time of surgical exposure of the valve. Because of these complexities, the correction factor and the hydraulic principles used in the Gorlin formula continue to be re-examined using in vitro methods, and theoretic modifications have been proposed (11–13). Despite these approximations, the valve orifice area calculated from the Gorlin equation is a measure of the hemodynamic behavior of a stenosed orifice even if it does not exactly measure the actual anatomic orifice area, and it continues to provide a useful **"functional" valve area** determination (13).

Dependence on Transvalvular Flow

A major criticism of the Gorlin formula calculated valve area has been that it varies with changes in transvalvular flow. The model on which the Gorlins based their calculation of valve area is the Torricelli principle of laminar flow through a flat orifice. In this model, for valve area to remain constant with changes in transvalvular flow, the pressure gradient must be proportional to the square of flow ($(P_1 - P_2) \propto F^2$). As stated, the Gorlin formula requires an empiric constant (C) to account for blood viscosity, density, turbulence, and the ratio of the valve area to the vena contracta, or the narrowest part of the stream that passes through the orifice (4). Evidence suggests that this constant may be variable at differing flow rates (11). Clearly, if the "constant" varies with changes in flow, then the calculated valve area may also change. In fact, by exercising patients and using pharmacologic manipulations, several investigators have shown that the Gorlin calculated valve area is variable with changes in transvalvular flow (11, 14–21). Because of the flow dependence of the Gorlin formula, other measures of stenosis severity have been proposed that may vary less with changes in transvalvular flow. However, because of familiarity and that it is an anatomic description in easily understood units (cm²), valve area has remained the most commonly used index of stenosis severity.

Valvular Resistance

The concept of valvular resistance was actually developed before the Gorlins published their formula for calculating valve area (22, 23). Resistance is simply defined as the mean pressure gradient divided by the mean transvalvular flow:

$$R = (P_1 - P_2)/F \qquad (11)$$

where R = valvular resistance in dynes × sec × cm^{-5}, $(P_1 - P_2)$ = mean (time averaged) pressure gradient, and F = flow in mL/sec. Flow can be calculated in the same manner as in the Gorlin formula; for the aortic valve, Equation 11 can be rewritten as:

$$R = (1333(P_1 - P_2) \times HR \times SEP)/CO \qquad (12)$$

where HR = heart rate in beats per minute, SEP = systolic ejection period in seconds per beat, CO = cardiac output in mL/min, and 1333 converts millimeters of mercury to dynes · seconds × cm^{-5}.

For valvular resistance to remain constant with changes in transvalvular flow, the pressure gradient must be proportional to the first power of flow (($P_1 - P_2$) ∝ F). Therefore, it is obvious that the Torricelli and resistance models cannot both be correct. A theoretic advantage of the valvular resistance model is that it does not require

an empiric constant that may vary with changes in transvalvular flow. In fact, many investigators have found resistance to be less flow dependent than the Gorlin formula calculated valve area (15, 18, 21, 24–26). Others have shown that resistance also varies with changes in transvalvular flow (16, 27). Despite the fact that resistance does not incorporate an assumed constant, and may be less flow dependent than valve area, it has not gained widespread use as an index of stenosis severity.

Percent of Left Ventricular Stroke Work Loss

To calculate the aortic valve area or valvular resistance, it is necessary to measure cardiac output. Without strict attention to detail, and at low flow rates, the determination of cardiac output may be imprecise. This fact may add to the apparent variation of these indices at differing flow rates. To avoid this source of error, percent of left ventricular stroke work loss has been proposed as an index of aortic stenosis severity, which is dependent on only the most accurate measurements obtainable at left-sided heart catheterization, namely the pressures. This value is a function of the left ventricular pressure–volume work per stroke dissipated in ejecting blood across a stenotic orifice (28, 29).

Total left ventricular stroke work is equal to the product of left ventricular pressure and the volume of blood ejected, integrated over the systolic ejection period:

$$SW_{TOTAL} = \int_0^T P_{LV} \times dV/dt \times dt \qquad (13)$$

where SW_{TOTAL} = total left ventricular stroke work, T = the systolic ejection period, P_{LV} = systolic left ventricular pressure, dV/dt = the infinitesimal volume (dV) ejected in the infinitesimal time interval (dt). By approximating the derivative, this formula can be simplified to:

$$SW_{TOTAL} = mean\ P_{LV} \times SV \qquad (14)$$

where SV = stroke volume, and mean P_{LV} = mean systolic left ventricular pressure.

The effective stroke work delivered to the circulation can be similarly estimated as:

$$SW_{EFF} = mean\ P_{Ao} \times SV \qquad (15)$$

where mean P_{Ao} = mean systolic aortic pressure.

Percent of left ventricular work loss (the difference between the total stroke work and the effective stroke work expressed as a percentage of the total) can then be calculated as:

$$\%LVSWL$$
$$= ((SW_{TOTAL} = SW_{EFF}))/SW_{TOTAL} \times 100\%$$
$$\%LVSWL$$
$$= (((mean\ P_{LV} \times SV)$$
$$- (mean\ P_{Ao} \times SV))$$
$$/ (mean\ P_{LV} \times SV)) \times 100\%$$
$$\qquad (16)$$

where $\%LVSWL$ = percent left ventricular stoke work loss. This formula can be simplified to:

$$\%LVSWL$$
$$= (mean\ aortic\ valve\ gradient/mean\ PLV)$$
$$\times 100\%$$
$$\qquad (17)$$

Although this index of stenosis severity uses no empiric constants, and it is not subject to the inaccuracies of the measured cardiac output, it has still been shown to vary with changes in transvalvular flow (15, 16, 27). Because of this finding, and the fact that mean systolic left ventricular pressure is not commonly measured, the percent of left ventricular stroke work loss has not gained widespread use as a measure of stenosis severity.

VALVULAR INSUFFICIENCY

Functional Problems Caused by a Regurgitant Cardiac Valve

In contrast to a stenotic cardiac valve, which directly affects only the chamber immedi-ately upstream from it, a regurgitant valve always affects at least two chambers. One of the affected chambers is always a ventricle.

The fundamental physiologic conse-quence of a regurgitant cardiac valve is that the regurgitant volume (the blood that the valve allows to regurgitate) moves uselessly back and forth between the cardiac cham-bers upstream and downstream from the re-gurgitant valve. Thus, both chambers are subjected to an increased volume load, which requires both affected chambers to be distended to larger than normal volumes during their respective filling periods. This also requires that the ventricle affected by the regurgitant valve generate a stroke vol-ume, which is the sum of the net forward and regurgitant volumes.

Valvular insufficiency also differs from stenosis in that **insufficiency can develop acutely.** Disorders such as ineffective endo-carditis, rupture of chordae tendinae, and aortic dissection can cause severe, acute val-vular insufficiency. The hemodynamic con-sequences of abruptly developing insuffi-ciency are different from those of gradually developing insufficiency because the heart does not have time to develop an appropri-ate hypertrophic response to deal with the abnormal loading condition (30–33).

Determinants of the Severity of Valvular Insufficiency

The biophysics of antegrade flow across ste-notic orifices should also apply to regurgi-tant flow across incompetent valves. Thus, the quantitative severity of insufficiency through a cardiac valve should be deter-mined by the pressure gradient between the two chambers during the period of insuffi-ciency and by the size of the regurgitant ori-fice. Accordingly, attempts have been made to extend the principle of the Gorlin equa-tion to calculate an effective regurgitant ori-fice area to explain the behavior of regurgi-tant cardiac valves (34, 35). Ideally, the size of the regurgitant orifice area should pre-dict the performance of the heart under all conceivable hemodynamic conditions. Un-fortunately, this concept has not worked well in clinical practice because the nature of the pathology of many regurgitant valves causes regurgitant orifices that vary in size with changes in hemodynamic conditions (36).

Implications of Regurgitant Volume as a Quantification of the Severity of Valvular Insufficiency

The total stroke volume of the ventricle, which is directly affected by a regurgitant valve, is the sum of the effective stroke volume (the net forward stroke volume) and the regurgitant stroke volume (the volume of blood that travels retrogradely across the regurgitant valve). Thus, if systemic cardiac output (and, consequently, effective stroke volume) is to remain in the normal range, the total stroke volume must be increased by the regurgitant volume. Two other consequences are derived from this principle.

1. The peak volume of both of the affected chambers must equal the sum of the total stroke volume and the volume at the point of maximal emptying. Thus, the increase in ventricular volume required by valvular insufficiency is determined by the magnitude of the regurgitant volume and by the quality of ventricular ejection performance.
2. The magnitude of chamber cavity pressure at the point of maximal filling is one of the determinants of the impact of the insufficiency on the overall performance of the heart. This pressure is determined by the chamber's pressure–volume relationship and the volume to which it must be distended.

Thus, the effect of valvular insufficiency on the circulation is determined by regurgitant volume, ventricular ejection performance, and the pressure–volume relationships of the affected cardiac chambers.

Regurgitant volume is not constant. Many changes in the operating parameters of the circulatory system can change the magnitude of the regurgitant volume (37–39). Changes in heart rate alter the amount of time available for insufficiency. Changes in arterial pressure can change the driving pressure responsible for the insufficiency. Changes in ventricular volume and contractile state can change the actual geometry of the regurgitant orifice (35).

Measurement of the Severity of Valvular Insufficiency

Regurgitant Volume and Regurgitant Fraction

The most rigorous way to quantify the severity of valvular insufficiency is technically the most difficult (i.e., to measure the regurgitant volume). No practical technique exists to measure regurgitant volume directly in intact humans. Therefore, indirect measures are employed. Aortic regurgitant volume has been measured in humans by using catheter-mounted flow velocity transducers and scaling the velocity signal by measuring the **aortic cross-sectional area** (40). However, this technique is difficult to perform with precision, and it is not practical for routine clinical catheterization. The most practical technique is to measure the total stroke volume of the affected ventricle by quantitative angiography (see Chapter 15), and the net forward stroke volume by measuring cardiac output either by the Fick or the indicator-dilution technique (see Chapter 11). The regurgitant volume is then given by the difference between the total stroke volume and the regurgitant stroke volume (41).

$$RV = SV_{ANGIO} - SV_{CO} \qquad (18)$$

where RV = regurgitant volume (mL), SV_{ANGIO} = ventricular stroke volume (mL) measured from ventriculography, and SV_{CO} = net forward stroke volume (mL) measured from a cardiac output determination.

The regurgitant volume index may be calculated by normalizing the regurgitant volume-to-body surface area in the same manner as cardiac output is normalized to body surface area to calculate the cardiac index.

$$RVI = RV/BSA \qquad (19)$$

where RVI = regurgitant volume index (mL/min/m^2), and BSA = body surface area (m^2).

In general, a regurgitant volume index

less than 700 mL/min/m^2 represents mild insufficiency, 700 to 1700 mL/min/m^2 represents moderate insufficiency, 1700 to 3000 mL/min/m^2 represents moderately severe insufficiency, and more than 3000 mL/min/m^2 represents severe insufficiency (42, 43).

The regurgitant volume may be normalized to total stroke volume by dividing the former by the latter, yielding the regurgitant fraction.

$$RF = RV/SV_{ANGIO} \qquad (20)$$

where RF = regurgitant fraction (%).

The regurgitant fraction, as with the ejection fraction, is a dimensionless variable that is the percent of the total stroke volume that regurgitates through the incompetent valve. In general, a regurgitant fraction of 0 to 20% represents mild insufficiency, 20 to 40% represents moderate insufficiency, 40 to 60% represents moderately severe insufficiency, and greater than 60% represents severe insufficiency (43).

Measurements of regurgitant volume and regurgitant fraction are not widely used in routine clinical cardiac catheterization because of the complexity of making accurate measurements. Several potential sources of error exist that must be carefully controlled. The independent determinations of cardiac output and stroke volume cannot be made simultaneously but must be made as close together in time as possible. The accuracy of determination of left ventricular volume is dependent on having optimal radiographic image quality, optimal chamber opacification, precise identification of chamber borders, normal chamber geometry, a representative cardiac cycle for analysis, and accurate magnification correction.

Because many of the conditions necessary for optimal ventricular volume measurement are compromised by the enlargement and distortion of the left ventricle, which occurs in chronic aortic and mitral insufficiency, precise determination of regurgitant volume and regurgitant fraction is difficult.

Qualitative Angiographic Assessment

Insufficiency severity may also be judged by a qualitative assessment of a properly performed angiogram. This method is less rigorous, but it is convenient, pragmatically useful, and, hence, most commonly used clinically. A qualitative system for assessing insufficiency has been in place essentially unmodified since 1964 (44). The system is as follows:

1+ (mild): A trace of contrast agent is visible in the receiving chamber, but it clears out during the emptying phase of the cardiac cycle.

2+ (moderate): Regurgitant contrast agent is visible within the entire receiving chamber, and it does not clear during the emptying phase of the cardiac cycle.

3+ (moderately severe): Regurgitant contrast agent opacifies the receiving chamber, and the opacification becomes more dense with each cardiac cycle.

4+ (severe): Regurgitant contrast agent completely opacifies the receiving chamber during the first cardiac cycle after full opacification of the injected chamber.

In general, these qualitative grades correspond roughly to the quantitative ranges of insufficiency severity outlined above. However, it is important to bear in mind that this system is qualitative and that the grading of a particular angiogram is influenced by a variety of other factors not directly related to the quantitative severity of the insufficiency. These include (*a*) the volume of the chamber into which the contrast agent is injected, (*b*) the volume of the chamber that receives the regurgitant volume, (*c*) the heart rate and the systemic cardiac output, and (*d*) observer bias. Each of these factors affects the degree of dilution of the regurgitant contrast agent and, as a result, the extent of opacification of the chamber that receives it. These factors must be taken into account when assessing angiograms for insufficiency.

Studies that have examined the validity of this system have shown a reasonable semiquantitative relationship between the angiographic grade of insufficiency and a quantitative measure of insufficiency (42, 43). However, within any particular angiographic grade of insufficiency severity, a substantial scatter of the measured regurgitant volume index is found (Figs. 25.4 and 25.5).

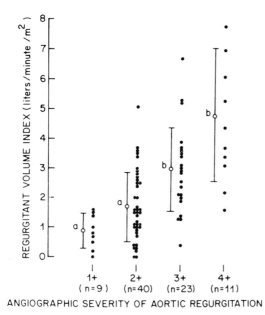

ANGIOGRAPHIC SEVERITY OF AORTIC REGURGITATION

Figure 25.4. Aortic insufficiency. Relationship between qualitative angiographic grade and quantitative measured regurgitant volume index. Each dot represents data from an individual patient (*n*), and the mean + 1 standard deviation (SD) is shown to the left of each set of dots. Mean values of groups marked with the same letter are statistically indistinguishable. Mean values of groups marked with different letters are statistically different (*P* < 0.05). Note that although there is a statistical relationship between increasing grade of insufficiency and increasing regurgitant volume index, considerable scatter of the data is present. (Reprinted with permission from Croft CH, Lipscomb K, Mathis K, et al. Limitations of qualitative grading in aortic or mitral regurgitation. Am J Cardiol 1984; 53:1593–1598. Reproduced with permission of the American Journal of Cardiology.)

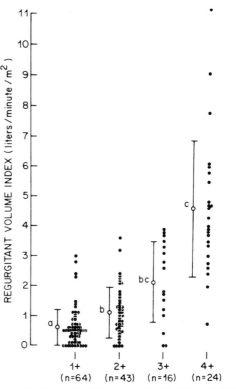

ANGIOGRAPHIC SEVERITY OF MITRAL REGURGITATION

Figure 25.5. Mitral insufficiency. Relationship between qualitative angiographic grade and quantitative measured regurgitant volume index. Format of the graph is identical to that of Figure 25.4. Note that the same semiquantitative relationship exists as for aortic insufficiency. For mitral insufficiency, the quantitative magnitude of insufficiency in the lower angiographic grades is slightly less than for aortic insufficiency. (From Croft CH, Lipscomb K, Mathis K, et al. Limitations of qualitative grading in aortic or mitral regurgitation. Am J Cardiol 1984;53:1593–1598. Reproduced with permission of the American Journal of Cardiology.)

AORTIC VALVE

Aortic Stenosis

Hemodynamic Assessment

Aortic stenosis is usually valvular, but occasionally it is subvalvular, and rarely supravalvular. The hemodynamic alterations of aortic stenosis include the aortic valve pressure gradient, an elevated left ventricular systolic pressure, a variable elevation of left ventricular filling pressure, and a slowing of the rate of the aortic pressure upstroke during systole. It is important to bear in mind that hypertrophic obstructive cardiomyopathy is another potential cause of a left ventricular outflow gradient.

The quantitative severity of aortic stenosis is most commonly assessed by calcula-

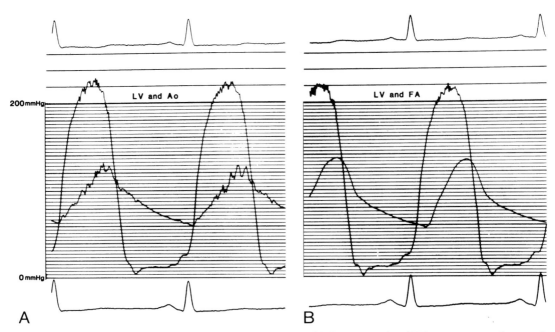

Figure 25.6. Aortic stenosis. Simultaneous recordings of left ventricular (*LV*) pressure and central aortic (*Ao*) pressure (**A**), and left ventricular and femoral arterial (*FA*) pressure (**B**) from the same patient. Note that the femoral arterial pressure has a phase lag and that the systolic peak is artifactually elevated by summation of the antegrade pulse wave with reflected waves. To determine a valid aortic valve gradient using a peripheral arterial pressure recording, the recording must first be corrected for phase lag and downstream distortion. (See text for details.)

tion of the aortic valve area. This requires simultaneous measurement of left ventricular pressure, aortic pressure, and cardiac output. Optimally, the aortic pressure recording should be obtained from the ascending aorta rather than from a peripheral arterial site. This is because the peripheral arterial pulse waveform is delayed by the time required for pulse wave transmission from the central aorta, and it is distorted by reflected pulse waves (Fig. 25.6) (45). If a peripheral arterial pressure is used, it should also be recorded simultaneously with central aortic pressure to judge the magnitude of phase delay and pulse amplification. The peripheral arterial waveform can then be corrected to approximate the central aortic waveform. Simply using a simultaneous left ventricular–femoral artery gradient tends to underestimate the true left ventricular-central aortic gradient, and aligning the two waveforms tends to overestimate the true gradient (46).

Catheterization Technique

Two principal techniques are employed for obtaining left ventricular pressure recordings. The left ventricle may be entered either retrogradely across the aortic valve (47) or antegradely across the mitral valve via the transseptal route (48). A third, infrequently used technique for obtaining left ventricular pressure is direct left ventricular puncture. This technique is reserved for selected cases such as patients with prosthetic mechanical mitral valves and is discussed in Chapter 9.

The retrograde approach is most commonly used, but occasionally it can be difficult in a patient with extreme poststenotic aorta dilation or an eccentrically located valve orifice. Occasionally, retrograde crossing of a stenotic aortic valve dislodges calcific fragments that embolize. In patients with extremely tight aortic stenosis, the cross-sectional area of the catheter shaft occasionally can constitute a significant fraction of the aortic valve orifice area. In this circumstance, the catheter shaft's presence in the aortic valve orifice reduces the effective cross-sectional area of the valve orifice. In such circumstances, the aortic pressure has been observed to rise after catheter withdrawal (49). The aortic pressure may be measured from a second retrograde catheter positioned in the ascending aorta or the peripheral arterial pressure may be measured from the side port of the sheath used to introduce the retrograde catheter into the arterial system. If a peripheral arterial pressure is used, it should be corrected as described above. If the side port of the arterial introducing sheath is used as a source of the pressure signal, the inside diameter of the sheath should be a full French size larger than the outside diameter of the catheter within it.

The transseptal approach has the advantage of not having to cross the aortic valve and of using the retrograde aortic catheter, inserted for aortography and coronary arteriography, to obtain a high-quality central aortic pressure. On the other hand, the transseptal approach is dangerous in inexperienced hands and should be employed only by those who have mastered the technique.

When measuring left ventricular pressure with a multiple-hole catheter (e.g., a pigtail), one should be careful to be certain that all of the holes are fully in the left ventricle. Otherwise, depending on the route of access, a hybrid left ventricular–left atrial pressure or a hybrid left ventricular–aortic pressure will be obtained that superficially appears to be a valid left ventricular pressure, but which gives an inappropriately low value for pressure during systole, causing an underestimation of the aortic valve pressure gradient (Figs. 25.7 and 25.8).

Determination of Severity

Aortic stenosis becomes hydraulically significant when the aortic valve area approaches 1 cm^2. Normal resting aortic valve flow rates are approximately 200 mL/sec of systole. During moderately intense exercise, aortic valve flow rates increase to 300 mL/sec of systole. A valve area of 1.0 cm^2 can transmit a flow of 200 mL/sec of systole at a pressure gradient of 21 mm Hg and a flow of 300 mL/sec of systole at a pressure gradient of 47 mm Hg. As valve area is progressively reduced below 1.0 cm^2, the parabolic relationship between valve pressure gradient and flow rate requires a large pressure gradient increase (Fig. 25.2). A valve area of 0.5 cm^2 requires a pressure gradient of 84 mm Hg to transmit a flow of 200 mL/sec of systole and 188 mm Hg to transmit a flow of 300 mL/sec of systole. An aortic valve pressure gradient greater than 150 mm Hg is probably unattainable because the left ventricle typically cannot generate a systolic pressure greater than 300 mm Hg. Thus, an aortic valve area of 0.5 mm Hg constitutes "critical" aortic stenosis. At this valve area, a large resting pressure gradient is required to maintain a normal resting cardiac output, and the ability to increase cardiac output is severely limited or absent.

One should be cautious not to be misled by an apparently small systolic pressure gradient in patients with congestive heart failure and low cardiac output. A patient with an aortic valve pressure gradient of only 25 mm Hg and a cardiac output of 3.0 L/min may have an aortic valve area of 0.5 cm^2. An accurate valve area determination should be performed in all patients who have an aortic valve pressure gradient greater than 10 mm Hg.

Although other measures of stenosis severity are not commonly used, they have been compared with the Gorlin calculated aortic valve area. A valvular resistance of 300 dynes $\times$ sec $\times$ cm^{-5} or greater has been shown to correlate with a valve area 0.7 cm^2 or less (24, 50). A percent stroke work loss of 30% or more has been associated with a valve area of 1.0 cm^2 (28).

Aortic Insufficiency

Hemodynamic Assessment

Hemodynamic assessment of aortic insufficiency requires measurement of central aortic pressure, left ventricular pressure, right side heart pressures, and cardiac output. The severity of the insufficiency is assessed

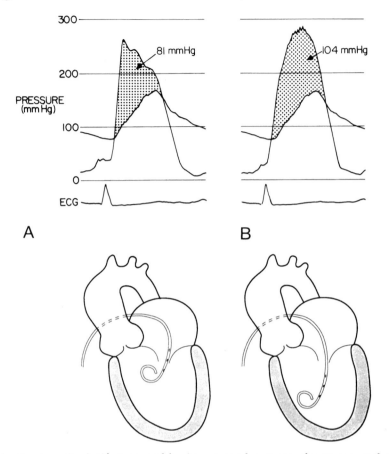

Figure 25.7. Aortic stenosis. Artifact caused by incorrect placement of a transseptal catheter in the left ventricle. **A.** Central aortic pressure recording and an inaccurate left ventricular pressure recording obtained from an improperly positioned pigtail catheter. The left ventricular catheter is positioned such that some of its proximal holes are on the atrial side of the mitral valve. (See corresponding diagram immediately below pressure recording.) This produces a recording that superficially appears to be a valid left ventricular pressure but actually underestimates the peak value of left ventricular systolic pressure. Consequently, it underestimates the aortic valve pressure gradient. **B.** Central aortic pressure recording and an accurate left ventricular pressure recording in the same patient, obtained by advancing the transseptal catheter until all of its holes are on the left ventricular side of the mitral valve. (See text for details.)

by aortic root angiography. Because the aortic valve is not obstructive, no particular obstacle is presented to gaining access to the left ventricle by the retrograde route. In pure aortic insufficiency, the left ventricular systolic pressure should be nearly equal to aortic systolic pressure.

Chronic Aortic Insufficiency

The hemodynamic alterations of chronic severe aortic insufficiency include a large aor-

tic pulse pressure, a low aortic diastolic pressure (Fig. 25.9A) (37), and depending on the severity of insufficiency and the quality of left ventricular function, a variable elevation of left ventricular filling pressure.

Acute Aortic Insufficiency

The hemodynamics of acute severe aortic insufficiency differ substantially from those of long-standing aortic insufficiency (Fig.

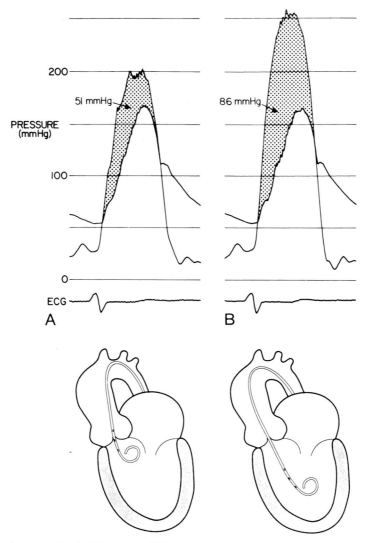

Figure 25.8. Aortic stenosis. Artifact caused by incorrect placement of a retrograde catheter in the left ventricle. The format of this figure is identical to that of Figure 25.7. **A.** Central aortic pressure recording and an inaccurate left ventricular pressure recording obtained from an improperly positioned pigtail catheter. The left ventricular catheter is positioned such that some of its proximal holes are on the aortic side of the aortic valve. (See corresponding diagram immediately below the pressure recording.) As in Figure 25.7, this produces a recording that underestimates the peak left ventricular systolic pressure and, accordingly, the aortic valve pressure gradient. **B.** Central aortic pressure recording and an accurate left ventricular pressure recording in the same patient, obtained by advancing the retrograde catheter until all of its holes are on the left ventricular side of the aortic valve. (See text for details.)

25.9*B*) (30). When severe aortic insufficiency develops acutely, the left ventricle cannot accept a large regurgitant volume at a normal or even moderately elevated filling pressure. Patients with acute severe aortic insufficiency are generally acutely ill

with tachycardia, narrow aortic pulse pressure, and a normal aortic diastolic pressure. The aortic diastolic pressure is not low because it is supported by equilibration with a greatly elevated left ventricular end-diastolic pressure. Left ventricular end-dia-

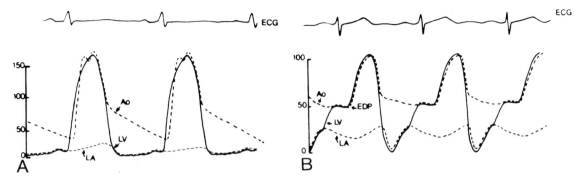

Figure 25.9. Aortic insufficiency. Representative recordings of aortic (*Ao*) and left ventricular (*LV*) pressure in chronic severe aortic insufficiency (**A**), and acute severe aortic insufficiency (**B**). A representation of left atrial (*LA*) pressure has been drawn into the figures to illustrate the behavior of the mitral valve in the two conditions. In the example of chronic aortic insufficiency, note the large aortic pulse pressure, low aortic diastolic pressure, and relatively normal left ventricular filling pressure and left atrial pressure. In the example of acute aortic insufficiency, note the normal aortic pulse pressure, normal aortic diastolic pressure, and strikingly elevated left ventricular filling pressure that equilibrates with aortic pressure and, during the latter portion of diastole (*EDP*), exceeds left atrial pressure, passively closing the mitral valve. *ECG*, electrocardiograph. (Modified from Morganroth J, Perloff JK, Zeldis SM, et al. Acute severe aortic regurgitation: pathophysiology, clinical recognition, and management. Ann Intern Med 1977;87:223–232.)

stolic pressure frequently exceeds left atrial pressure, causing premature closure of the mitral valve.

Catheterization Technique

Contrast aortography is performed by injecting 40 to 60 mL of contrast agent into the aortic root at 20 to 30 mL/sec. Cinefilming should be carried out with the patient positioned so that the ascending aorta, the entire left ventricle, and the left atrium are included in the image. If the procedure is being performed with single-plane radiographic equipment, the left anterior oblique projection is preferable to the right anterior oblique because it is the optimal projection to demonstrate the anatomy of the aortic root. An interpretable study must provide rapid dense opacification of the aortic root without the catheter touching the aortic valve. Accordingly, the catheter should be positioned with its tip just above the aortic valve. During the injection, the catheter should be allowed neither to recoil into the upper ascending aorta nor to advance into contact with the aortic valve. In patients with severe aortic insufficiency who are he-

modynamically precarious and can only tolerate a single contrast agent injection, this study, if properly executed, will both define the severity of the aortic insufficiency and opacify the left ventricle sufficiently to assess its function and the mitral valve competence.

MITRAL VALVE

Mitral Stenosis

Hemodynamic Assessment

The hemodynamics of mitral stenosis are characterized by the mitral valve pressure gradient and elevated left atrial pressure. Chronic left atrial hypertension causes reactive pulmonary arteriolar vasoconstriction, which may lead to chronic obliterative destruction of the pulmonary arterioles. Consequently, patients with mitral stenosis can have both a reactive and a fixed elevation of pulmonary vascular resistance. The left ventricle is underfilled because of the valvular obstruction to filling, and its function is affected only by whatever distortion of its geometry is caused by enlargement and hypertrophy of the right ventricle (51). Pulmonary artery pressure and left atrial pressure are variably elevated, and cardiac output is normal or variably reduced (52). This wide variation in hemodynamic profile, in which some patients have normal cardiac output and substantially elevated left atrial and right side heart pressures, while others have reduced cardiac output and normal or only slightly elevated left atrial and right side heart pressures, provided the original stimulation for the research that led to the Gorlin valve orifice area formula.

As with aortic stenosis, mitral stenosis severity is most commonly quantified by the calculation of the mitral valve area. This requires simultaneous measurement of left atrial pressure, left ventricular pressure, and cardiac output. Optimally, the left atrial pressure should be obtained directly from the left atrium rather than indirectly from a pulmonary–capillary wedge recording. However, in practice, the pulmonary–capillary wedge pressure is frequently substituted for the direct left atrial pressure.

Catheterization Technique

The mitral valve pressure gradient is determined by simultaneously recording left atrial and left ventricular pressures (Fig. 25.10). If a pulmonary–capillary wedge recording is to be used, great care must be taken to maximize the fidelity of the recording. This may be difficult in patients with mitral stenosis because right side heart enlargement frequently complicates catheter manipulation. The pulmonary–capillary wedge pressure is damped and has a phase lag compared with the directly recorded left atrial pressure. The damping attenuates the y descent of left atrial pressure and the phase lag delays it. Both of these phenomena can cause an incorrect overestimation of the mitral valve pressure gradient (Fig. 25.11). Ideally, the recording should be

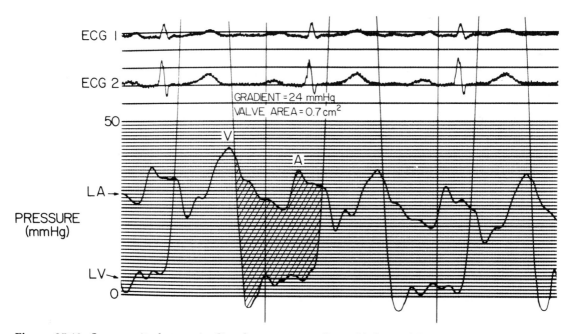

Figure 25.10. Severe mitral stenosis. Simultaneous recording of left atrial (*LA*) and left ventricular (*LV*) pressure illustrating the mitral valve pressure gradient. Note that the descent of the *V* wave begins promptly at the time of the early diastolic pressure crossover. Note also that the stenotic mitral valve impedes transmission of the *A* wave of left atrial systole to the left ventricle. Thus, during atrial systole the pressure gradient increases.

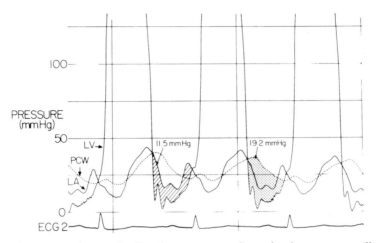

Figure 25.11. Moderate mitral stenosis. Simultaneous recording of pulmonary–capillary wedge pressure (*PCW*), left atrial (*LA*) pressure, and left ventricular (*LV*) pressure to illustrate the relationship between pulmonary–capillary wedge pressure and the directly recorded left atrial pressure. The pulmonary–capillary wedge pressure recording is shown by a *dashed line* to distinguish it from the left atrial recording. Mitral valve pressure gradients determined from the two recordings are shaded in different beats, and their planimetered values are indicated. Note that, compared with the left atrial recording, the pulmonary–capillary wedge pressure has a phase lag and that oscillations are damped. Damping attenuates the rate of the y descent from the peak of the V wave, causing overestimation of the mitral valve pressure gradient. The degree of overestimation could be even greater if a poor quality pulmonary–capillary wedge recording were used. Note also that, in this case of moderate mitral stenosis, the left atrial A wave is partially transmitted to the left ventricle. *ECG*, electrocardiograph.

made with a standard end-hole catheter, such as a Cournand or Goodale-Lubin or Lehman catheter. If a flow-directed, balloon-tipped catheter is used it should be one with a large internal lumen such as an Arrow Wedge catheter. Recordings from a standard Swan-Ganz balloon-tipped catheter may be unacceptably damped and will have an even greater phase lag than seen with an end-hole catheter. When the pulmonary–capillary wedge pressure is used in place of direct left atrial pressure, especially if it is from a balloon-tipped catheter, the phase lag (Fig. 25.11) should be corrected by aligning the peak of the V wave slightly to the left of the rapid downstroke of left ventricular pressure decline on the left ventricular pressure recording (53). Patients with mitral stenosis are frequently in atrial fibrillation, and, accordingly, at least 10 consecutive cardiac cycles should be averaged to determine the mean diastolic gradient. Left ventricular pressure is generally obtained by retrograde catheterization using standard techniques. A technique for antegrade crossing of the mitral valve, using a balloon-tipped catheter introduced through a transseptally placed sheath, has been developed (54). Because left atrial pressure can then be measured using the side port of the sheath, a simultaneous measurement can be made of left ventricular pressure and left atrial pressure from a single venous entry. However, because most assessments of mitral stenosis require a separate arterial entry, left ventricular pressure is most commonly recorded from a retrograde entry into the left ventricle.

Determination of Severity

Mitral stenosis becomes hydraulically significant when mitral valve area approaches 1.5 cm^2, and it becomes critical at a valve area of 1.0 cm^2. This is a larger area than the corresponding range for the aortic valve because the maximal mitral valve pressure gradient that can be tolerated is substantially lower than the corresponding gradient for the aortic valve. Because the lungs generally do not tolerate a pulmonary–capillary wedge pressure greater than 30 mm Hg, the maximal tolerable mean mitral valve pressure gradient is approximately 20 mm Hg.

Normal resting mitral valve flow rates are approximately 150 mL/sec of diastole. Because diastole duration is abbreviated as heart rate increases, mitral valve flow rate must increase markedly when heart rate and cardiac output increase. A mitral valve area of 1.5 cm^2 requires a pressure gradient of 7 mm Hg to transmit a flow rate of 150 mL/sec of diastole. If left ventricular filling pressure is normal, a mean left atrial pressure of 15 mm Hg would be required. At the maximal allowable pressure gradient of 20 mm Hg, a mitral valve area of 1.5 cm^2 can transmit a flow rate of 250 mL/sec of diastole. However, if mitral valve area is reduced to 1.0 cm^2, a 16 mm Hg pressure gradient is required to transmit the normal resting flow rate of 150 mL/sec of diastole. This requires a resting left atrial pressure of 20 to 25 mm Hg. The parabolic relationship between valve pressure gradient and transvalvular flow (Fig. 25.12) dictates that, at a valve area of 1.0 cm^2, the transvalvular flow rate is essentially fixed. Thus, a mitral valve area of 1.0 cm^2 represents critical mitral stenosis.

Mitral Insufficiency

Hemodynamic Assessment

The hemodynamic assessment of mitral insufficiency requires measurement of left ventricular pressure, left atrial or pulmonary–capillary wedge pressure, aortic pressure, right side heart pressure, and cardiac output. Mitral insufficiency severity is assessed by left ventriculography.

Chronic Mitral Insufficiency

The hemodynamics of chronic severe mitral insufficiency are characterized by a brisk

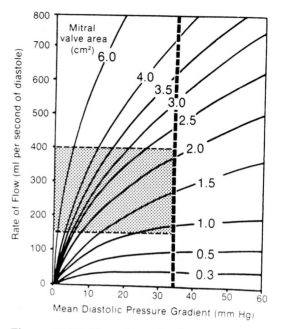

Figure 25.12. Hemodynamic characteristics of mitral stenosis. Graph of a family of curves illustrating quadratic relationship between mitral valve pressure gradient (*mm Hg*) and the transvalvular flow rate (*mL/sec of diastole*) for different mitral valve orifice areas. The two *horizontal lines* represent the normal mitral valve flow rate at rest and the flow rate achieved during moderately intense exercise, respectively. The *vertical line* represents the upper limit of allowable left atrial pressure. The *stippled area* enclosed by the lines illustrates boundaries within which the heart must operate. Note the parabolic shape of the curves and that the curves become increasingly horizontal as valve area decreases. This relationship demonstrates why a mitral valve of 1.0 cm^2, which only enters the lower right corner of the operating range, represents critical mitral stenosis. (Modified from Wallace AG. Pathophysiology of cardiovascular disease. In: Smith LH, Thier SO, eds. Pathophysiology. The biological principles of disease. Philadelphia: WB Saunders, 1981:1192.)

systolic upstroke of aortic pressure (55, 56), and by highly variable elevations of left atrial pressure and left ventricular filling pressure (57). The striking variation in left atrial pressure and left ventricular filling pressure is attributable to variations in intravascular volume, left atrial compliance, left ventricular function, and systemic vascular resistance. Similarly, the prominence of the left atrial V wave is variable. It is important to emphasize that the V wave of left atrial pressure is neither a sensitive nor a specific criterion for including or excluding the presence of chronic mitral insufficiency of any severity (58).

Acute Mitral Insufficiency

The hemodynamics of acute severe mitral insufficiency differ from those of the chronic severe form of the disease. The aortic pressure is generally low, left atrial pressure is generally elevated and has a prominent V wave, and left ventricular filling pressure is variably elevated (Fig. 25.13). Patients with acute severe mitral insufficiency are generally acutely ill with tachycardia, pulmonary vascular congestion, and reduced forward cardiac output. In this circumstance, the reflex elevation of systemic vascular resistance is detrimental to the generation of systemic cardiac output. Such

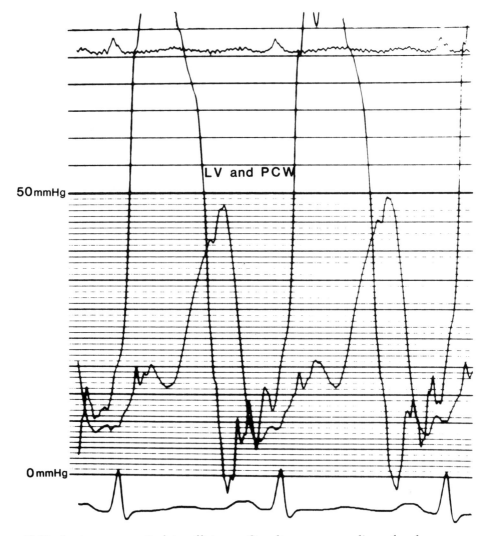

Figure 25.13. Acute severe mitral insufficiency. Simultaneous recording of pulmonary–capillary wedge (*PCW*) and left ventricular (*LV*) pressures. Note the large V wave, which frequently occurs in acute severe mitral insufficiency. The apparent early diastolic mitral valve pressure gradient is attributable to a somewhat damped pulmonary–capillary wedge tracing and rapid diastolic transmitral flow velocity, which is required by the insufficiency.

patients often exhibit dramatic acute hemodynamic improvement when treated with vasodilators (59).

Catheterization Technique

Contrast ventriculography is performed by injecting 40 to 50 mL of contrast agent into the left ventricle at 10 to 14 mL/sec. Care should be taken to position the catheter within the left ventricle not too close to the mitral valve and to select an injection rate that provides satisfactory opacification but does not cause ventricular ectopia. If the study is performed with single-plane radiographic equipment, the right anterior oblique projection should be used. The degree of obliquity should be slightly greater than usual to separate the left atrium from the thoracic spine. If biplane radiographic equipment is used, the left anterior oblique projection should be sufficiently steep to separate the left atrium from the thoracic spine and should be cranially angulated to separate the left atrium from the left ventricle. The angiographic study should, if properly executed, quantify left ventricular size and function and the severity of the mitral insufficiency.

PULMONIC VALVE

Pulmonic Stenosis

Hemodynamic Assessment

Pulmonic stenosis is almost invariably congenital. The stenosis can be either at the level of the pulmonic valve itself, above or below the valve, or at multiple locations. The most common form of pulmonic stenosis is the combination of valvular and subvalvular (or infundibular) stenosis. The hemodynamics of pulmonic stenosis are characterized by the pulmonic valve pressure gradient and the right ventricular response to the pressure load. The pulmonary artery pressure is invariably normal or low.

Therefore, the right ventricular pressure is an accurate reflection of the severity of the obstruction.

Catheterization Technique

The three purposes of the catheterization study in pulmonic stenosis are to localize the obstruction, to quantify its severity, and to identify any other congenital abnormalities. Accordingly, the pressure gradient across the pulmonic valve is measured by simultaneous recording of right ventricular and pulmonary artery pressures, and cardiac output is determined.

Particular care must be taken to localize the obstruction by pressure recording during a careful pullback across the pulmonary outflow tract. Subvalvular obstruction can be identified by finding a zone in the right ventricular outflow tract in which the pressure contour is clearly ventricular but has a lower systolic peak than does the body of the ventricle (Fig. 25.14). Right ventricular angiography delineates the anatomy of the right ventricular outflow tract. This also helps to localize the obstruction.

Determination of Severity

Although the valve area concept should apply to the pulmonic valve, it is rarely used in specifying pulmonic stenosis severity. In general, mild pulmonic stenosis is defined by a right ventricular outflow gradient of more than 50 mm Hg, and severe pulmonic stenosis, a gradient of more than 75 mm Hg (60).

TRICUSPID VALVE

Tricuspid Stenosis

Hemodynamic Assessment

Tricuspid stenosis hemodynamics are characterized by the tricuspid valve pressure

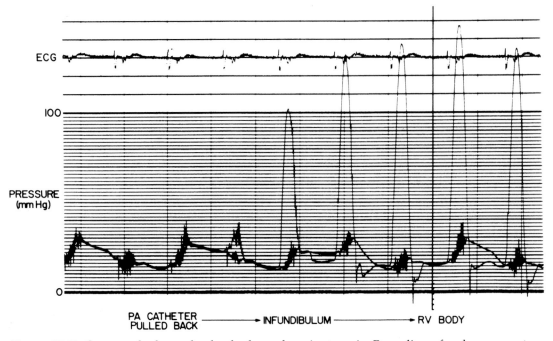

Figure 25.14. Severe valvular and subvalvular pulmonic stenosis. Recording of pulmonary artery (*PA*) pressure with two catheter-mounted micromanometers. During the recording, one of the two micromanometers was gradually pulled back across the pulmonic valve into the right ventricle (*RV*). During one cardiac cycle, it was located in the subvalvular infundibular chamber where it recorded a right ventricular pressure with a peak systolic pressure 30 mm Hg below the systolic pressure recorded in the body of the ventricle. This demonstrates the two zones of obstruction to right ventricular outflow.

gradient and consequent elevation of right atrial pressure and relative underfilling of the right ventricle. Tricuspid stenosis, which is almost invariably a sequella of rheumatic fever, almost always coexists with disease of other cardiac valves. Consequently, the other right heart pressures will be influenced by the severity and type of other valve disease.

Catheterization Technique

The tricuspid valve must be crossed to measure the gradient. This may be technically difficult because patients with tricuspid stenosis frequently have very large right atria, which makes catheter manipulation difficult. The difficulty of crossing the tricuspid valve generally discloses the presence of previously unrecognized tricuspid stenosis.

Because the degree of pressure elevation tolerable is less for the right atrium than for the left atrium, the magnitude of the pressure gradient found across a stenotic tricuspid valve is less than that commonly found across a stenotic mitral valve. Patients with tricuspid stenosis frequently have atrial fibrillation. The combination of atrial fibrillation and the small pressure gradient makes simultaneous right atrial and right ventricular pressure recording essential to the detection and accurate assessment of tricuspid stenosis.

The tricuspid valve area can be calculated using the same equation as for the mitral valve.

Determination of Severity

As mentioned above, tricuspid stenosis is clinically significant at a larger valve area than is mitral stenosis. Thus, a tricuspid valve area as large as 1.5 cm^2 constitutes severe tricuspid stenosis.

Acknowledgments

The authors would like to thank Howard C. Herrmann, MD, William G. Kussmaul, MD, and Warren K. Laskey, MD, and their colleagues on the faculty of the Cardiac Catheterization Laboratory at the Hospital of the University of Pennsylvania for contributing some of the pressure recordings used in this chapter; and John H. Miller, MD, faculty of the Clinical Electrophysiology Laboratory at the Hospital of the University of Pennsylvania, for assistance in preparing illustrations.

References

1. Murgo J, Altobelli S, Dorethy J, et al. Normal ventricular ejection dynamics in man during rest and exercise. Circ Res 1975;46:92–101.
2. Nichols W, Pepine C, Geiser E, et al. Vascular load defined by the aortic input impedance spectrum. Fed Proc 1980;39:196–201.
3. Murgo J, Westerhof N, Giolma J, et al. Effects of exercise on aortic input impedance and pressure wave forms in normal humans. Circ Res 1981; 48:334–343.
4. Gorlin R, Gorlin SG. Hydraulic formula for calculation of the area of the stenotic mitral valve, other cardiac valves, and central circulatory shunts. I. Am Heart J 1951;41:1–29.
5. Hammermeister K, Murray J, Blackmon J. Revision of Gorlin constant for calculation of mitral valve area from left heart pressures. Br Heart J 1972; 35:392–396.
6. Cohen M, Gorlin R. Modified orifice equation for the calculation of mitral valve area. Am Heart J 1972;84:839–840.
7. Young J, Quinones M, Waggoner A, et al. Diagnosis and quantification of aortic stenosis with pulsed Doppler echocardiography. Am J Cardiol 1980; 45:487–494.
8. Holen J, Aaslid R, Landmark K, et al. Determination of pressure gradient in mitral stenosis with noninvasive ultrasound Doppler technique. Acta Med Scand 1976;199:455–460.
9. Hakki A-H, Iskandrian A, Bemis C, et al. A simplified valve formula for the calculation of stenotic cardiac valve areas. Circulation 1981;63: 1050–1055.
10. Angel J, Soler-Soler J, Anivarro I, et al. Hemodynamic evaluation of stenotic cardiac valves. II. Modification of the simplified valve formula for mitral and aortic valve area calculation. Cathet Cardiovasc Diagn 1985;11:127–138.
11. Cannon SR, Richards KL, Crawford M. Hydraulic estimation of stenotic orifice area: a correction of the Gorlin formula. Circulation 1985; 71:1170–1178.
12. Flachskampf F, Weyman A, Guerrero J, et al. Influence of orifice geometry and flow rate on effective valve area: an in vitro study. J Am Coll Cardiol 1990;15:1173–1180.
13. Gorlin R. Calculations of cardiac valve stenosis: restoring an old concept for advanced applications. J Am Coll Cardiol 1987;10:920–922.
14. Bache RJ, Wang Y, Jorgensen CR. Hemodynamic effects of exercise in isolated valvular aortic stenosis. Circulation 1971;49:1003–1013.
15. Blitz LR, Herrmann HC. Hemodynamic assessment of patients with low-flow, low-gradient valvular aortic stenosis. Am J Cardiol 1996; 78:657–661.
16. Burwash IG, Pearlman AS, Kraft CD, et al. Flow dependence of measures of aortic stenosis severity during exercise. J Am Coll Cardiol 1994; 24:1342–1350.
17. Segal J, Lerner DJ, Miller C, et al. When should Doppler-determined valve area be better that the Gorlin formula? Variation in hydraulic constants in low flow states. J Am Coll Cardiol 1987; 9:1294–1305.
18. Martin TW, Moody JM Jr, Bird JJ, et al. Effects of exercise on indices of valvular aortic stenosis. Cathet Cardiovasc Diagn 1992;25:265–271.
19. Paulus WJ, Sys SU, Heyndrickx GR, et al. Orifice variability of the stenotic aortic valve: evaluation before and after balloon aortic valvuloplasty. J Am Coll Cardiol 1991;17:1263–1269.
20. Anderson FL, Tsagaris TJ, Tikoff G, et al. Hemodynamic effects of exercise in patients with aortic stenosis. Am J Med 1969;46:872–885.
21. Casale PN, Palacios IF, Abascal VM, et al. Effects of dobutamine on Gorlin and continuity equation valve areas and valve resistance in valvular aortic stenosis. Am J Cardiol 1992;70:1175–1179.
22. Dow JW, Levine HD, Elkin M, et al. Studies of congenital heart disease. IV. Uncomplicated pulmonic stenosis. Circulation 1950;1:267–287.
23. Silber EN, Prec O, Grossman N, et al. Dynamics of isolated pulmonary stenosis. Am Heart J 1951; 10:21–26.
24. Ford LE, Feldman T, Chiu YC, et al. Hemodynamic resistance as a measure of functional impairment in aortic valvular stenosis. Circ Res 1990;66:1–7.
25. Cannon JD, Zile MR, Crawford FA, et al. Aortic valve resistance as an adjunct to the Gorlin formula in assessing the aortic stenosis in symptomatic patients. J Am Coll Cardiol 1992;20:1517–1523.
26. Bermejo J, García-Fernández MA, Torricilla EG, et al. Effects of dobutamine on Doppler echocardiographic indexes of aortic stenosis. J Am Coll Cardiol 1996;28:1206–1213.
27. Voelker W, Reul H, Nienhaus G, et al. Comparison of valvular resistance, stroke work loss, and Gorlin valve area for the quantification of aortic stenosis: an in vitro study in a pulsatile aortic flow model. Circulation 1995;91:1196–1204.

28. Tobin JR, Rahimtoola SH, Blundell PE, et al. Percentage of left ventricular stroke work loss: a simple hemodynamic concept for estimation of severity in valvular aortic stenosis. Circulation 1967; 35:868–879.

29. Sprigings DC, Chambers JB, Cochrane T, et al. Ventricular stroke work loss: validation of a method of quantifying the severity of aortic stenosis and derivation of an orifice formula. J Am Coll Cardiol 1990;16:1608–1614.

30. Morganroth J, Perloff J, Zeldis S, et al. Acute severe aortic regurgitation: pathophysiology, clinical recognition, and management. Ann Int Med 1977; 87:223–232.

31. Auger P, Wigle E. Sudden severe mitral insufficiency. Can Med Assoc J 1967;96:1493–1503.

32. Braunwald E. Mitral regurgitation: physiological, clinical and surgical considerations. N Engl J Med 1969;281:425–433.

33. Sasayama S, Takahashi M, Osakada G, et al. Dynamic geometry of the left atrium and left ventricle in acute mitral regurgitation. Circulation 1979; 60:177–186.

34. Gorlin R, Dexter L. Hydraulic formula for the calculation of the cross sectional area of the mitral valve during regurgitation. Am Heart J 1952; 43:188–205.

35. Yellin E, Yoran E, Sonnenblick E, et al. Dynamic changes in the canine mitral regurgitant orifice area during ventricular ejection. Circ Res 1979; 45:677–683.

36. Yoran C, Yellin E, Becker R, et al. Dynamic aspects of acute mitral regurgitation: effects of ventricular volume, pressure and contractility on the effective regurgitant orifice area. Circulation 1979; 60:170–176.

37. Judge T, Kennedy J, Bennett L, et al. Quantitative hemodynamic effects of heart rate on aortic regurgitation. Circulation 1971;44:355–367.

38. Dehmer GJ, Firth EG, Hillis LD, et al. Alterations in left ventricular volumes and ejection fraction at rest and during exercise in patients with aortic regurgitation. Am J Cardiol 1981;48:17–27.

39. Yoran C, Yellin E, Becker R, et al. Mechanism of reduction of mitral regurgitation with vasodilator therapy. Am J Cardiol 1979;43:773–777.

40. Nichols W, Pepine C, Conti C, et al. Quantitation of aortic insufficiency using a catheter-tip velocity transducer. Circulation 1981;64:375–380.

41. Sandler H, Dodge H, Hay R, et al. Quantitation of valvular insufficiency in man by angiocardiography. Am Heart J 1963;65:501–513.

42. Hunt D, Baxley W, Kennedy J, et al. Quantitative evaluation of cineaortography in the assessment of aortic regurgitation. Am J Cardiol 1973; 31:696–700.

43. Croft CH, Lipscomb K, Mathis K, et al. Limitations of qualitative grading in aortic or mitral regurgitation. Am J Cardiol 1984;53:1593–1598.

44. Sellers R, Levy M, Amplatz K, et al. Left retrograde cardioangiography in acquired cardiac disease. Am J Cardiol 1964;14:437–447.

45. Murgo J, Westerhof N, Giolma J, et al. Aortic input impedance in normal man: relationship to pressure wave forms. Circulation 1980;62:105–116.

46. Folland E, Parisi A, Carbone C. Is peripheral arterial pressure a satisfactory substitute for ascending aortic pressure when measuring aortic valve gradients? J Am Coll Cardiol 1984;4:1207–1212.

47. Laskey W, Hirshfeld J, Untereker W, et al. A safe and rapid technique for retrograde catheterization of the left ventricle in aortic stenosis. Cathet Cardiovasc Diagn 1982;8:429–435.

48. Laskey W, Kusiak V, Untereker W, et al. Transseptal left heart catheterization: utility of a sheath technique. Cathet Cardiovasc Diagn 1982;8:535–542.

49. Carabello B, Barry W, Grossman W. Changes in arterial pressure during left heart pullback in aortic stenosis; a sign of severe aortic stenosis. Am J Cardiol 1979;44:424–427.

50. Kegel JG, Schalet BD, Corin WJ, et al. Simplified method for calculating aortic valve resistance: correlation with valve area and standard formula. Cathet Cardiovasc Diagn 1993;30:15–21.

51. Ahmed S, Regan T, Fiore J, et al. The state of the left ventricular myocardium in mitral stenosis. Am Heart J 1977;94:28–36.

52. Hugenholtz P, Ryan T, Stein S, et al. The spectrum of pure mitral stenosis. Hemodynamic studies in relation to clinical disability. Am J Cardiol 1962; 10:773–784.

53. Grossman W. Calculation of stenotic valve orifice area. In: Grossman W, Baim D, eds. Cardiac catheterization, angiography and intervention. Philadelphia: Lea and Febiger, 1991:156–157.

54. Lam W, Jones J, Pietras R. Transseptal balloon catheterization of the left ventricle in adult valvular heart disease. Am Heart J 1984;107:147–152.

55. Braunwald E, Welch G, Sarnoff S. Hemodynamic effects of quantitatively varied experimental mitral regurgitation. Circ Res 1957;5:539–545.

56. Ross J, Braunwald E, Morrow A. Clinical and hemodynamic observations in pure mitral insufficiency. Am J Cardiol 1958;2:11–23.

57. Braunwald E, Awe W. The syndrome of severe mitral regurgitation with normal left atrial pressure. Circulation 1963;27:29–35.

58. Fuchs R, Heuser H, Yin F, et al. Limitations of pulmonary wedge V waves in diagnosing mitral regurgitation. Am J Cardiol 1982;49:849–854.

59. Harshaw C, Grossman W, Munro A, et al. Reduced systemic vascular resistance as therapy for severe mitral regurgitation of valvular origin. Ann Int Med 1975;82:312–316.

60. Johnson L, Grossman W, Dalen J, et al. Pulmonic stenosis in the adult: long term followup results. N Engl J Med 1972;287:1159–1163.

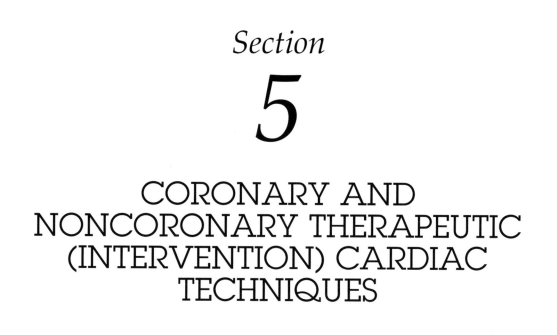

Section

5

CORONARY AND NONCORONARY THERAPEUTIC (INTERVENTION) CARDIAC TECHNIQUES

26
Indications and Contraindications: Patient Selection for Coronary Artery Interventions

Charles R. Lambert, MD, PhD
James A. Hill, MD
Carl J. Pepine, MD

INTRODUCTION

In the previous edition of this textbook, the statement was made that "current day-to-day practice of interventional cardiologists often requires evaluation and treatment of certain patients for which precise indications or guidelines for a particular procedure may not yet have been established." This statement is just as true today as it was then despite a great deal of clinical investigation done in past years to define appropriate indications for use of various devices.

A subcommittee of the American Heart Association (AHA) and the American College of Cardiology (ACC) Task Force to assess diagnostic and therapeutic cardiovascular procedures was established in 1987 to address the issue of percutaneous transluminal angioplasty (PTCA utilization, and guidelines for use of this procedure were published in 1988 (1). A second subcommittee revised these guidelines in 1993 (2). Those guidelines have been widely applied to establishing standards of care by healthcare planning groups, legal concerns, and physicians involved in performance of PTCA and other interventional procedures. Although these guide-

lines have not been revised since 1993, in our opinion, they remain appropriate to guide clinical practice in most cases and can be applied to patient selection regardless of interventional device or a combination thereof. The guidelines for coronary angiography have recently been revised (Chapter 15) and have been broadened to cover indications involving certain aspects of PTCA performance, such as in the setting of acute myocardial infarction. As in the previous edition, this chapter mainly covers indications for balloon angioplasty as defined by the ACC/AHA Task Force. Special considerations given to selection of patients for atherectomy, laser angioplasty, and stenting are covered in Chapters 29–32.

ACC/AHA TASK FORCE GUIDELINES FOR PTCA (2)

Definition of a Successful Procedure

A successful angioplasty procedure is defined as one in which a 20% increase in lumenal diameter is achieved, with the final diameter stenosis less than 50%, and without death, acute myocardial infarction, or need for emergency bypass operation. Standard practice suggests that a residual diameter stenosis less than 30% without complications is most desirable. Objective measurement of coronary narrowing by caliper technique is readily available, and these data correlate closely with more laborious and time-consuming computer-based quantitative methods. In some laboratories intravascular ultrasound offers more precision in assessing lumenal dimensions and morphology. For this chapter, a significant stenosis is defined as one that results in a 50% reduction in coronary lumen diameter as determined by caliper method.

Another consideration affecting judgment of procedural adequacy has been the advent and proliferation of coronary stenting. As covered in Chapters 31–33, stenting has taught interventional cardiologists to strive for an optimal result in terms of lumen diameter and morphology than is often achieved with conventional PTCA alone. Indeed, most operators strive for a slightly negative residual stenosis with placement of intracoronary stents. Such a target is not advisable with conventional PTCA, and it stresses the importance of understanding differences in applying different interventional techniques.

An important part of the 1988 Task Force guidelines involved an attempt to estimate anatomic lesion type to better predict outcome and, therefore, use this information to formulate indications based on angiographic appearance. This lesion classification scheme is summarized below, although its importance in day-to-day practice has been altered somewhat by the widespread use of stenting, which allows optimal results to be obtained in less optimal lesions.

Lesion Classification

Type A Lesions

These are lesions in which the anticipated success rate should be 85% and the risk of abrupt vessel closure is low because they

are discrete (length < 10 mm), concentric lesions and demonstrate all of the following characteristics: ready accessibility, location in a nonangulated segment (< 45°), smoothness of contour, little or no calcification, absence of total occlusion, nonostial location, and absence of major branch involvement apparent thrombus.

Type B Lesions

These are lesions in which the anticipated success rate ranges from 60 to 85% or the risk of abrupt vessel closure is moderate, or both. They include all lesions that are neither type A nor type C, and they are usually identified by such characteristics as, but not limited to, tubular shape (length 10–20 mm), eccentricity, accessibility influenced by moderate proximal segment tortuosity, location in a moderately angulated segment (> 45°,< 90°), contour irregularity, moderate or severe calcification, thrombus, ostial location, bifurcation lesions requiring double guidewires, and total occlusions less than 3 months old. It is recognized that lesions with these characteristics, although associated with some increase in abrupt vessel closure, may, in certain instances, be associated with a comparatively low likelihood of a major complication. This is often the case, for example, in unsuccessful attempts to dilate total occlusions that are less than 3 months old, or in the dilation of some type B lesions in which the distal vessel is supplied by abundant collaterals.

Type C Lesions

These are lesions in which the anticipated success rate is less than 60% or the risk of abrupt vessel closure is high, or both, because they demonstrate any of the following characteristics: diffuse disease (> 2 cm in length), excessive proximal segment tortuosity, location in an extremely angulated segment (> 90°), total occlusion more than 3 months old (and/or bridging collaterals), inability to protect major side branches, or degeneration of older vein grafts with friable lesions. Attempts to dilate such lesions should not be undertaken when they are present in vessels supplying large or moderate areas of viable myocardium.

Classification Scheme

As outlined in Chapter 15 on diagnostic catheterization, a classification scheme was adopted to grade indications for PTCA as follows:

Class I: Conditions for which there is general agreement that coronary angioplasty is justified. A class I indication should not be taken to mean that coronary angioplasty is the only acceptable therapy or that it must be done in this condition.

Class II: Conditions for which coronary angioplasty is performed but there is divergence of opinion with respect to its justification in terms of value and appropriateness.

Class III: Conditions for which there is general agreement that coronary angioplasty is not ordinarily indicated. A class III indication should not be taken to mean that coronary angioplasty is never indicated in these conditions.

Indications for PTCA

Single Vessel Coronary Artery Disease

Asymptomatic or Mildly Symptomatic (Functional Class I) Indications for PTCA are for patients with or without medical therapy.
Symptoms are defined in accordance with the Canadian Cardiovascular Society Classification

Class I   Class I category applies to patients who have a significant lesion in a major epicardial artery that subtends a large area of viable myocardium and who

1. Show evidence of severe myocardial ischemia during laboratory testing, i.e., ischemia induced by low-level exercise (Bruce stage 1 or less or < 4.0 METS, or heart rate < 100 beats per minute) and manifested by: (*a*) ischemic ST segment depression ≥ 1 mm in multiple leads or lasting ≥ 3 minutes into recovery, or (*b*) systolic hypotension during exercise, or, (*c*) evidence of a significant area of ischemia on nuclear, echocardiographic, or radionuclide angiographic stress testing or a moderate area of ischemia with increased lung thallium-201 uptake, or (*d*) exercise-induced reduction in the ejection fraction or wall motion abnormalities on radionuclide ventriculographic studies, or both, or
2. Have been resuscitated from either cardiac arrest or sustained ventricular tachycardia in the absence of acute myocardial infarction, or
3. Must undergo high-risk noncardiac surgery, such as repair of aortic aneurysm, iliofemoral bypass, or carotid artery surgery, if angina is present or there is objective evidence of ischemia as defined above.

All of these patients should have a lesion or lesions associated with a high likelihood of successful dilation, and be at low risk for morbidity and mortality.

Class II   This category (mild or no symptoms, single vessel coronary disease) applies to patients who have a significant lesion in a major epicardial artery that subtends at least a moderate-sized area of viable myocardium and who

1. Show objective evidence of myocardial ischemia during laboratory testing, and (*a*) have at least a moderate likelihood of successful dilation, (*b*) a low risk of abrupt vessel closure, and (*c*) are in the low risk group for morbidity and mortality.

Class III   This category (mild or no symptoms, single vessel coronary disease) applies to all other patients with single vessel disease and mild or no symptoms who do not fulfill the preceding criteria for class I or class II. It includes, for example, patients who

1. Have only a small area of viable myocardium at risk, or
2. Do not manifest evidence of myocardial ischemia during laboratory testing, or
3. Have borderline lesions (50 to 60% diameter reduction) and no inducible ischemia, or

4. Are in the moderate or high-risk group for morbidity and mortality.

COMMENTS In some patients, circumstances of occupation or employment may result in a class II indication being viewed as a class I category. Such patients would include individuals whose occupation involves the safety of others (e.g., airline pilots, bus drivers, truck drivers, air traffic controllers), and those in certain occupations that frequently require sudden vigorous activity (e.g., fire fighters, police officers, athletes). However, class III indications for asymptomatic or mildly symptomatic individuals with single vessel disease pertain to a risk profile that precludes the patient's suitability as a class I or II indication.

Symptomatic Patients with Angina Pectoris (Functional Classes II to IV, Unstable Angina) with Medical Therapy and Single Vessel Disease

Class I This category applies to patients who have a significant lesion in a major epicardial artery that subtends at least a moderate-sized area of viable myocardium and who

1. Show evidence of myocardial ischemia while receiving medical therapy (including ECG monitoring at rest), or
2. Have angina pectoris that has proved inadequately responsive to medical treatment. Inadequately responsive is taken to mean that patient and physician agree that angina significantly interferes with the patient's occupation or ability to perform his or her usual activities, or
3. Are intolerant of medical therapy because of uncontrollable side effects.

All of these patients should have at least a moderate likelihood of successful dilation and be in the low risk group for morbidity and mortality.

Class II This category (symptomatic, single vessel coronary disease) applies to patients who have a significant lesion in a major epicardial artery that subtends at

least a moderate-sized area of viable myocardium and who

1. Show evidence of myocardial ischemia during laboratory testing and (*a*) have one or more complex (type B or C morphology) in the same vessel or its branches, or (*b*) are in the moderate risk group for morbidity, or
2. Have disabling symptoms and a small area of viable myocardium at risk, and (*a*) at least a moderate likelihood of successful dilation, and (*b*) are in the low risk group for morbidity and mortality, or
3. Have at least moderately severe angina on medical therapy with equivocal or nondiagnostic evidence of myocardial ischemia on laboratory testing and who prefer treatment with coronary angioplasty to medical therapy, and (*a*) have at least a moderate likelihood of successful dilation, (*b*) are in the low risk group for morbidity and mortality.

Class III This category (symptomatic, single vessel, coronary disease) applies to all other symptomatic patients with single vessel disease who do not fulfill the preceding criteria for class I or class II. It includes, for example, patients who

1. Have only a small area of viable myocardium at risk in the absence of disabling symptoms, or
2. Have clinical symptoms not likely indicative of ischemia, or
3. Have a low likelihood of successful dilation, or
4. Are in the high-risk group for morbidity and mortality, or
5. Have no symptoms or objective evidence for myocardial ischemia during high-level stress testing (more than 12 METS).

COMMENTS Patients with single vessel disease who have significant symptoms constitute one of the largest groups of patients undergoing angioplasty. However, the generally excellent prognosis for patients with single vessel disease must be a paramount consideration before undertaking an interventional procedure in these patients. It is imperative that there be some assurance that the significant symptoms are indeed caused by the coronary lesion proposed for dilation. Although significant symptoms may justify a lower tolerance for the risk of abrupt vessel closure or subsequent restenosis, one cannot compromise on the risk for significant mortality or morbidity. In view of evidence that angina can diminish, or even disappear, in many patients with occlusive coronary disease, especially those with single vessel disease, patients should be informed before angioplasty of the possibility that their symptoms may improve spontaneously on medical treatment alone.

Multivessel Coronary Artery Disease

Asymptomatic or Mildly Symptomatic (Functional Class I) Patients With or Without Medical Therapy

Class I This category applies to patients who have one significant lesion in a major epicardial artery that could result in nearly complete revascularization because the additional lesion(s) subtends a small viable or nonviable area of myocardium. Additionally, patients in this category must

1. Have a large area of viable myocardium at risk, and
2. Show evidence of severe myocardial ischemia while receiving medical therapy during laboratory testing, or
3. Have been resuscitated from either cardiac arrest or sustained ventricular tachycardia in the absence of acute myocardial infarction, or
4. Be undergoing high-risk noncardiac surgery and demonstrate objective evidence of ischemia.

All of these patients should have one or more lesions that would be expected to have a high success rate and whose successful dilation would provide relief to all major regions of potential ischemia, and they should be in the low risk group for morbidity and mortality.

Class II This category (mild to no symptoms, multivessel coronary disease) applies to patients who

1. Are similar to patients in class I but who (*a*) have a moderate-sized area of viable myocardium at risk, or (*b*) have objective evidence of myocardial ischemia during laboratory testing, or

2. Have significant lesions in two or more major epicardial arteries, each of which subtends at least a moderate-sized area of viable myocardium or
3. Have a subtotally occluded vessel requiring angioplasty wherein the development of total occlusion of the vessel would result in severe hemodynamic collapse because of left ventricular dysfunction.

All of these patients should show evidence of myocardial ischemia while receiving medical therapy during laboratory testing, and have one or more lesions with at least a moderate likelihood of successful dilation (type A or B lesions) whose successful dilation would provide relief to all major regions of potential ischemia, and be in the low or moderate risk group for morbidity and mortality.

Class III This category (mild to no symptoms, multivessel disease) applies to all other patients with multivessel disease and mild or no symptoms who do not fulfill the above criteria for class I or class II. It includes, for example, patients who

1. Have only a small area of viable myocardium at risk, or
2. Have chronic total occlusions in major epicardial vessels subtending moderate or large areas of viable myocardium, or
3. Are at high risk for morbidity or mortality.

Symptomatic Patients with Angina Pectoris (Functional Classes II to IV, Unstable Angina) with Medical Therapy and Multivessel Disease

Class I This category applies to patients who have significant lesions in each of two major epicardial arteries, both subtending at least moderate-sized areas of viable myocardium and who

1. Show evidence of myocardial ischemia while receiving appropriate medical therapy during laboratory testing, or
2. Have unstable angina or angina pectoris that has proved inadequately responsive to medical therapy, or
3. Are intolerant of medical therapy because of

uncontrollable side effects that are unacceptable to the patient.

All of these patients should have lesion morphology associated with a high success rate and (type A and B lesions) whose successful dilation would be expected to provide relief of all major regions of potential ischemia, and be in the low risk group for morbidity and mortality.

Class II This category (symptomatic, multivessel disease) applies to patients who have significant lesions in two or more major epicardial arteries that subtend at least moderate-sized areas of viable myocardium and who

1. Are similar to patients in class I but who are in the moderate risk group for morbidity and mortality, or
2. Have angina pectoris but do not necessarily have objective evidence of myocardial ischemia while receiving medical therapy during laboratory testing.

All of these patients should have lesion morphology associated with a high success rate and (type A and B lesions) whose successful dilation would be expected to provide relief of all major regions of potential ischemia, and be in the moderate risk group for morbidity and mortality.

Patients in this category are also those who

3. Have disabling angina that has proved inadequately responsive to medical therapy, and (*a*) are considered poor candidates for surgery because of advanced physiologic age or coexisting medical disorders, (*b*) have lesions with at least a moderate likelihood of successful dilation, and (*c*) are in the moderate risk group for morbidity and mortality.
4. Have a subtotally occluded target vessel for angioplasty wherein the development of total occlusion of the vessel would result in severe hemodynamic collapse because of left ventricular dysfunction.

Class III This category (symptomatic, multivessel coronary disease) applies to all other symptomatic patients with multivessel disease who do not fulfill the preceding criteria summarized in class I or class II. It includes, for example, patients who

1. Have only a small area of myocardium at risk in the absence of disabling symptoms, or

2. Have lesion morphology with a low likelihood of successful dilation (type C lesions in major epicardial vessels) serving moderate or large areas of viable myocardium, or
3. Are in the high-risk group for morbidity or mortality, or both.

COMMENTS It is to be stressed that risk assessment is different in patients with multivessel, as compared with single vessel, obstruction. In single vessel obstruction, ideally a high probability for anatomically complete revascularization should be present, but with multivessel obstruction the probability for complete revascularization using PTCA is markedly reduced. It is recognized that adequate functional revascularization can be achieved without necessarily being anatomically complete. In every instance, the goal is to achieve relief of ischemia at an acceptable risk. In estimating this risk in patients with multivessel disease, it is imperative that each lesion be considered in the context of all other lesions present. Some assessment must then be made of the consequences likely to ensue should any one of the attempted dilations fail and result in abrupt vessel closure. For example, it may be inappropriate to attempt dilation of a proximal high-grade left anterior descending artery lesion if that vessel was supplying many collateral vessels to a large area of viable myocardium in the distribution of totally occluded right and left circumflex coronary arteries.

Direct PTCA for Acute Myocardial Infarction

Class I This category applies to dilation of a significant lesion in the infarct-related artery only in patients who can be managed in the appropriate laboratory setting and who

1. Are within 0–6 hours of onset of myocardial infarction as an alternative to thrombolytic therapy, or
2. Are within 6–12 hours of onset of myocardial infarction, but who have continued symptoms of ongoing myocardial ischemia, or
3. Are in cardiogenic shock with or without previous thrombolytic therapy and within 12 hours of the onset of symptoms.

Class II This category applies to patients who

1. Are within 6–12 hours of the onset of an acute myocardial infarction and have no symptoms of myocardial ischemia, but who have a large area of myocardium at jeopardy or are in a higher risk clinical category, or
2. Are within 12–24 hours of the onset of an acute myocardial infarction, but who have continued symptoms of ongoing myocardial ischemia, or
3. Have received thrombolytic therapy and have continuing or recurrent symptoms of active myocardial ischemia.

Class III This category applies to

1. Angioplasty of a noninfarct related artery at the time of acute myocardial infarction, or
2. Patients who are more than 12 hours after the onset of infarction at the time of admission and who have no symptoms of myocardial ischemia, or
3. Patients who have had successful thrombolytic therapy within the past 24 hours and have no symptoms of myocardial ischemia.

As noted in the introduction to this chapter, these guidelines were published in 1993. Despite that fact, they are fully applicable to current practice and to a variety of different devices. In terms of acute myocardial infarction, the new guidelines for coronary angiography (Chapter 15) bridge angiography and intervention to offer indications in the setting of acute myocardial infarction and the subsequent hospitalization that go beyond and complement the PTCA guidelines outlined herein. Further comments regarding patient selection in the setting of acute infarction, indications other than from the ACC/AHA Task Force, and outcomes can be found in Chapter 37 on unstable ischemic syndromes.

Although a specific guidelines document has not been published for coronary stent implantation, an ACC Expert Consensus paper has been published (3). The clinical studies supporting this document are discussed in Chapters 32 and 33. Briefly, recommendations for use of coronary stents include improvement of short-term outcome in patients with short non-restenotic lesions in large native coronary arteries, in threatened or actual acute closure, and in certain patients with suboptimal angioplasty results. Presumably, these patients would have been preselected using the PTCA criteria outlined above. In addition, value was found for preventing restenosis in large coronary arteries and in selected patients with saphenous vein bypass graft lesions that are short, non-restenotic, and not associated with thrombus and nonostial.

Patient selection for rotational, extraction, and directional atherectomy has not been distilled into a set of Task Force guidelines; however, the PTCA document described above also applies to these patients. The particular lesion subsets and clinical selection criteria useful for these modalities are described in Chapter 29. In general, directional atherectomy has found continued use in eccentric noncalcified lesions, and it may be of particular use in ostial locations. Rotational atherectomy may be particularly useful in diffusely diseased and calcified vessels and extraction atherectomy may be useful for thrombus-associated lesions or in diffusely diseased saphenous bypass grafts.

Patient selection for combination therapy with two or more devices, such as atherectomy and stent implantation or laser angioplasty followed by balloon dilation, may seem obvious in particular clinical situations, and combination therapy is becoming more common. Such practices may not, however, be supported by randomized trials or specific rigorous guidelines for patient selection. In any event, regardless of the therapeutic device or devices, the guidelines developed by the ACC/AHA Task Force are useful in patient selection because of their basis in functional anatomy and risk stratification.

Contraindications to PTCA

As with diagnostic catheterization, a universal contraindication to PTCA is lack both of an appropriately trained and skilled interventional cardiologist and of high-quality cardiac catheterization facilities and staff. In addition, many of the contraindications outlined in Chapter 15 on diagnostic catheterization also apply to PTCA.

Absolute contraindications include (*a*) no significant obstructing lesion; (*b*) a significant obstruction (> 50%) in the left main coronary artery and this main segment is not protected by at least one completely patent bypass graft to either the left anterior descending or left circumflex artery; and (*c*) no formal cardiac surgical program within the institution.

Relative contraindications include (*a*) a coagulopathy is present; (*b*) the patient has diffusely diseased saphenous vein grafts without a focal dilatable lesion; (*c*) the patient has diffusely diseased native coronary arteries with distal vessels suitable for bypass grafting; (*d*) the vessel in question is the sole remaining circulation to the myocardium; (*e*) the patient has chronic total occlusions with clinical and anatomic features that result in a low anticipated success rate of dilation; (*f*) the lesion under consideration is a borderline stenotic lesion (usually < 50% stenosis); and (*g*) the procedure is proposed for a noninfarct related artery in patients with multivessel disease who are undergoing direct angioplasty for acute myocardial infarction.

In addition to these generally accepted relative contraindications, other conditions exist in which clinicians have considerable reservation about the risk:benefit ratio of angioplasty. Over and above a finite risk of mortality and morbidity, present is an added dimension of risk if associated with failure of the procedure as a result of either early closure or development of restenosis. Risks are viewed as a continuum, and it is their aggregate weight that should ultimately determine whether a specific procedure should or should not be undertaken in any patient.

Although these contraindications are derived from the 1988 Task Force recommendations, they generally hold today. Some patients do, however, currently undergo PTCA in circumstances where a relative contraindication may exist as defined by these guidelines. An example of such a case would be the unstable patient in whom an artery supplies a large amount of viable myocardium and the lesion is a type C or other variant felt to be high risk by early standards. The advent of percutaneous bypass, perfusion balloons, high-pressure systems, backup atherectomy, and intracoronary stents make such cases routine in certain experienced hands. Despite this reality and the changing face of interventional cardiology, the indications and contraindications reviewed seem appropriate for most hospitals and operators performing PTCA.

References

1. Guidelines for percutaneous transluminal coronary angioplasty. A report of the American College of Cardiology-American Heart Association task force on assessment of diagnostic and therapeutic cardiovascular procedures (subcommittee on percutaneous transluminal coronary angioplasty) J Am Coll Cardiol 1988;12:529–545.
2. ACC/AHA task force report: guidelines for percutaneous transluminal coronary angioplasty. J Am Coll Cardiol 1993;22:2033–2054.
3. ACC expert consensus document: coronary artery stents. J Am Coll Cardiol 1996;28:782–794.

27
Introduction to Coronary Angioplasty

George W. Vetrovec, MD

INTRODUCTION

Coronary angioplasty has made a major impact on the management of coronary artery disease. Beginning as a procedure for patients with discrete, focal lesions, the technique has evolved dramatically (1). With the availability of more sophisticated equipment (including nonballoon devices) and increased operator experience, angioplasty rapidly became much more applicable to the management of complex artery disease including (2) patients with multiple vessel disease, total occlusions, tandem lesions, and complex branch disease. Operator experience and skill and the availability of new devices, particularly coronary stents, contribute to the high success rates in treating complex coronary anatomy (3). However, important to successful angioplasty is appropriate case selection based on coronary anatomy, lesion morphology, and left ventricular function. Thus the outcome of coronary angioplasty is the product of multiple factors, including (*a*) operator technical skill, (*b*) appropriate case selection, (*c*) familiarity in equipment use to expedite and facilitate the procedure, and (*d*) high-quality angiographic techniques used to identify vessel anatomy and lesion morphology.

This chapter describes the basic considerations for case selection, equipment utilization, and patient management during coronary angioplasty. Complex angioplasty is discussed in Chapter 28, whereas other chapters (29–33) describe the use of nonballoon devices.

REQUISITES FOR ANGIOPLASTY TRAINING

Coronary angioplasty is a technique that requires both technical and cognitive skills. Today these skills are acquired in a formal training program (see Chapter 3). The cardiology trainee in interventional cardiology must therefore have basic and clinical knowledge of ischemic heart disease management as well as proficiency in performing coronary angiography. This includes a basic understanding of radiation physics and safety, catheter selection and manipulation, anatomically appropriate views, and critical film review (3, 4). Coronary angioplasty training requires the melding of these requisites with the additional cognitive and technical knowledge acquired during laboratory-based training that exposes the candidate to a wide variety of cases in an educational environment.

PATIENT SELECTION

Coronary angioplasty has expanded into the management of complex, multivessel

551

Table 27.1.
Coronary Applications: Clinical and Angiographic Factors

Indications[a]
    Angina/anginal equivalent symptoms/ischemia
        Stable
        Unstable
    Significant, viable myocardium at jeopardy
    Acute myocardial infarction
    Postmyocardial infarction
        Ischemia
        Vessel patency
Major contraindications
    Significant left main coronary obstruction
    Unprotected left main angioplasty
    Single artery to remaining viable myocardium
Relative contraindications[b]
    Severe left ventricular dysfunction
    Occlusive multivessel disease with complex collaterals creating an unprotected left main equivalent
    Nonideal lesion(s) supplying significant myocardial segment
    Unable to provide complete or nearly complete revascularization
    Unstable/uncontrolled systemic or metabolic abnormality (i.e., renal insufficiency, and so forth)

[a] All clinical indications require favorable vessel, and lesion anatomy.
[b] Decisions in this category require weighing risks versus benefits of angioplasty, other catheter-based revascularization, surgery, or continued medical therapy for an individual patient, most often in consultation with a cardiac surgeon and the patient's primary physician.

Table 27.2.
Balloon Angioplasty: Nonideal Lesions

Y-branch
Heavily calcified
Eccentric
Total occlusions (particularly long and/or
    nonacute)
Thrombus associated
Long
Extreme vessel tortuosity and/or stenosis in
    a bend
Old vein graft lesions, particularly diffuse

disease (5). However, certain basic principles remain critical to optimize patient outcomes. Table 27.1 summarizes the **clinical and angiographic lesion factors** important in patient selection; Table 27.2 lists nonideal, but not absolute, contraindications to angioplasty. Patients with single or multiple vessel disease with individual lesions amenable to dilation are potential anatomic candidates for angioplasty in the absence of unprotected left main coronary obstruction, which remains a lesion of unacceptable risk even with the availability of stents. Clinical indications include significant effort-limiting angina or equivalent symptoms such as dyspnea or exercise fatigue (6, 7). Patients with ischemia without symptoms but with significant myocardial jeopardy are also potential candidates, in the setting of an active lifestyle with incomplete medical alleviation of ischemia. Because of a high incidence of acute and subacute failure of medical management, patients with high- or intermediate-risk unstable angina frequently undergo diagnostic coronary angiography and angioplasty, when feasible. Currently, revascularization requires specific goals aimed at treating documented ischemic symptoms or prognostically important ischemia as opposed to treating anatomy only (8).

In addition to left main obstruction, other relative contraindications to angioplasty include severe left ventricular dysfunction, particularly with complex collaterals such that dilation of a single lesion potentially affects a large multivessel distribution relative to ventricular function. Likewise, patients with limited potential to achieve complete revascularization with angioplasty are better candidates for bypass surgery. Results of randomized trials comparing bypass surgery with angioplasty in patients with multivessel disease amenable to either therapy have shown no overall difference in 2–5 year survival (9). The National Institutes of Health-sponsored Bypass Angioplasty Revascularization Investigations (BARI) Trial (10), which randomized over 1800 patients, showed no statistically significant overall difference in survival free of myocardial infarction (MI), although treated diabetics (not one of the predetermined subgroups) had better survival with bypass surgery compared with angioplasty. Patients undergoing angioplasty had more total procedures, mostly in the first year secondary to restenosis. However, the BARI Trial did not include use of intracoronary stents, which could potentially reduce the risk of restenosis. With angioplasty, overall median return to work was earlier with angioplasty and total costs were slightly less (11). In complex, high-risk multivessel cases, joint review between the interventionalist and the cardiac surgeon is useful to determine the relation risk/benefit and, thus, the most ideal strategy.

Management of the patient with an acute myocardial infarction requires special considerations because of the urgency of initial treatment. Primary angioplasty, a method of revascularization in the absence of thrombolytic therapy, has theoretic advantages over thrombolytics, and it has grown in popularity in some institutions (12). The theoretic advantage of primary angioplasty is the greater probability of achieving thrombolysis in myocardial infarction (TIMI) 3 flow, which appears to decrease mortality (13). Furthermore, angioplasty has a lower risk of hemorrhagic stroke. Because many localities lack facilities to provide angioplasty urgently, however, current recommendations are for decisions on therapy to be made on the basis of the most immediate form of reperfusion (14). Special consideration for primary angioplasty includes patients who have contraindications to thrombolytic therapy or those who have failed to reperfuse with thrombolytic therapy and continue to have significant ischemic pain and electrocardiographic (ECG) changes of infarct evolution involving a large segment of myocardium (i.e., anterior) or are hemodynamically un-

stable. Finally, patients with cardiogenic shock appear to benefit with early revascularization (15). All emergency angioplasty should be done only in hospitals performing more than 200 procedures per year and by operators performing more than 75 interventions per year (4).

Secondary indications for angioplasty in a recent myocardial infarction relate to residual stenoses or occlusions in the infarct-related artery, particularly in the setting of recurrent ischemia. Multivessel angioplasty is beneficial in selected patients with multivessel disease and continued postinfarction ischemia (16). However, results of both TIMI IIA (17) and TAMI (18) indicate that urgent postthrombolytic angioplasty is not indicated because it increases the risk of acute, often serious, complications. Cardiologists have generally performed early angiography to assess risk of postinfarction patients. Revascularizartion has been performed on patients with severe residual stenoses, suspected viable myocardium, and persistent total occlusions, whereas patients with noncritical residual disease in the infarct-related artery or with moderate obstruction (i.e., 70% obstruction) undergo stress testing to demonstrate ischemia before dilation is considered. In the absence of angiography, risk stratification includes stress testing followed by angiography and potential intervention for patients with continued ischemia, unstable angina, or exercise-induced ischemia. In general, current evidence-based medicine dictates angioplasty for specific ischemic rather than anatomic indications (8). Table 27.3 summarizes indications for percutaneous transluminal coronary angioplasty (PTCA) in acute MI.

SIGNIFICANCE OF CORONARY ANGIOGRAPHY

As noted, angiographic assessment of lesion morphology, overall coronary anatomy, and ventricular function is important for patient and device selection. Tables 27.4 and 27.5 summarize angiographic features that are most important in assessing patients

Table 27.3.
Applications of Coronary Angioplasty in Acute Myocardial Infarction

Primary (immediate)
  Primary contraindication(s) to thrombolytic therapy
Primary strategy for reperfusion
  Failure to reperfuse with thrombolytic therapy
  Cardiogenic shock
Secondary (during hospitalization)
  Anatomy
    Severe stenosis or occlusion in infarct-related artery
  Ischemia
    Infarct-related artery and/or additional lesions in coronary circulation

Table 27.4.
Angiographic Assessment Before Angioplasty

Lesion severity
  Degree of stenosis, length
Lesion morphology
  Eccentricity, thrombus, calcium, complexity
Branches
  Lesion-associated branches with or without associated stenosis
  Vessel-associated branches potentially affecting guidewire passage
Collateral supply
  Presence and extent of collaterals
  Presence and extent of disease in collaterals supplying the target artery
Proximal artery characteristics
  Origin, size, and course of artery containing lesion potentially influences guide catheter selection
  Tortuosity, which may affect balloon, atherectomy device, or stent delivery

Table 27.5.
Angiographic Assessment After Angioplasty[a]

Resultant lesion
  Percent residual stenosis with or without contrast flow compromise (e.g., TIMI grade)
Lesion morphology
  Split or dissection
  Thrombus
Distal/adjacent vessels
  Associated branch damage
  Emboli

[a] Position of lesion, particularly related to tortuosity, distal vessel, vessel size.
TIMI, thrombolysis in myocardial infarction.

Table 27.6.
Supplemental Views Helpful in Angiographic Assessment of Lesions Before and After Coronary Angioplasty

Coronary Zone	Views
Proximal-mid LAD and diagonals	90°–110° LAO
	RAO/cranial
	AP/cranial, shallow RAO, steep cranial
	AP or steep RAO caudal
Proximal intermediate marginal	LAO/caudal
	LAO 110°/caudal
Proximal and mid marginals	RAO/caudal
	AP/caudal
Ostial and proximal RCA	LAO/caudal
Proximal-mid RCA	Lateral
Distal RCA and PDA–PLB bifurcation	AP/cranial
	Lateral/cranial

AP, anterior-posterior; LAO, left anterior oblique; RAO, right anterior oblique; LAD, left anterior descending.

pre- and postangioplasty. Because angiography is limited by the fact that it only provides a luminogram, in selected cases intravascular ultrasound can provide additional information regarding absolute vessel size, plaque and vessel wall composition, stenosis severity in eccentric lesions, stent deployment adequacy, and local dissection extent postintervention.

Other sections of this text address the importance of angiography and intravascular ultrasound for optimal safety, and the results of interventional therapy. However, multiple angiographic views are important to identify associated branch disease and lesion eccentricity to enhance both patient selection and guidewire manipulation. Table 27.6 summarizes supplemental angiographic views, which are frequently helpful in coronary angioplasty procedures.

CLINICAL RESULTS

Overall success rates for coronary angioplasty exceed 95% for patients with ideal lesions, but it is nearer to 90% for patient populations with multivessel disease. However, compared with bypass surgery in randomized trials, angioplasty is associated with less complete revascularization (10).

Although early results of angioplasty for unstable angina have been associated with more acute complications, current use of abciximab has improved acute outcomes.

RESTENOSIS

Restenosis remains the major current limitation to wider applicability of coronary angioplasty for revascularization. Symptoms with angiographic evidence of restenosis (19, 20) occur in 25 to 30% of patients with balloon alone. Studies using angiography as an end point demonstrate even higher rates of angiographic (20) restenosis. However, clinical correlation suggests that angiographically less severe restenotic lesions are more likely to be asymptomatic (21). With the greater use of intracoronary stents, restenosis is significantly reduced in lesions treated with one or two stents (22).

Table 27.7 summarizes anatomic and angiographic factors associated with restenosis with balloon only, which appears to have reduced restenosis with stenting using two or fewer stents. Currently, no drug therapy has been unequivocally shown to reduce restenosis. Thus, postballoon angioplasty medical treatment consists of daily aspirin and antianginals for possible continued angina only in patients with incomplete revascularization or suspected spasm. For patients receiving stents, ASA plus ticlopidine (for 1 month) is used to prevent stent thrombosis.

Finally, although subacute (0–9 months) angioplasty outcomes are determined predominantly by the presence or absence of restenosis, late results for patients not experiencing restenosis appear to be affected predominantly by native vessel disease progression. This latter fact may be a major late benefit of angioplasty as compared with bypass surgery, which is affected late by progressive vein graft disease as well as by native vessel disease.

FACILITATING THE PROCEDURE

Patient Preparation

Although single vessel dilation of an isolated proximal stenosis may require minimal time, more complex angioplasty—including multiple devices—can be time consuming, requiring special attention toward patient anxiety and comfort. An effective preprocedure sedative regimen is 1–2 mg of lorazepam in conjunction with parental morphine, which is similar to preinduction for patients undergoing cardiac surgery. Once in the laboratory, sedation may be extended and enhanced by incremental dosages of intravenous morphine or fentanyl. Other premedications should include aspirin and a calcium channel antagonist. Systemic heparinization is important during the procedure, guided by activated clotting time (ACT) measurements every 20–30 minutes to maintain the ACT longer than 300 seconds.

In patients with unstable syndromes, recent myocardial infarction, angiographic evidence of recent clot, or diffuse disease in old vein grafts, pretreatment with abciximab (23) significantly reduces the risk of acute or subacute complications. In patients receiving abciximab, lower heparin dosages used to maintain an ACT longer than 200 seconds are associated with lower bleeding complications with equal or improved coronary outcome. Finally, intracoronary or intravenous nitroglycerin may be used prophylactically or in response to spasm or ischemia. In patients not receiving abciximab, 24 hours of heparin before the procedure appears to reduce complications (24).

Table 27.7.
Restenosis: Predictive Factors (Balloon Only—Versus Stenting)

Anatomic Factors (all reduced with Palmaz-Schlatz stenting)
   Proximal LAD Lesions
   Aorto-ostial native or vein graft lesions
   Vein bypass grafts (body of graft)
Angiographic Factors
   Small vessels (2.5–3 mm)
   Incomplete dilatation (>10% residual; "non–stent-like results" by balloon only)
   Elastic recoil

Because of financial insurance pressures as well as patient preference, many patients having elective angiography undergo ad hoc angioplasty at the time of diagnostic catheterization. However, exclusion of additional lesions or other important angiographic findings requires careful angiographic review before dilation. Furthermore, prior to the diagnostic study patients should have a clear understanding of the additional goals and risks associated with angioplasty and agree to proceed based on the judgment of the operator. If the operator is unsure regarding the risk/benefits or optimal devices required for the intervention based on the diagnostic digital or tape replay, it is clearly preferable to delay the procedure and either leave the sheaths in place until later in the day or remove the sheaths and perform a diagnostic procedure only.

Dilation

Arterial access is obtained by techniques described in Chapter 9. Effective local anesthesia is important for patient comfort. Some operators do not obtain venous access in low-risk procedures, whereas in other cases venous access is obtained, if necessary, for use in situations such as when a temporary pacing wire is needed during rotational atherectomy of the right coronary artery. For hemodynamically unstable patients, a right-sided heart catheter is often helpful to optimize hemodynamics.

Arterial access sites include the groin, brachial, and radial sites. Radial access is popular in Europe, where unsheathed stents are placed via 6 F guiding catheters. The radial site is attractive for early ambulation and ease of compression. Percutaneous left brachial access allows use of the Judkins-shaped guides, whereas right brachial access is required for multipurpose or the Amplatz-style guide catheters. Using 8 F catheter and sheath systems is associated with a modest risk of brachial arterial complications. The groin is the most frequent site for arterial access. Because of the relative stiffness and lack of tip tapering, guide catheters should always be advanced through a sheath and over a supporting wire passed around the arch.

Once the guide catheter is seated in the ostium of the target vessel, the balloon catheter with guidewire is advanced. The guidewire should always be advanced beyond the balloon catheter by several centimeters in the over-the-wire systems to provide maximal flexibility of the wire. Some operators pass a "bare" wire across the lesion first, and then advance the balloon. However, when traversing tortuous coronary vessels, an over-the-wire balloon system can be converted into a "fixed" wire system by advancing the balloon and the extended guidewire as a single unit while steering the guidewire. This technique enhances steerability. Once the guidewire or "steerable balloon" reaches the lesion, it is important to advance the wire slowly with gentle rotation so that the true lesion lumen is crossed. With markedly eccentric lesions, it is useful to work in a projection that identifies the course of the lesion channel to aid in steering the guidewire.

Advancing the balloon itself across the lesion may require considerable guiding catheter support in severely stenotic lesions. In some instances, the guiding catheter must be advanced deep into the coronary ostium to achieve adequate support. By so doing, it is important to advance the guiding catheter slowly and to be certain that it is advancing coaxially over the balloon system to provide maximal stability while minimizing the risk of arterial dissection. Care should be taken to observe arterial pressure from the tip of the guide catheter to be sure that "damping" does not occur. If either "damping" or "ventricularization" occurs, the balloon should be advanced quickly across the stenosis and the guiding catheter withdrawn immediately to a more proximal or ostial position to reestablish adequate coronary flow. If the balloon does not cross promptly, the guide must be withdrawn and an alternate strategy considered.

With the balloon in place across the stenosis, a 2-atm inflation is performed under fluoroscopy to confirm the position noted by balloon indentation. Subsequently, the balloon is slowly inflated to higher pressures, sufficient to provide its full expansion. However, full inflation may not be necessary on the first inflation, and it may be achieved with subsequent inflations to higher pressures. Operators use a variety of inflation strategies, from slow to rapid increases. However, no documented difference in outcome is known. Balloon inflations are usually maintained for 60 seconds unless hemodynamic compromise occurs. Longer, frequently lower, pressure inflations can be used to "mold" lesions following acute closure or for stabilizing local dissection. Maximal balloon pressure should be limited to the value that achieves an adequate angiographic result, as higher pressures increase the probability of greater dissection. Likewise, longer inflations may be used in an attempt to prevent reclosure and to improve the angiographic result. Prolonged inflations frequently require a perfusion balloon to reduce ischemia, although in high flow states or in segments supplied by a major branch, perfusion balloons may not completely prevent ischemia. With the greater use of abciximab and intracoronary stents, the need for prolonged inflations as a strategy to prevent acute closure has markedly decreased. Furthermore, the actual balloon procedure is modified in patients selected for initial stenting. In these circumstances, balloon inflation is often used to lower pressure to retain some lesion identity, thus making stent positioning easier in a more obvious residual area of stenosis. Likewise, inflations are for 10–15 seconds only.

Balloon sizing is an important consideration. Even if a small or low profile balloon is required for initial lesion crossing, the final balloon used should have an inflated diameter similar to the estimated diameter of the native coronary artery. Restenosis rates are higher in lesions having incomplete dilation, whereas oversizing balloons is associated with higher initial complication rates.

Finally, an optimal result includes the best angiographic outcome feasible with minimal vessel damage. Ideally, the lowest restenosis is seen with a stentlike balloon result of less than 10% residual. In unstable lesions, in-lab sequential angiographic observation for 10 minutes is recommended to identify threatened reclosure. This practice allows the operator an opportunity to either perform repeat angioplasty or use alternative techniques to stabilize the lesion before acute closure occurs.

EQUIPMENT SELECTION

Angioplasty equipment continues to evolve as manufacturers develop newer products aimed at improving the safety and ease of the procedure. An outline of some of the types and characteristics of guiding catheters, balloon dilation catheters, and guidewires currently in use appears in Tables 27.8–27.10. Appropriate equipment choice and use is important for optimal angioplasty results with the least risk and least procedure cost.

Guiding Catheters

Guiding catheters are important for coronary access and backup support. The first factor in guiding catheter selection is choosing a French size that has an adequate internal diameter to allow good coronary visualization with guidewire(s) and balloon(s) in place, including circumstances in which simultaneous or dual balloon access for complex Y-lesions is anticipated. Thus, diameter sizing of a guide catheter depends primarily on the anticipated balloon or stent equipment needed, whereas, to some degree, sizing may be dictated by peripheral vascular status and coronary ostium size. In most instances, because of today's high stent utilization, most operators start with stent-compatible equipment. Thus, an 8-F guide catheter offers optimal support and torque ability, and has an internal diameter that allows maximal visualization with a variety of balloon and stent choices.

Most of the standard guide catheter shapes parallel diagnostic coronary angiographic catheters (Table 27.8). However, certain differences exist; for example, left Judkins guide curves tend to be more "open" and thus may require a smaller curve size to access the coronary ostium than is required for a diagnostic catheter. If a 4-cm left Judkins diagnostic catheter is

Table 27.8.
Guiding Catheter Selection from Femoral Approach

Vessel	Catheters	Curves	Comments
Left coronary artery	Left Judkins	3.5–6 cm	Easy left coronary access; good backup for LAD in most patients; less ideal for circumflex
	Left Amplatz	I–IV	Occasionally needed for access and support in LAD; often helpful for support in distal and/or tortuous circ lesions
	Multipurpose		Helpful in "high takeoff" left main
Right coronary artery	Right Judkins	3.5–5 cm	Familiar access for operator, but frequently lacks support
	Williams Right		Easy access; avoids catheter torquing
	Internal mammary artery		Useful for upward directed proximal right
	Left Amplatz	0.75, I, II	Excellent for improved support
	Right Amplatz		Useful for downward directed proximal RCA
	Hockey stick		May aid in difficult access or provide improved support in special circumstances
	El Ganal		
	Arani		
	Multipurpose		
Internal mammary artery (left and right)	Internal mammary artery		May require initial subclavian access via a diagnostic catheter with a long wire exchange
Vein bypass grafts	Right Judkins		Left grafts
	Right bypass		Excellent for right graft
	Left bypass		Left grafts only
	Multipurpose		Right grafts
	Left Amplatz		Left grafts
	Right Amplatz		Right grafts

Table 27.9.
Steerable Coronary Angioplasty Guidewire Characteristics

Size
  Diameter: 0.010″, 0.012″, 0.014″, 0.016″, 0.018″, 0.021″
  Length: 180 cm; 360 cm
Tip shapes
  Straight; preshaped "J"
Tip stiffness
  Very flexible or "floppy"
  Flexible or "intermediate" stiffness
  Limited flexibility—"standard"

difficult to engage because of a relatively small aortic root, it may be wise to choose a 3.5-cm left Judkins guide catheter, which often more easily accesses the ostium. For dilation of the left circumflex artery, left Amplatz-type catheters frequently provide the greatest backup support.

Access to the right coronary artery with a standard right Judkins guiding catheter frequently requires more patience and skill in torquing the catheter into the right coronary ostium. Rotation can be facilitated by gently moving the guiding catheter backward and forward in the sheath while transmitting torque to the catheter. Likewise, wetting the catheter with saline at the entrance to the sheath decreases friction, which reduces the possibility of catheter kinking. Special consideration must be

Table 27.10.
Coronary Angioplasty Balloon Characteristics

Delivery
  Over-the-wire
  Monorail
  Nonover-the-wire
Material
  Compliant, noncompliant, semicompliant
Performance
  Profile
  Pushability
  Trackability
Rewrap characteristic
Resistance to rupture
Size
  Inflated diameter 1.5–4 cm in 0.25 cm
  Available lengths 1.0 to 4 cm
Inflation Pressures
  Nominal size 5–8 atm; variable growth with
    increasing pressures up to 0.5 cm maximal
    growth
  Maximal burst 12–25 atm
Special characteristics
  Perfusion, passive and active

given to the tortuous or **"shepherd's crook"** right coronary artery. To enhance support and "straighten" the vessel for guidewire and balloon passage, a left Amplatz (0.75, I, or II curve), Arani, or multipurpose catheter is often helpful.

Use of a guiding catheter with side holes is particularly helpful for the right coronary artery. Compared with the left, the right coronary ostium is frequently smaller and requires deeper access. Blocking antegrade coronary flow with a guide catheter results in ischemia, marked bradycardia, or ventricular fibrillation, the latter secondary to stagnation of injected contrast material. A right coronary artery guide catheter with side holes frequently prevents these complications. Conversely, side holes are rarely needed for left coronary artery angioplasty unless the left main coronary artery is exceedingly small. In such circumstances, a guiding catheter with side holes may be misleading (i.e., arterial pressure in the catheter may appear normal, but left main flow is inadequate, leading to severe ischemia). Furthermore, left coronary guide catheter-related flow reduction may be limited by slightly removing the guiding cathe-

ter from the ostium once the guidewire and balloon catheter are in position, except during contrast injections. Coronary visualization may be reduced by side hole contrast leakage during coronary injection. Thus, to prevent bradycardia, arrhythmias, and ischemia, side holes are useful for right coronary angioplasty wherein guide catheter retraction is often difficult, but side holes are rarely necessary for left coronary artery angioplasty.

Inexperienced operators frequently begin with the standard Judkins catheters and only go to other more specialized catheters if these are not satisfactory for access or support. More experienced operators tend to choose first the catheter most likely to provide the most efficient dilation success. Although Amplatz catheters may be associated with a minimally higher risk of coronary vessel dissection, in experienced hands this risk is low and is compensated for by assuring the highest probability of success in crossing the lesion on the first attempt or providing adequate support for stent delivery. Amplatz-type guiding catheters should be removed from the coronary artery under fluoroscopy because, during withdrawal, the Amplatz guiding catheter may, paradoxically, advance further down the coronary artery. When this occurs, the guide catheter should be advanced with counterclockwise rotation, which will cause the catheter to "fall" out of the coronary ostium, frequently into the left ventricle from which it can be safely withdrawn.

Guidewires

Guidewires are available with a variety of tip configurations and sizes (Table 27.9). In general, the larger the wire the more steerable it is and the greater the push for crossing total occlusions. The smaller (0.010 and 0.012) wires are highly torquable, and they are potentially useful in crossing more distal or severe lesions. However, the smaller wires tend to provide less support for balloon tracking.

Guidewires also vary according to tip stiffness. The more rigid, steerable wires are particularly useful for steering (torque ability) and for crossing total occlusions and re-canalized channels that often require greater force in crossing the lesion. Conversely, the more flexible and floppy wires are less steerable, but they are also less traumatic in crossing complex unstable lesions, graft stenoses, or in recrossing lesions immediately after dilation. Another advantage of the extremely flexible wires is that the floppy tip can avoid some of the difficulty associated with traversing multiple branches by forming a **tip loop,** which then passes freely down the vessel.

A guidewire complication may occur if the tip of the guidewire becomes inadvertently lodged in a small distal vessel segment; continuing to force the wire forward may cause it to become embedded in the vessel wall. If this occurs, retracting the wire may fracture the tip ribbon. The wire will then begin to uncoil and, if pulled briskly, may fracture, leaving behind a distal wire fragment. **Tip ribbon fracture** is easily recognized by failure to visualize movement of the wire tip on withdrawal of the guidewire. Once this is recognized, the balloon catheter should be advanced as far as possible to the tip end of the wire. The balloon and wire should then be retracted as a unit, with slow but firm force. This technique can prevent complete wire fracture. Should the wire fracture, surgical or percutaneous removal of the wire may be necessary. Large fragments need to be removed because of the risk of systemic or coronary emboli. Small, distal fragments have been left in place without late complication.

Exchange length or extendible guidewires allows exchange of balloon catheters for larger or smaller sizes without having to recross coronary lesions. An extendible or exchange wire also allows retraction of the balloon catheter after dilating, providing maximal contrast injection through the guiding catheter. This technique, which provides high-quality angiographic definition after dilation before guidewire removal, has become routine for many operators, particularly when using large balloons and/or smaller guiding catheters (6 or 7 F) with a small internal diameter.

The frequent use of stents has significantly influenced guidewire use. If stenting is anticipated, an exchange length extra support wire is used from the beginning of the procedure to alleviate need for extending the standard length wire and to support stent delivery. Because of poor steerability, maximal support stent wires are rarely used as a first wire, but are exchanged through the balloon system if needed for stent delivery.

One consequence of extra support wires is that in highly tortuous vessels, coronary wrinkling is seen, which may be confused with vessel dissection. Recognition is based on noting the wrinkling in an area, without prior disease, that is markedly straightened by a wire. A useful technique is to remove the guide until the flexible tip is at the questionable area. Doing so maintains access but allows the vessel to reform, which should confirm that the abnormality was a result of vessel straightening by the stiff wire.

It is important to recognize that extra support wires may make passage of the wire through highly tortuous vessels difficult. Thus, sometimes a standard support wire is required to access the vessel, and, if an extra support wire is necessary for stent delivery, exchange is accomplished through a balloon passed distally into the vessel.

Balloon Catheters

Balloon catheters are of three types (Table 27.10). **Over-the-wire** systems use freely movable, steerable guidewires that have the advantage of being exchangeable while maintaining translesion guidewire access. **Nonover-the-wire** or fixed-wire, steerable balloon systems tend to be lower profile, which enhances "crossability" of severe lesions while improving the ability to test-inject contrast material through a small, 6 or 7 F, guiding catheter with the balloon still across the stenosis. However, fixed-wire systems require recrossing lesions to upsize or downsize balloons. Although concern exists regarding the inability to recross a dilated lesion, in reality most lesions can be repeatedly crossed without complication. **Monorail balloon** systems use the benefits of steerable wires, but allow rapid exchange of balloons without extending the guidewire while maintaining lesion access. These systems are somewhat limited by less "pushability" than standard over-the-wire systems with relatively similar balloon profiles. The advantage is the ease of balloon exchange, potentially reducing operator radiation exposure. However, most operators today use an over-the-wire balloon because this system is compatible with current stents and these systems are more reliable and safer than systems that are not over-the-wire type.

Balloon material is another important distinguishing feature. Compliant balloons tend to have lower crossing profiles, excellent rewraps for subsequent crossing of another lesion, and grow with higher inflation pressures. Thus, greater size flexibility is possible if the exact size of a vessel is unclear or if two lesions of relatively similar size are to be dilated. The ability to use one balloon for both dilations is cost efficient. Balloons can inflate up to 0.25 mm in diameter from minimal to maximal inflation.

Conversely, noncompliant balloons are less "crossible" (larger profile), rewrap less well, and decrease ability to recross lesions, but they maintain diameter with minimal growth despite high pressures. Thus, noncompliant balloons have become popular for poststent deployment because compliant balloons are a cross between the two, having some features of each. Therefore, in an effort to economize, noncompliant balloons are used for initial dilation when stenting is anticipated. The noncompliant balloon can be inflated to low pressures to predilate a lesion and then inflated to high pressures poststent deployment.

Special feature balloons include perfusion balloons used when long balloon inflation is both required and associated with either severe ischemic pain or hemodynamic compromise. Long balloons (30–40 cm in length) potentially provide efficient dilation of long or diffuse lesions, and they may minimize trauma to lesions dilated on an angle.

STENTS VERSUS BALLOONS

In the current era of high stent use for predictable outcomes with a low risk of acute occlusions and a reduced risk of restenosis, what is the role of balloon only angioplasty? (See Chapters 31–33.) Although oral anticoagulants are no longer a major issue, the cost of stents remains a concern. Based on available data, particularly from the STRESS trial (22), multiple stents, nonleft anterior descending (LAD) lesions, and larger vessels ($\geq$ 3.0 mm) appeared to have no significant benefit from stenting with regard to restenosis. Thus, if an excellent balloon result is obtained in larger ($\geq$ 3.0 mm), non-LAD vessels expected to require more than two stents, the advantages of coronary stenting to prevent restenosis remain less clear.

Long balloons in sizes of 30–40 cm in length potentially provide efficient dilation of long or diffuse lesions and minimize trauma to lesions being dilated on an angle. With complex angioplasty, these balloons appear to facilitate the procedure as well as potentially add safety.

Complications

Major cardiac complications associated with coronary angioplasty include myocardial infarction, urgent bypass surgery, and death. The risk of major complications is 4 to 5%. Death occurs in 1% or less, whereas acute myocardial infarction occurs in approximately 3 to 4% of patients, many of which are nontransmural (see also Chapter 8).

Acute Closure

Acute closure represents the major reason for urgent coronary artery bypass surgery after angioplasty. Acute closure risk is associated with a major coronary dissection or lesion thrombus (25) (Table 27.11). Recognition of patients at risk, based on clinical and angiographic findings, often allows acute closure to be anticipated and treated in the laboratory. If acute closure is identified, most lesions can be recrossed with subsequent successful angioplasty or stenting. Acute and threatened closure represent prime indications for stent use (see Chap-

Table 27.11.
Predictors of Acute Closure

Clinical
  Recent lesion-associated unstable ischemia or
    myocardial infarction (Consider IIb/IIIa
    antagonists)
Angiographic
  Pre-PTCA
    Complex lesions, thrombus (consider IIb/
      IIIa antagonists)
  Post-PTCA
    Thrombus (consider IIb/IIIa antagonists)
    Large dissections, particularly with flow
      compromise (stent; Cook or Palmaz-
      Schlatz)

Table 27.12.
Peripheral Vascular Complications

Puncture site bleeding, hematoma
Retropentoneal hemorrhage
Pseudoaneurysm
AV fistula
Arterial occlusion
Distal embolism
Infection; hematoma
Cholesterol emboli (atheroemboli)

ters 31–33). The use of abciximab reduces acute closure related to thrombolytic lesions (23). In patients who are not candidates for stents or IIB, IIIA antagonists, longer inflations—often at low pressures—may result in a stable angiographic result.

Peripheral Vascular Complications

Peripheral vascular complications are unfortunately a frequent adverse event in coronary interventional therapy, and studies (26, 27) have addressed the incidences and causes (Table 27.12). A frequently associated factor is persistent postprocedure heparinization (28). The primary vascular complication is development of a femoral artery **pseudoaneurysm.** Recognition and assessment of the size are important. Small pseudoaneurysms frequently heal without treatment, whereas larger ones require either percutaneous compression for closure or surgical repair. Carefully titrated heparin and restricted ambulation while on heparin reduce the risk of groin complications. With the greater use of IIB, IIIA antagonists associated with shorter duration heparin and with poststent anticoagulation limited to aspirin and ticlopidine, the incidence of anticoagulation-related groin complications has diminished.

Other complications include an infected groin hematoma, which rarely occurs except in repeated vascular access in the same groin over a short time span. Collagen vascular plug device use appears to enhance early ambulation, but its impact on groin infection needs to be monitored over time.

SUMMARY

Coronary angioplasty continues to evolve. Although new devices appear to increase the application and safety of nonsurgical revascularization in selected patients, balloon angioplasty alone, or in conjunction with other devices, remains the basic device consistently used as primary or adjunctive treatment. The technical descriptions in this chapter provide an introduction and basic understanding of coronary angioplasty, as well as a background for safe and efficient extension into nonballoon device applications, which are discussed in the following chapters.

References

1. Gruentzig AR, Senning A, Siegenthaler WE. Nonoperative dilatation of coronary artery stenosis: percutaneous transluminal coronary angioplasty. N Engl J Med 1979;301:61–68.
2. DiSciascio G, Cowley MJ, Vetrovec GW, et al. Triple vessel coronary angioplasty: acute outcome and long-term results. J Am Coll Cardiol 1988;12:48.
3. ACC/AHA Task Force Report. Guidelines for percutaneous transluminal angioplasty. A report of the American College of Cardiology/American Heart Association Task Force on Assessment of Di-

agnostic and Therapeutic Cardiovascular Procedure (Committee on Percutaneous Transluminal Coronary Angioplasty. 1993; J Am Coll Cardiol 22(7):2033–2054.

4. Cowley MJ, King SB III, Baim D, et al. Guidelines for credentialing and facilities for performance of coronary angioplasty. Cathet Cardiovasc Diagn 1988;15:136–138.

5. Detre K, Holubkov R, Kelsey S, et al. Percutaneous transluminal coronary angioplasty in 1985–1986 and 1977–1981. The National Heart, Lung, and Blood Institute Registry. N Engl J Med 1988;318:265–270.

6. Holmes DR Jr, Vlietstra RE. Balloon angioplasty in acute and chronic coronary artery disease. JAMA 1989;261:2109–2115.

7. Prisi AF, Folland ED, Hartigan P, on behalf of the Veterans Affairs ACME Investigators. A comparison of angioplasty with medical therapy in the treatment of single-vessel coronary artery disease. N Engl J Med 1992;326:10–16.

8. Guidelines. Committee on Coronary Angiography. ACC/AHA Guidelines for Coronary Angiography: A report of the ACC/AHA Task Force. J Am Coll Cardiol 1998.

9. Pocock SJ, Henderson RA, Richards AF, et al. Meta analysis of randomized trials comparing coronary angiography and bypass surgery. Lancet 1995;346:1184–1189.

10. The Bypass Angioplasty Revascularization Investigations (BARI) Investigators. Comparison of coronary bypass surgery with angioplasty in patients with multivessel disease. N Engl J Med 1996;335:217–225.

11. Weintraub WS, Mauldin PD, Becker E, et al. A comparison of the cost of and quality of life after coronary angioplasty or coronary surgery for multivessel coronary artery disease. Circulation 1995;92:2831–2840.

12. Grines CL, Browne KF, Marco J, et al. A comparison of immediate angioplasty with thrombolytic therapy for acute myocardial infarction. N Engl J Med 1993;328:673–679.

13. Gibbons RJ, Holmes DR, Reeder GS, et al. Immediate angioplasty compared with the administration of thrombolytic agent followed by conservative treatment for myocardial infarction. N Engl J Med 1993;328:685–691.

14. Committee on Management of Acute Myocardial Infarction. ACC/AHA Guidelines for Management of Patients with Acute Myocardial Infarction Executive Summary. A report of the American College of Cardiology/American Heart Association Task Force on Practice Guideline. Circulation 1996;94:2341–2350.

15. Lee L, Erbel R, Brown TM, et al. Multicenter registry of angioplasty therapy of cardiogenic shock: initial and long-term survival. J Am Coll Cardiol 1991;17:599–603.

16. Nath A, DiSciascio G, Vetrovec GW, et al. Multivessel coronary angioplasty after acute myocardial infarction. J Am Coll Cardiol 1990;16:545–550.

17. Topol EJ, Califf RM, George BS, et al. A randomized trial immediate versus delayed elective angioplasty after intravenous tissue plasminogen activator in acute myocardial infarction. N Engl J Med 1987;317:581–588.

18. The TIMI Study Group. The thrombolysis in myocardial infarction (TIMI) trial. N Engl J Med 1985;312:932–936.

19. Serruys PW, Luijten HE, Beatt KJ, et al. Incidence of restenosis after successful coronary angioplasty: a time-related phenomenon. A quantitative angiographic study in 342 consecutive patients at 1, 2, 3, and 4 months. Circulation 1988;77:361–371.

20. Hirshfeld JW, Schwartz JS, Jugo R, et al. Restenosis after coronary angioplasty. A multivariate analysis of lesion and procedure variables related to the restenosis rate. J Am Coll Cardiol 1991;18:647–656.

21. Vetrovec GW, DiSciascio G, Jugo R, et al. Comparative clinical and angiographic findings in patients with symptomatic and asymptomatic restenosis following angioplasty [abstract]. J Am Coll Cardiol 1990;15 (Suppl A):59A.

22. Fishman DL, Leon MB, Baim DS, et al. for the Stent Restenosis Study Investigators. A randomized comparison of coronary-stent placement and balloon angioplasty in the treatment of coronary artery disease. N Engl J Med 1994;331:496–501.

23. EPIC Investigators. Use of a monoclonal antibody directed against the platelet glycoprotein IIb/IIIa receptor in high-risk coronary angioplasty. N Engl J Med 1994;330:956–961.

24. Laskey MAL, Deutsch E, Hirshfeld JW Jr, et al. Influence of heparin therapy on percutaneous transluminal coronary angioplasty outcome in patients with coronary arterial thrombus. Am J Cardiol 1990;65:179–182.

25. Goldbaum TS, Cowley MJ, DiSciascio G, et al. Clinical and angiographic markings of early occlusion following successful PTCA. Cathet Cardiovasc Diagn 1989;17:22–27.

26. Wyman RM, Safian RD, Portway V, et al. Current complications of diagnostic and therapeutic cardiac catheterization. J Am Coll Cardiol 1988;12:1400.

27. Kresowik TF, Khoury MD, Miller BV, et al. A prospective study of the incidence and natural history of femoral vascular complications following percutaneous transluminal coronary angioplasty. J Vasc Surg 1991;13:328–333.

28. Oweida SW, Roubin GS, Smith III RB, et al. Postcatheterization vascular complications associated with percutaneous transluminal coronary angioplasty. J Vasc Surg 1990;12:310–315.

28

Complex Coronary Angioplasty

John S. Douglas, Jr, MD
Spencer B. King III, MD

INTRODUCTION

The interventional cardiologist approaching the new millennium has the ability to offer percutaneous catheter-based myocardial revascularization to many patients who previously required coronary bypass surgery or, in some cases, were denied attempts at revascularization because of complex anatomic or comorbid conditions. The development of tools for atherectomy and stent implantation, refinement of techniques, and evolution of new adjunctive strategies, although permitting management of increasingly complex patients, have placed considerable demands on the interventional operator whose wish is to provide the patient with the best that contemporary interventional cardiology has to offer. This chapter addresses the selection of patients, devices, and technical strategy for the performance of percutaneous coronary intervention in complex clinical and anatomic subsets.

General Considerations

The growth of percutaneous coronary intervention, which approaches 1,000,000 cases per year worldwide, has been fueled by improved angioplasty technology, the availability of stents, and recently developed antithrombotic measures (1). Rational patient selection, however, requires an analysis of multiple clinical variables, including a risk-to-benefit assessment of each target lesion with respect to the probability of successful intervention, the likelihood and consequences of complications, and restenosis and incomplete revascularization compared with other possible treatments. **In the current climate of cost awareness one must also consider, relative to other treatment options, the comparative costs of the initial treatment and any subsequent interventions.** Understandably, the durability of percutaneous revascularization has become an increasingly important issue as more complex clinical and anatomic subsets of patients are considered. A detailed analysis of some of these considerations is provided in the American College of Cardiology/American Heart Association (ACC/AHA) Guidelines for Percutaneous Transluminal Coronary Angioplasty (2, 3) and in Chapter 26.

COMPLEX CLINICAL SUBGROUPS

Unstable Angina

Acute coronary syndromes have a common pathophysiology of plaque disruption and partially or completely occlusive thrombus (4, 5) that is demonstrated dramatically by in vivo angioscopy (6, 7). Suspected myocardial ischemic pain at rest, without ST segment elevation, is a common syndrome in clinical practice, accounting for more than 750,000 hospital admissions in the United States. Unstable angina and non–Q-wave myocardial infarction, conditions not distinguishable clinically or angiographically without measurement of serum creatine kinase or other markers of myocardial necrosis, have been considered together in many clinical trials (8, 9). Increased complications—particularly abrupt closure—have been reported with coronary angioplasty (2, 3, 10) in these patients, presumably related to increased procoagulant activity, leading many operators to defer percutaneous coronary intervention for several days while instituting aggressive antianginal, heparin, and aspirin therapy (11, 12), particularly when there is obvious

thrombus on angiography (13, 14) (see *Thrombus* below). Other operators have pursued a more aggressive strategy of early intervention based on the encouraging results of angioplasty within 18–48 hours after hospitalization in randomized trials comparing early invasive and conservative management in this patient subgroup. The early invasive strategy yielded 96% angioplasty success, 2.9% myocardial infarction, 0.7% emergency bypass surgery, 2.2% abrupt closure, and fewer later repeat hospitalizations compared with the conservative strategy group (26 versus 33%, $P < .0001$) (8, 9). Early intervention is especially appealing when there is a perception of increased risk of an impending coronary event—that is, in those with medically refractory or postinfarction angina (Fig. 28.1) or malignant arrhythmias (15, 16). Cardiac-specific tropo-

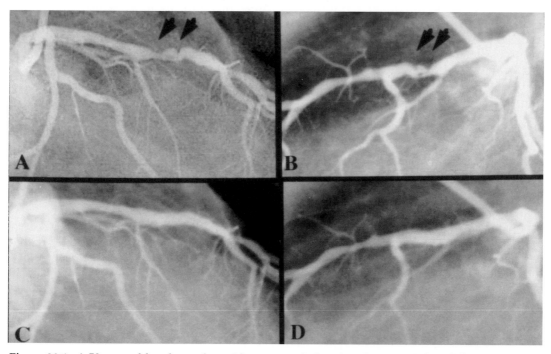

Figure 28.1. A 53-year-old male smoker with recurrent ischemic pain at rest 3 days following non–Q-wave myocardial infarction (creatinine kinase 450, MB34) in spite of intravenous heparin, nitroglycerin, and β-blockers. Left ventriculogram was normal; coronary arteriography revealed a complex ulcerated lesion of the left anterior descending (LAD) coronary artery with intraluminal filling defects (**A,** 30° right anterior oblique view; **B,** 90° left lateral; *arrows* denote lesion preintervention). Following predilation with a 3.5 mm balloon, a 4.0 × 15 mm Palmaz-Schatz stent (Johnson & Johnson, Warren, NJ) was implanted and expanded with a 4.0-mm balloon to 15 bar with an excellent angiographic result (**C, D**). Postintervention treatment include IIb/IIIa platelet receptor blockade, ticlopidine, and aspirin.

nin use to achieve early identification of unstable patients at high risk and those with micronecrosis appears promising (17–19) and merits further study. In patients with unstable angina who stabilize on medical therapy, risk stratification with noninvasive testing or coronary arteriography is carried out in most centers, and coronary revascularization is recommended for those with severe ischemia and obstructive lesions in important coronary arteries that are anatomically suitable for bypass.

Platelet glycoprotein IIb/IIIa receptor antagonist use is effective in reducing ischemic complications of coronary intervention in unstable angina in the EPIC, Impact II, RESTORE, and EPILOG studies (20–23) (see Chapter 34). Interim results from CAPTURE (c7E3 antiplatelet therapy in unstable angina) testing this agent in refractory unstable angina led to premature termination of the study because of a significant reduction of death, myocardial infarction (MI), and urgent intervention (10.8 versus 16.4% in the placebo group) (23). A meta-analysis of approximately 1200 patients with unstable angina indicated a 40 to 50% reduction in the composite of death, re-infarction, and refractory ischemia with use of GPIIb/IIIa antagonists, whereas direct antithrombins have proved much less effective (22, 23), and the routine administration of thrombolytic agents has reduced the thrombus burden, but with increased in-hospital ischemic complications of coronary intervention when studied in a randomized trial (12.9 versus 6.3% without thrombolytics, *P* = .02) (24). At Emory University Hospital, approximately 20% of patients undergoing coronary intervention receive GPIIb/IIIa inhibitors because of unstable ischemic syndromes and this factor, along with stents and other innovations such as the avoidance of nonionic contrast agents (25), has contributed to a reduced complication rate also noted in other active centers (26).

The choice of devices to accomplish percutaneous catheter-based revascularization in unstable angina is, for the most part, unencumbered. **Rotational atherectomy is contraindicated in the presence of lesion-associated thrombus,** but results in unstable angina have been reported to be similar to those in stable patients (27, 28). Some

have noted increased slow or no reflow in patients with rest pain (29). At Emory University, lesions with filling defects, haziness, and those treated early postinfarction are not usually selected for rotational atherectomy. On the contrary, directional atherectomy has been used commonly and with good success to treat such lesions in unstable patients in our hospital and in others (30). There are, however, reports of increased complications and lower event-free survival in these patients (31–33). The use of stents electively and to treat unfavorable results of other interventional strategies has expanded to include patients with unstable ischemic syndromes. Although unstable angina has been documented to be a predictor of stent thrombosis with a reported tenfold increase in some studies (34, 35), small single-center reports have indicated excellent outcome of stenting in this patient subgroup (36, 37). **We commonly use stents to treat unstable patients with lesions that appear unfavorable for other interventional strategies, and often use adjunctive antithrombotic measures such as IIb/IIIa inhibitors** in these patients (Fig. 28.1).

Advanced Age

Life expectancy at age 75 to 80 in the United States is approximately another 10 years, and among the 25% at this age with symptomatic cardiovascular disease, an increasing number prove refractory to medical therapy and require coronary revascularization (38–43). Compared with patients aged 65–70 years, those aged 80 years or older undergoing bypass surgery have much higher in-hospital mortality (11.5 versus 4.4%), costs ($48,200 versus $38,000), and 3-year mortality (28.8 versus 13.1%) (42). Percutaneous coronary intervention, when feasible, is an attractive, less-invasive alternative, although complications are more frequent and revascularization less complete than in younger patients. Percutaneous intervention is commonly feasible even in those very elderly patients who may not be candidates for surgical revascularization (Fig. 28.2). When a group of 192 patients aged 75 years or older,

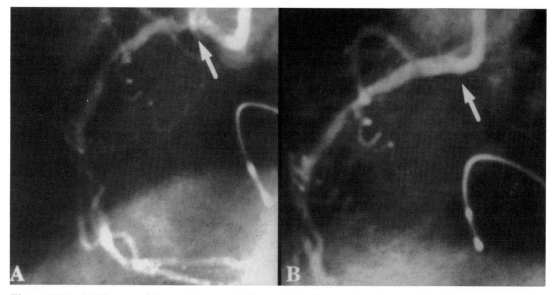

Figure 28.2. A 100-year-old retired automobile assembly line worker presented with severe chest pain and dyspnea. Cardiac catheterization confirmed the suspected presence of moderate aortic stenosis (65 mm Hg aortic value gradient) and coronary arteriography revealed moderate diffuse left coronary artery disease and severe calcific stenosis of the right coronary artery ostium (**A,** left anterior oblique review, *arrow* indicates ostial stenosis). Rotational atherectomy (1.5 mm and 20 mm burrs) followed by placement of a 3.0 × 15 mm Palmaz-Schatz (Johnson and Johnson Interventional Systems, Warren, NJ) stent expanded by a 20-bar balloon inflation yielded an excellent angiographic result (**B**). The patient became asymptomatic and was able to return to his apartment where he lives alone and functions independently.

who underwent percutaneous coronary intervention, were matched for gender, angina class, left ventricle function, number of vessels diseased, and prior MI with control patients aged 40–65 years, long-term follow-up for a mean of 40 months showed freedom from angina was less frequent (55 versus 75%, $P = .03$) as was freedom from cardiac death (92 versus 98%, $P = .05$), but when completely revascularized matched patients were compared, very little difference was found in long-term outcome (41). Complete revascularization, a laudable goal, is simply not feasible, however, in many older patients who may benefit symptomatically from a limited percutaneous revascularization.

Rotational atherectomy is used more often in elderly patients to treat fibrocalcific lesions, and increasingly stents are applied as an adjunct to rotational atherectomy (Fig. 28.2) or as primary therapy. In a contemporary series of 245 patients aged more than 75 years treated with stents, 3% died within

1 month, 1.6% had myocardial infarction, 0.4% stroke, 1.6% experienced stent thrombosis, and none required emergency surgery (a composite of adverse outcomes of 5%) (44).

Diabetes Mellitus

Approximately 10 to 20% of patients currently undergoing myocardial revascularization procedures are diabetic, a group of patients with accelerated vascular disease as well as a host of hematologic and metabolic factors that significantly complicate coronary revascularization (45–47). In most published series, diabetic patients requiring coronary revascularization were older; they had more diffuse proximal and distal coronary artery disease, more triple-vessel disease, and they had experienced more short and long-term risk. Diabetic patients in the 1985–1986 percutaneous transluminal coronary angioplasty (PTCA) Registry had a greater than sixfold increased risk of in-hospital death and the subsequent 9-year mortality rate was twice as high as in nondiabetics (35.9 versus 17.9%) (47), whereas at Emory University the in-hospital mortality rates of insulin requiring, noninsulin requiring, and nondiabetics undergoing coronary angioplasty between 1980–1990 were 0.8%, 0.26%, and 0.26%, respectively (45). Interest in diabetes as a possible predicator of poor angioplasty outcome relative to surgery was heightened by the disturbing report from the Bypass Angioplasty Revascularization Investigation (BARI), which between 1988 and 1991 randomized 1829 patients including 353 treated diabetics with a near twofold increased 5-year mortality in diabetics treated with PTCA (35 versus 19%, $P = .02$) (48). In nondiabetics, the 5-year mortality rates following PTCA and coronary artery bypass graft (CABG) were similar, 9%. The poorer long-term outcome of diabetics treated with PTCA, which were not attributable to differences in in-hospital mortality (1.2% for CABG, 0.6% for PTCA), led to reanalysis of BARI, which revealed that the benefit of CABG was limited to patients receiving an internal mammary artery (IMA) graft (5-year mortality with IMA = 13% versus 45% for saphenous vein graft [SVG] only), and greater for patients with four or more significant lesions (5-year mortality: with ≥ 4 lesions, CABG 21.6 versus PTCA 43.4% and 17.1 versus 24.6%, respectively, for patients with less than four significant lesions) (49). In contrast, the mortality rate of PTCA-treated diabetics in the smaller Emory Angioplasty versus Surgery Trial (EAST) was not higher than in the CABG group (50), and analyses of the Duke and Emory cardiac data banks comparing nonrandomized contemporaneous diabetic patients treated with PTCA and CABG revealed similar outcomes (51–53). These findings did not support the conclusion that diabetic status alone should determine revascularization method. Other recently reported comparisons of PTCA outcomes of matched diabetics and nondiabetics (54) and an analysis of data from seven multicenter trials of more than 6000 patients (55) also suggest that the negative impact of diabetes is not so great as BARI indicated, and that it is reasonable to offer percutaneous intervention to diabetics with suitable anat-

omy. Diabetic patients in whom PTCA is especially favored over surgery (56), in our practice, include those patients with three or fewer suitable target lesions, and those who have good recognition of ischemic symptoms, the relief of which will be beneficial and whose return would signal the need for reevaluation. Given the prothrombotic milieu present in diabetic vessels and the greater extent of disease, we use stents (Fig. 28.3) and IIb/IIIa inhibitors frequently (57, 58), especially in acute coronary symptoms where shock, heart failure, and in-hospital mortality are common in diabetics (59–62). Renal insufficiency in diabetic patients has important procedural and long-term implications (see *Renal Insufficiency* below).

Acute Myocardial Infarction

The recognition that coronary artery reperfusion strategies can save approximately 21 deaths per 1000 patients treated (35/1000 when seen within 1 hour) has revolutionized the treatment of acute myocardial infarction, the topic of a recently published ACC/AHA Guideline statement (63). Thrombolytic therapy, the simplest, most widely available method, is applicable in only half of patients with acute myocardial infarction (64); in those who are candidates for thrombolytic therapy, the results are not completely satisfactory. With the aggressive front-loaded use of t-PA, patency rates of 80% and TIMI-3 flow rates of only 50 to 60% were reported at 90 minutes and ischemia or stroke recurred in 10 to 15% of patients during the hospitalization, and late reocclusion in 30% (63, 65, 66). Early recognition of the lack of optimal reperfusion with thrombolytic therapy led to a series of trials of adjunctive angioplasty, which showed that routine PTCA up to 48 hours after t-PA resulted in better infarct-artery patency, but higher mortality, abrupt closure, and reocclusion without improving left ventricular function (67–69). Identification of patients who fail to reperfuse with thrombolytic therapy is difficult because complete chest pain relief and ST segment normalization occur in a minority of patients. When thrombolytic failures have been identified,

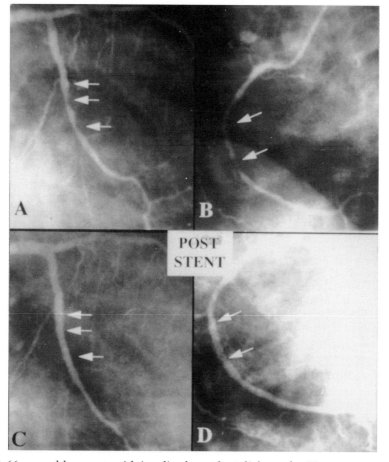

Figure 28.3. A 66-year-old woman with insulin-dependent diabetes for 20 years presented with chest pain and pulmonary edema. Cardiac catheterization revealed moderate anterior hypokinesis, severe stenosis (*arrows*) of the midcircumflex (**A**) and mid right coronary (**B**), 100% occlusion of diagonal, and moderate diffuse left anterior descending (LAD) disease. All distal vessels were diffusely diseased. Angioplasty followed by placement of a 3.0 × 20 mm Gianturco-Roubin stent yielded an excellent angiographic result in the circumflex (*arrows*, **C**) and a 3.0 × 15 mm Palmaz-Schatz (Johnson and Johnson Interventional Systems, Warren, NJ) stent (*arrows*, **D**) yielded a similarly good result in the right coronary artery. The patient is doing well 3 months postprocedure.

the results achieved with catheter-based reperfusion were suboptimal; angiographic success rate was only 80%, and 33% of angioplasty failures died (70–72).

Direct infarct-artery recanalization without adjunctive thrombolytic therapy when performed within 6 hours of symptom onset was reported in early experiences to result in angioplasty success rates of over 90%, fewer episodes of recurrent ischemia, and no strokes (73–76). Primary PTCA and thrombolytic therapy were compared in a series of randomized trials that showed

that PTCA was more successful in achieving vessel patency, in restoring normal TIMI-3 flow, which was the only independent predictor of in-hospital survival and preservation of ventricular function, and in meta-analyses reduced in-hospital death and re-infarction (Fig. 28.4), and the incidence of rehospitalization and costs largely by reducing recurrent ischemia (77–84). Mortality was 8.8%, 7.0%, and 3.7% for TIMI grades 0/1, 2, and 3 respectively (83). In the PAMI-I Trial, survival without recurrent infarction was 86% with primary PTCA com-

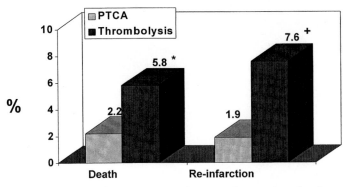

In-hospital Death and Re-Infarction in Three Randomized Trials of PTCA and Thrombolysis in Acute Myocardial Infarction

Figure 28.4. In-hospital death and reinfarction in three randomized trials of percutaneous transluminal coronary angioplasty (PTCA) and thrombolysis in acute myocardial infarction: odds ratio for in-hospital mortality with thrombolysis versus angioplasty = 2.68 (95% confidence limits, 1.16–6.92; P = .023). Odds ratio for in-hospital reinfarction with thrombolysis versus angioplasty = 4.22 (95% confidence limits; 1.82–11.46; P = .0008). Data obtained from meta-analysis by Simari et al. (81) of 640 patients in three trials (77, 78, 79).

pared with 79% with thrombolytic therapy at 2 years (80).

Subsequent reports have indicated that the excellent results reported with primary PTCA were dependent on short door-to-balloon time (ideally < 60 minutes), a feat not attainable in all centers (85). In 19 Seattle hospitals, 14 of which were community hospitals, between 1988 and 1994, the mean interval from emergency room arrival to balloon inflation was 1.7 ± 1.2 hours (2.3 hours in low volume hospitals) compared with 1.0 ± 1.0 hours to receive thrombolytic therapy and, in this nonrandomized comparison of strategies, there was no difference in in-hospital or long-term mortality (mortality during hospitalization 5.6 versus 5.5%; adjusted hazard ratio for risk of death within 3 years after primary PTCA, 0.95; 95% confidence interval; 0.8–1.2) (86). This study, which may be influenced by selection bias in the physician choice of reperfusion method, prompted considerable debate on the merits of the two reperfusion strategies (65, 87).

Whereas there may be debate regarding the degree of superiority, or the equivalence, of primary angioplasty compared with thrombolytic therapy in the treatment of acute MI, no evidence is found that

thrombolytic therapy is superior to a timely angioplasty performed by skilled operators. Patents most likely to benefit from primary PTCA as seen in the PAMI Trial include those aged more than 65 years (mortality rate 5.7 versus 15% with thrombolytics), with anterior infarction (mortality 1.4 versus 11.9%, P = .01), patients with prior bypass surgery (see *Prior Bypass Surgery*) and high-risk patients such as those with inferior infarction with anterior ST segment depression, and patients in cardiogenic shock, in whom mortality is reduced from the 70% reported with thrombolytic therapy to approximately 50% (63, 65, 88). Improvement in clinical outcome has also been reported with adjunctive intra-aortic balloon pumping in high-risk patients undergoing primary PTCA (89). Other advantages of primary PTCA include the avoidance of the risk of thrombolytic therapy in the 5 to 10% of patients with no high-grade lesions and the ability to risk stratify patients and to make early assignment to appropriate therapies, which range in acute myocardial infarction from bypass surgery in approximately 5% of patients to early discharge (day 3) in low-risk patients resulting in a $4000.00 reduction in hospital charges (65).

Although it appears that the benefit of primary PTCA over thrombolytic therapy may have narrowed when front-loaded t-PA and primary PTCA are compared in community hospitals, it should be recognized that primary PTCA is currently being revolutionized and enhanced as a result of a much more aggressive use of stents and IIb/IIIa receptor inhibitors, both of which appear to reduce acute events and restenosis (21, 90–93). The place of extraction atherectomy in primary PTCA, evaluated recently in 100 patients (94), remains to be determined, but this strategy may be helpful in heavily thrombotic lesions in large vessels that are free of sharp angulations.

What should be done for the patient with an occluded infarct artery discovered a few days postinfarction? The answer is simple in the presence of documented ischemia where elective PTCA is indicated (63). However, recent provocative studies suggest that late (up to 2 weeks) opening of totally occluded infarct arteries may also be beneficial in selected patients who are at risk for ventricular dilation, especially those with anterior Q-wave infarction and reduced ejection fraction (95, 96).

Prior Coronary Bypass Surgery

Early Postoperative Ischemia

Severe myocardial ischemia manifests as unstable angina or evolving myocardial infarction occurs in at least 3 to 5% of patients within a few hours or days of coronary bypass surgery, most often because of venous graft occlusion, and immediate coronary arteriography should be considered to pinpoint the problem (97–99). Although a quarter of ischemic patients catheterized within a few hours of surgery have normal grafts and no apparent cause for ischemia, most have remedial problems requiring emergency PTCA (98, 100–103) or reoperation (99). Targets for PTCA include narrowed vein graft or internal mammary artery (IMA) anastomotic sites (97, 98, 100), IMA trunk lesions (101), kinked vein grafts (102), and ungrafted (97, 98) and grafted

vessels with occluded grafts (Fig. 28.5). Shock caused by occlusion of a critically important graft is not rare and immediate action can be lifesaving (98, 103). Although angioplasty of anastomotic lesions has been safe in our experience and in that of others within a week of surgery (97, 98, 100), we are aware of unreported cases of suture line disruption and hemorrhagic shock that may have been related to guidewire and, subsequently, balloon catheter passage through the suture line. These observations engender a cautious approach to these lesions, including conservative balloon sizing. Whether thrombolytic agent use early postoperatively is safe, as has been suggested (100), requires further study. In an early experience with intragraft thrombolysis in the immediate postoperative period, Rentrop reported mediastinal bleeding requiring drainage in approximately one third of patients (personal communication).

Recurrent angina between 1 and 6 months following surgery is commonly caused by to perianastomotic graft stenosis, graft occlusion, or mid-SVG stenoses caused by fibrous intimal hyperplasia and rarely related to atherosclerotic plaque rupture or progression. Angina recurrence at precisely 3 months strongly suggests a distal venous or arterial graft anastomotic lesion in our experience (Fig. 28.6), and should lead to coronary arteriography in most patients given the excellent results with PTCA at this site (see below).

Late Recurrent Ischemia Post-CABG

When angina recurs months or years following surgery, venous graft disease and native vessel progression are common. In approximately 100 patients presenting with unstable angina many months following surgery, paired coronary arteriograms were carefully analyzed to assess disease progression. A culprit lesion was identified in over 80% of patients: in a vein graft in 54%, in an ungrafted coronary artery in 18%, and a grafted artery proximal or distal to graft insertion in 9%. Total occlusion was present in half of the culprit vein grafts and 25% of ungrafted coronary arteries whereas the presence of thrombus was more common in vein grafts than in native coronary arteries (37 versus 12%, $P = .04$) (104). This observation that unstable angina in post-CABG patients is most often caused by thrombotic venous graft disease, a difficult condition to treat effectively, parallels our Emory University experience.

Following bypass surgery, approxi- mately 3% of patients experience acute myocardial infarction annually (105), and adverse outcomes related to reperfusion strategies are relatively common, because of increased prevalence of multivessel disease and poor left ventricular function (106–110). In patients with evolving myo- cardial infarction, the culprit lesion has been reported to be a vein graft in up to two thirds of patients (109). In the PAMI trials of primary PTCA, the infarct vessel was a

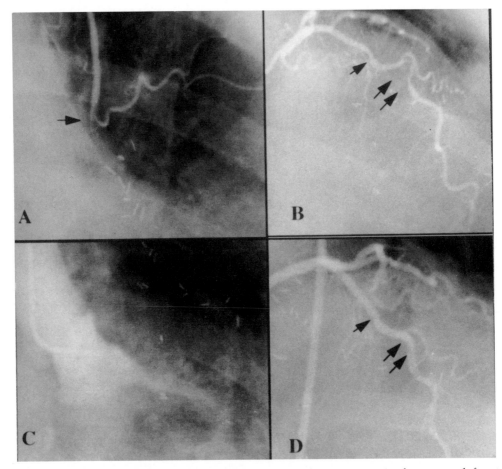

Figure 28.5. A 78-year-old woman with refractory angina and severe stenosis of a tortuous left anterior descending (LAD) artery was referred for minimally invasive direct coronary bypass surgery (mid-CABG). The left internal mammary artery was anastomosed to the LAD via the left fourth intercostal incision without cardiopulmonary bypass. Within a few hours following surgery, the patient complained of recurrent angina and the ECG had anterior T-wave inversion. Recatheterization 2 days following mid-CABG revealed an occluded left internal mammary artery (LIMA) graft approximately 4 cm from its LAD insertion (*arrow*, **A**). The LAD was patent but tortuous with multiple severe stenosis (*arrows*, **B**). Left ventriculogram was normal (**C**). Following placement of three intracoronary stents (*arrows*) expanded by a 16-bar balloon inflation, the angiographic result was excellent (**D**). The patient has remained free of angina subsequently.

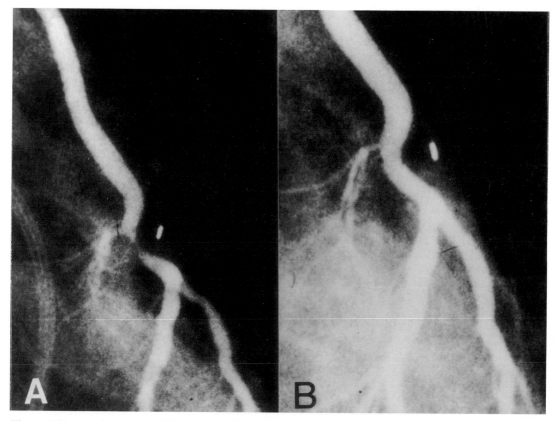

Figure 28.6. Angina recurred 3 months following saphenous vein bypass to the left anterior descending (LAD) and right coronary arteries. Coronary arteriography revealed severe stenosis at the anastomosis of the saphenous vein graft to the LAD (**A**). Balloon angioplasty was successful and repeat angiography 12 years later revealed a widely patent percutaneous transluminal coronary angioplasty (PTCA) site (**B**). Lesions at this site appearing 3–6 months postoperatively have an excellent long-term patency.

venous graft in 45% of patients (111) and the PTCA outcome was similar to that obtained in patients with no prior surgery (TIMI-3 flow in 88 versus 95%, $P = .06$; no difference in mortality, reinfarction, recurrent ischemia). In contrast, reperfusion of venous grafts with thrombolytic therapy was successful in few as 25% of patients in observational studies (109). In the GUSTO-1 ANGIO Trial, angiography at 90–180 minutes after thrombolytic treatment showed that TIMI grade 2 or 3 flow was achieved in only 48% of SVGs (112). These observations strongly support aggressive intervention in post-CABG patients with acute MI when feasible, and thrombolytic therapy when prompt catheter-based intervention is not available (63, 113).

Revascularization Choices Post-CABG

As in initial revascularization procedures, selection of a percutaneous approach in the post-CABG patient frequently yields a less complete and less durable revascularization result and subsequent procedures are frequently necessary, but this is offset by the fact that reoperations are two to three times more likely to lead to in-hospital death or infarction, and are more costly and less effective in relieving symptoms than first operations (114–117). This choice, which can be difficult (118), resulted in PTCA in 63% of more than 4000 post-bypass patients undergoing repeat revascularization at

Emory University, whereas 37% underwent re-CABG with a 1.2% and 6.8% ($P < .001$) in-hospital mortality rate, respectively, and in-hospital costs of $8500 versus $24,200 ($P < .001$) (119). Among 632 post-bypass patients treated at the Mid-American Heart Institute in 1987–1988 and followed for 4 years, the 74% who underwent PTCA had lower in-hospital death than those who had repeat surgery (0.3 versus 7.3%, $P < .0001$) and Q-wave MI (0.9 versus 61%, $P < .0001$), but less complete revascularization (38 versus 92%, $P < .0001$), more subsequent interventions (64 versus 8%, $P < .0001$), and similar angina relief, actuarial 6-year survival, and MI-free survival (120).

Among the factors that influence revascularization choices, the status of the left anterior descending (LAD) artery and its graft are perhaps the most important. A patent LIMA graft to the LAD has been shown to enhance event-free survival for up to 20 years (121–124). Reoperative CABG to treat ischemia in non-LAD territories offers no survival benefit (125, 126), may jeopardize patent arterial grafts; these concerns favor percutaneous intervention whereas LAD ischemia, multiple vessel involvement, severe venous graft disease, small number of patent grafts, and poor left ventricle function frequently lead to surgical revascularization in our practice and in that of others (127). Importantly, catheter revascularization can be offered to many post-bypass patients who are not candidates for repeat surgery because of medical comorbidity, inadequate target vessels, absent conduits, or limited myocardium in jeopardy. Both the short- and long-term outcomes of catheter revascularization are significantly influenced by the conduit vessel (SVG versus native vessel versus IMA) and the specific location of the target lesion(s).

Native Vessel

Recurrent ischemia, which is often related to venous graft disease, can be ameliorated by native vessel intervention in many patients with more lasting benefit and less risk than with vein graft intervention. Targets include, in many cases, the lesions that led

to surgery (an unusually difficult collection of very old lesions), total occlusions, and new lesions distal to grafts and in ungrafted vessels. Effective intervention on these lesions may require cutting-edge technology (Fig. 28.7). Treatment of lesions distal to grafts can be challenging, especially when the location is in the native coronary artery proximal to graft insertion. In approaching this problem, incremental guidewire stiffening and high performance balloon catheters may be required to pass severely angulated segments (128).

The results of native vessel intervention were reported in 1987 for the initial Emory experience with 372 patients where angiographic success was achieved in 91%, death occurred in 0.3%, Q-wave myocardial infarction in 2%, and bypass surgery was required in 6% (129). Among 1543 post-bypass patients with native vessel intervention at Mid-America Heart Institute, most of whom had triple-vessel disease, angiographic success was 94%, in-hospital mortality 0.8%, Q-wave infarction 1.5%, and 1.0% required emergency CABG (130). Native coronary intervention in 2246 post-bypass patients at Emory University between 1980 and 1995 was performed with procedural success in 89%, in-hospital death in 1%, Q-wave myocardial infarction in 1%, non–Q-wave infarction (creatinine kinase three or more times normal) in 4%, and elective or emergency CABG in 2.8%. The definitions of outcomes were somewhat different in these series, but overall results were similar with a trend toward slightly higher mortality, because of selection of sicker patients, and a reduced need for in-hospital CABG in the more recent experience.

Venous Grafts

The results of saphenous vein graft interventions have been disappointing. Gruentzig et al. noted that among the first 50 patients treated with balloon angioplasty, 3 of 5 patients who had successful SVG dilation experienced restenosis, leading them to question "whether we should eliminate this lesion from consideration" (131). Subsequent reports indicated that in patients with

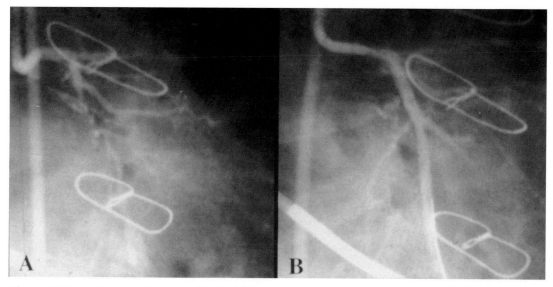

Figure 28.7. A 63-year-old man with disabling angina and a history of coronary bypass surgery 4 years earlier was found to have occlusion of the saphenous vein graft to the circumflex coronary artery and a patent left internal mammary artery (LIMA) to the left anterior descending artery. The circumflex was occluded (as it had been 4 years earlier), but was tapered at the point of occlusion (**A**). The total occlusion was crossed with a 0.010-inch steerable guidewire and following balloon dilation and stenting, a large lumen was recreated (**B**) that provided excellent symptomatic relief.

focal vein graft disease, balloon angioplasty yielded a high success rate of 90%, whereas approximately 2% or less experienced Q-wave MI, 2% required elective or emergency CABG, and 1% died (132–145). Non–Q-wave MI was the most common complication in early series occurring in 13% of 599 patients at Emory University (140). Late cardiac events and restenosis, unfortunately, were common. Important predictors of restenosis included the lesion site (proximal anastomosis 68%, mid-SVG 61%, distal anastomosis 45%, $P = .05$), and time since CABG (< 6 months 32%, 6–12 months 43%, 1–5 years 61%, and 64% for SVG age more than 5 years, $P = .02$). Distal anastomotic lesions treated within 1 year of surgery had a restenosis rate of 22% and excellent subsequent event-free survival. However, even when the angiographic outcome of balloon angioplasty of mid-SVG lesions was quite favorable (< 20% residual diameter stenosis), only approximately half of patients were event-free at 1 year, and, of the 40% of patients who required repeat

intervention, 90% were at the original PTCA site (146).

In an effort to blunt the aggressive restenosis process in SVGs, a number of nonballoon approaches were tried. Directional atherectomy appeared to be a promising method in early observational trials (147, 148). In our experience, directional atherectomy appeared effective in the initial treatment of bulky SVG lesions; however, a high rate of non–Q-wave MI of 48% was observed (149). In a randomized trial (CAVEAT II), balloon angioplasty and directional atherectomy were compared in the treatment of SVG lesions in approximately 300 patients (150). Eighty-six percent of lesions were in mid-SVG sites. The results were similar to CAVEAT I. Although angiographic success was a bit higher with directional coronary atherectomy (DCA), there were more non–Q-wave infarctions with DCA (16 versus 9.6%), and the 6-month restenosis rate was not different (45.6% with DCA, 50.5% for PTCA, $P = 0.49$). At 6 months, there was a trend toward more target lesion revascularization with PTCA (26 versus 19%, $P = .09$). Of some concern was the observation that distal embolization, which was twice as common with DCA (13.5% versus 5.1%), was associated with worse in-hospital and 12-month outcomes (151). This higher complication rate with DCA coupled with similar restenosis outcome and added cost and complexity have resulted in a dramatic decrease in the use of DCA for de novo SVG lesions and also for restenotic lesions where acute complications were less frequent but restenosis rates higher, approximately 80% (152, 153). Directional atherectomy continues to be a viable option for treatment of aorto-ostial SVG lesions: angiographic success 94%, major complications 5.9%, target lesion repeat interventions 42% at 12 months, compared with 33% with Palmaz-Schatz (Johnson and Johnson Interventional Systems, Warren, NJ) stents, $P = .05$ (154) and in nondilatable SVG lesions at ostial and mid-SVG sites.

The excimer laser has been applied in SVG angioplasty as a debulking technique, usually followed by balloon dilation or stent implantation. In a report of treatment of 545 lesions between 1989 and 1993, 91% followed by balloon angioplasty, 0.4% with DCA, and none with stenting, clinical success was achieved in 92%. At least one in-hospital complication occurred in 6.1% of patients: death (1%), CABG (1.6%), Q-wave (2.4%) or non–Q-wave (2.2%) MI (155). The highest success and lowest complication rates were in lesions at ostial sites, lesions less than 10 mm in length, and in SVGs with diameters less than 3 mm. Two earlier reports also confirmed high success rates with aorto-ostial laser angioplasty (156, 157). In multicenter experience with 106 consecutive patients treated with laser angioplasty for SVG lesions, quantitative analysis of procedural and follow-up angiograms revealed that minimum lumenal diameter (MLD) increased from 1.09 mm before treatment to 1.61 mm after laser to 2.18 mm after adjunctive balloon dilation (158). Angiographic success (< 50% diameter stenosis) was 54% after laser and 91% after adjunctive PTCA. In-hospital complications were death 0.9%, myocardial infarction (Q- and non–Q-wave) 4.5%, and bypass surgery 0.9%. Angiographic follow-up was ob-

tained in 83% of eligible patients; restenosis occurred in 52% and approximately half had total occlusion. Overall 1-year mortality was 8.6%. These results, comparable to balloon angioplasty alone, have not encouraged laser usage as an adjunct to balloon dilation of saphenous vein grafts. In some centers, however, laser angioplasty has been used as a debulking technique prior to stenting with good results in observation studies. Employing 2-mm catheters and a saline flush technique (159) to minimize laser trauma, favorable results were obtained by operators at the Washington Hospital Center in thrombus-containing and degenerated grafts in 81 patients (100% procedural success, 8.7% non-Q myocardial infarction, 0% no reflow) (160). Long-term outcome of this strategy is unknown.

A variety of stents have been implanted in saphenous vein grafts. The first was the Wallstent (Schneider, Zurich, Switzerland) (161) (Fig. 28.8) and subsequently its use has been associated with high initial success rates exceeding 95%, but stent thrombosis occurred in 4 to 10% and restenosis was reported in over 50% in some series (162–164). In an analysis of the outcome of 93 stent implantations (84 Wallstent and 9 Palmaz-Schatz) in 62 patients between 1986 and 1994, in-hospital complications occurred in 11%: death 3%, myocardial infarction 3%, CABG 5% reducing the initial clinical success to 89% (164). During follow-up (median 2.5 years, range 0–5.9), another 8% died, 23% sustained myocardial infarction, and 43% underwent repeat revascularization procedures yielding event-free survival rates at 1 and 5 years of only 46% and 30%, respectively. This disturbingly poor long-term outcome was achieved without routine high-pressure balloon expansion of the stents that has become standard contemporary practice and parallel results obtained with balloon angioplasty alone. Whether better results can be obtained with more optimal Wallstent expansion is under investigation. Also being studied is the perhaps overly optimistic application of long Wallstents (mean length 63 mm) to the treatment of diffuse vein graft disease (165).

The Palmaz-Schatz coronary stent has been used extensively in saphenous vein grafts, and the results of its use were re-

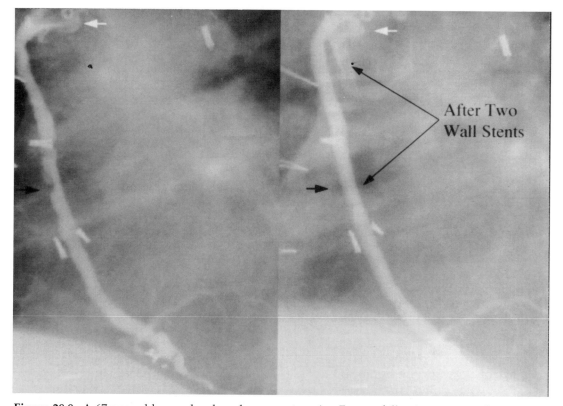

Figure 28.8. A 67-year-old man developed recurrent angina 7 years following coronary bypass surgery. Recatheterization revealed a patent left internal mammary artery (LIMA) graft to the left anterior descending (LAD) artery and severe focal disease in the midportion of the saphenous vein graft (SVG) to the right coronary artery, which was a small vessel. Because of the patent arterial graft to the LAD and poor distal right coronary artery, angioplasty and stenting of the SVG was carried out with a 5-mm diameter Wallstent (Schneider, Zurich, Switzerland) at the target site, and a second stent more proximally. The patient was treated with IIb/IIIa platelet receptor inhibitors and experienced a non–Q-wave myocardial infarction postprocedure.

ported for experience in observational registries (166–168), in comparisons with contemporaneously treated patients receiving balloon angioplasty (146, 169), in randomized trials of stenting versus balloon angioplasty (the SAVED Trial) (170), and in an observational trial of aspirin and ticlopidine in SVG stenting (RAVES) (171). In the United States Multicenter Palmaz-Schatz Registry, the results of vein graft stent implantation in 589 patients were more favorable than those reported in subsequent rigorous randomized trials: procedural success 97%, stent thrombosis 1.4%, death 1.7%, Q-wave myocardial infarction 0.3%, urgent CABG 0.9%, 6-month restenosis 18% for de novo and 46% for restenotic lesions, and 12-

month event-free survival 76% (166). Palmaz-Schatz coronary stent use in the treatment of aorto-ostial SVG lesions was reported in observational studies in 20 patients in whom restenosis developed in 7 (35%) (168), and in 29 patients event-free survival was 82% at 11 months (167).

When optimal angioplasty (< 20% residual stenosis) in 48 patients was compared with stenting of mid-SVG lesions in 41 patients in a retrospective analysis, the late outcome was more favorable in the stent patients: death, 2.4% versus 8.3%; reintervention, 4.9% versus 35% ($P < .01$); and freedom from events, 88% versus 54% ($P < .01$) (146).

The SAVED Trial compared initial and

6-month outcome of balloon angioplasty versus Palmaz-Schatz stenting in 220 randomized patients with angina pectoris or objective evidence of myocardial ischemia and new saphenous vein graft lesions (170). Patients with myocardial infarction within 7 days, lesion length more than two stents, and evidence of SVG thrombus were excluded. Stented patients received warfarin anticoagulation. Baseline characteristics were similar except that more diabetic patients were present in the angioplasty group (36 versus 23%, $P = 0.05$). The angiographic success rate was significantly higher in the stent group as was the postprocedural minimal lumen diameter (2.81 versus 2.16 mm, $P < .001$). The in-hospital complication rate was similar in the two groups. At 6 months, the cardiac event rate (death, myocardial infarction, repeat revascularization) was significantly lower in the stent group (26 versus 39%, $P = .04$), and Kaplan-Meier event-free survival at 240 days was 73% for the patients who received stents compared with 58% ($P = 0.03$) for the angioplasty group. The lack of a statistically significant difference in restenosis rates (37 versus 46%, $P = .24$) was caused by the greater late lumen loss in the stent group (1.1 versus 0.66 mm, $P < .01$) and to the fact that the sample size was underpowered to demonstrate a significant difference in angiographic restenosis. The 9% difference in restenosis rates in the SAVED Trial is similar to the difference observed in the larger Stress and Benestent trials of native vessel stenting.

Adjunctive anticoagulation, antiplatelet, and pharmacologic strategies are being evaluated. A trial of reduced anticoagulation trial in saphenous vein graft stent implantation (RAVES) was conducted during which 201 patients at 19 clinical sites underwent stenting of 231 lesions followed by aspirin and ticlopidine 250 mg twice daily for 1 month. Eighty percent of patients received a single stent, 14% two Palmaz-Schatz stents. A preliminary report at 30 days indicated that 8% of patients experienced acute or threatened closure or no reflow, and 21% of patients had Q- or non–Q-wave myocardial infarction: Q-wave 2.0%, non–Q-wave with CK-MB more than eight times normal in 6.5%, and non–Q-wave myocardial infarction with CK-MB three to eight times normal in 13% (171). Long-term outcomes

are being evaluated. Platelet IIb/IIIa receptor inhibitors, which have been shown to reduce evidence of distal embolization in saphenous vein graft intervention (172), and calcium channel blocking agents (173), which are effective in treatment of no reflow and are used with increasing frequency in our hospital, warrant further study.

The Palmaz-Schatz "biliary" stent has been used primarily in larger saphenous vein grafts (5–9 mm in diameter) where results have been similar to the coronary stent (174). The biliary stent has struts that are approximately twice as thick as the 0.0025-in struts of the coronary stent and this results in much greater visibility and radial compressive strength, but these stents are less flexible and deployment is therefore significantly more difficult. Wong et al. (174) treated 163 SVG lesions in 124 patients with this stent with 99% deployment success, 94% clinical success, one death, no Q-wave infarctions, and one CABG. These results were comparable to those obtained with the coronary stent in smaller vein grafts in their center. The Palmaz-Schatz biliary stent has been used successfully, either free-mounted on a suitable balloon catheter (106) or with a double guide catheter system to sheath the stent (175, 176).

Thrombus is common in SVG lesions associated with acute ischemic syndromes, and the presence of obvious thrombus has been regarded as an indicator of high risk and an exclusion for most trials of SVG intervention. The transluminal extraction catheter (TEC) has been used to debulk thrombus-laden and bulky SVG lesions prior to balloon angioplasty or stent implantation (160, 177–188). Some operators have used prolonged (8–24 h) intragraft urokinase infusions (50,000–100,000 U/h) prior to intervention to reduce thrombus (189–192), and others have delivered thrombolytic agents locally using the Dispatch catheter (Scimed-Boston Scientific, Maple Grove, MN) (193, 194). The primary disadvantage of prolonged urokinase infusion is bleeding complications (see below).

Use of TEC in 58 thrombus-containing vein graft lesions compared with 125 thrombus-free lesions resulted in lower clinical success (69 versus 88%, $P = .01$), higher no reflow (19 versus 5%), and more complications (composite end point of death, CABG and Q-wave myocardial infarction in 13 versus 2%, $P < .01$), but restenosis was similar, approximately 65% (180). In an experience with 127 TEC procedures in vein grafts in the New Approaches to Coronary Intervention (NACI) Registry, coronary embolization was experienced in 15.4% of patients with a 36.4% mortality rate (177). Although angioscopy has indicated relatively complete removal of thrombus from the treatment site (186,187,195), distal embolization of some of the thrombus and friable atheroma must be unavoidable as evidenced by significant non–Q-wave infarction rates in most series. In a Washington Hospital Center experience, treatment of 36 patients with complex vein graft lesions with TEC followed by immediate stent implantation resulted in 100% procedural success, 15% non–Q-wave myocardial infarction, 2.2% no reflow, and 2.9% abrupt closure (160). The definition of non–Q-wave myocardial infarction, however, was a rather high CPK-MB value of five times upper limit of normal. The place of TEC in the treatment of saphenous vein graft disease is not yet determined, but may be clarified by ongoing trials (183).

Successful recanalization of totally occluded saphenous vein grafts encountered apart from the setting of acute myocardial infarction (i.e., chronic or subacute occlusion) has been reported, but complications are frequent and long-term patency is low. Prolonged intragraft urokinase infusions were used most frequently (196–208), and in addition to puncture site bleeding complications, thromboembolic myocardial infarction (197, 199–202, 206, 208), intracranial bleeding (204, 207, 208), retroperitoneal bleeding (208), and intramyocardial hemorrhage (205) have been reported. Among 107 patients in multiple centers who received low-dose intragraft urokinase (100,000 U/h) for a mean infusion time of 25 hours, 69% their grafts were re-opened, but the following complications were experienced: Q-wave MI 5%, non–Q-wave MI 17%, emergency CABG 4%, stroke 3%, transfusion 19%, and 6.5% died in-hospital (208). On follow-up at 6 months, there were 2 additional deaths, 4 repeat revascularizations, and 16 (40%) of the 40 patients recatheterized had a patent graft. This relatively poor long-term outcome was mirrored in two single-center

reports. At a mean of 13 months after attempted recanalization of occluded vein grafts in 10 consecutive patients, Levine et al. found no patient was free of either reocclusion or a clinical end point of myocardial infarction, or death (198). In a Mayo Clinic experience with 77 consecutive patients with occluded SVGs, intervention was successful in 71% but 5.2% died and 8% underwent CABG within 30 days (209). Survival, event-free survival, and freedom from severe angina at 3-year follow-up were not different in patients with angiographic success and failure. Among the newer approaches to saphenous vein graft recanalization are the use of the Dispatch catheter to deliver urokinase locally (210, 211) and direct catheter recanalization using TEC (212, 213) or rheolytic thrombectomy devices (Fig. 28.9) followed by stent implantation. The benefit of recanalizing these occluded saphenous vein grafts, relative to complications and cost, however, has not been clearly established.

Arterial Grafts

Percutaneous intervention in arterial grafts to treat stenotic lesions is relatively uncommon because of their immunity from atherosclerosis. Lesions, when found, are most often at the anastomosis of arterial grafts with coronary arteries occurring within a few days (see *Early Postoperative Ischemia*), or more likely, a few months after surgery, but occasionally occur in midgraft or at ostial sites, owing apparently, in some cases, to catheter-related trauma (214–222). Intervention directed at lesions in the internal mammary and gastroepiploic artery grafts is usually carried out with 6–8 F catheters from the femoral artery, but a brachial approach may be helpful when IMA engagement is difficult or tortuous, or in the case of a difficult distal lesion or total occlusion. A novel catheter shape for a right brachial approach to right internal mammary artery (RIMA) lesions has been reported (214). Occlusive lesions in the subclavian or innominate arteries have been treated prior to or following CABG surgery using stents or conventional balloon angioplasty to improve IMA flow and to treat subclavian dissection complicating IMA angiography or angioplasty (223–228).

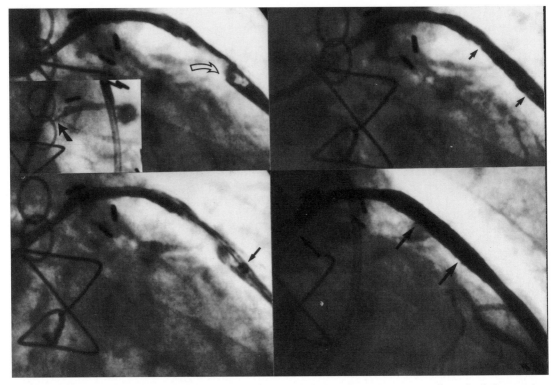

Figure 28.9. Following recanalization of a totally occluded saphenous vein graft to the left anterior descending artery (**insert**), a large filling defect consistent with thrombus was apparent (**upper left,** *open arrow*). Treatment with a rheolytic thrombectomy device (**lower left panel**) removed most of the thrombus (**upper right panel**) and, following stent deployment, an excellent lumen was created. (Courtesy of Dr. Donald Baim.)

Conventional balloon angioplasty is used for most anastomotic lesions, and an over-the-wire system is used for tortuous grafts or when total occlusions must be recanalized. Balloon-mounted stents have been used to treat dissections and as primary therapy for mid and proximal IMA lesions (229, 230). Ioxaglate, a low osmolar ionic dimer is the most frequently used contrast agent in our hospital for IMA intervention. This agent caused less discomfort than iopamidol in a double-blinded study (231). When approaching distal sites via tortuous grafts, it may be necessary to use extra long (145 cm) balloon catheters or short (80–90 cm) guide catheters to provide the extra length needed, or, if necessary, the guide catheter can be shortened using a flared, short sheath one size smaller to close the catheter end (232, 233).

The results of internal mammary graft intervention are highly dependent on case selection because extreme graft tortuosity may significantly reduce success rates. Among approximately 250 patients reported in seven series (215–221), the success rate was 89% and serious complications were rare: dissection 3.5%, Q-wave myocardial infarction less than 1%, bypass surgery less than 1%. In a recent report of 68 consecutive patients who underwent IMA PTCA, initial success was achieved in 89% and, with a mean angiographic follow-up of 8 months obtained in 78% of patients with successful procedures, restenosis occurred in 15% (6 of 40) of lesions at the anastomosis and in 43% (3 of 7) in the midgraft. After a mean interval of 14 months, 76% of patients were in class I or II, and event-free survival was high, 86% (221). The excellent outcome of PTCA of IMA anastomotic lesions is similar to the results following PTCA of distal anastomosis lesions in vein grafts. No large series or long-term outcome data are known regarding PTCA of gastroepiploic artery grafts (222).

Left Ventricular Dysfunction

Left ventricular function, an important correlate of survival in patients with coronary artery disease, is not surprisingly an important predictor of immediate and long-term outcome of coronary intervention (234). Patients with severe angina and an ejection fraction less than 25% or with a target vessel supplying more than 50% of the remaining viable myocardium were classified by Vogel et al. as high-risk (235). In the case of coronary bypass surgery, scoring systems have been devised that, with reasonable accuracy, predict the risk of surgery using preoperative variables (236). Left ventricular function is a core variable shown to be unequivocally related to operative mortality. Ellis et al. (237) applied the Jeopardy Score developed by Califf et al. (238) to estimate the mortality risk associated with a failed PTCA in more than 8000 patients among whom 32 died. Their analysis showed that patients with a large amount of viable myocardium potentially subject to acute ischemic dysfunction with a failed angioplasty had a mortality rate of 12 to 33%.

Analyzing patient outcomes of coronary intervention from four multicenter trials, Anderson et al. reported that ejection fraction and the presence of congestive heart failure (CHF) were powerful predictors of both early and late outcome (239). Thirty-day mortality rates for patients without CHF with ejection fractions of less than 30%, 30 to 40%, and more than 40% were 8%, 1%, and 1%, respectively, whereas the presence of heart failure increased 30-day mortality to 14%, 3%, and 2% for the three categories of ejection fraction. Patients with heart failure and an ejection fraction less than 30% had a 9-month mortality rate of 32% and a composite adverse outcome (death, MI, or repeat revascularization) of 64%. These sobering observations should not dissuade the interventional operator from offering percutaneous revascularization when it is appropriate, but they should engender a cautious analysis of options with the aim of obtaining the most complete and durable revascularization possible.

In an effort to mitigate the impact of periprocedural ischemia in the presence of baseline left ventricular dysfunction, a variety of strategies have been used ranging from perfusion balloon catheters to the intra-aortic balloon pump (IABP) (240), percutaneously inserted cardiopulmonary support (CPS) (241–243), and the Hemopump (244). Although these support devices appear to enhance the procedural safety of coronary intervention, death in high-risk patients frequently occurs several hours or days postprocedure at a time when the use of a support device is not feasible. In approximately 100 patients treated with CPS, Shawl et al. reported 5 in-hospital deaths after the procedure and 23 deaths between 1 and 23 months (243). In 35 high-risk patients in Germany who underwent coronary intervention with CPS (6 patients), CPS standby (21 patients), or Hemopump (8 patients), the in-hospital mortality rate was 8.6% and during the next 24 months, another 7 patients died (total mortality 28.6%) (244). These poor long-term results led the authors to recommend CABG surgery in those patients who are stabilized by supported PTCA and judged then to be surgical candidates. In the experience at Emory University, CPS has been needed in less than 0.05% of patients. Prophylactic IABP support is also rarely needed, but it is usually the method of choice in our experience. Whether the use of stents can provide a more durable result and improve long-term outcome in CPS-supported patients is a point of considerable interest. Circulatory support with a left ventricular assist device (LVAD) is occasionally required as a bridge to transplantation in suitable patients.

In patients with left ventricular dysfunction, special caution is warranted in selection of patients for SVG graft intervention when a high risk of major atheroembolization exists (bulky or thrombus-laden graft) and in the use of rotational atherectomy where regional left ventricular dysfunction induced by microembolization of atheromatous debris may, when added to existing left ventricular abnormalities, induce shock or acute pulmonary edema.

Medical Comorbidity

Renal Insufficiency

Patients with impaired renal function who undergo complex or multivessel intervention are at increased risk of acute renal failure, especially when diabetes mellitus is present. Among 1828 consecutive patients who underwent catheter-based intervention at William Beaumont Hospital in 1993–1994, 265 (14.5%) experienced a 25% increase in serum creatinine, whereas 15 (0.8%) required dialysis with an in-hospital mortality rate of 33.3% (245). No patient with baseline creatinine clearance greater than 47 mL/min (Cockcroft-Gault method) or contrast load less than 100 mL required dialysis; diabetics were at increased risk (odds ratio 5:12). Levy et al. reported the outcome of 183 patients with contrast-associated renal failure ($\geq$ 25% increase serum creatinine) compared with matched patients, noting a more than sixfold increase in-hospital death rate (246), highlighting the importance of avoiding this dangerous and costly complication (247, 248). An important impact on late mortality was noted in approximately 2000 patients following ablative new-device angioplasty at Washington Hospital Center where 6.9% developed acute renal failure, which was associated with a more than sixfold increase in late mortality (compared with no renal failure) (249).

Prior to coronary intervention in the patient with renal failure (serum creatinine > 1.5 mg/dL), a careful risk-benefit analysis should be carried out weighing the potentially life-threatening consequences of acute renal failure against the need to relieve symptoms of myocardial ischemia, realizing that reported outcome of catheter-based and surgical revascularization are not as favorable as in patients without renal insufficiency (250, 251). O'Keefe et al. reported 10-year survival of only 7% following PTCA in diabetics with serum creatinine level of 2.5 compared with 90% for nondiabetics with a creatinine level of less than 1; a linear inverse relationship existed between outcome and creatinine level throughout the range of creatinine levels (250).

The manner in which the patient is prepared and complex angioplasty conducted determines the risk of acute renal failure. Preprocedural hydration (saline 100 mL/hour for 12 hours before and after the procedure) without mannitol or diuretics (252), use of the smallest amount of low osmolar contrast agents possible (253, 254), and omission of nonsteroidal anti-inflammatory agents (255) and angiotensin-converting-enzyme inhibitors (248) are strongly recommended. We have found the following measures to be helpful in minimizing contrast agent usage: preferential use of stents, intravascular ultrasound guidance to monitor the procedure, identification of important anatomic landmarks such as surgical clips on vein grafts or coronary artery calcification, and use of guidewires with 15-mm interval markers (Stabilizer, Cordis Corp., Miami, FL) to assist in positioning balloons and stents without contrast injections. Complex intervention can frequently be conducted with use of less than 50 mL of contrast media (Fig. 28.10) and sometimes less than 10 mL. This approach dramatically alters the risk of complex angioplasty in such patients, making it available even to those at highest risk, the diabetic with a serum creatinine of more than 5 mg/dL.

Miscellaneous Comorbidity

Percutaneous revascularization has become an option for many symptomatic patients who would not be candidates for surgical revascularization because of pulmonary insufficiency, life-shortening process such as neoplasm, thrombocytopenia syndromes, stroke, and other debilitating chronic conditions (Fig. 28.11). It is in these patients that some of the most complex, high-risk procedures have been conducted in an effort to achieve palliation.

ANGIOGRAPHIC FEATURES DENOTING COMPLEXITY

Vessel and Lesion Characteristics

Vessel and lesion characteristics assessed angiographically have been important pre-

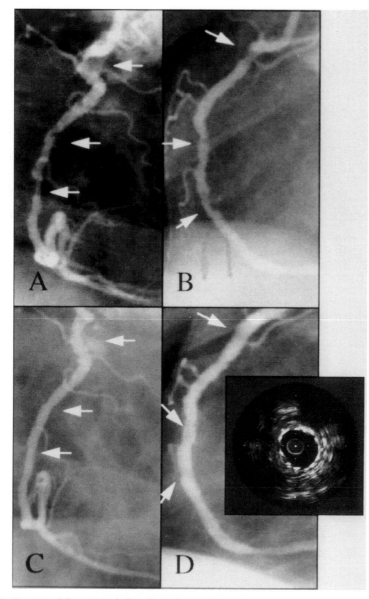

Figure 28.10. A 49-year-old man with familial glomerulonephritis (BUN 65, creatinine 3.2) developed unstable angina. Coronary arteriography revealed multiple stenoses in the proximal and midright coronary artery (**A** and **B**). By utilizing intravascular ultrasound (IVUS) guidance and by taking advantage of the radiopacity of the initial stent to position subsequent stents and balloons, it was possible to deploy and expand three Palmaz-Schatz stents achieving an excellent angiographic (**B** and **C**) and IVUS result (**insert**) using only 42 mL of low osmolar contrast media. No change occurred in BUN or creatinine. In simpler cases, we have used less than 10 mL of contrast to minimize risk of contrast nephropathy.

dictors of the outcome of coronary angio-plasty as reflected in the ACC/AHA PTCA Guideline "ABC" Classification (2, 3). The utility of this classification was confirmed for a variety of patient subgroups in the late 1980s, and in patients undergoing balloon angioplasty in the 1990s. Tan et al. recently reported balloon angioplasty success rates

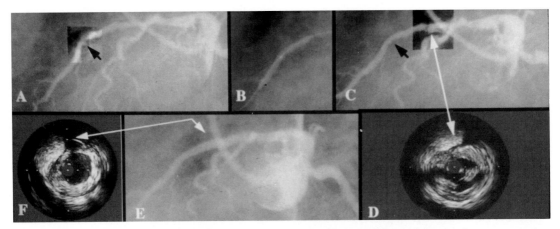

Figure 28.11. A 70-year-old patient with metastatic melanoma experienced a non–Q-wave anterior myocardial infarction (creatine phosphokinase, 290; MB, 42) and recurrent refractory angina subsequently. Coronary arteriography revealed severe stenosis of the midleft anterior descending artery (**A**) and global hypokinesis with an ejection fraction of 25%. Balloon inflations (**B**) improved the target site, but a more proximal site appeared to have thrombus or intimal disruption (**C**). Intravascular ultrasound (IVUS) revealed obvious localized vessel wall dissection (**D**), which was treated with stenting without aggressive antithrombotic measures (ASA + ticlopidine only). The angiographic and IVUS images (**E** and **F**) revealed excellent results. IVUS guidance was extremely helpful because we initially thought thrombus was the major problem and the treatment strategies were different.

of 96%, 93%, and 80% for A, B, and C lesions respectively, but noted that certain lesion characteristics (lesion length, calcification, angulated lesions, stenosis severity, and thrombus) had more value in predicting procedural success and complications (256). In a recently reported series of over 1000 lesions treated in the new-device era, procedural success was 100% for type A lesions, 97.3% for B, 97.1% for B_2, and 87.4% for C lesions. Predictors of procedural failure were noted to be lesion length greater than 20 mm, TIMI-1 flow, calcification, angle more than 90%, and chronic total occlusion (257). Although the ABC classification continues to be of some prognostic value, differences in outcome between A, B, and B_2 lesions have narrowed significantly with the use of improved technology and antithrombotic measures, and most operators find the use of specific angiographic characteristics to be more helpful than the ABC classification in assessing procedural strategy and outcome. Angiographic lesion characteristics associated with increased risk of restenosis include lesion length, thrombus, total occlusion, ostial location,

saphenous vein grafts, and prior PTCA to the same site.

Assessment of complex lesion morphology by intracoronary ultrasound has also been shown to have predictive value, to be useful in guiding intervention (Fig. 28.11), and in some centers is used routinely (see Chapter 18). In our hospital, the technical strategies used in complex coronary intervention are based primarily, but not exclusively, on angiographic features. A provisional stent strategy has been frequently employed whereby excellent results of balloon angioplasty were accepted, a strategy that is supported by the observation from the Benestent II pilot study that patients with less than 30% residual stenosis had outcomes comparable to those of stented patients (258). Increasingly, however, primary stent placement is used, particularly for complex anatomy unfavorable for balloon angioplasty. At Emory University Hospital in 1996, 33% of patients who underwent coronary intervention received stents, 5.5% rotational atherectomy, 1.2% directional atherectomy, 0.2% laser angioplasty, 0.9% extraction atherectomy, and 59% balloon angioplasty alone.

Long Lesions

Although there is little agreement to what constitutes a long lesion and its optimal management, it is clear that increasing length is associated with reduced initial success, more complications, and higher late cardiac events and restenosis. With balloon angioplasty, Tan reported procedural success in 95%, 85%, and 78% for lesions less than 10 mm, 10–20 mm, and greater than 20 mm, respectively (256). Tenaglia et al. reported use of long balloons (33% of lesions were > 20 mm) with procedural success in 97%, abrupt closure in 6%, complication-free success in 90%, and restenosis in 55% (259), results that mirror our experience at Emory University. Excimer laser angioplasty (260, 261) and rotational atherectomy (27) have been used to debulk long lesions prior to balloon angioplasty, but the advantages of these strategies are not certain, even in the case of laser angioplasty after a randomized trial (261). Rotational atherectomy in longer lesions was associated with no reflow and serious ischemic complications (Q-wave MI in 2.8 versus 0.7%, $P = .02$) (262). Columbo et al. used multiple stents to treat lesions greater than 20 mm in more than 100 patients with 93% initial success,

and in 77 patients who underwent recatheterization restenosis occurred in 27 (35%) (263). Using optimal stent implantation techniques (> 14 atm and < 20% residual stenosis) to treat long lesions, Eccleston et al. reported almost comparable 180-day outcome in 152 patients requiring multiple stents compared with 329 patients receiving single stents (composite adverse outcome in 21.8 versus 17.9%, $P = .43$) (264). Initial results at Emory University using long (39 mm) stents to treat long lesions have been favorable (Fig. 28.12), but late events and restenosis rates are not yet known.

Calcification, Undilatable Lesions

Angiographically visible target lesion calcification is a predictor of dissection, complications, and procedural failure with balloon angioplasty and directional atherectomy and when stent implantation is proceeded only by balloon dilation (2, 3, 10, 31, 256, 265). Tan et al. reported balloon angioplasty success in 74% of patients with calcified stenosis compared with 94% without calcification ($P < .001$) and an increased rate of abrupt closure (14 versus 2.5%, $P = .001$) (256). Dissection has been reported to occur

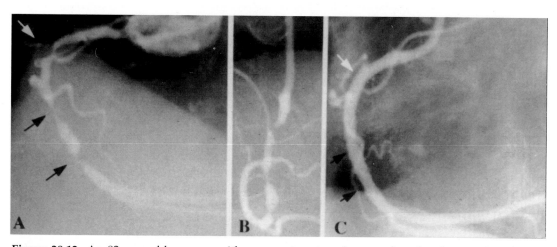

Figure 28.12. An 82-year-old woman with recurrent rest angina was found to have severe diffuse disease throughout the proximal and midright coronary artery (**A,** left anterior oblique; **B,** right anterior oblique). The right coronary artery was dilated with a 3.0 × 40 mm balloon (*white arrow*), and a 3.0 × 39 mm AVE stent was deployed and expanded (*black arrows*) with a 3.5 mm balloon inflated to 15 bar. The patient is doing well over 4 months postprocedure.

frequently at the junction of calcified tissue and soft plaque (266). However, intravascular ultrasound studies have shown that only approximately half of calcified target lesions are recognized by angiography. Among 110 patients undergoing coronary intervention, Mintz et al. reported that 50 (48%) had target lesion calcification by fluoroscopy whereas 84 (76%) had target lesion calcification by ultrasound (267). In another series of 183 patients, the sensitivity and specificity of angiography in identifying target lesion calcification were 40% and 80%, respectively (268). Although it is clear that angiographically occult calcification is common, it is less clear to what extent it should be searched for.

Rotational atherectomy has been shown to be successful in 94.3% of angiographically calcified lesions versus 95.2% of noncalcified lesions (269), and it is the treatment of choice for most interventionalists faced with an angiographically calcified stenosis (27, 28) (Fig. 28.13). The presence of superficial calcium over a wide vessel (180°–360°) by ultrasound, or the presence of an undilatable lesion suggests the need for rotational atherectomy. However, more studies are needed to determine ultrasound imaging criteria that would justify use of this more expensive strategy. In a relatively small series of 24 patients, elective stent implantation following rotational atherectomy of calcified lesions yielded favorable 30-day

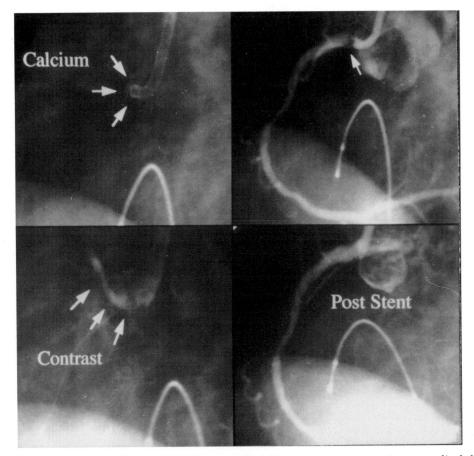

Figure 28.13. An 82-year-old woman with severe disabling angina unresponsive to medical therapy was found to have heavy calcification (**upper left panel**) and stenosis (**upper right panel**) of the right coronary ostium. Rotational atherectomy yielded an improved lumen, but contrast extravasation showed a small perforation (**lower left**) that was sealed with placement of a Palmaz-Schatz stent (**lower right**), producing an excellent result.

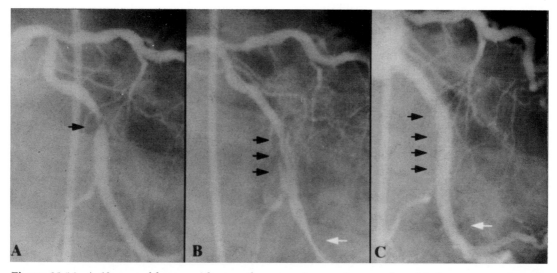

Figure 28.14. A 60-year-old man with recently worsening angina was found to have severe stenosis of the circumflex coronary artery (**A**) and referred for angioplasty. The lesion was on a bend and the vessel was quite rigid. Balloon dilation with an undersized 2.5-mm balloon produced an extensive distal dissection (**B**). Passage of a stent through the tortuous rigid proximal circumflex was not possible until two Platinum-Plus guidewires were introduced to straighten it. Placement of Palmaz-Schatz stents, beginning distally, yielded an excellent result (**C**). The appearance of the distal vessel (*white arrow*) was due to poor filling pressure rather than to dissection extension.

outcome: 100% procedural success, no stent thrombosis, 25% non–Q-wave myocardial infarction (CPK-MB > 5× normal), and no major complications (270). These results appear to be better than those reported with balloon angioplasty before stent implantation in calcified arteries (265).

Lesions on a Bend

Angioplasty of lesions in angulated segments has a lower procedural success and a higher rate of arterial dissection (Fig. 28.14), abrupt closure, and restenosis (2, 3, 10, 256, 257). With the improved balloon technology of the 1990s, Ellis and colleagues reported success in only 84% of lesions on bends of 45° (271). Tan et al. noted increasing abrupt closure in relation to the degree of angulation (2% risk in bends < 45°, 8.8% risk in bends 45°–90°, and 13% risk in bends > 90°, $P = .006$ (256). Whether the use of long, noncompliant balloons, which produce less straightening (272), influences outcomes fa-

vorably is uncertain but the use of long balloons is common.

Ablative technology (rotablator and excimer laser) use in angulated segments has been associated with unfavorable outcome. Chevalier et al. reported that rotational atherectomy in bends 45° or greater was associated with reduced success (86 versus 94%, $P < .001$), increased dissection (36 versus 16%, $P < .05$), and higher mortality (2.7 versus 0.3%, $P < .05$) (273), results similar to those of Ellis et al. (27) with the rotablator and Klein et al. who reported abrupt closure in 9% and perforation in 2.8% with excimer laser angioplasty in bends greater than 45° (274). Currently no excellent strategy exists for bend point lesions. Primary long-balloon angioplasty with stent backup using a stiff guidewire and strong guide catheter support (to ensure stent deployment if needed) will be expected to give way to primary stenting as more flexible, lower profile stents become available.

In the course of angioplasty, straightening of tortuous vessels frequently produces pseudostenoses, because of vessel wall invagination, that disappear when the stiff guidewire is removed or replaced with one that is more flexible.

Thrombus

Lesion-associated thrombus seen on angiography or by angioscopy, usually accompanying an acute ischemic syndrome (see *Unstable Angina* above), is a marker for increased complications of coronary intervention (2, 3, 10, 256, 275), but the optimal treatment is not clear. Whereas thrombus removal prior to intervention is desirable to reduce abrupt closure and distal embolization, each of the available approaches has major limitations: prolonged administration of heparin and aspirin (13, 14) escalates costs and may not be sufficiency effective, systemic thrombolytics expose the patient to risks of intracranial and other bleeding complications (189–192, 204, 207), local delivery of thrombolytic agents is not broadly applicable (193, 194), use of TEC in native coronary arteries and vein grafts is associated with a high complication rates (177, 180), mechanical thrombectomy devices are experimental (276) (Fig. 28.9), and platelet IIb/IIIa receptor inhibitors have not been well tested in this setting. Commonly, thrombus reduction with one of these methods is attempted and an ionic contrast agent

(25) and adjunctive use of a IIb/IIIa receptor blocker are employed periprocedure. Stenting, regarded by some as relatively safe even in the presence of thrombus (36, 37), should not be undertaken lightly (Fig. 28.15) because thrombus is a predictor of subacute thrombosis (34, 35).

Eccentricity, Complex Morphology

Angiographic lesion eccentricity, which is often not confirmed on intracoronary ultrasound, is not a predictor of adverse outcome with coronary intervention in most studies. Although eccentricity is the prototypic indication for directional atherectomy, the randomized Canadian atherectomy versus angioplasty trial showed that even patients with this lesion morphology had no advantage with directional atherectomy (277). In our practice, extremely eccentric, shelflike lesions, intimal flaps, and complex ulcerated lesions that were previously apparently effectively treated with directional atherectomy are increasingly treated with stent implantation, although definitive studies supporting this strategy have not been reported. Adjunctive use of platelet IIb/IIIa receptor inhibitors is considered when thrombus is present or suspected.

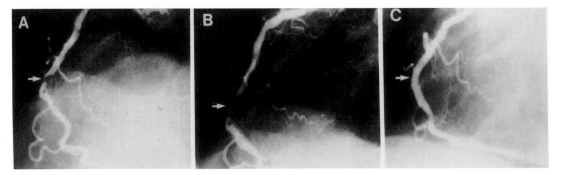

Figure 28.15. A 75-year-old pharmacist had incessant angina unresponsive to intensive medical therapy. Coronary arteriography revealed a severe, eccentric stenosis of the right coronary artery with a filling defect consistent with thrombus (**A**). Angioplasty, performed because of persisting symptoms, yielded a suboptimal result (**B**) even after local delivery of urokinase 150,000 units over 30 minutes via a 3.5-mm Dispatch catheter (Scimed, Maple Grove, MN). A 3.5-mm Palmaz-Schatz stent was implanted and dilated with a high pressure balloon. The patient has remain asymptomatic subsequently and a stress thallium scan at 7 months showed no ischemia.

Total Occlusion

Successful angioplasty of total occlusions, which has been shown both to reduce angina and the risk of PTCA of a contralateral vessel and to decrease need for subsequent CABG surgery, was significantly influenced by the duration of the occlusion and anatomic features such as vessel tapering and bridging collaterals, which impact guidewire passage (278–284). Suitability for intervention and choice of strategies are currently based on careful angiographic assessment of the shape and length of the occlusion and distal vessel characteristics using simultaneous contralateral coronary injections if necessary. Tapered occlusions can frequently be crossed with a 0.010-inch guidewire (Fig. 28.7) because the presence of nonvisualized recanalized channels (285), but an old nontapered occlusion with bridging collaterals usually demands a stiff or hydrophilic-coated wire (285, 286), or an experimental excimer laser guidewire (287). Although serious complications are less common than with subtotal occlusion (because of a reduced consequence of abrupt closure), coronary perforation resulting in cardiac tamponade occurred in 4 of 397 attempts (283), and interruption of bridging collaterals (288) or distal embolization (Fig. 28.16) may result in ischemia or infarction.

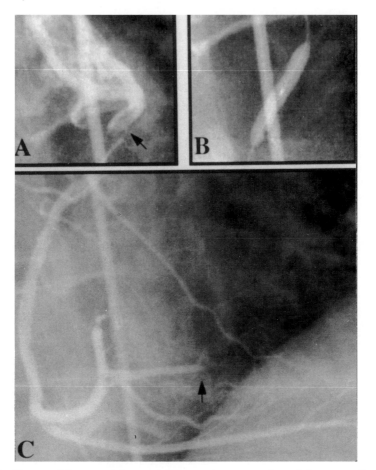

Figure 28.16. A 47-year-old man with worsening angina was referred for recanalization of a right coronary artery occlusion of uncertain duration. Proximal to the total occlusion, a thrombus appeared to be present (**A,** right anterior oblique view). Wire passage followed by balloon inflation was successful in reopening a large right coronary artery, but was complicated by embolization to the distal left ventricular branch (**C**). In most such cases, the thrombus is fragmented by a low-pressure balloon inflation and the proximal site is stented.

Proxima vessel dissection may occur related to guide catheter trauma contributing to a higher than expected mortality of approximately 1% in reported series (279–284). Worthy of attention is the observation that among 60 patients in whom guidewire passage was unsuccessful, 32 had successful angioplasty after an 8-hour urokinase infusion (289).

Because of high restenosis rates following balloon angioplasty of total occlusions, elective stent implantation was performed in observational and randomized studies with encouraging results (290–292). Among 119 randomized patients, Sirnes et al. reported more stented patients were angina-free (57 versus 24% in the PTCA group, $P < .001$) and restenosis was less frequent (32% versus 74%, $P < .001$) (292), whereas Goldberg et al. reported angiographic restenosis in 20% of 59 patients with stented occlusions (290).

Bifurcations

Lesions involving branch points continue to plague interventional operators who frequently use double-wire approaches to avoid side branch closure when the branch vessel ostium has significant stenosis. Elastic recoil at branch points is common with balloon angioplasty, leading many operators to attempt debulking with directional atherectomy (Fig. 28.17), a strategy supported by CAVEAT I (293) and the results of Altmann et al. (294) who recommended directional coronary athrectomy (DCA) of the parent vessel and of branch vessels 3 mm or greater diameter in that order. In smaller vessels ($\leq$ 3-mm diameter) and in the presence of calcification, rotational atherectomy is a viable option (295). Stenting, which is technically difficult, can be performed by stenting the branch vessel first and then bridging the branch with a second stent, or placing short stents just proximal and distal to the branch, but long-term results are not known.

Ostial Location

Because of poor initial and long-term outcome of balloon angioplasty at aorto-ostial sites, atherectomy and stent implantation currently account for most interventions (296). Even after debulking with atherectomy or laser and adjunctive balloon angioplasty, if needed, repeat interventions are common, leading to an increasing use of stents primarily or after debulking (Fig. 28.18) (296, 297). Intravascular ultrasound or a low pressure balloon inflation can be used to estimate the need for rotational atherectomy in lesions with less than moderate calcification. Nonaorto-ostial LAD lesions also have elastic recoil, limiting the effectiveness of balloon angioplasty. Although data from CAVEAT did not support DCA at this site (298), many operators use DCA or rotational atherectomy, and there is increasing use of stents, although the results are not clearly superior (299, 300), and there is some risk of jeopardy to the circumflex origin acutely and as a late "restenotic" event.

Multivessel Disease

Although angioplasty as first conceived was applied to patients with single obstructive lesions and most angioplasty continues to focus on alleviating lesions in a single vessel, multivessel disease patients are commonly treated with angioplasty. At Emory University Hospital in 1995, most patients had multivessel disease. This is colored somewhat by patients who had had prior bypass surgery, but excluding such patients, most patients without prior bypass surgery also had multivessel disease. Factors that impeded enthusiasm for angioplasty in multivessel disease included the potential for acute closure, which could result in massive areas of myocardium becoming ischemic, the ability of surgery to perform complete revascularization in most patients, and the previous documentation that surgery had been lifesaving in certain forms of multivessel disease.

Is Complete Revascularization Necessary?

Surgeons generally attempt to bypass as many distal vessels as possible, and incomplete revascularization has been associated

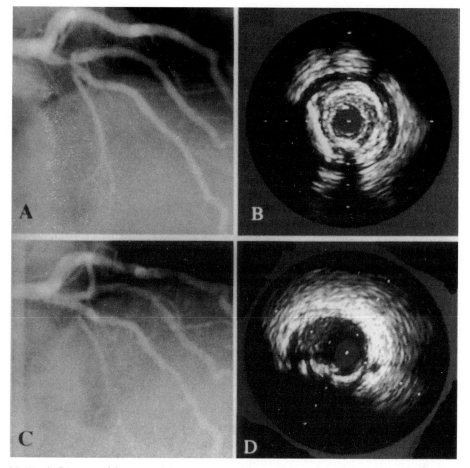

Figure 28.17. A 56-year-old man with angina and severe stenosis of the left anterior descending (LAD) artery at the diagonal bifurcation (**A**). Considerable vessel calcification was present, which on ultrasound appeared to be deep in the vessel wall (**B**). Directional atherectomy using a 7 F cutter was successful with an excellent angiographic result in the LAD and diagonal (**C**). However, intravascular ultrasound revealed considerable residual plaque (**D**).

with a poorer long-term symptomatic outcome in patients undergoing bypass surgery (301). This incomplete revascularization may be unavoidable because of the nature of the disease, but clearly it is associated with diminished long-term survival (302). Long-term follow-up of patients undergoing bypass surgery with complete and incomplete revascularization was studied at Emory University (303); 3481 patients had bypass surgery. Fewer grafts were placed in the patients with incomplete revascularization (2.6 per patient) as compared with those with complete revascularization (3.2 per patient). When these patients

were followed long term, both freedom from angina and survival were better in the patients who could have complete revascularization. Survival at 10 years was 81% in those with complete revascularization and 72% in those with incomplete. This difference in survival held even when correcting for all the baseline features; therefore, as nearly complete revascularization as possible has been the goal of bypass surgery. Another reason for this effort at completeness of revascularization is to avoid the necessity for a second operation, which carries a higher risk.

The evidence that complete revasculari-

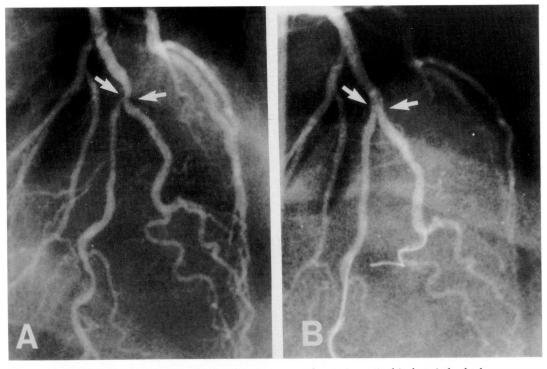

Figure 28.18. A 54-year-old man with angina pectoris and anterior septal ischemia had a long, severe stenosis in the midleft anterior descending artery involving the diagonal (**A**) and was treated with rotational atherectomy to both vessels followed by adjunctive balloon angioplasty. The angiographic result was excellent (**B**) and recatheterization 7 months later revealed excellent patency at the treatment site.

zation is required in coronary interventions is much less compelling. In an observational study conducted at Emory University looking at patients with two-vessel coronary artery disease who had either angioplasty or bypass surgery, 417 patients with angioplasty and 503 patients with surgery were followed for 5 years (304). They had different baseline features; the angioplasty patients were 3 years younger; fewer had diabetes, prior myocardial infarctions, class III and IV angina, and LAD disease; and the ejection fraction was higher in the angioplasty group. Complete revascularization was achieved in 26% of angioplasty patients and 92% of CABG patients, $P < .0001$. There were 3.4 grafts placed per patient in the surgery group and only 1.5 lesions per patient dilated in the angioplasty group. At 5 years, angina status was similar and survival data showed superiority of angioplasty (survival 93 versus 89%); however, when correcting for baseline features, no survival difference

was seen. The angioplasty patients underwent additional revascularization procedures over the follow-up period (43 versus 7%, $P < .001$).

This ability to reintervene on angioplasty patients who became symptomatic creates a major difference in attitude toward revascularization, particularly in regard to milder lesions that are not judged to be producing angina. One is likely to avoid addressing these lesions while opening lesions that are clearly flow limiting. Because angioplasty can be repeated without the morbidity attendant to surgery, one is less compelled to open the less severe stenoses. Such observational studies give us an impression of what has been done, but do not predict what would happen if complete or incomplete revascularization was attempted. Such prospective studies have never been done. However, randomized trials of angioplasty versus surgery have given us a clue regarding completeness of revascularization.

Evidence From Randomized Trials

The effectiveness of revascularization was judged in the Emory Angioplasty versus Surgery Trial (305). This study was a prospective trial of patients with multivessel coronary artery disease randomized to angioplasty or bypass surgery (306); 394 patients were randomized; all baseline features were comparable. The average age was 62 years, 60% of the patients had disease involving two of the vascular systems, and 40% had involvement of all three systems. The revascularization strategy was at the discretion of the surgeon in the case of the surgery patients and the angioplasty operator in the case of angioplasty. The coronary tree was divided into segments of the major coronary arteries so that measurement of revascularization effectiveness to each of these segments could be assessed. Following the baseline procedure, 71% of the obstructed index segments were revascularized by angioplasty as judged angiographically and virtually 100% of the index segments had bypass grafts placed. At 1-year follow-up, there was a significant difference in revascularization, with 88% of the index segments patent in the surgery group compared with 59% of the index segments patent in the angioplasty group. By 3 years, the difference had narrowed because repeat procedures in the angioplasty group (87% of the index segments in the surgery group were patent compared with 70% of index segments in the angioplasty group). These judgments were made by follow-up quantitative angiographic assessment and the difference would suggest that there was significantly decreased myocardial perfusion in the angioplasty group that was not apparent; however, the measurement used was 50% narrowing of the artery and, therefore, if the same measurements were made using more severe stenoses such as 70%, the difference between the surgery and angioplasty group narrows significantly. These 70% obstructed segments were revascularized 96% of the time in the angioplasty group at baseline; 90% of them were patent at 1 year and 93% at 3 years, no difference was found between angioplasty and surgery in this regard at 3 years.

The 3-year follow-up of the EAST patients showed no difference in survival (93.5%), but a difference in the occurrence of angina class II and above (12% with surgery and 20% with angioplasty). When studying the revascularization status at baseline, we could not correlate that with 1-year survival or myocardial infarction, but we did see a difference in the occurrence of angina 1 year later, with patients with complete revascularization having 13% incidence of angina, those with an intermediate revascularization status 20%, and those with poor revascularization 26%. This difference, however, did not hold at 3 years. Our conclusions from this study were that patients with multivessel stenosis suitable for angioplasty or surgery in the EAST trial had more complete revascularization with surgery. However, when physiologic priority and severity were considered, the advantage of surgery became less significant. This relatively comparable revascularization, which was achieved over time by repeat procedures in the angioplasty group, may have accounted for the comparable survival in the randomized trials that have been performed. Certainly the results of BARI mirror those of EAST in terms of the disparent completeness of revascularization initially (54% for PTCA versus 91% for CABG), more repeat revascularization with angioplasty (54 versus 8%), but comparable outcomes at 5 years (48). It would seem that with bypass surgery complete revascularization is a desirable goal, but it is predicted more by uncontrollable baseline features than by the surgeon's intention. Long-term outcomes with angioplasty may relate to completeness of revascularization, but multiple interventions common in angioplasty patients make this a difficult assessment.

One additional observation regarding completeness of revascularization may be pertinent. **The patients with diabetes observed in the BARI trial had a poorer outcome with angioplasty than with surgery** as mentioned earlier in this chapter (48, 49). The survival at 5 years was 80.6% in the surgery group and 65.5% in the angioplasty group. When these patients were studied in more detail, it was discovered that the greatest difference in survival occurred in those patients with more than four lesions, and these diabetic patients indeed frequently had more diffuse disease than the remainder of the population; therefore the need for revascularization and the amount of myocardium at risk was greater in the diabetic patients than the remainder of the population. Another feature that can only be speculated on is that diabetic patients sometimes have blunted symptomatic manifestations of coronary artery disease and, therefore, do not reliably perceive angina. It is possible that a more complete revascularization done at baseline is protective in these patients when compared with a strategy (angioplasty) that depends in part on repeat procedures to cope with the issue of restenosis.

The question of cost of subsequent revascularization procedures is an important issue, although the initial catheter-based revascularization in EAST was significantly less costly, the increased need for repeat revascularization, mostly related to restenosis, reduced the cost advantage of angioplasty and at 3 years the difference in total costs ($23,734 for PTCA and $25,310 for coronary surgery, $P < .0001$) had narrowed considerably (50). How the current use of stents, which increase initial costs but improve the durability of the revascularization, will alter the comparative cost-effectiveness of angioplasty and surgery in multivessel disease remains to be seen.

Technical Considerations

The approach to multivessel angioplasty has been driven by safety considerations. It was long felt that if one lesion was dilated and then others were attempted, one should be considering the consequence of acute closure at multiple sites on left ventricular perfusion. This led frequently to a staging approach to multivessel angioplasty in which one or two lesions were dilated at one sitting and additional lesions dilated a day or two later, depending on the maintained patency of the first lesion. In this strategy, the more severe lesion was usually opened first; if possible, the lesion serving an artery that receives collaterals would be opened first. An example would be a patient with a to-

tally occluded right coronary artery and a high-grade stenosis in the LAD. In this setting, if the right is opened first and the success of that procedure is documented by passage of some time, then the LAD could be opened with less risk to the patient.

This strategy was the one that was pursued on many patients throughout the recruitment period of the EAST trial (1987–1990). Patients who were randomized in that trial (60% two-vessel disease and 40% triple-vessel disease) frequently underwent staged procedures. By comparison, the eligible but not randomized patients seen during the same time frame had less frequent staged procedures. Nonetheless, staging in the randomized patients (40%) and in the registry patients (19%) was much more common than in our current practice. At the present time with the availability of stents for bailout and more reliable initial results of dilated lesions as well as the availability of potent antiplatelet agents, abrupt vessel closure has become less of a concern. Because of that, most patients are treated completely in one setting, although there remain high-risk patients who should undergo staged procedures. Much of the decision-making regarding staging or not staging must be made by an experienced operator, given experience and confidence in the stability of each lesion dilated, and issues such as total volume of contrast media and the length of the procedure.

SUMMARY

Percutaneous coronary intervention is an option for the treatment of many patients with coronary heart disease who have complex clinical and anatomic features. The success of the procedure, its associated risk, and the quality of long-term result, for the most part, will be determined by decisions made by the interventional operator whose relevant data base is constantly evolving. Issues in rapid transition include the place of stents and new antithrombotic strategies, and of nonangiographic methods of lesion assessment. At odds with this new technology is the increasing concern over health care resource utilization. This chapter addresses some of these issues with an eye toward safe, durable, and, hopefully, cost-effective interventional strategies for percutaneous revascularization of complex patients.

References

1. Bittl JA. Advances in coronary angioplasty. N Engl J Med 1996;335:1290–1302.
2. Ryan TJ, Faxon DP, Gunnar RM, et al. Guidelines for percutaneous transluminal coronary angioplasty. A report of the American College of Cardiology/American Heart Association Task Force on Assessment of Diagnostic and Therapeutic Cardiovascular Procedures (Subcommittee of Percutaneous Transluminal Coronary Angioplasty). J Am Coll Cardiol 1988;12:519–540.
3. Ryan TJ, Bauman WB, Kennedy JW, et al. Guidelines for percutaneous transluminal coronary angioplasty: a report of the American Heart Association/American College of Cardiology Task Force on Assessment of Diagnostic and Therapeutic Cardiovascular Procedures (Committee on Percutaneous Transluminal Coronary Angioplasty). Circulation 1993;88:2987–3007.
4. Fuster V, Badimon L, Badimon JJ, et al. The pathogenesis of coronary artery disease and acute coronary syndromes. N Engl J Med 1991;326:242–250; 320–328.
5. Davies MJ. Stability and instability: two faces of coronary atherosclerosis. Circulation 1996;94:2013–2020.
6. Mizuno K, Satomura K, Miyamoto A, et al. Angioscopic evaluation of coronary artery thrombi in acute coronary syndromes. N Engl J Med 1992;326:287–291.
7. Waxman S, Mittleman MA, Manzok, et al. Culprit lesion morphology in subtypes of unstable angina as assessed by angioscopy [Abstract]. Circulation 1995;92(Suppl I):I-79.
8. The TIMI IIIB Investigators. Effects of tissue plasminogen activator and a comparison of early invasive and conservative strategies in unstable angina and non-Q wave myocardial infarction. Circulation 1994;89:1545–1556.
9. Anderson HV, Cannon CP, Stone PH, et al. One-year results of the thrombolysis in myocardial infarction (TIMI) IIIB clinical trial. A randomized comparison of tissue-type plasminogen activator versus placebo and early invasive versus conservative strategies in unstable angina and non-Q wave myocardial infarction. J Am Coll Cardiol 1995;1643–1650.
10. Ellis SG, Roubin GS, King SB III, et al. Angiographic and clinical predictors of acute closure after native vessel coronary angioplasty. Circulation 1988;77:372–379.
11. Laskey MA, Deutsch E, Barnathan E, WKL. Influence of heparin therapy on percutaneous transluminal coronary angioplasty outcome in unstable angina pectoris. Am J Cardiol 1990;65:1425–1429.
12. Rosenman Y, Gilon D, Zelingher J, et al. Importance of delaying balloon angioplasty in patients with unstable angina pectoris. Clin Cardiol 1996; 19:111–114.
13. Douglas JS Jr, Lutz JF, Clements SD, et al. Therapy of large intracoronary thrombi in candidates for percutaneous transluminal coronary angioplasty [Abstract]. J Am Coll Cardiol 1988;11:238.
14. Laskey MA, Deutsch E, Hirshfeld JWJ, et al. Influence of heparin therapy on percutaneous transluminal coronary angioplasty outcome in patients with coronary arterial thrombus. Am J Cardiol 1990;65:179–182.
15. Ghigliotti G, Brunelli C, Corsiglia L, et al. Identification of high-risk patients with unstable angina [Abstract]. J Am Coll Cardiol 1996;27(Suppl A): 332A.
16. Cannon CP, McCabe CH, Stone PH, et al. Prospective validation of the Braunwald classification of unstable angina: results from the thrombolysis in myocardial ischemia (TIMI) III Registry [Abstract]. Circulation 1995; 92(Suppl I):I-19.
17. Lindahl B, Venge P, Wallentin L, et al. Relation between troponin T and the risk of subsequent cardiac events in unstable coronary artery disease. Circulation 1996;93:1651–1657.
18. Ohman EM, Armstrong PW, Christenson RH, et al. Cardiac troponin T levels for risk stratification in acute myocardial ischemia. N Engl J Med 1996; 335:1333–1341.
19. Antman EM, Tanasijevic MJ, Thompson B, et al. Cardiac-specific troponin I levels to predict the risk of mortality in patients with acute coronary syndromes. N Engl J Med 1996;335:1342–1349.
20. Schulman SP, Goldschmidt-Clermont PJ, Topol EJ. Effects of integrelin, a platelet glycoprotein IIb/IIIa receptor antagonist, in unstable angina. A randomized multicenter trial. Circulation 1996; 94:2083–2089.
21. The EPIC Investigators. Use of a monoclonal antibody directed against the platelet glycoprotein IIb/IIIa receptor in high-risk coronary angioplasty. N Engl J Med 1994;330:956–961.
22. Serruys PW, Herrman J-PR, Simon R, for the HELVETICA investigators. A comparison of hirudin with heparin in the prevention of restenosis after coronary angioplasty. N Engl J Med 1995;333: 757–763.
23. Ferguson JJ. EPILOG and CAPTURE trials halted because of positive interim results. Circulation 1996;93:637.
24. Ambrose JA, Almeida OD, Sharma SK, et al. for the TAUSA investigators. Adjunctive thrombolytic therapy during angioplasty for ischemic rest angina: results of the TAUSA trial. Circulation 1994;90:69–77.
25. Grines CL, Schreiber TL, Savas V, et al. A randomized trial of low osmolar ionic versus nonionic contrast media in patients with myocardial infarction or unstable angina undergoing percutaneous transluminal coronary angioplasty. J Am Coll Cardiol 1996;27:1381–1386.
26. Ellis SG, Whitlow PL, Guetta V, et al. A highly significant 40% reduction in ischemic complications of percutaneous coronary intervention in

1995: beginning of a new era? [Abstract]. J Am Coll Cardiol 1996;27(Suppl A):253A.

27. Ellis SG, Popma JJ, Buchbinder M, et al. Relation of clinical presentation, stenosis morphology, and operator technique to the procedural results of rotational atherectomy and rotational atherectomy-facilitated angioplasty. Circulation 1994;89:882–892.

28. Mojares JJ, Kaplan BM, O'Neill, et al. Clinical and angiographic predictors of adverse cardiac events after rotablator atherectomy. J Am Coll Cardiol 1996;27(Suppl A):168A.

29. Sharma SK, Duvvuri S, Mehran R, et al. What are the best predictors of slow flow during rotational atherectomy? Invasive Cardiol 1996;8:36.

30. Hugo L, de la Serna F, Juan T, et al. Transcatheter therapy in unstable angina: clinical, angiographic and procedural variables of directional atherectomy and elective stenting versus balloon angioplasty. Journal of Invasive Cardiology 1996;8:34.

31. Abdelmeguid A, Ellis S, Sapp S, et al. Directional coronary atherectomy in unstable angina. J Am Coll Cardiol 1994;24:46–54.

32. Ghazzal Z, Hinohara T, Vetter J, et al. Directional coronary atherectomy in patients with recent myocardial infarction. A NACI Registry Report. J Am Coll Cardiol 1993;21:32A.

33. Umans V, de Feyter P, Deckers J, et al. Acute and long-term outcome of directional coronary atherectomy for stable and unstable angina. Am J Cardiol 1993;74:641–646.

34. Mak K, Belli G, Ellis SG, et al. Subacute stent thrombosis: evolving issues and current concepts. J Am Coll Cardiol 1996;27:494–503.

35. Yokoi H, Nobuyoshi M, Nosaka H, et al. Coronary stent thrombosis: pattern, management and long-term follow-up result. Circulation 1996;94(Suppl I):I-332.

36. Mattos L, Chaves A, Feres F, et al. Safety of coronary stenting in acute coronary syndromes. J Invasive Cardiol 1996;8:52.

37. Robinson NMK, Thomas MR, Wainwright RJ, et al. Is unstable angina a contraindication to intracoronary stent insertion? J Invasive Cardiol 1996:8:351–356.

38. de Jaegere PPT, de Feyter PJ, van Domburg R, et al. Immediate and long-term results of percutaneous transluminal coronary angioplasty in patients aged 70 and over. Br Heart J 1992;167:138–143.

39. Imburgia M, King TR, Soffer AD, et al. Early results and long-term outcome of percutaneous transluminal coronary angioplasty in patients 75 years and older. Am J Cardiol 1989;63:1127–1129.

40. Buffet P, Danchin N, Juilliere Y, et al. Percutaneous transluminal coronary angioplasty in patients more than 75 years old: early and long-term results. Int J Cardiol 1992;37:33–39.

41. ten Berg JM, Voors AA, Sutorp MJ, et al. Long-term results after successful percutaneous transluminal coronary angioplasty in patients over 75 years of age. Am J Cardiol 1996;77:690–695.

42. Peterson ED, Cowper PA, Jollis JG, et al. Outcomes of coronary artery bypass graft surgery in 24,461 patients aged 80 years or older. Circulation 1995;92(Suppl II):II-85–II-91.

43. Laster SB, Rutherford BD, Giorgi LV, et al. Results of direct percutaneous transluminal coronary angioplasty in octogenarians. Am J Cardiol 1996;77:10–13.

44. Lefevre T, Morice M, Labrunie B, et al. Coronary stenting in elderly patients. Results from the stent without Coumadin French Registry [Abstract]. J Am Coll Cardiol 1996;27(Suppl A):252A.

45. Stein B, Weintraub WS, Gebhart SSP, et al. Influence of diabetes mellitus on early and late outcome after percutaneous transluminal coronary angioplasty. Circulation 1995;91:979–989.

46. Weintraub WS, Stein B, Gebhart SSP, et al. The impact of diabetes on the initial and long-term outcome of coronary artery bypass surgery [Abstract]. Circulation 1995;92(Suppl I):I-643.

47. Kip KE, Faxon DP, Detre KM, et al. Coronary angioplasty in diabetic patients. Circulation 1996;94:1818–1825.

48. The Bypass Angioplasty Revascularization Investigation (BARI) Investigators. Comparison of coronary bypass surgery with angioplasty in patients with multivessel disease. N Eng J Med 1996;335:217–225.

49. The BARI Investigators. The influence of diabetes on five year mortality and morbidity after angioplasty (PTCA) and bypass surgery (CABG) in the BARI randomized trial [Abstract]. Circulation 1996;94(Suppl I):I-318.

50. Weintraub WS, Mauldin PD, Becker E, et al. A comparison of the costs of and quality of life after coronary angioplasty or coronary surgery for multivessel coronary artery disease: results from the Emory Angioplasty Versus Surgery Trial (EAST). Circulation 1995;92:2831–2840.

51. Weintraub WS, King SB III Guyton RA, et al. Coronary surgery and PTCA in diabetics with multivessel disease: can the BARI results be generalized?[Abstract]. Circulation 1996;94(Suppl I):I-435.

52. Barsness GW, Peterson ED, Ohman EM, et al. The role of diabetes in long-term survival after coronary bypass and angioplasty [Abstract]. Circulation 1996;94(Suppl I):I-435.

53. Weintraub WS, Jones EL, Craver JM, et al. The choice of repeat CABG or PTCA in diabetics who have had previous CABG [Abstract]. Circulation 1996;94(Suppl I):I-435.

54. Hassinger NL, Grill DE, Holmes DR Jr. Outcomes and their predictors after PTCA in patients with type II diabetes mellitus [Abstract]. Circulation 1996;94(Suppl I):I-435.

55. Anderson RD, Wildermann NW, Harrington RO, et al. The association between a history of diabetes and outcome in patients undergoing percutaneous interventions [Abstract]. Circulation 1996;94(Suppl I):I-435.

56. James TW, Quinton HB, Birkmeyer JD, et al. Diabetes and coronary artery bypass graft surgery risk [Abstract]. Circulation 1996;94(Suppl I):I-412.

57. De Franco AC, Tuzcu EM, Ziada KM, et al. Intravascular ultrasound evidence for balloon oversizing in diabetics: a factor in higher complication rates?[Abstract]. J Am Coll Cardiol 1996;27(Suppl A):180A.

58. Goldberg S, Savage MP, Fischman DL. The interventional cardiologist and the diabetic patient.

Have we pushed the envelope too far or not far enough? Circulation 1996;94:1804–1806.

59. Stuckey TD, Brodie BR, Wall TC, et al. Significance of diabetes mellitus in patients with acute myocardial infarction receiving primary angioplasty [Abstract]. Circulation 1996;94(Suppl I):I-330.

60. Hildebrande P, Kaiser-Nielsen PK, Seibaek M, et al. Myocardial infarction in diabetic patients: presentation, residual systolic function and heart failure [Abstract]. Circulation 1996;94(Suppl I):I-610.

61. Emanuelsson H, Beatt KJ, Aytward P, et al. Diabetes in acute coronary syndromes—experience from the GUSTO IIb trial [Abstract]. Circulation 1996;94(Suppl I):I-610.

62. Paul SD, Lambrew CT, Rogers WJ, et al. A study of 118,276 patients with acute myocardial infarction in the United States in 1995: less aggressive care, worse prognosis and longer hospital length of stay for diabetics [Abstract]. Circulation 1996; 94(Suppl I):I-610.

63. Ryan TJ, Anderson JL, Antman EM, et al. ACC/AHA guidelines for the management of patients with acute myocardial infarction. A report of the American College of Cardiology/American Heart Association Task Force on Practice Guidelines (Committee on Management of Acute Myocardial Infarction). J Am Coll Cardiol 1996; 28:1328–1428.

64. Ellis CJ, French JK, Williams BF, et al. Thrombolytic therapy can be given to half of hospitalized patients with acute myocardial infarction [Abstract]. J Am Coll Cardiol 1996;27(Suppl A):249A.

65. Grines CL. Primary angioplasty—the strategy of choice. N Eng J Med 1996;335:1313–1317.

66. Meijer A, Verheugt FW, Werter CJ, et al. Aspirin versus coumadin in the prevention of reocclusion and recurrent ischemia after successful thrombolysis: a prospective placebo-controlled angiographic study: results of the APRICOT Study. Circulation 1993;87:1524–1530.

67. TIMI Research Group. Immediate versus. delayed catheterization and angioplasty following thrombolytic therapy for acute myocardial infarction: TIMI II A results. JAMA 1988;260:2849–2858.

68. Simoons ML, Arnold AER, Betriu A, et al. Thrombolysis with tissue plasminogen activator in acute myocardial infarction: no additional benefit from immediate percutaneous coronary angioplasty. Lancet 1988;197–203.

69. Topol EJ, Califf RM, George BS, et al. A randomized trial of immediate versus delayed elective angioplasty after intravenous tissue plasminogen activator in acute myocardial infarction. N Engl J Med 1987;317:581–588.

70. McKendall GR, Forman S, Sopko G, et al, and the Thrombolysis in Myocardial Infarction Investigators. Value of rescue percutaneous transluminal coronary angioplasty following unsuccessful thrombolytic therapy in patients with acute myocardial infarction. Am J Cardiol 1995;76:1108–1111.

71. Abbottsmith C, Topol E, George B, et al. Fate of patients with acute myocardial infarction with patency of the infarct-related vessel achieved with successful thrombolysis versus rescue angioplasty. J Am Coll Cardiol 1990;16:770–778.

72. Ellis S, Ribeiro-da Silva E, Heyndrickx G, et al. Randomized comparison of rescue angioplasty with conservative management of patients with early failure of thrombolysis for acute anterior myocardial infarction. Circulation 1994; 90:2280–2284.

73. O'Keefe J Jr, Rutherford BD, McConahay DR, et al.: Early and late results of coronary angioplasty without antecedent thrombolytic therapy for acute myocardial infarction. Am J Cardiol 1989; 64:1221–1230.

74. Rothbaum DA, Linnemeier TJ, Landin RJ, et al. Emergency percutaneous transluminal coronary angioplasty in acute myocardial infarction: a 3 year experience. J Am Coll Cardiol 1987; 10:264–272.

75. O'Neill WW, Brodie B, Knopf W, et al. Initial report of the Primary Angioplasty Revascularization (PAR) Multicenter Registry [Abstract]. Circulation 1991;84(Suppl 2):II-536.

76. Lieu TA, Gurley RJ, Lundstrom RJ, et al. Primary angioplasty and thrombolysis for acute myocardial infarction: an evidence summary. J Am Coll Cardiol 1996;27:737–750.

77. Grines CL, Browne KF, Marco J, et al. A comparison of immediate angioplasty with thrombolytic therapy for acute myocardial infarction. N Engl J Med 1993;328:673–679.

78. Gibbons RJ, Holmes DR, Reeder GS, et al. Immediate angioplasty compared with the administration of a thrombolytic agent followed by conservative treatment for myocardial infarction. N Engl J Med 1993;328:685–691.

79. Zijlestra F, De Boer MJ, Hoorntje JCA, et al. A comparison of immediate coronary angioplasty with intravenous streptokinase in acute myocardial infarction. N Engl J Med 1993;328:680–684.

80. Nunn C, O'Neill W, Rothbaum D, et al. Primary angioplasty for myocardial infarction improves long-term survival: PAMI-1 follow-up [Abstract]. J Am Coll Cardiol 1996;27(Suppl A):153A.

81. Simari RD, Berger PB, Bell MR, et al. Coronary angioplasty in acute myocardial infarction: primary, immediate adjunctive, rescue, or deferred adjunctive approach? Mayo Clin Proc 1994; 69:346–358.

82. Lundergan CF, Reiner JS, Ross AM. Determinants of 30 day and one year mortality in acute myocardial infarction: benefit of early angiography [Abstract]. J Am Coll Cardiol 1996;27(Suppl A):153A.

83. Anderson JL, Karagounis LA, Califf RM. Meta-analysis of five reported studies on the relation of early coronary patency grades with mortality and outcomes after acute myocardial infarction. Am J Cardiol 1996;78:1–8.

84. Laster SB, O'Keefe JH, Gibbons RJ. Incidence and importance of thrombolysis in myocardial infarction grade 3 flow after primary percutaneous transluminal coronary angioplasty for acute myocardial infarction. Am J Cardiol 1996;78:623–626.

85. Cannon CP, Lambrew CT, Tiefenbrunn AJ, et al. Influence of door-to-balloon time on mortality in primary angioplasty results in 3,648 patients in the Second National Registry of Myocardial In-

farction (NRMI-1) [Abstract].J Am Coll Cardiol 1996;27(Suppl A):61A.

86. Every NR, Parsons LS, Klatky M, et al. A comparison of thrombolytic therapy with primary coronary angioplasty for acute myocardial infarction. N Eng J Med 1996;335:1253–1260.

87. Lange RA, Hillis LD. Should thrombolysis or primary angioplasty be the treatment of choice for acute myocardial infarction? N Engl J Med 1996; 335:1311–1312.

88. Stone GW, Grines CL, Browne KF, et al. Influence of acute myocardial infarction location on in-hospital and late outcome after primary percutaneous transluminal coronary angioplasty versus tissue plasminogen activator therapy. Am J Cardiol 1996;78:19–25.

89. Stone GW, Marsalese D, Brodie B, et al. The routine use of intra-aortic balloon pumping after primary angioplasty improves clinical outcome in very high risk patients with acute myocardial infarction: results of the PAMI-2 trial [Abstract]. Circulation 1995;92(Suppl I):I-139.

90. Schultz RD, Heuser RR, Hatler C, et al. Primary angioplasty in acute myocardial infarction. Use of c7E3 Fab in conjunction with primary coronary stenting for acute myocardial infarctions complicated by cardiogenic shock. Cathet Cardiovasc Diagn 1996;39:143–148.

91. Antoniucci D, Valenti R, Buonamici P, et al. Direct angioplasty and stenting of the infarct-related artery in acute myocardial infarction. Am J Cardiol 1996;78:568–571.

92. Benzuly KH, O'Neill WW. The relentless pursuit of sustained patency after acute myocardial infarction. Cathet Cardiovasc Diagn 1996; 39:155–156.

93. Le May MR, Labinaz M, Beanlands RSB, et al. Usefulness of intracoronary stenting in acute myocardial infarction. Am J Cardiol 1996; 78:148–152.

94. Kaplan BM, Larkin T, Safian RD, et al. Prospective study of extraction atherectomy in patients with acute myocardial infarction. Am J Cardiol 1996; 78:383–388.

95. Pizzetti G, Belotti G, Margonato, et al. Coronary recanalization by elective angioplasty prevents ventricular dilation after anterior myocardial infarction. J Am Coll Cardiol 1996;28:837–845.

96. Hockman JS. Has the time come to seek and open all occluded infarct-related arteries after myocardial infarction? J Am Coll Cardiol 1996; 28:846–848.

97. Douglas JS Jr. Percutaneous intervention in patients with prior coronary bypass surgery: In: Topol EJ, ed. Textbook of interventional cardiology. 2nd ed. Philadelphia: WB Saunders, 1993; 339–354.

98. Reifart N, Haase J, Storger H, et al. Interventional standby for cardiac surgery [Abstract]. Circulation 1996;94:(Suppl I):I-86.

99. Rasmussen C, Thiis JJ, Clemmensen, et al. Management of suspected graft failure in coronary artery bypass grafting [Abstract]. Circulation 1996; 94(Suppl I):I-413.

100. Cutlip DE, Dauerman HL, Carrozza JP. Recurrent ischemia within thirty days of coronary artery bypass surgery: angiographic findings and outcome of percutaneous revascularization [Abstract]. Circulation 1996;94(Suppl I):I-249.

101. Kollar A, Simonton CA, Thomley AM, et al. Balloon angioplasty of the internal mammary artery trunk for early postoperative ischemia: a case report. Cathet Cardiovasc Diagn 1996;37:49–51.

102. Broderick TM, Wolf RK. Coronary angioplasty to relieve a kinked venous bypass conduit. Cathet Cardiovasc Diagn 1995;35:161–164.

103. Macaya C, Alfonso F, Iniguez A, et al. Stenting for elastic recoil during coronary angioplasty of the left main coronary artery. Am J Cardiol 1992; 70:105–107.

104. Chen L, Theroux P, Lesperance J, et al. Angiographic features in vein grafts versus in ungrafted coronary arteries in patients with unstable angina and previous bypass surgery [Abstract]. J Am Coll Cardiol 1996;27(Suppl A):333A.

105. Coronary Artery Surgery Study (CASS) and Their Associates. A randomized trial of coronary artery bypass. Quality of life in patients randomly assigned to treatment groups. Circulation 1983; 68:951–956.

106. Maynard C, Weaver WD, Litwin P, et al. Acute myocardial infarction and prior coronary artery surgery in the Myocardial Infarction Triage and Intervention Registry: patient characteristics, treatment, and outcome. Coron Artery Dis 1991; 2:443–448.

107. Wiseman A, Waters DD, Walling A, et al. Long-term prognosis after myocardial infarction in patients with previous coronary artery bypass surgery. J Am Coll Cardiol 1988;12:873–880.

108. Little WC, Gwinn NS, Burrows MT, et al. Cause of acute myocardial infarction late after successful coronary artery bypass grafting. Am J Cardiol 1990;65:808–810.

109. Grines CL, Booth DC, Nissen SE, et al. Mechanism of acute myocardial infarction in patients with prior coronary artery bypass grafting and therapeutic implications. Am J Cardiol 1990; 65:1292–1296.

110. Kavanaugh KM, Topol EJ. Acute intervention during myocardial infarction in patients with prior coronary bypass surgery. Am J Cardiol 1990; 65:924–926.

111. Stone GW, Brodie B, Griffin J, et al. Primary angioplasty in patients with prior bypass surgery [Abstract]. Circulation 1996;94(Suppl I):I-243.

112. Reiner JS, Lundergan CF, Kopecky SL, et al. Ineffectiveness of thrombolysis for acute MI following vein graft occlusion [Abstract]. Circulation 1996; 94(Suppl I):I-570.

113. Kleiman NS, Berman DA, Gaston WR, et al. Early intravenous thrombolytic therapy for acute myocardial infarction in patients with prior coronary artery bypass grafts. Am J Cardiol 1989; 63:102–104.

114. Loop FD, Lytle BW, Cosgrove DM, et al. Reoperation for coronary atherosclerosis. Ann Surg 1990; 212:378–386.

115. Lytle BW, Loop FD, Cosgrove DM. Fifteen hundred coronary reoperations: results and determinants of early and late survival. J Thorac Cardiovasc Surg 1987;93:847–857.

116. Cameron A, Kemp HG Jr, Green GE. Reoperation for coronary artery disease: 10 years of clinical follow-up. Circulation 1988;78:1–158.

117. Weintraub WS, Jones EL, Craver JM, et al. In-hospital and long-term outcome after reoperative coronary artery bypass graft surgery. Circulation 1995;92(Suppl II):II-50–II-57.

118. Mills RM, Kalan JM. Developing a rational management strategy for angina pectoris after coronary bypass surgery: a clinical decision analysis. Clin Cardiol 1991;14:191–197.

119. Weintraub WS, Mauldin PD, Becker E, et al. Cost versus. outcome for redo coronary surgery vs. coronary angioplasty for clinical recurrence after coronary surgery [Abstract]. J Am Coll Cardiol 1996;27(Suppl A):318A.

120. Stephan WJ, O'Keefe JH Jr, Piehler JM, et al. Coronary angioplasty versus repeat coronary artery bypass grafting for patients with previous bypass surgery. J Am Coll Cardiol 1996;28:1140–1146.

121. Loop FD, Lytle BW, Cosgrove DM, et al. Influence of internal-mammary-artery graft on 10-year survival and other cardiac events. N Engl J Med 1986;314:1–6.

122. Cameron A, Davis KB, Green G, et al. Coronary bypass surgery with internal-thoracic-artery grafts—effects on survival over a 15-year period. N Engl J Med 1996;334:216–219.

123. Loop FD. Internal-thoracic-artery grafts. N Engl J Med 1996;334:263–265.

124. Cameron AAC, Green GE, Brogno DA, et al. Internal thoracic artery grafts: 20-year clinical follow-up. J Am Coll Cardiol 1995;25:188–192.

125. Lytle BW, Loop FD, Taylor PC, et al. The effect of coronary reoperation on the survival of patients with stenoses in saphenous vein to coronary bypass grafts. J Thorac Cardiovasc Surg 1993;105:605–614.

126. Lytle BW. The clinical impact of the atherosclerotic saphenous vein to coronary artery bypass grafts. Semin Thorac Cardiovasc Surg 1994;6:81–86.

127. Brener SJ, Ellis SG, Dykstra DM, et al. Cleveland Clinic Foundation, Cleveland OH. Determinants of the key decision for prior CABG patients facing need for repeat revascularization: PTCA or CABG? [Abstract]. J Am Coll Cardiol 1996;27(Suppl A):45A.

128. Kahn JK, Hartzler GO. Retrograde coronary angioplasty of isolated arterial segments through saphenous vein bypass grafts. Cathet Cardiovasc Diagn 1990;20:88–93.

129. Douglas JS Jr, King SB III, Roubin GS, et al. Native coronary artery angioplasty in patients with previous coronary bypass surgery: update of in-hospital and long term results [Abstract]. Circulation 1987;76(Suppl IV):IV-465.

130. Miranda CP, Rutherford BD, McConahay DR, et al. Elective PTCA in post-bypass patients: comparison between those undergoing native artery dilatations and those undergoing bypass graft dilatations [Abstract]. Circulation 1992;86:I-457.

131. Gruentzig AR, Senning A, Siegenthaler WE. Nonoperative dilatation of coronary artery stenosis: percutaneous transluminal coronary angioplasty. N Engl J Med 1979; 303:61–68.

132. Douglas JS Jr, Gruentzig AR, King SB III, et al. Percutaneous transluminal coronary angioplasty in patients with prior coronary bypass surgery. J Am Coll Cardiol 1983;2:745–754.

133. Douglas J, Robinson K, Schlumpf M. Percutaneous transluminal angioplasty in aortocoronary venous graft stenoses: immediate results and complications [Abstract]. Circulation 1986;74:II-281.

134. Cote G, Myler RK, Stertzer SH, et al. Percutaneous transluminal angioplasty of stenotic coronary artery bypass grafts: 5 years' experience. J Am Coll Cardiol 1987;9:8–17.

135. Pinkerton CA, Slack JD, Orr CM, et al. Percutaneous transluminal angioplasty in patients with prior myocardial revascularization surgery. Am J Cardiol 1988;61:15G–22G.

133. Dorros G, Lewin RF, Mathiak LM, et al. Percutaneous transluminal coronary angioplasty in patients with two or more previous coronary artery bypass graft operations. Am J Cardiol 1988;61:1243–1247.

136. Reed DC, Beller GA, Nygaard TW, et al. The clinical efficacy and scintigraphic evaluation of post-coronary bypass patients undergoing percutaneous transluminal coronary angioplasty for recurrent angina pectoris. Am Heart J 1989;117:60.

137. Platko WP, Hollman J, Whitlow PL, et al. Percutaneous transluminal angioplasty of saphenous vein graft stenosis: long-term follow-up. J Am Coll Cardiol 1989;7:1645–1650.

138. Plokker HW, Meester BH, Serruys PW. The Dutch experience in percutaneous transluminal angioplasty of narrowed saphenous veins used for aortocoronary arterial bypass. Am J Cardiol 1991;67:361–366.

140. Douglas JS Jr, Weintraub WS, Liberman HA, et al. Update of saphenous graft (SVG) angioplasty: restenosis and long term outcome [Abstract]. Circulation 1991;84:II-249.

141. Webb JG, Myler RF, Shaw RE, et al. Coronary angioplasty after coronary bypass surgery: initial results and late outcome in 422 patients. J Am Coll Cardiol 1990;16:812–820.

142. Reeves F, Bonan R, Cote G, et al. Long-term angiographic follow-up after angioplasty of venous coronary bypass grafts. Am Heart J 1991;122:620–627.

143. Morrison DA, Crowley ST, Veerakul G, et al. Percutaneous transluminal angioplasty of saphenous vein grafts for medically refractory unstable angina. J Am Coll Cardiol 1994;23:1066–1070.

144. Douglas JS Jr, Weintraub WS, King SB III. Changing perspectives in vein graft angioplasty [Abstract]. J Am Coll Cardiol 1995;25(Suppl A):78A.

145. De Feyter PJ, Van Suylen R, De Jaegere PPT, et al. Balloon angioplasty for the treatment of lesions in saphenous vein bypass grafts. J Am Coll Cardiol 1993;21:1539–1549.

146. Abhyankar A, Bernstein L, Harris PJ, et al. Reintervention and clinical events after saphenous vein graft angioplasty—a comparison of optimal PTCA versus stenting [Abstract]. Circulation 1996;94(Suppl I):I-686).

147. Garratt KN, Holmes DR, Bell MR, et al. Results of directional atherectomy of primary atheromatous

and restenosis lesions in coronary arteries and saphenous vein grafts. Am J Cardiol 1992; 70:449–454.

148. Pomerantz RM, Kuntz RE, Carrozza JP, et al. Acute and long-term outcome of narrowed saphenous vein grafts treated by endoluminal stenting and directional atherectomy. Am J Cardiol 1992; 70:161–167.

149. Waksman R, Scott NA, Douglas JS Jr, et al. Distal embolization is common after directional atherectomy in coronary arteries and vein grafts [Abstract]. Circulation 1993; 88(Suppl I):I-299.

150. Holmes DR, Topol EJ, Califf RM, et al. A multicenter, randomized trial of coronary angioplasty versus directional atherectomy for patients with saphenous vein graft lesions. Circulation 1995; 91:1966–1974.

151. Lefkovits J, Holmes DR, Califf RM, et al. Predictors and sequelae of distal embolization during saphenous vein graft intervention from the CAVEAT-II Trial. Circulation 1995;92:734–740.

152. Hinohara T, Robertson GC, Selmon MR, et al. Restenosis after directional coronary atherectomy. J Am Coll Cardiol 1992;20:623–632.

153. Meany T, Kramer B, Knopf W, et al. Multicenter experience of atherectomy of saphenous vein grafts: immediate results and follow-up. J Am Coll Cardiol 1992;19:262.

154. Wong SC, Popma JJ, Hong MK, et al. Procedural results and long term clinical outcome in aorto-ostial saphenous vein graft lesions after new device angioplasty [Abstract]. J Am Coll Cardiol 1995;25(Suppl A):394A.

155. Bittl JA, Sanborn TA, Yardley DE, et al. Predictors of outcome of percutaneous excimer laser coronary angioplasty of saphenous vein bypass graft lesions. Am J Cardiol 1994;74:144–148.

156. Eigler NL, Weinstock B, Douglas JS Jr, et al. Excimer laser coronary angioplasty of aorto-ostial stenoses. Results of the Excimer Laser Coronary Angioplasty (ELCA) Registry in the first 200 patients. Circulation 1993;88:2049–2057.

157. Douglas JS Jr, Ghazzal ZMB, Balalbaki HA, et al. Excimer laser coronary angioplasty of ostial lesions. Cathet Cardiovasc Diagn 1991;23:74.

158. Strauss BH, Natarajan MK, Batchelor WB, et al. Early and late quantitative angiographic results of vein graft lesions treated by excimer laser with adjunctive balloon angioplasty. Circulation 1995; 92:348–356.

159. Deckelbaum LI, Natarjan K, Bittl JA, et al. Effect of intracoronary saline infusion on dissection during excimer laser coronary angioplasty: A randomized trial. J Am Coll Cardiol 1995;26:1264–1269.

160. Hong MK, Wong SC, Popma JJ, et al. Favorable results of debulking followed by immediate adjunct stent therapy for high risk saphenous vein graft lesions [Abstract]. J Am Coll Cardiol 1996; 27(Suppl A):A179.

161. Urban P, Sigwart U, Golf S, et al. Intravascular stenting for stenosis of aortocoronary venous bypass grafts. J Am Coll Cardiol 1994;23:1296–1304.

162. de Scheerder JK, Strauss BH, De Feyter PJ, et al. Stenting of venous bypass grafts: a new treatment modality of patients who are poor candidates for reintervention. Am Heart J 1992;23:1296–1304.

163. Strauss BH, Serruys PW, Bertrand ME, et al. Qualitative angiographic follow-up of the coronary Wallstent in native vessel bypass grafts. Am J Cardiol 1992;69:475–481.

164. De Jaegere PP, Van Domburg RT, De Feyter PJ, et al. Long-term clinical outcome after stent implantation in saphenous vein grafts. J Am Coll Cardiol 1996;28:89–96.

165. Colombo, Itoh A, Hall P, et al. Implantation of the Wallstent for diffuse lesions in native coronary arteries and venous bypass grafts without subsequent anticoagulation. J Am Coll Cardiol 1996; 53A.

166. Wong SC, Baim DS, Schatz RA, et al. Acute results and late outcomes after stent implantation in saphenous vein graft lesions: the multicenter USA Palmaz-Schatz stent experience. J Am Coll Cardiol 1995;26:704–712.

167. Rechavia E, Litvack F, Macko G, et al. Stent implantation of saphenous vein graft aorto-ostial lesions in patients with unstable ischemic syndromes: Immediate angiographic results and long-term clinical outcome. J Am Coll Cardiol 1995;25:866–870.

168. Rocha-Singh K, Morris N, Wong SC, et al. Coronary stenting for treatment of ostial stenoses of native coronary arteries or aortocoronary saphenous venous grafts. Am J Cardiol 1995;75:26–29.

169. Brenner SJ, Ellis SG, Apperson-Hansen C. Compared with balloon angioplasty of saphenous vein grafts, stenting is associated with highly favorable results. J Invasive Cardiol 1996;8:38.

170. Savage MP, Douglas JS Jr, Fischman DL, et al. A randomized trial of coronary stenting and balloon angioplasty in the treatment of aortocoronary saphenous vein bypass graft disease. N Eng J Med 1997; in press.

171. Leon MB, Ellis SG, Moses J, et al. Interim report from the reduced anticoagulation vein graft stent (RAVES) study [Abstract]. Circulation 1996; 94(Suppl I):I-683.

172. Challapalli RM, Eisenberg MJ, Sigmon K, et al. Platelet glycoprotein IIb/IIIa monoclonal antibody (c7E3) reduces distal embolization during percutaneous intervention of saphenous vein grafts [Abstract]. Circulation 1995;92(Suppl I):I-607.

173. Kaplan BM, Benzuly KH, Kind J, et al. Treatment of no-reflow in degenerated saphenous vein graft interventions: comparison of intracoronary Verapamil and nitroglycerin. Cathet Cardiovasc Diagn 1996;39:113–118.

174. Wong SC, Popma JJ, Pichard AD, et al. Comparison of clinical and angiographic outcomes after saphenous vein graft angioplasty using coronary versus biliary tubular slotted stents. Circulation 1995;91:339–350.

175. Nunez BD, Simari RD, Keelan ET, et al. A novel approach to the placement of Palmaz-Schatz biliary stents in saphenous vein grafts. Cathet Cardiovasc Diagn 1995;35:350–353.

176. Linnemeier TJ. Biliary stents for saphenous vein grafts: reducing the risk of stent implantation. Cathet Cardiovasc Diagn 1995;35:354.

177. Moses JW, Teirstein PS, Sketch MH Jr, et al. Angiographic determinants of risk and outcome of

coronary embolus and myocardial infarction (MI) with the transluminal extraction catheter (TEC): a report from the New Approaches To Coronary Intervention (NACI) Registry [Abstract]. J Am Coll Cardiol 1994;220A.

178. Safian RD, Grines CL, May MA, et al. Clinical and angiographic results of transluminal extraction coronary atherectomy in saphenous vein bypass grafts. Circulation 1994;89:302–312.

179. Meany TB, Leon MB, Kramer BL, et al. Transluminal extraction catheter for the treatment of diseased saphenous vein grafts: a multicenter experience. Cathet Cardiovasc Diagn 1995;34:112–120.

180. Dooris M, Hoffmann M, Glazier S, et al. Comparative results of transluminal extraction coronary atherectomy in saphenous vein graft lesions with and without thrombus. J Am Coll Cardiol 1995; 25:1700–1705.

181. Al-Shaibi KF, Goods CM, Jain SP, et al. Does transluminal extraction atherectomy reduce distal embolization in saphenous vein grafts? [Abstract]. Circulation 1995;92:I-329.

182. Hong M, Pichard A, Kent K, et al. Assessing a strategy of stand-alone extraction atherectomy followed by staged stent placement in degenerated saphenous vein graft lesions [Abstract]. J Am Coll Cardiol 1995;25:394A.

183. Parks JM. TEC before stent implantation. J Invasive Cardiol 1995;7(Suppl D):10D–13D.

184. Kramer B. Optimal Therapy for degenerated saphenous vein graft disease. J Invasive Cardiol 1995;7(Suppl D):14D–20D.

185. George BS. TEC for old grafts, TEC for new clots: if you don't like it, you're not using it right. J Invasive Cardiol 1995;7(Suppl D):21D–24D.

186. Kaplan BM, Safian RD, Goldstein JA, et al. Efficacy of angioscopy in determining the effectiveness of intracoronary urokinase and TEC atherectomy thrombus removal from an occluded saphenous vein graft prior to stent implantation. Cathet Cardiovasc Diagn 1995;36:335–337.

187. Kaplan BM, Safian RD, Grines CL, et al. A prospective study of stent implantation in high risk lesions utilizing adjunctive extraction atherectomy and angioscopy guidance. J Invasive Cardiol 1996;8:38.

188. Hong MK, Mintz GS, Popma JJ, et al. Angiographic results and late clinical outcomes utilizing a stent synergy (pre-stent atheroablation) approach in complex lesion subsets. J Invasive Cardiol 1996;8:15–22.

189. Chapekis AT, George BS, Candela RJ. Rapid thrombus dissolution by continuous infusion of urokinase through an intracoronary perfusion wire prior to and following PTCA: results in native coronaries and patent saphenous vein grafts. Cathet Cardiovasc Diagn 1991;23:89–92.

190. Cundey PE, Whitlock RR, Norman J, et al. Prolonged intragraft urokinase with a new infusion wire: improved short-term results. Cathet Cardiovasc Diagn 31:150–152.

191. Denardo SJ, Teirstein PS. Urokinase infusion and stenting of older saphenous vein grafts. J Invasive Cardiol 1995;7(Suppl E):26E–35E.

192. Denardo SJ, Morris NB, Rocha-Singh KJ, et al. Safety and efficacy of extended urokinase infu-

sion plus stent deployment for treatment of obstructed, older saphenous vein grafts. Am J Cardiol 1995;76:776–780.

193. McKay RG. Site-specific, catheter-based thrombolysis: a new technique for treating intracoronary thrombus and thrombus-containing stenosis. J Invasive Cardiol 1995;7:36E–43E.

194. Mitchel JF, Fram DB, Palme DF, et al. Enhanced intracoronary thrombolysis with urokinase using a novel, local drug delivery system. Circulation 1995;91:785–793.

195. Annex BH, Larkin TJ, O'Neill WW, et al. Evaluation of thrombus removal by transluminal extraction coronary atherectomy by percutaneous coronary angioscopy. Am J Cardiol 1994;74:606–609.

196. Frumin H, Goldbert MJ, Rubenfire M, et al. Late thrombolysis of an occluded aortocoronary saphenous vein graft. Am Heart J 1983; 106:401–403.

197. De Feyter PJ, Serruys P, Van Den Brand M, et al. Percutaneous transluminal angioplasty of a totally occluded bypass graft: a challenge that should be resisted. Am J Cardiol 1989;64:88–90.

198. Levine DJ, Sharaf BL, Williams DO. Late follow-up of patients with totally occluded saphenous vein bypass grafts treated by prolonged selective urokinase infusion [Abstract]. J Am Coll Cardiol 1992;19:292A.

199. Hartmann J, McKeever L, Teran J, et al. Prolonged infusion of urokinase for recanalization of chronically occluded aortocoronary bypass grafts. Am J Cardiol 1988;61:189–191.

200. Marx M, Armstrong W, Brent B, et al. Transcatheter recanalization of a chronically occluded saphenous aortocoronary bypass graft. AJR 1987; 148:375–377.

201. Gurley JC, MacPhail BS. Acute myocardial infarction due to thrombolytic reperfusion of chronically occluded saphenous vein coronary bypass grafts. Am J Cardiol 1991;68:274–275.

202. McKeever LS, Hartman JR, Bufalino VJ, et al. Acute myocardial infarction complicating recanalization of aortocoronary bypass grafts with urokinase therapy. Am J Cardiol 1989;64:683–685.

203. Margolis JR, Mogensen L, Mehta S, et al. Diffuse embolization following percutaneous transluminal coronary angioplasty of occluded vein grafts: the blush phenomenon. Clin Cardiol 1991; 14:489–493.

204. Pitney MR, Cumpston N, Mews GC, et al. Use of twenty-four hour infusions of intracoronary tissue plasminogen activator to increase the application of coronary angioplasty. Cathet Cardiovasc Diagn 1992;26:255–259.

205. Bedotto JB, Rutherford BD, Hartzler GO. Intramyocardial hemorrhage due to prolonged intracoronary infusion of urokinase into a totally occluded saphenous vein bypass graft. Cathet Cardiovasc Diagn 1992;25:52–56.

206. Blankenship JC, Modesto TA, Madigan NP. Acute myocardial infarction complicating urokinase infusion for total saphenous vein graft occlusion. Cathet Cardiovasc Diagn 1993;28:39–43.

207. Taylor MA, Santoian EC, Ali J, et al. Intracerebral hemorrhage complicating urokinase infusion into

an occluded aortocoronary bypass graft. Cathet Cardiovasc Diagn 1994;31:206–210.

208. Hartmann JR, McKeever LS, O'Neill WW, et al. Recanalization of chronically occluded aortocoronary saphenous vein bypass grafts with long-term, low dose direct infusion of urokinase (ROBUST): a serial trial. J Am Coll Cardiol 1996; 27:60–66.

209. Berger PB, Bell MR, Simari R, et al. Immediate and long-term clinical outcome in patients undergoing angioplasty of occluded vein grafts [Abstract]. J Am Coll Cardiol 1996;76(Suppl A): 180A.

210. Glazier JJ, Bauer HH, Kiernan FJ, et al. Recanalization of totally occluded saphenous vein grafts using local urokinase delivery with the Dispatch catheter. Cathet Cardiovasc Diagn 1995; 36:326–332.

211. Heuser RR. Recanalization of occluded SVGs: is there light at the end of the graft? Cathet Cardiovasc Diagn 1995;36:333–334.

212. Sullebarger JT, Puleo J. Extraction atherectomy for the recanalization of totally occluded aortocoronary saphenous vein grafts. Cathet Cardiovasc Diagn 1995;36:339–343.

213. Margolis JR, Mahta S, Kramer B, et al. Extraction atherectomy for the treatment of recent totally occluded saphenous vein grafts [Abstract]. J Am Coll Cardiol 1994;(Suppl A):405A.

214. Brown RIG, Gilligan L, Penn IM, et al. Right internal mammary artery graft angioplasty through a right brachial artery approach using a new custom guide catheter. A case report. Cathet Cardiovasc Diagn 1992;25:42–45.

215. Webb JG, Myler RF, Shaw RE, et al. Coronary angioplasty after coronary bypass surgery: initial results and late outcome in 422 patients. J Am Coll Cardiol 1990;16:812–820.

216. Dimas AP, Arora RR, Whitlow PL, et al. Percutaneous transluminal angioplasty involving internal mammary artery grafts. Am Heart J 1991; 122:423–429.

217. Sketch MH, Quigley PJ, Perez JA, et al. Angiographic follow-up after internal mammary artery graft angioplasty. Am J Cardiol 1992;70:401–403.

218. Shimshak TM, Giorgi LV, Johnson WL, et al. Application of percutaneous transluminal coronary angioplasty to the internal mammary artery graft. J Am Coll Cardiol 1988;12:1205–1214.

219. Hill DM, McAuley BJ, Sheehan DJ, et al. Percutaneous transluminal angioplasty of internal mammary artery bypass grafts [Abstract]. J Am Coll Cardiol 1989;13:221A.

220. Shimshak TM, Rutherford BD, McConahay DR, et al. PTCA of internal mammary artery (IMA) grafts procedural results and late follow-up [Abstract]. Circulation 1991;84:II-590.

221. Hearne SE, Wilson JS, Harrington J, et al. Angiographic and clinical follow-up after internal mammary artery graft angioplasty: a 9-year experience [Abstract]. J Am Coll Cardiol 1995;25(Suppl A): 139A.

222. Isshiki T, Yamaguchi T, Tamura T, et al. Percutaneous angioplasty of stenosed gastroepiploic artery grafts. J Am Coll Cardiol 1993;22:727.

223. Ernst S, Bal E, Plokker T, et al. Percutaneous balloon angioplasty (PBA) of a left subclavian artery stenosis or occlusion to establish adequate flow through the left internal mammary artery for coronary bypass purposes. Circulation 1991;84:II-591.

224. Shapira S, Braun S, Puram B, et al. Percutaneous transluminal angioplasty of proximal subclavian artery stenosis after left internal mammary to left anterior descending artery bypass surgery. J Am Coll Cardiol 1991;18:1120–1123.

225. Kugelmass AD, Kim D, Kuntz RE, et al. Endoluminal stenting of a subclavian artery stenosis to treat ischemia in the distribution of a patent left internal mammary graft. Cathet Cardiovasc Diagn 1994;33:175–177.

226. Sullivan TM, Bacharach JM, Childs MB. PTA and primary stenting of the subclavian and innominate arteries [Abstract]. Circulation 1995;92(Suppl I):I-383.

227. Kumar K, Dorros G, Bates MC, et al. Primary stent deployment in occlusive subclavian artery disease. Cathet Cardiovasc Diagn 1995;34:281–285.

228. Galli M, Goldberg SL, Zerboni S, et al. Balloon expandable stent implantation after iatrogenic arterial dissection of the left subclavian artery. Cathet Cardiovasc Diagn 1995;35:355–357.

229. Almagor Y, Thomas J, Colombo A. Balloon expandable stent implantation of a stenosis at the origin of the left internal mammary artery graft. Cathet Cardiovasc Diagn 1991;24:256–258.

230. Bajaj RK, Roubin GS. Intravascular stenting of the right internal mammary artery. Cathet Cardiovasc Diagn 1991;24:252–255.

231. Miller RM, Knox M. Patient tolerance of ioxaglate and iopamidol in internal mammary artery arteriography. Cathet Cardiovasc Diagn 1992; 25:31–34.

232. Stratienko AA, Ginsberg R, Schatz RA, et al. Technique for shortening angioplasty guide catheter length when therapeutic catheter fails to reach target stenosis. Cathet Cardiovasc Diagn 1993; 30:331–333.

233. Satler LF. The advantage of anticipating the need for a short guiding catheter [Abstract]. Cathet Cardiovasc Diagn 1996;37:76.

234. Holmes DR Jr, Detre KM, Williams DO, et al. Long-term outcome of patients with depressed left ventricular function undergoing percutaneous transluminal coronary angioplasty: the NHLBI PTCA Registry. Circulation 1993; 87:21–29.

235. Vogel RA, Shawl F, Tommaso CL, et al. Initial report of the national registry of elective cardiopulmonary bypass supported coronary angioplasty. J Am Coll Cardiol 1990;15:23–29.

236. Jones RH, Hannan EL, Hammermeister KE, et al. Identification of preoperative variables needed for risk adjustment of short-term mortality after coronary artery bypass graft surgery. J Am Coll Cardiol 1996;28:1478–1487.

237. Ellis SG, Myler RK, King SB, et al. Causes and correlates of death after unsupported coronary angioplasty. Implications for use of angioplasty and advanced support techniques in high-risk settings. Am J Cardiol 1991;68:1447–1451.

238. Califf RM, Philips HR, Hindman MC, et al. Prog-

nostic value of a coronary artery jeopardy score. J Am Coll Cardiol 1988;5:1055–1063.

239. Anderson RD, Wildermann NM, Holmes DR Jr, et al. Prognostic value of a history of congestive heart failure in patients undergoing percutaneous coronary interventions [Abstract]. J Am Coll Cardiol 1996;27(Suppl A):180A.

240. Aguirre FV, Kern MJ, Bach R, et al. Intraaortic balloon pump support during high-risk coronary angioplasty. Cardiology 1994;84:175–186.

241. Tommaso CL, Vogel RA. National Registry for Supported Angioplasty: Results and follow-up of three years of supported and standby supported angioplasty in high-risk patients. Cardiology 1994;84:238–244.

242. Tommaso CL. Supported angioplasty: another look. Cathet Cardiovasc Diagn 1996;38:249–250.

243. Shawl FA, Quyyumi AA, Bajaj, et al. Percutaneous cardiopulmonary bypass-supported coronary angioplasty in patients with unstable angina pectoris or myocardial infarction and a left ventricular ejection fraction ≤ 25%. Am J Cardiol 1996;77:14–19.

244. Ferrari M, Scholz H, Figulla HR. PTCA with the use of cardiac assist devices: risk stratification, short- and long-term results. Cathet Cardiovasc Diagn 1996;38:242–248.

245. McCullough PA, Wolyn R, Rocher LL, et al. Acute contrast nephropathy after coronary intervention: incidence, risk factors, and relationship to mortality [Abstract]. J Am Coll Cardiol 1996;27(Suppl A):304A.

246. Levy EM, Viscoli CM, Horwitz RI. The effect of acute renal failure on mortality. A cohort analysis. JAMA 1996;275:1489–1494.

247. Turney JH. Acute renal failure—a dangerous condition. JAMA 1996;275:1516–1517.

248. Thadhani R, Pascual M, Bonventre JV. Acute renal failure. N Engl J Med 1996;334:1448–1460.

249. Redwood SR, Popma JJ, Kent KM, et al. Predictors of late mortality following ablative new-device angioplasty in native coronary arteries [Abstract]. J Am Coll Cardiol 1996;27(Suppl A):167A.

250. O'Keefe JH, McCallister BD, Blackstone EH, et al. The effects of diabetes and renal function on long-term outcome after coronary angioplasty [Abstract]. Circulation 1996;94(Suppl I):I-717.

251. Rao V, Christakis GT, Weizel RD, et al. Effect of renal insufficiency on the results of coronary bypass surgery [Abstract]. Circulation 1996; 94(Suppl I):I-571.

252. Solomon R, Werner C, Mann D, et al. Effects of saline, mannitol, and furosemide on acute decreases in renal function induced by radiocontrast agents. N Engl J Med 1994;331:1416–1420.

253. Rudnick MR, Goldfarb S, Wexler L, et al. Nephrotoxicity of ionic and nonionic contrast media in 1196 patients: a randomized study. Kidney Int 1995;47:254–261.

254. Barrett BJ, Carlisle EJ. Metaanalysis of the relative nephrotoxicity of high- and low-osmolality iodinated contrast media. Radiology 1993;188:1: 171–178.

255. Gutch, CF. Nonsteroidal anti-inflammatory agents and acute renal failure. Arch Intern Med 1996;156:2414.

256. Tan K, Sulke N, Taub N, et al. Clinical and lesion morphologic determinants of coronary angioplasty success and complications: current experience. J Am Coll Cardiol 1995;25:855–865.

257. Fry ET, Hermiller JB, Peters TF, et al. Is ACC/AHA classification predictive of successful coronary intervention in the era of new devices? [Abstract]. J Am Coll Cardiol 1996;27(Suppl A):152A.

258. Serruys PW, Azar AJ, Sigwrt U, et al. Long term follow-up of "stent-like" (≤ 30% diameter stent post) angioplasty: a case for provisional stenting [Abstract]. J Am Coll Cardiol 1996;27(Suppl A): 15A.

259. Tenaglia AN, Zidar JP, Jackman JD, et al. Treatment of long coronary artery narrowings with long angioplasty balloon catheters. Am J Cardiol Coll 1993;71:1274–1277.

260. Appelman YE, Piek J, Redekop WK, et al. Excimer laser angioplasty versus balloon angioplasty in longer coronary lesions: a multivariate analysis. Circulation 1995;92:I-74.

261. Foley DP, Appleman YE, Piek JJ, et al. Comparison of angiographic restenosis propensity of excimer laser coronary angioplasty and balloon angioplasty in the Amsterdam Rotterdam (AMRO) trial [Abstract]. Circulation 1995;92:I-477.

262. Reisman M, Cohen B, Warth D, et al. Outcome of long lesions with high speed rotational ablation [Abstract]. J Am Coll Cardiol 1993;443A.

263. Akira I, Hall P, Maiello L, et al. Coronary stenting of long lesions greater than 20 mm—a matched comparison of different stents [Abstract]. Circulation 1995;92:I-688.

264. Eccleston DS, Belli G, Penn IM, et al. Are multiple stents associated with multiplicative risk in the new stent era? [Abstract]. Circulation 1996; 94(Suppl I):I-454.

265. Yokoi H, Nobuyoshi M, Mosaka H, et al. Palmaz-Schatz stent implantation in calcified lesions: immediate and follow-up results [Abstract]. Circulation 1996;94(Suppl I):I-453.

266. DeFranco AC, Nissen SE, Tuzcu EM, et al. Ultrasound plaque morphology predicts major dissections following stand-alone and adjunctive balloon angioplasty [Abstract]. Circulation 1994; 90(Suppl I):I-90.

267. Mintz GS, Douek P, Pichard AD, et al. Target lesion calcification in coronary artery disease: an intravascular ultrasound study. J Am Coll Cardiol 1992;20:1149–1150.

268. Tuzcu EM, Berkalp B, De Franco AC, et al. The dilemma of diagnosing coronary calcification: angiography versus intravascular ultrasound. J Am Coll Cardiol 1996;27:832–838.

269. MacIsaac AI, Bass TA, Buchbinder M, et al. High speed rotational atherectomy: outcome in calcified and non-calcified coronary artery lesions. J Am Coll Cardiol 1995;26:731–736.

270. Hong MK, Mintz GS, Popma JJ, et al. Safety and efficacy of elective stent implantation following rotational atherectomy in large, calcified coronary arteries [Abstract]. Cathet Cardiovasc Diagn 1996; Suppl 3:50–54.

271. Ellis SG, Cowley MJ, Whitlow PL, et al. Prospective case-control comparison of percutaneous transluminal coronary revascularization in pa-

tients with multivessel disease treated in 1986–1987 versus 1991: improved in-hospital and 12-month results. J Am Coll Cardiol 1995; 25:1137–1142.

272. Barasch E, Conger JL, Kadipasaoglu KA, et al. PTCA in angulated segments: effects of balloon material, balloon length, and inflation sequence in straightening forces in an in vitro model. Cathet Cardiovasc Diagn 1996;39:207–212.

273. Chevalier B, Commeau P, Favereau X, et al. Limitations of rotational atherectomy in angulated coronary lesions [Abstract]. J Am Coll Cardiol 1994;285A.

274. Klein LW, Litvack F, Holmes D, et al. Prospective multicenter analysis of excimer laser coronary angioplasty (ELCA) in stenoses with complex morphology [Abstract]. J Am Coll Cardiol 1994;448A.

275. White CJ, Ramee SR, Collins TJ, et al. Angioscopically detected coronary thrombus correlates with adverse PTCA outcome [Abstract]. Circulation 1993;88(Suppl I):I-596.

276. Ramee SR, Kuntz RE, Schatz RA, et al. Preliminary experience with the POSSIS coronary angiojet rheololytic thrombectomy catheter in the VEGAS 1 PILOT Study [Abstract]. J Am Coll Cardiol 1996;27(Suppl A):69A.

277. Kimball BP, Cohen EA, Adelman AG, for the Canadian Coronary Atherectomy Trial Investigators. Influence of stenotic lesion morphology on Immediate and long-term (6 months) angiographic outcome: comparative analysis of directional coronary atherectomy versus standard balloon angioplasty. J Am Coll Cardiol 1996; 27:543–551.

278. Stone GE, Rutherford BD, McConahay DR, et al. Procedural outcome of angioplasty for total coronary artery occlusion: an analysis of 971 lesions in 905 patients. J Am Coll Cardiol 1990;15:849–856.

279. Ivanhoe RJ, Weintraub WS, Douglas JS Jr, et al. Percutaneous transluminal coronary angioplasty of chronic total occlusions. Circulation 1992; 85:106–115.

280. Bell MR, Berger PB, Bresnahan JF, et al. Initial and long term outcome of 354 patients following coronary balloon angioplasty of total coronary artery occlusions. Circulation 1992;85:1003–1011.

281. Ruocco NA, Ring ME, Holubkov R, et al. Results of coronary angioplasty of chronic total occlusions (the National Heart, Lung, and Blood Institute 1985–1986 Percutaneous Transluminal Angioplasty Registry). Am J Coll Cardiol 1992; 69:69–76.

282. Haine E, Urban P, Dorsaz PA, et al. Outcome and complications of 500 consecutive chronic total occlusion angioplasties [Abstract]. J Am Coll Cardiol 1993;21:138A.

283. Kinoshita I, Katoh O, Nariyama J, et al. Coronary angioplasty of chronic total occlusions with bridging collateral vessels: immediate and follow-up outcome from a large single-center experience. J Am Coll Cardiol 1995;26:409–415.

284. Puma JA, Sketch MH, Tcheng JE, et al. Percutaneous revascularization of chronic coronary occlusions: an overview. J Am Coll Cardiol 1995; 26:1–11.

285. Katsuragawa M, Fujiwara H, Miyamae M, et al.

Histologic studies in percutaneous transluminal coronary angioplasty for chronic total occlusion: comparison of tapering and abrupt types of occlusion and short and long occluded segments. J Am Coll Cardiol 1993;21:604–611.

286. Zimarino M, Rasetti G, Venarucci V, et al. Terumo glidewire. The wire of choice for chronic total occlusion. Cathet Cardiovasc Diagn 1995; 34:186–188.

287. Serruys PW, Leon M, Hamburger JN, et al. Recanalization of chronic total coronary occlusions using a laser guidewire: the Eu and US total experience [Abstract]. J Am Coll Cardiol 1996;27(Suppl A): 152A.

288. Pijls NHJ, Bracke FALE. Damage to the collateral circulation by PTCA of an occluded coronary artery. Cathet Cardiovasc Diagn 1995;34:61–64.

289. Zidar FJ, Kaplan BM, O'Neill WW, et al. Prospective, randomized trial of prolonged intracoronary urokinase infusion for chronic total occlusions in native coronary arteries. J Am Coll Cardiol 1996; 27:1406–1412.

290. Goldberg SL, Colombo A, Maiello L, et al. Intracoronary stent insertion after balloon angioplasty of chronic total occlusions. J Am Coll Cardiol 1995;713–719.

291. Thomas M, Hancock J, Holmberg S, et al. Coronary stenting following successful angioplasty for total occlusions: preliminary results of a randomized trial [Abstract]. J Am Coll Cardiol 1996; (Suppl A):153A.

292. Sirnes PP, Golf S, Myreng Y, et al. Stenting in chronic coronary occlusion (SICCO): a randomized, controlled trial of adding stent implantation after successful angioplasty. J Am Coll Cardiol 1996;28:1444–1451.

293. Brener SJ, Leya FS, Apperson-Hansen C, et al. A comparison of debulking versus dilatation of bifurcation coronary arterial narrowings (from a CAVEAT I Trial). Am J Cardiol 1996; 78:1039–1041.

294. Altmann DB, Popma JJ, Pichard AD, et al. Impact of directional atherectomy on adjacent branch vessels. Am J Cardiol 1993;72:351–353.

295. Whitlow PL, Cowley M, Bass T, et al. Risk of high speed rotational atherectomy in bifurcation lesions [Abstract]. J Am Coll Cardiol 1993;445A.

296. Kereiakes JD. Percutaneous transcatheter therapy of aorto-ostial stenoses. Cathet Cardiovasc Diagn 1996;38:292–300.

297. Jain SP, Liu MW, Babu R, et al. Balloon versus debulking devices versus stenting for right coronary ostial disease: acute and long-term results [Abstract]. Circulation 1996;94(Suppl I):I-248.

298. Boehrer JD, Ellis SG, Keeler GP, et al. Differential benefit of directional atherectomy over angioplasty for left anterior descending in proximal, non-ostial lesions: results from CAVEAT [Abstract]. J Am Coll Cardiol 1994;386A.

299. Tanaka S, Ueda K, Yung-Sheng H. Directional coronary atherectomy in ostial lesion of left anterior descending artery—comparison with stenting [Abstract]. Circulation 1996;94(Suppl I):I-258.

300. Chauhan A, Penn IM, Donald RR. Trial of angioplasty and stents in Canada (TASCI): is stent-

mania justified? A sobering insight from TASCI [Abstract]. Circulation 1996;94(Suppl I):I-324.

301. Cukingnan RA, Carey JS, Wittig JH, et al. Influence of complete coronary revascularization on relief of angina. J Thorac Cardiovasc Surg 1980; 79:188–193.

302. Lawrie GM, Morris GC, Silvers A, et al. The influence of residual disease after coronary bypass on the 5-year survival rate of 1274 men with coronary artery disease. Circulation 1982;66:717–723.

303. Jones EL, Craver JM, Guyton RA, et al. Importance of complete revascularization in performance of the coronary bypass operation. Am J Cardiol 1983;51:7–12.

304. Weintraub WS, King SB III, Jones EL, et al. Coronary surgery and coronary angioplasty in patients with two-vessel coronary artery disease. Am J Cardiol 1993;71:511–517.

305. Zhao X, Brown G, Stewart DK, et al. Effectiveness of revascularization in the Emory Angioplasty Versus Surgery Trial. A randomized comparison of coronary angioplasty with bypass surgery. Circulation 1996;93:1954–1962.

306. King SB III, Lembo NJ, Weintraub WS, et al. A randomized trial comparing coronary angioplasty with coronary bypass surgery. N Engl J Med 1994;331:1044–1050.

29

Coronary Atherectomy: Directional, Rotational, and Extraction Techniques

Richard A. Kerensky
Jay D. Schlaifer

INTRODUCTION

Although the exact mechanism of coronary angioplasty is the subject of ongoing debate, it appears that vessel stretching and plaque compression are the major mechanisms of balloon dilation. Thus, the luminal enlargement that occurs with percutaneous transluminal coronary angioplasty (PTCA) is modest, and it is not the result of any actual removal of the plaque. In addition, plaque fracture and dissection are common after balloon angioplasty. A procedure that actually removes plaque from the lumen of the artery, therefore, may have advantages over conventional angioplasty. It is this thinking that led to the development of atherectomy devices, designed to eliminate plaque from the lumen of the artery. Atherectomy procedures are distinctly different from PTCA in terms of mechanism of action and potential complications. The three atherectomy devices approved by the US Food and Drug Administration for use in the coronary arteries are the rotational atherectomy device (Rotablator, Boston Scientific), the directional atherectomy catheter (Atherocath DVI), and the transluminal extraction catheter (TEC) (TEC Interventional Technologies Inc.). The role of each of these catheters in the practice of interventional cardiology re-

mains unclear, and is the subject of ongoing debate. **The success of coronary stenting has reduced the overall use of atherectomy devices in many catheterization laboratories.** Study of the various atherectomy devices has, at least, increased our knowledge of both the mechanisms of coronary luminal enlargement after coronary interventions and the factors contributing to restenosis. Further study of each of these devices is required to determine their value in practice and to determine if theoretic advantages translate into clinical benefit. Continuous modification and refinement of these techniques has made it difficult to draw conclusions from many of the previous clinical trials. It is important, however, that interventional cardiologists objectively evaluate these tools in terms of cost, risk, and efficacy to determine their utility in an interventional practice. In this chapter we review the current knowledge and technical aspects of each of these atherectomy devices.

ROTATIONAL ATHERECTOMY

Basic Concepts

The rotational atherectomy device designed by David Auth works as a high speed rota-

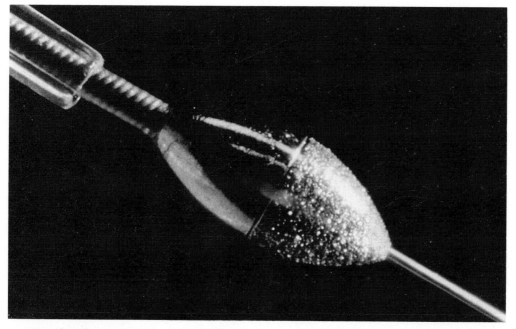

Figure 29.1. Stainless steel rotational atherectomy burr has its leading surface coated with diamond chips ranging in size up to 50 μ. The ablation drill and rotating drive shaft ride coaxially over a 0.009-inch steerable guidewire.

tional "drill" actually pulverizing the plaque, generating small particles that are dispersed distally into the coronary artery (Fig. 29.1). This is an over-the-wire device that is rotated at high speeds (usually 160,000–180,000 rpm) within the coronary artery. The lumen that is created by the use of this device is generally smooth and circular—a "cored out" appearance compared to the intimal disruption created by balloon angioplasty (1–4). The magnitude of luminal enlargement is limited by the relatively small size of the device (maximal burr size 2.5 mm) (5). Continuous saline flushing via an outer sheath extending to just proximal to the burr is used to minimize heat generation.

Differential Cutting and Plaque Ablation

The rotational atherectomy burr has a leading surface coated with diamond chips up to 50 μ (Fig. 29.1) The rotational atherectomy device works by a process called *differential cutting*. Theoretically, the rotating

burr deflects more elastic tissue (less diseased portions of the artery) and selectively drills and ablates the harder atheromatous material (Fig. 29.2). This design has led many operators to use this device as a "niche" device only for lesions that are heavily calcified by either ultrasound or angiography. The atheromatous plaque is pulverized into micro particles (generally under 5 μ) and dispersed into the distal circulation. Recently, increasing interest is found in performing rotational atherectomy in lesions containing soft plaque without calcification (6). In these lesions the differential cutting mechanism would be less important; however, uniform plaque ablation with a smooth circular lumen may offer some advantage.

Theoretic Advantages Over Conventional PTCA

Imaging Studies

Ultrasound, angiographic, and angioscopic studies have shown that after rotational ath-

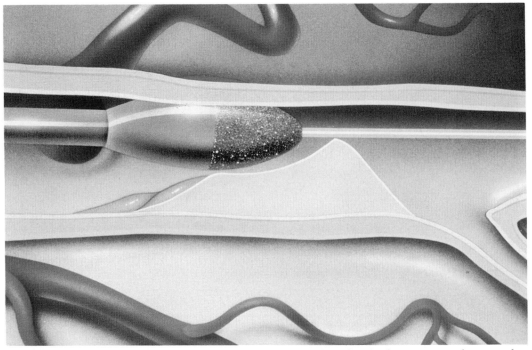

Figure 29.2. The high-speed rotating drill selectively ablates hard atheromatous plaque and relatively spares the softer, less diseased vascular luminal surface.

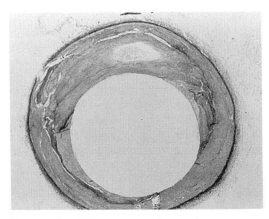

Figure 29.3. Necropsy specimen of a coronary artery following high-speed rotational ablation. The residual lumen appears smooth and circular, lacking the marked stretching and intimal disruption often noted following coronary balloon angioplasty.

erectomy the lumen is generally more circular and smoother than following balloon angioplasty (Fig. 29.3) (1, 2, 4). This is particularly true in the case of heavily calcified lesions, which have a high incidence of dissection with balloon dilation (6, 7). Theoretically, this round smooth lumen after rotational atherectomy may have improved flow characteristics per lumen area compared with the irregular lumen of PTCA. Also, injury of deep wall elements may be less because visually the deep wall appears to be spared with this device. On the other hand, the heat and vibration generated by the rotating burr may have effects on the vascular wall not encountered with conventional angioplasty.

Restenosis

None of the comparative studies or registry data have indicated that rotational atherectomy reduces restenosis compared with PTCA (8–10). However, the technique of rotational atherectomy has been far from standardized in previous studies and early use. Many operators use the device as an adjunct to PTCA (facilitated PTCA), simply debulking a small portion of the lesion before standard balloon dilations. Others have used rotational atherectomy as a "stand-alone" device, trying to achieve as large a lumen as possible with atherectomy and then very low pressure balloon inflations to further smooth the edges of the lumen without any balloon dilation. This aggressive approach of rotational atherectomy has not yet been systematically compared with PTCA or other devices, but trials are currently in progress. If the Rotablator has any potential to reduce restenosis it would appear that this aggressive burr sizing approach would most likely achieve this goal. Theoretically, the relative gain in the caliber of the artery may be achieved with less deep wall injury, reducing late loss in lumen diameter. As noted, however, the early gain in lumen caliber will generally be less with this device because of its relatively small size. Therefore, if restenosis rates are reduced with rotational atherectomy, late loss in lumen diameter will have to be reduced. This strategy is different from all previous strategies to reduce restenosis in which maximizing the initial gain in lumen caliber has been used to "outrun" the restenotic process.

Disadvantages and Complications

Technical Considerations

The technique of rotational atherectomy is markedly different from standard PTCA. Some new operators find the device user friendly; others find it difficult to master. Clearly a learning curve exists, and the aid of an experienced operator is crucial during initial use of the device. In contrast to balloon angioplasty where an experienced assistant is often not required, the help of a second operator familiar and experienced with the device is extremely beneficial during rotational atherectomy. Also, relatively frequent use of the device improves the expertise of the operator and the catheterization staff. Education, updates, and involvement of the catheterization staff in the use of rotational atherectomy will enhance the acceptance of this device into an interven-

tional practice. If complications occur during the first cases in a laboratory starting to use the device, the staff and physicians are often "soured" on its use and may discontinue the program. It is crucial, therefore, that appropriate training is taken prior to starting rotational atherectomy, and that an experienced proctor be involved in the first 5–10 cases. Selecting straightforward cases, with high expected success rates early in the experience, is important to ensure success of the new technique.

Cost

Rotational atherectomy using current technology is more expensive than standard PTCA (11). The cost of the burrs, often only two or more per case, is one factor in the increased cost. Catheterization laboratory time is usually increased compared with standard PTCA, especially early in the experience. The costs rise higher if multiple burrs or other adjunct devices such as stents are used. The use of this device in lesions with lower success rates or higher complication rates with standard PTCA, such as heavily calcified stenosis prone to dissection, could potentially reduce cost in some situations, but this is difficult to demonstrate. Many catheterization and hospital administrators are skeptical about the use of rotational atherectomy because of the perception that the device is costly without proved benefit.

Complications

No-Flow Phenomenon

Absent or markedly reduced distal flow in a coronary artery during intervention, in the absence of obstruction at the target site, is known as the no-flow or slow-flow phenomenon (10). Although, this phenomenon can be seen during balloon angioplasty, especially in patients with acute myocardial infarction (MI) or degenerated saphenous vein grafts (SVG), it is most often seen during rotational atherectomy (11). The mechanism of this phenomenon is not known, but it appears that it is not simply caused by mechanical obstruction of the distal vasculature by the particulate debris generated by the device. As noted, the microparticles generated by this device are smaller than red blood cells, making mechanical obstruction unlikely. Theoretic causes of this problem are platelet aggregation and activation, endothelial dysfunction, and vasospasm. The incidence of the no-flow or slow-flow phenomenon is difficult to determine because of varying definitions and incomplete reporting, but it probably occurs in 7 to 20% of patients undergoing rotational atherectomy (12–14). The incidence seems to have decreased with recent modifications of the technique, especially shorter ablation runs. Often this phenomenon is associated with severe chest discomfort, marked ST changes, arrhythmias, and, in some cases, severe hemodynamic compromise. Treatment, first and foremost, includes discontinuation of the use of the rotational atherectomy device. In addition, inflation of an appropriately sized PTCA balloon at and often distal to the target site seems to speed restoration of flow. Generous administration of intracoronary nitroglycerin is appropriate, depending on the systolic blood pressure. Other vasodilators, such as verapamil or adenosine, have been given, and they appear to be beneficial in some cases (15). Support of the patient with inotropes and intra-aortic balloon pumping is required in a small number of cases (12). "Bailout" stenting or emergent coronary artery bypass graft (CABG) are usually not beneficial, because the problem appears to be in the distal vasculature, and flow is usually not improved after these interventions. Fortunately, flow improves within minutes with medical treatment and balloon dilations in most cases. Various agents have been added to the flush solution administered via the outer Teflon sheath, including nitroglycerin, verapamil, adenosine, and heparin. The benefit of these "cocktails" is unclear. Prevention of this phenomenon is preferable, if at all possible, so that after every atherectomy sequence the flow in the distal vessel should be carefully assessed. If there is any hint of slow flow, then either rotational atherectomy should be stopped or adequate time should be allowed and vasodilators administered to restore flow to normal before proceeding. Patients often experience more chest pain with rotational atherectomy than with standard PTCA, but patients who experience severe pain appear to be at higher risk for the no-flow phenomenon. If severe chest pain occurs during the procedure, then more time should be taken between atherectomy sequences and flow assessed carefully. Use of the IIb/IIIa GP platelet receptor antagonists may reduce the incidence of no flow, but has is yet to be proved. Newer techniques, such as shorter atherectomy runs (15–30 seconds), and allowing less decrement of burr rotational speed (< 5000 rpm decrease), appear to have reduced the incidence of this phenomenon.

Cardiac Enzyme Elevation and Myocardial Infarction

The incidence of a rise in creatine kinase (CK) (> 2–3 × normal) or non–Q-wave myocardial infarction following rotational atherectomy ranges from 0 to 9.4% in a number of reported series (8, 10, 14, 16–18). In the report of the New Approaches to Coronary Intervention (NACI) registry, non–Q-wave MI occurred in 4.9% of the 266 patients undergoing rotational atherectomy (17). Although non–Q-wave MI rates appear higher in some series of patients treated with rotational atherectomy compared with standard PTCA case selection bias, varying definitions of non–Q-wave MI and lack of randomized data make comparison of results impossible. Clearly, more complex lesion morphology is present in many patients selected for treatment with rotational atherectomy, which may explain some of the apparent increase in ischemic complications with rotational atherectomy. MacIsaac et al. showed a trend toward an increase in non–Q-wave MI in patients with calcified versus noncalcified lesions (non–Q-wave MI 10% calcified; 7.7% noncalcified, $P = .054$) treated with rotational atherectomy (6). Long lesions and diffuse

Table 29.1.
Primary Success and Ischemia-Related Complications of Rotational Atherectomy

Report	NACI (17)	Warth et al. (10)	Ellis et al. (14)	Gilmore et al. (20)	Borrione et al. (18)	Guérin et al. (8)
Patients	266	709	316	108	166	32
Type	Registry	Registry	Registry	Single site case series	Single site case series	Randomized trial vs. PTCA
Definition non-Q MI	Not given	Persistent ST Δs or CK > 1.5× Normal †MB	CK > 2× normal ≥ 5% MB	CK > 3× baseline	Increased CK > 200 U/L + MB	CK > 2× normal
Non-Q MI (%)	4.9	5.2[a]	5.7	2.7	8.4	9.4
Q MI(%)	1.5	0.9	2.2	0.9	0.6	3.1
Death (%)	0.8	0.8	0.3	0.9	1.8	0
Procedural success (%)	94.3	94.7	89.8	92	95	94
Restenosis rate (%)	NA	37.7[b]	NA	NA	NA	39%

[a] Incomplete reporting.
[b] 64% angiographic follow-up.
MI, myocardial infarction; CK, creatine kinase; PTCA, percutaneous transluminal angioplasty; NA, not available.

disease are associated with a high incidence of non–Q-wave MI after rotational atherectomy (19). Randomized trials using newer techniques of atherectomy compared with PTCA are needed to assess the relative risk of ischemic complications with rotational atherectomy compared with other techniques.

A Q-wave infarction occurs in 0.9 to 3.3% of patients following rotational atherectomy in most series (10, 14, 16, 18, 20). Hetterich and McEniery reported right ventricular infarction due to occlusion of marginal side branches during successful rotational atherectomy of the right coronary artery (21). Table 29.1 shows the reported postprocedural non–Q-wave and Q-wave myocardial infarction rates for various series reported in the literature.

Coronary Perforation

The risk of coronary perforation is low with the use of rotational atherectomy, but it does occur and is likely under reported. Al-

juni et al. found a 0% incidence of perforations during 116 rotational atherectomy procedures, a 1.3% incidence during TEC, and a 0.25% incidence with directional atherectomy (22). The incidence of coronary perforation in a registry report by Ellis et al. was 1.5% (14). The highest risk for perforation during rotational atherectomy is in patients with severely angulated or branch point stenoses and even in these situations the risk is low with proper technique. A smaller burr size than usual is recommended in severely angulated or bifurcation stenoses.

Wire Fracture

Wire fracture may occur during rotational atherectomy, but it is uncommon. Safian et al. reported wire fracture in 3 of 104 patients (2.8%) undergoing rotational atherectomy (13). The risk of wire fracture is probably greater than for standard PTCA, because of the rotational device. Wire fracture can occur when the device is not coaxial with the artery, especially during atherectomy of right coronary ostial stenoses (23). Therefore, the right anterior oblique (RAO) projection should always be examined prior to activation of the device in ostial right coronary lesions. Wire fracture may also occur if the distal tip of the wire is not free during ablation.

Coronary Dissection

Coronary dissection occurs in approximately 10% of patients undergoing rotational atherectomy (10). The incidence of dissection is highest in American Heart Association/American College of Cardiology (AHA/ACC) type C lesions, where the incidence of dissection after standard PTCA is also highest. Many believe that the incidence of severe dissection is less with rotational atherectomy than with balloon angioplasty, especially in heavily calcified lesions. So-called wire bias may give the angiographic appearance of dissection, when in fact further atherectomy will yield excellent angiographic results. If dissection is encountered during the procedure or is present before the intervention, further ablation should be avoided. Bailout stenting for rotational atherectomy-induced dissections, which has been reported, is often successful (24).

Clinical Results

Primary Success

Primary success rates after rotational atherectomy are comparable to other interventional devices and standard PTCA (10, 14, 16, 18, 20). Greater than 90% primary success rates have been reported in most series. Table 29.1 shows primary success rates of rotational atherectomy in various series.

Complex Lesions and Calcification

In many of the registries' reports and case series, rotational atherectomy is used in more complex lesions than are often approached with standard PTCA. In the NACI registry report, rotational atherectomy was used in vessels with a relatively small reference diameter (2.8 mm) and a high incidence of calcification (49.8%) compared with other devices (17). A number of registry reports and single center series suggest that the complexity of the lesion (i.e., AHA/ACC lesion class) does not affect success rates with rotational atherectomy and that rotational atherectomy may have an advantage over PTCA in complex lesions. Initial experience with this device suggested that it may have a particular advantage over balloon dilation in heavily calcified lesions (17). MacIsaac et al. found primary success rates of 94.3% in calcified and 95.2% in noncalcified arteries in a comparative study from the Multicenter Rotational Atherectomy Registry (6). Major complication rates were similar in the calcified (4.1%) and noncalcified (3.1%) arteries in this nonrandomized comparison. There was, however, a trend toward a higher incidence of non-Q infarction (creatine kinase [CK] rise $> 2.5 \times$ normal) in the calcified (10.0%) versus noncalcified (7.7%) groups. In a randomized pilot study of rotational atherectomy-facilitated angioplasty versus standard balloon angioplasty in AHA/ACC class B2 lesions, Guérin et al. found similar primary success rates with both techniques (93.7% atherectomy and 87.5% PTCA P = NS) (8). A single moderate sized burr with a burr:artery ratio of 0.5:0.7 was used in most of the cases in this study, prior to standard balloon inflations. A stepwise aggressive burr sizing approach was not used. In the ERBAC trial, a randomized study comparing rotational atherectomy, excimer laser, and conventional PTCA in type B and C lesions, procedural success rates were highest in the rotational atherectomy (RA) group (91% RA versus 80% PTCA $P < .001$) (25). Again, the technique for rotational atherectomy varied in this trial, but most of the time a single moderate sized burr was used followed by balloon dilation. These data suggest that RA may offer an advantage in terms of procedural success in patients with calcified arteries, particularly smaller arteries prone to dissection. However, much of the data are nonrandomized, and variations in atherectomy technique make the data from these series difficult to interpret. We believe that heavy lesion calcification either by ultrasound or fluoroscopy is a relatively strong indication for the use of the rotational atherectomy device, particularly in vessels too small for coronary stenting. The current practice in many catheterization laboratories is to reserve the use of this device for heavily calcified stenoses (17). Intracoronary ultrasound use to detect lesion calcification prior to intervention is reviewed in Chapter 18.

Special Patient Groups

Rotational atherectomy has been used successfully in a number of relatively uncommon situations encountered in an interventional practice, including anomalous coronary arteries, distal saphenous vein graft anastomosis, undilatable lesions, and protected left main stenoses (24, 26–28). Many operators have performed rotational atherectomy successfully in patients with in-stent restenosis. Rotational atherectomy seems to effectively ablate restenotic lesions caused by intimal hyperplasia within well-expanded stents. The long-term success of RA for in-stent restenosis is not known.

Restenosis

There are no data to suggest that rotational atherectomy reduces the restenosis rate compared with balloon angioplasty or other devices. The few trials comparing RA and balloon angioplasty have shown similar restenosis rates (Table 29.1) (8, 10, 25). Many of the patients included in these series actually had rotational atherectomy-facilitated angioplasty so it is not surprising that the restenosis rates are so similar to PTCA. A number of trials comparing aggressive RA without adjunctive PTCA and conventional PTCA are ongoing. Because the acute luminal gain achieved with current burr sizes is moderate compared with stenting or directional atherectomy, any advantage that RA may have in terms of restenosis will have

to be because of a reduction in late loss. It remains to be seen if this device can remove plaque without deep wall injury because of heat, vibration, or other factors perhaps not apparent by ultrasound, angioscopy, or angiography.

Rotational Atherectomy Technique

Equipment

Guiding Catheters and Wires

The guiding catheters used in rotational atherectomy are the same as those used for balloon angioplasty. In general, rotational atherectomy does not require the guiding catheter "back-up" or support that is necessary for PTCA, but it is important that the guide "fit" the artery reasonably well to avoid acute angles when advancing the burr. Left coronary guides with gentler Judkins-type curves similar to left coronary directional atherectomy guides may make advancing the burr through the guide easier. The size of the guiding catheter required depends on the anticipated largest burr size to be used. Table 29.2 shows the minimal internal diameter and suggested guiding catheter sizes for the various burr sizes.

The wire used for rotational atherectomy is stiffer and less steerable than standard angioplasty guidewires. Until recently the diameter of the wire was 0.09 inches for most of its length, with a 0.017-inch distal flexible tip. The tips come in different stiffnesses from floppy (type C) to standard

Table 29.2.
Guiding Catheter Selection Based on Anticipated Burr Size for Rotational at Atherectomy

Internal Diameter	French Size (Large Lumen)	Maximal Burr Size
0.086	8	2.15
0.096	9	2.25
0.107	10	2.5

(type A). The type A wire was rarely used. Rotational atherectomy wires require a somewhat different advancement technique than do PTCA wires. The wire is steered with an external clip-on steering device rather than with a slide on a tighten-down device. The operator must shape the wire with a generous curve similar to the curve of a PTCA wire, with care being taken not to stretch the flexible tip. Wire advancement may take slightly more forward pressure than angioplasty wires; however, the wire should not be forced forward. Subtle steering turns often rotate the tip. Advancement of the free wire may be difficult in tortuous calcified coronary arteries. If the wire cannot be advanced, we frequently use a floppy PTCA wire to cross the lesion and then use a 0.018-inch internal diameter exchange or balloon catheter to place the rotational atherectomy wire in the distal vessel. The wire tip must be free in the distal vessel to avoid wire fracture. Alternatively, an exchange catheter (i.e., Buchbinder, Boston Scientific, Boston, MA) can be used to help steer the RA wire, which may be difficult to steer as a free wire. Recently, the design and terminology for the rotational atherectomy wire has changed. A more steerable and floppy version of the wire, RotoWire Floppy, has been developed. This wire has a smaller distal tip, so a 0.014-inch diameter catheter is all that is required for exchange. Although this wire is more steerable, it does not provide quite the support of the type C wire. The type C wire has been redesigned slightly; it has a 0.014-inch diameter tip and is now called the RotoWire Extra Support. **The most appropriate use of the new floppy wire is not clear.** Operators familiar with the type C wire must be aware that this new floppy wire does not provide strong support to direct the burr through the lesion, and the burr may tend to deviate "off line" in tortuous vessels. The risk of vessel perforation with this floppy wire may limit its use in vessels with marked angulation proximal to the lesion.

Power Source and Console

The rotational atherectomy burr is powered by a compressed gas-driven turbine that provides the rotary power. The drill speed is controlled by air pressure, which is measured and displayed by a fiberoptic digital tachometer. The speed of the device is displayed on the front of the power console. A foot pedal allows rapid activation and deactivation of the device. The rotational speed of the burr is adjusted by an assistant by turning the rpm control knob while observing the digital tachometer. Care must be taken to ensure that the tubing connecting the atherectomy device to the air power source is not kinked during connection. The gas reservoir (air tanks) should be checked prior to each case to ensure adequate gas pressure. The mode of the device is changed by a button control on the foot pedal and is displayed on the control panel. The atherectomy mode is for burr advancement whereas the dynaglide mode is for burr removal. The burr should never be advanced while in the dynaglide mode.

Rotational Atherectomy Device (Burr Selection)

The selection of burr size has been one of the major factors contributing to the widely variable technique of rotational atherectomy. Some operators intentionally undersize the burr ($\leq$ 0.6 burr:artery ratio), use a single burr, and then perform rotational atherectomy facilitated angioplasty. Other operators aggressively size the final burr (0.7–0.9 burr:artery ratio) and use a stepwise approach with multiple burrs. The operator should formulate a strategy of burr sizing prior to the procedure so that the maximal burr size to be used can be estimated. This is crucial because the larger burrs require larger guiding catheters. For example, if the target lesion is in a vessel with a reference segment of 3.25 mm and the operator is planning aggressive rotational atherectomy with a final burr:artery ratio of 0.8, the final burr size anticipated is 2.5 mm. This will require a 10 F guiding catheter, so the case would begin with a 10 F guide. During the procedure, the operator may decide to use a smaller final burr size if difficulties develop at smaller burr sizes;

but if a large burr is planned at the beginning of the case, an appropriately sized guide should be chosen. For an aggressive atherectomy strategy using a burr:artery ratio of greater than 0.8, we use a multiple burr strategy. In the example above with an estimated final burr size of 2.5 mm, we would begin with a 1.5-mm burr, followed by a 2.0-mm burr, and then if the case is proceeding as planned, the 2.5-mm burr. In general, we do not increase the size of the burr by more than 0.5 mm per burr except in straight forward lesions (i.e., short, moderately calcified) in large vessels (see *Atherectomy Strategies* below).

Patient Preparation

Prior to rotational atherectomy, patients should be prepared in a similar fashion to patients undergoing coronary angioplasty. Aspirin should be administered to all patients except those with true anaphylaxis who cannot be desensitized. Antianginal medications should be continued; many operators prefer to begin calcium antagonists in those patients not already receiving them. Large doses of intracoronary nitroglycerin are given during the procedure, so patients should be well hydrated to avoid hypotension. Volume depletion is a common problem in patients not permitted oral intake for procedures. Informed consent should be obtained for both rotational atherectomy and coronary angioplasty, and patients should be informed why rotational atherectomy was chosen over other techniques.

Patient and Lesion Selection

The use of rotational atherectomy instead of other revascularization techniques requires consideration of a number of factors. First, RA should only be used when it is felt to have an advantage over other percutaneous interventional techniques. Although there are few randomized data, it appears that rotational atherectomy may have an advantage in heavily calcified lesions, ostial steno-

Table 29.3.
Contraindications to Rotational Atherectomy

1	Angiographic evidence of thrombus pretreatment
2	Dissection at treatment site
3	Ejection fraction < 30%
4	Target vessel supplying ≥ 50% of viable myocardium
5	Unprotected left main stenosis
6	Saphenous vein graft stenosis
7	Inability to pass guidewire

ses (especially those that are calcified), and longer lesions (20–30 mm)—especially those in smaller vessels. Other possible indications for RA are restenosis within Palmaz-Schatz (Johnson and Johnson Interventional Systems, Warren, NJ) stents and stenoses at bifurcations with varying degrees of involvement of side branches. We use rotational atherectomy in many of the above lesions when there are no contraindications to its use. The relative contraindications to RA are shown in Table 29.3. Most operators avoid the use of rotational atherectomy in patients with acute ischemic syndromes or with angiographic or ultrasound evidence of lesion-associated thrombus because of the risk of the no-flow or slow-flow phenomenon in these patients. Similarly, culprit lesions of recent myocardial infarction are usually avoided. We have performed RA in the culprit lesion of recent myocardial infarction when the vessel was heavily calcified. In this situation, we perform the procedure more than 10 days after the acute event, and do not proceed if there is angiographic evidence of thrombus on the guiding angiograms. Patients with severe left ventricular dysfunction are not good candidates for RA, and many operators avoid patients with ejection fractions less than 30%. Also of concern is the situation in which the target vessel supplies the only source of collaterals to a second vascular distribution, and generally this vessel should be avoided. Vessels with poor distal flow at baseline also should be approached with caution with this device. Some operators employ this device for patients with long lesions, but complication rates clearly increase with increased lesion length (14). Recently there has been interest in rotational atherectomy for in-stent restenosis. This approach seems to be safe when adequate stent expansion is documented with intracoronary ultrasound. Excellent angiographic and intracoronary ultrasound results have been obtained in patients with intimal hyperplasia within stents treated with RA. Although nearly complete removal of the in-stent plaque is often achieved, restenosis rate is not known.

Temporary Pacing

Because of a high incidence of bradycardia caused by transient complete atrioventricular (AV) block, a temporary pacemaker should be placed in all patients undergoing rotational atherectomy of the right coronary artery. Heart block generally occurs shortly after engagement of the lesion with the rotating burr, and it usually resolves within 30 seconds of each ablation. Pretreatment with atropine and theophylline decreases the incidence of bradyarrythmias, but prophylactic pacing is still required. Prophylactic pacing is not required during atherectomy of the left coronary artery, but a venous sheath should be placed in case urgent pacing is necessary.

Anticoagulation and Vasodilator Treatment

A number of different intraprocedure regimens of anticoagulation and vasodilators aimed at preventing the no-flow phenomenon and other ischemic complications have been tried during rotational atherectomy. The efficacy of these various "cocktails" is not known. Calcium antagonists, nitroglycerin, adenosine, and heparin have been added to the saline flush solution that infuses through the sheath around the device. Alternatively, nitroglycerin can be administered via the guiding catheter at various times during the procedure. Heparin should be administered to elevate the activated clotting time (ACT) to more than 350 seconds as with any coronary intervention. The use of IIb/IIIa GP platelet receptor inhibitors may be helpful during RA considering the impressive results with these agents during balloon angioplasty and directional atherectomy (29, 30). It is not known, however, if platelet receptor antagonists will have similar effects during rotational atherectomy.

Burr Placement

Once the atherectomy wire is in position across the lesion, the burr is removed from its package and connected to the power source, the tachometer, and the outer sheath flush system. The device is then backloaded onto the wire and advanced to just outside of the rotating hemostatic valve. The clip is placed on the wire and the device is activated outside of the body. An assistant adjusts the speed of the device to the appropriate level (160,000–180,000 rpms). At this time, the wire brake is checked by pulling back on the wire. If the brake is functioning properly the wire will not move while the device is activated. Also, the flush is checked to ensure it is flowing at high rate during activation of the device. Once the system is checked, the device is advanced through the guide over the wire into the proximal vessel while it is inactivated. The technique for advancing the device is much different than advancing an angioplasty balloon. The assistant at the distal end of the device holds the guidewire and pulls vigorously on the wire, pulling the device forward. The front operator at the guiding catheter simply applies gentle forward pressure on the device, but most of the advancement comes from the pulling action of the back assistant. When the curved portion of the guide or a tortuous portion of the vessel is encountered, a fairly vigorous pulling action is needed to advance the catheter forward. This is usually accomplished by applying vigorous tension and intermittently releasing the tension, allowing the catheter to move slowly forward. Once the burr is in location proximal to the target lesion, it is important that the tension built up within the catheter is released so that the burr will not abruptly "jump" forward when the device is activated. This is done by loosening the rotating hemostatic valve and shaking both the device and the advancement control. Care should be taken not to nose the device into the lesion prior to activation, but instead to keep it well proximal to the lesion in a relatively disease-free segment where it will be activated and then advanced.

Ablation

Recently, the technique of atherectomy has been somewhat modified by decreasing both the time of each ablation run and the amount of decrease in rpms accepted as the lesion is engaged with the burr. After the burr is in position in the proximal artery and the tension in the catheter is released, the device is activated by the operator using the foot pedal. The technologist assisting then adjusts the speed control to the desired rpm. At this point, the device is gently advanced into the lesion using the advancing control knob. Care is taken not to let the rpm decrease by more than 5000 rpm during any ablation. Generally, short runs of 15 to 30 seconds are being used by many experienced operators with 1–2 minutes between ablations. Accordingly, it may take a number of ablations to advance the burr through the lesion into the distal vessel. The device should always be retracted into the proximal vessel and out of the lesion before it is deactivated. Once the lesion has been completely crossed with the device, the system is switched to dynaglide mode, and the device is turned on and gently retracted over the wire out of the guiding catheter. A second larger burr can be loaded onto the wire after the first is removed or balloon dilations can be performed.

Wire "Bias"

Wire "bias" is a term used to describe a phenomenon in which the relatively stiff atherectomy wire directs the burr to remove one portion of the plaque more vigorously than another. Wire bias may override the property of differential cutting because of the stiffness of the wire. For example, if the wire is pulled snugly against the inner curve of a vessel, the burr will tend to remove plaque along the inner curve more so than plaque along the outer curve. Wire bias may cause an unusual "burrowed out" appearance to the lesion, especially after small burrs, that can resemble dissections. Wire bias can be used to the operator's advantage to direct the burr to an eccentric lesion if the wire can be positioned in such a way that the path of the wire favors ablation of the eccentric plaque. The concept of wire bias is an oversimplification because angiographic estimates of eccentricity are frequently incorrect and estimates of plaque location by angiography are often inaccurate. Ultrasound studies are likely to define more clearly the concept of wire bias during rotational atherectomy. Operators, however, should be aware of this phenomenon and assess the path of the wire through the lesion prior to burr advancement.

Atherectomy Strategies

A number of rotational atherectomy strategies have been described in the literature. These range from a single burr with a small burr:artery ratio of 0.5 to 0.7 ratio (lesion debulking to facilitate PTCA) with standard balloon inflations to multiple burrs with large burr:artery ratios ($\geq$ 0.8) and no adjunctive PTCA.

When using the device as a debulking tool, a small single burr with a burr:artery ratio of 0.5 to 0.7 may be used to enlarge the lumen prior to balloon dilations (16, 31, 32). Guerin et al. compared this small burr approach followed by balloon dilation to standard PTCA in American College of Cardiology/American Heart Association (ACC/AHA) type B2 stenosis (8). In this randomized trial including 64 patients, the investigators found no advantage of the rotational atherectomy-facilitated angioplasty over standard PTCA. Primary success rates were high in both groups (94% RA versus 88% PTCA, P = NS). Restenosis rates were no different between the two strategies (39% RA versus 42% PTCA, P = NS).

Probably the most commonly employed use of rotational atherectomy is an approach using multiple burrs with a final burr:artery ratio of approximately 0.7–0.8. If the residual stenosis following atherectomy exceeds 30%, or there is irregularity or haziness at the lesion site, balloon dilations are performed to further enlarge the lumen (1, 2, 13, 14, 20). Using this strategy, approximately 70 to 80% of patients will have balloon dilations and most lesions will require at least two atherectomy burrs. In some cases, low-pressure balloon inflations are performed to simply "smooth" the plaque edges; in other cases, actual balloon dilation is performed. Thus, the patients treated in these series represent a "mixed bag" with varying degrees of actual atherectomy or balloon dilation as the primary mechanism of luminal enlargement in each case. Although this technique has yielded high initial success rates, no evidence shows that restenosis rates are reduced using this strategy. In fact, because balloon dilation is frequently used in these patients, it is not surprising that restenosis rates are not different from PTCA alone.

Recently there has been increased interest in more aggressive burr sizing strategies in an attempt to maximize the luminal gain from atherectomy and eliminate the need for adjunctive balloon dilations. Hope exists that, with this approach, some additional benefit in terms of restenosis may be achieved by avoiding balloon injury. This strategy is somewhat limited by the smaller size of even the largest burr (2.5 mm), leading to residual postintervention stenoses in patients with arteries larger than 3.25–3.5 mm. Theoretically, this aggressive burr sizing strategy could lead to improved results because of the smooth round lumen obtained with rotational atherectomy, even if the initial gain in lumen size is modest compared with stenting, or optimal with directional atherectomy. Trials of this more aggressive burr sizing approach are ongoing. The dilation versus ablation revascularization (DART) trial will compare standard PTCA versus aggressive ablation with burr: artery ratios of 0.7–0.9 in type A and B1 lesions. Aggressive ablation will be followed by low pressure (< 1 atm) oversized balloon inflation. Planned enrollment is 1000 pa-

tients with a restenosis substudy in 500 patients. The study to determine Rotablator and transluminal angioplasty strategy (STRATUS) will compare two different rotational atherectomy strategies. An aggressive strategy will employ a burr:artery ratio of 0.7–0.9, either as a stand-alone procedure or followed by less than 1 atm balloon inflations, compared with a strategy using a burr:artery ratio of 0.6–0.8 followed by routine postablation balloon inflations of 4 atm or more. Planned enrollment is 500 patients.

Combination With Other Devices

Directional Atherectomy

In a number of reports of the combined use of rotational and directional atherectomy in calcified stenoses, directional atherectomy was used instead of balloon dilation as an adjunct to rotational atherectomy (33, 34). These studies show that pretreatment with RA allows the use of directional atherectomy in calcified stenoses that otherwise would not be amenable to the directional atherectomy. The luminal gain with adjunctive directional atherectomy appears greater than that with PTCA. Further evaluation and randomized trials of this combined atherectomy technique are needed to determine if there is long-term advantage. Certainly procedural costs should be considered when evaluating this combined technique.

Coronary Stenting

Coronary stenting can be performed as an adjunct to rotational atherectomy to maximize postprocedural increase in luminal gain. Rotational atherectomy probably improves acute angiographic results with coronary stenting in some heavily calcified vessels in which stent deployment would be suboptimal if debulking was not accomplished prior to stenting.

Rotational atherectomy is often used in conjunction with balloon angioplasty for aorto-ostial lesions (35, 36). Many operators prefer RA with coronary stenting in patients with calcified ostial stenoses, especially of the right coronary artery. Acute angiographic results are usually excellent with this approach, but long-term follow-up data and restenosis rates are lacking.

Future Directions

The challenges for rotational atherectomy are to (*a*) standardize and optimize procedural technique based on the results of ongoing trials; (*b*) reduce procedural costs using replaceable burrs or other technical advancements; and (*c*) reduce complications, especially the no-reflow phenomenon. The role of rotational atherectomy in future interventional strategies depends, in large part, on the successful resolution of the problems discussed above.

Conclusions

Rotational atherectomy uses the property of differential cutting to ablate plaque from coronary arteries. Because of its unique mechanism of action this device has potential advantages over other interventional tools. Its use has been proved mostly in the treatment of heavily calcified stenoses that are undilatable or prone to severe dissection with other devices. Primary success rates with this device, comparable or superior to PTCA, are possible in certain complex lesions using this technique. Use of this device varies widely from an adjunctive debulking tool to a stand-alone interventional tool. Restenosis rates are similar to PTCA. The optimal strategy for the use of this device needs further clarification. Trials are ongoing to assess optimal burr:artery ratios, adjunctive balloon dilation, and other technical questions. Whether the theoretic advantages of rotational atherectomy will translate into benefit for a variety of patient and lesion subsets requires randomized trials with standardized techniques. Therefore, the role of this device in an interventional practice currently is not clearly defined.

DIRECTIONAL CORONARY ATHERECTOMY

The concept of **directional coronary atherectomy (DCA), a nonsurgical technique to remove atheroma** rather than compress it, was first pioneered by John Simpson in the early 1980s to overcome some of the complications of PTCA and perhaps reduce restenosis (37). It was hypothesized that atherectomy would provide a larger and smoother surfaced lumen with less dissection and thrombus formation, result in less stimulation of smooth muscle cell proliferation, and prevent the elastic recoil seen with PTCA.

The initial prototype was designed to emulate the mechanism of a Cope pleural biopsy needle and subsequently underwent multiple design modifications. Initial testing was performed in peripheral vessels in the intraoperative setting, but not until the guiding catheters were redesigned to accommodate the stiff cutting device could atherectomy be considered for the coronary arteries. In 1990, after premarket clinical trials were performed, DCA became the first nonsurgical coronary revascularization technique approved by the US Federal Drug Administration since PTCA. Over the course of the last 6 years, a number of studies have been performed to look at the effects of DCA on safety, acute outcome, and restenosis rates. Recent advances in intravascular ultrasound imaging have also provided much data regarding the mechanism of DCA and the type of lesions most appropriate for this technique.

DCA Equipment

Simpson Coronary Atherocath

The Simpson Coronary Atherocath (SA) is the most commonly used coronary atherectomy catheter (Fig. 29.4). The SA is designed as a side cutter enclosed in a housing to permit directional excision of the atheroma by

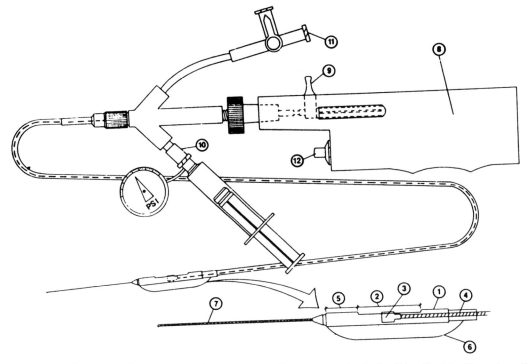

Figure 29.4. Simpson atherectomy catheter system. Components include: (*1*) cylindrical housing, (*2*) longitudinal opening, (*3*) cutter, (*4*) cutter drive cable (to motor), (*5*) specimen collection area, (*6*) balloon support mechanism, (*7*) fixed guidewire, (*8*) motor, (*9*) cutter-advance level, (*10*) balloon inflation port, (*11*) flush port, and (*12*) on-off switch for motor. PSI, pressure per square inch. (From Simpson JB, Selmon MR, Robertson GC, et al. Transluminal atherectomy for occlusive peripheral vascular disease. Am J Cardiol 1988;61:96G–101G. Reprinted with permission of the American Journal of Cardiology.)

aiming the cutter window toward the diseased segment. The housing is a metal cylindrical chamber 17 mm in length, with a rectangular window approximately 10 mm in length. The cutter rotates within the housing at approximately 2000 rpms. A low-pressure, noncompliant balloon is positioned 180° opposite the window to anchor the device and allow part of the lesion to protrude into the window. At the distal tip of the device is a more flexible nose cone that serves to collect the atheromatous debris and prevent distal embolization. It also allows retrial of the atheroma for examination and histologic analysis. The catheter shaft is 125 cm in length with a diameter of 2.3 mm (7 F), except for the distal 10 cm, which tapers to 6 F. The drive cable that rotates the cutter extends the length of the catheter and has a central lumen that accommodates a 0.014-inch guidewire. The drive cable is connected proximally to the

motor drive unit (MDU), which is battery operated and contains the on/off switch for the cutter. The proximal end of the catheter also has a rotator and an adaptor with two ports. The proximal port is fitted with a one-way valve and permits flushing with saline; the distal port is the balloon inflation/deflation port.

Catheters are available in four sizes (5, 6, 7, and 7 F graft); selection is based on the size of the vessel. It is recommended that the size of the catheter be decreased by one French size when any of the following characteristics are present in the target vessel: calcification, evidence of noncompliance, tortuosity, severe lesion angulation, distal vessel, or ostial location. As a general rule, we use a 7 F device if the vessel is 3 mm or greater. If the vessel is less than 3 mm, we often start with a 6 F cutter. The SA-EX catheter has replaced the SA-LP design, and it is equipped with a longer, more tapered tip to facilitate tracking in tortuous or non-compliant vessels.

Guiding Catheters

The guiding catheter required for directional atherectomy has been specifically designed to accommodate the large and rigid SA. The distal curve of the guide catheter is shaped like a large semicircle to provide good support for effective delivery of the device to the coronary artery. Currently, guide catheters come in three sizes (9.5 F for right coronary artery and 10 or 11 F for the left coronary artery) with 11 different tip shapes (Fig. 29.5, 29.6). The large diameter of the catheters mandates the use of soft, atraumatic tips and sideholes. The guides are 100 cm in length and have an internal diameter larger than 0.104 in. Either a 7 or 8 F introducer is used in association with the guide catheter to straighten the curve and prevent catheter kinking while it is advanced through the vascular sheath and into the ascending aorta.

DCA Technique

Catheter Advancement

With the cutter advanced distally and locked in place on the MDU, the SA can be

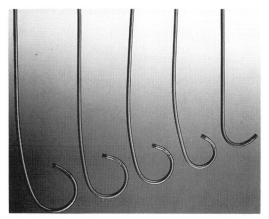

Figure 29.6. Directional coronary atherectomy (DCA) guiding catheters for use in native left coronary artery procedures are available in 10 and 11 F sizes. Five tip shapes are available for various aortic root sizes and anatomic takeoffs. *Left to right,* JL 5.0, JL 4.5, JL 4.0, JL 3.5, JL GRF.

advanced through the guide catheter over a 0.014-inch guidewire. Prior to advancing the catheter into the coronary artery, it is important that the distal guidewire be free of side branches because it rotates when the cutter is turned on. Because of the large profile of these catheters, the guide catheter should be optimally aligned coaxially with the vessel. Occasionally it is necessary to predilate the lesion using a 2.0-mm or less balloon prior to DCA to advance the device through the lesion. However, excessive predilation may interfere with maximal tissue retrieval with DCA. In the initial US Multicenter Registry, 20% of the lesions required predilation as did 15% of lesions in the CAVEAT I trial (54). With increased operator experience, it appears the need for predilation decreases.

Directional Atherectomy Technique

Following the placement of the device across the stenosis, the cutting chamber window is positioned facing the atheroma and the balloon is initially inflated using low pressure (5–15 psi) to minimize compressive effects and avoid deep cuts into the

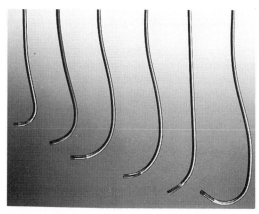

Figure 29.5. Directional coronary athrectomy guiding catheters (9.5 F) for use in native right coronary artery procedures. There are six tip shapes for various anatomic takeoffs. *Left to right,* Hockey stick, JR 4.0ST, JR 4.0, JR 4.0 inferior, multipurpose, JR GRF.

media. The cutter is then retracted and activated, followed by the slow advancement of the rotating cutter. The atheroma is excised and displaced into the nose cone. The MDU is turned off and the balloon deflated. The atherectomy device can then be reoriented, and the procedure repeated six to eight times before the device is removed from the coronary artery. The lesion is assessed angiographically and, if the result is not adequate, further cuts can be made using higher balloon inflation pressures (up to 60 psi) or a larger device. Adjunctive balloon PTCA can follow DCA to optimize results with or without the use of intravascular ultrasound to guide the intervention.

Mechanisms of Lumen Enlargement with DCA

Tissue Removal

Directional coronary atherectomy was designed for plaque removal to provide a smoother and larger lumen and thus decrease acute complication and restenosis rates. However, excision of atheroma is not the only mechanism responsible for lumen enlargement with DCA. Early observational studies of DCA noted the removal of only 18–20 mg of tissue using the SA, despite reduction in diameter stenosis from 80 to 5% and an increase in minimal lumen diameter from 0.6 to 2.9 mm. This degree of lumen enlargement should yield approximately 70 mg of tissue if the angiographic improvement was entirely due to plaque removal. Therefore, the remainder of the lumen enlargement must be secondary to mechanical dilation, either from a "Dotter" effect caused by the catheter or stretch from the low-pressure inflation used to anchor the cutter (38, 39). Using area-length calculations of volumetric lumen changes following intervention, it initially appeared that the major mechanism of DCA was vessel stretching. Penny et al. (39) hypothesized that discrete atherectomy cuts that extend to or through the internal or external elastic lamina increase the radial compliance of the vessel, therefore facilitating its mechanical

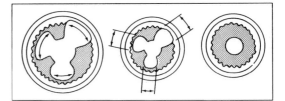

Figure 29.7. Mechanism of vessel expansion with directional coronary atherectomy. Discrete atherectomy cuts extend through the internal elastic lamina (*wavy line*), altering the radial compliance of the vessel. Further expansion can then occur following balloon angioplasty, preferentially at the bases of the original atherectomy cuts, providing a smooth lumen without dissection. (Reprinted with permission from Penny WF, Schmidt DA, Safian RD, et al. Insights into the mechanism of luminal improvement after directional coronary atherectomy. Am J Cardiol 1991;67:435–437.)

expansion, preferentially at the bases of the cuts (Fig. 29.7). This may account for the smooth angiographic appearance following atherectomy in contrast to balloon angioplasty, which transmits pressure indiscriminately, resulting in dissection. It may also account for the decrease in elastic recoil observed following DCA (40).

Ultrasound Studies

Intravascular ultrasound provides a unique opportunity to visualize the vessel wall in a tomographic cross-sectional view, providing accurate calculations of both lumen and plaque areas. Tenaglia et al. compared post-interventional results following PTCA and DCA using ultrasound (41). Following intervention, minimal lumen dimensions as well as percent of area narrowing were similar in patients undergoing PTCA and DCA. Dissection was identified in 50% of patients undergoing PTCA compared with only 8% of patients undergoing DCA (*P* < .01). Although the lumen plus plaque area (area inside the internal elastic lamina) was significantly greater at the treatment site compared with the reference segment site in patients undergoing PTCA, it was not significantly different between the treatment and reference sites in the DCA group. This suggests that vessel stretch is a major mechanism in PTCA, but not with DCA, contrasting with angiographic studies. Similar observations have been reported in other mechanistic studies of DCA using ultrasound before and after intervention (42–44). These studies demonstrated that 61 to 87% of lumen enlargement with DCA was due to plaque removal whereas only 13 to 39% of lumen gain was secondary to vessel expansion or stretch. Although vessel stretch appears to play a lesser role in DCA than in balloon angioplasty, angioscopic indices of intimal injury were similar in both treatment groups (44). Plaque reduction was more commonly seen when DCA was done in ultrasound-defined eccentric stenoses (42).

Although plaque removal appears to be the major mechanism of DCA and one typically sees angiographic reductions in percent of vessel stenosis from 70 to 19%, plaque area stenosis is only reduced from 83 to 61%. Only an average of 2.5 mm^2 of atheroma is removed, and a large plaque burden generally remains after DCA (43). DCA does not appear to cut atheroma uniformly, creating an eccentric morphology despite rotating the cutter radially and using intravascular ultrasound to redirect the device. Nakamura et al. (43) hypothesize that once the initial cut is made in the atheroma, the cutter may keep slipping back into the same trough previously created, limiting plaque removal. Plaque removal and final lumen area is also limited by the extent of superficial calcification. Lesions with 90° or greater arc of superficial calcification identified by intravascular ultrasound had significantly greater residual plaque and smaller residual lumens than did lesions with either less than 90° arc of calcium or no calcium (40).

Results

Immediate Outcome

Since its early use, atherectomy has been associated with a high degree of angiographic success. In the preapproval US Multicenter DCA Registry (45), the overall primary success rate—defined as less than 50% final stenosis—and the absence of a major complication (death, Q-wave infarction, or emergent bypass surgery) was 85% for 1015 lesions undergoing DCA. Of the DCA failures, most occurred because of failure to cross the target lesion with the atherectomy device. Primary success was highest in the proximal (not ostial) left anterior descending artery, in lesions less than 20 mm long, in restenosis lesions, and in noncalcified lesions. Similar findings have been reported in a number of subsequent observational studies demonstrating a primary angiographic success rate of 87 to 95% using DCA (40, 46–49). Hinohara et al. (46) reported a mean reduction in coronary stenosis from 75 to 13%, with less than 20% residual stenosis obtained in 79% of lesions. Again, the success rates were significantly higher and the complication rates lower for restenotic lesions compared with de novo lesions. The success rate was less than 80% in calcified lesions or in vessels that demonstrated significant tortuosity and more than 80% in eccentric, ostial, or irregular lesions.

Further clinical experience has identified a number of morphologic and clinical factors influencing the procedural outcome using DCA. Ellis et al. (47) showed that lesion success and complications were closely correlated with the ACC/AHA Task Force lesion morphological criteria similar to angioplasty. Class A stenoses were associated with 93% success rate and 3% complication rate; class B1 lesions, 88% success and 6% complication rates; and type B2 lesions, 75% success and 13% complication rates. Bend stenoses, proximal tortuosity, preatherectomy MLD, and lesion calcification were independent predictors of adverse outcome. Additionally, prior restenosis and complex, thrombus-containing lesions were independent predictors of successful DCA.

Angulated lesions, vessel tortuosity, and preatherectomy MLD are associated more with the success of delivering the atherectomy device to the lesion than with ability to remove plaque. Lesion length more than 10 mm and lesion calcification are significantly correlated with smaller final luminal cross-sectional areas (50). Robertson et al.

(51) compared the success rates of DCA in lesions with (n = 149) and without (n = 490) calcification and found that the success rate was significantly decreased in the presence of calcium (73% versus 93%). In fact, intravascular ultrasound studies show that the arc of superficial calcium measured is the single most consistent lesion characteristic that predicts DCA results (40, 52). Larger atherectomy catheter size has also been shown to be an independent predictor of percent of plaque volume removal, whereas atherectomy balloon pressure was not predictive (50, 52).

Comparison with PTCA

In 1993, the results of two large, multicenter, randomized trials were reported comparing PTCA and DCA. The Canadian Coronary Atherectomy Trial (CCAT) enrolled 274 patients with de novo lesions 60% or greater stenosis in the proximal one third (but not ostial) of the left anterior descending (LAD) artery (53). The CAVEAT enrolled 1012 patients from 35 centers who had 60% or greater diameter stenosis in any native coronary artery suitable for DCA or PTCA (54). Both trials showed that atherectomy was associated with a greater degree of initial angiographic success, defined as residual stenosis less than 50%, compared with angioplasty (98 versus 91% for CCAT; 89 versus 80% for CAVEAT). Compared with PTCA, atherectomy resulted in significantly greater initial lumen gain (1.02 mm versus 0.87 mm, $P = .0001$), larger lumen dimensions (1.88 versus 1.71 mm), and lower percent stenosis (33 versus 40%). However, the improvement in angiographic success seen with atherectomy in CAVEAT was associated with a significantly higher periprocedural complication rate than seen with conventional angioplasty (11 versus 5%). No difference was found in in-hospital mortality, but there was a trend toward a higher need for emergency bypass surgery (3.7% for DCA and 2.2% for PTCA) and a significantly greater incidence of abrupt closure and myocardial infarction with atherectomy. The increase in myocardial infarction with DCA was attributed primarily to an increase in non–Q-wave infarctions (19 versus 8%). In CCAT, no difference was found in complication rates between the two treatment strategies. However, this was a much smaller trial limited to proximal LAD stenosis, whereas CAVEAT included lesions in any native coronary segment, which may account for the discrepancy in complications.

Complications

The complications of DCA are similar to that seen with coronary balloon angioplasty. When combining a large number of single and multicenter studies of DCA, an estimated overall major complication (death, emergent bypass surgery, or Q–wave-myocardial infarction) rate of 0.5 to 11% is seen (46–49). The estimated rate of death is 0 to 3%, with more than 50% of the deaths felt to be directly attributable to DCA in the DVI multicenter registry. Q-wave myocardial infarctions occur in 2% or fewer cases, similar to the reported incidence in the PTCA arm of CAVEAT. The most common major complication is emergent bypass surgery occurring in 0.5 to 5.5% atherectomy procedures. In the DVI registry there was a 3.8% referral for emergent bypass surgery (46). Fifty-seven percent of cases were referred secondary to flow obstruction at the atherectomy site, 9% because of perforation, 13% guide catheter dissections, 8% device-related complications, and 11% PTCA-related complications. Lesions with ulceration or dissection appear to be at highest risk for requiring emergency surgery. With the increased use of intravascular ultrasound guidance to avoid deep cuts in normal tissue and the availability of stents for bailout purposes, the incidence of these major complications decreases.

Non–Q-Wave MI

Several early observational studies reported a 5 to 7.4% incidence of in-hospital non–Q-wave myocardial infarction in patients as a result of DCA. In CAVEAT, the incidence of MI, defined as an increase in creatine kinase-MB levels more than three times normal, was significantly greater in the DCA group (19 versus 8% for the PTCA group, $P < .001$). Furthermore, postprocedural myocardial infarction was highly predictive of mortality, bypass surgery, or repeat intervention within 30 days ($P < .0001$) (55).

Abrupt Closure

Observational studies suggest an incidence of abrupt closure that is similar to PTCA (3.7 to 6.9%) (46–49). However, the randomized data from CAVEAT indicates that abrupt closure is more common with DCA than with angioplasty (8.0 versus 3.8%, $P = .005$), and it is associated with a significant risk of myocardial infarction, emergent bypass surgery, and death (56). Lesions found to be at increased risk for abrupt closure include de novo stenoses as opposed to restenotic lesions, right coronary lesions as opposed to left coronary lesions, and native vessels as opposed to vein grafts. Eccentric, long, angulated ostial and bifurcating stenoses as well as preexisting thrombus are also associated with an increased risk (56, 57).

Dissections account for approximately 30% of abrupt closure in the US Multicenter Registry, whereas in CAVEAT dissections were identified in 68% of the patients with abrupt closure. Dissections occur at the atherectomy site in 1 to 11% of procedures and are associated with a 10-fold increase in the risk of abrupt closure. In addition to dissections at the site of DCA, dissections can occur distal to the stenosis because of nose cone trauma or proximally because of guide catheter injury. Because the guide catheters required for DCA are large, injury to the coronary ostia accounts for 9% of abrupt closures. The highest risk for guide catheter dissections occurs when there is ostial disease and in procedures involving the right coronary artery where inadvertent deep seating of the guiding catheter may occur. PTCA can reestablish flow in more than 60% of cases of abrupt closure when caused by thrombus formation, but is successful only in 27% of cases where DCA causes dissection (57).

Coronary Perforation

Coronary perforation is a major concern with excisional atherectomy, although it is rare. Perforation occurs in 0.5 to 0.8% of DCA procedures, and it is thought to result from deep cuts into the adventitia and cuts directed toward nondiseased portions of the vessel wall (46–49). Approximately 50% of perforations require emergent bypass surgery because of abrupt closure or pericardial tamponade. Late complications of perforation include coronary aneurysm or arteriovenous fistula formation.

Embolization

Distal coronary embolization is relatively rare in native coronary arteries, occurring in 2% of cases. Embolization can result from a variety of causes, including dislodgment of thrombus or friable plaque. Additionally, if the nose cone does not completely capture all the excised tissue, some may embolize downstream. Degenerated saphenous vein grafts, on the other hand, are at an extremely high risk for downstream embolization and the no-reflow phenomenon. In CAVEAT II, distal embolization occurred in 13.4% patients assigned to DCA compared with 5.1% patients assigned to PTCA for the treatment of saphenous vein graft lesions (58). This was associated with almost a 10-fold increase risk of in-hospital adverse event and a threefold increase in 12-month adverse event rate. No-reflow phenomenon caused by embolization may respond to intracoronary infusion of nitroglycerin or calcium channel blockers, but it often results in an increase in creatine kinase levels.

Miscellaneous

Side branch occlusion occurs in approximately 3% of cases and can usually be successfully treated with PTCA or even DCA if the vessel is 2.5 mm or greater in diameter. Coronary vasospasm occurs in an estimated 2% of DCA procedures. This usually occurs at the site of atherectomy but may also occur at the site of nose cone trauma or at the tip of the guidewire. Vasospasm usually responds promptly to 100–200 µg intracoronary nitroglycerin. DCA has been associated with a 0.6% greater risk of vascular complications than seen with PTCA because of the large vascular sheaths (> 10 F) required for DCA. A 3.7% incidence of groin complication requiring surgical repair and a transfusion rate of 2.6% have been reported following DCA (49). Because of their increased risk, larger sheaths should be removed the same day as the procedure, if possible. Atherectomy also proves to be much more time consuming than balloon angioplasty even for experienced operators. In both the CAVEAT and CCAT, DCA was associated with 20 minutes longer procedural time and 10 minutes longer fluoroscopic time compared with PTCA. DCA also requires an average of almost 100 mL more contrast dye than do angioplasty procedures (CCAT) (54, 55).

Long-term Outcome

Restenosis

It was initially believed that atherectomy would decrease the incidence of restenosis by creating a larger lumen to accommodate tissue growth, a smoother surface with less vessel injury, and less elastic recoil. However, early clinical experience made it obvious that DCA does not eliminate restenosis. Angiographic restenosis rates, defined as greater than 50% diameter stenosis at the DCA site, are 32 to 58% of patients within 6 months of the procedure (48, 49, 54, 55). In both CCAT and CAVEAT, the overall restenosis rates were extremely high compared with previous observations, and no significant difference was found in the restenosis rates between atherectomy and angioplasty (46 versus 43% in CCAT; 50 versus 57% in CAVEAT). Only for the

predefined subgroup in CAVEAT who underwent revascularization of a proximal LAD stenosis was there an advantage of DCA in reducing restenosis (51 versus 63% restenosis).

Initial Gain versus Late Loss

Intravascular ultrasound studies have demonstrated that restenosis following DCA results primarily from intimal hyperproliferation with minimal elastic recoil in contrast to PTCA (40). Proponents of the "bigger is better" theory suggest the a larger initial gain may overcome the increase in neointimal hyperplasia and result in a reduction in restenosis. Compared with PTCA, the initial greater gain with DCA was balanced by a greater late loss, resulting in a similar net gain (54). To differentiate the device specific mechanisms versus extent of immediate gain on restenosis, Umans et al. (59) compared matched procedural outcomes following DCA and PTCA in 160 lesions. By matching lesions with similar preprocedural and postprocedural MLD in both groups, the immediate lumen gain achieved with atherectomy was comparable with that achieved with angioplasty (1.15 versus 1.10 mm). The binary restenosis rate, defined as greater than 50% diameter stenosis, was similar between the two treatment groups (28 versus 22%). However, the atherectomy group demonstrated a significantly higher late loss during follow-up (0.53 versus. 0.26 mm, $P < .005$), resulting in a significantly smaller residual MLD after atherectomy than after PTCA. Multivariant analysis identified vessel size and immediate gain as determinants of optimal atherectomy whereas device type remained an independent predictor of late MLD and lumen loss. Because atherectomy is associated with an increased intimal hyperplastic response, an optimal lumen gain is required to limit restenosis. This may explain the high restenosis rates seen in CCAT and CAVEAT. Despite a predefined goal of greater than 20% residual stenosis, operators only achieved a mean residual stenosis between 25 and 33% after atherectomy in CCAT and CAVEAT.

Predictors of Restenosis

The only clinical predictor of restenosis that has been consistently demonstrated is a history of previous PTCA or DCA at the lesion site. The Sequoia Hospital Registry reported a restenosis rate for de novo lesions in native coronary arteries of 31%, whereas the restenosis rate for restenosed lesions was 41% overall; 28% for one previous PTCA, 49% for two previous PTCAs, and 44% for three or more PTCAs (46). The US Multicenter DCA Registry noted a restenosis rate of 46% in restenosis lesions versus 30% in primary lesions (45). Fishman et al. also demonstrated significantly higher restensosis rates for restenosis lesions compared with de novo lesions treated with DCA (39 versus 28%) (49).

Angiographic predictors of restenosis include small vessel size (< 3 mm) and lesions more than 10 mm in length (46, 60). Saphenous vein graft lesions have been associated with a greater risk of restenosis in several series (48, 49). Postprocedural MLD is the most consistent procedural factor associated with restenosis following DCA. Postprocedure lumen diameter greater than 3 mm is associated with significantly less restenosis (46, 49, 60) in observational studies. The incidence of restenosis was 41% if post-DCA diameter was less than 3 mm compared with 28% if a post-DCA diameter was greater than 3 mm in the Sequoia Hospital series (46). Similar results were reported by Fishman et al.; 39% restenosis if postprocedural MLD less than 3 mm and 24% if a diameter greater than 3 mm were achieved (49). Using a multivariant analysis model, post-DCA MLD and device:artery ratio were independent predictors of both follow-up MLD and late loss (60, 61).

Clinical Events

Observational studies have reported late clinical event rates following DCA of between 24 and 30%. Repeat PTCA or DCA was required for symptomatic recurrence in 10 to 17% of patients, and coronary artery bypass surgery was required in 13 to 19% of patients at 6-month follow-up (40, 46, 48). One-

year and 2-year mortality rates following DCA were reported to be 2 and 4%, respectively (49). Factors reported to be associated with late clinical events are diabetes mellitus, unstable angina, restenosis lesions, and saphenous vein graft disease (40, 60).

"Optimal" Atherectomy

Based on the concept of "bigger is better," the current strategy by many operators is to minimize the final diameter stenosis as much as possible using aggressive atherectomy techniques and adjunctive balloon angioplasty (Fig. 29.8). Early studies reported that deep, subintimal resection with atherectomy was associated with a higher incidence of restenosis (46, 62). However, contrasting data have been reported by several investigators (49, 63, 64). In one study of 225 atherectomy lesions, where recovery of deep wall components was frequent, medial resection was not associated with restenosis and recovery of adventitia actually was associated with reduced restenosis (24 versus 30% with no deep wall component recovery) (49).

Although postdilation was discouraged in CCAT and CAVEAT, it has been shown to safely improve the results of DCA. The Optimal Atherectomy Restenosis Study (OARS) assessed the early and late angiographic outcomes of 211 lesions in 199 patients treated with ultrasound-guided atherectomy (65). The goal was to achieve less than 10% visual residual stenosis using ultrasound-guided atherectomy and adjunctive balloon postdilation. Mean MLD increased from 1.19–2.73 mm following atherectomy. Balloon postdilation resulted in further improvement in lumen size with a final MLD of 3.15 mm and a 7% residual stenosis by quantitative analysis. This low residual percent stenosis using ultrasound-guided optimal atherectomy was associated with few (2%) major angiographic complications. Additionally, the 6-month follow-up MLD was 1.99 mm. The restenosis rate using a binary definition of 50% or greater diameter stenosis was 30%. Recent results from the randomized Balloon versus Optimal Atherectomy Trial (BOAT) showed a 32% restenosis rate for optimal DCA and

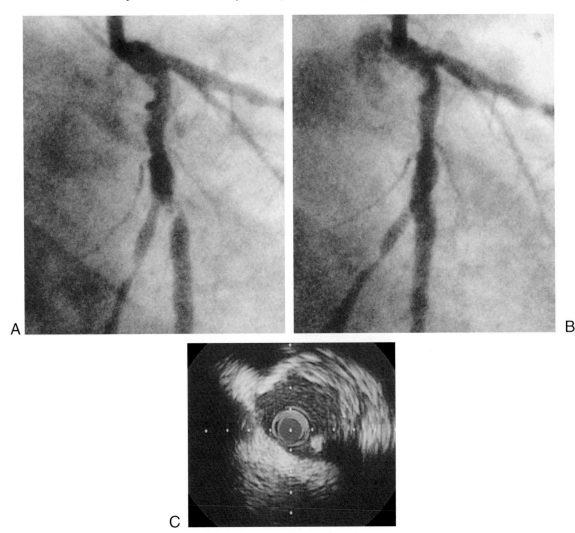

Figure 29.8. Optimal atherectomy of a marginal branch of the circumflex artery. **A.** A high-grade eccentric, ulcerated lesion at the marginal branch bifurcation (*arrow*). **B.** After multiple directional coronary atherectomy cuts and adjunctive balloon angioplasty, a good angiographic result is obtained at the previous lesion site. **C.** Postprocedure intravascular ultrasound shows mild amount of residual plaque burden with discrete atherectomy cuts (*arrows*) and focal area of calcification. Minimal lumen diameter was 3.5 mm.

a 40% restenois rate for PTCA, which was statistically different (66). Once again, DCA was associated with a significantly higher frequency of myocardial infarction compared with angioplasty (17 versus 5%). However, this did not result in a higher in-hospital or 1-year mortality rate. It remains unanswered whether optimal atherectomy has an advantage over other techniques in which an aggressive approach is also applied to achieve an optimal lumen diameter.

Potential Niches for DCA

Ostial and Proximal Left Anterior Descending Artery Lesions

Balloon angioplasty of ostial and proximal LAD lesions is associated with lower procedural success rates, higher incidence of complications, and high restenosis rates

(> 60%). Elastic recoil is believed to be the major mechanism behind the acute and long-term adverse outcome following PTCA of ostial lesions. Additionally, the potential for creating a dissection that propagates back into the main artery (i.e., left main for an LAD ostial stenosis) makes these lesions suboptimal for PTCA. By excising tissue and creating fewer dissections rather than stretching the vessel, DCA has a theoretic advantage over PTCA. DCA of ostial lesions has been associated with success rates of 82 to 100% achieving residual stenoses 16 to 17%, an acceptable degree of major complications (3 to 4%) and an angiographic restenosis rate of 39% (45, 46, 67). The CAVEAT database compared the two techniques in the treatment of 74 ostial LAD lesions (68). This retrospective subgroup analysis demonstrated a similar procedural success rate but a higher acute gain with atherectomy (1.13 versus 0.56 mm). However, DCA was also associated with a higher rate of non–Q-wave-myocardial infarctions (24 versus 13%) and no improvement in restenosis rates (48 versus 46%) in this subgroup. The lowest restenosis rates reported for DCA appear to occur in the proximal LAD (46). The CCAT, which randomized patients with lesions in the proximal one third of the LAD, obviously showed no difference in restenosis rates between DCA and PTCA. Whereas DCA resulted in less restenosis than PTCA (51 versus 66%) in a predefined subgroup of patients in CAVEAT with nonostial proximal LAD stenoses, this did not result in a reduction in clinical restenosis at 6 months (68).

Thrombus-associated Lesions

Intraluminal thrombus is associated with decreased procedural success and increased incidence of acute closure during angioplasty. DCA appears well suited for complex lesions with thrombus. In one study, DCA successfully treated 100% of the 35 thrombotic lesions, and thrombus was found to be an independent predictor of success (12). Umans et al. (69) demonstrated a procedural success rate of 88% for DCA in patients with unstable angina, which was similar to the 91% success rate in patients with stable angina. Additionally, there was no difference in in-hospital adverse events, including acute closure between stable and unstable angina groups. Thus, atherectomy appears to be performed effectively in unstable lesions. However, removal of the thrombotic material did not appear to affect the poor long-term clinical outcome seen in this subset of patients. The high incidence of non–Q-wave infarctions with DCA makes its use in thrombus-containing lesions of concern.

Bifurcation Lesions

Bifurcation lesions are associated with an increased risk of side branch compromise and ischemia during PTCA. The most common mechanism for side branch compromise is plaque redistribution or dissection into the branch while dilating the adjacent artery. Again, by excising rather than shifting plaque, as well as reducing the incidence of dissection, DCA has a theoretic advantage for treating bifurcation lesions if both vessels are greater than 2.5 mm in diameter. Double wiring the vessels for side branch protection is not an option with DCA as it is with PTCA because of the risk of guidewire fracture or entrapment. Thus, bifurcation lesions need to be debulked sequentially: major artery revascularization followed by revascularization of the side branch. In a small series of eight patients, Mansour et al. demonstrated successful atherectomy of both major and side branch vessels in 100% of cases (70).

Saphenous Vein Grafts

Restenosis rates following PTCA of aortocoronary vein grafts are markedly higher than seen in native coronary vessels, particularly in grafts older than 3 years or in lesions located at the ostium or in the body of the graft (71). Additionally, intervention within the vein graft is associated with a higher major complication rate because of distal embolization of atherosclerotic or thrombotic material. DCA can be applied relatively easily in most saphenous vein grafts because of their large size and nontortuous character. In the initial DVI registry, DCA of vein graft lesions was associated with an 85% success rate without major complications and a 57% restenosis rate overall (45). The restenosis rate was significantly lower with de novo graft lesions (38%) compared with restenosis lesions (75%). Similar findings have been reported by others (46–48, 67). In the only direct comparison between DCA versus PTCA in saphenous vein grafts, CAVEAT II randomized 305 patients with de novo vein graft lesions to atherectomy or angioplasty (72). Atherectomy resulted in higher procedural success rates (87 versus 79%) and acute lumen gain (1.45 versus 1.12 mm) at the cost of more distal embolization and a trend toward more non–Q-wave myocardial infarctions. Additionally, DCA did not result in any benefit with regard to the 6-month restenosis rates (46% DCA versus 51% PTCA).

DCA for Failed PTCA

In the early atherectomy experience, DCA appeared to be a valid technique for rescue therapy in the setting of failed angioplasty, thus avoiding myocardial infarction or emergent bypass surgery. Atherectomy has the ability to excise intraluminal dissection flaps and thrombus, which account for a most acute or threatened closure following angioplasty. In one retrospective analysis of 100 patients with 103 lesions with threatened or acute closure treated with DCA (73), failed PTCAs were principally due to dissection in 50%, recoil in 42%, and thrombus in 8% of the cases. DCA was successful in 91.3% of cases, defined as the establishment of thrombolysis in myocardial infarction (TIMI) grade 3 flow with greater than 20% stenosis reduction without death, Q-wave MI, or bypass surgery. Coronary perforation occurred in 1%, emergent bypass surgery in 6%, and death in 2%. Although a viable option in the setting of failed angioplasty, bailout stenting with 93 to 97% success rates has likely replaced rescue atherectomy.

Future of DCA

With the advent of stenting and the results of CAVEAT and CCAT, the enthusiasm that was initially present with directional atherectomy has dwindled. The recent results from BOAT are encouraging that we can reduce the restenosis rates using aggressive atherectomy techniques along with adjunctive angioplasty. However, it appears that this improvement in long-term angiographic restenosis comes at the cost of increased incidence of procedural myocardial infarctions. Perhaps with refinement in catheter design or with the use of intravascular ultrasound to guide therapy, further reductions in restenosis can be found while improving safety. An atherectomy device combined with an imaging transducer has been designed to allow the area of plaque being cut to be directly imaged (74). One could then assess the plaque burden prior to making additional cuts.

Some evidence is found that DCA may be an extremely effective adjunctive therapy to rotational atherectomy in calcified lesions (33). Additionally, specialized tungsten blade cutters are being designed to provide more effective atherectomy of calcified plaque or end-cutting to aid in crossing difficult lesions. Certainly the technique of directional atherectomy will continue to evolve.

TRANSLUMINAL EXTRACTION CATHETER (TEC) ATHERECTOMY

The transluminal extraction catheter (TEC) is one of three atherectomy devices approved by the US Food and Drug Administration for the treatment of atherosclerosis in human coronary arteries and saphenous vein grafts. This technique differs from other coronary interventional techniques in that it **simultaneously cuts tissue into small particles and then aspirates this tissue into an external reservoir,** thus potentially reducing the risk of distal embolization. Although it was initially conceived to reduce the restenosis rate in coronary arteries, it stands to reason that the greatest potential for TEC may be in degenerated saphenous vein grafts, which have an abundance of friable plaque and thrombus with a predisposition for distal embolization. Current evaluation of TEC atherectomy relies on observational studies, making comparison with other interventional strategies difficult.

TEC Atherectomy Equipment

The TEC catheter assembly comes in five sizes ranging from 5.5 to 7.5 F (1.83–2.5 mm). The TEC device consists of a distal cutting tip attached to a flexible, hollow tube that is then connected to a hand-held, battery-operated motor drive unit. Additionally, rear extension tubing connects the TEC catheter to special vacuum bottles, wherein the debris is collected. The distal tip is a conical-shaped rotational cutter consisting of two stainless steel blades rotating around a central guidewire. When activated by a trigger on the motor drive unit, suction is applied to the catheter and the cutter rotates at 750 rpms. Using the TEC device requires a special 300-cm, 0.014-inch extra support guidewire with a terminal 0.021-inch ball that prevents advancement of the cutter distal to the guidewire. The stiff guidewire is designed to straighten angulated segments of the vessel, theoretically decreasing the incidence of perforation during atherectomy. Other special equipment required includes a 10 F guide catheter designed to accommodate the TEC catheter and a "HemoValve" Toohy-Borst type hemostatic kit, which prevents air aspiration.

TEC Procedure

Preparation of the patient prior to TEC atherectomy is the same as for PTCA, including the administration of aspirin. Femoral artery access is achieved using a 10.5 F sheath and then the patient is systemically heparinized to maintain a therapeutic activated clotting time. The large (10 F) guide catheter is advanced into the ascending aorta using either a 0.063-inch J-tip guidewire or a 7 F tapered introducer catheter over a 0.035-inch J-tip guidewire to straighten the guide and avoid trauma to the aorta. Once the target vessel is engaged, the TEC guidewire can be advanced across the lesion with the tip positioned as far distally as possible. Vessel spasm often occurs in response to advancing this stiff guidewire and requires generous amounts of intracoronary nitroglycerin to reverse. The TEC device is then advanced over the guidewire, which was preloaded prior to introduction into the guide catheter, until the tip is several millimeters proximal to the target lesion. Prior to activating the cutter, continuous heparinized saline flush is started through the guide catheter to facilitate aspiration of tissue. The trigger on the motor drive is depressed to activate the suction and cutting device simultaneously. Once suction return is visualized in the rear extension tube, the cutting tip can be advanced across the lesion using a control device on the motor drive. Advancement of the TEC catheter across the lesion is similar to the technique used for rotational atherectomy. After several passes have been made, the assembly is removed from the guide catheter and angiographic assessment is made of the results. Further atherectomy can be performed using progressively larger cutter sizes, or adjunctive balloon angioplasty may be performed, if necessary, using the same wire. Cutter sizes are initially chosen based on size of target vessel, lesion severity, and thrombus presence. The device is generally best used for debulking rather than for definitive lumen enlargement. Therefore, a device:artery ratio of 0.5–0.7 is often chosen initially, but small devices are used if the stenosis is extremely severe and larger sizes used if the main goal is to excise thrombus.

Results

Procedural Success

The ability or inability of a device to be beneficial depends heavily on the context in which it is used (i.e., the complexity and morphologic features of the lesions). Because the various new interventional devices appear to have their own niches, it is very difficult to directly compare results. Currently there are no randomized trials evaluating TEC atherectomy. However, in the last few years, there have been several observational studies from which some conclusions can be drawn.

Initial observations of the US TEC Multicenter Registry indicate the extraction atherectomy can be performed with a high degree of procedural success in both native coronary arteries and saphenous vein grafts (75). Using data taken from 29 centers in the United States from July 1988 to January 1992, this registry analyzed 1318 lesions in 1147 patients who underwent TEC atherectomy, which represents the largest collective experience. Additionally, almost half the lesions (650/1318) were in saphenous vein grafts, making some comparisons between the two possible. The device success, defined as greater than 50% residual stenosis after TEC atherectomy, was 88% in native vessels and 86% in vein grafts. Of the treated lesions, 75% had adjunctive PTCA to increase the lumen diameter, which increased the lesion success rates to 95% and 96% for native arteries and vein grafts, respectively. TEC was associated with an overall 5.7% major complication rate (76). Major complications appeared to be more common when using the TEC catheter for native coronary arteries. Although the mortality rate was lower (1.6 versus 3.2%), the need for emergent bypass surgery was higher (3.6 versus 0.4%) for native arteries. Lesions that had been previously considered high risk for PTCA but responded well to TEC included SVG more than 3 years of age, native coronary lesions more than 10 mm in length, and lesions with thrombus.

Using a uniform method of recording procedural outcomes, the New Approaches to Coronary Intervention (NACI) Registry collected data on patients undergoing treatment with new or investigational devices from 36 participating centers (17). From November 1990 to November 1992, 14 sites enrolled 240 lesions from 211 patients undergoing TEC atherectomy; 64% of the lesions were in SVGs, 41% contained throm-

bus, and 34% had diffuse disease, indicating the high-risk nature of these lesions. The device success, defined as 20% or greater reduction in diameter stenosis and less than 50% residual stenosis, was only 48%. Adjunctive PTCA was performed in 89% of the cases, improving the procedural success to 80%. This compared less favorably with other new devices such as directional atherectomy, rotational atherectomy, or stents, which probably reflects the baseline high-risk nature of the lesions referred for TEC atherectomy. Additionally, TEC was associated with a 7.1% major complication rate (5.7% death, 1.4% Q-wave myocardial infarction, 0.9% emergent bypass surgery).

Native Coronary Arteries

The database from William Beaumont Hospital includes 181 native coronary artery lesions in 175 consecutive patients treated with TEC atherectomy (77). At this single center, 99% of the lesions were accessible to the device, verifying its flexibility and ease of use. However, only 29% of the lesions met the criteria for device success, defined as less than 50% residual stenosis following TEC atherectomy alone; 84% of the lesions required adjunctive PTCA, resulting in 84% procedural success without major complication. The MLD only increased from 1.0 to 1.3 mm following TEC, correlating with a decrease in diameter stenosis from 70 to 61%. Following adjunctive PTCA, the MLD increased to 2.1 mm and the diameter stenosis decreased to 36%. Thus, the final lumen diameter following the procedure is similar to that expected following PTCA alone. This disappointing degree of lumen enlargement following TEC is most likely secondary to the small catheter sizes available (≤ 2.5 mm) and to an extensive amount of recoil. Overall efficacy of lumen enlargement appears much less than with directional or rotational atherectomy. Furthermore, a 20% angiographic complication rate was reported from this database, including an 11% incidence of abrupt closure and a 2.2% incidence of perforation. Clinical complications included 2.3% in-hospital deaths, 3.4% Q-wave myocardial infarction, and 2.8% need for emergency bypass surgery.

Saphenous Vein Grafts

Percutaneous coronary angioplasty of saphenous vein graft lesions is associated with poor angiographic results and high degree of complications, presumably from distal embolization of atheromatous material and thrombus. From the early US TEC Multicenter Registry, TEC atherectomy appeared to be a promising alternative to PTCA for vein graft disease, especially that associated with thrombus (75). The William Beaumont database similarly looked at 158 SVG lesions in 146 consecutive patients undergoing extraction atherectomy (78). The mean age of the grafts was 8.3 ± 3.0 years, and 17% were considered degenerated, 6% had complex lesions, 64% had eccentric lesions, 18% had ulcerated plaques, and 28% had evidence of thrombus. In 9% of the cases, the lesion could not be crossed with the atherectomy catheter but was subsequently successfully dilated with a balloon. Similar to native coronary arteries, the device success rate (39.2%) was limited by the available catheter sizes and the large diameter of the vein conduits. The MLD increased from 0.9 to 1.5 mm and diameter stenosis decreased from 75 to 58% following TEC. Therefore, adjunctive PTCA was required in 91% lesions, improving the procedural success rate to 84%. After PTCA, the MLD further increased to 2.3 mm with a final diameter stenosis of 36%. Once again, there was a 21% angiographic complication rate immediately following the TEC procedure, with an additional 5% incidence of complications following PTCA. Where the major angiographic complication seen in native arteries was abrupt closure, most of the complications seen in saphenous vein grafts were distal embolization (11.9%) or the no-reflow phenomenon (8.8%) with no perforations and a 5% rate of abrupt closure. The clinical complications included 2.0% in-hospital death rate, 0.7% emergency bypass surgery, 2.0% Q-wave myocardial infarction, 2.7% non–Q-wave infarction, and 6.1% vascular injury.

These complications, however, must be considered in light of the complex nature of the lesions undergoing intervention. Hong et al. (79) looked at factors associated with distal embolization following TEC atherectomy in saphenous vein grafts. This study evaluated 86 vein graft lesions in 65 consecutive patients undergoing TEC atherectomy. Most of these patients underwent adjunctive balloon angioplasty with device and procedural success rates similar to the data reported above. Distal embolization occurred in 12.8% of the cases, but most cases of embolization (63%) occurred following balloon angioplasty rather than immediately after atherectomy. The lesion complexity defined by ACC/AHA criteria was similar in patients who developed embolization and in those who had not. However, thrombus was identified as an independent predictor of embolization, present in 82% of cases complicated by distal embolization versus 40% in those without distal embolization. Distal embolization resulted in significantly lower procedural success (55 versus 91%) and an increase in death and Q-wave and non–Q-wave myocardial infarctions (46 versus 2% complication rate).

Angioscopy was performed on 14 patients with acute coronary syndromes undergoing TEC atherectomy (80). Only 6 of the 12 lesions with thrombus before TEC had no residual thrombus detected after TEC, and 3 of the lesions had no thrombus removed at all. Globular thrombus was removed in all cases, but older, more laminated thrombus was difficult to remove with the TEC device. The failure of TEC to achieve 100% efficacy in thrombus removal and the forward cutting action of the device in otherwise degenerated or complex lesions may explain the increased angiographic and clinical complication rates observed. Whether pretreatment with GIIb/IIIa receptor antagonists such as abciximab will alter this complication rate remains unanswered.

Late Outcome

As with many of the other new percutaneous revascularization devices that improve the initial success of the procedure, TEC atherectomy is still limited by restenosis. In the US TEC Muticenter Registry, extraction atherectomy with or without adjunctive angioplasty was associated with a 51% restenosis rate for native coronary arteries and 60% restenosis in saphenous vein grafts (75). Safian et al. similarly reported an angiographic restenosis rate of 61% for native coronary arteries and 69% for saphenous vein grafts undergoing TEC atherectomy at a single center (77, 78). Six-month clinical restenosis (repeat intervention, late bypass surgery, myocardial infarction, or death) was 29% for native arteries and 42% for vein grafts.

The Duke Multicenter Coronary TEC Registry enrolled 313 patients with 351 lesions undergoing TEC atherectomy (81). Despite a 95% procedural success rate, the overall 6-month angiographic restenosis rate was 48% in 256 eligible patients, whereas lesion restenosis was similar between native arteries and vein grafts (45 versus 46%). Subgroup analysis suggested that optimal lumen enlargement (< 25% residual stenosis) using the TEC alone in native arteries led to improved restenosis rates (18%); however, patient sample size was too small to draw any conclusions.

SUMMARY

Although TEC atherectomy is associated with high procedural success rates, adequate lumen enlargement requires adjunctive PTCA in most cases. Unlike most other devices, the success rates of TEC in saphenous vein grafts appeared equal or superior to the success obtain in native coronary arteries. In both, the high success rates have been associated with relatively high frequency of angiographic and clinical complications. Additionally, the long-term restenosis following TEC is similar to the restenosis rates with PTCA. However, TEC was used in complex lesions that otherwise would be considered too risky to do PTCA. So without a head-to-head comparison in similar lesions, one cannot say that TEC is not beneficial. This technique's greatest niche may be in the setting of degenerated saphenous vein grafts, which are difficult to treat using PTCA. In the future, use of GIIb/IIIa agents may make atherectomy in these complex lesions safer with improved results.

References

1. Kovach JA, Mintz GS, Pichard AD, et al. Sequential intravascular ultrasound characterization of the mechanisms of rotational atherectomy and adjunct balloon angioplasty. J Am Coll Cardiol 1993;22: 1024–1032.
2. Mintz GS, Potkin BN, Keren G, et al. Intravascular ultrasound evaluation of the effect of rotational atherectomy in obstructive atherosclerotic coronary artery disease. Circulation 1992;86:1383–1393.
3. Farb A, Roberts DK, Pichard AD, et al. Coronary artery morphologic features after coronary rotational atherectomy: insights into mechanisms of lumen enlargement and embolization. Am Heart J 1995;129:1058–1067.
4. von Birgelen C, Umans VA, Di Mario C, et al. Mechanism of high-speed rotational atherectomy and adjunctive balloon angioplasty revisited by quantitative coronary angiography: edge detection versus videodensitometry. Am Heart J 1995;130: 405–412.
5. Safian RD, Freed M, Lichtenberg A, et al. Are residual stenoses after excimer laser angioplasty and coronary atherectomy due to inefficient or small devices? Comparison with balloon angioplasty. J Am Coll Cardiol 1993;22:1628–1634.
6. MacIsaac AI, Bass TA, Buchbinder M, et al. High speed rotational atherectomy: outcome in calcified and noncalcified coronary artery lesions. J Am Coll Cardiol 1995;26:731–736.
7. Mintz GS, Douek P, Pichard AD, et al. Target lesion calcification in coronary artery disease: an intravascular ultrasound study. J Am Coll Cardiol 1992; 20:1149–1155.
8. Guerin Y, Spaulding C, Desnos M, et al. Rotational atherectomy with adjunctive balloon angioplasty versus conventional percutaneous transluminal coronary angioplasty in type B2 lesions: results of a randomized study. Am Heart J 1996;131:879–883.
9. Koller PT, Freed M, Grines CL, et al. Success, complications, and restenosis following rotational and transluminal extraction atherectomy of ostial stenoses. Cathet Cardiovasc Diagn 1994;31:255–260.
10. Warth DC, Leon MB, O'Neill W, et al. Rotational atherectomy multicenter registry: acute results, complications and 6-month angiographic follow-up in 709 patients. J Am Coll Cardiol 1994;24: 641–648.
11. Nino CL, Freed M, Blankenship L, et al. Procedural cost of new interventional devices. Am J Cardiol 1994;74:1165–1166.
12. O'Murchu B, Foreman RD, Shaw RE, et al. Role of intraaortic balloon pump counterpulsation in high risk coronary rotational atherectomy. J Am Coll Cardiol 1995;26:1270–1275.
13. Safian RD, Niazi KA, Strzelecki M, et al. Detailed angiographic analysis of high-speed mechanical rotational atherectomy in human coronary arteries. Circulation 1993;88:961–968.
14. Ellis SG, Popma JJ, Buchbinder M, et al. Relation of clinical presentation, stenosis morphology, and operator technique to the procedural results of rotational atherectomy and rotational atherectomy-

facilitated angioplasty. Circulation 1994;89: 882–892.

15. Piana RN, Paik GY, Moscucci M, et al. Incidence and treatment of 'no-reflow' after percutaneous coronary intervention. Circulation 1994;89: 2514–2518.

16. Porter GF, Ormiston JA, Webster MW. Percutaneous rotational coronary atherectomy: initial Green Lane and Mercy hospitals' experience. N Z Med J 1996;109:203–205.

17. Baim DS, Kent KM, King SBR, et al. Evaluating new devices. Acute (in-hospital) results from the New Approaches to Coronary Intervention Registry. Circulation 1994;89:471–481.

18. Borrione M, Hall P, Almagor Y, et al. Treatment of simple and complex coronary stenosis using rotational ablation followed by low pressure balloon angioplasty. Cathet Cardiovasc Diagn 1993;30: 131–137.

19. Teirstein PS, Warth DC, Haq N, et al. High speed rotational coronary atherectomy for patients with diffuse coronary artery disease [see comments]. J Am Coll Cardiol 1991;18:1694–1701.

20. Gilmore PS, Bass TA, Conetta DA, et al. Single site experience with high-speed coronary rotational atherectomy. Clin Cardiol 1993;16:311–316.

21. Hetterich FS, McEniery PT. Right ventricular infarction following percutaneous coronary rotational atherectomy. Cathet Cardiovasc Diagn 1995; 34:321–324.

22. Ajluni SC, Glazier S, Blankenship L, et al. Perforations after percutaneous coronary interventions: clinical, angiographic, and therapeutic observations. Cathet Cardiovasc Diagn 1994;32:206–212.

23. Foster Smith K, Garratt KN, Holmes DR Jr. Guidewire transection during rotational coronary atherectomy due to guide catheter dislodgement and wire kinking. Cathet Cardiovasc Diagn 1995;35: 224–227.

24. McKenna CJ, McCann HA, Sugrue DD. Emergency bail-out stenting for major coronary dissection complicating rotational atherectomy. Ir Med J 1995; 88:32.

25. Vandormael M, Reifart N, Preusler W, et al. Six months follow-up results following excimer laser angioplasty, rotational atherectomy, and balloon angioplasty for complex lesions: ERBAC study [Abstract]. Circulation 1994;90:I-213A.

26. Bass TA, Gilmore PS, Ceithaml EL. Rotational atherectomy in anomalous coronary arteries. Cathet Cardiovasc Diagn 1992;27:322–324.

27. Brogan WCD, Popma JJ, Pichard AD, et al. Rotational coronary atherectomy after unsuccessful coronary balloon angioplasty [see comments]. Am J Cardiol 1993;71:794–798.

28. Cardenas JR, Strumpf RK, Heuser RR. Rotational atherectomy in restenotic lesions at the distal saphenous vein graft anastomosis. Cathet Cardiovasc Diagn 1995;36:53–57.

29. The EPIC Investigators. Use of a monoclonal antibody directed against the platelet glycoprotein IIb/ IIIa receptor in high-risk coronary angioplasty. The EPIC Investigation [see comments]. N Engl J Med 1994;330:956–961.

30. Moliterno DJ, Califf RM, Aguirre FV, et al. Effect of platelet glycoprotein IIb/IIIa integrin blockade on activated clotting time during percutaneous transluminal coronary angioplasty or directional atherectomy (the EPIC trial). Evaluation of c7E3 Fab in the Prevention of Ischemic Complications trial. Am J Cardiol 1995;75:559–562.

31. Safian RD, Freed M, Lichtenberg A, et al. Usefulness of percutaneous transluminal coronary angioplasty after new device coronary interventions. Am J Cardiol 1994;73:642–646.

32. Safian RD, Freed M, Reddy V, et al. Do excimer laser angioplasty and rotational atherectomy facilitate balloon angioplasty? Implications for lesion-specific coronary intervention. J Am Coll Cardiol 1996;27:552–559.

33. Dussaillant GR, Mintz GS, Pichard AD, et al. Mechanisms and immediate and long-term results of adjunct directional coronary atherectomy after rotational atherectomy. J Am Coll Cardiol 1996;27: 1390–1397.

34. Mintz GS, Pichard AD, Popma JJ, et al. Preliminary experience with adjunct directional coronary atherectomy after high-speed rotational atherectomy in the treatment of calcific coronary artery disease. Am J Cardiol 1993;71:799–804.

35. Sabri MN, Cowley MJ, DiSciascio G, et al. Immediate results of interventional devices for coronary ostial narrowing with angina pectoris. Am J Cardiol 1994;73:122–125.

36. Simarino M, Corcos T, Favereau X, et al. Rotational coronary atherectomy with adjunctive balloon angioplasty for the treatment of ostial lesions. Cathet Cardiovasc Diagn 1994;33:22–27.

37. Simpson JB. How atherectomy began: a personal history. Am J Cardiol 1993;72:3E–5E.

38. Safian RD, Gelbfish JS, Erny RE, et al. Coronary atherectomy: clinical, angiographic, and histological findings and observations regarding potential mechanisms. Circulation 1990;82:69–79.

39. Penny WF, Schmidt DA, Safian RD, et al. Insights into the mechanism of luminal improvement after directional coronary atherectomy. Am J Cardiol 1991;67:435–437.

40. Pompa JL, Mintz GS, Satler LF, et al. Clinical and angiographic outcome after directional coronary atherectomy: a qualitative and quantitative analysis using coronary arteriography and intravascular ultrasound. Am J Cardiol 1993;72:55E–64E.

41. Tenaglia AN, Buller CE, Kisslo DB, et al. Mechanisms of balloon angioplasty and directional coronary atherectomy as assessed by intracoronary ultrasound. J Am Coll Cardiol 1992;20:685–691.

42. Braden GA, Herrington DM, Downes TR, et al. Qualitative and quantitative contrasts in the mechanisms of lumen enlargement by coronary balloon angioplasty and directional coronary atherectomy. J Am Coll Cardiol 1994;23:40–48.

43. Nakamura S, Mahon DJ, Leung CY, et al. Intracoronary ultrasound imaging before and after directional coronary atherectomy: In vitro and clinical observations. Am Heart J 1995;129:841–851.

44. Baptista J, di Mario C, Ozaki Y, et al. Impact of plaque morphology and composition on the mechanisms of lumen enlargement using intracoronary ultrasound and quantitative angiography after balloon angioplasty. Am J Cardiol 1996;77:115–121.

45. Baim DS, Hinohara T, Holmes D, et al. for the US

DCA Investigator Group. Results of directional coronary atherectomy during multicenter preapproval testing. Am J Cardiol 1993;72:7E–11E.

46. Hinohara T, Rowe MH, Robertson GC, et al. Effect of lesion characteristics on outcome of directional coronary atherectomy. J Am Coll Cardiol 1991;17: 1112–1120.

47. Ellis SG, De Cesare NB, Pinkerton CA, et al. Relation of stenosis morphology and clinical presentation to the procedural results of directional coronary atherectomy. Circulation 1991;84:644–653.

48. Garratt KN, Holmes DR, Bell MR, et al. Results of directional atherectomy of primary atheromatous and restenosis lesions in coronary arteries and saphenous vein grafts. Am J Cardiol 1992;70: 449–454.

49. Fishman RF, Kuntz RE, Carrozza JP, et al. Long-term results of directional coronary atherectomy: Predictors of restenosis. J Am Coll Cardiol 1992; 20:1101–1110.

50. Pompa JJ, de Cesare N, Ellis SG, et al. Clinical, angiographic and procedural correlates of quantitative coronary dimensions after directional coronary atherectomy. J Am Coll Cardiol 1991;18: 1183–1189.

51. Robertson GC, Vetter JW, Selmon MR, et al. Directional coronary atherectomy is less effective for calcified primary lesions [Abstract]. Circulation 1991;84(4):II-520.

52. Matar FA, Mintz GS, Pinnow E, et al. Multivariate predictors of intravascular ultrasound end points after directional coronary atherectomy. J Am Coll Cardiol 1995;25:318–324.

53. Adelman AG, Cohen EA, Kimball BP, et al. A comparison of directional atherectomy with balloon angioplasty for lesions of the left anterior descending coronary artery. N Engl J Med 1993;329: 228–233.

54. Topol EJ, Leya F, Pinkerton CA, et al. A comparison of directional atherectomy with coronary angioplasty in patients with coronary artery disease. N Engl J Med 1993;329:221–227.

55. Harrington RA, Lincoff M, Califf RM, et al. Characteristics and consequences of myocardial infarction after percutaneous coronary intervention: insights from the coronary angioplasty versus excisional atherectomy trial (CAVEAT). J Am Coll Cardiol 1995;25:1693–1699.

56. Holmes DR, Simpson JB, Berdan LG, et al. Abrupt closure: the CAVEAT I experience. J Am Coll Cardiol 1995;26:1494–1500.

57. Pompa JJ, Topol EJ, Hinohara T, et al. Abrupt vessel closure after directional coronary atherectomy. J Am Coll Cardiol 1992;19:1372–1379.

58. Lefkovits J, Holmes DR, Califf RM, et al. Predictors and sequellae of distal embolization during saphenous vein graft intervention from the CAVEAT-II trial. Circulation 1995;92:734–740.

59. Umans VA, Keane D, Foley D, et al. Optimal use of directional coronary atherectomy is required to ensure long-term angiographic benefit: a study with matched procedural outcome after atherectomy and angioplasty. J Am Coll Cardiol 1994;24: 1652–1659.

60. Umans VA, Robert A, Foley D, et al. Clinical, histologic and quantitative angiographic predictors of restenosis after directional coronary atherectomy: a multivariate analysis of the renarrowing process and late outcome. J Am Coll Cardiol 1994;23:49–58.

61. Kuntz RE, Safiean RD, Carrozza JP, et al. The importance of acute luminal diameter in determining restenosis after coronary atherectomy or stenting. Circulation 1992;86:1827–1835.

62. Garrat KN, Holmes DR, Bell MR, et al. Restenosis after directional coronary atherectomy: differences between primary atheromatous and restenosis lesions and influence of subintimal tissue resection. J Am Coll Cardiol 1990;16:1665–1671.

63. Kuntz RE, Hinohara J, Safian RD, et al. Restenosis after directional coronary atherectomy. Effects of luminal diameter and deep wall excision. Circulation 1992;86:1394–1399.

64. Holmes DR, Garratt KN, Isner JM, et al. Effect of subintimal resection on initial outcome and restenosis for native coronary lesions and saphenous vein graft disease treated by directional coronary atherectomy. J Am Coll Cardiol 1996;28:645–651.

65. Pompa JJ, Baim DS, Kuntz RE, et al. Early and late quantitative angiographic outcomes in the Optimal Atherectomy Restenosis Study (OARS) [Abstract]. J Am Coll Cardiol 1996;27:291A.

66. Baim DS, Pompa JJ, Sharma SK, et al. Final results in the Balloon vs Optimal Atherectomy Trial (BOAT): 6 month angiography and 1 year clinical followup [Abstract]. Circulation 1996;94:I-436.

67. Stephan WJ, Bates ER, Garratt KN, et al. Directional atherectomy of coronary and saphenous vein graft ostial stenoses. Am J Cardiol 1995;75:1015–1018.

68. Boehrer JD, Ellis SG, Pieper K, et al. Directional atherectomy versus balloon angioplasty for coronary ostial and nonostial left anterior descending coronary artery lesions: results from a randomized multicenter trial. J Am Coll Cardiol 1995;25: 1380–1386.

69. Umans VA, de Feyter PJ, Deckers JW, et al. Acute and long-term outcome of directional coronary atherectomy for stable and unstable angina. Am J Cardiol 1994;74:641–646.

70. Mansour M, Fishman RF, Kuntz RE, et al. Feasibility of directional atherectomy for the treatment of bifurcation lesions. Coronary Artery Dis 1992;3: 761–765.

71. Platko WP, Hollman J, Whitlow P, Franco I. Percutaneous transluminal angioplasty of saphenous vein graft stenosis: long-term follow-up. J Am Coll Cardiol 1989;1645–1650.

72. Holmes DR, Topol, Califf RM, et al. A multicenter, randomized trial of coronary angioplasty versus directional atherectomy for patients with saphenous vein bypass graft lesions. Circulation 1995; 91:1966–1974.

73. McCluskey ER, Cowley M, Whitlow PL. Multicenter clinical experience with rescue atherectomy for failed angioplasty. Am J Cardiol 1993;72:42E–50E.

74. Fitzgerald PJ, Belef M, Connolly AJ, et al. Design and initial testing of an ultrasound-guided directional atherectomy device. Am Heart J 1995;129: 593–598.

75. O'Neill WW, Kramer BL, Sketch MH, et al. Mechanical extraction atherectomy: report of the U.S. Transluminal Extraction Catheter Investigation [abstract]. Circulation 1992;86:I-779.

76. Sutton JM, Gitlin JB, Casale PN. Major complications after TEC atherectomy: preliminary analysis derived from the multicenter registry experience [Abstract]. Circulation 1992;86:I-456.
77. Safian RD, May MA, Lichtenberg A, et al. Detailed clinical and angiographic analysis of transluminal extraction coronary atherectomy for complex lesions in native coronary arteries. J Am Coll Cardiol 1995;25:848–854.
78. Safian RD, Grines CL, May MA, et al. Clinical and angiographic results of transluminal extraction coronary atherectomy in saphenous vein bypass grafts. Circulation 1994;89:302–312.
79. Hong MK, Pompa JJ, Pichard AD, et al. Clinical significance of distal embolization after transluminal extraction atherectomy in diffusely diseased saphenous vein grafts. Am Heart J 1994;127: 1496–1503.
80. Annex BH, Larkin TJ, O'Neill WW, et al. Evaluation of thrombus removal by transluminal extraction coronary atherectomy by percutaneous coronary angioscopy. Am J Cardiol 1994;74:606–609.
81. Sketch MH, O'Neill WW, Galichia JP, et al. Restenosis following coronary transluminal extraction-endarterectomy: the clinical analysis of a multicenter registry [Abstract]. J Am Coll Cardiol 1992;19: 277A.

30

Laser Techniques for Coronary Artery Intervention, and Other Alternative Techniques

John A. Bittl, MD

INTRODUCTION

Laser angioplasty has evolved remarkably during the past 15 years. Based on the ability of laser energy to heat and ablate biologic tissue, several angioplasty systems were developed to overcome the limitations of conventional balloon angioplasty. Hot-tip lasers were introduced to recanalize total occlusions, laser-assisted balloon angioplasty was developed to weld vascular dissections, and excimer laser angioplasty was initially studied to reduce restenosis. Currently, excimer laser angioplasty remains the only active application of laser for the treatment of coronary artery disease. The current use of excimer laser angioplasty, however, is not based on its ability to reduce restenosis. Instead, excimer laser angioplasty is a versatile treatment whose use has evolved to expand the indications of cardiovascular interventions.

Excimer laser coronary angioplasty was initially approved by the US Food and Drug Administration in 1993 for six indications—saphenous vein graft lesions, total occlusions, calcified lesions, ostial lesions, lesions greater than 20 mm in length, and balloon dilation failures. The results of randomized clinical trials and other studies suggest, however, that excimer laser angioplasty may not be the optimal therapy for some of these lesion types. During the past

4 years, several other indications for laser angioplasty have emerged. **The most promising application is the use of a laser guidewire for chronic total occlusions** refractory to other types of treatment. Another promising indication is laser angioplasty used in conjunction with stenting, especially in saphenous vein graft lesions because of low rates of embolization after laser treatment. Much interest is also found in excimer laser angioplasty to treat restenosis within stents because of its ability to ablate the restenotic tissue and achieve lumens larger than those obtained with balloon angioplasty.

This chapter briefly reviews the fundamental mechanisms of laser angioplasty. Presented are the results of clinical trials, findings of several registries, and details of rapidly changing patient selection and techniques of excimer laser angioplasty.

HISTORICAL SURVEY

The first cardiovascular applications of lasers involved the percutaneous treatment of peripheral vascular disease and the intraoperative treatment of coronary artery disease. In 1984, Ginsburg (1) and Geschwind (2) successfully used argon and neodymium:

yttrium-aluminum-garnet (Nd:YAG) lasers attached to bare optical fibers to treat peripheral arterial disease; however, vessel perforation was a common complication (3). Choy et al. (4) used an argon laser with bare optical fibers in the coronary circulation at the time of bypass surgery, but reocclusion occurred in all treated vessels. Foschi et al. (5) used a laser delivery system based on a balloon-centering device to reduce the risk of vessel perforation seen with bare optical fibers. A single 200-μm quartz fiberoptic fiber was advanced through the central lumen of a conventional coronary balloon angioplasty catheter to align the optical fiber coaxially within the coronary artery. The balloon-centered system was designed to be used as an initial treatment before conventional balloon angioplasty in cases of total or subtotal occlusions refractory to crossing with conventional guidewires. In preliminary studies (5), procedural success was observed in 51 of the 67 lesions (76%) treated. Complications included one case of vessel perforation, two cases of abrupt vessel closure requiring emergency bypass surgery, and one case of distal embolization causing myocardial infarction. This argon-laser system was limited by its inefficient wavelength for plaque ablation, the inability to treat calcified or proximal lesions, and the need to treat relatively straight arterial segments.

Laser-induced fluorescence systems were developed to selectively ablate atherosclerotic tissue while minimizing injury to normal components of the arterial wall. During fluorescence feedback laser angioplasty, the target tissue was identified by its unique fluorescent characteristics. In response to illumination with low-power radiation transmitted via the fiberoptic catheter system, a fluorescence signal was detected by a computer that classified the signal as coming from normal or atherosclerotic tissue. If the target was classified as atherosclerotic, high-power laser light was transmitted through the same fiberoptic system to ablate the plaque. This test-and-ablate sequence was repeated until the plaque was removed and the underlying normal components of the arterial wall exposed, fluorescent recognition of which would inhibit further high-power laser output. Clinical studies in peripheral vascular disease were performed with a system incorporating a high-power, 480-nm pulsed-dye laser, and a low-power, 325-nm helium-cadmium laser for inducing fluorescence. A report (6) of 66 patients with refractory total occlusion of the iliofemoral artery showed a primary success rate of 82%, but 8 patients experienced vessel perforation. The efficacy of the fluorescence-feedback laser system in limited coronary testing was compromised by the presence of calcification, the slow response time of the algorithms used for tissue discrimination, and the likelihood of vessel perforation.

In an effort to solve the problems of vessel perforation with the bare fiber systems, Sanborn et al. (7) worked with a system that had a rounded metal cap placed on a laser fiber to eliminate direct interaction between laser energy and tissue. At the same time, Abela et al. (8) developed a similar system using a hybrid thermal probe system that also emitted a forward laser beam. Both systems were based on the rapid heating of the metal cap and surrounding tissue to more than 200°C. Investigation of this approach was abandoned because vessel perforation occurred with disturbing frequency. Other problems included the welding of the metal cap to the vessel wall as well as lack of benefit of thermal probe angioplasty over conventional mechanical approaches (9, 10).

Laser balloon angioplasty (11) was developed by Spears et al. (12) to prevent elastic recoil, weld vessel wall dissections, and reduce smooth muscle cell proliferation in an effort to treat abrupt vessel closure and reduce late restenosis. The laser balloon system consisted of a modified coronary angioplasty catheter and a Nd:YAG laser source. A helical diffusing fiber traversed the entire length of the angioplasty balloon, with two gold-leaf deflecting shields attached to the ends of the balloon to reduce laser radiation beyond the balloon and make laser energy distribution more uniform within the balloon. Use of the technique in elective settings was limited by restenosis rates consistently greater than 50% (13).

A pulsed dye laser system operating at 480 nm was developed by Gregory et al. (14) and investigated in a small clinical trial in patients with acute myocardial infarction who could not receive thrombolytic agents. The novel catheter system transmitted laser energy through radiographic contrast medium. The laser light was avidly absorbed by hemoglobin, whose ablation threshold is well below that of either normal arterial wall or atherosclerotic plaque (14). In the first clinical experience, laser thrombolysis was attempted in 18 patients with acute myocardial infarction. All patients had totally occluded infarct-related arteries. In six patients, the laser was not fired because of technical problems or failure to reach the occlusion. In 10 of the remaining 12 patients (83%), thrombus was ablated and coronary flow improved without evidence of perforation or dissection.

EXCIMER LASERS

The operation of an excimer laser is based on the formation of an excited dimer, created by a high-voltage electrical discharge in mixture of an inert gas such as xenon in the presence of highly dilute hydrogen chloride. The excited dimer (i.e., XeCl) dissociates and emits energy in the ultraviolet portion of the electromagnetic spectrum at 308 nm.

A single vendor exists for coronary excimer lasers and catheters (Spectranetics, Colorado Springs, CO). The catheters used for excimer laser coronary angioplasty are manufactured in diameters of 1.4, 1.7, or 2.0 mm. All laser catheters are advanced over a guidewire using either an over-the-wire or a monorail system. At the tip of the catheter, the wire lumen is surrounded by a concentric or eccentric array of densely packed 61-μm optical fibers.

The laser wire used for crossing refractory total occlusions has an outer diameter of 0.018 inch and contains twelve 61-μm optical fibers, as well as a shaping ribbon. After successful crossing, the wire is converted to a 300-cm exchange wire for adjunctive therapy with laser angioplasty, balloon angioplasty, or stenting. The stiffness of the laser wire is similar to that of a conventional high-torque standard guidewire.

Ablation of Tissue with Excimer Laser Radiation

The threshold energy density (fluence) for ablation of biologic tissue by 308-nm excimer laser light is approximately 30 mJ/mm^2 (15). Each pulse at this fluence will produce a crater about 40 μm deep. Thus, 25 pulses delivered over one second will produce a crater about 1.0 mm deep. The threshold for calcified atheroma, however, may exceed 60 mJ/mm^2 (15–17), which is the maximum fluence used clinically.

Clinical Results

Registry Reports

In a consecutive series of 3000 patients with a broad range of target lesions treated with excimer laser angioplasty, Litvack and colleagues (18) reported that the procedural success (final stenosis $\leq$ 50% without in-hospital Q-wave myocardial infarction, coronary artery bypass surgery, or death) was 90%. Complications included in-hospital bypass surgery (3.8%), Q-wave myocardial infarction (2.1%), and death (0.5%). Coronary artery perforation occurred in 1.2% of patients but significantly decreased to 0.4% in the last 1000 patients (0.3% of lesions). Angiographic dissection occurred in 13% of lesions, transient occlusion in 3.4%, and sustained occlusion in 3.1%. Success and complication rates were not related to lesion length or complexity.

In a separate consecutive series of 2041 patients with 2324 stenoses treated with excimer laser coronary angioplasty, Bittl and colleagues (19) reported that clinical success (final stenosis $\leq$ 50% stenosis and without in-hospital death, Q-wave or non–Q-wave myocardial infarction, repeat percutaneous transluminal coronary angioplasty, or need for bypass surgery) was achieved in 1814 patients (89%). The likelihood of clinical success ranged from 86 to 95% and depended on the phase of investigation. The incidence of vessel perforation fell significantly during the course of the study ($P =$

.02), but the rate of vessel dissection did not change (20). The risk of major complications increased with the presence of any complication (Table 30.1).

Multivariable analysis suggested that clinical success was related to multiple factors. Saphenous vein graft stenoses (n = 676) were associated with superior success rates (93%), whereas lesions longer than 20 mm (n = 224, success = 84%) and calcified lesions (n = 428, success = 83%) tended to be associated with decreased success (P < .001). Clinical success was associated with

Table 30.1.
Sequelae of Vessel Dissection During Excimer Laser Coronary Angioplasty

	Total Population	Any Dissection	P Value
N	2041	309	
Death	27 (1%)	3 (1%)	1.000
Q-wave MI	25 (1%)	26 (8%)	< 0.001
Non–Q-wave MI	48 (2%)	24 (8%)	< 0.001
Emergency bypass	92 (4%)	62 (20%)	< 0.001
Abrupt closure	121 (5%)	77 (25%)	< 0.001

Reprinted with permission from Bittl JA, Estella P, Abela GS. Complications of laser Coronary angioplasty. In: Lutz J, ed. Complications of interventional procedures. New York: Igoku-Shoin, 1995;186–207.

operator experience. Cardiologists performing more than 25 excimer laser cases had better success rates (success 91%, P = .003) than those performing 25 cases or less.

Randomized Controlled Trials of Excimer Laser Angioplasty

Two randomized studies comparing excimer laser with other treatments have been completed (21, 22). In the **Am**sterdam-**Rot**terdam (AMRO) trial, 308 patients with lesions greater than 10 mm in length were randomly allocated to treatment with either excimer laser coronary angioplasty or conventional balloon angioplasty. The baseline characteristics were identical between the two groups. Procedural success was achieved in 80% of the excimer laser angioplasty-treated patients and in 79% of the balloon angioplasty-treated patients, based on core laboratory angiographic criteria of less than 50% residual stenosis and the absence of major complication. The cumulative rates of major complications were identical at six months (Table 30.2). Subgroup analyses reportedly showed no benefit for total occlusions (23).

The decision to enroll patients with lesions greater than 10 mm in length in the

Table 30.2.
Multicenter Randomized Clinical Trials of Ablative Devices with Balloon Angioplasty

	AMRO (48)		AMRO Substudy (23)	
	Lesions > 10 mm in length in native coronary arteries		Total or subtotal occlusions in native coronary arteries	
End Points	PTCA n = 157	ELCA n = 151	PTCA n = 54	ELCA n = 49
Angiographic success (%)[a]	78.8	80.2	61.1	65.3
Final % stenosis	37.9	37.6	34.5	40.0
Restenosis rate (%)[b]	41.3	51.6	48.5	66.7
Myocardial infarction at 6 mo (%)	5.7	4.6	5.6	2.0
Death at 6 mo (%)	0.0	0.0	0.0	0.0

[a] Angiographic success = < 50% diameter stenosis and no major in-hospital complication such as death, myocardial infarction, or emergency bypass surgery.
[b] Restenosis rate = proportion of patients with > 50% diameter stenosis on coronary arteriography performed 3 to 6 months after initial treatment.
P = NS for all comparisons; AMRO, Amsterdam-Rotterdam Laser Study; CAVEAT, Coronary Angioplasty Versus Excisional Atherectomy Trial; ELCA, excimer laster coronary angioplasty; PTCA, percutaneous transluminal coronary angioplasty.

Table 30.3.
Randomized Comparison of Percutaneous Transluminal Coronary Angioplasty, Excimer Laser, and Rotational Atherectomy at a Single Center

	PTCA	ELCA	PTRA
N	210	195	215
Calcified lesions (%)	86 (41%)	84 (43%)	71 (33%)
Device success (%)	176 (84%)	172 (88%)	200 (93%)
Death, MI, or CABG (%)	10 (4.8%)	12 (6.2%)[a]	5 (2.3%)
Restenosis rate at 6 mo	51%	61%	56%
Clinical event rate at 6 mo	45%	49%	53%

Reprinted with permission from Vandormael M, Reifart N, Preusler W, et al. Six months follow-up results following excimer laser angioplasty, rotational atherectomy and balloon angioplasty for complex lesions: ERBAC study [abstract]. Circulation 1994;90(Suppl I):I213.
[a] P < 0.05, as compared with PTCA or PTRA.
[b] P < 0.05, as compared with PTCA.
PTCA, percutaneous transluminal coronary angioplasty; ELCA, excimer laser coronary angioplasty and adjunctive balloon angioplasty; PTRA, percutaneous transluminal rotational atherectomy plus adjunctive balloon angioplasty; Device success = < 50% diameter stenosis after device, balloon angioplasty, or both *plus* absence of major complication; MI, myocardial infarction; CABG, emergency bypass surgery; restenosis rate = angiographic restenosis; any clinical event = death, myocardial infarction, bypass surgery, or repeat intervention.

AMRO Trial was based on information available in 1991 when the study protocol was developed. Although excimer laser angioplasty was initially promoted for such lesions (24), later studies showed lower success and higher restenosis rates for long lesions than for discrete lesions (19, 25, 26). The current success rates of 87 to 88% (18, 19) for excimer laser angioplasty for lesions greater than 20 mm in length do not exceed the success rates for balloon angioplasty of 82 to 84% (27, 28) by a significant margin. Improvements in balloon catheters (long balloons and lower profile devices) and changes in conventional angioplasty technique (dilation with low pressures to avoid dissection), as well as the rapid development of coronary stenting for long lesions, have produced success rates as high as 96% with nonlaser approaches (29).

In the Excimer Laser Rotational Atherectomy Balloon Angioplasty Comparison (ERBAC Trial), 620 patients undergoing interventional therapy for type B and C lesions, including a high proportion of calcified lesions, were randomly treated with excimer laser angioplasty, conventional balloon angioplasty, or percutaneous transluminal rotational atherectomy (22). The procedural success rate was 84% for balloon angioplasty, 88% for excimer laser angioplasty, and 93% for rotational atherectomy (Table 30.3). The incidence of major complications (death, myocardial infarction, or bypass surgery) was greater after excimer laser angioplasty than after rotational atherectomy (6.2 versus 2.3%, P < .05), whereas the use of balloon angioplasty was associated with an intermediate rate of complications (4.8%). At 6-month follow-up, the incidence of clinical events (death, myocardial infarction, bypass surgery, or repeat intervention) was greater after treatment with rotational atherectomy than after balloon angioplasty (53 versus 45%, P < .05), whereas treatment with excimer laser angioplasty was associated with an intermediate rate of clinical events (49%).

The ERBAC Trial evaluated the success of conventional balloon angioplasty, excimer laser angioplasty, and rotational atherectomy for patients with complex lesions. The study did not specifically evaluate the relative success of the three devices for aorto-ostial stenoses or saphenous vein graft lesions—lesion types commonly selected for which excimer laser angioplasty has superior success rates. The ERBAC Trial confirms the results of recent analyses suggesting that calcified lesions may not be ideally suited for treatment with excimer laser angioplasty (19, 25).

During excimer laser angioplasty, light at a wavelength of 308 nm emitted from optical fibers at the catheter tip vaporizes atheromatous tissue. The failure of excimer laser angioplasty to achieve better clinical outcomes in the AMRO or ERBAC studies has been attributed to inadequate tissue removal (30), along with an increased risk of vessel dissection (31) and perforation (32) from the formation of intraluminal vapor bubbles in blood (33). The incidence of dissection may have been reduced by infusing saline through the guide catheter during excimer laser angioplasty (34).

Undilatable Lesions

Calcified and fibrotic lesions cannot always be dilated with conventional balloons, even at high pressures. Pulsed excimer laser radiation, however, results in the formation of transient, high-pressure stress waves, which may be responsible for the production of vessel dissection in coronary angioplasty but may be exploited for dilating resistant lesions. In a prospective series of 2432 patients undergoing excimer laser angioplasty, 37 patients (1.5%) with 38 lesions were enrolled for the primary indication of failure to dilate the target lesion with conventional balloon angioplasty (n = 24) at 16 ± 5 atm (range 14–25 atm), or inability to cross the target lesion with the balloon (n = 14) after successful wire placement (35). Of the 38 lesions, 14 (37%) were total occlusions crossable with a guidewire, and 14 (37%) were calcified stenoses. Excimer laser treatment successfully facilitated balloon dilation in 34 of 38 lesions (89%), leading to less than 50% diameter stenosis and no in-hospital complication. Complications included non–Q-wave myocardial infarction in 2 of 37 patients (5%), emergency bypass surgery in 1 (3%), and no deaths or Q-wave myocardial infarctions (Table 30.4). Evaluation of predictors of success suggested that excimer laser angioplasty for undilatable lesions was more successful for noncalcified lesions than for calcified lesions (96 versus 79%, $P < .05$). At 6-month follow-up in 33 patients, clinical or angiographic evidence of restenosis was detected in 43%. Thus, excimer laser angioplasty appears to be a safe and effective treatment for lesions not dilatable by balloon angioplasty alone. Through the mechanism of stress

Table 30.4.
Results of Excimer Laser Coronary Angioplasty for Undilatable Lesions

Angiographic success (38 lesions) (%)	34 (89)
Complications in hospital (%)	3 (8)
—Death	0
—Q-wave myocardial infarction	0
—Non–Q-wave myocardial infarction	2 (5)
—Coronary artery bypass graft	1 (3)
—Any major complication	2 (6)
Failure to cross lesion	4 (11)
Significant dissection	3 (8)
Minor dissection	10 (26)
Perforation	1 (3)
Spasm	1 (3)
Abrupt closure	1 (3)
Embolization	0
Aneurysm formation	0
Filling defect	1 (3)

Reprinted with permission from Ahmed WH, Al-Anazi MM, Bittl JA. Excimer laser facilitated angioplasty for undilatable coronary narrowings. Am J Cardiol 1996;78:1045–1047.

wave formation, this treatment overcomes the tensile strength of fibrotic lesions to facilitate dilation.

Laser Wire Angioplasty for Total Occlusions

In a multicenter study of the 0.018-inch excimer laser wire for total occlusions, 200 consecutive patients have been enrolled (36). The mean age of patients was 59 years. The minimal duration of total occlusion was 2 weeks with a median angiographic age of the occlusion of 12 weeks (range 2 to 540). The overall success of the laser wire was 57% (Fig. 30.1). Success was achieved in 65 of 116 patients (56%) in whom mechanical guidewires had failed to achieve recanalization. The risk of major complications was low, with death occurring in no patients, emergency surgery in no patients, and myocardial infarction in two (1%). Although the laser wire perforated the vessel in 48 cases (24%), hemopericardium and cardiac tamponade occurred in only 2 patients (1%). Perforation occurred after inadvertent advancement of balloon catheters over the perforated wire in two patients in whom

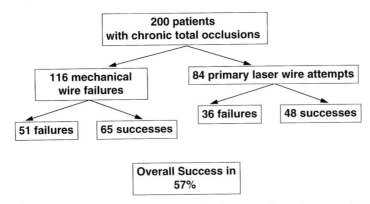

Figure 30.1. Laser wire for total occlusions. Two hundred patients have been enrolled in the European Multicenter Surveillance Study. In 116 patients, attempts with mechanical wires were unsuccessful, but subsequent use of the laser wire was successful in 65 patients (56%). In 84 patients, the laser wire was successful in 48 (57%). (Reprinted with permission from Hamburger JN, de Feyter PJ, Serruys PW. The laser guidewire experience: "crossing the Rubicon." Semin Intervent Cardiol 1996;1:163–171.)

wire perforation was unrecognized and who were successfully treated with pericardiocentesis and discontinuation of anticoagulation alone.

Once the laser wire is successfully positioned across the total occlusion, adjunctive therapy with a broad range of devices is possible. Laser-assisted laser angioplasty with adjunctive balloon angioplasty was used in 56 of 113 successfully treated patients, and stenting was used in 21 patients (36).

EXCIMER LASER ANGIOPLASTY TECHNIQUE

Conventional, commercially available guiding catheters are used for excimer laser angioplasty. Because laser catheters are stiffer than balloon catheters and have difficulty negotiating acute angles into the target vessel, coaxial alignment of guiding catheters is important. Firm guide support, however, is not usually needed to advance the activated laser catheter through the target lesion. Forceful advancement of the catheter across the lesion may increase the risk of vessel dissection.

A 7 F guiding catheter may be used for 1.4-mm laser catheters; an 8 F guiding catheter is required for 1.7-mm or 2.0-mm laser catheters. For excimer laser angioplasty of lesions in the left anterior descending artery, the Judkins configuration is the shape of choice. For laser angioplasty of lesions in the left circumflex coronary artery or obtuse marginal branches, an Amplatz shape may be selected for smoother passage of the laser catheter. For the 1.7- and 2.0-mm catheters, guidewires up to 0.018-inch in diameter can be used. For the 1.4-mm laser catheters, a 0.014-inch guidewire is required, although an "extra support" wire may help in cases involving proximal vessel tortuosity.

It is important to select a laser catheter with a diameter smaller than the reference diameter of the target vessel to reduce the risk of vessel perforation with excimer laser angioplasty. The laser catheter should be about 1.0 mm smaller than the reference diameter of the vessel (32), or about two thirds the size of the reference diameter of the target vessel (37). Thus, the 2.0-mm laser catheter should be reserved for treating vessels larger than 3.0 mm in diameter. For diffuse disease or total and subtotal occlusions, the 1.4-mm laser catheter is recommended.

Although currently available laser catheters are more flexible than the prototype catheters used several years ago, the relatively stiff laser catheters are still less likely than balloon catheters to negotiate an angle less than 90° and should not be used in tortuous or angulated anatomy. When laser

Table 30.5.
Technique for Saline Infusion During Excimer Laser Coronary Angioplasty

1. Position laser catheter in contact with target lesion.
2. Replace contrast syringe with a 20-mL saline-filled syringe.
3. Flush manifold and guide catheter with 20 mL saline to remove contrast.
4. Adjust O-ring on Y-adapter so laser catheter can be advanced without saline leak during injection.
5. Immediately before activating laser and advancing laser catheter, inject 10 mL bolus saline via guide catheter.
6. Upon advancing activated laser catheter, inject saline (1–3 mL/sec).
7. Repeat saline injection procedure for each laser train.

catheters are used in angulated segments, the stiff catheters may overdrive the guidewire and direct laser energy against the vessel wall, causing dissection or perforation.

After the target lesion is crossed with the guidewire, the laser catheter is advanced to the proximal end of the lesion. This catheter position should be documented on cine. Before activating the laser and beginning lesion ablation, every effort must be made to first remove all contrast medium from the target vessel by flushing the guide catheter with at least 30 mL of saline (Table 30.5). This is important because the interaction between excimer laser radiation and any retained contrast medium may increase the generation of shock waves with disruption of adjacent tissue planes (34, 38).

During pulsed excimer laser angioplasty, laser energy is delivered at a fluence of 40 to 60 mJ/mm^2 at a frequency of 25 to 40 Hz for 1 to 5 seconds as the end of the catheter is advanced through the lesion. For soft lesions such as saphenous vein graft lesions and restenosis lesions, laser treatment may commence at a fluence of 40 mJ/mm^2, but for calcified lesions and de novo lesions in the native coronary arteries, laser treatment should begin at 50 mJ/mm^2. As the laser is activated, the catheter is advanced slowly under fluoroscopic guidance through the lesion at an average rate of 0.5 to 1.0 mm/sec. Faster rates of advancement may exceed the rate at which excimer laser

irradiation can ablate atheromatous plaque (15) and should be avoided. After each train of laser pulses, the laser catheter should not be activated for 10 seconds to reduce the attenuation of energy transmission through the optical fibers. If the laser catheter meets resistance and cannot pass through the lesion at the initial fluence, the energy output should be increased to a maximum of 60 mJ/mm^2. If the laser catheter still cannot be advanced at higher fluence levels, the repetition rate should be increased to a maximum of 40 Hz. If the laser catheter still fails to make progress through a stenotic segment after 15 seconds of laser time, the temptation for forceful advancement of the catheter should be resisted. Repetitive, forceful advancement of the laser against a resistant lesion only increases the risk of vessel perforation. Once the laser catheter has been advanced completely through the stenotic segment, adjunctive balloon postdilation is required in about 90% of laser angioplasty procedures to reduce the residual stenosis below 30% (18, 25). Further improvement can be achieved by following excimer laser angioplasty with stent placement.

To reduce the likelihood of vessel spasm during excimer laser angioplasty, empiric treatment with intravenous nitroglycerin is recommended. If dissection occurs, it should be managed like dissection after balloon angioplasty, using either prolonged perfusion balloon inflation or coronary stenting. Embolization of particulate material is uncommon during excimer laser angioplasty, even in the setting of saphenous vein grafts (26).

If perforation occurs (Fig. 30.2), the treatment is straightforward (Table 30.6). A perfusion balloon catheter should be advanced over the guidewire and inflated at the perforation site to seal the leak in the vessel (39). In many cases, small perforations that present as localized contrast extravasation can be successfully treated with prolonged balloon inflation alone (32). Larger perforations communicating with the pericardial space, however, may require prompt and aggressive intervention beyond perfusion balloon treatment. If hemopericardium ensues, the cardiac silhouette border may cease to move under fluoroscopy. If this is associated with hypotension, emergency

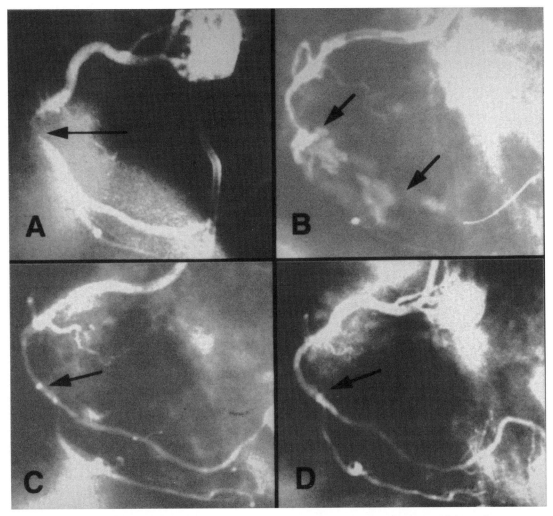

Figure 30.2. Coronary artery perforation. An angulated lesion in the midportion of the right coronary artery was treated with excimer laser angioplasty (**A,** *arrow*). After passage of the laser catheter, the patient complained of bilateral shoulder and chest pain. Coronary arteriography showed extravasation of contrast (**B,** *arrows*). A perfusion balloon was advanced over the guidewire and inflated for 20 minutes (**C,** *arrow*), heparin was discontinued, and protamine was administered. The final views 2 hours later (**D**) and 4 days later (not shown) showed no further extravasation but a widely patent vessel. (Reprinted with permission from Parker JD, Ganz P, Selwyn AP, et al. Successful treatment of an excimer laser-associated coronary artery perforation with the Stack perfusion catheter. Cathet Cardiovasc Diagn 1991;22:118–123.)

pericardiocentesis is essential. A free perforation communicating with the pericardial space that does not seal with prolonged balloon inflation alone may do so after reversal of anticoagulation; otherwise, emergency bypass surgery with oversewing of the perforation site is indicated. It is also important to be wary of the possibility of delayed cardiac tamponade (40).

Specific Lesion Types

Saphenous Vein Graft Lesions

Excimer laser angioplasty has been used extensively to treat lesions in saphenous vein grafts (Fig. 30.3), with success rates of ap-

Table 30.6.
Management of Vessel Perforation During Excimer Laser Coronary Angioplasty

If extravasation of contrast material noted...

1. Keep guide catheter in coronary artery and maintain guidewire position across lesion at all times.
2. Select perfusion balloon to match vessel diameter, advance balloon to site of perforation, and inflate to 2–4 atm to stabilize disruption and stop further extravasation.
3. Distinguish between contained perforations ("deep-wall dissections") versus free perforations communicating with pericardial space.
4. Use hemodynamic measurements to evaluate possibility of cardiac tamponade.
5. In hypotensive patient, emergently investigate possibility of tense hemopericardium by fluoroscopy in anteroposterior projection without magnification to evaluate motion of cardiac border.
6. Perform pericardiocentesis immediately if evidence of cardiac tamponade.
7. Discontinue all infusions of heparin and other antithrombotic therapies.
8. In stable patient, use echocardiography to evaluate presence of pericardial fluid.
9. Consult cardiac surgery and cardiac anesthiology.
10. If extravasation persists after 10 to 20 minutes of balloon inflation, reverse heparin with protamine, but flush guide catheter and perfusion balloon with saline at least every 2 minutes.
11. If free extravasation stops completely after catheter-based therapies, transfer patient with pulmonary artery line in place to intensive care unit for close observation and daily echocardiographic assessment for minimum of 2 to 3 days.
12. If free extravasation persists after reversal of heparin and prolonged treatment with balloon inflation, or if anticoagulation is required after free perforation with pericardial space, refer patient for cardiac surgery for direct control of perforation and coronary bypass.

proximately 92% (18, 26). In a series of 495 patients with saphenous vein graft lesions treated with excimer laser angioplasty, the following complications occurred: death in 1.0%, emergency bypass surgery in 0.6%, and Q-wave myocardial infarction in 2.4%. Angiographic complications included embolization in 3.3%, perforations in 1.3%, and dissections in 8.8% (26). A lower incidence of complications was seen for ostial lesions than for lesions in the body of the saphenous vein graft, for discrete lesions than for long lesions, and for lesions in vein grafts less than 3.0 mm in diameter than for lesions in large grafts. In this series where the mean graft age was more than 8 years, graft age did not affect the outcome of the procedure. The overall angiographic restenosis rate for saphenous vein graft lesions was approximately 55%, but was lower for discrete lesions in saphenous vein grafts more than 3.0 mm in diameter (26).

Excimer laser angioplasty has an important role in the treatment of saphenous vein graft lesions. Lesions in large saphenous vein grafts respond to stenting after excimer laser pretreatment, and lesions in small saphenous vein grafts have excellent success rates with excimer laser angioplasty and adjunctive balloon angioplasty. It is important to note that excimer laser angioplasty has the unique trait among interventional devices of achieving higher success rates in saphenous vein grafts than in native vessels (19, 25, 41). In spite of its unique capability for saphenous vein graft lesions, excimer laser angioplasty is not widely advocated as a first-line device for this indication because of concerns about embolization or inadequate dilation. Recent studies suggest that the risk of embolization with excimer laser angioplasty in saphenous vein grafts is low (18, 26) and, although restenosis rates after adjunctive balloon angioplasty alone may be higher than ideal (26, 42), adjunctive therapy after excimer treatment with stenting may result in more favorable long-term outcome (43, 44). Debulking of complex saphenous vein graft lesions with laser angioplasty before stenting is a strategy that has been compared with transluminal extraction atherectomy (45). In 81 consecutive patients treated with laser and stenting, the success rate was 100% and the incidence of non–Q-wave myocardial infarction was 8.7%. In 36 consecutive patients treated with transluminal extraction atherectomy and stenting, the success rate was also 100%, but the rate of myocardial infarction was 15.6% (45).

For laser angioplasty of left saphenous

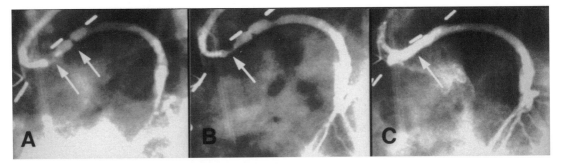

Figure 30.3. Complex lesions in saphenous vein graft. Several ulcerated stenoses were observed in the proximal segment of an 8-year-old saphenous vein graft in a patient with unstable angina (**A,** *arrows*). After a single passage of a 2-mm laser catheter, a lumen was formed (**B,** *arrow*) that permitted passage and deployment of a 5-mm stent (**C,** *arrow*).

vein graft lesions, left bypass graft guides or hockey stick-shaped guides are useful. For left saphenous vein graft bypass grafts with a severe initial upward course, internal mammary guides can provide ideal coaxial alignment. For left saphenous vein graft bypass grafts with an initial horizontal or downward course, left or right Amplatz or right Judkins guides are useful. For right saphenous vein bypass grafts with a downward course, either a multipurpose guide, right Judkins guide, or right Amplatz guide can be used. The results with excimer laser angioplasty have been increasingly improved with the adjunctive use of other devices, including atherectomy and stenting.

Ostial Stenoses

Because of the likelihood of elastic recoil after balloon dilation alone, ostial stenoses often require an ablative therapy, such as excimer laser angioplasty, for successful outcome (Fig. 30.4). In a total of 344 patients with aorto-ostial stenoses treated with excimer laser angioplasty, the success rate was 90 to 94% (46, 47). Complications included death in 0.6%, emergency bypass in 2.3%, and non-Q or Q-wave myocardial infarction in 2.3% of patients. The rates of angiographic restenosis have ranged from 39 to 41%.

For laser angioplasty of the ostium of the right coronary artery with a downward or horizontal proximal segment, a Judkins right guide is recommended. For the right coronary artery with a superiorly directed proximal segment, an Amplatz left 1.0 or 1.5 is the guide catheter of choice. In this setting, Amplatz left guides allow the greatest flexibility for coaxial alignment, which is achieved by withdrawing the guide to direct the tip downward and advancing the guide to point the tip upward.

Calcified Lesions

Calcified lesions were initially thought to be a suitable indication for excimer laser angioplasty (24, 25), but results of more recent studies have tempered the enthusiasm for this indication. In an analysis of 428 patients undergoing excimer laser angioplasty for calcified lesions (19), the success rate was 83%, which was lower than that for patients with noncalcified lesions ($P = .002$). The ERBAC Trial (Table 30.3) evaluated the success of conventional balloon angioplasty, excimer laser angioplasty, and rotational atherectomy for patients with complex lesions. Because the ERBAC study enrolled patients with a high proportion of calcified lesions, and because most of the failed laser procedures occurred with these lesions (22), the results support the conclusion that excimer laser angioplasty should not be considered for patients with significant lesion calcification.

Long Lesions

Although long lesions were initially identified as the most promising indication for excimer laser angioplasty because of success rates that are independent of lesion length (18, 25, 41), recent analyses have suggested that long lesions are associated with trends toward reduced success (19), and strategies using long balloons and selective use of coronary stent placement (29) may result in superior success rates.

In a randomized comparison of excimer laser angioplasty with balloon angioplasty for lesions greater than 10 mm in length in 308 patients, the AMRO Trial (Table 30.2) reported equivalent results for both types of treatment (48).

In-Stent Restenosis

The appeal of excimer laser angioplasty for in-stent restenosis is based on several factors. First, the limitations of vessel dissection and perforation are minimized within stented segments of coronary arteries. Second, the inability of balloon angioplasty to ablate the exuberant tissue within stents may be responsible for high repeat restenosis rates. Third, laser angioplasty is effective in removing tissue from within stents and in producing larger lumens than those achieved with balloon angioplasty alone (49).

Excimer laser angioplasty for in-stent restenosis involves the multiple passage of either the concentric laser catheter or, preferably, the eccentric laser catheter during saline infusion. It is important, however, to limit excimer laser treatment to stented segments and avoid the production of marginal dissections.

Laser Angioplasty for Total Occlusions

Total occlusions crossable with a guidewire are associated with procedural success rates of 84 to 90% with excimer laser angioplasty (25, 50). Although conventional excimer laser angioplasty requires that the lesion be crossed with a guidewire, it may facilitate subsequent dilation by ablating tissue. It must be emphasized, however, that excimer laser angioplasty is not being used extensively to treat total occlusions associated with acute myocardial infarction.

Many dissections that occur with excimer laser angioplasty, especially in the treatment of total occlusions, take place because the guidewire has traveled along an extraluminal course. It is important to ensure that the guidewire is in the true lumen of the vessel by frequent contrast media injections and by confirming that the distal tip remains mobile. The long-term success after excimer laser treatment of total occlusions is limited by the development of restenosis in approximately 46% of patients (25).

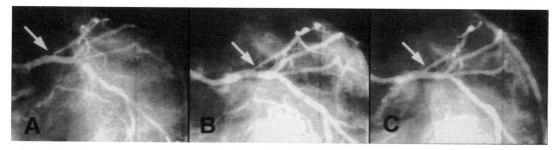

Figure 30.4. Ostial stenosis. A patient presented with unstable angina associated with an 80% stenosis at the ostium of a 2.2-mm left anterior descending artery (**A,** *arrow*). Because the vessel size and lesion location were unsuitable for treatment with stenting or atherectomy, a 1.4-mm laser catheter was used, leaving a 30% residual stenosis (**B,** *arrow*). This was followed with low-pressure balloon angioplasty, leaving no residual stenosis (**C,** *arrow*).

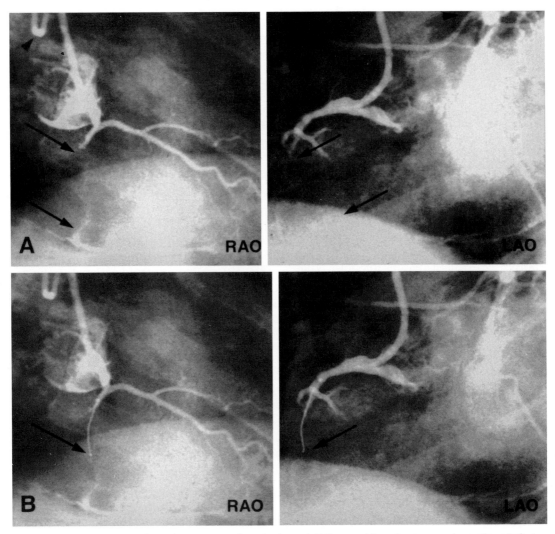

Figure 30.5. Laser wire for refractory total occlusion. A 56-year-old patient experienced an inferior myocardial infarction 20 years earlier, but developed worsening angina with increasingly frequent episodes of atrial flutter refractory to medical therapy. Biplane bilateral angiography showed complete occlusion of the right coronary artery (**A**, *large arrows*) with good visualization of the distal artery filling via collaterals from the left coronary artery injected simultaneously through a diagnostic catheter (**A**, *arrowheads*). Attempts at advancing high-torque standard and standard steerable guidewires were unsuccessful (**B**, *arrows*). The 0.018-inch laser wire easily gained passage to the distal vessel, and it was converted to an exchange wire for laser angiolasty with a 1.7 laser catheter, leaving a lumen (**C**, *arrowheads*). Placement of two and one-half slotted-tube stents resulted in no residual stenosis (**D**). *LAO*, left anterior oblique; *RAO*, right anterior oblique.

Laser Wire Angioplasty

For total occlusions that cannot be crossed with a conventional guidewire, the new approach with an excimer laser wire angioplasty has been successful (Table 30.1). The most important aspect of laser wire angioplasty is patient and lesion selection. The stump of the total occlusion can have a broad range of morphologies, including a tapered funnel or blunt stump with side branches, but the critical aspect of lesion selection that ensures success of laser wire angioplasty is the presence of the distal vessel conspicuously visualized by collateral flow. If the source of collaterals is from the contralateral coronary artery, a second femoral sheath and diagnostic coronary catheter should be used.

The second aspect of lesion selection that ensures success is that absence of angulation in the totally occluded segments. This is important in considering those patients with occlusions of the right coronary artery involving a sharply angulated Shepherd's crook or segment involving the inherent angulation of the crux.

Successful laser wire angioplasty performance is aided by the use of biplane angiography. By using biplane-bilateral angiogra-

phy during advancement of the laser wire, the operator can be assured that the laser wire is tracking in the correct plane at all times (Fig. 30.5). Saline infusion is not required during laser wire angioplasty.

SUMMARY

Careful patient and lesion selection optimizes the outcome of excimer laser angioplasty. Saline infusion should be used during conventional laser angioplasty because it has reduced the rate of vessel dissection. The lesions most likely to benefit from laser angioplasty include those in saphenous

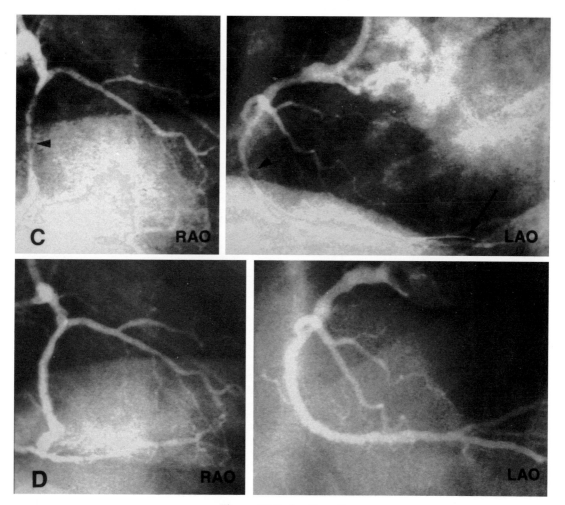

Figure 30.5. *(continued)*

vein grafts, ostial lesions, total occlusions, and balloon dilation failures. Calcified lesions have suboptimal success rates with excimer laser angioplasty, and they may respond better to treatment with alternative ablation devices. New techniques involving excimer laser angioplasty for saphenous vein graft lesions targeted for stenting, treatment of in-stent restenosis, and the excimer laser wire for total occlusions will increase the usefulness of excimer laser techniques in interventional cardiovascular medicine.

References

1. Ginsburg R, Kirr DS, Guthaner P, et al. Salvage of an ischemic limb by laser angioplasty: Description of a new technique. Clin Cardiol 1984;7:54–58.
2. Geschwind H, Boussignac G, Teisseire B. Percutaneous transluminal laser angioplasty in man [Letter]. Lancet 1984;2:844.
3. Ginsburg R, Wexler R, Mitchell RS, et al. Percutaneous transluminal laser angioplasty for treatment of peripheral vascular disease: clinical experience in 16 patients. Radiology 1985;156:619–624.
4. Choy DS, Stertzer SH, Myler RK, et al. Human coronary laser recanalization. Clin Cardiol 1984;7:377–381.
5. Foschi A, Myers G, Crick WF, et al. Laser angioplasty of totally occluded coronary arteries and vein grafts: preliminary report on a current trial. Am J Cardiol 1989;63 (Suppl F):9F–13F.
6. Geschwind HJ, Aptecar E, Boussignac G, et al. Results and follow-up after percutaneous pulsed laser-assisted balloon angioplasty guided by spectroscopy. Circulation 1991;83:787–796.
7. Sanborn TA, Faxon DP, Kellet MA, et al. Percutaneous coronary laser thermal angioplasty. J Am Coll Cardiol 1986;8:1437–1440.
8. Abela GS, Seeger JM, Pry RS. Percutaneous laser recanalization of totally occluded peripheral arteries: a technical approach. Dynamic Cardiovascular Imaging 1988;1:302–308.
9. Tobis JM, Conroy R, Deutsch L-S, et al. Laser-assisted versus mechanical recanalization of femoral arterial occlusions. Am J Cardiol 1991;68:1079–1086.
10. Belli AM, Cumberland DC, Procter AE, et al. Total peripheral artery occlusions: conventional versus laser thermal recanalization with a hybrid probe in percutaneous angioplasty: results of a randomized trial. Radiology 1991;181:57–60.
11. Hiehle JF. Nd:YAG laser fusion of human atheromatous plaque-arterial wall separations in vitro. Am J Cardiol 1985;56:953.
12. Spears JR, Reyes VP, Wynne J, et al. Percutaneous coronary laser balloon angioplasty: initial results of a multicenter experience. J Am Coll Cardiol 1990;16:293–303.
13. Kuntz RE, Safian RD, Levine MJ, et al. Novel approach to the analysis of restenosis after the use of three new coronary devices. J Am Coll Cardiol 1992;19:1493–1499.
14. Gregory KW, Block P, Knopf W, et al. Laser thrombolysis in acute myocardial infarction. Laser Surg Med 1993;51 (Suppl 5):13.
15. Grundfest WS, Litvack F, Forrester JS, et al. Laser ablation of human atherosclerotic plaque without adjacent tissue injury. J Am Coll Cardiol 1985;5:929–933.
16. Bonner R, Smith PD, Prevosti LD, et al. New sources for laser angioplasty: Er:YAG, excimer lasers, and nonlaser hot-tip catheters. In: Vogel JHK, King SBI, eds. Interventional cardiology: future directions, St. Louis: CV Mosby, 1989;101–118.
17. Litvack F, Forrester JS, Grundfest WS, et al. The excimer laser: from basic science to clinical application. In: Vogel JHK, King SBI, eds. Interventional cardiology: future directions, St. Louis: CV Mosby, 1989;170–181.
18. Litvack F, Eigler N, Margolis J, et al. Percutaneous excimer laser coronary angioplasty: results in the first consecutive 3,000 patients. J Am Coll Cardiol 1994;23:323–329.
19. Bittl JA, Brinker JA, Isner JM, et al. The changing profile of patient selection, techniques, and outcomes in excimer laser angioplasty. Journal of Interventional Cardiology; in press.
20. Bittl JA, Estella P, Abela GS. Complications of laser coronary angioplasty. In: Lutz J, ed. Complications of interventional procedures. New York: Igaku-Shoin, 1995;186–207.
21. Piek JJ, Appelman YE, Strikwerda S, et al. Excimer laser coronary angioplasty versus balloon angioplasty used in long coronary lesions: the in-hospital results of the AMRO-trial [Abstract]. Circulation 1994;90 (Suppl I):I-332.
22. Vandormael M, Reifart N, Preusler W, et al. Six months follow-up results following excimer laser angioplasty, rotational atherectomy and balloon angioplasty for complex lesions: ERBAC Study [Abstract]. Circulation 1994;90 (Suppl I):I-213.
23. Appelman YEA, Koolen JJ, Piek JJ, et al. Excimer laser angioplasty versus balloon angioplasty in functional and total coronary occlusions. Am J Cardiol 1996;78:757–762.
24. Cook SL, Eigler NL, Shefer A, et al. Percutaneous excimer laser coronary angioplasty of lesions not ideal for balloon angioplasty. Circulation 1991;84:632–643.
25. Bittl JA, Sanborn TA, Tcheng JE, et al. Clinical success, complications and restenosis rates with excimer laser coronary angioplasty. Am J Cardiol 1992;70:1533–1539.
26. Bittl JA, Sanborn TA, Yardley DE, et al. Predictors of outcome of percutaneous excimer laser coronary angioplasty of saphenous vein bypass graft lesions. Am J Cardiol 1994;74:144–148.
27. Ghazzal ZMB, Weintraub WS, Ba'albaki HA, et al. PTCA of lesions longer than 20 mm: initial outcome and restenosis [Abstract]. Circulation 1990; 82 (Suppl III):III-509.
28. Wolfe MW, Roubin GS, Schweiger M, et al. Length of hospital stay and complications after percutaneous transluminal coronary angioplasty: clinical

and procedural predictors. Circulation 1995;92: 311–319.

29. Cannon AD, Roubin GS, Hearn JA, et al. Acute angiographic and clinical results of long balloon percutaneous transluminal coronary angioplasty and adjuvant stenting for long narrowings. Am J Cardiol 1994;73:635–641.

30. Mintz GS, Kovach JA, Javier SP, et al. Mechanisms of lumen enlargement after excimer laser coronary angioplasty. Circulation 1995;92:3408–3414.

31. Baumbach A, Bittl JA, Fleck E, et al. Acute complications of coronary excimer laser angioplasty: analysis of two multicenter registries. J Am Coll Cardiol 1994;23:1305–1313.

32. Bittl JA, Ryan TJ Jr, Keaney JF Jr, et al. Coronary artery perforation during excimer laser coronary angioplasty. J Am Coll Cardiol 1993;21:1158–1165.

33. van Leeuwen TG, Meertens JH, Velema E, et al. Intraluminal vapor bubble induced by excimer laser causes microsecond arterial dilation and invagination leading to extensive wall damage in the rabbit. Circulation 1993;87:1258–1263.

34. Deckelbaum LI, Natarajan MK, Bittl JA, et al. Effect of intracoronary saline on dissection during excimer laser coronary angioplasty: A randomized trial. J Am Coll Cardiol 1995;26:1264–1269.

35. Ahmed WH, Al-Anazi MM, Bittl JA. Excimer laser facilitated angioplasty for undilatable coronary narrowings. Am J Cardiol 1996;78:1045–1047.

36. Hamburger JN, de Feyter PJ, Serruys PW. The laser guidewire experience: "crossing the Rubicon." Semin Intervent Cardiol 1996;1:163–171.

37. Holmes DR Jr, Reeder GS, Ghazzal ZMB, et al. Coronary perforation after excimer laser coronary angioplasty: the Excimer Laser Coronary Angioplasty Registry Experience. J Am Coll Cardiol 1994; 23:330–335.

38. Tcheng JE, Wells LD, Phillips HR, et al. Development of a new technique for reducing pressure pulse generation during 308 nm excimer laser coronary angioplasty. Cathet Cardiovasc Diagn 1994; in press.

39. Parker JD, Ganz P, Selwyn AP, et al. Successful treatment of an excimer laser-associated coronary artery perforation with the Stack perfusion catheter. Cathet Cardiovasc Diagn 1991;22:118–123.

40. Ellis SG, Ajluni S, Arnold AZ, et al. Increased coronary perforation in the new device era: incidence, classification, managment, and outcome. Circulation 1994;90:2725–2730.

41. Bittl JA, Sanborn TA. Excimer laser-facilitated coronary angioplasty: relative risk analysis of acute and follow-up results in 200 patients. Circulation 1992;86:71–80.

42. Strauss BH, Natarajan MK, Yardley DE, et al. Early and late quantitative angiographic results of vein graft lesions treated with excimer laser angioplasty. Circulation 1995;92:348–356.

43. Holmes DR Jr, Topol EJ, Califf RM, et al. A multicenter, randomized trial of coronary angioplasty versus directional atherectomy for patients with saphenous vein bypass graft lesions. CAVEAT-II Investigators. Circulation 1995;91:1966–1974.

44. Piana RN, Moscucci M, Cohen DJ, et al. Palmaz-Schatz stenting for treatment of focal vein graft stenosis: immediate results and long-term outcome. J Am Coll Cardiol 1994;23:1296–1304.

45. Hong MK, Wong SC, Popma JJ, et al. Favorable results of debulking followed by immediate adjunct stent therapy for high risk saphenous vein graft lesions [Abstract]. J Am Coll Cardiol 1996; 27(Suppl A):179A.

46. Eigler N, Weinstock B, Douglas JS Jr, et al. Excimer laser coronary angioplasty of aorto-ostial stenoses: results of the Excimer Laser Coronary Angioplasty (ELCA) Registry in the first 200 patients. Circulation 1993;88:2049–2057.

47. Tcheng JE, Bittl JA, Sanborn TA, et al. Treatment of aorto-ostial disease with percutaneous excimer laser coronary angioplasty [Abstract]. Circulation 1992;86 (Suppl I):I-512.

48. Appelman YEA, Piek JJ, Strikwerda S, et al. Randomised trial of excimer laser versus balloon angioplasty for treatment of obstructive coronary artery disease. Lancet 1996;347:79–84.

49. Mehran R, Mintz GS, Popma JJ, et al. Mechanisms of lumen enlargement during atheroablation of in-stent restenosis: a volumetric ultrasound analysis [Abstract]. J Am Coll Cardiol 1997;29 (Suppl A).

50. Holmes DR Jr, Forrester JS, Litvack F, et al. Chronic total obstruction and short-term outcome: The excimer laser angioplasty registry experience. Mayo Clin Proc 1993;68:5–10.

31
Introduction to Coronary Artery Stenting

Michael J.B. Kutryk, MD, PhD
Patrick W. Serruys, MD, PhD

INTRODUCTION: HISTORICAL OVERVIEW

Percutaneously introduced prosthetic devices use to maintain the luminal integrity of diseased blood vessels was initially proposed by Charles Dotter in 1964 when he speculated that the temporary use of a Silastic endovascular splint might maintain an adequate lumen following the creation of a pathway across a previously occluded vessel (1). Dotter and his colleagues were also the first to apply the term "stent" in their description of an experimental technique for the nonsurgical endarterial placement of tubular coiled wire grafts in the femoral and popliteal arteries of healthy dogs (2). These early stents were mounted coaxially on a guidewire and positioned with a pusher catheter. Because the pre- and postimplantation stent dimensions were identical, the graft diameter was limited by the size of the arteriotomy and the approach vessel, and only small coils could be passed percutaneously. Although these stents could be properly positioned, stent dislocations and significant narrowing within the stented segments occurred. These problems appeared to temporarily bridle any optimism that such a device might find clinical application in the treatment of vascular diseases.

In 1983 two preliminary reports were published demonstrating the feasibility of transcatheter arterial grafting, and they rekindled the interest in the nonsurgical placement of endovascular prostheses (3, 4). Using coil wire stents made of nitinol, a unique alloy of titanium and nickel, Dotter et al. (3) and Cragg et al. (4) described encouraging results of their transcatheter endoluminal placement in canine arteries. Nitinol has a unique heat-sensitive "memory" that allowed the coil stent to be straightened at room temperature and introduced through a catheter. When positioned properly, the coils were warmed to body temperature or higher, which caused the metal to lose its malleability and allowed the stent to return to its initially imparted configuration. The success of these devices in maintaining vessel patency at 4 weeks in nonheparinized dogs eslished the potential for its use in the nonsurgical treatment of vascular disease and provided the catalyst for experimentation with a variety of innovative devices.

Not long after the preliminary reports on the use of nitinol coils, Maass et al. reported the results of implanting expanding steel spirals in the aortae and vena cavae of dogs and calves (5). With the application of torque, the springs decreased in diameter, which allowed distal delivery, and, on release of the tension, they expanded to their predetermined dimensions. Although the spirals remained sle and did not cause perforation, thrombosis, or stenosis of the treated vessel, the large diameter of the applicator required to introduce and place them limited target lumen access. In 1985, the initial results of the implantation of spring-loaded self-expanding stents in dogs were described by Wright et al. (6). They appreciated the importance of oversizing the stent in relation to the size of the target vessel to prevent protheses migration.

The idea of a balloon-mounted stent for simultaneous dilation and stent delivery was introduced by Palmaz et al. (7). In 1985, they described preliminary results of the implantation of a balloon-expandable stainless steel wire mesh in canine peripheral arteries. The following year, Palmaz published the data on a larger group of 18 balloon-expandable stent implantations in canine femoral, renal, mesenteric, and carotid arteries (8). These early results foretold problems that would plague intravascular stent implantation for the coming decade. Four thrombotic occlusions occurred in the first group of treated animals emphasized the requirement for adequate antithrombotic and antiplatelet therapy at the time of stent deployment. Recognition by Palmaz's group that heparin therapy did not prevent late occlusion of stented segments with low flow and that the best results were obtained in those without flow restriction are now axioms of contemporary stenting. Finally, their observation of an overall patency rate of 77% at 35 weeks was surprisingly similar to the findings of subsequent stent trials.

With the refinement of equipment smaller vessels could be accessed and application of this technology to the coronary system became possible. Rousseau et al. tested a flexible, self-expanding stainless steel mesh stent that was restrained with a protective sheath (9). Forty-seven devices were implanted in 28 dogs, 21 of these devices in coronary arteries. No anticoagulant or antiplatelet agents were used, and partial or total thrombotic occlusion was seen in 8 animals (35%). Thrombus formation was recognized to occur at points of rapid reduction of vessel diameter, when the end of the prosthesis was impinging on a side branch

of a major vessel and when there was a high ratio of unconstrained to implant device diameter. Endothelialization and incorporation of the stent into the vessel wall by neo-intimalization occurred by the third week after implantation, consistent with the results of stainless steel stents previously reported (6, 7). The feasibility of balloon expandable stent implantation into canine coronary arteries was also demonstrated in the same year. Roubin et al. (10) described implantation in 39 animals of a balloon mounted interdigitating flexible coil stent with a novel design. Schatz et al. (11) reported the results of the percutaneous implantation of a nonarticulated, modified Palmaz-type stent in the coronary circulation of 20 dogs. No thrombotic events were observed in these animals. The publication of these two studies in the cardiovascular literature and not in a radiologic journal heralded the divorce of coronary stenting from the field of vascular radiology.

The early experience of Rousseau's group with the implantation of the self-expanding stent in coronary arteries provided the impetus for the implantation of a stent in an atheromatous human coronary artery. The first human implantation was performed by Jacques Puel (Toulouse, France) in 1986 (12), followed shortly after by Ulrich Sigwart (Lausanne, Switzerland). Subsequently, they reported the results of the implantation of 24 self-expanding mesh stents (Medinvent SA, Lausanne) in the coronary arteries of 19 patients (13). Three conditions were considered indications for stent insertion: (*a*) restenosis of a segment previously treated with angioplasty; (*b*) stenosis of aortocoronary bypass grafts; and (*c*) acute coronary occlusion secondary to intimal dissection following balloon angioplasty. Two complications related to stent thrombosis occurred (10.5%), and there were no cases of retensosis reported within the stented segment 9 weeks to 9 months after implantation. As a consequence of the encouraging results of this landmark study, the US Food and Drug Administration (FDA) approved phase I trials in the United States using the balloon expandable Gianturco- and Palmaz-Schatz (Johnson and Johnson Interventional Systems, Warren, NJ) intracoronary stents.

By the early part of 1988, 117 self-expanding intravascular stents, subsequently called the Wallstent (Schneider, Zurich, Switzerland), had been implanted in native coronary arteries (n = 94) or in aortocoronary bypass grafts (n = 23) of 105 patients (14). Stents were placed for dilation of a restenosis, acute vessel occlusion after angioplasty, chronic occlusion after angioplasty, and as an adjunct to primary angioplasty. The results of intermediate-term follow-up of this first series were sobering with four patient deaths before repeat angiography, complete stent occlusion of 27 stents in 25 patients (24%), and a long-term restenosis rate in those that remained patent of 14% (14). The overall mortality rate at 1 year was 7.6%. The results also emphasized the controversy that surrounded the choice of a suile anticoagulation regimen to minimize postprocedural complications and hemorrhagic side effects. These results, coupled with the comments found in a daunting editorial that accompanied the manuscript (15), allayed the initial optimism for the future of these new devices.

The potential benefit of intracoronary stenting for the treatment of acute and threatened closure complicating pertcutaneous transluminal coronary angioplasty (PTCA) was demonstrated by Roubin et al. (16). They reported on their experience during the years 1987–1989 using the balloon-expandable Gianturco-Roubin stent, which was designed specifically to control dissection and acute closure (Table 31.1). Stents

were successfully deployed in all of the 115 patients studied, and optimal results were obtained in 93% of the cases. Despite the emergent nature of the procedures, the number of complications was low with 4.2% of cases requiring coronary artery bypass graft (CABG), an overall myocardial infarction (MI) rate of 16%, a subacute thrombosis rate of 7.6%, and an in-hospital mortality rate of 1.7%. These results suggested that stenting for acute or threatened closure limited the need for emergency CABG and favorably impacted on the incidence of MI. The high incidence of restenosis (41%), similar to rates seen in acute closure successfully managed by balloon dilation alone, indicated that the stent conferred no benefit on late outcome when used for the treatment of acute closure.

More favorable were the results of a multicenter registry of elective stent placement in native coronary vessels (1987–1989). These results were presented in 1991 by Schatz et al. who reported the results of implantation of a balloon-expandable articulated Palmaz-type stent fashioned with a bridging strut between two shorter stainless steel slotted tubes (Palmaz-Schatz stent) (17). Of their patient population, 21% had total occlusion and 69% had a previously successful coronary angioplasty with clinical and angiographic restenosis. Successful delivery of 299 stents was accomplished in 230 lesions in 213 patients (93%). Failed delivery occurred with 22 stents, 11 of which were successfully withdrawn, 3 were partially deployed and 8 embolized systemically after failed withdrawal. Two anticoagulation regimens were employed in this patient registry. The first 17 stented patients were given procedural dextran and heparin and discharged on aspirin and dipyridamole only. No episodes of abrupt closure were seen in these patients. As the series of patients grew, a significant number of thrombotic episodes occurred and warfarin was added to the postprocedural regimen after the first 35 patients were treated. In the 174 patients receiving stents thereafter, warfarin was administered and continued for 1–3 months and a dramatic reduction in the incidence of occlusive thrombosis (0.6%) was observed. This low incidence of subacute thrombosis could not

Table 31.1.
Characteristics of the Cook Inc. Gianturco-Roubin Stents

	First Generation Flex-Stent	Second Generation GR II Stent
Balloon	Compliant	Noncompliant
Profile	High	Low
Delivery	Over-the-wire	Monorail and over-the wire
Vessel sizes	2.0–3.8 mm	2.0–5.0 mm
Lengths	12, 20 mm	12, 30, 40 mm
Radio-opaque markers	No	Yes

be confirmed in a retrospective analysis reported in the same year, using the same device (18). In the latter study, a subacute thrombosis rate of 14% was reported, although the studies were not directly comparable with respect to patient selection. Restenosis rates determined at follow-up angiography was 36% in the registry series of Schatz (19), whereas that observed by Haude et al. was 27% (18). A higher restenosis rate was seen in those lesions treated with multiple stents (19, 20) and in those with a history of restenosis in the stented segment (19).

The results of the first trial to focus specifically on stent implantation for the treatment of restenosis after angioplasty were reported in 1992 (20). In this article, de Jaegere et al. described their experience with the Medtronic Wiktor stent, a unique coil-like prosthesis made of a single loose interdigitating tantalum wire. Stents were successfully implanted in 59 patients. Thrombotic stent occlusion occurred in 10% of the treated patients, all of whom subsequently suffered a myocardial infarction. The restenosis rate, defined as a change in diameter stenosis to greater than 50% at follow-up, was 29%.

Together, these early observational trials highlighted problems concerning stent use. Subacute stent thrombosis was clearly a problem despite the aggressive anticoagulation regimens that were used in several of the registries. Rigorous anticoagulation resulted in longer hospitalization and in difficult to control and, occasionally, serious bleeding complications. Restenosis of the stented segment appeared also to be a problem, with rates comparable to those seen with angioplasty alone. Technical obstacles with stent deployment were encountered, which helped to define ideal stent characteristics (Table 31.2). A few fundamental questions were raised by these and other small observational trials. Were the disparate results from the various stent registries related to the clinical circumstances dictating stent implantation or were they because of properties inherent to the particular device? Was there a clinical situation for which stenting could provide the solution? What became clear from these early trials was that the utility of stenting for

Table 31.2.
Desirable Stent Characteristics

Flexible
Trackable
Low unconstrained profile
Radio-opaque
Thromboresistant
Biocompatable
Reliable expandability
High radial strength
Circumferential coverage
Low surface area
Hydrodynamic compatibility

the treatment of obstructive coronary artery disease remained to be determined.

The conviction of these pioneer investigators that coronary stenting could become a standard therapeutic modality in interventional cardiology through improved periprocedural patient management, better patient selection, and clearly defined clinical indications led to the initiation of two major important randomized trials comparing balloon angioplasty with elective Palmaz-Schatz coronary stenting. The European-based BENESTENT (21) and the North American STRESS (22) studies both commenced patient recruitment in 1991 (Tables 31.3, 31.4, and 31.5).

With the publication of the positive BENESTENT and STRESS trial results and the resultant acceptance of coronary stenting as a promising alternative to angioplasty, efforts focused on improving technical aspects of stent implantation and optimizing the adjunctive therapy to minimize complication rates. Thrombosis within the self-expanding stainless steel Medinvent stent was seen in the early animal experiments (9), prompting the use of intracoronary urokinase along with heparin, aspirin, dipyridamole, and coumadin in the first human coronary implants (13). Despite this aggressive regimen, thrombosis remained a problem, and the addition of both dextran and sulfinpyrazone (14) increased the number of agents to seven with inevitable bleeding and vascular complications and a prolonged hospital stay. These high early occlusion rates with these devices (14, 15) led to the inference that stents were

Table 31.3.
Design of the BENESTENT and STRESS Trials

	BENESTENT Study	STRESS Study
Study design	Open, multicenter, randomized	Open, multicenter, randomized
Randomization	Telephone Service	Sealed envelope
End point	Angiographic	Angiographic
	MLD at FU	MLD at FU
	Restenosis rate (≥ 50% DS at FU)	Restenosis rate (≥ 50% DS at FU)
	Clinical	Clinical
	Composite clinical endpoint analysis of the occurrence of death, CVA, AMI, CABG, repeat intervention	Composite clinical endpoint analysis of the occurrence of death, AMI, CABG, bail-out stent, repeat intervention
Type of analysis	Intention to treat	Intention to treat
Power calculation	Based on an assumed clinical event rate of 30% in the control group and a reduction of 40% in the stent group, power of 0.80	Based on an assumed restenosis rate of 30% after PTCA and of 15% after stent implantation, power of 0.90
Patient population	Stable angina *de novo* lesion in coronary artery	Symptomatic ischemic heart disease *de novo* lesion in coronary artery
Patients randomized	520	410
Final study population	516	407
Study period	June 1991–March 1993	January 1991–February 1993
Number of centers	28	20

AMI, acute myocardial infarction; CABG, coronary artery bypass graft; CVA, cerebrovascular accident; DS, diameter stenosis; FU, follow-up; MLD, minimal luminal diameter; PTCA, percutaneous transluminal coronary angioplasty.

Table 31.4.
Clinical Results of the BENESTENT and STRESS Trials

	BENESTENT Study			STRESS Study		
	Balloon (n = 257)	Stent (n = 259)	P	Balloon (n = 202)	Stent (n = 205)	P
Composite clinical endpoint analysis						
In-hospital period	6.2%	6.9%	NR	11.4%	5.9%	NR
—At 6 months	29.6%	20.1%	< .05	23.8%	19.5%	ns
6-month event-free survival	70.4%	79.9%	< .05	76.2%	80.5%	ns
1-year event free survival	68.5%	76.8%	< .05	71.5%[a]	80.3%[a]	< .05
Acute closure/stent thrombosis	2.7%	3.5%	NR	1.5%	3.4%	ns
Bleeding and vascular complications	3.1%	13.5%	< .05	4.0%	7.3%	ns
Hospital stay, days	3.1	8.5	< .05	2.8	5.8	< .05

[a] Combined STRESS I and II data.
ns, nonsignificant; NR, not reported.

highly thrombogenic foreign bodies and discouraged investigators from using coronary stents as a primary treatment for coronary artery stenosis. Attributes intrinsic to the stent devices were thought to contribute to their inherent thrombogenicity, properties such as stent composition (6), stent shape (4–6), stent wire thickness (7), and

Table 31.5.
Angiographic Results of the BENESTENT, STRESS, and START Trials

	BENESTENT Study			STRESS Study			START Study		
	Pre-intervention	Post-intervention	FU	Pre-intervention	Post-intervention	FU	Pre-intervention	Post-intervention	FU
Balloon									
—RD (mm)	3.01 ± 0.46	3.09 ± 0.44	3.05 ± 0.49	2.99 ± 0.50	2.99 ± 0.46	2.98 ± 0.49	NR	Nr	NR
—MLD (mm)	1.08 ± 0.31	2.05 ± 0.33	1.73 ± 0.55	0.75 ± 0.25	1.99 ± 0.47	1.56 ± 0.65	0.80 ± 0.3	2.28 ± 0.5	1.63 ± 0.7
—Diameter stenosis (%)	64 ± 10	33 ± 16	43 ± 16	75 ± 8	35 ± 14	49 ± 19	NR	NR	NR
Stent									
—RD (MM)	2.99 ± 0.45	3.16 ± 0.43	2.96 ± 0.48	3.03 ± 0.42	3.05 ± 0.40	3.00 ± 0.41	NR	NR	NR
—MLD (mm)	1.07 ± 0.33	2.48 ± 0.39	1.82 ± 0.64	0.77 ± 0.27	2.49 ± 0.44	1.74 ± 0.60	0.79 ± 0.3	2.85 ± 0.5	1.96 ± 0.8
—Diameter stenosis (%)	64 ± 10	22 ± 8	38 ± 18	75 ± 9	19 ± 11	42 ± 18	NR	NR	NR
Restenosis rate (%) (≥ 50% DS at FU)									
—Balloon			32			42			37%
—Stent			22			31			22%

DS, diameter stenosis; FU, follow-up; MLD, minimal luminal diameter; RD, reference diameter; NR, not reported.

stent surface (23). Antonio Colombo and his group focused attention on the modalities of stent deployment, and questioned the dogma of the intrinsic thrombogenic nature of the stents. The major contribution of these investigators was to assume that normalization of the rheology inside the stent as well as its inflow and outflow would render the anticoagulation treatment superfluous. Intravascular ultrasound (IVUS) imaging played a pivotal role in revealing that most of the angiographically satisfactory stent implantations were far from being optimal (24, 25). Incomplete stent apposition, persistence of residual luminal narrowing caused by incomplete or asymmetric stent expansion, and presence of significant disease of the proximal and distal reference segments could not be easily detected with angiography, and required IVUS for visualization. Using additional high-pressure noncompliant balloon angioplasty to fully expand the stent and IVUS-guided optimization of deployment, the postintervention anticoagulation regimen was progressively decreased and finally stopped with a low closure rate and with similarly low incidence of vascular complications (26). Using a strategy of stent deployment largely influenced by the Colombo approach, a multicenter French trial was initiated in 1992 that examined the feasibility of stenting without postprocedural vitamin-K antagonists and without mandatory ultrasound. With combined aspirin plus ticlopidine antiplatelet therapy and subcutaneous low molecular weight heparin treatment, they observed a significant reduction in the rate of subacute thrombosis (27). These results are being validated in a larger multicenter European prospective observational trial (28). The observation by Neumann et al. that platelet markers rather than the coagulation parameters indicated stent thrombosis risk supports antiplatelet use rather than anticoagulant postprocedural management (29). The benefits of combined antiplatelet therapy compared with anticoagulant treatment after coronary stenting were confirmed by a pivotal prospective randomized trial showing aspirin plus ticlopidine therapy reduced incidence of both hemorrhagic and vascular complications and cardiac events (30).

Today, full antiplatelet therapy, without additional subcutaneous heparin and without ultrasound guidance, has become routine clinical practice. Using this approach, the acute and subacute closure rates have become acceptably low while the search for a better antiplatelet agent continues. The problem of restenosis remains, however. All currently available stents are made of metal, and they induce significant intimal hyperplasia. New approaches are currently being tested to solve the problem of restenosis, which include particular coatings for metallic stents, stents made of biologic materials, biodegradable stents, drug-eluting stents, and radioactive stents. With continued developments and refinements, coronary stenting will remain an integral part of interventional cardiology. The different types of stents available are presented in Table 31.6 and Figure 31.1.

RANDOMIZED CLINICAL TRIALS

Numerous randomized trials have been reported. These results are summarized in Chapter 33. The trials underway or planned are outlined here.

Stenting Compared with PTCA

The role of stents to reduce recurrent restenosis compared with balloon angioplasty is being evaluated in the now completed REST (stent versus PTCA RESTenosis) trial (31). This is a multicentered randomized trial comparing the implantation of a single Palmaz-Schatz stent versus conventional angioplasty in patients with restenosis in native coronary arteries. The primary objectives of this trial are the assessment of the minimal luminal diameter (MLD) and late loss at 6-month follow-up angiography. Secondary objectives include clinical events in and out of the hospital. A total of 400 patients have been randomized. Interim analysis of the first 123 patients showed favorable results with respect to acute and follow-up angiographic lumen diameter and a reduced restenosis rate based on the necessity for re-intervention for stenting compared with angioplasty alone (31). These early positive results need final confirmation, and it remains to be determined whether patients with more complex restenotic lesions will show similar benefits. Patients receiving stents in this trial were given a vitamin K antagonist for postprocedural anticoagulation, and experienced increased bleeding complications, resulting in a longer hospital stay compared with those treated by balloon angioplasty.

Acute or Threatened Closure After PTCA

The GRACE (Gianturco-Roubin stent Acute Closure Evaluation) study randomized patients with true (thrombolysis in myocardial infarction [TIMI] O or 1 flow, or TIMI 2 flow with angina or electrocardiogram (ECG) evidence of ischemia) and threatened (TIMI 2 or 3 flow with greater than 50% residual stenosis or TIMI 3 flow with dissection) to either Gianturco-Roubin stent implantation or prolonged balloon angioplasty (32). Designed in 1992, this study was hindered by slow recruitment partly because of an unwillingness on the part of many interventionalists to subject their patients with acute and threatened closure to prolonged and repeated balloon dilations with the availability of stents and the ease of their use. Results of this trial will soon be published.

The STENT-BY trial is a recently completed study carried out in eight German centers in which immediate Palmaz-Schatz stent implantation was compared with conservative techniques (autoperfusion catheters, high pressure, longer inflation, emergency CABG) for the treatment of abrupt vessel closure (TIMI 0) or symptomatic dissections (TIMI 1 flow + angina + persistent ECG changes refractory to standard intravenous therapy with heparin, nitroglycerin, and calcium channel blockers) during coronary balloon angioplasty (33). The strict inclusion criteria required that the lesion be less than 15 mm long in a vessel larger than 2.5 mm suitable to receive a single stent. A total of 100 patients were randomized into this trial. Interim analysis of the results of the first 75 patients treated suggests improved stabilization, fewer complications, and a better short- and long-term outcome in patients with stent implantation compared with conservative strategies for the treatment of abrupt closure or symptomatic postintervention dissections (33).

Table 31.6.
Types and Characteristics of Coronary Stents

Stent Type	Composition	Radio-opacity of Stent	Radio-opaque Markers	Surface Area (%) [4 mm expanded stent]	Mechanism of Expansion
Coil					
—Cardiocoil	Nitinol	Moderate	On delivery catheter	12–15	Self-expanding
—Freedom	Stainless steel	Moderate	None	11	Balloon delivery
—Wiktor-GX, -i	Tantalum	High	On delivery balloon	7	Balloon delivery
—Cordis	Tantalum	High	On delivery balloon	18	Balloon delivery
—Crossflex	Stainless steel	Moderate	On delivery balloon	18	Balloon delivery
—Angiostent	Platinum (90%), Iridium (10%)	High	On balloon and sheath	9	Balloon delivery
—GR II	Stainless steel	High	On stent	16	Balloon delivery
Slotted Tube					
—ACT-One	Nitinol	High	None	28	Balloon delivery
—Radius	Nitinol	Moderate	On restraining sheath	20	Self-expanding
—Divysio	Phoshphorylcholine coated stainless steel	Moderate	None	14	Balloon delivery
—beStent	Stainless steel	Moderate	On stent	16	Balloon delivery
—IRIS	Stainless steel	Moderate-high	None	NA	Balloon delivery
—Tensum Biotronik	Silicon carbide coated tantalum	High	None	13	Balloon delivery
—Palmaz-Schatz (PS153, Spiral, Crown)	Stainless steel	Moderate	On delivery balloon	< 20	Balloon delivery
—Fischell IsoStent	Radio-isotope implanted stainless steel	Moderate	On delivery balloon	< 20	Balloon delivery
—JoStent	Heparin coated and naked stainless steel	Moderate	None	16	Balloon delivery
—IsoStent BX	Stainless steel	Moderate	None	NA	Balloon delivery
—PURA-A, -VARIO	Stainless steel	Moderate	None	20	Balloon delivery
—ACS Multilink	Stainless steel	Moderate	On delivery balloon	15	Balloon delivery
Ring					
—AVE Micro II, gfx	Stainless steel	Moderate	On stent	8	Balloon delivery
—X-trode	Stainless steel	High (spine only)	None		Balloon delivery
Multidesign					
—NIR	Stainless steel	Moderate	On stent	16	Balloon delivery
Mesh					
—Wallstent	Cobalt alloy with platinum core	Moderate	On delivery catheter	20	Self-expanding

NA, not applicable.

The FRESCO (Florence Randomized Elective Stenting in Acute Coronary Occlusions) trial is a single center trial undertaken by a group in Italy. In this trial, 150 patients will be randomized to either conservative treatment or stent placement after optimization of angiographic results with prolonged autoperfusion balloon treatment. Randomization into this trial is currently underway.

The GRAMI (GR-II in Acute Myocardial Infarction) trial was designed to determine whether implantation of the GR-II would improve outcome in patients undergoing percutaneous intervention during acute MI. Patients were randomized to either primary PTCA alone or PTCA plus stent implantation within 24 hours of the onset of an acute MI. Results of the first 65 patients treated

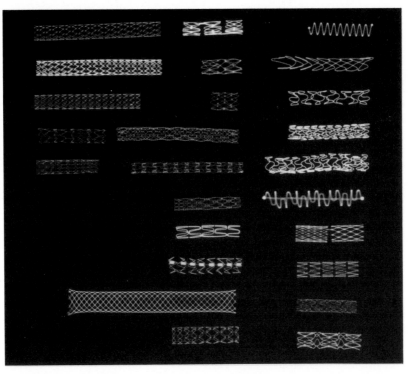

Figure 31.1. Composite radiograph of available stents showing radiopacity of each type. The order of the stents, top to bottom, left to right, is as follows: Column 1, abcde; column 2, fghijklmno; column 3, pqrstuvwxy. a, NIR stent; b, NIR Royal; c, JoStent; d, Divysio (open cell); e, Divysio (closed cell); f, Tensum Biotronik; g, Palmaz-Schatz Spiral; h, Palmaz-Schatz; i, Palmaz-Schatz Crown; j, beStent; k, IsoStent BX; l, Micro Stent II; m, Bard XT; n, Wallstent; o, IRIS; p, Coronary Cardiocoil; q, Freedom; r, Wiktor-*i*; s, CrossFlex; t, AngioStent; u, GR II; v, Act-One; w, Radius; x, Multilink; y, PURA-VARIO.

indicated that when used as a primary modality in an acute MI, coronary stenting was technically more successful with a better clinical outcome compared with PTCA alone (34).

The ESCOBAR trial is a single center trial being carried out in The Netherlands that is nearing completion (35). In this trial 93 patients were randomized to either PTCA or primary stent implantation. Preliminary results of this study indicate that primary stenting can be applied safely and effectively in the context of acute MI, and results in a better 6-month clinical outcome compared with angioplasty alone. Angiographic follow-up data from this trial are currently being analyzed. Also underway is the French STENTIM II trial, which will randomize patients with acute MI to either PTCA or PTCA plus stent implantation (36).

Evaluation of Adjunctive Therapy

Adjunctive Pharmacotherapy

Acute and Subacute Thrombosis

The high incidence of acute and subacute stent thrombosis seen in the early clinical stent trials and the publication of the results of the ISAR trial confirming that intense anticoagulation for the prevention of thrombosis may not be necessary (30), prompted the initiation of several randomized trials focused on the optimization of adjunctive pharmacotherapy. The STARS (Stent Anticoagulation Regimen Study) trial is a three-arm, multicenter, randomized trial (550 patients per arm designed to compare the

FDA-approved anticoagulation regimen of ASA [350 mg/day] plus coumadin [INR 2.0–2.5] with two antiplatelet regimens (ASA [350 mg/day] plus ticlopidine [250 mg twice daily for 4 weeks] and ASA [350 mg/day] alone) after optimal stent deployment (final angiographic stenosis < 10%; no major dissections or abrupt in-laboratory closure) of one or two Palmaz-Schatz stents in native coronary lesions (37). using high pressure ($\geq$ 16 atm) balloon deployment. The primary end point is a composite surrogate for "stent thrombosis" comprised of death, Q-wave MI, CABG, or repeat PTCA at 30 days. Both de novo and restenotic lesions are included. Enrollment in this trial is complete and preliminary results indicate a significant benefit of combination aspirin-ticlopidine therapy over aspirin alone and an aspirin-coumadin combination in the 30-day clinical outcome, with the benefit derived mainly from a reduction in the incidence of acute Q-wave MI.

The ENTICES (ENoxaprin, TIclopidine and aspirin versus the conventional Coumadin regimen after Elective Stenting) trial compares the use of enoxaprin (30–50 mg subcutaneously twice daily for 10 days), aspirin and ticlopidine with aspirin, dipyridamole, dextran, heparin and coumadin (38). One hundred and twenty patients will be randomized. Hematologic markers are measured 3 days after stent implantation, and will be correlated with clinical outcome at the trial's completion. Interim analysis of the results of the first 40 patients show that thrombin and fibrin activity are suppressed to a greater extent in those treated with enoxaprin, ticlopidine, and aspirin.

The EPILOG (Evaluation of PTCA to Improve Long-term Outcomes with c7E3 Glycoprotein IIb/IIIa-receptor blockade) stent study is a multicenter North American trial in which 3000 patients will be randomized to either balloon angioplasty with abciximab (c7E3, ReoPro), Palmaz-Schatz stent implantation with aspirin, or Palmaz-Schatz stent implantation with abciximab. Abciximab is a monoclonal Fab fragment directed against the glycoprotein IIb/IIIa (GPIIb/IIIa) receptor on the external surface of platelets. The GPIIb/IIIa receptors on adjacent platelets bind fibrinogen and von Willibrand factor, thereby mediating plate-let aggregation. The antithrombotic effect of abciximab is a result of direct inhibition of the binding of these proteins to the platelet receptors, which leads to a dose-dependent inhibition of platelet aggregation. The activity of abciximab is not limited to the GPIIb/IIIab receptor, and it may interact with vitronectin receptors on the vessel wall, which may account for the reduced clinical restenosis rate that was observed with its use in conjunction with coronary angioplasty (39). The EPILOG stent study will evaluate the effect of abciximab on both early and late clinical outcome of patients undergoing stent implantation. The aim of this study is to determine the potential complimentary action of abciximab with elective stenting for the reduction of clinical events.

Restenosis

The ERASER (Evaluation of ReoPro and Stenting to Eliminate Restenosis) study is a multicenter trial that will randomize 225 patients to placebo or one of two doses of abciximab. The primary objective of this trial is to determine if an absolute or dose-related difference exists in neointimal volume, as determined by IVUS, at 6 months poststent implantation between patients treated systemically with abciximab and placebo. The secondary end points of this trial include an assessment of major adverse cardiac events and angiographic outcome at 6 months. Enrollment in this study is proceeding.

The HIPS (Heparin Infusion Prior to Stenting) trial is a multicenter trial designed to test the hypothesis that local delivery of heparin prior to stent placement reduces subsequent restenosis. A total of 150 patients will be randomized to either a bolus of intracoronary heparin or heparin delivered using a local delivery catheter. In this trial, 5000 units of heparin will be given at the stented site using a LocalMed Infusa-Sleeve (LocalMed, Palo Alto CA) local delivery device. The primary end point is neointimal volume as measured by IVUS at 6 months. Secondary end points include angiographically determined restenosis at 6 months and the need for lesion revascularization. Enrollment into this trial is in progress.

The effect on restenosis of locally administered heparin delivered using the Dispatch (SciMED Life Systems, Maple Grove MN) is being assessed in a trial with a similar design. The DISTRESS (DISpatch STent REStenosis Study) is a single center, randomized pilot study being carried out at the Washington Cardiology Center. In total, 100 patients will be randomized to one of two arms. Patients in one arm of this trial will receive 6000 units of locally delivered heparin; patients randomized to the other arm will undergo conventional stent implantation. The primary end point of this trial is the difference in neointimal volume between the two groups at 6 months as assessed by IVUS. Secondary end points include the acute and late clinical events and the angiographically determined rate of restenosis.

An interesting single center trial is underway in The Netherlands examining locally delivered antisense oligonucleotides for the prevention of restenosis. The ITALICS (Investigation by the Thoraxcenter on Antisense DNA given by Local delivery and assessed by IVUS after Coronary Stenting) will examine the effects on restenosis of a synthetic 15-mer antisense phosphorothioate oligodeoxynucleotide directed against translation-initiation region of the c-*myc* nuclear proto-oncogene (40). In this trial 80 patients will be randomized, after successful placement of a Wallstent, to receive either placebo or the antisense compound via a local drug delivery catheter inside the stented segment. The primary end point for this trial is the in-stent neointimal volume at 6-month follow-up as assessed by IVUS. Secondary end points include angiographic assessment at 6-month follow-up and the adverse cardiac events. Randomization of patients into this trial is currently underway.

Another single center trial examining the local drug delivery after coronary stenting for the prevention of restenosis is underway in Milan, Italy. In this trial 200 patients will be randomized to stent only or the local delivery of long-acting steroid into the vessel wall using the Infiltrator (Interventional Technologies, San Diego CA) local drug delivery balloon prior to stent implantation. Primary end points for this trial are angiographic restenosis and target lesion revascularization at 6-month follow-up. Secondary end points include acute procedural complications, subacute stent thrombosis, major adverse cardiac events, and the degree of intimal hyperplasia at follow-up as determined by IVUS.

Bleeding and Vascular Complications

The FANTASTIC (Full ANticoagulation versus Ticlopidine plus Aspirin after STent Implantation) is a multicenter European trial designed to determine whether two-pronged antiplatelet therapy can significantly reduce bleeding complications seen with anticoagulation therapy (41). All patients undergoing Wiktor stent implantation were eligible for enrollment in this trial. After successful stent implantation, patients were randomized to receive either aspirin plus ticlopidine or aspirin plus coumadin (target INR of 2.5–3.0). A secondary end point of this trial was to establish if the antiplatelet regimen would compromise the patency of the stented segment. A total of 485 patients have been randomized, and enrollment has ended. Results of this trial will soon be made available.

Adjunctive Rotational Atherectomy

The RotaStent trial is a randomized trial to assess the safety and efficacy of stent placement with adjunctive atherectomy in patients with calcified lesions or diffuse lesions in native coronary arteries. In this trial, 400 patients will be randomized in 15 centers in the United States and Europe to either stent alone or stent plus pretreatment with rotational atherectomy. Primary and secondary end points include major adverse cardiac events at 30 days, angiographic restenosis, and the need for target vessel revascularization at 6-month follow-up. Patient inclusion in this trial is currently underway.

Adjunctive Radiotherapy

The IRIS (IsoStent for Restenosis Intervention Study) is designed to examine the safety and efficacy of low dose β-irradiation emitted from the surface of the radioactive Fischell IsoStent for the prevention of clinical and angiographic restenosis. In total, 1200 patients will be randomized to control non-radioactive stent implantation and to one of three activity ranges of ^{32}P. End points in this trial are clinical events, including target lesion revascularization and angiographic results determined at 6 month follow-up.

The SCRIPPS trial (Scripps Coronary Radiation to Prevent Restenosis), undertaken by the group at the Scripps Foundation in California, has been recently completed (42). In this trial, 55 patients with restenosis following PTCA who were candidates for Palmaz-Schatz stent implantation were randomized to conventional therapy or to treatment with intracoronary gamma irradiation using ^{192}Ir radiation. End points include angiographically determined late lumen loss. Final results of this trial should soon be made available.

Stenting Compared with Surgery

A randomized trial comparing coronary bypass surgery with coronary stent implantation employing the Cordis/Johnson and Johnson Crown stent for multiple vessel coronary disease is about to begin. This multicenter trial, given the acronym ARTS (Arterial Revascularization Therapies Study), will randomize a total of 1200 patients to either CABG or stent implantation. The primary objective of ARTS is an assessment of the effectiveness of each treatment as measured by freedom from major adverse cardiac and cerebrovascular events over a period of 1 year. Secondary objectives are to compare both strategies with respect to adverse events at 30 days, and at 3 and 5 years, and cost effectiveness and quality of life over 1-, 3-, and 5-year follow-up.

The SOS (Stent Or Surgery) trial is a large multicenter international trial currently underway. The trial plans to randomize 1800 patients with multivessel stenoses to either stent implantation or CABG to determine whether the benefits of stenting will translate to the management of multivessel coronary artery disease. Primary end points of this trial are myocardial infarction free survival at 1–4 years poststent implantation. Secondary end points include death, need for repeat revascularization, anginal symptoms, medication requirements, quality of life analysis, cognitive function, psychologic assessment, and cost analysis. Randomization is underway in Europe and is awaiting FDA approval in the United States.

Comparison of Stents

Several randomized trials are ongoing comparing various stent designs. The SMART (Study of Microstent's Ability to limit Restenosis Trial) study began randomization late in 1996. It is designed to compare the clinical and angiographic restenosis outcomes between the AVE Micro stent and the Palmaz-Schatz stent in native coronary arteries. The trial will randomize 650 patients, who will be followed clinically, with the end point being the clinically driven need for target site revascularization at 9 months postprocedure. Angiographic follow-up will be performed on a subgroup of 250 patient.

The ACT-One trial is an international randomized trial designed to compare the ACT-One stent with the Palmaz-Schatz coronary stent in terms of late-term clinical outcomes in de novo and restenotic lesions. In total, 800 patients will be randomized to implantation of either a Palmaz-Schatz or an ACT-One stent. Secondary objectives of this trial are the assessment of acute success rate, hemorrhagic and vascular complications, and angiographic restenosis. A registry will be maintained in parallel with this trial, which will include 300 patients, to examine the effectiveness of stenting with the ACT-One stent in saphenous vein grafts and in the setting of abrupt or threatened closure. The results of this registry series will be compared with the control arm of the randomized trial. Completion of this trial is expected to be 1998.

The second generation Gianturco-Roubin (GR-II) stent is being compared with the Palmaz-Schatz stent in the 31-site randomized GR-II (US) Study. A total of 700 patients will be randomized, with the primary end point being freedom from major cardiac events (death, MI, target vessel revascularization) at 6 months postprocedure. Secondary end points include angiographically determined rate of restenosis at 6 months, in-hospital procedural success, and major clinical events. The trial will include four registry series: saphenous vein graft lesions, lesions in small vessels, stenting for abrupt or threatened closure, and restenotic lesions. The aims of this trial are not only to compare the GR-II stent to the Palmaz-Schatz stent with respect to the four registry series listed, but also to compare the late clinical efficacy of GR-II stents versus Palmaz-Schatz stents in short (one Palmaz-Schatz stent) and long (two Palmaz-Schatz versus 40 mm GR-II stent) in de novo native coronary lesions. Enrollment in this trial is nearing completion.

The RACE (RAndomized trial of Cardiocoil for Equivalency with the Palmaz-Schatz stent) study is a multicenter trial that will randomize 600 patients in the United States to either Palmaz-Schatz or Cardiocoil stenting. The primary end point of this trial is a clinical event 9 months postprocedure. Secondary end points will include an angiographic analysis of a subpopulation of the patients randomized.

The ACS Multilink Stent Trial is being carried out in several centers in North America. A total of 1000 patients with focal, de novo lesions have been enrolled and randomized to elective stenting with either the ACS Multilink stent or the Palmaz-Schatz stent. Poststent treatment consisted of combined ticlopidine-aspirin antiplatelet therapy without oral anticoagulants. The primary end point of this trial is clinical restenosis at 6 months. An angiographic substudy of 500 patients is also being performed.

Assessment of the Role of Intravascular Ultrasound (IVUS)

The need for IVUS guidance of stent placement is being assessed in two studies in which patients are randomized to either IVUS or angiography-guided stent implantation and expansion. In the AVID (Angiography Versus Intravascular ultrasound Directed coronary stent placement) trial, patients are randomized to further angiographic guidance or IVUS guidance after obtaining an optimal angiographic result (< 10% diameter stenosis on visual estimate and full stent apposition) (43). In the angiography arm, blinded IVUS is performed and the patients are discharged on aspirin and ticlopidine. In the IVUS-directed arm, patients who fail the IVUS criteria (< 10% stenosis, absence of dissection, and full stent apposition) are treated with larger balloons. Patients who fulfill the IVUS criteria are discharged on aspirin and ticlopidine. Patients who fail angiographic or IVUS criteria receive enoxaprin for 2 weeks in addition to aspirin and ticlopidine. Enrollment is near completion, with a total of 800 patients planned for randomization. Preliminary results from the first 218 patients have been reported (44). In the angiography group, the IVUS results were unblinded in 2.6% of the patients and an additional stent placed for dissection. Results at 30 days indicate no difference in clinical outcome between the two groups. Stent thrombosis was observed in 1.8% of the angiography-guided group and in 1.9% in the IVUS-guided cohort. One patient (0.9%) in the angiography group and two patients (1.9%) in the IVUS group required CABG. These results were seen despite the observation that 33% of patients with optimal stenting by angiographic criteria failed to satisfy IVUS criteria. No complications from IVUS therapy were seen in this trial. These data suggest that IVUS-directed stent implantation can indeed improve acute stent dimensions (32% increase in cross-sectional area in those who underwent larger balloon inflation for an underdilated stent in the IVUS arm), but that it does not influence the 30-day clinical event rate. The OPTICUS (OPTimization with IntraCoronary UltraSound to reduces stent restenosis) is a multicenter, randomized study comparing the restenosis rate after IVUS-guided and angiography-guided stenting in 500 patients with stable or unstable angina (Braunwald class 1–2, A-C) and a single lesion suitable for Palmaz-Schatz stent implantation. Recruitment into this study is currently underway.

The aim of the single center randomized SIPS (Strategy of Intracoronary ultrasound guided PTCA and Stenting) trial is to determine if the everyday use of intracoronary ultrasound (ICUS) improves the acute and chronic outcome poststent placement at an acceptable cost. In all, 300 patients will be randomized. The primary angiographic end points of this trial are the acute MLD and the MLD at follow-up; the clinical end points are major cardiac events (death, MI, and repeat revascularization) at 6-month follow-up.

Comparison of Access Site

The BRAFE (Brachial Radial Femoral) trial is a multicenter trial that includes 150 patients at six different Belgian sites. Patients are being randomized to three different approaches for the elective implantation of Palmaz-Schatz stents (femoral puncture, brachial cutdown with 6 F guiding catheter, radial puncture with 6 F guiding catheter). The primary end point of this trial is the entry site complication rate and average poststent hospitalization. Secondary end points include success rate, failure rate, subacute thrombosis rate, and the clinical end points of death, MI, and the requirement for repeat revascularization. Preliminary results show that no patient required vascular surgery in any of the three groups. A trend was seen toward more technical difficulties and more failures in the brachial group; however, a greater subjective sense of comfort was found in the brachial and radial groups.

CURRENT INDICATIONS FOR STENTING

Coronary stent implantation as a primary treatment modality in interventional cardiology is increasing at a staggering rate. The rapid increase in the use of stents has come primarily in treatment categories not included in the few completed controlled randomized trials. In most interventional centers, stents are used in 50% or more of all coronary angioplasty procedures. This represents an enormous mismatch between clinical practice and trial based evidence. This 'stentomania' is driven both by the gratifying acute results seen by the interventionalist when using these devices and by results extrapolated from observational and randomized trials. The 'bigger is better' attitude first proposed by Kuntz et al. (45) has been adopted by many operators who feel that the greater the acute gain in lumen diameter, the smaller the chances of short- and long-term failure (46). Inherent in this concept is that the stent is merely a means to an end, and therefore, irrespective of the particular stent or other dilating or debulking device employed, success of the procedure is determined solely by the acute results. **Whether differences between various stent designs and materials are sufficient to have an impact their clinical effects remains to be demonstrated** in controlled stent versus stent trials.

The positive results of the few completed randomized trials have been enthusiastically applied to almost every other patient and lesion subcategory. The unequivocal indications for stenting are currently only those few that have been supported by observational and randomized trials, and they are limited to very few stent types. The definitive evidence for the use of stents for several specific clinical indications is still lacking. As results of the many ongoing randomized stent trials become available, the indications for stenting will have to be adapted accordingly.

Currently, solid evidence from observational and randomized trials support the use of coronary stents for two indications:

1. Treatment of abrupt or threatened vessel closure during angioplasty, and
2. Primary reduction in restenosis in de novo focal lesions in vessels greater than 3.0 mm in diameter.

Treatment of Abrupt or Threatened Vessel Closure During Angioplasty

Despite increased operator experience and improved catheter technology, abrupt ves-

Table 31.7.
Events Following Stent Implantation for Threatened or Acute Closure After Percutaneous Transluminal Coronary Angioplasty

Study	Study Period	Patients (n)	Implantation success (%)	Complications (%)			Occlusion (%)		Restenosis (%)
				Death	AMI	Urgent CABG	Incidence	Time interval	
Wallstent									
—Sigwart et al (50)	1986–1988	11	100	9	9	0	9	NR	—
—de Feyter et al (51)	1989–1990	15	100	7	13	60	20	Day 0–7	—
—Goy et al (52)	1986–1989	17	100	0	6	0	6	Day 0	25
—Eeckhout et al (53)	1986–1991	33	100	3	30	9	24	NR	9
Gianturco-Roubin									
—George et al (54)	1988–1991	518	95	2	6	7	9	Day 0–29	—
—Hearn et al (55)	1987–1990	116	89	4	4	28	9	NR	53
—Roubin et al (16)	1989–1991	115	96	2	7	4	8	NR	—
—Sutton et al (56)	1989–1991	415	NR	3	5	12	NR	NR	—
—Chan et al (57)	1991–1994	42	95	0	5	7	24	NR	—
Palmaz-Schatz									
—Haude et al (58)	NR	15	100	0	0	7	7	Day 0	21
—Hermann et al (59)	1988–1991	50	98	4	20	13	16	Day 1–10	—
—Maiello et al (60)	1990–1992	32	100	6	6	6	6	NR	54
—Kiemeneiji et a (61)	1990–1991	52	89	7	NR	15	23	NR	29
—Colombo et al (62)	1989–1992	56	100	4	4	5	2	NR	36
—Foley et al (63)	1990–1992	60	100	0	22	7	17	NR	50
—Schömig et al (64)	1989–1993	327	97	1	4	9	7	NR	30
—Alfonso et al (65)	1990–1993	42	93	0	5	3	5	NR	—
Wiktor									
—Vrolix and Piessens (66)	1991	119	95	3	NR	3	17	NR	—
Strecker									
—Reifart et al (67)	1990–1991	48	97	10	2	6	21	Day 0–19	—

AMI, acute myocardial infarction; CABG, coronary artery bypass graft; NR, not reported.

sel closure continues to limit the safety and efficacy of coronary angioplasty (Table 31.7). Acute closure is usually defined as TIMI grade 0 or 1 flow after PTCA. A consensus has not been reached for the definition of threatened closure, which may in-clude one or more of the following: 50% or greater residual stenosis, dissection 15 mm or longer, extraluminal contrast, angina, or electrocardiographic changes of ischemia. Overall, an incidence of acute or threatened closure of 4 to 10% has been reported, although the determination of its exact incidence is hampered by the use of different criteria to define acute occlusion as well as by differences in patient characteristics used in the various trials (47). The cause of abrupt closure is multifactorial; it includes arterial dissection, elastic recoil, thrombus formation, and intramural hemorrhage (48, 49). The clinical consequences of abrupt vessel closure are significant, leading to death in 5% of patients and myocardial infarction and urgent bypass surgery in 30 to 40%. Successful redilation can be achieved in approximately 44% of the patients, however, 4% of these still die, 20% sustain an acute myocardial infarction, and 7% require urgent bypass surgery, which after failed PTCA carries a perioperative mortality of 4.2% (47). In some of these cases, conventional balloon redilation may be effective, but in most instances prolonged inflation times with a autoperfusion balloon is necessary to avoid ischemic complications.

The rationale for using intracoronary stents as a bail-out technique in acute or threatened closure is based on their ability to scaffold the vessel from its endoluminal surface and, therefore, repair the dissected and reoccluded artery and reduce elastic recoil. Clinical experience with bail-out stent implantation was first reported by Sigwart et al. (13). The Wallstent was implanted in a limited number of patients, which resulted in immediate flow restoration, ECG normalization, and relief of symptoms with no evidence of acute MI. A larger experience, restricted to bail-out stenting, was subsequently reported by this group in 1988 (50). Since these early reports, several observational trials have been published using different stent types for the treatment of abrupt closure (16, 50–67). The technical success rate of these observational trials was high, although significant differences in the incidence of adverse events were apparent. These differences can be attributed to ambiguity in the definition of subacute closure, differences in the patient populations studied, and variability in the techniques for stent deployment and periprocedural pharmacotherapy. A French multicenter trial examining stent implantation without the use of postprocedural oral anticoagulant therapy in 529 consecutive patients treated since

November of 1993 was recently reported (68). In the subgroup of 112 patients receiving stents for bail-out indications, coronary events possibly related to stent thrombosis, recorded up to 30 days postprocedure, occurred in 5.4%. The overall cardiac complication rate, including the need for emergency CABG, in these patients was 18.8%, which compares favorably to the complication rate seen after autoperfusion balloon therapy.

Results of a case-control analysis comparing clinical outcome after stenting with that after conventional therapy for abrupt or threatened closure have been reported (69). For this analysis, 61 patients treated by stenting for acute closure were matched, according to angiographic features of closure and estimated left ventricular mass at risk for ischemia, with patients treated conventionally before stent availability. Despite better immediate angiographic results, no difference was found in the likelihood or severity of MI in patients with established vessel closure. In this patient subset, the need for urgent bypass surgery was significantly lower in those treated with stenting (4.9 versus 18% in the conventionally treated group, $P = .02$). Patients with threatened vessel closure could not be shown to benefit from stent treatment.

In contrast to the case-control study of Lincoff et al (69), registry results from The New York Hospital-Cornell Medical Center suggested a benefit of stenting for the treatment of acute vessel closure (70). Using registry data, angioplasty complication rates at this tertiary care referral center were compared before and after the availability of coronary stents in 2242 consecutive patients. Major complications (composite of in-hospital death, Q-wave MI, and need for emergency bypass surgery) occurred in 4.1% of patients treated before stent availability and 2.0% afterwards ($P < .01$), suggesting a benefit of coronary stenting.

Although the results of TASC II trial and preliminary results from the STENT-BY trial are suggestive of a benefit of stenting over other treatments for acute or threatened closure, the GRACE trial will provide clear information on the direct comparison between the two preferred treatment modalities, stent implantation and autoperfusion balloon treatment. Despite the lack of conclusive results from completed randomized trials, because of the additional catheterization time required with prolonged balloon inflation and the significant crossover to stenting with this strategy, early stenting for the treatment of acute and threatened closure may indeed be the preferred approach. The timing of stent implantation for abrupt closure also appears to be important. The risk of MI has been shown to be nearly threefold higher when stents are used for established acute closure than for threatened closure (71). Information on the long-term clinical outcome of stenting in this setting is still lacking.

Primary Reduction in Restenosis in De Novo Focal Lesions in Vessels Greater Than 3.0 mm in Diameter

Histologic studies have shown that irrespective of the type of vessel wall injury, neointimal hyperplasia as a nonspecific tissue reaction will occur and may lead to restenosis when excessive. Intracoronary stent implantation may reduce the restenosis rate by optimizing the acute angiographic results, allowing for greater accommodation of the neointimal tissue (72). One factor that may account for the improved immediate results is the prevention of elastic recoil. Elastic recoil has been reported to account for a 32 to 47% loss of the maximally achievable vessel diameter or cross-sectional area immediately after balloon angioplasty (73,74). In contrast, the recoil with Palmaz-Schatz stent implantation is 4 to 18% and 20 to 22% with Gianturco-Roubin or Wiktor stent implantation (75,76). In addition to preventing acute recoil, stent implantation may have favorable effects on vessel wall remodeling (77,78).

Four trials have been completed comparing stenting to PTCA in de novo lesions in the native circulation (21, 22, 79, 80). All of these trials show a significant benefit in the rate of restenosis seen at follow-up with Palmaz-Schatz stent implantation compared with balloon angioplasty alone. The favorable results of these trials have been used to justify the enormous increase in stent use as the first choice treatment strategy in patients referred for balloon angioplasty. Caution must be exercised, however, in the interpretation of the results of these trials. It must be recognized that the **observed benefits of stent implantation may only apply to a select group of patients** dictated by the inclusion and exclusion criteria of these studies. The conclusions of these trials may not pertain to patients with different lesion characteristics (long, multiple, mainstem) or in whom the technical approach differs (stent type, multiple stents, periprocedural management). In these subgroups, additional data are necessary. Prudence must also be exercised when considering the patient population included in these studies. For instance, meta-analysis of the BENESTENT and Stress I and II trials suggests that stent placement in vessels less than 2.6 mm in diameter and in those greater than 3.4 mm provides no advantage in either restenosis rates or in clinical events when compared with angioplasty alone (81). Similarly, working on the premise that "bigger is better," stratification of the patients in the BENESTENT trial based on acute angiographic results suggests that in those patients treated with balloon angioplasty in whom a 30% or less diameter stenosis was obtained at the time of the intervention, 1-year outcome was similar to stented patients with similar acute angiographic results (68). The expression "stentlike" has been coined in reference to such an agreeable angioplasty result. The strategy of striving for and accepting a "stentlike" result has been termed "provisional stenting" (82). In the BENESTENT trial, stentlike results were achieved in 35% of the patients treated with angioplasty alone. Thus, not all patients with the similar to those included in the BENESTENT study may benefit from primary stent implantation. A strategy of balloon angioplasty in vessels with a diameter less than 2.6 mm and acceptance of postprocedural results of a diameter stenosis 30% or less measured by on-line quantitative angiography in those above 2.6, may result in long-term outcomes comparable to primary stenting. The effectiveness of provisional stenting in terms of clinical outcome and cost needs to be assessed in a randomized trial before such a algorithm can be applied in the clinical arena.

Saphenous Vein Graft Disease

Ongoing randomized trials support encouraging observational data favoring the use of stents for the treatment of saphenous vein graft disease.

The management of patients with recurrent angina after coronary bypass surgery presents a very difficult problem. Attrition rates of saphenous vein grafts of 15 to 20% in the first year after bypass surgery, 1 to 2% per year 1–6 years after surgery, and 4% per year between years 6 and 10 have been reported (83). By 5 years, about 45% of the grafts are occluded. As a result of attrition and progression of coronary artery disease, 10 to 15% of bypass patients will require repeat surgery within 10 years after the initial operation. Reoperation is technically more difficult, and it is associated with a higher mortality (3 to 7%) and perioperative MI rate (3 to 12%) (83). It is for these reasons that percutaneous treatment modalities have been explored.

In selected cases, balloon angioplasty is associated with a high initial success rate of between 75 and 94%, with a combined overall success rate of 88% (83). The complication rate is relatively low, with a procedure-related death rate of less than 1%, a MI rate of approximately 4%, and a need for urgent surgery of less than 2%. These comparatively good immediate results are offset by a high restenosis rate and poor long-term clinical outcome. The reported restenosis rate is 28% for lesions in the distal end of the graft, but it is 58% for ostial or proximal lesions and 52% for lesions in the body of the graft. The reported 5-year survival rate and event-free survival (freedom from MI, repeat bypass surgery, and angioplasty) are 74 and 26%, respectively (84).

Results of several observational studies have shown a high procedural success rate for stenting of vein grafts and an improved long-term graft patency and in-hospital clinical outcome (85–99). The incidence of restenosis in the early observational trials was reported as high as 47% (87), whereas in the later studies, restenosis rates below 20% (91, 92) were reported. Similar to findings using balloon angioplasty, the restenosis rate after stenting of nonostial lesions is significantly lower (29%) compared with ostial lesions (60 to 62%) (100, 101). The first reported results of the SAVED study are in agreement with those of the observational studies, showing an improved clinical outcome at 6-month follow-up in patients with vein graft disease treated with stent implantation (102, 103). Based on the results of the observational trials and the SAVED study, stenting with **the Palmaz-Schatz stent in short, nonrestenotic, nonostial vein graft lesions is associated with better acute and intermediate-term outcomes compared with PTCA.**

Little data are available on the long-term results of stenting in saphenous vein graft disease. A single center observational trial recently reported 5-year follow-up results of 62 post-bypass patients treated with stent implantation (104). Overall survival at 5 years was 83%, whereas event-free survival was 30%. Analysis of pooled data from the literature shows similar results, with 5-year event-free survival of 26% after balloon angioplasty, 30% after stent implantation, and 63 to 76% after repeat surgery (104).

Preliminary data from randomized trials as well as observational studies and case reports indicate that a benefit may exist for the use of stents in the treatment of restenotic lesions, chronic total occlusions, osteal and left main artery disease, bifurcation lesions, and in the setting of an acute MI.

Restenotic Lesions after Previous Balloon Angioplasty

Irrespective of the definition of restenosis, it is estimated that approximately 25% of all PTCAs are performed for the treatment of restenosis (105) of a previously dilated lesion. The pathologic substrate of the restenotic lesion is different than that of a primary stenosis and, therefore, the favorable results of the primary restenosis prevention trials likely cannot be extrapolated to secondary restenosis prevention. Several reports have been published of observational studies that have addressed secondary restenosis prevention, although in many of these trials it was not the main focus and most were performed in the early days of stenting (17, 20, 53, 56, 106–110). Results of the most recently reported of these observational trials indicated that the number of balloon angioplasty procedures performed before stent implantation did not influence the risk for subsequent restenosis after stenting (110). The odds for restenosis in the situation of stent implantation for a second, third, or fourth restenosis compared with stent implantation for a first restenosis was 0.8 (95% confidence interval [CI] 0.4–1.8) according to the 0.72 mm criterion and 1.5 (95% CI 0.6–3.7) based on the 50% diameter stenosis criterion. The only significant predictor of recurrence of restenosis was the relative gain when it exceeded 0.48 (odds ratio 2.7, 95% CI 1.1–6.4) based on the 0.72 mm criterion. This result confirms earlier data indicating that deep arterial injury is associated with more extensive neointimal proliferation.

In a recently reported prospective analysis, the long-term outcome of some of the first patients to receive stents were reported (111). One hundred and thirteen stents (78 Wallstents, 29 Palmaz-Schatz, and 6 Wiktor) were implanted in 106 patients to treat restenosis following angioplasty both in native coronaries (86 cases) and in vein grafts (20 cases). Follow-up at 6 months showed a combined angiographic and restenosis rate of 18%, and a clinical event rate of 20%. Long-term follow-up at a mean of 65 months showed an additional 9% of patients experienced a clinical event and 14% exhibited angiographic restenosis, which occurred between 6 and 65 months.

The definitive answer to the question of whether stent implantation reduces recurrent restenosis compared with repeated balloon angioplasty will be answered by final analysis of the REST study (31). Interim analysis of the results of this trial suggests a more favorable intermediate-term clinical and angiographic outcome with stent implantation.

Chronic Total Occlusions

Balloon angioplasty of chronically occluded arteries is both technically demanding and associated with a high incidence of luminal renarrowing, reocclusion, and restenosis (112). Limited observational data exist suggesting that coronary stent implantation is feasible and that it may have a benefit with respect to reocclusion and restenosis when compared with historic data of standard angioplasty after resolution of flow in a previously occluded vessel (113–120). Preliminary results of three relatively small randomized trials show benefit of stent placement in the acute angiographic results; however, only the results of the stenting in chronic coronary occlusion (SICCO) trial indicate an advantage of stent implantation for the prevention of restenosis (121–123). Confirmation of these results is necessary in further randomized trials.

Acute MI

Balloon angioplasty has been introduced as an alternative to thrombolytic therapy for the treatment of patients with an acute MI (124–126). In selected patients, it may be superior to thrombolytic therapy for the restoration of TIMI 3 flow and for reducing mortality and the recurrence of MI (127). Despite these promising results, reocclusion of the infarct artery occurs in 5 to 10% of the patients before hospital discharge and 10 to 15% exhibit a total occlusion in the treated artery at 6-month follow-up (128–130). Concerns over the thrombogenicity of stents, resulted in an early reluctance to use them in acute MI. Several reports of stent implantation in the setting of failed primary PTCA for acute MI have shown that stenting is feasible, safe, and effective with low subacute occlusion rates comparable to those of bail-out stenting after elective balloon angioplasty (131–146). The advantages of antiplatelet therapy only after stent placement was suggested by a trial by Neumann et al. (131). In this trial, 80 patients with complicated angioplasty for acute MI were treated with stent implantation, the last 30 of whom were treated without postprocedural oral anticoagulants with good outcomes.

The low subacute occlusion rates observed with stent implantation in the setting of acute MI for bail-out purposes or for sub optimal results after PTCA prompted investigations that focus on their utility as primary treatment for acute MI. The results from a small, monocenter Italian registry were recently reported (147). In this trial, 22 patients with acute MI were treated with primary stenting. Inclusion criteria into this trial were very strict (< 6 hours after onset of chest pain, culprit vessel diameter > 3 mm, single vessel disease, target lesion length < 15 mm). Nevertheless, the results of this trial were good with all stents patent at 24 hours, and recurrence of symptoms in only one patient at intermediate-term follow-up. Postprocedure pharmacotherapy included intravenous (IV) heparin, aspirin, ticlopidine, and subcutaneous low molecular weight heparin. Angiographic follow-up was only performed in 50% of the patients, and restenosis was observed in only one patient studied. Subsequent reports from other observational trials with primary stent implantation in acute MI have also been favorable (148–153).

Results of the prospective pilot study STAMI (STenting in Acute Myocardial Infarction) were also encouraging (154, 155). The inclusion criteria in this trial were not as strict as in the Italian trial (chest pain < 12 hours, ST segment elevation, target vessel diameter ≥ 3.0 mm). Fifty-five patients were enrolled. In-hospital death occurred in 4.2% of patients. At 6-month follow-up, there was one additional death. Chest pain recurred in 33%, and MI in 4 and 15% required target vessel revascularization. All patients in this trial were treated with aspirin, ticlopidine, and coumadin.

The PAMI-Stent pilot study is a prospective pilot study examining the role of primary stenting as a reperfusion strategy for patients with acute MI. A total of 200 patients with stents will be enrolled at nine international sites, and they will undergo clinical and angiographic follow-up at 9 months. Preliminary results are encouraging, and they indicate that stent implantation is feasible in most instances (156, 157). Of the first 201 patients, 25% were considered ineligible for stent placement (target vessel diameter < 2.5 mm, requirement for more than two stents, large residual thrombus, ostial left anterior descending (LAD) artery or circumflex lesion, side branch jeopardy, inability to deliver or expand stent). Analysis of 151 patients who received stents showed in-hospital events of death, 0.7%; re-infarction, 1.4%; recurrent ischemia, 2.8%; predischarge re-PTCA, 1.4%. No out-of-hospital subacute thrombotic events had occurred. Final results of this trial, which was performed in preparation for the randomized PAMI-Stent trial, will soon be released. Despite these encouraging preliminary results, differences in outcome between the two groups could relate to differences in the patient population and to investigator bias. This underscores the need for results from a randomized trial designed to compare PTCA alone with stent implantation.

Three other randomized trials are underway comparing PTCA alone with PTCA plus stent implantation for primary treatment of acute MI: the GRAMI, STENTIM, and ESCOBAR trials (34–36). The final results of these trials should establish the role of primary stent implantation in patients undergoing catheter-based intervention for the treatment of acute MI.

Ostial and Left Main Disease

Aorto-ostial stenoses are not amenable to treatment with balloon angioplasty because of the elasticity of the aorta. Only a few, small, uncontrolled observational studies suggest that stent implantation is feasible, and that it has good angiographic results in aorto-osteal saphenous vein graft lesions (158–163) and osteal right coronary lesions (158, 160, 164). In these situations, results of observational series suggest that stenting may be superior to both directional atherectomy (163) and balloon angioplasty (164). Stent implantation in the aorto-osteal position is technically difficult, and this is a situation where IVUS may be beneficial in assessing the degree of calcification prestent, guiding proper stent sizing, and ensuring adequate stent expansion and apposition to the vessel wall.

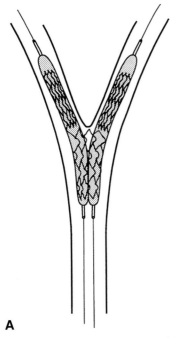

A

Figure 31.2. A, The Colombo "Inverted Y" technique. Three stents are mounted on suitably long balloons, one stent being mounted on both balloons. The entire "bifurcation stent" is placed in one maneuver. *(continues)*

Two trials report on stent placement in the ostium of the LAD (158, 165) that show encouraging results. In a small trial, analyzing Palmaz-Schatz stent placement in 23 ostial LAD lesions, no acute adverse events occurred. There was one case of subacute thrombosis and at follow-up the restenosis rate was 22% (165). The anatomic characteristics differ between aorto-osteal vein graft lesions, aorto-osteal right coronary artery lesions, and osteal circumflex and LAD lesions, which likely contributes to differences in behavior poststenting with restenosis rates as high as 62% in osteal vein-graft stents. Although the results to date look promising, large registry series or randomized trials are necessary to support conclusively stent use for osteal stenoses.

Left main disease has been thought of as not being amenable to percutaneous treatment, because of poor results obtained in the 1980s. With improved techniques and operator experience, this contraindication to stenting is being re-evaluated. Only a few observational trials are reported on stenting for left main artery disease (166–170). In these small trials, stenting has been shown to be technically feasible with high procedural success rates and low in-hospital and long-term complication rates relative to medical or surgical therapy. Currently, however, CABG surgery remains the treatment of choice for all patients with significant left main artery disease other than those who are clearly not surgical candidates. In this patient population, left main artery stent placement may be a reasonable option. In those who are good surgical candidates, these data indicate that randomized trials are needed to compare left main coronary artery stenting to surgical management for those patients who are good surgical candidates. The 16-center ULTIMA (Unprotected Left Main Trunk Intervention Multicenter Assessment) registry is currently underway, which will collect data on consecutive unprotected left main transcatheter treatments from 1994 to the present (171). Results from this registry will provide further information on the feasibility and success of this mode of treatment for left

Figure 31.2. B, The "Culotte" technique. (*a*) The first coil stent is placed in the main artery and the side branch and post-dilated. This temporarily traps the main vessel guidewire (*b*) which is retracted and readvanced through the stent struts. The stent is further post-dilated to further open the struts (*c*). A second stent is placed in the main vessel across the bifurcation, with proximal overlap of the two stents (*d*), which traps the side branch wire. The wire is removed and repositioned (*e*), and the bifurcation is then appropriately post-dilated. **C**, The "Monoclonal Antibody" technique. (*a*) Guidewires are placed in the two vessels and a "kissing balloon" pre-dilatation is performed. A stent is then placed in the main vessel with entrapment of the side branch wire (*b*). The side branch wire is withdrawn and reintroduced through the stent struts (*c*). The stent struts are separated with balloon inflation (*d*). A short balloon with a crimped stent is introduced through the stent struts (*e*), and a second balloon is introduced and inflated in the main vessel (*f*). The side branch balloon is then pulled against this balloon and inflated as appropriate to deploy the second stent.

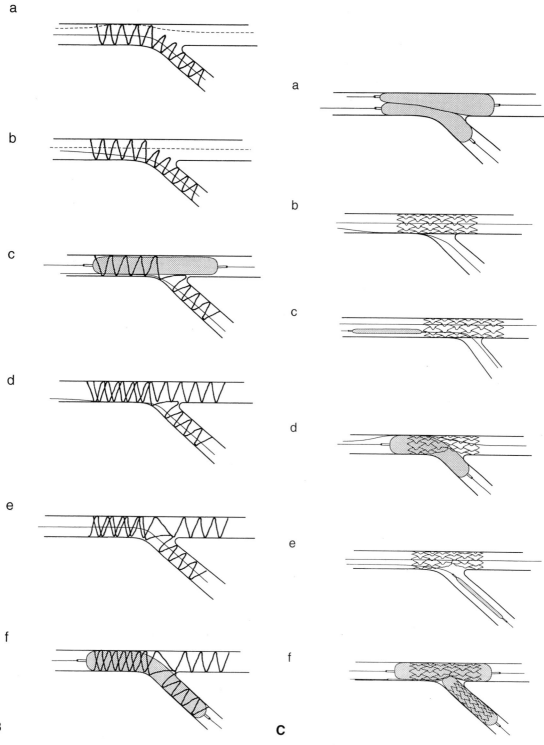

B

C

main coronary artery disease and may prompt further trials.

Bifurcation Lesions

A bifurcation lesion is defined as the presence of greater than 50% stenosis involving both a parent vessel and the ostium of its side branch. Balloon angioplasty of such stenoses is associated with a significant risk of side branch occlusion (172) and several techniques have been developed to reduce the complication rate. If a stent has been deployed in the parent vessel, several stent designs allow passage of a second balloon and stent through the struts of the first (173), and experimental studies have identified a number of balloons that will pass through a deployed Palmaz-Schatz stent and return intact without damaging the stent (174). Borrowing from the experience with angioplasty, new stenting techniques are being investigated for the treatment of bifurcation stenosis. A 'kissing stent' procedure has been described (175, 176), which is analogous to the 'kissing balloon' technique introduced by Gruentzig in 1981, and presented by Meier in 1984 (177). This procedure involves simultaneous inflation of two separate balloons, one in the parent vessel and one in the side branch, followed by simultaneous stent deployment. Other approaches that have been recently described include the 'Y' technique, a 'T' technique, the 'Culotte' technique, and a 'Monoclonal Antibody' technique. The 'Y' technique involves simultaneous deployment of stents at the ostium of the side branch and in the parent vessel distal to its take-off, followed by stent placement proximal to the ostium of the side branch (178). None of the stents in the resultant Y configuration are over-lapping. The T-stenting technique involves placing a stent first in the side branch followed by stenting of the major vessel across the side branch (179). The Culotte technique employs two Freedom or GR-II stents that allow interlocking of the devices without an undue excess of metal (180, 181). In this method, the side branch is stented first, with the stent extending into the main vessel, which is subse-

quently stented with proximal overlapping of the two stents. The Monoclonal Antibody approach involves stenting of the main vessel followed by a T-stenting technique of the side branch with an inflated balloon in the main vessel stent (180) (Fig. 31.2). All of these methods are technically demanding and their success is dependant on the skill of the operator. Controlled studies must be performed to confirm the feasibility and long-term success of such treatments.

STENT GUIDANCE AND ADJUNCTIVE APPROACHES

Coronary Angiography

Coronary angiography has been the mainstay not only in guiding intracoronary stenting procedures, but for all coronary interventional procedures. Visual estimation of dimensions from the angiogram or "eyeballing" has been shown to be notoriously inaccurate by a limited number of studies, but proof of point comes mostly from the personal experiences of interventionalists (182). In particular, minor residual narrowings ($< 20\%$ residual stenosis) are often overlooked with visual assessment. A precise and accurate delineation of angiographic contours can be provided by algorithms widely available on-line in digital angiographic systems. The accuracy and reproducibility of such systems have been repeatedly demonstrated (183–185). Using automated edge detection algorithms, the goal of treatment is for a complete absence of residual stenosis or the presence of a "negative diameter stenosis" within the stent when visualized in multiple views. In most cases, the detection of residual in-stent narrowing is possible with quantitative coronary angiography, and these systems, therefore, can provide a relatively inexpensive means for the guidance and the optimization of coronary stent implantation. Angiography has several limitations however. Angiographic techniques determine only lumen size and not vessel size; therefore, severe and diffuse involvement of an entire artery may not be recognized and the severity of a lesion may be substantially underestimated (186–189). These limitations are particularly important in the context of coronary stent implantation, because in diffusely diseased vessels the sole use of angiography carries the risk of inappropriate sizing of the stent on a falsely normal reference segment. A prerequisite for optimal stent implantation with high-pressure dilation is that the stent should cover the entire stenotic region up to a relatively disease-free proximal and distal segment. With IVUS, it is relatively easy to identify a relatively plaque-free reference segment. Poststenting, angiography typically overestimates the increase in lumen area after stent deployment because it does not distinguish stent diameter and lumen diameter in patients with suboptimal stent expansion. The discrepancy between IVUS-determined diameter and that determined angiographically has been shown to decrease with progressively higher inflation pressures (190). In addition, angiographic techniques do not offer much information on stent-to-strut contact with the vessel wall, the degree of stent symmetry, or the adequacy of stent expansion. Detailed information on complicating marginal dissections at the proximal inflow or distal outflow of stented segments is also not obtainable using current quantitative angiography algorithms. The full extent of intimal dissections and their subsequent management may be better defined with IVUS than with angiography. Hoyne et al. reported that an1giographically visualized dissections suggested a much larger cross-sectional lumen than that measured with IVUS, and that coronary dissections and intimal flaps were more often identified with ultrasound (191). In a provocative report, it has been shown that the correlation between angiographically determined MLD and IVUS, MLD varies considerably depending on the stent design with 'less strut, less metal' stents showing a particularly poor correlation with IVUS (192) (Table 31.8). This suggests that information obtained by IVUS may be favored with the use of particular stent types. Moderately radio-opaque stents, such as the Wallstent, might be adequately assessed by angiographic means alone. The reliability of quantitative coronary angiography can be expected to improve with the introduction of the gradient field transform algorithm for the tracking of dissections and complex lesions (193) and with the application of dynamic algorithms with adaptive weighting of the first and second derivatives to address the issues of overestimation of small lumen diameters and the underestimation of large luminal diameters, and thus the underestimation of acute luminal gain and recoil (194). Whether more detailed information on prestent lesion morphology and poststent characteristics will translate into improved short- and long-term outcomes after stenting has not yet been answered, and such is the focus of the randomized trials AVID, OPTICUS and SIPS, which compare angiographic with IVUS-guided stent implantation.

Role of Intravascular Ultrasound

Without a doubt, the amount of information gained by intravascular ultrasound (IVUS) far exceeds that of angiographic measurements. Intracoronary measurement enables visualization of a full 360° circumference. Preintervention IVUS provides information on lesion morphology and the extent of atherosclerotic disease, and allows direct measurements of inner dimensions, including minimal and maximal diameter and cross-sectional area, which may assist in device selection and balloon sizing. Additional information that can be obtained using IVUS before stent implantation include an assessment of balloon angioplasty adequacy, identification or exclusion of thrombus, and determination of stent size. Poststent IVUS can be used to identify the adequacy of lesion coverage by the stent and plaque prolapse, as well as to assess the parameters for optimal stent implantation. A question arises to whether the benefit of this additional information, which complements angiographic findings, outweighs the additional cost of the procedure using IVUS.

The age of IVUS in coronary stenting was heralded by provocative reports from Antonio Colombo and his group from Milan. Initial IVUS observations by this group showed that in using the traditional

Table 31.8.
Coating Material Considered for Use with Metal Intracoronary Stents

Synthetic Substances/Reference	Naturally Occurring Substances/Reference
—Polyurethane (233–235)	—Collagen/lamanin (241)
—Segmented poluurethaneurea/heparin (236)	—Heparin (242–244)
—Poly-L-lactic acid (237)	—Fibrin (245, 246)
—Cellulose ester (238)	—Phosphorylcholine (231)
—Polyethylene glycol (239)	—AZ1 adsorbed to cellulose (247, 248)
—Polyphosphate ester (240)	AZ1/UK absorbed to cellulose (248, 249)

AZ1, monoclonal antibody directed against rabbit platelet integrin $\alpha_{IIb}\beta_3$; AZ1/UK, monoclonal antibody directed against rabbit platelet integrin $\alpha_{IIb}\beta_3$/urokinase conjugate

stent deployment techniques employed at that time, which resulted in an acceptable angiographic appearance, approximately 80% of stents were under-expanded by criteria which they described (minimal intrastent cross-sectional area < 70% of balloon cross-sectional area, with the balloon size being 0.5 mm larger than the reference vessel diameter (24, 25). They also demonstrated that the use of larger balloons and higher pressures resulted in increased cross-sectional areas. These observations led to the hypothesis that stent thrombosis was more likely caused by stent under-expansion rather than a property inherent to the stent itself, the under-expanded stent struts serving as a nidus for thrombus formation. This hypothesis was later tested in a prospective clinical trial that began in 1993 (26). In this observational study, 334 consecutive patients underwent Palmaz-Schatz stent implantation. Routine high-pressure balloon angioplasty was carried out and IVUS was used to confirm and document optimal stent deployment. Postprocedural treatment consisted of antiplatelet agents alone. At 1 month the incidence of stent thrombosis was 0.9%. At the time of the report from Colombo's group, both low and high pressure balloon stent deployment was being performed using oversized balloons. The approach outlined by these investigators stressed the achievement of a vessel lumen of uniform caliber in the reference and stented segments with high-pressure dilation using a minimally compliant or a noncompliant balloon matching the size of an angiographically normal segment.

The Colombo et al. report (26) suggested two novel elements in their strategy for stent implantation: high-pressure in-stent dilation and ultrasound guidance. The result was "optimized" stent implantation, abolishing the need for postprocedural anticoagulation. In this series, patients who did not meet the ultrasound criteria despite high-pressure balloon dilation were subsequently anticoagulated with coumadin. Therefore, it was not clear from the study of Colombo et al. whether high-pressure balloon inflation without ultrasound would suffice to reduce the risk of subacute stent thrombosis. The necessity for ultrasound guidance was put into question by several observational trials that adopted the technique described by Colombo's group but used angiography instead of ultrasound to guide optimal implantation. A large French trial evaluated the 30-day clinical outcome of a prospective registry of 2900 patients in whom successful coronary artery stenting was performed without coumadin anticoagulation (195). Angiographically guided stent implantation was done using relatively high-pressure in-stent postdilation, with 82% of the patients receiving Palmaz-Schatz stents. Postprocedural treatment included aspirin and ticlopidine. Low molecular weight heparin treatment was progressively reduced in four consecutive stages from 1-month treatment to none. Overall, subacute stent thrombosis occurred in 1.8% of patients, indicating that IVUS was not necessary to reduce the rate of subacute occlusion. Using a regimen of aspirin, ticlopidine, and periprocedural dextran therapy without IVUS guidance, Lablanche et al. reported their results of stent implantation in 529 consecutive patients (68). Palmaz-

Schatz, Wiktor, Gianturco-Roubin, and AVE stents were implanted as bailout therapy for failed angioplasty, for suboptimal results after angioplasty, and electively. Stent thrombosis occurrence was 5.4% of the patients stented as a bail-out procedure and 1.8% in patients stented for a suboptimal result with no thrombotic events occurring in those treated electively. In 1.8% of the patients, ticlopidine treatment had to be stopped prematurely because of the development of adverse effects.

The applicability of the high-pressure stent dilation technique introduced by Colombo's group for the implantation of coil stents was shown in a study reported by Goods et al. (196). Intravascular ultrasound was not used to guide stent deployment in this study, and a poststent protocol of aspirin and ticlopidine was employed in 264 patients with angiographically determined successful stent implantation. During the 30-day follow-up, stent thrombosis occurred in only 0.9% of patients, which indicated that, without IVUS, patients receiving the balloon expandable coil stent with optimal angiographic results can be managed safely with a combination of aspirin and ticlopidine without anticoagulation.

Currently, the issue of the routine use of IVUS to guide stenting procedures has divided the interventional cardiology community. The favorable results of the observational trials in which high-pressure balloon optimization of stent implantation was performed without adjunctive IVUS examination has led many to conclude that IVUS is not essential for a favorable poststent outcome. Supporters of routine IVUS contend that IVUS is necessary prior to stent implantation for information on the plaque quality and, therefore, on the compliance of the lesion to facilitate the device selection (197). They also maintain that when examined with ultrasound, echo-free spaces, oblique strut position, and stent asymmetry are often seen in stents implanted with high-pressure balloon after treatment (198), with more than 40% of stents with an acceptable angiographic result after high-pressure expansion still requiring additional dilation with higher pressures or a larger balloon for ultrasound optimization (26), and they present these findings as arguments against the use of a "blind" angiography only approach. The basis of the current controversy is whether optimal stent deployment should be defined based on clinical outcome or on intravascular ultrasound confirmation. This controversy will not be solved until the final results of the randomized trials AVID, OPTICUS, and SIPS, which compare angiography alone to IVUS guidance, are reported. Until these results are available, the use of IVUS for routine stent deployment should be discouraged. It is expensive to perform, increases the catheterization laboratory time, and is not without risk. In addition, the IVUS defined criteria for optimal stent deployment touted by the supporters of the routine use of the technique are arbitrary and have not been tested in a controlled manner. This may account in part for the similarity in clinical outcome between the two groups in the early reports of the AVID trial (44).

Doppler Flow

Details of the use of Doppler flow are addressed in Chapter 18. There is no current application specific to stents.

Angioscopy

The use of angioscopy has been described for the identification of incomplete stent apposition and residual dissection (199). It has been shown, however, that IVUS is superior to angioscopy for the assessment of stent expansion and stent symmetry, and to indicate optimal implantation (200). A role for angioscopy has been proposed for the evaluation of thrombus after transluminal extractional (TEC) atherectomy or intracoronary thrombolysis prior to stent implantation (201), and for interventions in saphenous vein bypass grafts (202).

Atherectomy Devices

Directional atherectomy (DCA), Rotablator atherectomy, transluminal extraction (TEC) atherectomy, and laser atherectomy (ELCA) have all been successfully used as adjuncts to coronary stenting. DCA followed by coronary stenting has been shown to result in a larger lumen immediately after the procedure than DCA followed by PTCA (203). Whether this will result in a better long-term outcome (bigger is better contention), or a device-specific effect will have an impact on the results has yet to be shown. In heavily calcified lesions, where optimal stent expansion is often difficult, Rotablator atherectomy followed by Palmaz-Schatz stenting was shown to be superior to a Rotablator and PTCA combination, resulting in larger postprocedural lumen area and a lower residual stenosis as assessed by IVUS (204). The procedural complication rate was similar in this series. Both TEC (201, 205–207) and ELCA (206) have been used in the setting of stent implantation in high-risk (totally occluded, thrombus containing, or degenerated) saphenous vein grafts with favorable results. **A larger body of supportive data is needed for firm conclusions to be made concerning the benefits of these new technologies over more conventional therapies.**

COMPLICATIONS OF CORONARY STENTING

Subacute Stent Thrombosis

The Problem

Despite a high rate of procedural success, the early experience with stenting was confounded by a unacceptably high (ca. 25%) rate of stent thrombosis (14, 17). Although increased operator experience and evolution in the indications for stent implantation have contributed to a decrease in the rate of stent thrombosis, two pivotal changes in clinical practice have had the greatest impact on the incidence of this complication: the implementation of high-pressure balloon expansion of stents and the simultaneous finding of the benefits of enhanced antiplatelet therapy. With these improvements

in stent deployment and periprocedural management, recent studies have reported thrombosis rates of less than 2% when stents are implanted electively (68, 195, 196) and 5% in treatment of abrupt closure (196). Although the rates are low compared with the results from the early series, stent thrombosis is a disastrous complication that carries with it a high rate of ischemic sequelae. The pooled data from numerous trials show rates of MI and death of 61 and 12%, respectively (208). This devastating outcome has bolstered the continued investigations to solve this complication.

Acute stent thrombosis occurs within hours of the stenting procedure and is almost always caused by incomplete stent expansion and vessel dissection. Patients are still hospitalized, and, therefore, diagnosis and treatment are usually rapid. With routine high-pressure balloon expansion, acute thrombosis is rare, complicating less than 1% of stent procedures (208). Subacute thrombosis, on the other hand, is a more common occurrence with a less easily defined cause. It can occur up to 30 days after the stent procedure with the modal presentation being between days 5 and 6 for both the Wiktor and the Palmaz-Schatz stents (22, 209, 210). In their experience with the Palmaz-Schatz stent used as a bail-out device, Schömig et al. observed that 43% of patients with subacute stent thrombosis present within the first week and 80% in the first two weeks (64). Therefore, patients with subacute occlusion have commonly been discharged the from hospital and ischemic sequelae and death are common.

Factors Affecting Stent Thrombosis

Device-Related Factors

Foreign material within the vascular system increases the risk of thrombosis through several inter-related mechanisms. These can be broadly classified as surface interactions and rheologic factors.

Surface Interactions Stent implantation initiates an complex interaction between the blood components and the metallic surface of the stent. Endothelialization of implanted stents is a relatively slow process that is completed only 2–3 months after implantation (211, 212). The clinical observation that the risk for thrombotic occlusion is maximal in the first 2 weeks after stenting illustrates that passivation of the stented surface can occur despite only partial endothelial coverage. Adsorption of the plasma proteins to the surface of the stent to form a monolayer occurs immediately on stent deployment (213). The nature of the component proteins forming this monolayer is determined by the concentration of the various constituents in the plasma and the affinity of each of the proteins for the metal surface. Protein collisions with subsequent adsorption to the stent surface are most likely to be dominated by albumin, as this is the most abundant plasma protein, and, therefore, it displays a competitive advantage. However, other proteins such as fibrinogen, complement factors, fibronectin, and high molecular weight kininogen have a higher affinity for the metal surface and will soon displace the preadsorbed albumin from the stent (the Vroman effect) (214). Composition of the stent and the character of its surface can influence its ability to selectively adsorb and conformationally change plasma proteins. The adsorption of these proteins influences the subsequent interaction with the cellular components of circulating blood. In stented segments, circulating platelets can adhere not only to the exposed collagen of the underlying damaged vessel wall, but also to the protein adsorbed to the stent surface. Platelet adherence results in their activation and in the release of chemoattractant molecules from their granules and the subsequent formation of a platelet aggregate.

The coagulation cascade also plays an important role in stent thrombosis. Activation of the coagulation sequence results in the formation of fibrin clot by the enzymatic cleavage of fibrinogen to fibrin by thrombin. The coagulation cascade can be initiated through both the extrinsic and the intrinsic pathways. The extrinsic pathway is initiated by the contact of factor VII with thromboplastin released by the injured vessel. The intrinsic pathway is triggered by the adsorption of factor XII to the foreign surface and its conversion to factor XIIa.

Characteristics of the stent itself have been shown to influence the adsorption of proteins to the surface, the subsequent activation of circulating platelets, and the proclivity for thrombosis (23). Results of in vitro experiments suggest that metals possessing a higher surface potential cause pronounced attraction of negatively charged platelets and plasma proteins (215, 216). A rough surface texture has also been thought to promote stent thrombosis (217) In a rabbit model, stent surface charge was not seen to contribute to thrombogenicity whereas surface texture was an important factor in determining the bicompatibility of coated Palmaz-Schatz stents (218), perhaps by providing more surface area to circulating blood components. In this regard, electrochemical polishing of stainless steel devices has been shown to result in a less thrombogenic surface (Y. de Scheerder, personal communication). The rapidity of the binding of fibrinogen and platelets to stainless steel surfaces on contact with blood has prompted the search for a more biocompatible alternative to bare stainless steel. Initial evaluation of stents made of tantalum metal suggested that they were less thrombogenic than stainless steel (219, 220); however, controlled evaluation in the porcine coronary model concluded that no difference existed in the thrombogenicity of tantalum wire and stainless steel coil stents (221). Comparison between stainless steel and nitinol slotted tube stents in the rabbit carotid artery model showed stainless steel to be more thrombogenic and caused more extensive vascular injury than nitinol (222, 223). Platinum and gold coatings are currently being considered for coronary stents. These metals are particularly resistant to corrosion and may be less thrombogenic than their stainless steel counterparts. Gold also has the added advantage of possessing antibacterial properties and may exhibit antiproliferative effects (217).

Interest in the use of polymers is mounting, either as the sole material of stent construction, as a component of polymer-metal composite stents, as a surface coating for metal stents, or as a means to decrease the thromogenicity of implanted devices. Many different biodegradable and inert synthetic polymers have been tested in animal models as the lone component of coronary stents, including polyethylene terephthalate (Dacron) (224, 225), polyhydroxybutyrate valerate (226), poly-L-lactic acid (227), polyglycolic acid(228, 229), and a copolymer of polyglycolic and polylactic acid (230). Although often contradictory, overall the results of the use of these polymeric stents in animal models have been disappointing. The inconsistencies of the results has made it apparent that the reaction to the polymeric materials differs not only across species, but also in different vascular beds within the same animal, making a direct extrapolation of the results to the human condition extremely difficult. A polymer-metal composite stent design has recently been described. The device is an ACS locking stent backbone between a poly-L-lactic acid and polycaprolactone laminate. The stent is designed to provide mechanical hoop strength as well as a platform for local drug delivery through impregnation of the bioabsorbable polymer. This stent design is currently in the research and development stage.

The list of materials used to coat metal stents in an attempt to reduce their inherent thrombogenicity is long and ever increasing (231–249). A few, however, deserve special attention. Most coatings tested are placed mainly to provide a biologically inert barrier between the stent surface and the circulating blood. In contrast, heparin surface coatings have been studied as a means of providing a biologically active surface that interacts with the circulating blood. Many techniques have been applied to attach heparin to synthetic surfaces; however, the description of a process for end point attachment of heparin to polymer coated surfaces that preserves the activity of the antithrombin binding site made the production of heparin-coated stents feasible (250). Heparin-coated stents were shown to be effective in reducing thrombosis in rabbit peripheral vessels (242) and in porcine coronary arteries (243, 244). These encouraging results led to the evaluation of the high activity end point attached heparin-coated stents in the BENESTENT II pilot study. In this nonrandomized trial, no incidence of subacute oc-

clusion occurred (251). Currently, several commercial heparin-coated stents are available, which are assessed for clinical use.

Fibrin coating of intravascular stents has been proposed as a means of passivating the stent surface and providing a platform for the recolonization of endothelial cells (245). Fibrin-coated Palmaz-Schatz stents were shown to be free of thrombus and foreign body reaction when examined 8 weeks after implantation in peripheral arteries of dogs (246). This was compared with 45% incidence of thrombosis seen with the implantation of naked stents. More notable was the finding of endothelialization of 96% of surface of the fibrin-coated stents, whereas the uncoated controls were covered with endothelial cells over only 18% of their surface.

Phosphorylcholine-coated stents are being evaluated in clinical trials in Europe for their ability to reduce the incidence of subacute occlusion and improve the long-term outcome in stented coronary segments. Phosphorylcholine is the major phospholipid component of biologic membranes. Based on promising results in vitro (231) and in vivo in animal models it is anticipated that these coated devices will behave as intact tissue elements, a form of biomimicry, and result in a reduction in the incidence of subacute occlusion and an improvement in the long-term patency rates of treated segments.

Polymeric coating of the stent in situ has also been shown to be feasible, a technique referred to a "gel paving" (252). In a recently reported trial, the application of polyethelene-glycol-lactide hydrogel polymers to the surface of Palmaz stents implanted in the porcine femoral artery model has been described (252). The applied polymer is then photopolymerized in situ to form a short-term, semipermeable barrier. Stented segments treated in such a manner showed less gross thrombosis, less microscopic platelet adherence, and enhanced vessel patency compared with control stented segments. Much more animal data must be collected before this type of technology can be considered for clinical application.

The seeding of intravascular stents with endothelial cells to passivate the stent surface has been an area of ongoing research for over 9 years. Both self-expanding (253) and balloon expandable (254) stents have been successfully seeded with endothelial cells, and they have been shown to retain a significant number of viable cells after deployment in vitro (253, 254a). In these early experiments, the stents were precoated with fibronectin matrix as a foundation for the endothelial cells. Although endothelial seeding was shown to be feasible, the clinical utility of such an approach was questionable. Fibronectin itself is thrombogenic and the loss of attached cells on stent deployment would expose this thrombogenic surface to the circulating blood if used in vivo. The source of the endothelial cells also presents a problem. Homologous tissue would be necessary to prevent acute rejection of the grafted tissue on transplantation. Recent reports have addressed these two problems. Using autologous endothelial cells derived from sheep saphenous veins, a group at the National Heart, Lung, and Blood Institute (NHLBI) has successfully seeded metallic stents and implanted the stents into the femoral arteries of the donor animals (255). The transplanted endothelial cells could be detected in six of nine animals treated in this manner 10 days after stent implantation. Scott et al also were successful in identifying endothelial cells on seeded stents 3 hours after intracoronary implantation in pigs (256). These investigators used immortalized human microvascular cells that retain the phenotypic characteristics of endothelial cells after more than 50 passages (257). These cells were successfully seeded in vitro on an uncoated tantalum wire coil stent prior to deployment. One stent had been frozen for 2 months, and then thawed prior to use. On explantation, retained endothelial cells could be seen predominantly on the lateral aspects of the stent. Another approach that has been taken for the passivation of the stent surface by endothelial cells has been called cell "sodding" (258). This strategy involves the local delivery of homologous or autologous endothelial cells via a local delivery catheter to the site of stent implantation. In both pig coronaries and rabbit iliac arteries, greater than 75% of the stent surface was covered with endothelial cells 4 hours after stent deployment. By 14 days, the coverage had increased to more than 90% (258).

Genetic manipulation of the seeded endothelial cells is currently being investigated, both as a means to increase the retention of the transplanted cells (259), and as a means of introducing genetic material to produce bioactive proteins for the prevention of local thrombosis and late restenosis (260, 261). The local delivery of plasmid DNA encoding vascular endothelial growth factor (phVEGF$_{165}$) has recently been shown to increase stent endothelialization in situ and to reduce stent thrombosis and intimal thickening in the rabbit model (262). Recent successes in this area of research has renewed interest in endothelial passivation of stents.

A novel approach to stent passivation is being applied in Greece by Stefanadis and Toutouzas. Their approach involves passivation of the stent surface by applying a segment of autologous vascular tissue. The technique uses a segment of cephalic vein or ulnar artery to cover the stent. An appropriate size portion of the graft is explanted at the time of the stent procedure, and cleaned of boundary tissue to obtain a thin-walled segment. It is then introduced into the lumen of a Palmaz-Schatz stent, the ends of the graft reversed on the metallic stent struts, and sutured on the external surface of the stent. The result is that both the internal and external surfaces of the stent are totally covered by the graft. The results of implantation of a device with a vein graft covering only the external surface of the stent have been reported, both for elective indications (263, 264), and in the setting of an acute MI (265). Further studies are necessary to clarify the potential of this technique.

Although the data are limited, the results of several studies indicate that long stent use may increase the risk for stent thrombosis. The use of a 20 mm long coil stent as opposed to a stent 12 mm in length was associated with a higher incidence of stent thrombosis in a recently reported observational study that included 288 patients stented for various indications (266) (9.4% versus 3.1%, $P < .3$). Similar results were reported for 115 patients treated for acute or threatened vessel closure with 20 and 12 mm coil stents with a 10% incidence of stent thrombosis in the long stent group compared with 0% in group receiving the short stent (16). The presence of more metal, providing a greater thrombogenic surface in the longer stents, has been proposed as one of the factors contributing to a higher incidence of thrombosis; however, other factors, such as the indication for the longer stent must be considered. Long stents are often chosen for the treatment of long or spiral dissections, as well as for long, tortuous, and ulcerated lesions. It may be that the characteristics of the lesion itself contribute more to the thrombogenicity of the stented site than does the metal of the stent.

Whether the implantation of multiple stents carries with it an increased risk of thrombosis over single stent implantation is still an area of controversy. Three early investigations have shown that the placement of multiple stents significantly increases the incidence of thrombosis (33, 266, 267, 268), whereas several other trials have not demonstrated a difference in the results using single and multiple stents (54, 59, 62, 63, 209, 269). A recently reported observational trial, comparing the clinical outcome after single and multiple stent implantation with high-pressure poststent balloon dilation technique, also did not demonstrate a difference with optimal multiple stent deployment (270). In contrast to these results is the report of an observational trial examining the outcome between patients treated with one or two stents and those treated with three or more (271). In this analysis, the patients receiving more than two stents showed a significantly higher rate of restenosis and need for target vessel revascularization because of subacute thrombosis and late restenosis. Whereas intuitively one may think that multiple stent deployment will present a greater thrombogenic surface, it has been proposed that technical difficulties with the placement of single short stents may result in suboptimal final results and a greater likelihood of persistent dissections that may counter the thrombogenic effects of more metal presence. Clearly, further trials are necessary to address this important controversy.

Rheologic Factors The nature of the flow in a vessel determines the degree to which blood elements interact with the structures on the vessel wall. Under laminar flow conditions, blood moves in a well-defined, streamlined fashion, with mass transfer of materials occurring by diffusion through the fluid. The presence of a stent in a vessel lumen may induce blood flow disturbances, and the 'hydrodynamic compatibility' of a stent is slowly becoming recognized as an important feature of ideal stent design. In vitro assessment of fluid dynamics in a stented artery model has shown that immediately before and behind the expanded stent wires is a region of low velocity flow, whereas maximal turbulence was seen directly over the stent struts (272). These stagnant flow areas are the site of fibrin and platelet deposition, whereas enhanced shear stress can act as a platelet agonist, causing aggregation (273). As the ratio of the distance between stent struts and the profile of the stent is reduced (the pitch: height ratio of coil stents), the peristrut stagnation and maximal turbulence of the flow increase (272). These findings suggest that a stent designed with optimal strut spacing and thin stent struts would result in less disturbed flow when deployed. These results may also account for the empiric findings of Colombo's group concerning optimal apposition of the stent to the vessel wall using high-pressure balloon inflation. A poorly deployed stent would have a smaller fraction of the stent strut embedded and thus present a higher profile to the flowing blood (a lower pitch:height ratio). The greater amount of exposed metal in this circumstance may also contribute to the observed high thrombotic potential.

Further evidence shows that stent design and configuration can influence stent thrombosis. With deployment techniques held constant, in vitro studies have shown that increases in flow velocity and turbulence are highest with wire loop stents and that single articulation slotted tube stents actually decreased both flow velocity and turbulence. Helically wound wire stents resulted in changes intermediate between the two other designs (274). These findings have been supported by findings in an animal model where a significantly higher incidence of stent thrombosis was seen in arterial segments stented with a corrugated ring stent compared with a slotted tube device (23). A small retrospective trial failed to show any differences between the Palmaz-Schatz, Wiktor, or Gianturco Roubin stents with respect to stent thrombosis; however, the retrospective nature and the small size of this trial limit the interpretation (275).

Two small randomized trials have been reported comparing stents of two different designs (276, 277). No differences were seen in the incidence of thrombosis, however, the trials were not powered to show small differences in the already low incidence. The results of larger randomized trials are needed to conclusively show that stent configuration affects device thrombogenicity in clinical applications.

Patient-Related Factors

Vessel Characteristics The anatomic location of coronary lesions and their characteristics are important determinants of their propensity to thrombose after coronary stenting. These characteristics may be independent of the lesion (e.g., reference vessel diameter), or they may indicate stent placement (e.g., bail-out), or they be a result of the intervention (e.g., presence of thrombus before stent placement).

Vessel Size An increase thrombotic risk when stents were deployed in small caliber vessels (< 3 mm) was seen early in the clinical use of coronary stents (14), which led to the exclusion of patients with lesions in small vessels from many of the subsequent stent trials. This finding was supported by several subsequent observational studies (16, 54, 266). Thrombosis rates of 9.5% have been reported for vessels stented with a 2.5 mm device (16), and rates as high as 25% have been reported for stented vessels with a diameter of 2.0 mm (54). Results of more recent studies, using higher balloon pressure inflation to optimize stent delivery, are more encouraging. With the use of a Gianturco-Roubin Flex-Stent in bail-out situations after failed angioplasty, a thrombosis rate of below 5% was reported (57). Better results were seen with stent placement for elective situations in small vessels (193,

278–281). Despite this improvement, **vessel size less than 3.0 mm remains an important predictor of stent thrombosis,** likely as a result of the presence of relatively more metal per lumen area and less flow in smaller vessels.

Lesion Characteristics Several reports evaluating the predictors of stent thrombosis using multivariate analysis have identified lesion characteristics that are independent predictors for higher risk of stent thrombosis. The characteristics found to be predictive of poststent thrombosis include lesion eccentricity (209), amount of atherosclerotic plaque (269), AHA/ACC (American Heart Association/American College of Cardiology) lesion type B2 or C (63, 269), lesion length (269, 282), residual dissection poststent placement (63, 269, 283), bail-out indication after failed PTCA (195, 209, 268, 269, 282, 284, 285), presence of intracoronary thrombus (59, 266, 282, 285); and, in vessels with poor distal run-off, presence of collaterals; or vessels supplying akinetic or severely kinetic regions of myocardium (14). Many of the predictors of thrombosis are subject to some controversy. Prestent thrombus presence is an example. Several reports indicate that the presence of thrombus has not resulted in a greater risk of acute and subacute closure poststent (54, 131, 286). Broad classification of lesion morphology has also been suggested not to correlate with risk of thrombosis (287). Much of these data were accumulated in the era of low-pressure stent deployment. Preliminary unpublished data using high-pressure balloon expansion without anticoagulation suggest that low ejection fraction, residual dissection presence, multiple stents per lesion, and small diameter remain as predictors of thrombosis, whereas bail-out stenting and prestent lesion characteristics are not predictive (197). These findings suggest that the final result obtained poststent is the key factor in determining predisposition to stent thrombosis. In addition to these lesion-related characteristics, stent implantation in patients with acute coronary syndromes has been shown to be associated with a higher incidence of thrombosis (195, 209, 269, 281, 282). As the techniques of stent implantation evolve and the poststent management improves, these markers for risk need to be reassessed to determine whether they are still valid predictors of stent thrombosis.

Anatomic Location of Stent Placement Stent location in the coronary arterial system has been shown to influence the thrombosis rate. Thrombosis risk has repeatedly been shown to be highest in the LAD (64, 283, 288) and lowest in stents deployed in saphenous vein grafts (266, 283). These differences may be a result of more turbulent flow in the LAD as a result of frequent branch points and tortuosity of the vessel. The stented saphenous vein graft, on the other hand, may be more resistant to thrombosis because of its large diameter and the absence of branch points.

Hemostatic Predictors The recognized importance of the GPIIb/IIIa fibrinogen receptor on platelets in the development of thrombotic complications led to the hypothesis that a certain subpopulation of patients may be at risk of developing thrombosis based on alterations in the expression or activation of this platelet glycoprotein. This theory has recently undergone prospective evaluation in a study examining the hemostatic markers in 140 patients undergoing Palmaz-Schatz implantation for suboptimal PTCA results (29). Stents were expanded with high inflation pressures and all patients were treated with anticoagulation after the procedure. The expression of the GPIIb/IIIa was found to have a positive correlation with the occurrence of stent thrombosis. In this trial, neither plasma fibrinogen levels nor the change in level with time showed a significant relation to the risk of stent thrombosis. Similarly, the level of prothrombin fragment 1 + 2, a marker of thrombin formation, or conventional hemostatic monitoring parameters were not related to the risk of subsequent stent thrombosis. The results of this trial are important in several respects. First, the results emphasize the importance of platelet activity on the thrombotic system relative to the coagulation system, a finding that has been realized in practice with the introduction of postprocedural ticlopidine. These data also demonstrate for the first time, that a patient-

related variable can modulate the risk of stent thrombosis. In clinical practice, this implies that it might be possible to identify patients who are at risk for developing stent thrombosis before the interventional procedure and treat them more aggressively to prevent this complication.

Technique-Related Factors

The greatest impact on the prevention of stent thrombosis has come with the improvement of stent deployment techniques and in poststent pharmacologic management. The thrombogenicity of the stent was shown to be largely a consequence of disturbed blood rheology resulting from stent asymmetry and gaps between the stent struts and the vessel wall. The need for anticoagulation appears to be abolished when stents are optimally deployed, with the stent struts well apposed to the vessel wall and in full expansion providing a favorable milieu for laminar flow, which can be achieved with appropriate balloon deployment. Stent implantation pressures below 12 atm have been shown to significantly increase the risk of stent thrombosis (289). An optimally deployed stent should restore the anatomy of the vessel as close as possible to the normal state, both in dimension and geometry, and this is the focus of research into device design and deployment.

Because platelets have been shown to be the primary participants in stent thrombosis (290), it has been proposed that with optimal stent deployment proper antiplatelet therapy should be sufficient to prevent thrombosis until neointima formation is complete. More than 35 trials have reported using reduced anticoagulation regimens after coronary stenting (26, 27, 30, 130, 195, 196, 279–281, 291–318). Each of these trials employed aspirin and high-pressure balloon inflation poststent implantation, with different stent types and for different clinical indications. The subacute thrombosis rates in these trials ranged from 0 to 3.6%. From these trials, it is apparent that the regimen of aspirin plus ticlopidine in combination with high-pressure deployment techniques has resulted in a significantly lower incidence of stent thrombosis compared with earlier anticoagulation regimens, with a concomitant significant reduction in bleeding and vascular complications. What remains to be answered is whether different antiplatelet agents or adjunctive therapy with antithrombins will result in a better outcome without significantly increasing hemorrhagic side effects.

Ticlopidine expresses its antiplatelet activity via adenosine diphosphate-mediated inhibition of platelet-fibrinogen binding, and works in synergy with aspirin (319). Although certainly effective, ticlopidine use is not without its problems. In most instances, ticlopidine is started on the day of the stent procedure and its maximal pharmacologic effect occurs only at 4–8 days of treatment. This is after the occurrence of the peak incidence of subacute thrombosis. It is interesting to note, however, that when used in combination with aspirin, the anti-adenosine diphosphate (ADP) activity is seen to be maximally expressed only after 2 days of therapy, which is in keeping with the favorable clinical data found on use of this drug (320). The major concern regarding the use of ticlopidine, however, relates to its side effect profile. Ticlopidine therapy causes gastrointestinal symptoms, cutaneous rashes, and elevations in liver function tests. However, the most significant of its toxicities is the unpredictable occurrence of granulocytosis, neutropenia, and thrombocytopenia, which generally happens at about the third week of therapy (321). It is, therefore, recommended that white blood cell and platelet counts be performed 2 weeks after initiating therapy and at regular intervals beyond that if treatment is continued beyond 1 month. As a result of the delayed onset of action, the side effects and the persistent, albeit low, incidence of stent thrombosis with ticlopidine use, considerable efforts are underway to identify a better postprocedural medication regimen to further decrease the incidence of stent thrombosis. Despite the shortcomings of combined aspirin and ticlopidine therapy, this regimen has been supported by the Expert Consensus Committee of the American College of Cardiology in patients undergoing elective stent implantation with 3 mm or larger diameter arteries without evidence of

thrombus in whom the stent has been optimally deployed (103). **Full anticoagulation is recommended for high-risk patients.** This advice has been recently challenged by Schühlen et al., who reported that the clinical outcome was better and the rate of subacute thrombosis was lower in high-risk patients treated with antiplatelet therapy compared with those treated with an aspirin-anticoagulant combination (322). This must be assessed in a controlled manner before definite conclusions can be drawn.

Whether aspirin therapy alone is adequate antiplatelet coverage has been addressed in several trials, with conflicting results. In the Multicenter Ultrasound Intracoronary Stent (MUSIC) study, stents are implanted according to strict ultrasound guidance criteria (293). Aspirin only therapy is given to those patients meeting the MUSIC criteria, whereas aspirin and intravenous anticoagulation poststenting is given to those not meeting the criteria. Preliminary results from 160 patients show that one patient experienced a subacute thrombosis (0.6%); one Q-wave MI (0.6%) occurred; one patient required CABG (0.6%); and two patients required repeat PTCA (1.3%) by 30 day follow-up. Similarly favorable clinical outcomes were seen in another small series (323). In contrast to these promising results was the report of a trial that prospectively assigned 342 patients to aspirin or aspirin plus ticlopidine therapy after native coronary artery stent implantation. IVUS was not used to assess stent deployment. In this trial, stent thrombosis and death were significantly higher in the aspirin-alone treatment arm compared with the aspirin plus ticlopidine treated group (6.6 versus 0.7%; $P = .2$, 4.4 versus 0.3%; $P = .3$, respectively). The only reported randomized trial failed to show a difference between the aspirin-alone and in combination with ticlopidine, which may be a result of its small size (291). The results of the STARS trial may answer the question whether aspirin therapy alone is better than the combination of aspirin and ticlopidine or coumadin (37).

Several other adjunctive therapies are being considered. The benefit of subcutaneously administered low molecular weight heparin with aspirin and ticlopidine therapy is being compared with a standard anti-coagulation regimen in the ENTICES trial (38). Results from the IMPACT II (Integrelin to Manage Platelet Aggregation to Prevent Coronary Thrombosis) trial, which examined the use of integrelin, a GPIIb/IIIa inhibitor, in 4000 high-risk patients undergoing percutaneous intervention, indicate that GPIIb/IIIa inhibition may be of benefit in the prevention of stent thrombosis. In this trial, 160 patients required bail-out stent implantation for failed PTCA. Integrelin use was associated with a lower rate of MI at 30-day clinical follow-up than the placebo-treated group (16 versus 32%; $P = .01$). The EPILOG stent trial is specifically designed to assess the clinical effects of adjunctive GPIIb/IIIa inhibition in coronary stenting.

Treatment

The importance of avoiding stent thrombosis cannot be overemphasized. Careful attention must be paid to stent deployment technique and antithrombotic with or without anticoagulant therapy. Residual filling defects within the stent, which might represent extruded atheromatous tissue or thrombus, should be treated with additional high-pressure balloon inflations. Marginal dissections at inflow or outflow of the stent should be corrected with the placement of additional stents. Patients who receive stents for high-risk indications should be considered for more intense antithrombotic or prolonged anticoagulant therapy. It is important to realize that no antithrombotic or anticoagulant regimen has been identified to prevent thrombosis of a suboptimally deployed stent (324).

The clinical features of stent thrombosis usually include chest pain and ECG changes suggestive of ischemia. Thrombosis of a previously occluded artery, however, may be clinically silent. Prompt vessel recanalization is central to the effective management of acute or subacute thrombosis. Catheter-based therapies have been most commonly employed with the goal of identifying potential causes such as inadequate stent expansion, improper stent sizing, persistent dissections, or the presence of intimal flaps protruding from the stent struts. These frequently are managed by repeat balloon dilation with or without concomitant intracoronary thrombolytic therapy; however, the support for such management comes from a relatively low number of small trials (63, 209, 269). In the reported series, the successful restoration of flow was achieved in 41 to 80% of instances, those that were not successfully managed percutaneously, however, had severe adverse clinical outcomes. In a recently reported trial, the outcome of those treated with angioplasty-based procedures for stent thrombosis were retrospectively analyzed (210). In this trial, 23 patients were treated with catheter-based therapies (angioplasty alone in 14, angioplasty and intracoronary urokinase in 7, and intracoronary urokinase alone in 2). TIMI grade 3 flow was restored in 21 of these patients; however, only 11 had no angiographic evidence of thrombus. Of the 23 patients, 2 died and 9 were referred for emergent or urgent bypass surgery because of refractory angina and residual thrombosis threatening reclosure. Despite restoration of flow in most patients, 20 of the 23 patients (87%) developed an acute MI. These findings certainly suggest that alternative or adjunctive therapies are needed to treat this disastrous complication.

Other therapies for the treatment of subacute thrombosis are being investigated. The local delivery of urokinase via local infusion or on a urokinase-hydrogel coated balloon has been proposed (325), and uncontrolled anecdotal evidence suggests benefit for intracoronary administration of platelet disaggregators, such as GPIIb/IIIa inhibitors (326). A newly introduced thrombectomy catheter (327), which removes thrombus by means of high velocity saline jets, has also proved to be effective in our hands (unpublished data). Further investigations must be performed before any newer therapy can be recommended.

Restenosis

The Problem

Restenosis is the decrease in the vessel lumen at the site of the catheter-based intracoronary therapies. With the failure of both systemic and conventional drug therapies to significantly reduce the restenosis rate after successful balloon angioplasty, newer technologies were touted as possibly providing the solution to this enormous problem. The demonstration by the BENE-STENT (21) and the STRESS (22) trials that the rates of restenosis could be significantly, although modestly, reduced was considered a major advance in the push to reduce and ultimately eliminate restenosis. What became quickly apparent after the release of the BENESTENT and STRESS results was that the beneficial effects of stent implantation on restenosis could be attributed to larger acute lumen dimensions achieved compared with balloon angioplasty and the elimination of vessel recoil after intervention (45, 328). More recently, the beneficial effects of coronary stent implantation on preventing late remodeling has been demonstrated (329, 330). What stents have failed to improve upon is the neointimal proliferative response to vessel injury, seen both with balloon angioplasty (plain old balloon angioplasty [POBA], as it is now called) and in stented vascular segments, and may actually stimulate neointimal formation (331). Intimal hyperplasia has been shown to be the major component of late lumen loss following stent implantation (332, 333). This has stimulated research into the pathobiology of the stent restenosis process, which has revealed interesting findings that will certainly guide its clinical management and prevention. The response to vascular injury resulting from the placement of an indwelling endovascular stent differs from that caused by balloon angioplasty alone in at least four ways (334).

Type of Injury

Through histologic examination of porcine coronary arteries, it has been shown that the site of neointimal proliferation in the setting of balloon angioplasty alone occurs at the site of disruption of the internal elastic lamina (335). When a stent is placed with the appropriate size in the pig model, the stent struts abut the vessel wall and compress the media without fracturing the internal elastic lamina. The result is little neointima formation. With stent strut penetration of the elastic lamina, neointimal proliferation is stimulated commensurate with the depth of strut penetration. It is tempting to extrapolate this finding to the clinical situation, and to suggest that intentional oversizing and high-pressure balloon postdilation techniques would result in increased rates of restenosis. This, however, may not be the case. One study has been reported in which high-pressure balloon inflation with pressures up to 24 atm reduced the incidence of thrombotic events without increasing the clinical restenosis rate as determined by need for revascularization (289). This may reflect enlargement of the lumen with higher pressures with accommodation of the greater neointimal burden. Angioscopic, IVUS, or postmortem studies need to be performed to answer the question of what is the ideal balloon inflation pressure needed to optimize stent expansion at minimal trauma to the vessel.

Pattern of Cell Response

The early events after the acute injury of the intervention differ between angioplastied lesions and stented vessels (334–336). The stent struts provide a scaffold for the formation of platelet-rich thrombi, into which inflammatory cells from the circulation migrate. The inflammatory cell component plays a much greater role in stented lesions than in those treated with balloon angioplasty alone. Smooth muscle cells then migrate to the neointimal layer where mural thrombi function as a substrate for smooth muscle cell migration and proliferation. The degree of neointimal formation and the proliferative rate of the smooth muscle cells is proportional to the early inflammatory cell involvement (23, 334).

Prolonged Radial Strain

Balloon angioplasty applies a transient strain to the vessel wall, whereas permanent strain is produced by an implanted stent, which may result in a prolonged stimulus for neointimal formation. Animal studies in a porcine coronary model demonstrate that, with both coil and slotted tube designs, histologically determined vessel wall injury progressed between weeks 1 and 12 after implantation. This change was manifest as progressive laceration of the internal elastic laminal and a deeper penetration of the struts through the media. This phase of chronic injury also typically involved a chronic inflammatory response in the media and, occasionally, in the intima. These inflammatory changes were never observed in balloon-treated vessels, and they are thought to contribute to derangements in endothelial lining integrity (337).

Presence of Foreign Material

The most apparent difference between balloon angioplasty and stenting may also be the most critical. A foreign body in the lumen of the vessel serves as a stimulus for intimal hyperplasia, and stent design and composition can greatly influence this process as has been shown in animal models (23). In vessels stented with devices with a single articulation, the pattern of lumen loss is not uniform along the stent, but it increases significantly at the central articulation (330, 333, 338, 339). When two stents are placed in sequence without overlapping, no corresponding increase in tissue accumulation is seen (334). The presence of a bridge, constraining one degree of freedom for the stent, seems to contribute to the restenosis process, indicating that stent design may affect restenosis in humans as well. Low electropositivity of the stent metal has also been shown to exaggerate neointimal proliferation (218).

The result of stent implantation is the production of a proliferative neointima. The layer that forms above the stent struts in humans has been shown, using atherectomy samples, to be relatively acellular, composed predominantly of extracellular matrix (340). This is similar to what has been seen in animal models where most of the late cellular activity in stented vessels can be found in the areas immediately around

and beneath the stent struts (334). The course of the stent restenosis process has been shown to be similar to that reported for PTCA, with almost no significant renarrowing occurring beyond 6 months (341).

Risk Factors

Several risk factors for the development of stent restenosis have been determined by univariate and multivariate analysis of several stented patient populations.

History of Restenosis

Stent implantation at the site of a restenotic lesion has been shown to be associated with a greater likelihood of stent restenosis (19, 109, 342, 343). This is similar to the situation seen with PTCA (344). Arterial trauma results in a change of the smooth muscle from contractile to an organelle-rich synthetic phenotype (345, 346), and it has been suggested that trauma to an area containing many phenotypically synthetic smooth muscle cells may heighten the risk of restenosis. It should be noted, however, that multivariate analysis in a recently reported trial using high-pressure balloon stent implantation and only antiplatelet therapy with aspirin plus ticlopidine poststent deployment failed to show a history of restenosis as a risk factor for subsequent clinical stent restenosis (347).

Multiple Stents

Multiple stent implantation has been shown to be a significant risk factor for stent restenosis in several trials (18, 19, 271, 342, 343). It has been hypothesized that stent-on-stent trauma may prevent passivation of the stent surface and thereby promote thrombus formation and stimulate restenosis. A recent IVUS study, however, demonstrated that tissue growth, late lumen loss, and chronic lumen dimensions were similar at the junction of two stents regardless if they were overlapping or not, suggesting that stent overlap is not responsible for the observed increase in risk (330). Supporting this suggestion was a recently reported trial that failed to show a difference in the clinically determined restenosis rate between patients treated with a single stent and those receiving multiple stents (270).

Extent of Residual Stenosis

The extent of residual stenosis after stenting has been shown to be correlated with the likelihood of subsequent restenosis (19, 343). This is likely a result of less encroachment of myointima being necessary to result in a greater than 50% reduction in lumen diameter, to meet the angiographic definition of restenosis, if a significant narrowing is already present.

Stenting of Total Occlusions

Stent placement in totally occluded vessels has been shown to be a risk factor for restenosis (19). Reported angiographic rates of restenosis from observational trials range from 19 to 76% (113–120), and seem to depend on the clinical situation, the type of stent implanted, and the location. Although not specifically addressed, it is likely that stent placement at the site of a chronic total occlusion will remain a significant independent predictor of restenosis using currently employed stenting techniques.

Other Risk Factors

Stent placement in vessels with an angiographically determined reference diameter of less than 3.0 mm has been shown to be a risk factor for restenosis (19, 81, 342). One explanation for this observation is that the absolute amount of neointima required to result in a greater than 50% stenosis is lower for vessels of smaller caliber. Stent deployment with a balloon pressures below 12 atm has also been found to be a risk factor for

restenosis (342), although this has not been corroborated (289).

Prevention

The discouraging results of most trials examining the systemic administration of pharmacologic agents to prevent restenosis in the setting of balloon angioplasty (348–351) has impacted on the focus of therapies directed at improving the long-term outcome of stent implantation. Few systemically administered agents have been shown to have some influence on clinical and angiographic rates of restenosis after PTCA. These include the prostacyclin analogue ciprostene (352), GPIIb/IIIa inhibitors (353, 354), omega-3 fatty acid (355), trapidil (356), and angiopeptin (357). These agents are also being investigated for their ability to prevent restenosis in the setting of stent implantation. The local delivery of heparin, steroids, and antisense oligonucleotides at the time of stent implantation are also being examined as a means of preventing subsequent restenosis.

As a result of their long residence times, attention has become focused on endovascular stents as a platform to deliver therapies for the prevention of restenosis. One such approach uses the stent as a reservoir for prolonged local drug administration. This can be accomplished by coating metallic stents with drug-containing polymer or incorporating a pharmacologically active compound into a biodegradable polymeric stent or in a polymer-metal composite stent. Several candidate drugs for stent coatings have been considered. Heparin-coated stents are now undergoing clinical assessment and a coating capable of delivering other agents is an area of active investigation. Incorporation of pharmacologically active agents into biodegradable stents is also a challenging area of active research (358). To be effective, a drug-releasing biodegradable stent must be biocompatible, not cause an inflammatory reaction, and the breakdown products must be nontoxic. Stent delivery must be reliable and the devices must have high radial strength. A device that seems to meet all of the necessary character-

692 / *Coronary and Noncoronary Therapeutic Techniques*

istics is the Duke Biodegradable stent, which is made from a specialized form of polylactic acid (PLLA) (359). PLLA has been shown to be useful for the local delivery of several pharmacologic agents (360). Self-expanding versions of the Duke stent have been successfully implanted in peripheral arteries of dogs and a balloon expandable version is currently undergoing evaluation (358).

Low-dose external beam irradiation has been shown to be a safe and effective means to treat several benign proliferative disorders. The success of this approach has led to the hypothesis that brachytherapy might also result in a reduction in intimal hyperplasia when administered after percutaneous revascularization. Early results from the balloon-injured swine model of restenosis demonstrated the efficacy of the gamma emitter iridium-192 (^{192}Ir) in limiting the formation of neointima in this model (361, 362). Endoluminal radiation in this model was delivered transiently immediately after injury, and effects of the radiation therapy persisted to 6 months after injury. Similarly favorable results were seen with both gamma and β-irradiation was applied transiently before stent implantation in the porcine model of vascular injury (363). It was also shown that neointimal proliferation could be inhibited in animal models with gamma and β-particle emitting stents (364), which led to the development of a pure β-emitting device (365–369). β-irradiation has the theoretic advantage of having a limited range in tissue, and the ^{32}P isotope used in the current designs has the added advantages of a short half-life and no associated gamma radiation. It is believed that radioactive stents act by culling the smooth muscle cell population as these cells pass through the 'electron fence' at the plane of the stent wires (368). Endothelialization of the stent proceeds normally, presumably because of the enhanced sensitivity of the actively proliferating smooth muscle cells to the ionizing radiation. Clinical trials are underway using both transiently applied gamma irradiation and the β-emitting stents to determine whether they are effective in preventing restenosis in humans. The feasibility of the implantation of a β-emitting strontium-90/yttrium-90 source (Novoste Corpora-

tion, Norcross, GA) has also been recently demonstrated in humans.

Treatment

The best management of patients with symptomatic in-stent restenosis has not been completely established. Reports have supported the use of conventional balloon angioplasty (18, 107, 332, 370–378), as well as the debulking techniques of directional atherectomy (379–381), rotational atherectomy (382), and excimer laser (383, 384) procedures. The mechanism underlying the beneficial effect of the debulking procedures is relatively straightforward, whereas that of balloon angioplasty is less clear. One quantitative angiographic study performed before the routine use of high-pressure stent deployment techniques demonstrated that 85% of the luminal enlargement produced by balloon dilation within stenotic stents was caused by compression of protruding tissue and extrusion of hyperplastic tissue through the stent interstices, and only 15% was related to additional stent expansion (385); however, the relative contribution of each mechanism seems to be device specific (376). It must be kept in mind that all of the treatment modalities have their own, often serious, complications. Balloon angioplasty of the stented segment is no exception, and serious dissections can result, which may require emergency surgery or, as has recently been described, stent deployment in the previously stented site (386). Follow-up angiography results are available from several of the series of patients treated for in-stent restenosis. Follow-up angiographic results at 7 months after stent redilation of 48% of the 105 patients in the US Multicenter Palmaz-Schatz Registry documented restenosis recurrence in 54% (377). Only one small study has reported the long-term outcome of patients treated with balloon angioplasty of stent restenosis (387). In this trial, 31 patients underwent balloon angioplasty for stent restenosis. The mean follow-up period in this trial was 43 ± 22 months, and 22% of patients treated with balloon angioplasty for stent restenosis required target vessel revascularization procedures. Using quantitative angiographic techniques, three patterns of stent restenosis have been described: diffuse in stent, focal stent border, and focal in-stent, with the diffuse pattern showing the greatest recurrence of stent restenosis after balloon angioplasty (388). This finding suggests that stent restenosis is not a single entity and a particular treatment may not be ideal for all patterns. Although all of the techniques for the treatment of stent restenosis have been shown to be feasible, no studies have been reported comparing the techniques head-to-head, so the best therapeutic approach has not yet been determined.

Bleeding and Vascular Injury

In the large randomized STRESS I and BENESTENT I trials, significant bleeding or vascular complications occurred in 7.3 and 13.5% of the stented patients, respectively, largely because of the intensive anticoagulation regimens that were employed (21,22). Reduced anticoagulation regimens have had a profound impact on reduction of local vascular complications. Major bleeding occurred in only 0.4% and major vascular complications requiring surgical repair occurred in 0.3% of 1157 patients treated without warfarin or postprocedural heparin after high-pressure stent deployment (195). The risk factors for vascular complications that have been identified include age more than 75 years, female gender, sheath size larger than 8 F, indwelling sheath and procedure durations, postprocedural use of heparinoids, saphenous vein graft stenting, hypertension, and stenting for bail-out indications (195, 389–393).

In addition to reduced anticoagulation regimens, several other approaches have been tried in an attempt to further reduce the vascular complication rate. Alternatives to the routine femoral access site is one strategy that has been considered. Historically, the first cardiac catheterization was performed through brachial access, isolated through brachial artery cutdown (394). One of the advantages of this approach was that the artery could be repaired with direct vis-

ualization after the procedure. The possibility of radial nerve damage and the potentially tragic consequences of damage to the brachial artery led to the development of the femoral access technique for cardiac catheterization by Judkins, which became the favored approach for angioplasty techniques. The large number of femoral access site complications after stent deployment with postprocedural anticoagulation led to an assessment of the feasibility of the brachial technique for stent implantation (395). Although the incidence of vascular complications was felt to be reduced using the brachial access site, compromise of blood flow to the hand, the consequence of brachial artery damage, limited the popularity of this technique.

The transradial approach for coronary stenting, first introduced in 1994 (396), has several advantages over femoral and brachial routes. The radial artery is superficial and, therefore, easily accessible and not located near important veins or nerves. A further advantage is that occlusion of the artery does not result in significant clinical sequelae in patients who demonstrate a normal Allen's test (397). In a comparative study between the transradial, transbrachial, and femoral approach for coronary angioplasty in 900 patients (the ACCESS study), no entry site complications were observed in the radial group whereas the incidence of complications in the brachial and femoral site groups were 2.3 and 2.0%, respectively (398). An observational analysis of 377 patients comparing radial and femoral access sites for stent implantation treated with either postprocedural anticoagulation or antiplatelet therapy only was recently reported (399). Vascular complications occurred in 6% of the patients treated with femoral access in both anticoagulant and antiplatelet treated group, whereas none of the patients in whom the radial approach was used showed access site complications. With increased operator experience, the radial approach for coronary stent implantation is gaining acceptance and has encouraged the development of lower profile devices and stents.

Percutaneous vascular closure devices have also been used in patients undergoing stent implantation via the femoral route in an attempt to reduce the vascular complication rate and promote early ambulation. The results of these devices on the vascular complication rates have been equivocal (400–405), and further trials are necessary to demonstrate their advantage.

Stent Embolization

Stent dislodgement from the delivery catheter may occur during the introduction of the stent, and it can result in stent embolization. The stent may embolize to the distal native coronary artery (406) or saphenous vein graft (407), or to peripheral vessels, including the aorta (408), iliac (409), or femoral (410) arteries. Fortunately, serious sequelae of such stent embolization appear to be rare. Several successful retrieval techniques have been described involving the use of additional balloon catheters (407), biopsy forceps and retrieval devices (408, 411, 412), and coaxial wires (406, 409, 413). Although feasible, these techniques are difficult, more so for radiolucent stents, and require considerable operator experience.

Side Branch Occlusion

Side branch occlusion is an infrequent occurrence complicating coronary stenting (414), with an incidence of less than 10% in one clinical series (415). The risk of side branch occlusion is related both to the luminal diameter of the side branch and to the extent of disease within its origin. Occlusion occurs by a shift of the atherosclerotic plaque from the parent vessel into the orifice of the side branch, dissection at the side branch ostium, or by mechanical obstruction of the side branch by the stent struts (415, 416). The clinical significance of the side branch occlusion relates to the size of the side branch and to the amount of myocardium supplied by the vessel. Surprisingly, coronary stent implantation for acute or threatened closure has been shown to restore the patency of side branches occluded by angioplastty (417). This is thought to be a result of the reapproximation of the dis-

sected and displaced intima toward it original position away from the ostium of the side branch that it is obstructing. The management of side branch occlusion involves passage of a balloon or stent through the struts of the stent in the parent vessel. Some stent designs facilitate the passage of angioplasty and stent systems through their struts (173), whereas others require selected devices (174).

Coronary Perforation

With the introduction of high-pressure balloon deployment and oversized balloon strategies for adequate stent expansion, the frequency of coronary perforation has increased, complicating 1.0 to 2.5% of stent procedures (24, 26, 418, 419). Features that appeared to be associated with perforation include complex lesion morphology, small vessel diameter, balloon:artery ratio 1.2:1 or greater, tapering vessel, need to recross a dissection with a guidewire, and heavy calcifications (26, 418, 420). Reduction of the ultrasound-determined balloon artery ratio from 1.2 to 1.05 has been shown to decrease the incidence of coronary perforation from 1.2% (4 ruptures in 339 lesions treated) to 0% (113 lesions treated) in one clinical series (26). Many localized perforations can be managed with prolonged balloon inflation, and they may require the administration of protamine in some instances. In the event of frank or threatened tamponade, pericardiocentesis may be necessary. Despite these interventions, emergency surgery may be necessary in up to 50% of perforations, and clinical sequelae include myocardial infarction and death in 40 and 30% of perforations, respectively (419).

Infection

Stent abscess occurrence is an extremely rare, but potentially catastrophic complication after coronary artery stenting. Only one report is found in the literature of a fatal perivascular myocardial abscess resulting from the implantation of a Palmaz-Schatz stent in the right coronary artery (421). Although there are no data to suggest the benefit of routine antibiotics in patients receiving intravascular stents, experimental data indicate that prophylactic antibiotics be given to those patients who at risk for transient bacteremia (422). In a porcine stent model, systemic bacterial challenge was administered immediately after stent deployment. When sacrificed at 72 hours, 80% of the animals showed positive stent cultures, whereas at 3 weeks 60% of the cultures were positive (422). Although not conclusive, these data support antibiotic prophylaxis for those patients who undergo dental procedures, endoscopic examinations, or other invasive procedures within 3 months of stent implantation (when neointimalization is complete).

LONG-TERM FOLLOW-UP

Although the number of stenting procedures is increasing at an alarming rate, little information is available on the long-term outcome of these patients and the integrity of the implanted devices. Serial angiographic studies with long-term follow-up clinical data have recently been reported. In one study, 143 patients were followed for up to 3 years, with angiography being performed at 6, 12, and 36 months after Palmaz-Schatz stent implantation in native coronary arteries (423). Complete angiographic data were available in roughly half of the patients at all time points. Follow-up coronary angiography revealed a decrease in minimal luminal diameter from 2.54 ± 0.44 mm immediately after stent implantation to 1.87 ± 0.56 mm at 6 months. Significant late improvement in luminal diameter was observed at 3 years (1.94 ± 0.48 mm at 6 months and 2.09 ± 0.48 mm at 3 years, $P < .001$ in patients with paired angiograms). Survival rate free of myocardial infarction, bypass surgery, and repeat coronary angioplasty at 3 years in this group of patients was 74.6%, which compared well with similar follow-up data for balloon angioplasty (424). Later lumen enlargement at the stented site was also noted in two other series (425, 426). Three-year event-free survival results have also been presented for

65 patients treated with elective Palmaz-Schatz stent implantation (427). Three-year event-free survival was 56% in this group, with most events occurring within the first year after stenting. Long-term clinical follow-up results up to 104 months have also been reported for patients with stents (Palmaz-Schatz, Wiktor, and Wallstent) implanted for the treatment of restenosis (111). In this series, 70% of the patients remained event free, with a survival rate of 95%. Long-term follow up results 9 years after implantation of the Wallstent for restenosis, bail-out indications, and in saphenous vein grafts demonstrated a 75% event-free survival rate in 131 stents implanted in 105 patients (428). Although these first results are encouraging, the number of reports is small and the patient population consists of those patients stented with early low-pressure balloon dilation techniques. More data at longer follow-up periods are required to advocate the continued long-term efficacy of coronary stent implantation.

FUTURE TRENDS

It is clear that the use of coronary stents will continue to increase in the near future as the indications expand and the results of randomized trials become available. Advances in device technology will certainly play a major part in determining the future role of stenting techniques. The field of stent coatings is a subject of intense investigation with new biocompatible polymers and drug-eluting polymers being developed for application to metal stent scaffold. Polymeric stents are also being developed, with the search for a biocompatible and biodegradable polymer capable of being loaded with antiproliferative or antithrombotic drugs an area being of intense interest. Composite stents, composed of metal-augmented polymers are also being developed in an attempt to combine the mechanical strength of a metal stent with biocompatible or drug-eluting properties of a polymer to minimize local tissue reaction. A promising advance has been the development of stents that provide locally active ionizing radiation. These devices have the potential to completely inhibit the restenosis process, although long-term effects of these devices must be carefully analyzed. Modifications in stent design are also proceeding at an unprecedented rate. Novel rotating and locking mechanisms are being incorporated into stent designs, affording them high flexibility when unexpanded and remarkable rigidity when expanded. Eagerly awaited is the first true bifurcation stent for use in lesions with significant side branch stenosis. This Y-shaped stent, currently being tested in animal models, will soon be available for testing in humans. Also very active is the search for a adjunctive pharmacologic or gene therapy to address the problem of stent restenosis. With these continued developments and refinements, it is possible that stenting will be the coup over angioplasty and surgery for coronary artery revascularization.

References

1. Dotter CT, Judkins MP. Transluminal treatment of arteriosclerotic obstruction. Circulation 1964;30:654–670.
2. Dotter CT. Transluminally placed coil spring end arterial tube grafts: long term patency in canine popliteal artery. Invest Radiol 1969;4:329–332.
3. Dotter CT, Buschmann PAC, McKinney MK, et al. Transluminal expandable nitinol coil stent grafting: preliminary report. Radiology 1983;147:259–260.
4. Cragg A, Lund G, Rysavy J, et al. Nonsurgical placement of arterial endoprostheses: a new technique using nitinol wire. Radiology 1983;147:261–263.
5. Maass D, Zollikofer CHL, Largiadèr F, et al. Radiological follow-up of transluminally inserted vascular endoprostheses: an experimental study using expanding spirals. Radiology 1984;152:659–663.
6. Wright KC, Wallace S, Charnsangavej C, et al. Percutaneous endovascular stents: an experimental evaluation. Radiology 1985;156:69–72.
7. Palmaz JC, Sibbit RR, Reuter SR, et al. Expandable intraluminal graft: a preliminary study. Radiology 1985;156:73–77.
8. Palmaz JC, Sibbit RR, Tio FOR, et al. Expandable intraluminal vascular graft: a feasibility study. Surgery 1986;99:199–205.
9. Rousseau H, Puel J, Joffre F, Sigwart U, et al. Self-expanding endovascular prosthesis: an experimental study. Radiology 1987;164:709–714.
10. Roubin GS, Robinson KA, King III SB, et al. Early and late results of intracoronary arterial stenting after coronary angioplasty in dogs. Circulation 1987;76:841–897.
11. Schatz RA, Palmaz JC, Tio FOR, et al. Balloon-expandable intracoronary stents in the adult dog. Circulation 1987;76:450–457.
12. Puel J, Joffre F, Rousseau H, et al. Endo-prothèses coronariennes auto-expansives dans la prévention des resténoses après angioplastie transluminale. Arch Mal Coeur Vaiss 1987;8:1311–1312.
13. Sigwart U, Puel J, Mirkovitch V, et al. Intravascular stents to prevent occlusion and restenosis after transluminal angioplasty. N Eng J Med 1987;316:701–706.
14. Serruys PW, Strauss BH, Beatt KJ, et al. Angiographic follow-up after placement of a self-expanding coronary artery stent. N Eng J Med 1991;324:13–17.
15. Block PC. Coronary-artery stents and other endoluminal devices. N Eng J Med 1991;324:52–53.
16. Roubin GS, Cannon AD, Agrawal SK, et al. Intracoronary stenting for acute and threatened closure complicating percutaneous transluminal coronary angioplasty. Circulation 1992;85:916–927.
17. Schatz RA, Baim DS, Leon M, et al. Clinical experience with the Palmaz-Schatz coronary stent. Initial results of a multicenter study. Circulation 1991;83:148–161.
18. Haude M, Erbel R, Straub U, et al. Short and long term results after intracoronary stenting in human coronary arteries: monocentre experience with the balloon-expandable Palmaz-Schatz stent. Br Heart J 1991;66:337–345.
19. Ellis SG, Savage M, Fischman D, et al. Restenosis after placement of Palmaz-Schatz stents in native coronary arteries. Initial results of a multicenter experience. Circulation 1992;86:1836–1844.
20. de Jaegere PP, Serruys PW, Bertrand M, et al. Wiktor stent implantation in patients with restenosis following balloon angioplasty of a native coronary artery. Am J Cardiol 1992;69:598–602.
21. Serruys PW, de Jaegere P, Kiemeneij F, et al; for the Benestent Study Group. A comparison of balloon-expandable-stent implantation with balloon angioplasty in patients with coronary artery disease. N Engl J Med 1994;331:489–495.
22. Fischman DL, Leon MB, Baim DS, et al; for the Stent Restenosis Study investigators. A randomized comparison of coronary-stent placement and balloon angioplasty in the treatment of coronary artery disease. N Engl J Med 1994;331:496–501.
23. Rogers C, Edelman ER. Endovascular stent design dictates experimental restenosis and thrombosis. Circulation 1995;91:2995–3001.
24. Goldberg SL, Colombo A, Nakamura S, et al. Benefit of intracoronary ultrasound in the deployment of Palmaz-Schatz stents. J Am Coll Cardiol 1994;24:996–1003.
25. Nakamura S, Colombo A, Gaglione S, et al. Intracoronary ultrasound observations during stent implantation. Circulation 1994;89:2026–2034.
26. Colombo A, Hall P, Nakamura S, et al. Intracoronary stenting without anticoagulation accomplished with intravascular ultrasound guidance. Circulation 1995;91:1676–1688.
27. Morice MC, Zemour G, Beneviste E, et al. Intracoronary stenting without coumadin: one month

results of a French multicenter study. Cathet Cardiovasc Diagn 1995;35:1–7.

28. Morice M-C. Preliminary results of the MUST trial. Journal of Invasive Cardiology 1996:8(Suppl E):8E-9E.

29. Neumann FJ, Gawaz M, Ott I, et al. Prospective evaluation of hemostatic predictors of subacute stent thrombosis after coronary Palmaz-Schatz stenting. J Am Coll Cardiol 1996;27:15–21.

30. Schömig A, Neumann FJ, Kastrati A, et al. A randomized comparison of antiplatelet and anticoagulant therapy after the placement of coronary-artery stents. N Engl J Med 1996;334:1084–1089.

31. Erbel R, Haude M, Höpp HW, et al. Rutsch W, Herrmann G; on behalf of the REST Study Group. REstenosis ST (REST)-Study: randomized trial comparing stenting and balloon angioplasty for treatment of restenosis after balloon angioplasty. J Am Coll Cardiol 1996;27(Suppl A):139A.

32. Keane D, Roubin G, Marco J, et al. GRACE, Gianturco Roubin stent Acute Closure Evaluation. Substrate, challenges and design of a randomized trial of bailout management. Journal of Interventional Cardiology 1994;7:333–339.

33. Haude M, Erbel R, Hoepp HW, et al, and the STENT-BY Study group. STENT-BY Study: a prospective randomized trial comparing immediate stenting versus conservative treatment strategies in abrupt vessel closure or symptomatic dissections during coronary balloon angioplasty [Abstract]. Eur Heart J 1996;17(Suppl):172.

34. Rodriguez A, Fernandez M, Bernardi V, et al; on behalf of the GRAMI investigators. Coronary stents improved hospital results during coronary angioplasty in acute myocardial infarction: preliminary results of a randomized controlled study (GRAMI Trial) [Abstract]. J Am Coll Cardiol 1997; 29(Suppl A):221A.

35. Hoorntje JC, Suryapranata H, de Boer M-J, et al. ESCOBAR: primary stenting for acute myocardial infarction: preliminary results of a randomized trial [Abstract]. Circulation 1996;94(Suppl):I-570.

36. Monassier JP, Elias J, Meyer P, et al. STENTIM I: the French registry of stenting at acute myocardial infarction [Abstract]. J Am Coll Cardiol 1996; 27(Suppl):68A.

37. Baim D, Leon M, Gordon P, Giambartolomei A, et al. The effect of different anticoagulation strategies on early clinical outcomes after optimal stent implantation: results from the Stent Anticoagulation Regimen Study (STARS) [Abstract]. J Am Coll Cardiol 1998.

38. Kruse KR, Greenberg CS, Tangueay J-F, et al. Thrombin and fibrin activity in patients treated with enoxaprin, ticlopidine and aspirin versus the conventional coumadin regimen after elective stenting: the ENTICES trial. J Am Coll Cardiol 1996;27(Suppl A):334A.

39. The EPIC Investigators. Use of a monoclonal antibody against the platelet glycoprotein IIb/IIIa receptor in high-risk coronary angioplasty. N Engl J Med 1994;330:956–961.

40. Kutryk MJB, Serruys PW. Antisense oligonucleotide therapy for the prevention of stent restenosis. The ITALICS trial. Thoraxcenter Journal 1996;8: 46–48.

41. Bertrand M, Legrand V, Boland J, et al. Full anticoagulation versus ticlopidine plus aspirin after stent implantation: a randomized multicenter European study: the FANTASTIC trial [Abstract]. Circulation 1996;94(Suppl):I-685.

42. Teirstein PS, Massullo V, Jani S, et al. Radiation therapy following coronary stenting—6 month follow-up of a randomized clinical trial. Circulation 1996;94(Suppl):I-210.

43. Russo RJ, Teirstein PS; for the AVID Investigators. Angiography versus intravascular ultrasound-directed stent placement [Abstract]. J Am Coll Cardiol 1996;27(Suppl A):306A.

44. Russo RJ, Teirstein PS; for the AVID Investigators. Angiography versus intravascular ultrasound-directed stent placement [Abstract]. Circulation 1996;94(Suppl):I-263.

45. Kuntz RE, Gibson CM, Nobuyoshi M, et al. Generalized model of restenosis after conventional balloon angioplasty, stenting and directional atherectomy. J Am Coll Cardiol 1993;21:15–25.

46. Macaya C, Serruys PW, Ruygrok P, et al. Continued benefit of coronary stenting versus balloon angioplasty: one year clinical follow-up of Benestent trial. J Am Coll Cardiol 1996;27:255–261.

47. de Feyter PJ, de Jaegere PPT, Serruys PW. Incidence, predictors and management of acute coronary occlusion after coronary angioplasty. Am Heart J 1994;127:643–651.

48. Lincoff AM, Popma JJ, Ellis SG, et al. Abrupt vessel closure complicating coronary angioplasty: clinical, angiographic and therapeutic profile. J Am Coll Cardiol 1992;19:926–935.

49. Ellis SG, Roubin GS, King III SB, et al. Angiographic and clinical predictors of acute closure after native vessel coronary angioplasty. Circulation 1988;77:372–379.

50. Sigwart U, Urban P, Golf S, et al. Emergency stenting for acute occlusion after coronary balloon angioplasty. Circulation 1988;78:1121–1127.

51. de Feyter PJ, de Scheerder IK, van den Brand M, et al. Emergency stenting for refractory acute coronary occlusion during coronary angioplasty. Am J Cardiol 1990;66:1147–1150.

52. Goy JJ, Sigwart U, Vogt P, et al. Long-term clinical follow-up after of patients treated with the self-expanding coronary stent for acute occlusion during balloon angioplasty of the right coronary artery. J Am Coll Cardiol 1992;19:1593–1596.

53. Eeckhout E, Goy JJ, Vogt P, et al. Complications and follow-up after intracoronary stenting: critical analysis of a 6-year single-center experience. Am Heart J 1994;127:262–272.

54. George BS, Voorhees WD III, Roubin GS, et al. Multicenter investigation of coronary stenting to treat acute or threatened closure after percutaneous transluminal coronary angioplasty: clinical and angiographic outcomes. J Am Coll Cardiol 1993;22:135–143.

55. Hearn JA, King SB III, Douglas JS, et al. Clinical and angiographic outcomes after coronary artery stenting for acute or threatened closure after percutaneous transluminal coronary angioplasty. Initial results with a balloon-expandable, stainless steel design. Circulation 1993;88:2086–2096.

56. Sutton JM, Ellis SG, Roubin GS, et al; for the

Gianturco-Roubin Intracoronary Stent Investigator Group. Major clinical events after coronary stenting. The multicenter registry of acute and elective Gianturco-Roubin stent placement. Circulation 1994;89:1126–1137.

57. Chan CNS, Tan ATH, Koh TH, et al. Intracoronary stenting in the treatment of acute or threatened closure in angiographically small coronary arteries (< 3.0 mm) complicating percutaneous transluminal coronary angioplasty. Am J Cardiol 1995;75:23–25.

58. Haude M, Erbel R, Straub U, et al. Results of intracoronary stents for the management of coronary dissection after balloon angioplasty. Am J Cardiol 1981;67:691–696.

59. Herrmann HC, Buchbinder M, Clemen MW, et al. Emergent use of balloon-expandable coronary artery stenting for failed percutaneous transluminal angioplasty. Circulation 1992;86:812–819.

60. Maiello L, Columbo A, Gianrossi R, et al. Coronary stenting for treatment of acute or threatened closure following dissection after balloon angioplasty. Am Heart J 1993;125:1570–1575.

61. Kiemeneij F, Laarman GJ, van der Wieken R, et al. Emergency coronary stenting with the Palmaz-Schatz stent for failed transluminal coronary angioplasty: results of a learning phase. Am Heart J 1993;126:23–31.

62. Colombo A, Goldberg SL, Almagor Y, et al. A novel strategy for stent deployment in the treatment of acute or threatened closure complicating balloon coronary angioplasty. Use of short or standard (or both) single or multiple Palmaz-Schatz stents. J Am Coll Cardiol 1993;22:1887–1891.

63. Foley JB, Brown RIG, Penn IM. Thrombosis and restenosis after stenting in failed angioplasty: comparison with elective stenting. Am Heart J 1994;128:12–20.

64. Schömig A, Kastrati A, Mudra H, et al. Four-year experience with Palmaz-Schatz stenting in coronary angioplasty complicated by dissection with threatened or present vessel closure. Circulation 1994;90:2716–2724.

65. Alfonso F, Hernandez R, Goicolea J, et al. Coronary stenting for acute coronary dissection after coronary angioplasty: implications of residual dissection. J Am Coll Cardiol 1994;24:989–995.

66. Vrolix M, Piessens J. Usefulness of the Wicktor stent for treatment of threatened or acute closure complicating coronary angioplasty. Am J Cardiol 1994;73:737–741.

67. Reifart N, Langer A, Storger H, et al. Strecker stent as a bailout device following percutaneous transluminal coronary angioplasty. Journal of Interventional Cardiology 1992;5:79–83.

68. Lablanche J-M, McFadden EP, Bonnet J-L, et al. Combined antiplatelet therapy with ticlopidine and aspirin. A simplified approach to intracoronary stent management. Eur Heart J 1996;17:1373–1380.

69. Lincoff AM, Topol EJ, Chapekis AT, et al. Intracoronary stenting compared with conventional therapy for abrupt vessel closure complicating coronary angioplasty: a matched case-control study. J Am Coll Cardiol 1993;21:866–875.

70. Altmann DB, Racz M, Battleman DS, et al. Reduction in angioplasty complications after the introduction of coronary stents: results from a consecutive series of 2242 patients. Am Heart J 1996;132:503–507.

71. Agrawal S, Liu M, Hearn J, et al. Can preemptive stenting improve the outcome of acute closure? [Abstract] J Am Coll Cardiol 1993;21(Suppl):291A.

72. de Jaegere PPT, Hermans WR, Rensing BJ, et al. Matching based on quantitative coronary angiography. A surrogate for randomized studies? Comparison between stent implantation and balloon angioplasty of a native coronary lesion. Am Heart J 1993;125:310–319.

73. Rensing BJ, Hermans WR, Strauss BJ, et al. Regional differences in elastic recoil after percutaneous transluminal coronary angioplasty: a quantitative angiographic study. J Am Coll Cardiol 1991;17:34B–38B.

74. Hanet C, Wijns W, Michel X, et al. Influence of balloon size and stenosis morphology in immediate and delayed elastic recoil after percutaneous transluminal coronary angioplasty. J Am Coll Cardiol 1991;18:506–511.

75. Haude M, Erbel R, Issa H, et al. Quantitative analysis of elastic recoil after balloon angioplasty and after intracoronary implantation of balloon-expandable Palmaz-Schatz stents. J Am Coll Cardiol 1993;21:26–34.

76. de Jaegere P, Serruys PW, van Es GA, et al. Recoil following Wiktor stent implantation for restenotic lesions of coronary arteries. Cathet Cardiovasc Diagn 1994;32:147–156.

77. Mintz GS, Kovach JA, Pichard AD, et al. Geometric remodelling is the predominant mechanism of clinical restenosis after coronary angioplasty [Abstract]. J Am Coll Cardiol 1994;25(Suppl):138A.

78. Brott BC, Labinaz M, Culp SC, et al. Vessel remodelling after angioplasty: comparative anatomic studies [Abstract]. J Am Coll Cardiol 1994;25(Suppl):138A.

79. Masotti M, Serra A, Fernandez-Avilés F, et al. Stent versus angioplasty restenosis trial (START). Angiographic results at six month follow-up [Abstract]. Eur Heart J 1996;17(Suppl):120.

80. Penn IM, Ricci DR, Almond DG, et al. Coronary artery stenting reduces restenosis: final results from the Trial of Angioplasty and Stents in Canada (TASC) I [Abstract]. Circulation 1995;92(Suppl I):I-279.

81. Azar AJ, Detre K, Goldberg S, et al; on behalf of the Benestent and Stent Restenosis Study. A meta-analysis on the clinical and angiographic outcomes of Stents vs PTCA in the different coronary vessel sizes in the Benestent-1 and Stress-1/2 trials [Abstract]. Circulation 1995;92(Suppl):I-475.

82. Foley DP, Serruys PW. Provisional stenting—"stent-like" balloon angioplasty. Evidence to define the continuing role of balloon angioplasty for percutaneous coronary revascularization; submitted for publication.

83. de Feyter PJ, van Suylen RJ, de Jaegere PPT, et al. Balloon angioplasty for the treatment of lesions in saphenous venous bypass grafts. J Am Coll Cardiol 1993;21:1539–1549.

84. Plokker HWT, Meester BH, Serruys PW. The Dutch experience in percutaneous transluminal angioplasty of narrowed saphenous veins used for aortocoronary bypass. Am J Cardiol 1991;67:361–366.

85. Stewart J, Williams M, Goy JJ, et al. Stenotic disease of saphenous vein coronary artery bypass grafts treated by self expanding stents [Abstract]. J Am Coll Cardiol 1992;19(Suppl):49A.

86. Urban P, Sigwart U, Golf S, et al. Intravascular stenting for stenosis of aortocoronary venous bypass grafts. J Am Coll Cardiol 1989;13:1085–1091.

87. de Scheerder IK, Strauss BH, de Feyter PJ, et al. Stenting of venous bypass grafts: a new treatment modality of patients who are poor candidates for reintervention. Am Heart J 1992;23:1046–1054.

88. Strauss BH, Serruys PW, Bertrand ME, et al. Qualitative angiographic follow-up of the coronary Wallstent in native vessel and bypass grafts (European experience: March 1986-March 1990). Am J Cardiol 1992;69:475–481.

89. Eeckhout E, Goy JJ, Stauffer JC, et al. Endoluminal stenting of narrowed saphenous vein grafts: long-term clinical and angiographic follow-up. Cathet Cardiovasc Diagn 1994;32:139–46.

90. Leon MB, Wong SC, Pichard AD. Balloon expandable stent implantation in saphenous vein grafts. In: Herrmann HC, Hirshfeld JW, eds. Clinical use of the Palmaz-Schatz Intracoronary Stent. Mount Kisco, NY: Futura Publishing Company, 1993:111–121.

91. Strumpf RK, Mehta SS, Ponder R, et al. Palmaz-Schatz stent implantation in stenosed saphenous vein grafts: clinical and angiographic follow-up. Am Heart J 1992;123:1329–1336.

92. Piana RN, Moscucci M, Cohen DJ, et al. Palmaz-Schatz stenting for treatment of focal vein graft stenosis: immediate results and long-term outcome. J Am Coll Cardiol 1994;23:1296–1304.

93. Maiello L, Colombo A, Gianrossi R, et al. Favourable results of treatment of narrowed saphenous vein grafts with Palmaz-Schatz stent implantation. Eur Heart J 1994;15:1212–1216.

94. Wong SC, Popma JJ, Pichard AD, et al. Comparison of clinical and angiographic outcomes after saphenous vein graft angioplasty using coronary versus 'biliary' tubular slotted stents. Circulation 1995;91:339–350.

95. Carrozza JP, Kuntz RE, Levine MJ, et al. Angiographic and clinical outcome of intracoronary stenting: immediate and long-term results from a large single center experience. J Am Coll Cardiol 1992;20:328–337.

96. Fenton SH, Fischman DL, Savage MP, et al. Long-term and clinical outcome after implantation of balloon expandable stents in aortocoronary saphenous vein grafts. Am J Cardiol 1994;74:1187–1191.

97. Wong SC, Baim DS, Schatz RA, et al; for the Palmaz-Schatz Stent Study Group. Acute results and late outcomes after stent implantation in saphenous vein graft lesions: the multicenter US Palmaz-Schatz stent experience. J Am Coll Cardiol 1995;26:704–712.

98. Fortuna R, Heuser RR, Garratt KN, et al. Wiktor intracoronary stent: experience in the first 101 vein graft patients [Abstract]. Circulation 1993;88(Suppl I):308.

99. Bilodeau L, Iyer S, Cannon AD, et al. Flexible coil stent (Cook Inc.) in saphenous vein grafts: clinical and angiographic follow-up [Abstract]. J Am Coll Cardiol 1992;19(Suppl):264A.

100. Fenton S, Fischman D, Savage M, et al. Does stent implantation in ostial saphenous vein graft lesions reduce restenosis [Abstract]? J Am Coll Cardiol 1994;25(Suppl):118A.

101. Wong SC, Hong MK, Popma JJ, et al. Stent placement for the treatment of aorto-ostial saphenous vein graft lesions [Abstract]. J Am Coll Cardiol 1994;25(Suppl):118A.

102. Douglas JS, Savage MP, Bailey SR, et al, Saved Trial Investigators. Randomized trial of coronary stent and balloon angioplasty in the treatment of saphenous vein graft stenosis [Abstract]. J Am Coll Cardiol 1996;27(Suppl A):178A.

103. Pepine CJ, Holmes DR, Block PC, et al; and the Cardiac Catheterization Committee. ACC Expert Consensus Document: coronary artery stents. J Am Coll Cardiol 1996;28:782–794.

104. de Jaegere PP, van Domburg R, de Feyter PJ, et al. Long-term clinical outcome after stent implantation in saphenous vein grafts. J Am Coll Cardiol 1996;28:89–96.

105. Califf RM, Fortin DF, Frid DJ, et al. Restenosis after coronary angioplasty: an overview. J Am Coll Cardiol 1991;17:2B-13B.

106. Sigwart U, Kaufman U, Goy JJ, et al. Prevention of coronary restenosis by stenting. Eur Heart J 1988;9:31–37.

107. Levine MJ, Leonard BM, Burke JA, et al. Clinical and angiographic results of balloon-expandable intracoronary stents in right coronary stenoses. J Am Coll Cardiol 1990;16:332–339.

108. Colombo A, Almagor Y, Maiello L, et al. Results of coronary stenting for restenosis [Abstract]. J Am Coll Cardiol 1994;25(Suppl):118A.

109. Savage MP, Fischman DL, Schatz RA, et al. Long-term angiographic and clinical outcome of a balloon-expandable stent in the native coronary circulation. J Am Coll Cardiol 1994;24:1207–1212.

110. de Jaegere P, Serruys PW, Bertrand M, et al. Angiographic predictors of recurrence of restenosis after Wiktor stent implantation in native coronary arteries. Am J Cardiol 1993;72:165–170.

111. Debbas NMG, Sigwart U, Eeckhout E, et al. Intracoronary stenting for restenosis: long-term follow-up: a single center experience. J Invas Cardiol 1996;8:241–248.

112. Hamburger JN, de Feyter PJ, Serruys PW. The laser guidewire experience: "crossing the Rubicon." Semin Interven Cardiol 1996;1:163–171.

113. Medina A, Melian F, Suarez de Lezo J, et al. Effectiveness of coronary artery stents for the treatment of chronic total occlusion in angina pectoris. Am J Cardiol 1994;73:1222–1224.

114. Ozaki Y, Violaris AG, Hamburger J, et al. Short- and long-term clinical and quantitative angiographic results with the new less shortening Wallstent for vessel reconstruction in chronic total occlusion: a quantitative angiographic study. J Am Coll Cardiol 1996;28:354–360.

115. Goldberg SL, Colombo A, Maiello L, et al. Intra-

coronary stent insertion after balloon angioplasty of chronic total occlusions. J Am Coll Cardiol 1995;26:713–719.

116. Almagor Y, Borrione M, Maiello L, et al. Coronary stenting after recanalisation of chronic total coronary occlusions [Abstract]. Circulation 1993; 88(Suppl):I-504.

117. Bilodeau L, Iyer SS, Cannon AD, et al. Stenting as an adjunct to balloon angioplasty for recanalization of totally occluded coronary arteries: clinical and angiographic follow-up [Abstract]. J Am Coll Cardiol 1993;21(Suppl):292A.

118. Etsuo T, Osamu K, Masanobu F, et al. Impact of stenting on PTCA of chronic total occlusions [Abstract]. Circulation 1996;94(Suppl):I-249.

119. Sultorp MJ, Mast G, Plokker HWT, et al. Primary coronary stenting after successful balloon angioplasty of chronic total occlusions: a single-center experience [Abstract]. Circulation 1996;94(Suppl): I-687.

120. Nienaber CA, Fratz S, Lund GK, et al. Primary stent placement or balloon angioplasty for chronic coronary occlusions: a matched pair analysis in 100 patients [Abstract]. Circulation 1996; 94(Suppl):I-686.

121. Sirnes PA, Golf S, Myreng Y, et al; for the SICCO Study Group. Stenting in chronic coronary occlusion (SICCO): a multicenter, randomized, controlled study [Abstract]. J Am Coll Cardiol 1996; 27(Suppl):139A.

122. Thomas M, Hancock J, Holmberg S, et al. Coronary stenting following successful angioplasty for total occlusions: preliminary results of a randomized trial [Abstract]. J Am Coll Cardiol 1996; 27(Suppl):153A.

123. Sato Y, Nosaka H, Kimura T, et al. Randomized comparison of balloon angioplasty versus coronary stent implantation for total occlusion [Abstract]. J Am Coll Cardiol 1996;27(Suppl):152A.

124. Grines CL, Browne KR, Marco J, et al; for the Primary Angioplasty in Myocardial Infarction Study Group. A comparison of primary angioplasty with thrombolytic therapy for acute myocardial infarction. N Engl J Med 1993;328:673–679.

125. Zijlstra F, de Boer MJ, Hoorntje JCA, et al. A comparison of immediate coronary angioplasty with intravenous streptokinase in acute myocardial infarction. N Engl J Med 1993;328:680–684.

126. Gibbons RJ, Holmes DR, Reeder GS; for the Mayo Coronary Care Unit and Catheterization Laboratory Groups. Immediate angioplasty compared with the administration of a thrombolytic agent followed by conservative treatment for myocardial infarction. N Engl J Med 1993;328:685–691.

127. Michels KB, Yusuf S. Does PTCA in acute myocardial infarction affect mortality and reinfarction rates? A quantitative overview of the randomized clinical trials. Circulation 1995;91:476–485.

128. O'Neill WW, Weintraub R, Grines CL, et al. A prospective placebo controlled randomized trial of intravenous streptokinase and angioplasty versus lone angioplasty therapy of acute myocardial infarction. Circulation 1992;86:1710–1717.

129. O'Neill WW, Brodie RR, Ivanhoe R, et al. Primary coronary angioplasty for acute myocardial infarction. Am J Cardiol 1994;73:627–634.

130. Brodie RR, Grines CL, Ivanhoe R, et al. Six-month clinical and angiographic follow-up after direct angioplasty for acute myocardial infarction. Final results from the primary angioplasty registry. Circulation 1994;90:156–162.

131. Neumann F-J, Walter H, Richardt G, et al. Coronary Palmaz-Schatz stent implantation in acute myocardial infarction. Heart 1996;75:121–126.

132. Eeckhout E, Stauffer J-C, Vogt P, et al. Unplanned use of intracoronary stents during rescue or direct PTCA following acute myocardial infarction [Abstract]. Transcatheter Cardiovascular Therapeutics 1996;8:43.

133. Lefèvre T, Morice M-C, Karrillon G, et al. Coronary stenting during acute myocardial infarction. Results from the stent without coumadin French registry [Abstract]. J Am Coll Cardiol 1996; 27(Suppl):69A.

134. Savalle LH, Schalij MJ, Jukema W, et al. The Micro Stent in acute myocardial infarction. Quantitative angiographic and procedural results [Abstract]. Transcatheter Cardiovascular Therapeutics 1996; 8:57.

135. Steinhubl SR, Moliterno DJ, Teirstein PS, et al. Stenting for acute myocardial infarction: the early United States multicenter experience [Abstract]. J Am Coll Cardiol 1996;27(Suppl):279A.

136. Garcia-Cantu E, Spaulding C, Corcos T, et al. Stent implantation in acute myocardial infarction. Am J Cardiol 1996;77:451–454.

137. Rodriguez AE, Fernandez M, Santaera O, et al. Coronary stenting in patients undergoing percutaneous transluminal coronary angioplasty during acute myocardial infarction. Am J Cardiol 1996;77:685–689.

138. Walton AS, Oesterle SN, Yeung AC. Coronary artery stenting for acute closure complicating primary angioplasty for acute myocardial infarction. Cathet Cardiovasc Diag 1995;34:142–146.

139. Ahmad T, Webb JG, Carere RR, et al. Coronary stenting for acute myocardial infarction. Am J Cardiol 1995;76:77–80.

140. Wong PH, Wong CM. Intracoronary stenting in acute myocardial infarction. Cathet Cardiovasc Diagn 1994;33:39–45.

141. Benzuly KH, Goldstein JA, Almany SL, et al. Feasibility of stenting in acute myocardial infarction [Abstract]. Circulation 1995;92(Suppl):I-616.

142. Iyer S, Bilodeau L, Cannon A, et al. Stenting the infarct related artery within 15 days of the acute event: immediate and long term outcome using the flexible metallic coil stent [Abstract]. J Am Coll Cardiol 1993;21(Suppl):291A.

143. Capers Q, Thomas C, Weintraub W, et al. Emergent stent placement: worse outcome in the patients with a recent myocardial infarction [Abstract]. J Am Coll Cardiol 1994;23(Suppl):71A.

144. Levy G, De Boisgelin X, Volpiliere R, et al. Intracoronary stenting in direct angioplasty: is it dangerous? [Abstract] Circulation 1995;92:I-139.

145. Katz S, Green SJ, Ong LY, et al. Intracoronary stenting in direct infarct angioplasty: experience with 117 consecutive cases [Abstract]. Circulation 1996;94(Suppl):I-576.

146. Hans-Jürgen R, Thomas V, Jürgen R, et al. Short and long-term results of stent implantation within

12 hours after failed PTCA in acute myocardial infarction [Abstract]. Circulation 1996;94 (Suppl): I-577.

147. Sheiban I, Tonni S, Chizzoni A, et al. Coronary stenting in primary angioplasty for acute myocardial infarction [Abstract]. Transcatheter Cardiovascular Therapeutics 1996;8:57.

148. Takayama M, Imaizumi T, Aoki S, et al. Favorable progress on coronary stent implantation as an early treatment in patients with acute myocardial infarction [Abstract]. Circulation 1996;94(Suppl): I-576.

149. Medina A, Hernández E, Suárez de Lezo J, et al. Primary stent treatment for acute evolving myocardial infarction [Abstract]. Circulation 1996; 94(Suppl):I-576.

150. Katz S, Chepurko L, Ong LY, et al. Is stent deployment during acute myocardial infarction superior to balloon angioplasty? [Abstract]. Circulation 1996;94(Suppl):I-576.

151. Ong LY, Katz S, Green SJ, et al. Routine stenting for acute myocardial infarction results in 6 month outcomes comparable to patients with elective stenting [Abstract]. Circulation 1996;94(Suppl):I-577.

152. Glatt B, Diab N, Chevalier B, et al. Prospective primary stenting in acute myocardial infarction [Abstract]. Circulation 1996;94(Suppl):I-577.

153. Valeix BH, Labrunie PJ, Massiani PF. Systematic coronary stenting in the first eight hours of acute myocardial infarction [Abstract]. Circulation 1996;94(Suppl):I-577.

154. Benzuly KH, O'Neill WW, Gangadharan V, et al. Stenting in acute myocardial infarction (STAMI): six month follow-up [Abstract]. J Am Coll Cardiol 1997;29(Suppl A):456A.

155. Benzuly KH, Guido-Allen D, Mason D, et al. A prospective pilot study of primary stenting for acute myocardial infarction (STAMI): preliminary results [Abstract]. Transcatheter Cardiovascular Therapeutics 1996;8:38.

156. Grines CL. Aggressive intervention for myocardial infarction: angioplasty, stents, and intra-aortic balloon pumping. Am J Cardiol 1996;78(Suppl 3A):29–34.

157. Stone GW, Brodie B, Griffin J, et al. A prospective, multicenter trial of primary stenting in acute myocardial infarction—the PAMI Stent Pilot Study [Abstract]. Circulation 1996;94(Suppl):I-570.

158. Rocha-Singh K, Morris N, Wong SC, et al. Coronary stenting for treatment of ostial stenoses of native coronary arteries or aortocoronary saphenous venous grafts. Am J Cardiol 1995;75:26–29.

159. Rechavia E, Litvack F, Macko G, et al. Stent implantation of saphenous vein graft aorto-ostial lesions in patients with unstable ischemic syndromes: immediate angiographic results and long-term clinical outcome. J Am Coll Cardiol 1995;25:866–870.

160. Zampieri P, Colombo A, Almagor Y, et al. Results of coronary stenting of ostial lesions. Am J Cardiol 1994;73:901–903.

161. Wong SC, Hong M, Popma J, et al. Stent placement for the treatment of aorto-osteal saphenous vein graft lesions [Abstract]. J Am Coll Cardiol 1994;23(Suppl):118A.

162. Fenton S, Fischman D, Savage M, et al. Does stent implantation in osteal saphenous vein graft lesions reduce restenosis? [Abstract] J Am Coll Cardiol 1994;23(Suppl):118A.

163. Wong SC, Popma J, Hong M, et al. Procedural results and long term clinical outcomes in aorto-osteal saphenous vein graft lesions after new device angioplasty [Abstract]. J Am Coll Cardiol 1994;25(Suppl):394A.

164. Jain SP, Liu MW, Babu R, et al. Balloon vs debulking devices vs stenting for right coronary osteal disease: acute and long term results [Abstract]. Circulation 1996;94(Suppl):I-248.

165. De Cesare NB, Bartorelli AL, Galli S, et al. Treatment of osteal lesions of the left anterior descending coronary artery with Palmaz-Schatz coronary stent. Am Heart J 1996;132:716–720.

166. Fajadet J, Brunel P, Jordan C, et al. Is stenting of left main coronary artery a reasonable procedure [Abstract]. Circulation 1995;92(Suppl):I-74.

167. Hausleiter J, Dirschinger J, Schühlen H, et al. Left main stenting [Abstract]. Circulation 1996; 94(Suppl):I-331.

168. Tamura T, Nobuyoshi M, Nosaka H, et al. Palmaz-Schatz stenting in unprotected and protected left main coronary artery: immediate and follow-up results [Abstract]. Circulation 1996;94(Suppl): I-671.

169. Barragan P, Silvestri M, Simeoni JB, et al. Stenting in unprotected left main coronary artery: immediate and follow-up results [Abstract]. Circulation 1996;94(Suppl):I-672.

170. Karam C, Jordan C, Fajadet J, et al. Six-month follow-up of unprotected left main coronary artery stenting [Abstract]. Circulation 1996;94(Suppl):I-672.

171. Ellis SG, Moses J, White HJ, et al. Contemporary percutaneous treatment of unprotected left main stenosis—a preliminary report of the ULTIMA (unprotected left main trunk intervention multicenter assessment) registry. Circulation 1996; 94(Suppl):I-671.

172. Meier B, Gruentzig AR, King III SB, et al. Risk of side branch occlusion during coronary angioplasty. Am J Cardiol 1984;53:10–14.

173. Nakamura S, Hall P, Maiello L, et al. Techniques for Palmaz-Schatz stent deployment in lesions with a large side branch. Cathet Cardiovasc Diagn 1995;34:353–361.

174. Erminia M, Sklar MA, Russo RJ, et al. Escape from stent jail: an in vitro model [Abstract]. Circulation 1995;92(Suppl):I-688.

175. Colombo A, Gaglione A, Nakamura S. "Kissing" stents for bifurcation coronary lesion. Cathet Cardiovasc Diagn 1993;30:327–330.

176. Colombo A, Maillo L, Itoh A, et al. Coronary stenting of bifurcation lesions immediate and follow-up results [Abstract]. J Am Coll Cardiol 1996; 27(Suppl):277A.

177. Meier B. Kissing balloon coronary angioplasty. Am J Cardiol 1984;54:918–920.

178. Fort S, Lazzam C, Schwartz L. Coronary 'Y' stenting: a technique for angioplasty of bifurcation stenoses. Can J Cardiol 1996;12:678–682.

179. Carlson TA, Guarneri EM, Stevens KM, et al. "T

stenting": the answer to bifurcation lesions? [Abstract]. Circulation 1996;94(Suppl):I-86.

180. Foley DP, Serruys PW. Bifurcation lesion stenting. Thoraxcenter Journal 1996;8:32–36.

181. Chevalier B, Glatt B. Kissing stenting in bifurcation lesions [Abstract]. Eur Heart J 1996;17(Suppl): 218.

182. Zir LM, Miller SW, Dinsmore RE. Intraobserver variability in coronary angiography. Circulation 1976;53:672–632.

183. Di Mario C, Haase J, den Boer A, et al. Edge detection versus densitometry in the quantitative assessment of stenosis phantoms: an in vivo comparison in porcine coronary arteries. Am Heart J 1992;124:1181–1189.

184. Foley DP, Escaned J, Strauss BH, et al. Quantitative coronary angiography in interventional cardiology: application to scientific research and clinical practice. Prog Cardiovasc Dis 1994;36: 363–384.

185. Keane D, Haase J, Slager C, et al. Comparative validation of quantitative coronary angiographic systems: results and implications from a multicenter study using standardized approach. Circulation 1995;91:2402–2412.

186. Arnett EN, Isner JM, Redwood DR, et al. Coronary artery narrowing in coronary heart disease: comparison of cineangiographic and necropsy findings. Ann Intern Med 1979;91:350–356.

187. Grondin CM, Dyrda I, Pasternac A, et al. Discrepancies between cineangiographic and postmortem findings in patients with coronary artery disease and recent myocardial revascularization. Circulation 1974;49:703–708.

188. Schwartz JN, Kong Y, Hackel DB, et al. Comparison of angiographic and postmortem findings in patients with coronary artery disease. Am J Cardiol 1975;36:174–178.

189. Yamagishi M, Miyatake K, Tamai J, et al. Intravascular ultrasound detection of atherosclerosis at the site of focal vasospasm in angiographically normal or minimally narrowed coronary segments. J Am Coll Cardiol 1994;23:352–357.

190. Blasini R, Schuhlen H, Mudra H, et al. Angiographic overestimation of lumen size after coronary stent placement: impact of high pressure dilation [Abstract]. Circulation 1995;92(Suppl):I-223.

191. Hoyne J, Mahon DJ, Tobis JM. Intravascular ultrasound imaging. Trends in Cardiovascular Medicine 1991;1:305–311.

192. Itoh A, Hall P, Moussa I, et al. Comparison of quantitative angiography and intravascular ultrasound after coronary stent implantation with 6 different stents [Abstract]. Circulation 1996; 94(Suppl):I-263.

193. van der Zwet PMJ, Reiber JHC. A new approach for the quantification of complex lesion morphology. The gradient field transform: basic principles and validation results. J Am Coll Cardiol 1994;24: 216–224.

194. Keane D, Gronenschild E, Slager CJ, et al. In vivo validation of an experimental adaptive quantitative coronary angiography algorithm to circumvent overestimation of small lumen diameters. Cathet Cardiovasc Diagn 1995;36:17–24.

195. Karrillon GJ, Morice MC, Benveniste E, et al. Intracoronary stent implantation without ultrasound guidance with replacement of conventional anticoagulation therapy by antiplatelet therapy: 30-day clinical outcome of the French Multicenter Registry. Circulation 1996;94: 1519–1527.

196. Goods CM, Al-Shaibi KF, Yadav SS, et al. Utilization of the coronary balloon-expandable coil stent without anticoagulation or intravascular ultrasound. Circulation 1996;93:1803–1808.

197. Moussa I, Di Mario C, Francesco LD, et al. Stents don't require systemic anticoagulation . . . but the technique (and results) must be optimal. Journal of Invasive Cardiology 1996;8(Suppl E):3E-7E.

198. Görge G, Haude M, Ge J, et al. Intravascular ultrasound after low and high inflation pressure coronary stent implantation. J Am Coll Cardiol 1995; 26:725–730.

199. Teirstein P, Schatz R, Wong C, et al. Coronary stenting with angioscopic guidance. Am J Cardiol 1995;75:344–347.

200. Shaknovich A, Lieberman S, Kreps E, et al. Qualitative comparison of intravascular ultrasound and angioscopy with angiographic assessment of Palmaz-Schatz (PS) coronary stents [Abstract]. J Am Coll Cardiol 1994;23(Suppl):72A.

201. Kaplan BM, Safian RD, Grines CL, et al. Usefulness of adjunctive angioscopy and extraction atherectomy before stent implantation in high-risk aortocoronary saphenous vein grafts. Am J Cardiol 1995;76:822–824.

202. Annex BH, Ajluni SC, Larkin TJ, et al. Angioscopic guided interventions in a saphenous vein bypass graft. Cathet Cardiovasc Diagn 1994; 31:330–333.

203. Mintz G, Pichard A, Dussalilant G, et al. Acute results of adjunct stents following directional coronary atherectomy [Abstract]. Circulation 1995; 92(Suppl):I-328.

204. Mintz G, Dussalilant G, Wong SC, et al. Rotational atherectomy followed by adjunct stents: the preferred therapy for calcified lesions in large vessels? [Abstract] Circulation 1995;92(Suppl):I-329.

205. Hong MK, Pichard A, Kent KM, et al. Assessing a strategy of stand-alone extraction atherectomy followed by staged stent placement in degenerated saphenous vein graft lesions [Abstract]. J Am Coll Cardiol 1995;25(Suppl):394A.

206. Hong MK, Wong SC, Popma JJ, et al. Favorable results of debulking followed by immediate adjunct stent therapy for high risk saphenous vein graft lesions [Abstract]. J Am Coll Cardiol 1996; 27(Suppl):179A.

207. Labib A. TEC before stenting in acute myocardial infarction. Journal of Invasive Cardiology 1996;8: 235–238.

208. Mak K-H, Belli G, Ellis SG, et al. Subacute stent thrombosis: evolving issues and current concepts. J Am Coll Cardiol 1996;27:494–503.

209. Nath FC, Muller DWM, Ellis SG, et al. Thrombosis of a flexible coil coronary stent: frequency, predictors and clinical outcome. J Am Coll Cardiol 1993; 21:622–627.

210. Hasdai D, Garratt K, Holmes DR, et al. Coronary angioplasty and intracoronary thrombolytics are

of limited value in resolving intracoronary stent thrombosis. J Am Coll Cardiol 1996;28:361–367.

211. van Beusekom HMM, van der Giessen WJ, van Suylen RJ, et al. Histology after stenting of human saphenous vein bypass grafts: observations from surgically excised grafts 3 to 320 days after stent implantation. J Am Coll Cardiol 1993;21:45–54.

212. Ueda Y, Nanto S, Komamure K, et al. Neointimal coverage of stents in human coronary arteries observed by angioscopy. J Am Coll Cardiol 1994;23:341–346.

213. Williams DF. Surface interactions. In: Sigwart U, ed. Endoluminal stenting. Philadelphia: WB Saunders, 1996:45–51.

214. Andrade JD, Hlady V. Plasma protein adsorption. The big twelve. In: Leonard EE, Turitto VT, Vroman L, eds. Blood in contact with natural and artificial surfaces. New York: New York Academy of Science, 1987:158–172.

215. Baier R. Initial events in interaction of blood with a foreign surface. J Biomed Mater Res 1969;3:191–206.

216. De Palma VE, Baier RE. Investigation of three-surface properties of several metals and their relation to blood biocompatibility. J Biomed Mater Res 1972;6:37–75.

217. Zitter H, Plenk H Jr. The electrochemical behavior of metallic implant material as an indicator of their biocompatibility. J Biomed Mater Res 1987; 21:881–896.

218. Hehrlein C, Zimmerman M, Metz J, et al. Influence of surface texture and charge on the biocompatibility of endovascular stents. Coron Artery Dis 1995;6:581–586.

219. Hearn JA, Robinson KA, Roubin GS. In-vitro thrombus formation of stent wires: role of metallic composition and heparin coating [Abstract]. J Am Coll Cardiol 1991;17(Suppl):302A.

220. van der Giessen WJ, Serruys PW, van Beusekom HMM, et al. Coronary stenting with a new radiopaque, balloon-expandable endoprosthesis in pigs. Circulation 1991;83:1788–1798.

221. Scott NA, Robinson KA, Nunes GL, et al. Comparison of the thrombogenicity of stainless steel and tantalum coronary stents. Am Heart J 1995;129:866–872.

222. Sheth S, Litvack F, Dev V, et al. Subacute thrombosis and vascular injury resulting from slotted-tube nitinol and stainless steel stents in a rabbit carotid artery model. Circulation 1996;94:1733–1740.

223. Sheth S, Dev V, Fishbein MC, et al. Reduced thrombogenicity of nitinol vs. stainless steel slotted stents in rabbit carotid arteries [Abstract]. J Am Coll Cardiol 1995;25(Suppl):240A.

224. Murphy JG, Schwartz RS, Edwards WD, et al. Percutaneous polymeric stents in porcine coronary arteries: initial experience with polyethylene terephthalate stents. Circulation 1992;86:1596–1604.

225. van Beusekom HMM, van der Giessen WJ, van Ingen Schenau D, et al. Synthetic polymers as an alternative to metal stents? In-vivo and mechanical behavior of polyethylene-terephthalate [Abstract]. Circulation 1992;86(Suppl):I-731.

226. Lincoff AM, Schwartz RS, van der Giessen WJ, et al. Biodegradable polymers can evoke a unique inflammatory response when implanted into the coronary artery [Abstract]. Circulation 1992; 86(Suppl):I-801.

227. Zidar JP, Gammon RS, Chapman GD, et al. Short- and long-term vascular tissue response to the Duke bioabsorbable stent [Abstract]. J Am Coll Cardiol 1993;21(Suppl):439A.

228. Tamai H, Doi T, Hsu YS, et al. Initial and long-term results of biodegradable polymer stent in canine coronary artery [Abstract]. Journal of Invasive Cardiology 1995;7:9A.

229. Susawa T, Shiraki K, Shimizu Y. Biodegradable intracoronary stents in adult dogs [Abstract]. J Am Coll Cardiol 1993;21(Suppl):483A.

230. Chapman GD, Gammon RS, Baumann RP, et al. A bioabsorbable stent: initial experimental results [Abstract]. Circulation 1990;82(Suppl III):III-72.

231. Chronos NAF, Robinson KA, Kelly AB, et al. Thromboresistant phosphorylcholine coatings for coronary stents [Abstract]. Circulation 1995;92 (Suppl I):I-685.

232. Kruse KR, Tanguay J-F, Williams MS, et al. A polymer-metal composite stent. Seminars in Interventional Cardiology 1996;1:46–48.

233. De Scheerder IK, Wilczek K, Van Dorpe J, et al. Ampiphilic polyurethane coating of intracoronary stents decreases mortality due to subacute thrombosis in porcine coronary model [Abstract]. Circulation 1993;88(Suppl):I-645.

234. De Scheerder IK, Wilczek K, Verbeken E, et al. Ampiphilic polyurethane coating of intracoronary stents decreases mortality due to subacute thrombosis in porcine coronary model [Abstract]. J Am Coll Cardiol 1994;23(Suppl):186A.

235. Holmes DR, Camrud AR, Jorgenson MA, et al. Polymeric stenting in the porcine coronary artery model: differential outcome of exogenous fibrin sleeves versus polyurethane-coated stents. J Am Coll Cardiol 1994;24:525–31.

236. Sheth S, Dev V, Jacobs H, et al. Prevention of subacute stent thrombosis by polymer-polyethylene oxide-heparin coating in the rabbit carotid artery [Abstract]. J Am Coll Cardiol 1995;25(Suppl): 348A.

237. Staab ME, Holmes DR Jr, Schwartz RS. Polymers. In: Sigwart U, ed. Endoluminal stenting. Philadelphia: WB Saunders, 1996:34–44.

238. Cox DA, Anderson PG, Roubin GS, et al. Effects of local delivery of heparin and methotrexate on neointimal proliferation in stented porcine coronary arteries. Coron Artery Dis 1992;3:237–248.

239. Slepian MJ, Roth L, Wesselcouch E, et al. Gel paving of intra-arterial stents: a method for reducing stent and adjacent arterial wall thrombogenicity [Abstract]. J Invasive Cardiol 1995;7:5A.

240. Schwartz RS, Murphy JG, Edwards WD, et al. Bioabsorbable, drug-eluting, intracoronary stents: design and future applications. In: Sigwart U, Frank GI, eds. Coronary stents. Berlin: Springer-Verlag, 1992:135–154.

241. van Beusekom HMM, van Vleit HHDM, van der Giessen WJ. Fibrin and basement membrane components, as a biocompatible and thromboresistant coating for metal stents. Circulation 1993; 88(Suppl):I-645.

242. Bailey SR, Paige S, Lunn A, et al. Heparin coating of endovascular stents decreases subacute thrombosis in a rabbit model [Abstract]. Circulation 1992;86(Suppl):I-186.

243. van der Giessen WJ, Härdhammar PA, van Beusekom HMM, et al. Prevention of (sub)acute thrombosis using heparin-coated stents [Abstract]. Circulation 1994;90(Suppl):I-650.

244. Härdhammar PA, van Beusekom HMM, Emanuelsson HU, et al. Reduction in thrombotic events with heparin-coated Palmaz-Schatz stents in normal porcine coronary arteries. Circulation 1996; 93:423–430.

245. Kipshidze N, Baker JE, Nikolaychik V. Fibrin coated stents as an improved vehicle for endothelial cell seeding [Abstract]. Circulation 1994; 90(Suppl):I-597.

246. Baker JE, Horn JB, Nikolaychik V, et al. Fibrin stent coatings. In: Sigwart U, ed. Endoluminal stenting. Philadelphia: WB Saunders, 1996:84–89.

247. Aggarwal RK, Martin W, Ireland DC, et al. Effects of polymer-coated stents eluting antibody to platelet integrin glycoprotein IIb/IIIa on platelet deposition and neointima formation [Abstract]. Eur J Cardiol 1996;17(Suppl):176.

248. Aggarwal RK, Martin WA, Azrin MA, et al. Effects of platelet GPIIb/IIIa antibody and antibody-urokinase conjugate adsorbed to stents on platelet deposition and neointima formation [Abstract]. Circulation 1996;94(Suppl);I-258.

249. Aggarwal RK, Ireland DC, Ragheb A, et al. Reduction in thrombogenicity of polymer-coated stents by immobilization of platelet-targeted urokinase [Abstract]. Eur J Cardiol 1996;17(Suppl):177.

250. Larm O, Larsson R, Olsson P. A new non-thrombogenic surface prepared by selective covalent binding of heparin via a reducing terminal residue. Biomat Med Dev Artif Org 1983;11:161–174.

251. Serruys PW, Emanuelsson H, van der Giessen W, et al; on behalf of the BENESTENT II Study Group. Heparin Coated Palmaz-Schatz stents in human coronary arteries. Early outcome of the BENESTENT II Pilot Study. Circulation 1996; 412–422.

252. Slepian MJ, Khosravi F, Massia SP, et al. Gel paving of intrarterial stents in vivo reduces stent and adjacent arterial wall thrombogenicity [Abstract]. J Vasc Interven Radiol 1995;6:50.

253. van der Giessen WJ, Serruys PW, et al. Endothelialization of intravascular stents. Journal of Interventional Cardiology 1988;1:109–120.

254. Dichek DA, Neville RF, Zwiebel JA, et al. Seeding of intravascular stents with genetically engineered endothelial cells. Circulation 1989;80: 1347–1353.

254a. Flugelman MY, Virmani R, Leon MB, et al. Genetically engineered endothelial cells remain adherent and viable after stent deployment and exposure to flow in vitro. Circ Res 1992;70:348–354.

255. Flugelman MY, Rome JJ, Virmani R, et al. Detection of genetically engineered endothelial cells seeded on endovascular prosthesis ten days after in vivo deployment [Abstract]. J Mol Cell Cardiol 1993;25 (Suppl)I-S-83.

256. Scott NA, Candal FJ, Robinson KA, et al. Seeding of intracoronary stents with immortalized human microvascular endothelial cells. Am Heart J 1995; 129:860–866.

257. Ades EW, Candal FJ, Swerlick RA, et al. HMEC-1: establishment of an immortalized human microvascular endothelial cell line. J Invest Dermatol 1992;99:683–690.

258. Bailey SR. Endothelial "SODDING": intraprocedural replacement of endothelial cells on endovascular stents [Abstract]. Circulation 1996: 94(Suppl):I-261.

259. Vinogradsky B, Sawa H, Guala A, et al. Seeding of stents with genetically modified endothelial cells: overexpression of urokinase receptor results in increased seeded cell retention [Abstract]. Circulation 1996:94(Suppl):I-261.

260. Dichek DA, Nussbaum O, Degen SJF, et al. Enhancement of the fibrinolytic activity of sheep endothelial cells by retroviral vector-mediated gene transfer. Blood 1991;77:533–541.

261. Flugelman MY. Inhibition of intravascular thrombosis and vascular smooth muscle cell proliferation by gene therapy. Thromb Haemost 1995;74: 406–410.

262. Van Belle E, Chen D, Tio FO, et al. Accelerated endothelialization improves stent biocompatibility: feasibility and effects of VEGF-gene transfer. Circulation 1996;94(Suppl):I-259.

263. Stefanadis C, Toutouzas P. Percutaneous implantation of autologous vein graft stent for the treatment of coronary artery disease. Lancet 1995;345: 1509.

264. Stefanadis C, Eleftherios T, Toutouzas K, et al. Autologous vein graft-coated stent for the treatment of coronary artery disease: immediate results after percutaneous placement in humans [Abstract]. J Am Coll Cardiol 1996;27(Suppl): 179A.

265. Toutouzas K, Stefanadis C, Tsiamis E, et al. Primary autologous vein graft-coated stent in acute myocardial infarction: immediate and short-term results [Abstract]. Circulation 1996;94(Suppl):I-576.

266. Agrawal SK, Ho DSW, Lie MW, et al. Predictors of thrombolytic complications after placement of the flexible coil stent. Am J Cardiol 1994;73: 1216–1219.

267. Doucet S, Fajadet J, Cassagneau B, et al. Early thrombotic occlusion following coronary Palmaz-Schatz stent implantation: frequency and clinical or angiographic predictors [Abstract]. Eur Heart J 1992;13(Suppl):4.

268. Fry ET, Hermiller JB, Peters TF, et al. Risks, treatment, and outcome of acute stent closure [Abstract]. Circulation 1994;90(Suppl):I-650.

269. Haude M, Erbel R, Issa H, et al. Subacute thrombotic complications after intracoronary implantation of Palmaz-Schatz stents. Am Heart J 1993; 126:15–22.

270. Eccleston DS, Belli G, Penn IM, et al. Are multiple stents associated with multiplicative risk in the optimal stent era? [Abstract] Circulation 1996; 94(Suppl):I-454.

271. Pulsipher MW, Baker WA, Sawchak SR, et al. Outcomes in patients treated with multiple coronary stents [Abstract] Circulation 1996;94(Suppl):I-332.

272. Xu XY, Collins MW. Fluid dynamics in stents. In:

Sigwart U, ed. Endoluminal stenting. Philadelphia: WB Saunders, 1996:52–59.

273. Brown CH, Leverett LB, Lewis CE. Morphological, biochemical and functional changes in human platelets subject to shear stress. J Lab Clin Med 1975;86:462–71.

274. Woscoboinik JR, Gordov EP, Boussignac G, et al. Difference in flow characteristics for different stent models: implications for stent design from results of an vitro study [Abstract]. Circulation 1996;94(Suppl):I-260.

275. Macisaac AI, Ellis SG, Muller DW, et al. Comparison of three coronary stents: clinical and angiographic outcome after elective placement in 134 patients. Cathet Cardiovasc Diagn 1994;33:199–204.

276. Goy JJ, Eeckhout E, Debbas N, et al. Stenting of the right coronary artery for de novo stenosis. A comparison of the Wicktor and the Palmaz-Schatz stents [Abstract]. Circulation 1995;92 (Suppl I):I-596.

277. Goy J-J, Eeckhout E, Stauffer J-C, et al. Emergency endoluminal stenting for abrupt vessel closure following coronary angioplasty: a randomized comparison of the Wiktor and Palmaz-Schatz stents. Cathet Cardiovasc Diagn 1995;34:128–132.

278. Teirstein P, Schatz R, Russo R, et al. Coronary stenting of small diameter vessels: is it safe? [Abstract] Circulation 1995;92(Suppl):I-281.

279. Hall P, Colombo A, Itoh A, et al. Gianturco-Roubin stent implantation in small vessels without anticoagulation [Abstract] Circulation 1995;92(Suppl):I-795.

280. Koning R, Cribier A, Chan C, et al. Palmaz-Schatz coronary stenting for de novo lesions in small coronary arteries: clinical and quantitative angiographic results of a prospective pilot study [Abstract]. Circulation 1996;94(Suppl):I-685.

281. Morice M-C, Amor M, Beneviste E, et al. Coronary stenting without coumadin phase II, III, IV, V [Abstract]. Circulation 1995;92(Suppl):I-795.

282. Yokoi H, Nobuyoshi M, Nosaka H, et al. Coronary stent thrombosis: pattern, management and long-term follow-up result [Abstract]. Circulation 1996;94(Suppl):I-332.

283. Liu MW, Voorhees WD, Agrawal S, et al. Stratification of the risk of thrombosis after intracoronary stenting for threatened or acute closure complicating coronary balloon angioplasty: a Cook registry study. Am Heart J 1995;130:8–13.

284. Shaknovich A, Moses JW, Bailey S, et al; for STRESS Investigators. Subacute stent thrombosis in the STent REStenosis Study (STRESS): clinical impact and predictive factors [Abstract]. Circulation 1994;90(Suppl):I-650.

285. Schömig A, Kastrati A, Dietz R, et al. Emergency coronary stenting for dissection during percutaneous transluminal coronary angioplasty: angiographic follow-up after stenting and after repeat angioplasty of the stented segment. J Am Coll Cardiol 1994;23:1053–1060.

286. Grinstead WC, Raizner AE, Churchill DA, et al; for the Cook Stent Investigators. J Am Coll Cardiol 1993;21(Suppl):30A.

287. Rocha-Singh KJ, Fischman DL, Savage MP, et al. Influence of angiographic lesion characteristics on early complication rates after Palmaz-Schatz stenting [Abstract]. J Am Coll Cardiol 1993;21(Suppl):292A.

288. Eeckhout E, Stauffer J-C, Vogt P, et al. Can early closure and restenosis following endoluminal stenting be predicted from clinical and angiographic variables at the time of intervention? [Abstract]. Journal of Invasive Cardiology 1995;7:7A.

289. Waksman R, Shen Y, Ghazzi Z, et al. Optimal balloon inflation pressures for stent deployment and correlates of stent thrombosis and in-stent restenosis [Abstract]. Circulation 1996;94(Suppl):I-258.

290. Jeong MH, Owen WG, Srivatsa SS, et al. Platelets are the primary component of acute stent thrombosis [Abstract]. J Invasive Cardiol 1995;7:11A.

291. Hall P, Nakamura S, Maiello L, et al. A randomized comparison of combined ticlopidine and aspirin therapy versus aspirin therapy alone after successful intravascular ultrasound-guided stent implantation. Circulation 1996;93:215–222.

292. Morice MC, Valeix B, Marco J, et al. Preliminary results of the MUST trial. Major clinical events during the first month [Abstract]. J Am Coll Cardiol 1996;27(Suppl):137A.

293. de Jaegere P, Mudra H, Almagor Y, et al; for the Music Study Investigators. In-hospital and 1-month clinical results of an international study testing the concept of IVUS guided optimized stent expansion alleviating the need of systemic anticoagulation [Abstract]. J Am Coll Cardiol 1996;27(Suppl):137A.

294. Morice MC, Breton C, Bunouf P, et al. Coronary stenting without intravascular ultrasound. Results of the French Registry [Abstract]. Circulation 1995;92(Suppl):I-796.

295. Goods CM, Al-Shabi KF, Iyer SS, et al. Flexible coil stenting without anticoagulation or intravascular ultrasound: a prospective observational study [Abstract]. Circulation 1995;92(Suppl):I-795.

296. Wong SC, Hong MK, Chuang YC, et al. The *Anti-PL*atelet treatment *A*fter intravascular *U*ltrasound guided optimal *S*tent *E*xpansion (APPLAUSE) trial [Abstract]. Circulation 1995;92(Suppl):I-795.

297. Fernández-Avilés F, Alonso J, Durán JM, et al. Subacute occlusion bleeding complications, hospital stays, and restenosis after Palmaz-Schatz stenting using a new antithrombotic regimen. J Am Coll Cardiol 1997;27:22–29.

298. Blasini R, Mudra H, Schühlen H, et al. Intravascular ultrasound guided optimized emergency coronary Palmaz-Schatz stent placement without post procedural systemic anticoagulation [Abstract]. J Am Coll Cardiol 1995;25(Suppl):197A.

299. Colombo A, Nakamura S, Hall P, et al. A prospective study of Gianturco-Roubin coronary stent implantation without anticoagulation [Abstract]. J Am Coll Cardiol 1995;25(Suppl):197A.

300. Russo R, Schatz RA, Sklar MA, et al. Ultrasound guided coronary stent placement without prolonged systemic anticoagulation [Abstract]. J Am Coll Cardiol 1995;25(Suppl):197A.

301. Colombo A, Nakamura S, Hall P, et al. A prospective study of Wicktor coronary stent implantation without anticoagulation [Abstract]. J Am Coll Cardiol 1995;25(Suppl):239A.

302. Van Belle E, McFadden EP, Bauters C, et al. Com-

bined antiplatelet therapy without anticoagulation: an effective alternative to prevent subacute thrombosis after coronary stenting? A 3 month follow-up [Abstract]. J Am Coll Cardiol 1995; 25(Suppl):197A.

303. Barragan P, Silvestri M, Sainsous J, et al. Prevention of subacute occlusion after coronary stenting with ticlopidine regimen without intravascular ultrasound guided stenting [Abstract]. J Am Coll Cardiol 1995;25(Suppl):182A.

304. Buszman P, Clague J, Gibbs S, et al. Improved post stent management: high gain at low risk [Abstract]. J Am Coll Cardiol 1995;25(Suppl):182A.

305. Van Belle E, McFadden EP, Lablanche J-M, et al. Two-pronged antiplatelet therapy with aspirin and ticlopidine without systemic anticoagulation: an alternative therapeutic strategy after bailout stent implantation. Coron Artery Dis 1995;6: 341–345.

306. Lablanche J-M, Grollier G, Bonnet J-L, et al. Ticlopidine aspirin stent evaluation (TASTE): a French multicenter study [Abstract]. Circulation 1995;92(Suppl):I-476.

307. Lablanche J-M, Bonnet J-L, Grollier G, et al. Combined antiplatelet therapy without anticoagulation after stent implantation: the Ticlopidine Aspirin Stent Evaluation (TASTE) Study [Abstract]. J Am Coll Cardiol 1996;27(Suppl):137A.

308. Belli G, Whitlow P, Gross L, et al. Intracoronary stenting without oral anticoagulation: the Cleveland Clinic Registry [Abstract]. Circulation 1995; 92(Suppl):I-796.

309. Saito S, Kim K, Hosokawa G, et al. Primary Palmaz-Schatz stent implantation without coumadin in acute myocardial infarction [Abstract]. Circulation 1995;92(Suppl):I-796.

310. Haase J, Reifart N, Baier T, et al. Bail-out stenting (Palmaz-Schatz) without anticoagulation [Abstract]. Circulation 1995;92(Suppl):I-795.

311. Galli S, Trabattoni D, Loaldi A, et al. Comparison of anticoagulation, combined ticlopidine and aspirin, and aspirin alone therapy following coronary stenting [Abstract]. Circulation 1996; 94(Suppl):I-684.

312. Sainsous J, Silvestri M, Bayet G, et al. Coronary artery stenting without anticoagulation, intravascular ultrasound or high pressure balloon: immediate results of one month follow-up [Abstract]. Circulation 1996;94(Suppl):I-262.

313. The STRESS Investigators. Early outcomes after coronary stent placement with high pressure inflation and antiplatelet therapy: interim results of the STRESS III Trial [Abstract]. Circulation 1996; 94(Suppl):I-684.

314. Lablanche J-M, Gauthier L, McFadden EP, et al. In-hospital and six month outcome after bailout stenting managed with antiplatelet therapy alone [Abstract]. Circulation 1996;94(Suppl):I-684.

315. Leon MB, Ellis SG, Moses J, et al. Interim report from the reduced anticoagulation VEin Graft Stent (RAVES) Study [Abstract]. Circulation 1996; 94(Suppl):I-683.

316. Dirschinger J, Schühlen H, Walter H, et al. Intracoronary stenting and antithrombotic regimen trial: one year clinical follow-up [Abstract]. Circulation 1996;94(Suppl):I-683.

317. Hong MK, Wong SC, Pichard AD, et al. Long-term results of patients enrolled in the anti-platelet treatment after intravascular ultrasound guided optimal stent expansion (APPLAUSE) trial [Abstract]. Circulation 1996;94(Suppl):I-686.

318. Strain JE, Rehman DE, Fischman D, et al; for the STRESS III Investigators. STRESS III: preliminary acute results of IVUS vs. non-IVUS stenting [Abstract]. Circulation 1996;94(Suppl):I-686.

319. Darius H, Veit K, Rupprecht H-J. Synergistic inhibition of platelet aggregation by ticlopidine plus aspirin following intracoronary stent placement [Abstract]. Circulation 1996;94(Suppl):I-257.

320. Preiss JP, Lecompte T, Alnot Y, et al. Serial antiplatelet effects of combined treatment with ticlopidine and aspirin after stent implantation [Abstract]. Circulation 1996;94(Suppl):I-685.

321. Rodriguez JN, Fernandez-Jurado A, Dieguez JC, et al. Ticlopidine and severe aplastic anemia [Letter]. Am J Hematol 1994;47:332.

322. Schühlen H, Hadamitzky M, Kastrati A, et al. Grading the risk for restenosis after coronary stent placement. Analysis of a prospective risk stratification protocol in the ISAR-trial [Abstract]. Circulation 1996;94(Suppl):I-91.

323. Mehan VK, Salzmann C, Kaufmann U, et al. Coronary stenting without anticoagulation. Cathet Cardiovas Diagn 1995;34:137–140.

324. Bittl JA. Coronary stent occlusion: thrombus horribilis [Editorial]. J Am Coll Cardiol 1996;28: 368–370.

325. Mitchel JF, McKay RG. Treatment of acute stent thrombosis with local urokinase therapy using catheter based, drug delivery systems: a case report. Cathet Cardiovasc Diagn 1995;39:149–154.

326. Robinson NMK, Thomas MR, Wainwright RJ, Jewitt DE. Is unstable angina a contraindication to intracoronary stent insertion. Journal of Invasive Cardiology 1996;8:351–356.

327. Hamburger JN, de Feyter PJ, de Mario C, et al. Preliminary experience with the coronary angiojet rheolytic thrombectomy catheter: a preamble to the Euro-ARTS study [Abstract]. Eur Heart J 1996;17(Suppl):181.

328. Kuntz RE, Safian RD, Carozza JP Jr, et al. The importance of acute luminal diameter in determining restenosis after coronary atherectomy or stenting. Circulation 1992;86:1827–1835.

329. Painter JA, Mintz GS, Wong SC, et al. Serial intravascular ultrasound studies fail to show evidence of chronic Palmaz-Schatz stent recoil. Am J Cardiol 1995;75:398–400.

330. Hoffmann R, Mintz GS, Dussaillant GR, et al. Patterns and mechanisms of in-stent restenosis. A serial intravascular ultrasound study. Circulation 1996;94:1247–1254.

331. Schwartz RS. Characteristics of an ideal stent based upon restenosis pathology. J Invasive Cardiol 1996;8:386–387.

332. Gordon PC, Gibson CM, Cohen DJ, et al. Mechanism of restenosis and redilatation within coronary stents: quantitative angiographic assessment. J Am Coll Cardiol 1993;21:1166–1174.

333. Dussaillant GR, Mintz GS, Pichard AD, et al. Small stent size and intimal hyperplasia contribute to restenosis: a volumetric intravascular ultra-

sound analysis. J Am Coll Cardiol 1995;26:720–724.

334. Edelman ER, Rogers C. Hoop dreams. Stents without restenosis [Editorial]. Circulation 1996;94:1199–1202.

335. Schwartz RS, Huber KC, Murphy JG, et al. Restenosis and proportional neointimal response to coronary artery injury: results in a porcine model. J Am Coll Cardiol 1992;19:267–274.

336. Carter AJ, Laird JR, Farb A, et al. Morphological characteristics of lesion formation and time course of smooth muscle proliferation in a porcine proliferative restenosis model. J Am Coll Cardiol 1994;24:1398–1405.

337. van Beusekom HMM, Whelan DM, Hofma SH, et al. Stents but not balloon angioplasty induce chronic neointimal permeability [Abstract]. Circulation 1995;92(Suppl):I-87.

338. Penn IM, Galligan L, Brown RIG, et al. Restenosis at the stent articulation: is this a design flaw? [Abstract] J Am Coll Cardiol 1992;19(Suppl):291A.

339. Ikari Y, Hara K, Tamura T, et al. Luminal loss and site of restenosis after Palmaz-Schatz coronary stent implantation. Am J Cardiol 1995;76:117–120.

340. Chung I-M, Reidy MA, Schwartz SM, et al. Enhanced extracellular matrix synthesis may be important for restenosis of arteries after stent deployment [Abstract]. Circulation 1996;94(Suppl):I-349.

341. Kastrati A, Schömig A, Dietz R, et al. Time course of restenosis during the first year after emergency coronary stenting. Circulation 1993;87:1498–1505.

342. Lablanche J-M, Danchin N, Grollier G, et al. Factors predictive of restenosis after stent implantation managed by ticlopidine and aspirin [Abstract]. Circulation 1996;94(Suppl):I-256.

343. Mittal S, Weiss DL, Hirshfield JW, et al. Restenotic lesions have a worse outcome after stenting [Abstract]. Circulation 1996;94(Suppl):I-131.

344. Black AJR, Anderson HV, Roubin GS, et al. Repeat coronary angioplasty: correlates of a second restenosis. J Am Coll Cardiol 1988;11:714–718.

345. Manderson JA, Mosse PRL, Safstrom JA, et al. Balloon catheter injury to rabbit carotid artery. I. Changes in smooth muscle phenotype. Arteriosclerosis 1989;9:289–298.

346. Simon M, Leclerc G, Safian RD, et al. Relation between activated smooth-muscle cells in coronary artery lesions and restenosis after atherectomy. N Eng J Med 1993;328:608–613.

347. Hong MK, Kent KM, Satler LF, et al. Are long-term results different when stents are used in de novo versus restenotic lesions? [Abstract] Circulation 1996;94(Suppl):I-131.

348. Herrman J-PR, Hermans WRM, Vos J, Serruys PW. Pharmacological approaches to the prevention of restenosis following angioplasty. The search for the Holy Grail? (Part I). Drugs 1993;46:18–52.

349. Herrman J-PR, Hermans WRM, Vos J, Serruys PW. Pharmacological approaches to the prevention of restenosis following angioplasty. The search for the Holy Grail? (Part II). Drugs 1993;46:249–262.

350. Kutryk MJB, Serruys PW. Prevention of restenosis after PTCA. Vessels 1996;2:4–12.

351. Dangas G, Fuster V. Management of restenosis after coronary intervention. Am Heart J 1996;132:428–436.

352. Labinaz M, Zidar JP, Stack RS, et al. Biodegradable stents: the future of interventional cardiology? J Interventional Cardiol 1995;8:395–405.

353. Raizner AE, Hollman J, Abukhail J, et al. for the Ciprostene Investigators. Ciprostene for restenosis revisited: quantitative analysis of angiograms. J Am Coll Cardiol 1993;21:321A.

354. Darius H, Nixdorff U, Zander J. Effects of ciprostene on restenosis rate during therapeutic transluminal coronary angioplasty. Agents Action (Suppl)1992;37:305–311.

355. Topol EJ, Califf RM, Weisman HF, et al. on behalf of the EPIC Investigators. Randomized trial of coronary intervention with antibody against platelet IIb/IIIa integrin for reduction of clinical restenosis: results at six months. Lancet 1994;343:881–886.

356. Maresta A, Balducelli M, Cantini L, et al. for the STARC Investigators. Trapidil (Triazolopyrimidine), a platelet-derived growth factor antagonist, reduces restenosis after percutaneous transluminal coronary angioplasty. Results of the randomized, double-blind STARC study. Circulation 1994;90:2710–2715.

357. Emanuelsson H, Beatt KJ, Bagger JP, et al. for the European Angiopeptin Study Group. Long-term effects of angiopeptin treatment in coronary angioplasty. Circulation 1995;91:1689–1696.

358. Labinaz M, Zidar JP, Stack RS, et al. Biodegradable stents: the future of interventional cardiology? J Interventional Cardiol 1995;8:395–405.

359. Gammon RS, Chapman GD, Agrawal GM, et al. Mechanical features of the Duke biodegradable intravascular stent [Abstract]. J Am Coll Cardiol 1991;17(Suppl):235A.

360. Tanguay J-F, Kruse KR, Phillips III HR, et al. The polymer stent. In: Sigwart U, ed. Endoluminal stenting. Philadelphia: WB Saunders, 1996:216–224.

361. Waksman R, Robinson KA, Crocker IR, et al. Endovascular low-dose irradiation inhibits neointima formation after coronary artery balloon injury in swine: a possible role for radiation therapy in restenosis prevention. Circulation 1995;91:1553–1559.

362. Mazur W, Ali MN, Dabaghi SF, et al. High dose rate intracoronary radiation suppresses neointimal proliferation in the stented and ballooned model of porcine restenosis [Abstract]. Circulation 1994;90(Suppl):I-652.

363. Waksman R, Robinson KA, Crocker IR, et al. Intracoronary radiation before stent implantation inhibits neointima formation in stented porcine coronary arteries. Circulation 1995;92:1383–1386.

364. Hehrlein C, Zimmerman M, Metz J, et al. Radioactive coronary stent implantation inhibits neointimal proliferation in non-atherosclerotic rabbits [Abstract]. Circulation 1993;88(Suppl):I-651.

365. Hehrlein C, Gollan C, Donges K, et al. Low-dose radioactive endovascular stents prevent smooth muscle cell proliferation and neointimal hyperplasia in rabbits. Circulation 1995;92:1570–1575.

366. Hehrlein C, Stintz M, Kinscherf R, et al. Pure β-

particle-emitting stents inhibit neointima formation in rabbits. Circulation 1996;93:641–645.

367. Laird JR, Carter AJ, Kufs WM, et al. Inhibition of neointimal proliferation with low-dose irradiation from a β-particle-emitting stent. Circulation 1996;93:529–536.

368. Fischell TA, Kharma BK, Fischell DR, et al. Low-dose β-particle emission from "stent" wire results in complete, localized inhibition of smooth muscle proliferation. Circulation 1994;90:2956–2963.

369. Fischell TA, Carter AJ, Laird JR. The β-particle-emitting radioisotope stent (Isostent): animal studies and planned clinical trials. Am J Cardiol 1996;78(Suppl 3A):45–50.

370. Fajadet JC, Marco J, Cassagneau G, et al. Restenosis following successful Palmaz-Schatz intracoronary stent implantation [Abstract]. J Am Coll Cardiol 1991;17(Suppl):346A.

371. Roubin G, Hearn J, Carlin S, et al. Angiographic and clinical follow-up in patients receiving a balloon-expandable, stainless steel stent (Cook, Inc.) for prevention or treatment of acute closure after PTCA [Abstract]. Circulation 1990;82(Suppl):III-191.

372. Colombo A, Maiello L, Almagor Y, et al. Coronary stenting: single institutional experience with the initial 100 cases using the Palmaz-Schatz stent. Cathet Cardiovasc Diagn 1992;26:171–176.

373. Levine M, Lemen M, Schatz R, et al. Management of restenosis following Palmaz-Schatz intracoronary stenting: multicenter results [Abstract]. Circulation 1990;82(Suppl):III-657.

374. Macander PJ, Agrawal SK, Cannon AD, et al. Is PTCA within the stenotic coronary stent safer than routine angioplasty [Abstract]. Circulation 1991;84(Suppl):II-199.

375. Garratt K, Holmes D, Schwartz R, et al. Balloon dilatation of restenotic lesions within metallic coronary stents: initial clinical and histopathologic observations [Abstract]. J Am Coll Cardiol 1992;19(Suppl):109A.

376. Macander PJ, Roubin GS, Agrawal SK, et al. Balloon angioplasty for treatment of in-stent restenosis: feasibility, safety, and efficacy. Cathet Cardiovasc Diagn 1994;32:125–131.

377. Baim DS, Levine MJ, Leon MB. Management of restenosis within the Palmaz-Schatz coronary stent (the U.S. multicenter experience). Am J Cardiol 1993;71:364–366.

378. Tan H-C, Sketch MH, Tan ME, et al. Is there an optimal treatment strategy for stent restenosis? [Abstract]. Circulation 1996;94(Suppl):I-91.

379. Bowerman RE, Pinkerton CA, Kirk B, et al. Disruption of a coronary stent during atherectomy for restenosis. Cathet Cardiovasc Diagn 1991;34:248–251.

380. Sharma SK, Duvvuri S, Kakarala V, et al. Rotational atherectomy (RA) for in-stent restenosis (ISR): intravascular ultrasound (IVUS) and quantitative coronary analysis (QCA) [Abstract]. Circulation 1996;94(Suppl):I-454.

381. Strauss B, Umans V, van Suylen R-J, et al. Directional atherectomy for treatment of restenosis within coronary stents: clinical, angiographic and histologic result. J Am Coll Cardiol 1992;20:1465–1473.

382. Buchbinder M, Goldberg SL, Fortuna R, et al. Rotational atherectomy for intra-stent restenosis: initial experience [Abstract]. Circulation 1996;94(Suppl):I-621.

383. Goy J-J, Sigwart U, Vogt P, et al. Long-term follow-up of the first 56 patients treated with intracoronary self-expanding stents (the Lausanne experience). Am J Cardiol 1991;67:569–572.

384. Köster RP, Koschyk DH, Kähler J, et al. Laser angioplasty of in-stent restenosis [Abstract]. Circulation 1996;94(Suppl):I-621.

385. MacDonald RG, O'Neill BJ, Creighton JE, et al. Is coronary stent expansion the mechanism for the successful dilatation of stent restenosis? A quantitative angiographic study [Abstract]. Circulation 1991;84(Suppl):II-196.

386. Morís C, Alfonso F, Lambert J, et al. Stenting for coronary dissection after balloon dilatation of in-stent restenosis: stenting a previously stented site. Am Heart J 1996;131:834–836.

387. Sridhar K, Teefy PJ, Almond DG, et al. Long-term clinical outcomes of patients with in-stent restenosis [Abstract]. Circulation 1996;94(Suppl):I-454.

388. Yokoi H, Kimura T, Nobuyoshi M. Palmaz-Schatz coronary stent restenosis: pattern and management [Abstract]. J Am Coll Cardiol 1994;25(Suppl):117A.

389. Oweida SW, Roubin GS, Smith RB III, et al. Postcatheterization vascular complications associated with percutaneous transluminal coronary angioplasty. J Vasc Surg 1990;12:310–315.

390. McCann RL, Schwartz LB, Pieper KS. Vascular complications of cardiac catheterization. J Vasc Surg 1991;14:375–381.

391. Muller DW, Shamir KJ, Ellis SG, et al. Peripheral vascular complications after conventional and complex percutaneous coronary interventional procedures. Am J Cardiol 1992;69:63–68.

392. Berge PG, Winter UJ, Hoffmann M, et al. Local vascular complications in heart catheter studies. Z Kardiol 1993;82:449–456.

393. Mansour KA, Moscucci M, Kent C, et al. Vascular complications following directional coronary atherectomy or Palmaz-Schatz stenting [Abstract]. J Am Coll Cardiol 1994;23(Suppl):136A.

394. Sones FM Jr, Shirey EK, Proudfit WL, et al. Cinecoronary arteriography [Abstract]. Circulation 1959;20(Suppl):773.

395. Resar JR, Wolff MR, Blumenthal RS, et al. Brachial approach for intracoronary stent implantation: a feasibility study. Am Heart J 1993;126:300–304.

396. Kiemeniej F, Laarman GJ. Bailout techniques for failed coronary angioplasty using 6 french guiding catheters. Cathet Cardiovasc Diagn 1994;32:359–366.

397. Kiemeniej F. Transradial artery coronary angioplasty and stenting: history and single center experience. J Invasive Cardiol 1996;8(Suppl D):3D-8D.

398. Arnold AM. Hemostasis after radial artery cardiac catheterization. J Invasive Cardiol 1996;8(Suppl D):26D-29D.

399. Mann JT III, Cubeddu G, Schneider JE, et al. Clinical evaluation of current stent deployment strategies. J Invasive Cardiol 1996;8(Suppl D):30D-35D.

400. Bartorelli AL, Sganzerla P, Fabbiocchi F, et al.

Prompt and safe femoral hemostasis with a collagen device after intracoronary implantation of Palmaz-Schatz stents. Am Heart J 1995;130:26–32.

401. Kiemeniej F, Laarman GJ. Improved anticoagulation management after Palmaz Schatz coronary stent implantation by sealing the arterial puncture site with a vascular hemostasis device. Cathet Cardiovasc Diagn 1993;30:317–322.

402. Webb JG, Carere RA, Dodek AA. Collagen plug hemostatic closure of femoral arterial puncture sites following implantation of intracoronary stents. Cathet Cardiovasc Diagn 1993;30:314–316.

403. von Hoch F, Neumann F-J, Theiss W, et al. Efficacy and safety of collagen implants for hemostasis of the vascular access site after coronary balloon angioplasty and coronary stent placement. A randomized study. Eur Heart J 1995;16:640–646.

404. Camenzind E, Grossholz M, Urban P, et al. Mechanical compression (Femostop) alone versus combined collagen application (Vasoseal) and Femostop for arterial puncture site closure after coronary stent implantation: a randomized trial [Abstract]. J Am Coll Cardiol 1994;25(Suppl): 355A.

405. Sridhar K, Porter K, Gupta B, et al. Reduction in peripheral vascular complications after coronary stenting by the use of a pneumatic vascular compression device [Abstract]. Circulation 1994; 90(Suppl):I-621.

406. Veldhuijzen FLMJ, Bonnier HJRM, Michels HR, El Gamal MIH, et al. Retrieval of undeployed stents from the right coronary artery: report of two cases. Cathet Cardiovac Diagn 1993;30:245–248.

407. Rozenman Y, Burstein M, Hasin Y, et al. Retrieval of occluding unexpanded Palmaz-Schatz stent from a saphenous aorto-coronary vein graft. Cathet Cardiovasc Diagn 1995;34:159–161.

408. Berder V, Bedossa M, Gras D, et al. Retrieval of a lost coronary stent from the descending aorta using a PTCA balloon and biopsy forceps. Cathet Cardiovasc Diagn 1993;28:351–353.

409. Cishek MB, Laslett L, Gershony G. Balloon catheter retrieval of dislodged coronary artery stents: a novel technique. Cathet Cardiovasc Diagn 1995; 34:350–352.

410. Mohiaddin RH, Roberts RH, Underwood R, et al. Localization of a misplaced coronary artery stent by magnetic resonance imaging. Clin Cardiol 1995;18:175–177.

411. Eeckhout E, Stauffer JC, Goy JJ. Retrieval of a migrated coronary stent by means of an alligator forceps catheter. Cathet Cardiovasc Diagn 1993; 30:166–168.

412. Foster Smith KW, Garratt KN, Higano ST, et al. Retrieval techniques for managing flexible intracoronary stent misplacement. Cathet Cardiovasc Diagn 1993;30:63–68.

413. Wong PH. Retrieval of undeployed intracoronary Palmaz-Schatz stents. Cathet Cardiovasc Diagn 1995;35:218–223.

414. Iniguez A, Macaya C, Alfonso F, et al. Early angiographic changes of side branches arising from a Palmaz-Schatz stented segment: results and clinical implications. J Am Coll Cardiol 1994;23: 911–913.

415. Fischman DL, Savage MP, Leon MB, et al. Fate of lesion-related side branches after coronary artery stenting. J Am Coll Cardiol 1993;22:1641–1646.

416. Pan M, Medina A, Suarez de Lezo J. Follow-up patency of side branches covered by intracoronary Palmaz-Schatz stent. Am Heart J 1995;129: 436–440.

417. Mazur W, Grinstead C, Hakim A, et al. Fate of side branches after intracoronary implantation of the Gianturco-Roubin flex-stent for acute or threatened closure after percutaneous transluminal coronary angioplasty. Am J Cardiol 1994;74: 1207–1210.

418. Benzuly KH, Glazier S, Grines CL, et al. Coronary perforation: an unreported complication after intracoronary stent implantation [Abstract]. J Am Coll Cardiol 1996;27(Suppl):252A.

419. Hall P, Nakamura S, Maiello L, et al. Factors associated with procedural complications during high pressure optimized Palmaz-Schatz intracoronary stent implantation [Abstract]. Circulation 1994; 90(Suppl):I-612.

420. Reimers B, von Birgelen C, van der Giessen WJ, et al. A word of caution on optimizing stent deployment in calcified lesion: acute coronary rupture with cardiac tamponade. Am Heart J 1996; 131:192–194.

421. Gunther HU, Strupp G, Volmar J, et al. Koronare stentimplantation: infektion und abszedierung mit lentalem ausgang. Z Kardiol 1993;82:521–525.

422. Thibodeaux LC, James KV, Lohr JM, et al. Infection of endovascular stents in a swine model. Am J Surg 1996;172:151–154.

423. Kimura T, Yokoi H, Nakagawa Y, et al. Three-year follow-up after implantation of metallic coronary artery stents. N Eng J Med 1996;334:561–566.

424. King SB III, Schlumpf M. Ten-year completed follow-up of percutaneous transluminal coronary angioplasty: the early Zurich experience. J Am Coll Cardiol 1993;22:353–360.

425. Foley JB, White J, Teefy P, et al. Late angiographic follow-up after Palmaz-Schatz stent implantation. Am J Cardiol 1995;76:76–77.

426. Hermiller JB, Fry ET, Peters TF, et al. Late coronary artery stenosis regression with the Gianturco-Roubin intracoronary stent. Am J Cardiol 1996;77:247–251.

427. Klugherz BD, DeAngelo D, Kim BK, et al. Three-year clinical follow-up after Palmaz-Schatz stenting. J Am Coll Cardiol 1996;27:1185–1191.

428. Debbas N, Sigwart U, Eeckhout E, et al. Late clinical follow-up 9 years after intra-coronary stenting with the Wallstent [Abstract]. Circulation 1995; 92(Suppl):I-280.

32
Stents for Coronary Artery Intervention: Types, Technical Issues, and Clinical Examples

Paul Kelly, MD
Ulrich Sigwart, MD

INTRODUCTION

Following the introduction of balloon angioplasty in 1978 (1), it soon became apparent that a number of technical limitations of this procedure existed. Suboptimal outcomes would often result, for example, in dissection of the vessel wall and acute or threatened closure; and, on follow-up, unacceptably high rates of restenosis, usually with recurrence of symptoms. It became clear that an adjuvant technique would be required to augment the results of the original interventional procedure.

The concept of an intravascular stent had been proposed as early as 1912 (2), but it was Charles Dotter in 1968 who first implanted metal spirals in animal arteries (3). The first stent used in peripheral and coronary arteries in humans was the self-expanding Wallstent (Schneider, Zurich, Switzerland) (4). Early results appeared favorable, but following the publication of multicenter experience with this device (5), it became apparent that a number of technical issues had to be addressed if this exciting development was going to add significantly to the nonsurgical management of coronary artery disease.

After the development of the Wallstent, and the demonstration that a stent could be deployed within a human coronary artery with significant clinical benefit both acutely and on follow-up, assessment of a limited number of stent types followed. After the publication of a number of trials on the elective use of single stents, in particular the BENESTENT (6) and STRESS (7) studies, the benefit of stenting compared with balloon angioplasty alone in the management of coronary artery disease was demonstrated definitively. The realization that this technology could be applied to a huge number of patients resulted in a rapid increase in the number and types of stents available to the interventional cardiologist.

As the use of stents increased, it also became apparent that a large number of technical issues needed to be considered. The individual characteristics of each stent varies according to the metal used, stent configuration, delivery mode, and presence of adjuvant materials.

The biologic response to stent implantation includes thrombus formation on the stent struts (8), smooth muscle cell proliferation, and neointimal hyperplasia as a result of expansion of the arterial lumen (9).

Modifications to the anticoagulation regimen after stent deployment, in particular, recognition that the use of antiplatelet therapy (ticlopidine and aspirin) is better than anticoagulation with warfarin, have

710

resulted in a reduced incidence of subacute thrombosis and significantly less local complications at the femoral puncture site (10, 11). A comparison of the same stent design when composed of different metal (stainless steel and tantalum stents) showed no difference in thrombogenicity in either a baboon or pig model (12). **Stents have been manufactured to produce as smooth a surface as possible,** usually with electrochemical polishing. Scanning electron micrographs have shown that this indeed results in a smoother surface, and appears to reduce the amount of thrombus formation.

Although a large number of stents are available, there are only a few classes of stent design. A comparison of a stainless steel slotted tube and corrugated ring stent showed that, although there was no difference in the total surface area occupied by metal (30%), the uncoated corrugated ring stent caused 38% less neointimal hyperplasia, as well as less thrombosis in comparison with the slotted tube stent (13). Currently, no data are available to compare the other classes of stent type, although this is likely to change for reasons to be discussed.

Inevitably, stents that have appeared on the market more recently were developed under the umbrella of the results of earlier trials, with manufacturers extrapolating data from these studies to their new products. The use of stents in Europe allowed the deployment of stent types as yet unproved in clinical trials. The Food and Drugs Administration (FDA) in the United States is less tolerant and consequently a number of direct stent-to-stent comparisons have to be performed against the original Palmaz-Schatz (Johnson and Johnson Interventional Systems, Warren, NJ) stent with its delivery system, which was the device used in the earlier clinical trials. Consequently, **the "best" stent for any particular situation has not been defined,** which has resulted in at least 22 stent types being available with considerable confusion and debate on which device to use for any given clinical situation.

TYPES OF STENTS

The following classification attempts to define the types of stents available, but consid-

ering the rapid changes in this field, inevitably this information will become outmoded with new developments.

Permanent Stents, Self-expanding Stents

Wallstent (Schneider)

The first stent used in human coronary and peripheral arteries was the self-expanding Wallstent (4). This elastic woven, wire mesh tube consists of metal braids of approximately 80 μm thickness. The spring type metal results in self-expansion as the stent is released from a constrained to an unconstrained form. **The Wallstent is geometrically stable, has a very large expansion ratio, remains flexible when compressed (allowing good trackability), and conforms to structures of different diameter.** The stent is delivered on a 5 F coaxial catheter on which the stent is restrained by a doubled-over membrane. The stent is deployed by retraction of the membrane; once deployment has begun, the stent can be pulled proximally in the artery but cannot be passed distally. Considerable shortening of the stent occurs as it is deployed from a constrained to an unconstrained form; consequently, ensuring correct positioning of the Wallstent does require some experience with its use.

A modification to the stent affected the braiding angle and stent strut, producing a system that shortens less on expansion, has greater radio-opacity, less radial force, and a lower metallic surface area than previously.

The combination of length, large diameter, and trackability make the Wallstent particularly suitable for tortuous native vessels and for degenerate vein grafts. The latter can be stented without predilation so reducing the risk of embolization (14, 15). Also, long segments of disease, for example, in previously occluded vessels can be treated with the Wallstent (16).

Recently, a development of the Wallstent, the "Magic Wallstent" has become available. The stent itself has been modified, with a different braiding angle, which renders it softer and less shortening, and a platinum core that makes it more radio-opaque. Instead of using a doubled-over membrane, it has a retractable sheath that constrains the stent. The middle marker of the rolling membrane delivery system has been removed from this new device, and an indication of the degree of shortening to be expected is achieved by examining the distance between the end of the stent and the marker that indicates its distal end in the constrained position. Consequently, as the sheath is retracted and the stent begins to expand, it shortens and, by assessing the amount of shortening distally and estimating the equivalent effect of this proximally, the position of the fully deployed stent can be determined. If the operator decides that the stent will not be positioned correctly, the stent can be recaptured by advancing the sheath (as long as the sheath has only been withdrawn up to two thirds of the stent length), the delivery system can then be moved and the process repeated. The main advantage to this system is the fact that it can be advanced distally after the initial attempt, a feature not available in its predecessor. However, the physical properties of the sheath in comparison with the doubled-over membrane will inevitably make the delivery system less flexible. This may reduce the unsurpassed trackability of the original Wallstent device.

Cardiocoil (In-stent)

The Cardiocoil is a device that utilizes the metallurgical thermoelastic shape memory properties of nitinol (nickel-titanium alloy) (17). Nitinol is unique among metal alloys in that it exists in two crystalline phases, martensitic and austenitic. The stent is inserted in the martensitic form. Nitinol can be deformed with relatively low pressures, which causes less vessel wall trauma and may result in a reduced incidence of subacute thrombosis (18). The Cardiocoil stent consists of a coil with one ball at each end, which is designed to ensure that no sharp

ends are on the coil when released from the delivery system.

In addition to being implanted, due to the properties of nitinol, the stent can be recovered at a later procedure. Thus, if a coaxial balloon system is used to deliver a small volume of fluid (Ringer's solution) at the transition temperature, the stent undergoes a rapid thermoelastic phase change to a different crystalline form (austinitic), whereby it collapses and resumes its pre-expanded geometry and can be removed with the retrieval catheter. Although not primarily designed for this purpose, in vitro studies in dogs and humans has shown that the stent can be safely removed at 24 hours, and that the angiographic appearances are favorable at this stage (19). Early results suggest that this combination may reduce the development of neointimal hyperplasia, but preserve the original gain in luminal diameter (20).

Scimed Radius Stent

The Scimed Radius (Boston Scientific, Boston, MA) stent is made from nitinol. The design and manufacture have features similar to the ACS Multi-Link stent. It has a sheathed delivery system, with markers indicating stent position. The strut thickness of 115 μm imparts good radial strength, and accurate positioning is facilitated by the degree of radio-opacity. Metal:surface ratio is 22%, with minimal shortening. The Radius stent is available in diameters of 2.75–4.25 mm and lengths of 14–31 mm.

Angiomed Memotherm Stent

The Angiomed Memotherm (Bard) stent is also made of nitinol. It has a slotted tube in its compressed (martensitic) state. After deployment at body temperature (austenitic state), it has features similar to the Wallstent, except for the overlapping wire construction. It shows minimal shortening on expansion. To date, this stent has been available in relatively large diameters and lengths (4–14 mm diameter and 30–120 mm length), although it is likely that stent sizes for coronary intervention will be available (21).

Balloon Expandable Stents, Flexible Wire Stents

Gianturco-Roubin Stent

The original version (GR-I) (Cook, Indianapolis) of this stent was the first stent to be approved for use by the FDA. A registry of patients receiving the device following a suboptimal percutaneous transluminal angioplasty (PTCA) result showed significant clinical benefit, with a stent thrombosis rate of 16.7% in the high-risk group (22). Another study revealed an in-hospital complication rate of 26%, and a follow-up restenosis rate of 50% (23). When used in patients with old saphenous vein grafts, patency was demonstrated in 99% of grafts that had been stented (24).

However, overall the initial and clinical outcomes were not without problems. This may have been related to (*a*) the delivery system that rendered many lesions inaccessible, (*b*) the fact that the wires were relatively thick with a diameter of 150 μm, and (*c*) the gaps between the wires were large, which resulted in plaque protrusion. This has previously been suggested as a factor that predisposed to increased restenosis (25). The structure of the stent also makes it prone to recoil.

Later work has shown that in favorable angiographic and clinical situations the GR-I stent can be used with aspirin and ticlopidine alone, with low subacute thrombosis and major clinical event rates (26).

The GR-II version modified the shape of the wire with a flat design to reduce flow turbulence generated by the wire stent. A unilateral spine was incorporated into the design to make the structure more stable; to assist in placement of the stent, a radio-opaque marker has been placed at each end. To date, no clinical trials with this device have been published.

Wiktor Stent (Medtronic)

The Wiktor (Medtronic) is a wire stent made of tantalum, which increases its radio-opacity and makes positioning within the artery easier (27). Previous claims that tantalum would give a more favorable biologic medium than stainless steel do not appear to have been realized. Tantalum is more brittle, and some authors have noted that deformation of the stent often results in major adverse outcomes (28). The spacing between the wires is large, and the radial strength is low. Early clinical experience suggested relatively high rates of subacute thrombosis and restenosis of 10 to 20% and 30 to 50%, respectively (29–31). Recently, a newer version has become available but there are no new data to show whether this new design will have improved clinical results.

Cordis Stent

The Cordis is a coil stent also made from tantalum wire, 130 μm in diameter, wound into a helical coil. The stent was premounted on balloons 3.0–4.0 mm in diameter, and was 18 mm long, shortening to 15 mm after expansion. Early clinical experience showed high rates of successful deployment (32), and approximately 30% patients had restenosis demonstrated angiographically at 6 months (33).

The successor of this original stent, the Crossflex Stent is made from stainless steel wire, 150 μm in diameter. Stainless steel is used because radio-opacity is too high with tantalum for this particular stent. It is premounted on a Worldpass balloon, and is available in 15 mm length. The single strand, helical coil design gives a relatively low profile that also provides good trackability and sidebranch access and patency for bifurcation lesions. Metal:artery ratio is 15%. Balloon sizes are 3.0–4.0 mm in diameter.

Angio Stent (Angiodynamics)

The Angio (Angiodynamics) wire stent is made from a combination of 90% platinum and 10% iridium. It has a high radio-opacity. The single wire, 127 μm in diameter is woven into seven segments; within each segment the wire is wound in a sinusoidal fashion. A longitudinal wire runs from one end of the stent to the other. The stent is premounted on a high-pressure balloon with a platinum band at each end of the balloon to facilitate positioning. The stent is covered with a sheath, and is available in 3.0–4.0 mm diameters, and 15 mm length. Lengths from 20–40 mm will be available. Early animal data have shown results comparable to similar devices (34).

Freedom Stent (Global Therapeutics, Inc.)

The Freedom (Global Therapeutics, Inc.,) is a 316LVM stainless steel wire stent, folded in bent concentric loops (fish scale design), which is available in both premounted and unmounted forms. The stent can be used in vessels of 2.5–4.5 mm diameter, and is available in lengths of 12–40 mm. It has been shown to be suitable for both long and bifurcation lesions, as well as standard indications. However, the low metal:surface ratio may predispose to insufficient wall support, and the design of the stent makes maneuvering the stent within the target vessel and recrossing with balloons and other devices more difficult than for other stents. However, early clinical trials have shown good procedural success with satisfactory early and late outcomes (35).

Slotted Tube Stents

Palmaz-Schatz Stent

This stent is the prototype of all slotted tube stents (36, 37, 38). Multiple rows of rectangles are excised from a tube of stainless steel. When the stent expands, these gaps become diamond shaped, permitting expansion to a maximal diameter of 5–6 mm for the coronary model. It has a relatively wide pore size, and also shortens with expansion; this can cause problems with coverage in vessels greater than 4 mm in diameter. The delivery system designed for these stents has a protective sheath with radio-opaque markers to assist in stent placement. However, the balloon does not allow for high-pressure inflation.

Serial intravascular ultrasound runs before and after stent deployment and subsequent high-pressure inflation have resulted in a number of criteria being established as optimal for "ideal" stent implantation (39). Consequently, the requirement to use a short, noncompliant high-pressure balloon is a recognized feature of using the Palmaz-Schatz stent.

Some shortcomings are found with the delivery system and, consequently, most of operators in Europe choose to use the stent in an unmounted form and crimp it onto a balloon to allow it to be deployed. Palmaz-Schatz stents are available in a variety of lengths, the shortest nonarticulated version of 8 mm, and the longest (consisting of three elements connected by a spiral articulation) of 21 mm.

Initially, when availability of other stents was low, coverage of long lesions or of extensive dissection led to the use of multiple stents within a single vessel. Some reports have suggested that this caused excessive amounts of restenosis (40–43). Deploying two stents on the same balloon helps to eliminate the gap between two stents positioned independently; thus, removing the possibility of an unstented segment of disease, a factor thought to increase restenosis.

The articulated design of the PS153 allowed for easier positioning of the stent, but the central articulation inevitably produced an area within the stent that did not experience the radial force of the remainder of the stented segment. Angiographic follow-up revealed that restenosis was prone to occur at this site in comparison with the remainder of the stent (44).

Palmaz-Schatz Crown Stent

This stent is the successor to the original Palmaz-Schatz stent. It is made from 70 μm diameter 316L stainless steel. The longitudinal slots are more intricate, and provide good wall coverage as well as increasing the flexibility of the stent delivery system. The stent is premounted on a low profile system, and is available in lengths of 15 mm, 22 mm, and 30 mm, and balloon diameters of 3.0–4.0 mm. The Crown stent will be used in the ARTS (stenting versus coronary artery bypass grafting) trial. To date, there are no data available from clinical experience with this device.

Tensum Coronary Stent (Biotronik)

This stent has a tubular slotted design made from Tantalum material, 80 μm in diameter. The stent to artery ratio is 13.7%. Tantalum has high radio-opacity and this assists in stent placement. In an attempt to reduce thrombogenicity, the stent is coated with silicon carbide (SiC) which is claimed to reduce the activation of fibrinogen. Each of the tubular segments is 4.2 mm long and they are connected by bridges 0.5 mm in length. The various stent lengths are dependent upon the number of segments joined together and are currently available in 8.9 mm, 13.6 mm and 18.3 mm lengths. The stents are premounted on balloons of 3.0–4.5 mm diameter.

ACT-One Stent (Progressive Angioplasty Systems Inc)

This slotted tube design stent is made from a martensitic nitinol material. Nitinol is a nickel-titanium alloy which expands uniformly at low pressures. The stent can be deployed at 4 atm irrespective of vessel diameter. It has been suggested that this will cause less vessel injury during stent deployment and hence less thrombus formation, and so, possibly less neointimal hyperplasia (45, 46). A comparison of stainless steel (Palmaz-Schatz) and nitinol slotted tube stents in a rabbit carotid artery model showed significantly less thrombus on the nitinol stents

at 4 days, there was no long-term follow-up to assess neointimal hyperplasia formation and instent restenosis (18). The stent is premounted on a balloon delivery system and when deployed has 36% wall coverage, the slot length of the ACT-One stent being twice as long as the Palmaz-Schatz stent.

Balloon-Expandable, Multiple Cell Stents

ACS Multi-Link Stent System (Guidant)

This stent design was based on the results of early stent experience, to provide a number of features considered necessary for successful clinical use. In particular, good structural support, flexibility, and easy delivery (47). In contrast to flexible metal stents constructed from wires, the Multi-Link stent is made from a stainless steel tube with a strut thickness of 50 μm. The mesh of the stent was modified to reduce the metal:air ratio by 35% in comparison to the Palmaz-Schatz stent. Despite this, the collapse pressure of the Multi-Link stent is higher than that of the self-expanding and wire stents, and only a little less than the Palmaz-Schatz stent. The stent is composed of individual metal rings connected by a number of bridges. The gaps between the struts are smaller than in other stents to reduce flow turbulence, and the reduced gap size allows improved tacking up of dissections. Despite this reduction in gap size, the design of the stent allows for easy access to side branches and so makes this stent particularly suitable for bifurcation lesions. Equally, the flexibility of the stent allows for relatively easy passage through tortuous vessels, and when positioned on a curved section of artery, the stent conforms to the anatomy of the vessel in which it is placed.

The original design was a coaxial system with a 15 mm long stent covered with a retractable sheath. In this, the stent is premounted on a stretchable elastic sleeve which covers the balloon. This sleeve encourages even expansion of the stent and helps to prevent stent dislodgement from the delivery system. The first balloon used for the delivery system was designed to be inflated to 9 atm to result in the stent diameter of nominal value. However, this can be exceeded where the vessel diameter allows to permit complete apposition of the stent to the wall of the artery. As recognized from studies using intravascular ultrasound it is important to use sufficiently high pressures to optimize stent deployment (48). Therefore, a new balloon material is now available with the Multi-Link stent. The ACS Multi-Link was the stent used in the WEST study (49). This was a trial of primary stenting in vessels with single lesions. The rate of subacute thrombosis was low, and restenosis rate was 12%.

There is now a monorail delivery system with an unsheathed stent that retains the feature of the sleeve between stent and balloon. As well as a 15 mm long stent, there are also 25 and 35 mm stent lengths available. These stents come in a variety of balloon sizes, and the advantages of the design as described above, allow for relatively easy accessibility to most lesions in native vessels and vein grafts despite the increased length of the stent and delivery balloon. At the time of writing, the Multi-Link stent is the leading stent in several European countries.

NIR Stent (Boston Scientific)

This stent has a multicellular design that confers a number of useful properties. As the stent is deployed, within a range of 3–5 mm diameter vessels, the cells conform to the vessel anatomy without shortening the overall stent length. The NIR stent is made from 316 stainless steel, and consequently is only faintly radio-opaque. It is currently available only in an unmounted form, but is available in 3 lengths, 9, 16, and 32 mm, the combination of variety of length, fairly good trackability and flexibility within the coronary vasculature make it useful for a large number of stenting indications. The stent provides an 11 to 18% surface area coverage and confers fairly high radial strength.

AVE Micro Stent and Micro Stent II (Arterial Vascular Engineering)

To date, there has been a large experience with AVE stents, both the Micro Stent, and its successor, the AVE Micro Stent II (50). The Micro Stent was formed of 4 mm segments, whereas the Micro Stent II consists of 3 mm segments, each connected by a single weld. Both stents were made from 200 μm diameter wire, and offered 15% wall coverage. The Micro Stent II is premounted, polished and provides high radial support and minimal recoil. It is moderately radiopaque which assists in positioning before deployment. It is available in balloon sizes from 2.5–4.0 mm, and lengths from 6–39 mm.

AVE GFX Stent (Arterial Vascular Engineering)

This stainless steel stent differs significantly from its predecessors. The number of loops (or crowns) within each 2 mm segment is increased to 6, making expansion more uniform and increasing radial strength. The strut design has also changed from round to ellipto-rectangular wire geometry in an attempt to improve stent/vessel wall apposition, with wire thickness of 130 μm diameter. Due to the design with a variable number of segments joined together by single welds the longitudinal flexibility persists. The stent is moderately radio-opaque, which assists in placement, and is available in lengths of 8–40 mm, and balloon diameters of 2.5–4.0 mm. At present, there are no data from clinical trials with this device.

JoStent (Jomed International)

This is a stainless steel stent with a multiple closed cell design, similar to the NIR stent. The stent has a low profile when crimped, and a high degree of longitudinal flexibility which allows easy tracking through tortuous vessels. On deployment, there is minimal foreshortening (3%), and a moderately high radial strength. It is available in an unmounted and premounted format, as well as having 3 different systems: small (< 3 mm) vessels, standard (3–5 mm diameter), and large (for vein grafts). The stent is available in lengths of 9–46 mm, and is also provided with a heparin coated where required.

Pura-Vario Stent (Devon Medical)

This stent is made from stainless steel 316L. It has a multiple cell design with minimal shortening (< 3%) on expansion. The stent is highly polished in an attempt to reduce thrombogenicity, and is available premounted, with a crimped diameter of 1.6 mm. The stent can be used in vessels of 3–5 mm diameter, and comes in lengths of 10–40 mm.

Be-Stent (Medtronic)

This stent has a similar geometry to the NIR stent. To date, there are no clinical trial data.

Coated Permanent Stents

Irrespective of the type of metal used, or the degree of polishing, all stents attract thrombin and platelets and initiate a thrombotic reaction and subsequent stimulate the development of neointimal hyperplasia (51). The concept of coating the stent with a polymer to enable other agents to be incorporated into the polymer matrix has been suggested for some time (52). Initially, work concentrated on the incorporation of specific thrombin inhibitors in an attempt to limit the problem of subacute thrombosis (53, 54). At present, most data is available for heparin coated stents.

Prior to the French experience and the randomized study of Schömig et al. (10) which showed a reduction in the incidence of subacute thrombosis with aspirin and ticlopidine compared to warfarin, the requirement of systemic anticoagulation with warfarin was responsible for an unacceptably high rate of local complications at the femoral puncture site. The concept of local as opposed to systemic drug delivery had been proposed as a means of reducing these unwanted side effects while maintaining potential benefit of the administered drug (55). The role of heparin in reducing the amount of stent thrombosis and so possibly the degree of neointimal hyperplasia had also been demonstrated (56, 57). The BENESTENT-I trial showed a significant improvement for stenting compared to balloon angioplasty (6), and the BENESTENT-II trial was designed to determine the clinical effect of a heparin-coated stent. Animal studies had shown that heparin-coated stents reduced acute thrombus formation in a rabbit model (58). The early BENESTENT-II results showed that it was safe to use ticlopidine and aspirin instead of warfarin, and that the subacute thrombosis rate was 0%. The overall event free rate was 86% (59). Further longer term follow-up data regarding instent restenosis rates for heparin-coated versus noncoated stents are awaited.

As described above, the Biotronik Tensum stent, made from tantalum, is coated with silicon carbide in an attempt to reduce activation of fibrinogen. The coating of tantalum stents with fibrin and deployment in a porcine coronary model showed favorable rates of restenosis in comparison to a polyurethane coated stainless steel stent model (60).

Future developments in this field are likely to include platelet glycoprotein IIb/IIIa inhibitors (61), antithrombins and possibly cells with the ability to express or produce substances such as tissue plasminogen activator.

Radioactive Permanent Stents

The problem of restenosis following balloon angioplasty or insertion of an intracoronary stent is the main limitation to its success (62). Studies in a porcine overstretch model have suggested that intracoronary radiation will reduce restenosis following coronary intervention (63, 64). Initial work used gamma radiation, but due to a number of procedural difficulties associated with this, it is now likely that a beta source would be more practical. The use of a beta emitting stent in porcine iliac arteries inhibited neo-intimal proliferation (65). Provisional work in man has demonstrated the feasibility of delivering appropriate doses of beta radiation to a coronary artery, to date there is insufficient data to comment on the long-term success of this therapy. At present two methods of radiation delivery are being evaluated. Radioactive stents, which will provide an equal circumferential dose, and brachytherapy provided by a removable source delivered via a catheter. This technique has the advantage of retaining the radioactive source within a confined system, however, the problem of centering the catheter within the vessel and ensuring that an equal dose is delivered to all parts of the vessel may prove to be a technical limitation. The long-term effects of the use of high-dose local radiation are also unknown.

Temporary Stents

Permanent stents provide a continuous mechanical stimulus to the vessel wall following implantation. As detailed above, this is likely to contribute to the development of neointimal hyperplasia. Temporary stents will provide benefit at the time of PTCA by sealing dissection flaps and preventing vessel recoil, however, their temporary presence may reduce the unwanted effect of restenosis. Temporary stents can be considered in 3 forms.

Catheter Mounted Perfusion Balloons

In principle, a perfusion balloon acts as a temporary stent (66). However, they only provide limited flow to the distal vessel and do not allow blood to pass into side branches. Consequently, they can only be used for a limited time period.

ACS Flow Support Catheter

This stent is no longer available. It was a wire stent which provided temporary support with good distal and side branch perfusion. Overall clinical experience is fairly limited, with results from an observational study showing significant improvement in angiographic appearance in about 40% of cases (67).

Retrievable Temporary Stents

HARTS Device (Advanced Coronary Technologies)

This temporary stent employs the metallurgical thermo-elastic shape memory properties of nitinol (nickel-titanium alloy) (17). The stent is inserted in the martensitic form, and when deployed, in the usual fashion on a balloon mounted catheter. However, the stent can be recovered at a later procedure because of the properties of nitinol. Thus, if a coaxial balloon system is used to deliver a small volume of fluid (Ringer's solution) at the transition temperature, then the stent undergoes thermo-elastic phase change to a different crystalline format and collapses onto the retrieval catheter (68, 69). This can only be performed up to 6 weeks after the initial implantation because of fibrous overgrowth preventing removal (70). In a canine coronary model in which the deployment, retrieval and angiographic appearances of 78 stents were assessed, all stents were successfully deployed and removed, and mean vessel diameter remained enlarged after stent removal (69).

Experience in an animal model of local drug delivery with a polymer-coated removable metallic stent has been described (71). Forskolin exerted vasodilating and antiplatelet actions during the time of stent deployment, and tissue levels were shown to decline rapidly after stent removal 24 hours following their initial implantation.

Biodegradable Stents

It is well recognized that the presence of a metal stent provides a stimulus to the formation of neointimal hyperplasia (51). The concept of a temporary stent that provides sufficient support, and allows the possibility of local drug delivery to modify the biologic response to stent implantation, (but does not require a further procedure to remove it), is therefore attractive.

Biodegradable Mesh Stents

A number of polymers and stent designs have been tested in this role. Thus, self-expanding braided or mesh stents with a design similar to the Wallstent (72), and a number of balloon-expandable stents (either polymer alone or a composite of polymer and metal) have been described (73). Of the various polymers reported to date, poly-L-lactic acid (PLLA) and polyglycolic acid (PGA) in particular have been studied extensively. Results are variable.

In a polymer only stent of PLLA, a significant amount of neointima formation was seen (74), whereas with a composite PLLA/tantalum stent, no inflammatory response was identified (75). In a stent made from PGA tested in a canine coronary artery model, rapid biodegradation of polymer fibers was seen, with some foreign body reaction. However, stents in all 15 dogs remained patent at 2 months (76). An early study by Murphy et al. showed that it was technically feasible to deploy stents made of polyethylene terephthalate but that an exaggerated proliferative response was observed (77). A study in swine of a polymeric stent made of strands 150 μm in diameter, showed that at 2 weeks a significant degree of endothelialization of the artery was observed, but there were significant uncovered areas also. The inflammatory response seemed to be related to the rate of absorption of the stent, however the proliferative response was not excessive (78).

From a technical viewpoint, the prospect of biodegradable stents appears to be varied. Because they are made from a polymer, and the requirement for sufficient mechanical support is paramount, the thickness of the stent filaments is larger than for metal stents. This induces greater amounts of turbulence and consequently enhances the possibility of thrombosis. Other technical issues such as the mechanism of deployment, and means of sterilization without affecting the properties of the polymer have yet to be fully characterized. However, the possibility of using a polymer matrix to deliver drugs and other moderators of the biologic response locally is potentially exciting and a feature that distinguishes polymer stents from metal stents at present.

SPECIFIC CLINICAL STATES AND PROBLEMS: CASE EXAMPLES

It is apparent that the range of stents currently available is extensive. The manufacturers make a number of claims as to the relative merits of their product in comparison to others but during an interventional procedure a particular stent is usually chosen because of previous experience in the a similar clinical situation, rather than for theoretic reasons.

Below we give a few examples of the use of stents in our everyday practice. These examples have been selected because they illustrate some of the technical difficulties that the interventional cardiologist will encounter. It follows from above that it is seldom, if ever, the case that there will be only one choice of stent for a particular situation. However, in our experience **the principles of stenting such as length, trackability, conformability, access to a side branch, etc. should be considered when deciding upon the required stent for each individual case.**

Case #1 (Figures 32.1, 32.2)

A 47-year-old woman presenting with acute inferior myocardial infarction treated with streptokinase. Recurrence of chest pain resulted in early angiography. Normal left coronary artery.

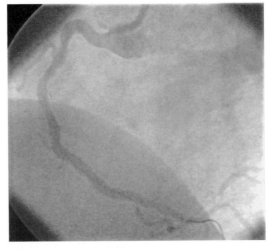

Figure 32.2. Postdeployment of 3.5 mm × 15 mm ACS Multilink stent (30 seconds at 14 bar).

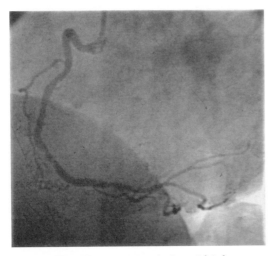

Figure 32.1. Severe stenosis in midright coronary artery.

Procedure

- A tortuous shepherd's crook proximal right coronary artery
- 8 F Judkins R4 guide catheter
- 0.014″ extra support guidewire
- Lesion predilated with 2.5 mm "Goldie" balloon

Author's note

Although the vessel is severely stenosed, the lesion is not long and therefore a standard length (15 mm) stent will be sufficient. The main issue in this case is the proximal tortuosity. The Judkins R4 gave good support, and an extra support guidewire was selected to further enhance support. An ACS multilink stent was selected because of its conformability and trackability, and because it was felt that this stent would have the required properties, once deployed, in particular, a low restenosis rate. The monorail delivery system was passed to the stenosis without difficulty, and the final angiogram confirms the satisfactory appearance of the stented vessel.

Case #2 (Figures 32.3, 32.4))

A 68-year-old woman with crescendo angina. Angiography: Normal right coronary artery. Mild diffuse disease in circumflex artery.

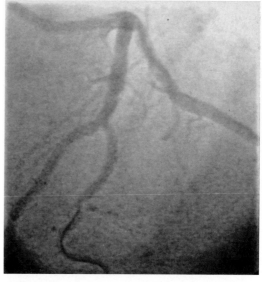

Figure 32.4. Final result after balloon inflation within stent; 0.014″ extra support guidewire in diagonal artery.

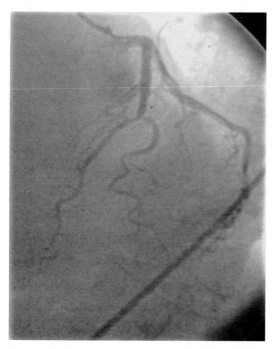

Figure 32.3. Severe stenosis in midleft anterior descending artery at bifurcation with diagonal.

Procedure

- 8 F Judkins L4 short tip guiding catheter
- 0.014″ extra support guidewire positioned in the left anterior descending *(LAD)* artery
- ACS Multilink 3.0 mm × 15 mm stent positioned in the LAD (across bifurcation), after predilation with 2.5 mm Schneider "Goldie" balloon
- 0.014″ extra support guidewire passed through the stent into the diagonal branch
- 2.5 mm "Goldie" balloon passed through stent and inflated (60 seconds at 8 bar) at the bifurcation stenosis

Author's note

It was felt that the diagonal branch was of sufficient size that it should not be "sacrificed" and that following stent deployment, balloon angioplasty and even stent deployment to the diagonal should be considered. An ACS Multilink stent was chosen because this allows the relatively easy passage of a guidewire, balloon and even a stent, through the stent into a side branch. In this case, the LAD was stented, the guidewire passed into the diagonal, and the balloon used for the LAD pre-dilation was used to dilate the bifurcational disease. It was not felt necessary to proceed to stenting of the diagonal artery.

Case #3 (Figures 32.5–32.7)

A 65-year-old man. Coronary artery bypass grafting 9 years previously. Angiography: Severe disease in all three native vessels. Satisfactory vein grafts to circumflex and left anterior descending arteries.

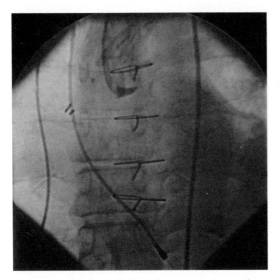

Figure 32.5. Occluded saphenous vein graft to intermediate artery

Procedure

- 8 F Judkins R4 guide catheter
- 0.014″ standard wire and 2.0 mm Scimed "Cobra" balloon

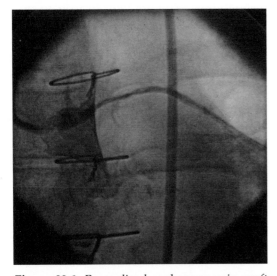

Figure 32.6. Recanalized saphenous vein graft with diffuse disease.

Procedure

- 0.014″ extra support wire inserted into saphenous vein graft via Cobra balloon

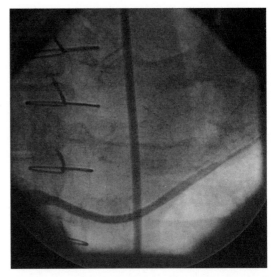

Figure 32.7. Final result after deployment of 4.5 mm × 44 mm Schneider Wallstent, and high-pressure inflation with 3.5 mm Schneider "Goldie" balloon (repeated inflations at 15 bar).

Author's note

The management of patients with severely stenosed, and even occluded saphenous vein grafts is an increasing problem for the interventional cardiologist. In this case, recent angiography had demonstrated severe stenoses at the ostium and in the body of the graft to the intermediate artery. When the patient presented for elective PTCA to this graft it was occluded. In this situation, it is often difficult to get a satisfactory position with the guide catheter. Frequently, this may only be achieved after a wire is advanced down the graft. A standard wire was required to cross the occlusion. Once the wire was passed down the graft, an over-the-wire balloon was also advanced and the standard wire exchanged for a 300 cm extra support wire. Unless necessary, we do not predilate severely diseased SVG because of the likelihood of embolization of degenerate material and the creation of a no-reflow situation.

We chose a long Wallstent to cover as much of the graft as possible, including the ostium. Although positioning the Wallstent requires more experience than using balloon-mounted stents, the advantages of large diameter, easier trackability and small pore size make it particularly suitable for this situation. Once deployed, high pressure balloon inflation can be performed to achieve good apposition of the stent to the wall of the vein graft.

Case #4 (Figures 32.8–32.10)

A 55-year-old man with crescendo angina, admitted for elective PTCA. Normal left coronary artery.

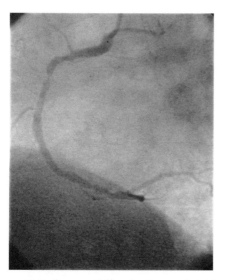

Figure 32.8. Severe, diffusely diseased right coronary artery.

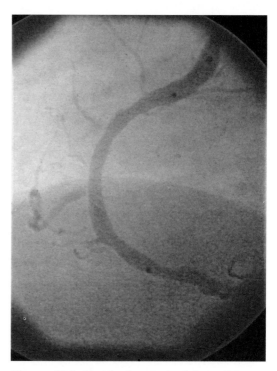

Figure 32.9. Postdeployment of long 5.0 mm Schneider Magic Wallstent.

Procedure

- 8 F Judkins R4 guiding catheter
- 0.014'' exchange length extra support guidewire
- Predilation with 3.0 mm × 20 mm ACS ''Concorde'' balloon

Procedure

- High pressure inflation with 4.5 mm Scimed ''Big'' balloon.

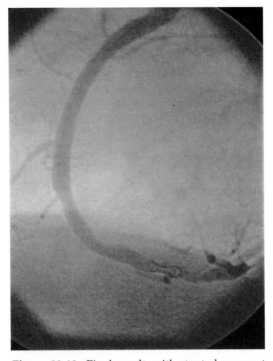

Figure 32.10. Final result, with stented segment of the vessel oversized in relation to the distal right coronary artery.

Author's note

It is generally accepted that restenosis is more likely if atheromatous disease is left uncovered at a stent margin. In this case, in addition to the long segment of diseased vessel there is proximal tortuosity. Although a long balloon-mounted stent may have been used, it was felt that it would be easier to deliver a self-expanding stent. The Magic Wallstent tracks easily and can cover long segments of diseased vessel. It shortens less than the classic Wallstent, and precise positioning of the stent at the ostium of the RCA was considered to be important. Post-deployment high pressure balloon inflation improves the angiographic appearance, decreases the possibility of stent thrombosis and may decrease the likelihood of restenosis.

Case #5 (Figures 32.11, 32.12)

A 60-year-old man. Acute inferior myocardial infarction, thrombolyzed but persistent chest pain and ST elevation. Angiography: Normal left coronary artery

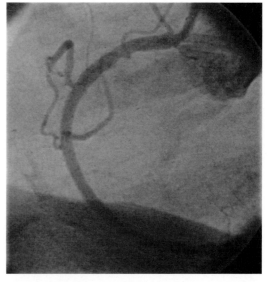

Figure 32.12. Final result. Reconstructed right coronary artery.

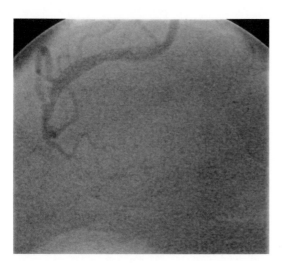

Figure 32.11. Occluded right coronary artery.

Procedure

- 8F Judkins R4 guide catheter
- 0.014″ high torque floppy guidewire
- 3.0 mm × 20 mm Scimed "Bandit" balloon inflated ×2
- 32 mm × 3.5 mm Scimed NIR stent deployed (at 12 bar) to distal right coronary artery on 36 mm × 3.5 mm Scimed "Viva Primo" balloon
- 15 mm × 3.5 mm ACS Multilink stent deployed in proximal right coronary artery at 14 bar

Author's note

The lack of proximal tortuosity and satisfactory guide catheter position were felt sufficiently positive characteristics in this case that it was not considered necessary to change to an extra support guidewire. A long NIR stent was chosen because of its conformability once deployed, and because it was unlikely that we would not be able to deliver the stent to the required part of the vessel. The NIR stent tracked easily and a satisfactory angiographic appearance was achieved. However, this highlighted the diffuse disease of the proximal vessel and it was felt that this area should also be stented. An ACS Multilink was chosen, but any tube stent would have been likely to give a favorable end result.

Case #6 (Figures 32.13, 32.14)

A 65-year-old man with unstable angina. Single vessel disease (right coronary artery).

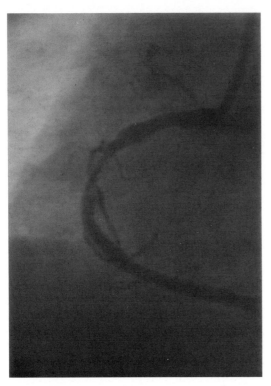

Figure 32.13. Severe long stenosis in right coronary artery.

Procedure

- GR-II stent with high-pressure inflation.

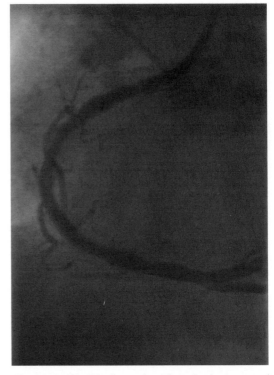

Figure 32.14. Final result: After deployment of 40 mm × 3.5 mm Cook GR-II stent.

Authors' note

There is a long segment of disease that required to be covered. Although the proximal vessel is not particularly tortuous, a coil stent is flexible and conforms to the vessel geometry. In the presence of diffuse disease and in the absence of severe discreet stenoses, the GR-II stent was chosen. This tracked easily down the artery and a good angiographic result was obtained.

References

1. Gruentzig A. Transluminal dilatation of coronary artery stenosis. Lancet 1978;1:263.
2. Carrel A. Results of the permanent intubation of the thoracic aorta. Surg Gyn Obstet 1912;16:245–248.
3. Dotter CT. Transluminally placed coil spring arterial tube grafts: long term patency in canine popliteal artery. Invest Rad 1969;4:329–332.
4. Sigwart U, Puel J, Mirkovitch V, et al. Intravascular stents to prevent occlusion and restenosis after transluminal angioplasty. N Engl J Med 1987;316:701–706.
5. Serruys PW, Strauss BH, Beatt KJ, et al. Angiographic follow-up after placement of a self-expanding coronary artery stent. N Engl J Med 1991;324:13–17.
6. Serruys PW, de Jaegere P, Kiemeneil C, et al. A comparison of balloon expandable stent implantation with balloon angioplasty in patients with coronary artery disease. N Engl J Med 1994;331:489–495.
7. Fischman DL, Leon MB, Baim DS, et al. A randomized comparison of coronary stent placement and balloon angioplasty in the treatment of coronary artery disease. N Engl J Med 1994;331:496-501.
8. Nath FC, Muller DWM, Ellis SG, et al. Thrombosis of a flexible coil coronary stent: frequency, predictors and clinical outcome. J Am Coll Cardiol 1993;21:622–627.
9. Karas SP, Gravanis MB, Santoian EC, et al. Coronary intimal proliferation after balloon injury and stenting in swine: an animal model of restenosis. J Am Coll Cardiol 1992;20:467–474.
10. Schomig A, Neumann F-J, Kastrati A, et al. A randomized comparison of antiplatelet and anticoagulant therapy after the placement of coronary artery stents. N Engl J Med 1996;334:1084–1089.
11. Karrillon GJ, Morice MC, Benveniste E, et al. Intracoronary stent implantation without ultrasound guidance and with replacement of conventional anticoagulation by antiplatelet therapy. Circulation 1996;94:1519–1527.
12. Scott NA, Robinson KA, Nunes GL, et al. Comparison of the thrombogenicity of stainless steel and tantalum coronary stents. Am Heart J 1995;129:866–872.
13. Rogers C, Edelman ER. Endovascular stent design dictates experimental restenosis and thrombosis. Circulation 1995;91:2995–3001.
14. Urban P, Sigwart U, Golf S, et al. Intravascular stenting for stenosis of aortocoronary venous bypass grafts. J Am Coll Cardiol 1989;13:1085–1089.
15. Kelly PA, Kurbaan A, Sigwart U. Total endovascular reconstruction of occluded saphenous vein grafts using coronary or peripheral Wallstents. Circulation 1996;94(Suppl I):258.
16. Ozaki Y, Violaris AG, Hamburger J, et al. Short- and long-term clinical and quantitative angiographic results with the new, less shortening Wallstent for vessel reconstruction in chronic total occlusion: a quantitative angiographic study. J Am Coll Cardiol 1996;28:354–360.
17. Shetky LM. Shape memory alloys. Sci Am 1979;241:74–83.
18. Sheth S, Litvack F, Dev V, et al. Subacute thrombosis and vascular injury resulting from slotted-tube nitinol and stainless steel stents in a rabbit carotid artery model. Circulation 1996;94:1733–1740.
19. Beyar R, Henry M. Removable self-expanding nitinol coil stent: initial report on in vitro, canine and human results. J Am Coll Cardiol 1993;21:439A.
20. Grenadier E, Shofti R, Beyar M, et al. Self-expandable and highly flexible nitinol stent: immediate and long term results in dogs. Am Heart J 1994;128:870–878.
21. Laeveren F, Zschegg H. The Angiomed memotherm stent. In: Sigwart U, ed. Endoluminal stenting. Philadelphia: WB Saunders, 1996: 246–248.
22. Liu MW, Voorhees WD III, Agrawal S, et al. Stratification of the risk of thrombosis after intracoronary stenting for threatened or acute closure complicating coronary balloon angioplasty: a Cook registry study. Am Heart J 1995;130:8–13.
23. Dorros G, Bates MC, Iyer S, et al. The use of Gianturco-Roubin flexible metallic coronary stents in old saphenous vein grafts: in-hospital outcome and 7 day angiographic patency. Eur Heart J 1994;15:1456–1462.
24. Roubin GS, King SB III, Douglas JS Jr, et al. Intracoronary stenting during percutaneous transluminal coronary angioplasty. Circulation 1990;81:92–100.
25. Hirshfield JW, Schwartz JS, Jugo R. Restenosis after coronary angioplasty: a multivariate statistical model to relate lesion and procedure variables to restenosis. J Am Coll Cardiol 1991;18:647–656.
26. Goods CM, Al-Shaibi KF, Yadav SS, et al. Utilization of the coronary balloon-expandable coil stent without anticoagulation or intravascular ultrasound. Circulation 1996;93:1803–1808.
27. White CJ, Ramee SR, Banks AK, et al. A new balloon-expandable tantalum coil stent: angiographic patency and histologic findings in an atherogenic swine model. J Am Coll Cardiol 1992;19:870–876.
28. Vogt P, Eeckhout E, Stauffer JC, et al. Stent shortening and elongation: pitfalls with the Wiktor coronary endoprosthesis. Cathet Cardiovasc Diagn 1994;31:233–235.
29. de Jaegere PP, Serruys PW, Bertrand M, et al. Wiktor stent implantation in patients with restenosis following balloon angioplasty of a native coronary artery. Am J Cardiol 1992;69:598–602.
30. Goy J-J, Eeckhout E, Stauffer JC, et al. Emergency endoluminal stenting for abrupt vessel closure following coronary angioplasty: a randomised comparison of the Wiktor and Palmaz-Schatz stents. Cathet Cardiovasc Diagn 1995;34:128–132.
31. de Jaegere PP, Serruys PW, Bertrand M, et al. Wiktor stent implantation in patients with restenosis following balloon angioplasty of a native coronary artery. Am J Cardiol 1992;69:598–602.
32. Penn IM, Barbeau G, Brown RIG, et al. Initial human implants with a flexible radio-opaque tantalum stent. J Am Coll Cardiol 1995;228A:773–776.
33. Hamasaki N, Nosaka H, Nobuyoshi M. Initial experience of Cordis stent implantation. J Am Coll Cardiol 1995;329A:967–917.
34. Hijazi ZM, Homoud M, Aronovitz MJ, et al. A new

platinum balloon-expandable stent (Angiostent) mounted on a high pressure balloon: acute and late results in an atherogenic swine model. Journal of Invasive Cardiology 1995;7:127–134.

35. Descheerder IK, Wang K, Kerdsinchai P, et al. Clinical and angiographic experience with coronary stenting using the Freedom stent. Journal of Invasive Cardiology 1996;8:418–427.

36. Schatz RA, Palmaz JC, Tio FO, et al. Balloon-expandable intra-coronary stents in the adult dog. Circulation 1987;76:450-457.

37. Schatz RA. An introduction to intravascular stents. Cardiol Clinic 1988;6:357–372.

38. Schatz RA, Baim DS, Leon M, et al. Clinical experience with the Palmaz-Schatz coronary stent. Circulation 1991;83:148–161.

39. Colombo A, Hall P, Nakamura S, et al. Intracoronary stenting without anticoagulation accomplished with intravascular ultrasound guidance. Circulation 1995;91:1676–1688.

40. Fajadet J, Marco J, Cassagneau B, et al. Multiple intra-coronary balloon expandable stent: early experience. Eur Heart J 1990;11:370.

41. Fajadet J, Marco J, Cassagneau B, et al. Coronary stenting with the Palmaz-Schatz stent: the Clinique Pasteur Interventional Cardiology Unit experience. In: Sigwart U, Frank GI, eds. Coronary stents. Berlin, Heidelberg, New York: Springer-Verlag, 1992:57–77.

42. Colombo A, Goldberg SL, Almagor Y, et al. A novel strategy for stent deployment in the treatment of acute or threatened closure complicating balloon coronary angioplasty. J Am Coll Cardiol 1993;22:1887–1991.

43. Eeckhout E, van Melle G, Stauffer J-C, et al. Can early closure and restenosis be predicted from clinical, procedural and angiographic variables at the time of intervention? Br Heart J 1995;74:592–597.

44. George G, Erbel R, Ge T, et al. Intravascular ultrasound after stent implantation: can stent recoil or compression occur? Eur Heart J 1992;13:308–312.

45. Sarembock IL, Laveau PJ, Sigal SL, et al. Influence of inflation pressure and balloon size on the development of intimal hyperplasia after balloon angioplasty. Circulation 1989;80:1029-1033.

46. Schwartz RS, Huber KC, Murphy JG, et al. Restenosis and the proportional neointimal response to coronary artery injury: results in the porcine model. J Am Coll Cardiol 1992;19:267–271.

47. Sigwart U, Khosravi F, Virmani R, et al. Bronco: ein neuer, balloon-expandierbarer, flexibler stent. Z Kardiol 1993;71:219–224.

48. Hall P, Colombo A, Almagor Y, et al. Preliminary experience with intravascular ultrasound guided Palmaz-Schatz coronary stenting. Journal of Interventional Cardiology 1994;7:141–159.

49. van der Giessen W, Emanuelsson H, Dawkins D, et al. Six month clinical outcome and angiographic follow-up of the West study. Eur Heart J 1996;(Suppl 17):2219.

50. Ozaki Y, Keane D, Ruygrok P, et al. Acute clinical and angiographic results with the new AVE micro coronary stent in bail out management. Am J Cardiol 1995;76:112–116.

51. Roubin GS, Robinson KA, King SB III, et al. Early

and late results of intracoronary arterial stenting after coronary angioplasty in dogs. Circulation 1987:76:891–897.

52. Sigwart U. Coronary stents: will they survive? In: Sigwart U, Frank GI, eds. Coronary stents. Berlin, Heidelberg, New York: Springer-Verlag, 1992:169–177.

53. Edelman ER, Adams DH, Karnovsky MJ. Effects of controlled adventitial heparin delivery on smooth muscle cell proliferation following endothelial injury. Proc Natl Acad Sci USA 1991;87:3773–3777.

54. Rogers C, Edelman ER. Controlled release of heparin reduces neointimal hyperplasia in stents in rabbit arteries: ramifications for local therapy. Journal of Interventional Cardiology 1992;5:195–202.

55. Hoefling B, Huehns TY. Intravascular local drug delivery after angioplasty. Eur Heart J 1995;16:437–440.

56. Morimoto S, Mizuno Y, Hiramitsu S, et al. Restenosis after percutaneous transluminal angioplasty in human beings. N Engl J Med 1981;305:382–386.

57. Cheeseboro JH, Lam JYT, Badimon L, et al. Restenosis after arterial angioplasty: a hemorrheological response to injury. Am J Cardiol 1987;60:10B-16B.

58. Bailey SR, Paige S, Lunn AC, et al. Heparin coating of endovascular stents decreases subacute thrombosis in a rabbit model. Circulation 1992;86(Suppl I):I-186.

59. Serruys PW, Emanuelson H, van der Giessen W, et al. Heparin-coated Palmaz-Schatz stents in human coronary arteries. Early outcome of the BENESTENT-II pilot study. Circulation 1996;93:412–422.

60. Holmes DR, Camrud AR, Jorgenson MA, et al. Polymeric stenting in the porcine coronary artery model: differential outcome of exogenous fibrin sleeves versus polyurethane-coated stents. J Am Coll Cardiol 1994;24:525–531.

61. Aggraval RK, Ireland DC, Ezekowitz MD, et al. Antiplatelet glycoprotein IIb/IIIa antibody adsorbed onto polymer coated stents reduces platelet deposition and abolishes cyclical flow variation. Eur Heart J 1995;16:1406A.

62. Pocock SJ, Henderson RA, Rickards AF, et al. Meta-analysis of randomised trials comparing coronary angioplasty with bypass surgery. Lancet 1995;346:1184–1189.

63. Waksman R, Robinson KA, Crocker IR, et al. Endovascular low dose irradiation inhibits neointima formation after coronary artery balloon injury in swine: a possible role for radiation therapy in restenosis prevention. Circulation 1995;91:1533–1539.

64. Wiedermann JG, Marboe C, Schwartz A, et al. Intracoronary irradiation reduces restenosis after balloon angioplasty in a porcine model. J Am Coll Cardiol 1994;23:1491–1498.

65. Laird JR, Carter AJ, Kufs WM, et al. Inhibition of neointimal proliferation with low-dose irradiation from a beta-particle emitting stent. Circulation 1996;93:529–536.

66. Hinohara T, Simpson JB, Phillips HR, et al. Transluminal catheter reperfusion: a new technique to reestablish blood flow after coronary occlusion during percutaneous transluminal coronary angioplasty. Am J Cardiol 1986;57:684–686.

67. Whitlow P, Gaspard P, Kent K, et al. Improvement

of coronary dissection with a removal flow support catheter. J Am Coll Cardiol 1992;19:217.

68. Mehran JK, Neal LE, Robert L, et al. Implantation and recovery of balloon delivered stents. J Am Coll Cardiol 1992;19:218–223.

69. Eigler NL, Khorsandi MJ, Forrester JS, et al. Implantation and recovery of temporary metallic stents in canine coronary arteries. J Am Coll Cardiol 1993;22:1207–1213.

70. Khorsandi MJ, Eigler NL, Lambert T, et al. Temporary stenting with heat activated recoverable temporary stent: implantation up to 6 weeks. Circulation 1992;86:I-800.

71. Lambert TL, Dev V, Rechavia E, et al. Localized arterial wall drug delivery from a polymer-coated removable metallic stent. Kinetics, distribution and bioactivity of forskolin. Circulation 1994;90: 1003–1011.

72. Zidar JP, Lincoff AM, Stack RS. In: Topol EJ, ed. Textbook of interventional cardiology, 2nd ed. Philadelphia: WB Saunders, 1994:784–802.

73. Tanguay J, Kruse KR, Phillips HR III, et al. The polymer stent. In: Sigwart U, ed. Endoluminal stenting. Philadelphia: WB Saunders, 1996: 216–224.

74. Lincoff AM, van der Giessen WJ, Schwartz RS, et al. Biodegradable and biostable polymers may both cause vigorous inflammatory responses when implanted in the porcine coronary artery [Abstract]. J Am Coll Cardiol 1993;21(Suppl 1):179.

75. Lincoff AM, Furst JG, Ellis SG, et al. Sustained local drug delivery by a novel intravascular eluting stent to prevent restenosis in the porcine coronary artery [Abstract]. J Am Coll Cardiol 1994;23 (Suppl 1):18.

76. Susawa T, Shiraki K, Shimizu Y. Biodegradable intracoronary stents in adult dogs [Abstract]. J Am Coll Cardiol 1993;21 (Suppl 1):483.

77. Murphy JG, Schwartz RS, Edwards WD, et al. Percutaneous polymeric stents in porcine coronary arteries. Initial experience with polyethylene terephthalate stents. Circulation 1992;86: 1596–1604.

78. Van der Giessen WJ, Slager CJ, van Beusekom H, et al. Development of a polymer endovascular prosthesis and its implantation in porcine arteries. Journal of Interventional Cardiology 1992;5: 175–185.

33
Angiographic and Clinical Results Using Coronary Stents

Sheldon Goldberg, MD
David L. Fischman, MD
Michael P. Savage, MD

INTRODUCTION

Metallic coronary stents were introduced into clinical cardiology to improve on long-term patency compared with standard balloon angioplasty. A plethora of different stents are being developed (see Chapters 31 and 32), however, the clinician should keep in mind several basic principles in evaluating the results of each particular stent. The device should (*a*) improve on the acute results of percutaneous transluminal coronary angioplasty (PTCA); (*b*) restenosis should be reduced; (*c*) complications related to the procedure should be acceptably low; and (*d*) stent implantation should be cost-effective in the long term. In this chapter, we describe the clinical and angiographic outcomes in a variety of patient populations and examine results for established and expanding indications for stent implantation.

STENTS FOR ABRUPT OR THREATENED CLOSURE

When balloon angioplasty results in threatened or abrupt closure, as has been de-

scribed in 2 to 10% (1–4) of angioplasty attempts, the risk of acute myocardial infarction (MI) and death rise substantially, even when emergent surgery is undertaken (5–7). An important use of the metallic implants has been to provide a predictable, stable lumen and thereby limit myocardial necrosis and avoid emergency bypass operations in this setting.

Several early studies have reported on the outcomes when stents are placed for this "bail-out" indication. Sigwart et al. (8) first reported encouraging results in a series of 11 patients in whom the self-expanding Wallstent (Schneider, Zurich, Switzerland) was placed. Subsequently, Hermann et al. examined the outcomes of emergency stenting in 56 consecutive patients treated with the Palmaz-Schatz (Johnson and Johnson Interventional Systems, Warren, NJ) stent between 1988–1991 (9). Whereas initial success rate was high at 98%, by 1 month, the clinical success rate had declined to only 71% with subsequent stent thrombosis complicating the clinical course in 16% of patients. Patients with frank abrupt closure were at higher risk for subsequent stent thrombosis. Colombo et al. reported outcomes in patients in whom single, multiple, or half stents were employed to seal coronary dissections (10). Although the primary success rate was 88%, subsequent major car-

Acute vs. Elective Stenting
Major cardiac events* at 90 days

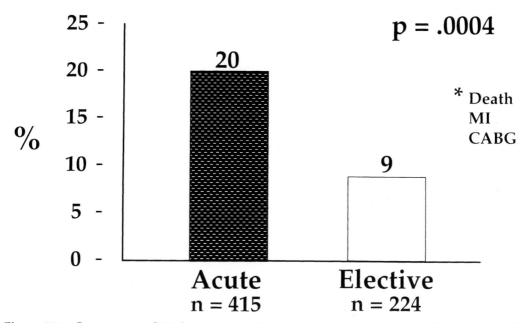

Figure 33.1. Comparison of 90-day major cardiac event rates (death, myocardial infarction [*MI*], coronary artery bypass graft surgery [*CABG*]) when the Gianturco-Roubin stent was placed for the acute bailout situation, versus elective implantation. (Adapted from Sutton JM, Ellis SG, Roubin GS, et al. Major clinical events after coronary stenting. The multicenter registry of acute and elective Gianturco-Roubin stent placement. The Gianturco-Roubin Intracoronary Stent Investigator Group. Circulation 1994;89:1126–1137.)

diac events occurred in 12.5% of patients at 10-month follow-up.

Results with the Gianturco-Roubin coil stent were assessed by Sutton et al., who compared elective placement (n = 224) with emergency stenting (n = 415) (11). All patients were treated with aspirin, heparin, and postprocedure warfarin. A marked difference was seen in the composite clinical end point, which included death, MI, or coronary artery bypass graft surgery at 90 days, between the emergent and elective groups (20 versus 9%, P = .0004) (Fig. 33.1). The incidence of acute myocardial infarction was 5% in the emergent group and 0.5% in the elective patients (P = .002), whereas the bypass surgery rate was 12 versus 6%

for the emergent and elective groups, respectively (P = .02). Thus, **bail-out stenting appears to be highly effective in salvaging failed angioplasty procedures.** However, complications associated with stenting appear to be significantly higher with emergent, bail-out procedures than with elective use.

It should be emphasized that these studies occurred in the early era of stent implantation under the most unstable circumstances, before the importance of current deployment techniques and optimal antithrombotic therapy were fully understood. Several caveats need to be kept in mind when extensive coronary dissection occurs. First, the clinician should make every attempt to scaffold the disrupted segment completely and assure proper inflow and outflow. Second, current high-pressure deployment (vide infra) should be used with proper sizing of the devices in relation to the reference vessel, as undersizing is a strong risk factor for subsequent thrombosis (11). Finally, optimization of the antithrombotic regimen (see below) may attenuate the late complications of emergency stent placement. Using current techniques, it is estimated that more than 90% of patients with abrupt or threatened closure can avoid a major cardiac complication.

Recently, the Canadian TASC-II (Trial of Angioplasty and Stents in Canada) randomized 43 patients with failed PTCA to Palmaz-Schatz stent or prolonged autoperfusion balloon angioplasty. The results showed higher clinical success (90 versus 47%) and superior angiographic results in patients receiving stents (11A). Several other randomized trials are ongoing (see Chapter 31).

STENTS TO REDUCE RESTENOSIS RATES

The clinical utility of stents in maintaining long-term arterial patency was examined by investigators in the initial Palmaz-Schatz stent registry. Three hundred consecutive patients with discrete lesions requiring a single, 15 mm stent in large ($\geq$ 3.0 mm) native vessels were enrolled in this study. Angiographic follow-up was performed at 6 months in 90% of eligible patients, and clinical events were assessed after 1 year in all patients (12). Using a pharmacologic regimen of postprocedure heparin and warfarin in conjunction with low molecular weight dextran and aspirin, the stent thrombosis rate was 4.7% at 5 $\pm$ 3 days after implantation. Restenosis by the binary definition ($\geq$ 50% diameter narrowing at 6-month angiographic follow-up) occurred in 14% of new lesions compared with 39% of restenotic lesions ($P < .001$). In addition, 87% of patients with new lesions were free of major cardiac events, whereas 77% of patients with restenotic lesions were event-free at 1-year follow-up. These encouraging registry results led to randomized studies directly comparing stent placement with balloon angioplasty in the treatment of new lesions.

Two landmark randomized trials were performed comparing placement of the Palmaz-Schatz stent with balloon angioplasty: The **ST**ent **RES**tenosis **S**tudy (STRESS) and the **BE**lgium **NE**therland **STENT** (BENESTENT) trial (13, 14). In STRESS, patients with new discrete lesions in larger (3–4 mm) native coronary arteries were randomly assigned to undergo either elective stent placement or elective balloon angioplasty with stent availability for bail-out. The primary end point of the trial was angiographic restenosis at 6 months by the 50% or greater binary definition. Major cardiac events and target lesion revascularization were tabulated as well as the incidence of bleeding and vascular complications and length of hospital stay. After the original STRESS I study, which enrolled 410 patients, enrollment continued for a total of 596 patients (STRESS I + II) and clinical follow-up was performed at 1 year (15).

Analysis of the angiographic results showed that patients' reference vessels were well-matched at approximately 3.0 mm (Fig. 33.2). Baseline minimal luminal diameter (MLD) was also similar for the two groups. Stent implantation was associated with a larger final MLD by nearly 0.5 mm. At 6 months (Fig. 33.3), patients randomized to stenting continued to have a larger MLD at follow-up. The restenosis rate was 45.5% in the PTCA group, and it was significantly reduced to 30.4% in the stent group (Fig. 33.4), a relative reduction of 33%. This reduction in restenosis was accompanied by a significant reduction in 1-year clinical events, including symptom-driven target vessel revascularization (Fig. 33.5).

In BENESTENT, 516 patients with stable angina and new lesions in large, native coronary arteries were similarly randomized to stent placement or to balloon angioplasty. Again, restenosis was reduced from 33 to 22%, while the composite clinical end point was also lowered from 30 to 20% (Fig. 33.6), mainly as a result of a reduced need for repeat PTCA in the patients randomized to stent implantation.

The results in the STRESS and BENESTENT trials (Table 33.1) were achieved, however, at the price of unacceptable rates

Stress I+II
Cumulative Frequency Distributions

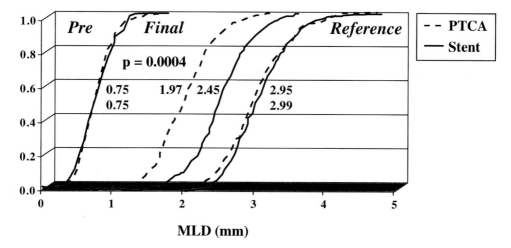

Figure 33.2. Cumulative frequency curves of minimal lumen diameter. The reference vessels are similar, as are the baseline (preprocedure minimal lumen diameter). Immediately following the procedure, the group assigned to stenting had a significantly greater minimal lumen diameter compared with the balloon group. (Adapted from Wong SC, Zidar JP, Chuang YC, et al. Stents improve late clinical outcomes: results from the combined (I + II) stent REStenosis Study. Circulation 1995;92:I-281.)

of stent thrombosis (2.6 to 3.5%), bleeding and vascular complications (7.3 and 13.5%), and prolonged length of in-hospital stay (5.8–8.5 days) compared with balloon angioplasty. It should be noted that in both trials, the implantation technique had not yet been standardized with respect to balloon inflation pressure. Furthermore, an intense anticoagulation regimen was employed, which consisted of a combination of preprocedure low molecular weight dextran and aspirin, intra- and postprocedure heparin, and postprocedure warfarin for 1 month along with long-term aspirin. Preliminary results from 452 patients randomized in the START (Stent versus Angioplasty Restenosis Trial) and 270 patients randomized in the Trial of Angioplasty and Stents in Canada (TASC-I) also show that restenosis rates are lower in stented patients.

Because the stent is a permanent im-

plant, the long-term safety and efficacy are of particular concern. Accordingly, long-term angiographic patency has been studied and the findings show no temporal delay in restenosis when stents are placed in native coronary arteries and no evidence of perforation, migration, or aneurysm formation (16). Thus, Kimura et al. (16), assessed angiographic and clinical results up to 3 years. Minimal lumen diameter at baseline, immediately after stent placement; at 6 months, 1 year, and 3 years was measured (Fig. 33.7). Importantly, an actual improvement was found in MLD at 3 years compared with the 6-month angiographic findings. These investigators concluded that, from a clinical standpoint, **borderline lesions in relatively asymptomatic patients were best left alone, if patients are recatheterized at 6 months and found to have only moderate degrees of intimal hyperplasia.**

Stress I+II
Cumulative Frequency Distributions

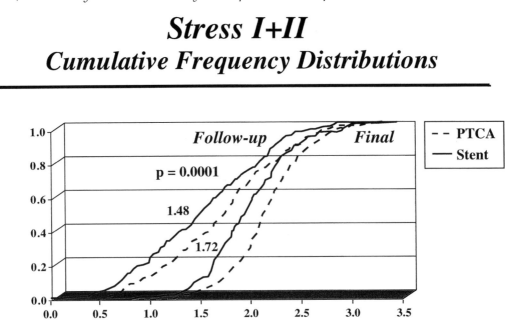

Figure 33.3. Cumulative frequency curves showing 6-month follow-up results for stents and angioplasty. Note that the stented group continues to show a significantly larger minimal lumen diameter at 6 months. (Adapted from Wong SC, Zidar JP, Chuang YC, et al. Stents improve late clinical outcomes: results from the combined (I + II) STent REStenosis Study. Circulation 1995;92:I-281.)

Late Clinical Outcomes: Stress I+II
Follow-Up Angiographic Findings

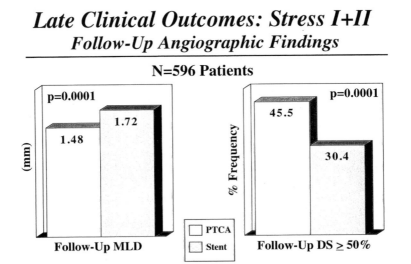

Figure 33.4. Follow-up minimal lumen diameter and angiographic restenosis rates. A 33% relative reduction was found in restenosis from 45.5% in the balloon group to 30.4% in the stent group. (Adapted from Wong SC, Zidar JP, Chuang YC, et al. Stents improve late clinical outcomes: results from the combined (I + II) STent REStenosis Study. Circulation 1995;92:I-281.)

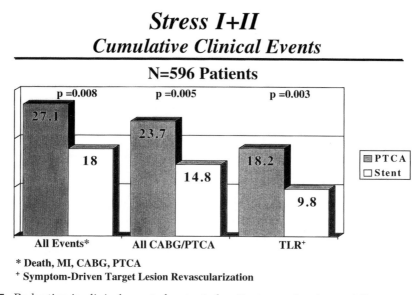

Figure 33.5. Reduction in clinical events for stented patients noted at 1-year follow-up. (*, Death, MI, CABG, PTCA; +, symptom-driven target lesion revascularization.) (Adapted from Wong SC, Zidar JP, Chuang YC, et al. Stents improve late clinical outcomes: results from the combined (I + II) STent REStenosis Study. Circulation 1995;92:I-281.)

IMPROVEMENTS IN DEPLOYMENT TECHNIQUE

The major drawback of stent implantation until the mid 1990s was the rate of subacute thrombosis. This complication, which occurred on average 5–6 days after stent placement, was associated with myocardial infarction and death in a large proportion of cases. That the complex problem of stent thrombosis could be alleviated by optimizing strut apposition to the vessel wall was first demonstrated by Colombo, et al. (17), who performed ultrasound-guided high pressure expansion of stents after initial deployment (Fig. 33.8). The ultrasound criteria used to judge optimal stent expansion in-

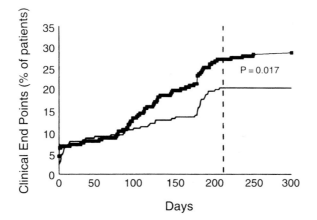

Figure 33.6. Reduction in composite clinical event rate from BENESTENT I in stented patients. (Reprinted with permission from Serruys P, De Jaegere P, Kiemeneji F, et al. A comparison of balloon expandable-stent implantation with balloon angioplasty in patients with coronary artery disease. N Engl J Med 1994;331:489–495.)

Table 33.1.
Randomized Trials of Single Stents for New Lesions in Native Coronary Arteries (14, 15)

	Stress I + II (n = 596)			Benestent (n = 516)		
	PTCA	STENT	P	PTCA	STENT	P
Restenosis (%)	45.5	30.4	0.0001	32	22	0.02
Clinical Events (%)	27.1	18	0.008	30	20	0.017
SAT (%)	—	2.6	—	—	3.5	—
Bleeding/vascular (%)	4.8	8.5	0.07	3.1	13.5	0.001
Length of stay (days)	2.9	9.3	0.0001	3.1	8.5	0.001

cluded (*a*) qualitative assessment of strut apposition to the vessel wall; (*b*) a quantitative criterion for the stented segment of 60% of the average of the proximal and distal cross-sectional areas (CSA) (this was later changed to an intrastent CSA equal to or larger than the distal reference vessel to assure adequate stent outflow); and (*c*) the absence of a significant lesion at the stent margins, defined as a CSA stenosis greater than 60% of the adjacent reference segment. Using strict criteria for ultrasound-guided placement, and an average inflation pressure of 15 atm, these investigators also eliminated postprocedure heparin and warfarin and used a simplified antiplatelet regimen of aspirin and ticlopidine (Table 33.2). The stent thrombosis rate was reduced to 1.6%

with this methodology. Subsequently, other investigators have performed high-pressure inflation without intravascular ultrasound guidance and have found similarly low thrombosis rates, with a marked reduction in bleeding and vascular complications.

IMPROVEMENTS IN ADJUNCTIVE PHARMACOLOGIC REGIMEN

A variety of regimens have been used in conjunction with stent implantation. The previously discussed regimen, which used postprocedure heparin and warfarin in addition to aspirin, was associated with stent thrombosis rates ranging from 2.6 to 4.7%,

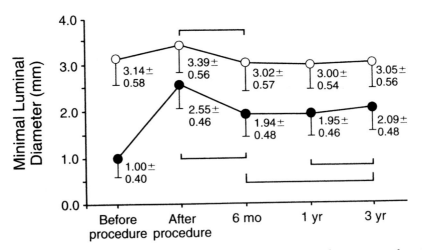

Figure 33.7. Plot of minimal lumen diameter at baseline, after stent placement and at 6 month, 1 year, and 3 years after the procedure. Note regression of intimal hyperplasia at 3 years. ○, Reference segment; ●, Stented segment; points linked by brackets (⌐‾⌐ or ∟__∟) are p < 0.001. (Reprinted with permission from Kimura T, Yokoi H, Nakagawa Y, et al. Three-year follow-up after implantation of metallic coronary artery stents. N Engl J Med 1996;334:561–566.)

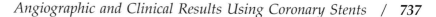

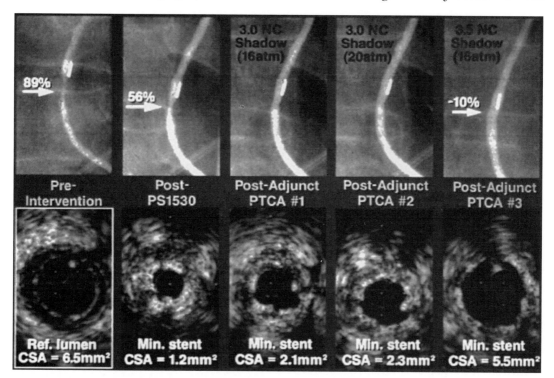

Figure 33.8. Example of ultrasound-guided stent deployment. Note that an angiographically satisfactory image (PTCA 1 and 2) is accompanied by suboptimal strut expansion by IVUS. Use of a larger balloon at high pressure fully expands the struts and increases the stent cross-sectional area from 2.1–6.5 mm. (Courtesy of G. Mintz: Washington Hospital Center.)

Table 33.2.
Outcomes Utilizing Ultrasound-Guided Stent Placement (17)

Stent Deployment Technique	
Coronary stenting without anticoagulation using IVUS guidance	
359 patients/452 lesions/ 864 stents	
IVUS criteria	
Stent CSA CSA of (Prox + Distal)/2 or	
Stent CSA CSA of distal vessel	
Inflation pressure	14.9 ± 3.0 atm
Balloon/artery ratio	1.17 ± 1.9
Stent thrombosis	5 (1.6%)
Death/MI/CAGB	1.9%/5.7%/6.4%
Any event at 6 months	21.7%

whereas bleeding and vascular complications occurred in up to 13.5%. In the multicenter French Registry, Morice et al. used a simplified regimen of aspirin (100 mg/day) + ticlopidine (250 mg/day), and low molecular weight heparin was given for progressively shorter periods in four phases: for 1 month, 2 weeks, 1 week, and finally omission of low molecular weight heparin. Of 2900 patients who had stent placement, thrombosis occurred in only 51 (1.8%) and bleeding and vascular complications in 55 (1.9%). In that study, predictors of stent thrombosis included small stent size (< 3.0 mm), use of stenting as a bail-out procedure, presence of unstable angina or acute MI, and low volume operators (18).

In the STRESS III trial, the investigators used the identical entry criteria as in the original STRESS study, but required high-pressure deployment of 14 atm or greater in conjunction with aspirin (325 mg/day)

+ ticlopidine (500 mg/day) for 1 month. Compared with the original STRESS trial, follow-up of 239 patients at 1 month showed a low rate of stent thrombosis of 1.3%, bleeding and vascular complications of only 1.7%. Length of hospital stay of 1.6 days was a far more acceptable (19).

In the Intracoronary Stenting and Antithrombotic Regimen (ISAR) trial, patients with who had Palmaz-Schatz stent placement for suboptimal balloon angioplasty results were randomized to receive antiplatelet therapy (ASA (aspirin) + ticlopidine) (n = 257) or anticoagulant therapy (heparin, warfarin, and ASA) (n = 260) (20). Of the patients assigned to receive antiplatelet therapy, only 1.6% reached a major cardiac end point (death, MI, coronary artery bypass graft [CABG], or repeat PTCA), whereas 6.2% of patients assigned to anticoagulants reached the composite end point (relative risk = 0.25). Patients receiving antiplatelet therapy had an 82% lower risk of an acute myocardial infarction and a 78% reduction in the need for early repeat intervention. Stent thrombosis occurred in only 0.8% of patients treated with antiplatelet agents versus 5.4% of patients in the anticoagulant group. Bleeding and vascular complications were also dramatically reduced in the patients assigned to antiplatelet therapy—an 87% reduction in peripheral vascular events (Fig. 33.9) (Table 33.3).

The comparative efficacy of three strategies was tested in 1650 patients in the STent Antithrombotic Regimen Study (STARS): anticoagulation with aspirin and warfarin, aspirin only, and aspirin plus ticlopidine. Preliminary analysis showed the combination of aspirin and ticlopidine to be associated with the lowest cardiac event rate (0.6% thrombosis) (21). Several other randomized trials are underway, including ENTICES (ENoxaprin, TIcopidine and aspirin versus Coumadin after Elective Stenting) and their results are eagerly awaited.

The physiologic basis for the efficacy of the approach with antiplatelet agents was elegantly elucidated by the work of Neumann et al. (22) who noted that increased surface expression of the platelet IIb/IIIa fibrinogen receptor was predictive of stent thrombosis (Fig. 33.10A), rather than the usual measures of anticoagulation, such as

level of international normalized ratio (INR) (Fig. 33.10B).

Given the current information available from several large series, including two randomized prospective trials, it is reasonable to recommend a regimen consisting of aspirin indefinitely in conjunction with ticlopidine for 1 month. No rational basis appears to be seen for the use of postprocedural heparin and warfarin, even in the bail-out setting. Some suggest that the use of IIb/IIIa receptor antagonists in conjunction with emergent stent placement may be beneficial. Preliminary results from the Impact II trial indicate that the rate of major cardiac events—most notably acute myocardial infarction—was reduced significantly when integrelin was administered in conjunction with stent placement (23). Future prospective studies evaluating the utility of IIb/IIIa antagonists in conjunction with stenting are underway.

HEPARIN-COATED STENTS

The concept of preventing or even eliminating stent thrombosis has given rise to the use of a heparin coating of the stent, which was clinically evaluated in the BENESTENT II pilot study (24). Serruys et al. implanted heparin coated Palmaz-Schatz stents in 207 patients with stable angina and new lesions in large, native coronary arteries. Postprocedure heparin was deferred progressively for 6, 12, and 36 hours in the first three phases of the trial and then given in conjunction with warfarin. In the fourth phase, aspirin (100 mg) and ticlopidine (250 mg/day) was substituted for postprocedure heparin and warfarin. Stent thrombosis was 0% in all four phases, whereas bleeding and vascular complications declined from 7.9 to 0% in the group treated with aspirin and ticlopidine. Angiographic restenosis was 13% for all four phases and a remarkable 6% in the last phase (Fig. 33.11). It should be emphasized that the excellent clinical results obtained in this pilot trial do not prove that the heparin coating per se was responsible for the low rates of thrombosis, restenosis, and bleeding and vascular complications noted. It must be realized that the

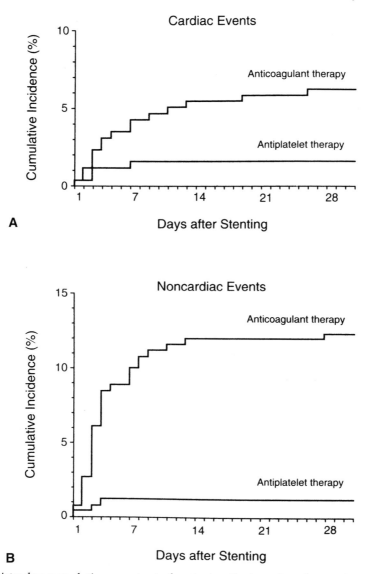

Figure 33.9. Thirty-day cumulative event rate for stent patients assigned to anticoagulation or antiplatelet therapy. (Reprinted with permission from Schomig A, Neumann FJ, Kastrati A, et al. A randomized comparison of antiplatelet and anticoagulant therapy after the placement of coronary artery stents. N Engl J Med 1996;334:1084–1089.)

patient population in the BENESTENT II pilot was at low risk for thrombosis and rates below 1% have been reported with nonheparin-coated stents. Furthermore, this study used the new high-pressure deployment technique with either ultrasound guidance or on-line quantitative coronary angiography (QCA). The low restenosis rates noted in this pilot study may have been in large part because of optimal stent deployment by ex-

perienced operators. Therefore, **although these pilot study results are encouraging, a more realistic test of heparin coating will be in higher risk populations (i.e., patients with acute MI, unstable angina, and smaller coronary arteries).**

The BENESTENT II trial has completed randomization of 827 patients at 40 sites to either a heparin-coated Palmaz-Schatz stent or conventional balloon angioplasty. Pa-

Table 33.3.
Comparison of Outcomes in the ISAR Study: A Randomized Comparison of Antiplatelet Versus Anticoagulant Therapies

Event (%)	Antiplatelet (n = 257)	Anticoagulation (n = 260)	Relative Risk
Reintervention	1.2	5.4	0.22
MI	0.8	4.2	0.18
Cardiac end point	1.6	6.2	0.25
Bleeding	0	6.5	0
Vascular access	0.8	6.2	0.13

tients were rerandomized to either clinical and angiographic follow-up or to clinical follow-up only. Results will be available after 12 months of follow-up.

EXPANDING INDICATIONS

The exponential growth in stent placement has come about as a result of the use of these devices for off-label or unapproved indications. Sawada et al.. compared outcomes for stent placement for STRESS/BENESTENT (S/B) type patients with non-S/B patients (25) (Table 33.4). Of note, only about 20% of the patients receiving stents in that series met the S/B criteria. Furthermore, the outcomes in these higher risk groups were not as favorable. Therefore, the results obtained in the randomized STRESS and BENE-STENT trials cannot be extrapolated to these higher risk subgroups. That outcomes are not as favorable in higher risk patients is not surprising. Hence, an important question concerns the efficacy and safety of stents relative to balloon angioplasty in these high-risk subgroups. We will review available data describing results for specific populations not included in the original STRESS/BENESTENT reports.

Small Vessels

An important group of patients who comprise approximately 30% of the angioplasty population are those with smaller coronary arteries (< 3.0 mm). The results of stenting versus balloon angioplasty were retrospectively evaluated in this population by exam-

ining this cohort of patients in the STRESS I + II trial (26).

Although the inclusion criteria for STRESS required a vessel size of 3.0 mm or larger, 55% of the patients had reference vessel sizes smaller than 3.0 mm when measured by quantitative coronary analysis. The reference diameters were 2.64 mm in the balloon group and 2.69 mm in the stent group. Procedural success was 92% in the PTCA group and 100% in the stent group ($P < .0001$). Restenosis was significantly reduced from 54 to 33% ($P < .001$) (Fig. 33.12A) with a concomitant reduction in target lesion revascularization from 31 to 19% ($P = .019$) (Fig. 33.12B). On the basis of these preliminary results, a prospective, randomized trial with a specifically designed stent for smaller coronary arteries (2.25–2.75 mm) (STRESS IV) is planned with 6-month follow-up quantitative coronary analysis and 1-year clinical event rates as end points.

Diffuse Disease

The presence of long lesions or multiple lesions in the same coronary vessel is particularly problematic for standard balloon angioplasty (Fig. 33.13). We recently retrospectively analyzed the outcomes in 41 patients with lesions larger than 3.0 mm or three or more lesions per vessel (27). The average lesion length was 42 ± 11 mm with a range of 28–71 mm. Multiple Palmaz-Schatz or biliary stents were used (an average of 3.7 stents per vessel). Clinical follow-up at 1 year showed no deaths, two myocardial infarctions (4.9%), no CABG, and seven (17%) repeat PTCA. Freedom from any

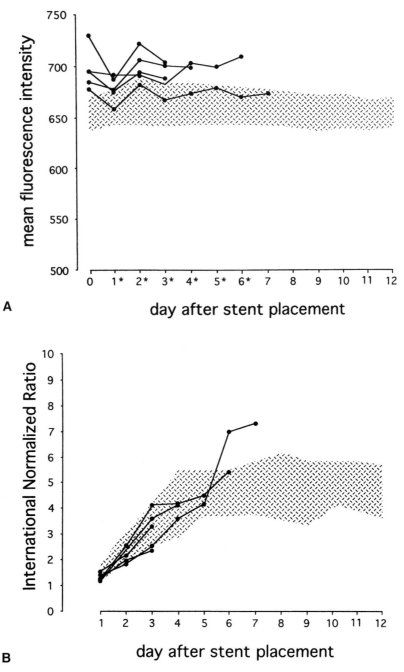

Figure 33.10. A. The predictive value of increased expression of the platelet IIb/IIIa receptor on development of subsequent stent thrombosis. **B.** The lack of predictive value of International Normalized Ratio (INR) level on development of stent thrombosis. This further implicates platelet-mediated events on development of stent thrombosis. (Reprinted with permission from Neumann FJ, Gawaz M, Ott I, et al. Prospective evaluation of hemostatic predictors of subacute stent thrombosis after coronary Palmaz-Schatz stenting. J Am Coll Cardiol 1996;27:15–21.)

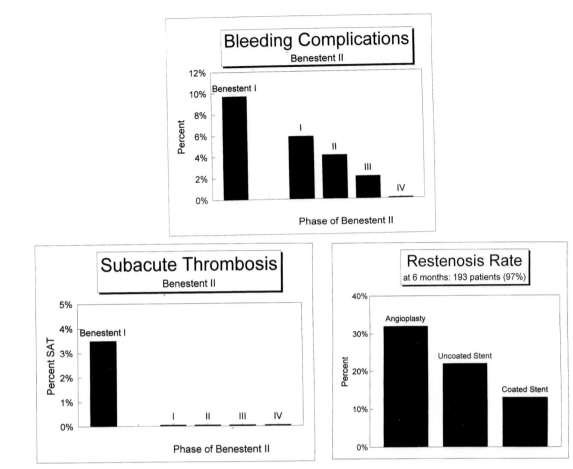

Figure 33.11. The efficacy of the heparin-coated stent. **A.** The rate of bleeding complications in BENES-TENT II declines progressively as postprocedure heparin is delayed for 6, 12, and 36 hours in phases I to III, and is omitted completely in phase IV. Warfarin was given in phases I to III, but omitted in phase IV, when only aspirin and ticlopidine were used. **B.** Stent thrombosis rates. The uncoated stent used in BENESTENT I in conjunction with postprocedure heparin and warfarin and aspirin compared with the heparin-coated stent. The thrombosis rate was 3.5% in BENESTENT I and 0% in BENESTENT II. **C.** Restenosis rates at 6 months (193 patients [97%]). The restenosis rates in the balloon and stent arms of BENESTENT I compared with restenosis rates in BENESTENT II (coated stent). The restenosis rate was reduced to 13% with the use of the coated stent. (Reprinted with permission from Serruys PW, Emanuelsson H, van der Giessen W, et al. Heparin-coated Palmaz-Schatz stents in human coronary arteries: Early outcome of the Benestent-II pilot study. Circulation 1996;93:412–422.)

event was found in 78% of the patients. However, examination of the procedural features showed a catheterization laboratory utilization time of 200 minutes (range: 99–360 minutes); fluoroscopic time of 67 mm (23–240 minutes), and a contrast volume of 605 mL (300–1465). Thus, although clinical outcome was reasonable, the resource utilization was unacceptable with current generation stents. **The develop-**

ment of longer, flexible stents might make the approach to diffuse disease a more practical, cost-effective therapy.

Saphenous Vein Grafts

The concept of stent placement for aged bypass grafts is particularly appealing given the relatively poor outcomes with both balloon angioplasty (28–34) and directional atherectomy (35). A major drawback of vein graft intervention is distal embolization of fragile atheromatous material, with resultant no reflow and myocardial infarction, a risk that increases with vein grafts older than 3–5 years (30). Another serious limitation is the high rate of restenosis, which may exceed 50% for lesions in the body of the vein graft, and is even higher for ostial stenoses (36). Furthermore, the temporal course of restenosis may be prolonged beyond the usual 6-month time frame noted in native vessels. In addition, disease may progress within a long graft at a nontarget lesion site.

Several multicenter registries have reported relatively favorable results with vein graft stenting. For example, in the multicenter Palmaz-Schatz registry, 589 patients with 624 focal stenosis were enrolled (37). Procedural success rate was 98.8%. Major in-hospital complications occurred in only 2.9%, with stent thrombosis being documented in only 1.4% of patients. Bleeding and vascular complications were frequent at 14.3%, because of full anticoagulation use with post-procedure heparin and warfarin. Coronary angiographic analysis of the first 198 patients in this registry showed an overall restenosis rate of 34, with 22% for new lesions versus 51% for restenotic lesions (Fig. 33.14).

Table 33.4.
Clinical Events at 6 Months in STRESS/BENESTENT-Type Lesions Versus Other Types

	STRESS/BENESTENT Type vs. Others at 3 to 6 Months			
	SAT (%)	Death/MI/CABG (%)	Restenosis (%)	TLR (%)
S/B (n = 152)	1.3	6.6	11	8.6
Non S/B (n = 593)				
Small	1.5	8.0	30[a]	19[a]
Long	1.6	4.8	32[a]	15
Ostial	2.1	11[a]	40[a]	14
Total	0	2.5	40[a]	7.5
SVBG	0	5.8	34[a]	21[a]
Restenotic	1	4.0	27[a]	15[a]
Poor LV	3.1	14	19	14

[a]$p < 0.05$ compared with S/B.
SAT, subacute thrombosis; MI, myocardial infarction; CABG, coronary artery bypass grafting; TLR, target lesion revascularization; SB, STRESS/BENESTENT.

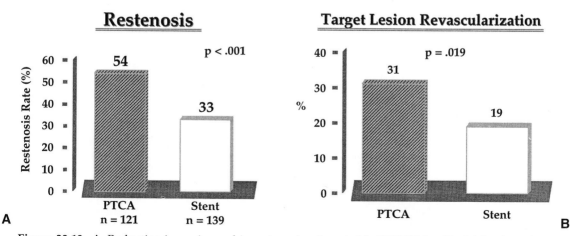

Figure 33.12. **A.** Reduction in angiographic restenosis rate noted in STRESS I + II trial for the cohort of patients with small vessels (< 3.0 mm in diameter). **B.** Concomitant reduction in target lesion revascularization for the patient group with smaller coronary arteries.

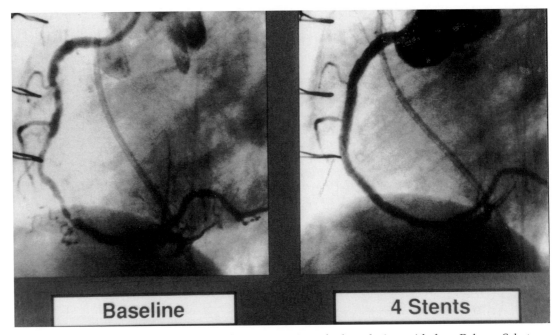

Figure 33.13. Example of endoluminal reconstruction of a long lesion with four Palmaz-Schatz stents before (**left**) and after (**right**) stent placement.

Furthermore, restenosis rates for stented ostial lesions were a disappointing 61% (36).

Biliary stents have been utilized by some groups for larger vein grafts (> 4 mm diameter) with results similar to coronary stents (38). This application has been limited to relatively straight grafts, which can be reached by guiding catheters without excessive curves.

The efficacy of stent placement versus PTCA was directly compared in the prospective randomized **SA**phenous **VE**in De novo (SAVED) trial (39). Two hundred twenty patients with focal, new lesions in aged bypass grafts were randomized to conventional PTCA or Palmaz-Schatz stent placement. Average graft age was approximately 10 years in each group. Procedural success (angiographic success without a major cardiac event) was markedly better in the stent group (92 versus 69%, $P < .001$) (Fig. 33.15). Angiographic restenosis by the binary definition was reduced from 47% in the PTCA group to 36% in the group receiving stents ($P = .11$) (Fig. 33.16). Furthermore, patients in the stent arm had a greater net gain at 6 months compared with PTCA. A composite clinical end point of major cardiac events at 6 months showed a reduction in the stent arm from 38 to 26% (Fig. 33.17). Importantly, a strong trend was found toward fewer non–Q-wave myocardial infarctions in the stented patients compared with the balloon group (Table 33.5).

Acute Myocardial Infarction

Patient with acute myocardial infarction were initially excluded from stent trials because of the thrombogenic milieu present in this clinical scenario. However, with improvements in deployment technique and more effective antithrombotic therapy, investigators began to evaluate stent placement in this challenging group of patients. Table 33.6 lists several observational trials of stenting for acute MI. Although overall success rate appears high with acceptable reocclusion and mortality figures, approximately 25% of patients with acute myocardial infarction actually received stents (40–45).

In the PAMI (**P**rimary **A**ngioplasty in **M**yocardial **I**nfarction) stent pilot study,

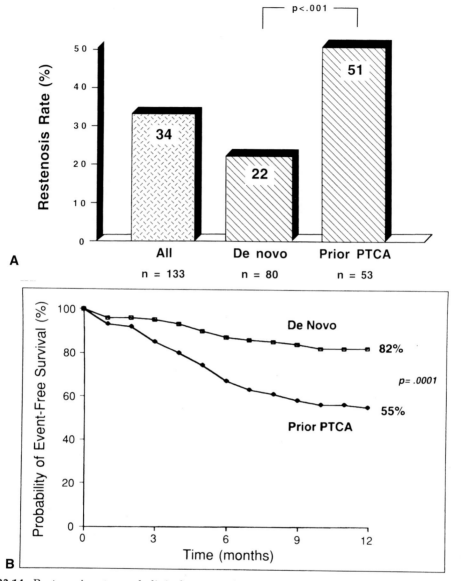

Figure 33.14. Restenosis rates and clinical events after stent placement in saphenous vein grafts. **A.** Restenosis rates after stent placement in degenerated saphenous vein bypass grafts. The restenosis rate was markedly lower in patients with new lesions as compared with those with previously treated stenoses. **B.** Kaplan-Meier survival curves for patients with new lesions and with previously dilated stenoses in saphenous vein bypass grafts. Freedom from death, myocardial infarction, coronary bypass surgery, or repeat angioplasty is substantially higher in patients with de novo lesions as compared with restenotic lesions. (Reprinted with permission from Fenton SH, Fischman DL, Savage MP, et al. Long-term angiographic and clinical outcome after implantation of balloon-expandable stents in aorto-coronary saphenous vein grafts. Am J Cardiol 1994;74:1187–1191.)

201 patients were enrolled within 12 hours of symptom onset. In this group, stenting was performed in 151 patients (75%), with small vessel size (< 2.5 mm) being the most common exclusion criterion for stent placement. Patients were treated with aspirin, ticlopidine, and heparin for 48 hours. thrombolysis in myocardial infarction

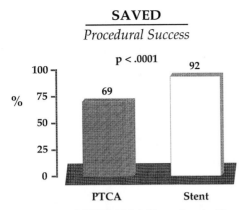

Figure 33.15. SAVED Trial. Procedural efficacy, i.e., success of the intended therapy and no in-hospital major adverse cardiac events. The failure rate of PTCA is about four times the failure rate of stents. (Reprinted with permission from Savage MP, Douglas J, Fischman D, et al. A comparison of stent placement with balloon angioplasty for stenosis of coronary bypass grafts. N Engl J Med 1997;337(11):740–747.)

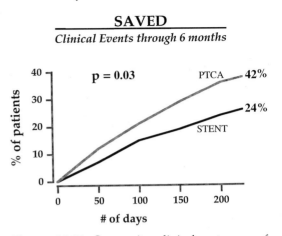

Figure 33.17. Composite clinical outcome of major cardiac events at 6 months. (Reprinted with permission from Savage MP, Douglas J, Fischman D, et al. A comparison of stent placement with balloon angioplasty for stenosis of coronary bypass grafts. N Engl J Med 1997; 337(11):740–747.)

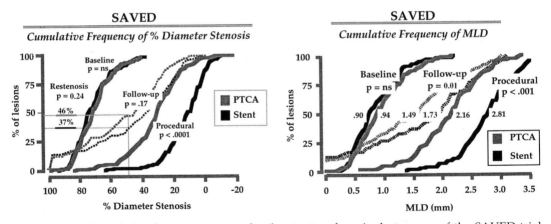

Figure 33.16. Cumulative frequency curves for the stent and angioplasty arms of the SAVED trial. The degree of narrowing was similar in the two groups at baseline. There is a strong trend toward reduction in angiographic restenosis and a larger follow-up minimal lumen diameter in the stent group. MLD, minimum lumen diameter. (Reprinted with permission from Savage MP, Douglas J, Fischman D, et al. A comparison of stent placement with balloon angioplasty for stenosis of coronary bypass grafts. N Engl J Med 1997;337(11):740–747.).

(TIMI) 3 flow was established in 98%. In-hospital events in stented patients included death in 0.7% and reinfarction in 1.4% (46). Because of these encouraging preliminary results, a prospective randomized trial, PAMI 3, is underway in which 900 patients

will be allocated either to PTCA or a new heparin-coated stent. End points will include qualitative coronary analysis and clinical events at 6 months, in addition to a cost-to-benefit analysis. The GRAMI (**Gi**anturco **R**oubin Stent II in **A**cute **M**yo-

Table 33.5.
Clinical Events at 240 Days in the SAphenous VEin De novo (SAVED) Trial (39)

Cumulative Events	PTCA (n = 107) n/%	Stent (n = 108) n/%	p
Death	9 (8)	7 (7)	NS
Q wave MI	4 (4)	5 (5)	NS
Non Q wave MI	11 (11)	6 (6)	0.13
CABG	12 (11)	7 (7)	NS
Repeat angioplasty	16 (16)	13 (13)	NS
Any event	39 (38)	26 (26)	0.04

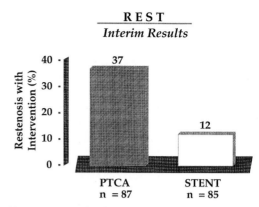

Figure 33.18. Preliminary results of the REST trial—a randomized comparison of stent versus angioplasty for restenotic lesions. A significant reduction is seen in restenosis with reintervention in the stented patients. (Adapted from Erbel R, Haude M, Hopp HW, et al. REstenosis STent (REST) Study: randomized trial comparing stenting and balloon angioplasty for treatment of restenosis after balloon angioplasty. J Am Coll Cardiol 1996; (Suppl) 27:139A.)

cardial Infarction) reported on the initial 65 patients randomized to either the GR-II stent or PTCA alone (45a). Stenting appeared to yield better results. Another trial (ESCOBAR) also favored stenting.

Restenotic Lesions

Patients with restenosis have a higher rate of recurrence after stent implantation compared with patients with new lesions (12). However, a direct comparison of a single Palmaz-Schatz stent with balloon angioplasty for restenotic lesions has been recently completed. The **RE**stenosis **ST**ent study (REST) has enrolled 400 patients with focal restenosis in native coronary vessels. The primary outcome variable is MLD and late loss at 6 months. Interim analysis (Fig. 33.18) of the initial 123 patients analyzed showed a reduction in restenosis with reintervention from 37 to 12% (46). Furthermore, in a consecutive group of 111 patients

with refractory restenosis (three or more prior PTCA attempts), placement of Palmaz-Schatz stents was associated with a favorable 78% 1-year event-free survival (46a). Stented patients in REST received warfarin and had increased bleeding complications with a longer hospitalization than patients randomized to balloon angioplasty alone. The effectiveness of the Wallstent to reduce restenosis after treatment of de novo and restonotic lesions is undergoing evaluation in the **W**allstent **I**n **N**ative vessel trial (WIN). A total of 514 patients will be randomized to either Wallstent or balloon angioplasty alone.

Table 33.6.
Trials of Stenting for Acute Myocardial Infarction

Study	AMI n	Stented n (%)	Success	Reocclusion	Mortality
Garcia-Cantu (40)	138	35 (25%)	100%	0	5.7%
Rodriquez (41)	140	30 (21%)	100%	3.3%	3.3%
LeMay (42)	—	32 (—)	81%	3.1%	6.2%
Antoniucci (43)	118	31 (26%)	100%	3.2%	—
Neumann (44)	375	80 (21%)	99%	8.5%	8.8%
Saito (45)	143	74 (52%)	97%	1.4%	1.4%
Pooled	—	282 (27%)	97%	4.0%	5.2%

AMI, acute myocardial infarction.

Chronic Total Occlusion

Observational reports have shown promise for stenting improving on the patency rates of chronically occluded coronary arteries. For example, in one series of 59 patients with 60 chronic occlusions longer than 3 months duration in half the patients, stents were successfully placed in 59 of 60 lesions (98%). Thrombosis occurred in three patients (5%). There was an angiographic restenosis rate of 20% (10/51) and 77% were event-free at 14-month follow-up (47).

More recently, a randomized trial of Stent in Chronic Coronary Occlusion (SICCO) was completed (48). One hundred nineteen patients in whom PTCA successfully recanalized a coronary artery were randomized to no further intervention or placement of a Palmaz-Schatz stent. No deaths occurred in either group, and one patient in the stent group had an acute MI. Subacute occlusion developed in four patients in the stent group and in three patients in the angioplasty arm. At follow-up, 57% in the stent group were angina free compared with 24% in the angioplasty group ($P < .001$). Angiographic restenosis occurred in 74% of angioplasty patients and in 32% of the stented patients ($P < .001$) (Fig.

33.19). This reduction in angiographic restenosis was accompanied by a reduction in target lesion revascularization from 42 to 22% ($P = .025$).

Preliminary results of a smaller (n = 60) randomized trial were reported by Thomas et al. (48a), and they supported those of the SICCO study (e.g., larger MLD, 2.8 versus 3.3 mm $P < .01$) and a trend toward lower restenosis rate, 30 versus 20% in stented patients.

SUMMARY AND FUTURE IMPLICATIONS

Coronary stents represent a significant advance in the treatment of patients with obstructive coronary artery disease. The major drawback of stenting—subacute thrombosis—has been reduced to approximately 1% by the meticulous deployment technique and the substitution of antiplatelet agents i.e, aspirin and ticlopidine) for postprocedure heparin and warfarin. Elimination of warfarin has also had the beneficial effect of reducing peripheral vascular complications and length of hospital stay. Restenosis for new discrete lesions seems to be reduced by approximately one third, as does the need for repeat intervention. Randomized trials of stents in patients with saphenous vein bypass graft lesions and restenotic native lesions have shown lower rates of complications and restenosis.

Coronary stent implantation will continue to evolve and become more practical with technologic refinements of the stents themselves. In addition, coupling of the mechanical scaffolding properties of the stent with biologic approaches designed to limit intimal proliferation and matrix deposition will be explored.

Accordingly, **customized stents (e.g., longer devices for diffuse disease, and radiopaque devices with greater radial strength for ostial lesions) will be developed for niche uses in specific situations.** Furthermore, systemic drugs, local drug delivery of antiproliferative compounds (49), and local irradiation by catheter-based sources (50) or radioactive stents (51) will

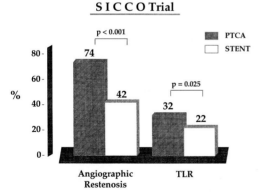

Figure 33.19. Results of the SICCO (Stenting In Chronic Coronary Occlusion) study. A significant reduction is seen in restenosis in patients randomized to the stent arm of the trial. TLR, target lesion revascularization. (Adapted from Sirnes PA, Golf S, Myreng Y, et al. Stenting in chronic coronary occlusion (SICCO): a randomized, controlled trial of adding stent implantation after successful angioplasty. J Am Coll Cardiol 1996;28:1444–1451.)

be tested in clinical trials with the goal to reduce restenosis even further, especially in high-risk patients.

References

1. Bredlau CE, Roubin GS, Leimgruber PP, et al. In-hospital morbidity and mortality in patients undergoing elective coronary angioplasty. Circulation 1985;72:1044–1052.
2. Simpfendorfer C, Bilardi, J, Bellamy G, et al. Frequency, management and follow-up of patients with acute coronary occlusions after percutaneous transluminal coronary angioplasty. Am J Cardiol 1987;59:274–276.
3. Cowley MJ, Dorros G, Kelsey SF, et al. Emergency coronary artery bypass surgery after coronary angioplasty: The National Heart and Lung Institute percutaneous transluminal angioplasty registry experience. Am J Cardiol 1984;52:22–26.
4. Black AJR, Namay DL, Neiderman AL, et al. Tear or dissection after coronary angioplasty: morphologic correlates of an ischemic complication. Circulation 1989;79:1035–1042.
5. Ellis SG, Roubin GS, King SB III, et al. Angiographic and clinical predictors of acute closure after native vessel coronary angioplasty. Circulation 1988;77:372–379.
6. Tebbe U, Ruchewski W, Knake W, et al. Will emergency coronary bypass grafting after failed elective percutaneous transluminal coronary angioplasty prevent myocardial infarction? J Thorac Cardiovasc Surg 1989;37:308–312.
7. Page US, Okies JE, Colburn LQ, et al. Percutaneous transluminal coronary angioplasty: a growing surgical problem. J Thorac Cardiovasc Surg 1986;92:847–852.
8. Sigwart U, Urban P, Golf S, et al. Emergency stenting for acute occlusion after coronary balloon angioplasty. Circulation 1988;78:1121–1127.
9. Hermann H, Buchbinder M, Cleman M, et al. Emergent use of balloon-expandable coronary artery stenting for failed percutaneous coronary angioplasty. Circulation 1992;86:812–819.
10. Colombo A, Goldberg SL, Almagor Y, et al. A novel strategy for stent deployment in the treatment of acute or threatened closure complication balloon coronary angioplasty. Use of short or standard (or both) single or multiple Palmaz-Schatz stents. J Am Coll Cardiol 1993;22:1887–1891.
11. Sutton JM, Ellis SG, Roubin GS, et al. Major clinical events after coronary stenting. The multicenter registry of acute and elective Gianturco-Roubin stent placement. The Gianturco-Roubin Intracoronary Stent Investigator Group. Circulation 1994;89:1126–1137.
11a. Penn IM, Ricci DR, Brown RI, et al. Randomized study of stenting versus balloon dilatation in failed angioplasty (PTCA): preliminary data from the trial of angioplasty and stents in Canada (TASC-II). Circulation 1993;88:I-601.
12. Savage MP, Fischman DL, Schatz RA, et al. Long-term angiographic and clinical outcome after implantation of a balloon-expandable stent in the native coronary circulation. Palmaz-Schatz Stent Study Group. J Am Coll Cardiol 1994;24:1207–1212.
13. Fischman D, Leon M, Baim D, et al. A randomized comparison of coronary-stent placement and balloon angioplasty in the treatment of coronary disease. N Engl J Med 1994;331:496–501.
14. Serruys P, De Jaegere P, Kiemeneji F, et al. A comparison of balloon expandable-stent implantation with balloon angioplasty in patients with coronary artery disease. N Engl J Med 1994;331:489–495.
15. Wong SC, Zidar JP, Chuang YC, et al. Stents improve late clinical outcomes: results from the combined (I + II) STent REStenosis Study. Circulation 1995;92:I-281.
16. Kimura T, Yokoi H, Nakagawa Y, et al. Three-year follow-up after implantation of metallic coronary artery stents. N Engl J Med 1996;334:561–566.
17. Colombo A, Hall P, Nakamura S, et al. Intracoronary stenting without anticoagulation accomplished with intravascular ultrasound guidance. Circulation 1995;91:1676–1688.
18. Karrillon GJ, Morice MC, Benveniste E, et al. Intracoronary stent implantation without ultrasound guidance and with replacement of conventional anticoagulation by antiplatelet therapy: 30-day clinical outcome of the French multicenter registry. Circulation 1996;94:1519–1527.
19. STRESS III Investigators. Early outcomes after coronary stent placement with high pressure inflation and antiplatelet therapy: interim results of the STRESS III trial. Circulation 1996;94(Suppl):I-684.
20. Schomig A, Neumann FJ, Kastrati A, et al. A randomized comparison of antiplatelet and anticoagulant therapy after the placement of coronary artery stents. N Engl J Med 1996;334:1084–1089.
21. Leon MB, Baim DS, Gordon P, et al. Clinical and angiographic results from the STent Anticoagulation Regimen Study (STARS). Circulation 1996;94(Suppl):I-685.
22. Neumann FJ, Gawaz M, Ott I, et al. Prospective evaluation of hemostatic predictors of subacute stent thrombosis after coronary Palmaz-Schatz stenting. J Am Coll Cardiol 1996;27:15–21.
23. Zidar JP, Kruse KR, Thel MC, et al. Integrelin for emergency coronary artery stenting. J Am Coll Cardiol 1996;27 (Suppl A): 138A.
24. Serruys PW, Emanuelsson H, van der Giessen W, et al. Heparin-coated Palmaz-Schatz stents in human coronary arteries: Early outcome of the Benestent-II pilot study. Circulation 1996;93:412–422.
25. Sawada Y, Nosaka H, Kimura T, et al. Initial and six months outcome of Palmaz-Schatz stent implantation: STRESS/BENESTENT equivalent vs non-equivalent lesions. J Am Coll Cardiol 1996;27 (Suppl A): 252A.
26. Savage M, Fischman D, Rake R, et al. Elective coronary stenting versus balloon angioplasty in smaller native coronary arteries: results from STRESS [Abstract]. J Am Coll Cardiol 1996;27 (Suppl A): 253A.
27. Savage M, Fernandes L, Fischman D, et al. Radical endoluminal reconstruction of diffusely diseased

coronary arteries using multiple stents [Abstract]. Circulation 1996;94 (Suppl I:I-25.

28. de Feyter PJ, van Suylen RJ, De Jaegere PPT, et al. Balloon angioplasty for the treatment of saphenous vein bypass grafts. J Am Coll Cardiol 1993;21:1539–1549.

29. Douglas JS Jr, Gruentzig AR, King SB III, et al. Percutaneous transluminal coronary angioplasty in patients with prior coronary bypass surgery. J Am Coll Cardiol 1983;2:745–754.

30. Dorros G, Johnson WD, Tector AJ, et al. Percutaneous transluminal coronary angioplasty in patients with prior coronary artery bypass grafting. J Thorac Cardiovasc Surg 1984;87:17–26.

31. Platko WP, Hollman J, Whitlow PL, et al. Percutaneous transluminal coronary angioplasty of saphenous vein graft stenosis: long-term follow-up. J Am Coll Cardiol 1989;14:1645–1650.

32. Reeves F, Bonan R, Cote H, et al. Long-term angiographic follow-up after angioplasty of venous coronary bypass grafts. Am Heart J 1991;122:620–627.

33. Webb JG, Myler RK, Shaw RE, et al. Coronary angioplasty after coronary bypass surgery: Initial results and late outcome in 422 patients. J Am Coll Cardiol 1990;16:812–820.

34. Plokker HWT, Meester BH, Serruys PW. The Dutch experience in percutaneous transluminal angioplasty of narrowed saphenous veins used for aortocoronary arterial bypass. Am J Cardiol 1991;67:361–366.

35. Holmes DF Jr, Topol EJ, Califf RM, et al. A multicenter, randomized trial of coronary angioplasty versus directional atherectomy for patients with saphenous vein bypass graft lesions. Circulation 1995;91:1969–1974.

36. Fenton SH, Fischman DL, Savage MP, et al. Long-term angiographic and clinical outcome after implantation of balloon-expandable stents in aortocoronary saphenous vein grafts. Am J Cardiol 1994;74:1187–1191.

37. Wong SC, Baim DS, Schatz RA, et al. Acute results and late outcomes after stent implantation in saphenous vein graft lesions: the multicenter USA Palmaz-Schatz stent experience. J Am Coll Cardiol 1995;26:704–712.

38. Wong SC, Popma JJ, Pichard AD, et al. Comparison of clinical and angiographic outcomes after saphenous vein graft angioplasty using coronary versus 'biliary' tubular, slotted stents. Circulation 1995;91:339–350.

39. Savage MP, Douglas J, Fischman D, et al. A comparison of stent placement with balloon angioplasty for stenosis of coronary bypass grafts. N Engl J Med 1997;337:740–741.

40. Garcia-Cantu E, Spaulding C, Corcos T, et al. Stent implantation in acute myocardial infarction. Am J Cardiol 1996;77:451–454.

41. Rodriquez AE, Fernandez M, Santaera O, et al. Coronary stenting in patients undergoing percutaneous transluminal coronary angioplasty during acute myocardial infarction. Am J Cardiol 1996;77:685–689.

42. LeMay MR, Labinaz M, Beanlands RSB, et al. Usefulness of intracoronary stenting in acute myocardial infarction. Am J Cardiol 1996;78:148–152.

43. Antoniucci D, Valenti R, Buonamici P, et al. Direct angioplasty and stenting of the infarct-related artery in acute myocardial infarction. Am J Cardiol 1996;78:568–571.

44. Neumann FJ, Walter H, Richardt G, et al. Coronary Palmaz-Schatz stent implantation in acute myocardial infarction. Heart 1996;75:121–126.

45. Saito S, Hosokawa G, Kim K, et al. Primary stent implantation without coumadin in acute myocardial infarction. J Am Coll Cardiol 1996;28:74–81.

45a. Fernández A, Goicolea J, Perez-Vizcayno MJ, et al. Late Clinical and angiographic outcome of bailout coronary stenting. A comparison study between Gianturco-Roubin and Palmaz-Schatz stents. J Am Coll Cardiol 1996;27 (Suppl):111A .

46. Erbel R, Haude M, Hopp HW, et al. REstenosis STent (REST) Study: randomized trial comparing stenting and balloon angioplasty for treatment of restenosis after balloon angioplasty. J Am Coll Cardiol 1996; (Suppl) 27:139A.

46a. Savage MP, Fischman DL, Fenton SH, et al. Coronary stents may be the preferred therapy for refractory restenosis after three or more prior PTCA [Abstract]. Circulation 1994;90:I-322.

47. Goldberg SL, Colombo A, Maiello L, et al. Intracoronary stent insertion after balloon angioplasty of chronic total occlusions. J Am Coll Cardiol 1995;26:713–719.

48. Sirnes PA, Golf S, Myreng Y, et al. Stenting in chronic coronary occlusion (SICCO): a randomized, controlled trial of adding stent implantation after successful angioplasty. J Am Coll Cardiol 1996;28:1444–1451.

48a. Thomas M, Hancock J, Holmberg S, et al. Coronary stenting following successful angioplasty for total occlusions: preliminary results of a randomized trial. J Am Coll Cardiol 1996;27 (Suppl):153A.

49. Rogers C, Karnovsky MJ, Edelman ER. Inhibition of experimental neointimal hyperplasia and thrombosis depends on the type of vascular injury and the site of drug administration. Circulation 1993;88:1215–1221.

50. Teirstein PS, Massullo V, Jani S, et al. Radiation therapy following coronary stenting: 6 month follow-up of a randomized clinical trial [Abstract]. Circulation 1996;94:I-222.

51. Fischell TA, Kharma BK, Fischell DR, et al. Low-dose B-particle emission from ''stent'' wire results in complete, localized inhibition of smooth muscle cell proliferation. Circulation 1994;90:2956–2963.

34
Antithrombotic Therapy During Percutaneous Coronary Intervention

Christopher B. Granger, MD
Robert A. Harrington, MD

INTRODUCTION

Two major limitations to current techniques of percutaneous coronary intervention exist: abrupt vessel closure and late restenosis (1, 2). Together they account for most of the acute and chronic morbidity and mortality associated with the procedure. The economic implications of both abrupt vessel closure (3) and a 20 to 40% restenosis rate are considerable (4). Although these two processes are much different with regard to their temporal occurrence, at least in part, they share a common pathophysiologic mechanism: platelet-dependent thrombosis. Both mechanical dissection of disrupted atherosclerotic plaque and elastic vessel recoil contribute to the problem of abrupt vessel closure, but because the freshly ruptured plaque with exposure of the subendothelium is such an intense thrombogenic stimulus, clearly the platelet-driven hemostatic response to injury must also be key. Likewise, restenosis following successful coronary intervention is a complex, multifactorial process. Part of the stimulation to intimal proliferation is the mitogenic properties of both platelets, with the production and release of growth factors such as PDGF (platelet derived growth factors), and thrombin. Modulation of the hemostatic process that occurs naturally as a response to vascular injury, therefore, may have a favorable impact on percutaneous intervention outcomes.

Based on empiric observation, **Gruentzig et al. liberally used both antiplatelet and antithrombin agents in the early balloon angioplasty experience (5).** Bull et al. had described the usefulness of the activated clotting time (ACT) to guide heparin anticoagulation during cardiopulmonary bypass (6). Heparin use during percutaneous coronary procedures was also empiric and relied on observational data from the surgical experience. More recent work has demonstrated a relationship between the ACT and clinical outcomes (7, 8). With regard to standard antiplatelet therapy, randomized trials have demonstrated the benefits of aspirin in this patient population (9). Although novel antithrombins, such as hirudin and hirulog, have not been shown to improve percutaneous transluminal coronary angioplasty (PTCA) outcomes beyond heparin and aspirin, the introduction of platelet glycoprotein (GP) IIb/IIIa receptor inhibitors has led to significant clinical benefits (10–14), and they represent a major advance in our understanding of interventional cardiology.

In this chapter, we discuss the rationale for the use of and experience with both antithrombin and antiplatelet therapies in percutaneous coronary intervention. Recommendations for antithrombotic therapy during the interventional procedure will be supported by clinical trial outcome data and expert consensus opinion (15).

ANTITHROMBIN THERAPY

Rationale

Coronary angioplasty has been recognized since its inception (5) as thrombogenic and thus has always been performed with antiplatelet and anticoagulant therapy. Pathologic (16) and ultrasound studies (17) have demonstrated the common occurrence of subintimal exposure of thrombogenic material and thrombus formation. One small study found that in patients who die early, despite heparin and aspirin use, platelet-rich thrombi predominate during the first 12 hours, whereas fibrin thrombi are more common thereafter (18). Hematologic studies measuring peptide markers and protein markers of platelet activity have demonstrated thrombin activation (19, 20), which may be suppressed with aspirin and high-dose heparin (21), although reactivation may occur on discontinuing heparin (22). Thus, the ample **evidence for thrombin activation and thrombosis resulting from the vascular injury provides a target for antithrombin therapy.**

Heparin

Although intravenous heparin is standard treatment during percutaneous coronary interventions, no randomized trials have specifically addressed the optimal dose or the degree of anticoagulation. A series of observational studies, however, all found that lower levels of anticoagulation are associated with higher incidences of complications (Table 34.1) (7, 8, 23).

One study evaluated patients undergoing coronary angioplasty who received a 10,000 U bolus followed by additional heparin according to the discretion of the investigator (24). Of the 1469 consecutive patients undergoing angioplasty, the 103 patients who died or underwent urgent or emergency bypass surgery were compared with 400 patients without complications. ACTs during the procedure, measured by the Hemochron device, were 30 to 60 seconds lower in patients with complications, and complications occurred in only 0.3% of patients with a final ACT of greater than 300 seconds. A second study used a case-control design to assess the relationship between degree of anticoagulation and outcome (8). ACT measured by the Hemochron device was compared both in 63 patients with abrupt closure, defined as documented vessel occlusion prior to discharge, and in 124 patients without complications who were matched for other major predictors of abrupt closure. Procedural ACTs were 25 to 30 seconds lower among patients with abrupt closure, and logistic regression anal-

Table 34.1.
Median Activated Clotting Time (Seconds) during Coronary Angioplasty According to Presence or Absence of Thrombotic Complications

	ACT Device	Complication[a]	No Complication	p
Narins et al. (8)				
Initial ACT (median)	HemoTec	350	380	0.004
Minimal ACT (median)		345	370	0.014
Ferguson et al. (7)				
ACT after heparin (mean)	Hemochron	229	259	< 0.0001
ACT at end of procedure (mean)		232	303	< 0.0001

[a] For Narins, angiographically documented abrupt closure before hospital discharge; for Ferguson, death or emergency coronary bypass surgery.
ACT, activated clotting time

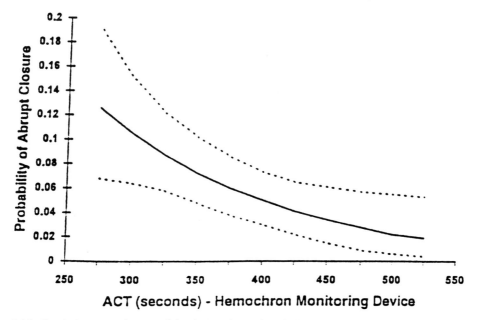

Figure 34.1. Logistic regression model relationship of probability of abrupt closure with initial activated clotting time. (Reprinted with permission from Narins CR, Hillegass WB, Nelson CL, et al. Activated clotting time predicts abrupt closure risk during angioplasty. Circulation 1996;93:667–671.)

ysis demonstrated a strong continuous relationship between the degree of ACT prolongation and the probability of abrupt closure ($P = .015$) (Fig. 34.1). No apparent relationship was found between ACT prolongation and subsequent bleeding. These two studies have led to the recommendation that intravenous heparin be administered before angioplasty as a bolus of at least 10,000 U, with additional boluses to keep the ACT at least 300 (HemoTec) to 350 (Hemochron) seconds (15). An alternative, and the standard approach in some clinical trials, is to give an initial weight-adjusted bolus of 100 U/kg (10, 11), with the same target ACT.

The heparin plasma levels and anticoagulant effect during angioplasty, similar to during coronary artery bypass surgery, are above the level at which the heparin versus activated partial thromboplastin time (APTT) response curve provides meaningful discrimination in heparin levels. Therefore, ACT, which has a stable response to changes in heparin at these higher levels, is the standard measure. The two commonly used devices to measure ACT vary considerably, with the Hemochron device giving values approximately 50 seconds higher

than the HemoTec with ACTs in the 300 second range (24).

Heparin need not be given routinely following the angioplasty procedure, based on two small randomized studies that found no difference in thrombotic complications among patients randomized to 24 hours of continuous intravenous heparin versus no additional heparin (15, 25, 26). Furthermore, a randomized trial (27) has shown reduced complications of groin bleeding when heparin is discontinued and the femoral artery sheath removed early following the procedure. Whether heparin should be continued following angioplasty with high-risk features for abrupt closure (such as unstable angina or suboptimal angiographic results) is not clear.

Together, the EPIC and EPILOG trials show that the heparin dose should be decreased when given with abciximab. The EPIC trial showed that full-dose heparin (given as 10 to 20,000 U initial bolus, ACT target of 300 to 350 seconds, followed by 12-hour heparin infusion) in combination with abciximab doubled the incidence of major bleeding (from 7 to 14%) compared with heparin without abciximab. On the other hand, in the EPILOG trial, abciximab used with lower dose heparin (70 U/kg bolus, a target ACT of at least 200 seconds, and no heparin after the procedure) was associated with a lower risk of major bleeding (2%) compared with full dose heparin alone (3.1%). When used with full dose heparin, abciximab is accompanied by ACT prolongation by 35 seconds on average (28).

Although prolonged heparin therapy and coumadin had been the standard approach following stent placement, in light of several trials showing equal or better outcomes with ticlopidine and aspirin alone (12, 29, 30), routine postprocedural heparin and coumadin use has been abandoned (31). Low molecular weight enoxaparin heparin use for patients with stent deployment who are at high risk for thombotic complications is being studied in a randomized trial.

Direct Thrombin Inhibitors

Although heparin is the established approach toward antithrombin therapy (32), its use is limited by indirect action through antithrombin III, relative ineffectiveness in inhibiting clot-bound thrombin (33), inconsistent anticoagulant effect due to circulating inhibitors such as platelet factor 4, and tendency to cause thrombocytopenia. **Direct thrombin inhibitors, on the other hand, are potent and predictable inhibitors of thrombin activity,** and therefore, considerable enthusiasm is found for their potential role in coronary intervention.

Hirulog

An analogue of hirudin, hirulog (bivalirudin) is a potent, synthetic bivalent molecule that has been studied in two clinical trials. A phase II trial of 129 patients undergoing elective coronary angioplasty (34) studied five doses of a 4-hour infusion of hirulog. The abrupt closure rate within 24 hours of the procedure tended to be lower in the two higher doses (3.9%) com-

pared with the three lower doses (11.3%). A phase III, double-blind controlled trial randomized 4098 patients to a 24-hour infusion of either hirulog (initial 1.0 mg/kg bolus) or heparin (initial 175 U/kg bolus) (35). The primary end point of in-hospital death, myocardial infarction, abrupt closure, or cardiac decompensation was not reduced by hirulog ($P = .44$). It was reduced, however, in a predefined subset of 704 patients with postinfarction angina, where the event rate was 9.1% versus 14.2% with heparin, $P = .04$, although the difference did not maintain statistical significance at 6-month follow-up ($P = .17$). Major bleeding was less than half in the hirulog group compared with heparin ($P = .001$).

Hirudin

The prototypic direct thrombin inhibitor, derived from the saliva of *Hirudo medicinalis*, hirudin has been tested in two trials of coronary angioplasty. In a phase II trial (36), 113 patients were randomized to a 24-hour infusion of hirudin or heparin. More cardiac complications were found with heparin (4 of 39 versus 1 of 74) and more bleeding with hirudin (4 of 74 versus 0 of 39). Hirudin was more effective at inhibiting thrombin activity as measured by fibrinopeptide A, and it resulted in more predictable and stable APTTs. The HELVETICA trial (37) randomized 1141 patients with unstable angina who were scheduled for angioplasty to one of three treatments: 24 hours of intravenous heparin (10,000 U initial bolus), 24 hours of intravenous hirudin (40 mg initial bolus), or 24 hours of intravenous hirudin followed by subcutaneous hirudin for 3 days. At the primary end point follow-up at 7 months, no difference was seen in event-free survival ($P = .61$), despite a significant reduction in early cardiac events (5.6% hirudin infusion and subcutaneous dosing versus 11% heparin, at 96 hours, $P = .023$). ACTs were not measured, and bleeding rates were similar in all three groups.

The combined experience of the direct thrombin inhibitors demonstrates a consistent modest early effect, which is not sustained. **More potent thrombin inhibition during and shortly following angioplasty, therefore, appears to reduce ischemic events during antithrombin treatment, but it does not prevent the clinical manifestations of restenosis.**

Low Molecular Weight Heparin

Low molecular weight heparin has relatively less antithrombin activity because of the certain length of the saccharide chain required for this activity, which is not necessary for anti-Xa activity. This gives low molecular weight heparin relatively more potency against factor Xa. This potency may provide an advantage of better inhibition of thrombin generation, which is relatively unaffected by unfractionated heparin (38) and hirudin (39). The potential for low molecular weight heparin to provide an advantage over unfractionated heparin in preventing ischemic events was highlighted by the results of the ESSENCE trial (40), in which 3173 patients with unstable angina were randomized to enoxaparin or heparin. Enoxaparin reduced death, myocardial infarction, and refractory ischemia by 16.7% ($P = .019$) with no increase in bleeding. Twice daily subcutaneous administration without need for anticoagulation monitoring also allows low molecular weight heparin to be administered to outpatients. This may be important if longer duration antithrombin therapy is necessary for a sustained effect.

One phase II trial studying enoxaparin for prevention of stent thrombosis randomized 122 patients undergoing elective stent placement to enoxaparin, ticlopidine, and aspirin versus heparin, coumadin, and aspirin. The enoxaparin group had fewer thrombotic events ($P = .01$) and less bleeding ($P = .05$) (41). A 2000-patient phase III trial will compare a 14-day regimen of enoxaparin with placebo, in addition to aspirin and ticlopidine, following stent placement in a population at high risk for stent thrombosis.

ANTIPLATELET THERAPY

Rationale

Platelets play a primary role in the hemostatic response to vascular injury. Following atherosclerotic plaque disruption by balloon angioplasty, directional or rotational atherectomy, or stent implantation, circulating platelets adhere to the injured surface via interaction between platelet surface receptors (GPIb) and subendothelial adhesive proteins such as Von Willebrand factor (42). A monolayer of platelets adherent to the injured surface forms the initial response to injury. Platelets are then activated by both humoral and mechanical (i.e., shear forces) stimuli, secrete vasoactive substances to promote vasoconstriction and further hemostasis, and express other surface receptors, namely GPIIb/IIIa, capable of binding fibrinogen between adjacent platelets and leading to a platelet aggregate (14). The rich phospholipid surface of this platelet aggregate participates in the formation of the prothrombinase complex, where coagulation, thrombin formation, and the subsequent conversion of fibrinogen to fibrin can occur. Steele et al. (43) have shown in a porcine model of carotid balloon angioplasty injury that platelet deposition at the site of vascular injury is intense, immediate, and persistent for at least 24 hours following injury.

Thus, the platelet and coagulation system responses to injury are tightly intertwined and effects on one may affect the other (44).

Aspirin

Given the prominent role that platelets play in the vascular response to injury, it is no surprise that treatment with the antiplatelet agent aspirin is beneficial to patients undergoing percutaneous coronary procedures. Four placebo-controlled trials with aspirin alone or in combination with dipyridamole have demonstrated an overwhelming benefit to antiplatelet therapy with regard to reducing the ischemic complications (e.g., death, myocardial infarction, need for urgent procedures, including coronary bypass surgery and repeat PTCA) of the percutaneous procedure (9).

Aspirin's advantages are its proved benefits, safety profile, ease of use, and low cost. All patients undergoing percutaneous coronary intervention need to be treated with aspirin prior to the procedure and indefinitely afterward, unless a true contraindication, such as an allergy manifested by urticaria, bronchospasm, or anaphylaxis, exists. Relative contraindications to aspirin use (e.g., gastrointestinal intolerance) need to be weighed against its impressive clinical benefits.

Dipyridamole and Ticlopidine

Most clinical trials of dipyridamole in PTCA have examined it in combination with aspirin and have compared it with aspirin alone and placebo. **No evidence has been found that dipyridamole adds incrementally to the benefits of aspirin** when given to patients undergoing angioplasty. Its use cannot be recommended for these patients.

Ticlopidine is another widely used oral antiplatelet agent. Although its mechanism of action is still not completely understood (45), it does weakly inhibit adenosine diphosphate (ADP)-induced ex vivo platelet aggregation probably by interfering with the ability of the GPIIb/IIIa receptor to bind fibrinogen. Randomized trials of patients with unstable angina and with symptomatic cerebrovascular disease (46–48) undergoing PTCA, have shown ticlopidine to have benefits at least comparable to aspirin. In coronary stenting, the combination of ticlopidine and aspirin has become the standard of postprocedure care with reasonable evidence that this combination is superior to warfarin plus aspirin (30) and more limited evidence that combination benefit exceeds aspirin alone (29). Patients who have received coronary stents should be treated with ticlopidine and aspirin for 1 month and then aspirin indefinitely. Whether less time with ticlopidine is equally beneficial is unknown but worthy of investigation.

Ticlopidine is a reasonable alternative to use in the patient with an aspirin contraindication, but a few caveats must be kept in mind. The maximal antiplatelet effect requires 3–5 days of therapy and so, if possible, ticlopidine should be given in advance of the procedure; some data support more immediate effects following a loading dose. Neutropenia is an uncommon but recog-

nized complication of ticlopidine therapy, and patients should be appropriately monitored after institution of therapy. Gastrointestinal side effects, including nausea and dyspepsia, are not uncommon. Finally, **the cost of ticlopidine far exceeds aspirin and, therefore patients who can take aspirin should not be given ticlopidine as a substitute.**

Glycoprotein IIb/IIIa Inhibition

Although oral antiplatelet therapy with aspirin or ticlopidine is associated with substantial clinical benefits, both agents are relatively weak platelet inhibitors. More potent platelet inhibition may be associated with even greater clinical benefits. **Platelets aggregate via ligand binding (predominantly fibrinogen) to the GPIIb/IIIa receptor complex. Binding to this receptor complex represents the "final common pathway" of platelet aggregation.** Because aspirin inhibits only the thromboxane A_2 activating pathway, platelets can still aggregate via a number of other pathways despite the presence of aspirin. Blockade of GPIIb/IIIa may offer an opportunity to test whether substantial inhibition of platelet aggregation offers benefits beyond those provided by less intense platelet inhibition.

Recognizing the pivotal role of the GPIIb/IIIa receptor complex in the aggregation of platelets, Coller developed a monoclonal antibody to the receptor (49) that demonstrated intense platelet inhibitory effects. Modifications to decrease immunogenicity while maintaining platelet inhibitory action resulted in a monoclonal chimeric antibody fragment against GPIIb/IIIa. Known as abciximab (ReoPro, Centocor, Malvern, PA), this chimeric antibody fragment was the first GPIIb/IIIa inhibitor to be tested clinically.

Percutaneous coronary intervention was chosen for the initial testing of this unique therapeutic concept because of (*a*) the prominent role platelets seemed to play in both the acute and chronic complications of the procedure, (*b*) the potential widespread applicability of the therapy if successful, and (*c*) the ease with which large clinical trials can be rapidly performed in this patient population. Initial dose-finding studies demonstrated that abciximab could be safely given to patients undergoing coronary interventional procedures with a drug bolus producing 80% inhibition of ADP-induced platelet aggregation and a 12-hour infusion sustaining that degree of inhibition for approximately 18–20 hours (50, 51). This degree of platelet inhibition requires approximately 80% receptor blockade by abciximab.

EPIC

The EPIC (Evaluation of 7E3 (abciximab) for the Prevention of Ischemic Complications) trial was the first large-scale clinical trial of platelet GPIIb/IIIa inhibition (10). In this trial, patients undergoing high-risk balloon angioplasty or directional atherectomy were randomized to one of three treatment strategies: abciximab bolus plus 12-hour infusion, abciximab bolus plus placebo infusion, or placebo bolus plus placebo infusion. High risk was defined by a variety of clinical or angiographic characteristics (Table 34.2) that indicated an increased risk for abrupt vessel closure. All patients received aspirin and heparin at the investigator's discretion with a recommended ACT of 300–350 seconds. The trial's primary end point was a 30-day composite of the ischemic complications of the procedure: death, myocardial infarction, coronary artery bypass surgery, repeat coronary intervention, bail-out coronary stenting, or

Table 34.2.
High-Risk Characteristics as Defined in the EPIC Trial

Clinical
  Unstable angina
  Acute myocardial infarction within 12 hours
Angiographic
  Two type B lesion characteristics
  Female $\geq$ 65 years with B_1 lesion
  Diabetic with B_1 lesion
  Patient with type C lesion

placement of an intra-aortic balloon pump to treat refractory ischemia.

The abciximab bolus plus infusion regimen was associated with a highly significant 35% reduction in the primary end point compared with placebo, demonstrating the effectiveness of platelet GPIIb/IIIa inhibition during high-risk coronary intervention. The patient subgroups with unstable angina or recent myocardial infarction derived the greatest clinical benefit from abciximab (in excess of 60% risk reduction), suggesting that **those with the highest thrombogenic stimuli achieve the greatest benefit from potent platelet inhibition** (52, 53).

This impressive clinical benefit was not without risk; patients receiving abciximab had a major bleeding event (including need for blood transfusion) at a rate two times that of placebo-treated patients (14 versus 7%). Patients at the greatest bleeding risk included lightweight, elderly women (54). Additionally, because heparin was not weight adjusted in EPIC, its dosage was significantly associated with an increased risk of bleeding. These analyses suggest that the high bleeding rate seen in EPIC could be reduced, perhaps through more judicious use of concomitant heparin therapy.

EPIC was also noteworthy for demonstrating that **abciximab may have a long-term beneficial effect.** Compared with placebo, treatment with abciximab bolus plus infusion resulted in a 23% reduction in the 6-month composite of death, nonfatal myocardial infarction, and the need for repeat revascularization (35.1 versus 27.0%, $P < .001$) (55). Given the impressive benefits of abciximab as seen in the EPIC trial, the US Food and Drug Administration (FDA) approved abciximab for use in high-risk percutaneous intervention in December 1994. Further studies (11, 12) expanded the patient population that would benefit from abciximab and demonstrated that the major bleeding problem could be satisfactorily addressed.

EPILOG and CAPTURE

EPILOG (Evaluation of PTCA to Improve Long-term Outcomes by c7E3 Glycoprotein IIb/IIIa receptor blockade) was designed to test whether abciximab was beneficial in a broader population of patients undergoing coronary intervention and whether the clinical benefit could be maintained while bleeding was decreased with lower heparin dosing. Initial plans were to randomize approximately 4800 patients to one of three treatment strategies: abciximab bolus plus infusion with standard heparin (ACT > 300 seconds), abciximab bolus plus infusion with lower-dose heparin (ACT 200–250 seconds), or standard dose heparin. Patients not considered to be high risk (as defined by EPIC) were eligible for enrollment if they were undergoing coronary intervention with any FDA-approved device other than planned coronary stenting or rotational atherectomy. Enrollment was terminated after approximately 2700 patients had been randomized when review of the data on the first 1500 patients demonstrated an overwhelmingly positive treatment effect in favor of abciximab, with the 30-day incidence of death or myocardial infarction being reduced in excess of 60% (11).

Final data on the 2792 randomized patients have shown a highly significant reduction in the risk of death or myocardial infarction at 30 days that is sustained to 6-month follow-up. Patients across all risk groups benefitted, and the results, therefore, extended the observation of EPIC to non–high-risk patients as well. Target vessel revascularization, a marker of clinical restenosis, was not affected by abciximab treatment, raising questions about the ability of potent platelet inhibition to reduce restenosis.

Most impressive, however, was the lower rate of bleeding seen in the group treated with abciximab and lower-dose heparin: major bleeding 3.9, 2.4, and 3.8%, respectively, for heparin, abciximab and low-dose heparin, and abciximab and standard heparin. EPILOG clearly showed that the beneficial effects of abciximab could be preserved, and even improved on, while decreasing serious bleeding.

CAPTURE (c7E3 Antiplatelet Therapy in Unstable Refractory Angina) tested the hypothesis that abciximab would be beneficial to patients with unstable angina who are to undergo PTCA after 24 hours of treatment with this potent antiplatelet therapy

(12). Patients who had refractory unstable angina despite medical therapy, and who had a coronary lesion amenable to percutaneous intervention, were eligible for randomization to treatment with abciximab bolus plus 24-hour infusion, or placebo, prior to angioplasty. As with EPILOG, CAPTURE was terminated prematurely on recommendation of an independent data and safety monitoring board after an interim analysis demonstrated a highly significant benefit of abciximab in decreasing death or myocardial infarction. At 30 days, the incidence of death, myocardial infarction, or need for urgent intervention was 16.4% in the placebo group compared with 10.8% in the abciximab-treated patients. Particularly intriguing is that abciximab appeared to have a beneficial effect even before the procedure, suggesting a possible role for this agent in the medical treatment of unstable angina.

IMPACT and RESTORE

Integrilin (COR Therapeutics, South San Francisco, CA), a peptide GPIIb/IIIa inhibitor, and tirofiban (Merck & Co., West Point, PA), a nonpeptide GPIIb/IIIa inhibitor, have also been studied in large trials of patients undergoing percutaneous intervention. Differing from the antibody inhibitor, these agents are synthetic, small molecules with high specificity for the GPIIb/IIIa receptor, and they have a rapid on/off rate, making their antiplatelet action immediately effective and readily reversible. Whether these characteristics of the small molecules are clinically desirable is unclear.

Integrilin has been studied in three clinical trials of percutaneous coronary intervention: IMPACT (56), IMPACT HIGH/LOW (57), and IMPACT II (13). The largest of these, IMPACT II, was a phase III, randomized clinical trial designed to test whether Integrilin administered to all patients undergoing percutaneous intervention could reduce the acute ischemic complications of the procedure. Two doses of Integrilin were studied in this clinical trial: a common bolus dose of 135 µg/kg followed by an infusion of either 0.5 or 0.75

µg/kg per minute for 20–22 hours. The strategy was to have complete platelet inhibition at the time the procedure was performed and to have one infusion strategy of potent antiplatelet activity whereas the second strategy allowed gradual restoration of platelet function in an effort to minimize bleeding complications.

Patients were eligible for enrollment in the trial if they were undergoing either elective or urgent intervention and were allowed to be treated with any interventional device that was FDA approved at the time, other than primary elective stenting. Bailout stenting was allowed in this protocol. The primary end point of the trial was a 30-day composite of the acute ischemic complications of angioplasty, including death, myocardial infarction, or need for urgent intervention (including urgent bypass surgery, urgent repeat angioplasty, or stent placement for abrupt closure). All patients were treated with aspirin and heparin, with a recommended ACT during the procedure of 300–350 seconds.

A total of 4010 patients were enrolled in IMPACT II, evenly divided among the three treatment groups. Of these, 139 patients did not receive the study drug, although they had been randomized in the study, mainly because after initial cine shots had been obtained in the angioplasty laboratory, the decision was made that percutaneous intervention and, therefore, treatment with the study drug were not appropriate. In the group of patients treated with the 135/0.5 Integrilin dosage, a 22% reduction occurred in the primary composite end point at 30 days compared with placebo (P = .035). In the 135/0.75 treatment group, a 14% reduction was found in the primary end point, compared with placebo at 30 days (P = .179). This compared to reductions of 19 and 13% in the randomized patients' analysis.

No bleeding concerns were found in this trial, with an equal incidence of major bleeding across all three treatment groups: 4.5 in placebo, 4.4 in 135/0.5, and 4.7% in the 135/0.75. Also, a similar need for transfusion was found among the three treatment groups. The benefit of Integrilin therapy was particularly noticeable early, with a 31% relative reduction in the primary end point at 24 hours and a 25% reduction in

the primary end point at 48 hours in the group of patients treated with Integrilin 135/0.5. This early benefit was sustained at 30 days and, in fact, the absolute benefit was sustained to 6 months, although it was no longer statistically significant at this point. Finally, the treatment benefit of Integrilin was particularly strong with regard to the reduction in death or myocardial infarction, the most important parts of the end point composite.

Although the trial achieved a statistically significant result, the magnitude of the benefit was less than had been seen in the trials with abciximab. Further exploration of some of the dosing issues suggested that the measurement of the antiplatelet effect of Integrilin in sodium citrate anticoagulant may have overestimated the platelet inhibitory effects of Integrilin, because its binding to the GPIIb/IIIa receptor is a calcium-dependent process and sodium citrate is a calcium-chelating agent (personal communication, David Phillips, COR Therapeutics). It is possible that higher doses of Integrilin with a subsequent greater degree of platelet inhibition may give results similar to abciximab, and this concept is being studied in additional clinical trials.

Tirofiban was studied in a situation similar to Integrilin in percutaneous coronary intervention (RESTORE), with the exception that the angioplasty population was a high-risk one. Just over 2100 patients were enrolled in this trial (12). At day 2, a 38% reduction (P ≤ .005) was found in the primary end point, which was similar to IMPACT II and EPIC. At day 7, the reduction was 27%, and at day 30, there was a 16% reduction, with an event rate of 12.2% in the placebo group and 10.3% in the tirofiban group (P = 0.16). The findings here are strikingly similar to those in IMPACT II, and they suggest the possibility of a common issue with the shorter-acting, small molecules compared with the monoclonal antibody fragment. It may be that the rapid "off" of the molecules from the receptor, which allows for rapid restoration of platelet function, is less clinically advantageous than the more prolonged duration of action seen with the monoclonal antibody. This hypothesis is untested, but certainly sug-

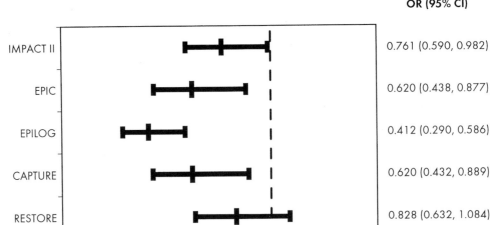

Figure 34.2. Odds ratio plot summarizing the randomized clinical trials of GPIIb/IIIa inhibition.

gests the possibility of beneficial orally active GPIIb/IIIa inhibitors that can be administered chronically beyond the initial periprocedural period.

Much evidence supports the use of platelet GPIIb/IIIa inhibition, during both high-risk and elective percutaneous coronary interventions (Fig. 34.2). The monoclonal antibody fragment is the only agent currently approved for use in percutaneous intervention, and issues need to be better defined as the use of this drug extends widely into clinical practice. Among these issues is **thrombocytopenia,** which has been reported to occur with a low but real incidence following the acute administration of abciximab (58). **Another issue is of readministration of a monoclonal antibody fragment, because of human antichimeric antibodies, which formed in a small population following initial administration of the agent.** A clinical registry of patients being readministered abciximab is currently underway to explore issues of efficacy and safety.

Costs of these agents and the incremental costs that they add to the angioplasty procedure also need to be taken into consideration. In the EPIC trial, where abciximab had a powerful effect in reducing not only death and MI, but repeat revascularization procedures after 6 months, a favorable cost benefit was found in the use of the drug during the index interventional procedure (3). Although a less powerful effect was found on revascularization procedures in the EPILOG trial, the overall cost benefit of abciximab is not known. Argument exists for the use of IIb/IIIa inhibition during all interventional procedures because preventing death and myocardial infarction has clearly been demonstrated with this class of drugs.

Whether GPIIb/IIIa inhibition adds clinical benefit incrementally to patients being treated with coronary stenting is another unknown area. The situation of bail-out stenting appears to be one where GPIIb/IIIa inhibition is favorable. Results from the IMPACT II trial suggest that myocardial infarctions that accompany bail-out stenting can be attenuated by one of these agents (59). Although primary coronary stenting has reduced the incidence of restenosis and the need for subsequent repeat interventional procedures, it has not eliminated myocardial infarction following the procedure (60, 61). At least suggestive evidence is found, therefore, that GPIIb/IIIa inhibition may add to the benefits of coronary stenting. This is currently being studied in a randomized trial of abciximab given with or

Table 34.3.

Agents	Patients
Antiplatelet therapy[a]	
Aspirin	All
Ticlopidine	All stents ×4 weeks; consider in ASA allergy
Abciximab	High risk; consider for all
Antithrombin therapy	
Heparin	All; ACT 300–350 without abciximab and 200–250 with abciximab

[a] Integrilin and tirofiban are not yet FDA approved. ACT, activated clotting time.

without coronary stenting versus stenting alone.

Finally, the broader question whether GPIIb/IIIa inhibition may be beneficial outside the realm of percutaneous intervention is currently being studied in both unstable angina and acute myocardial infarction. The results of several large clinical trials all contain information to address this situation and should be known sometime in 1997. To this end, PRISM (Platelet Receptor Inhibition for Ischemic Syndrome Management) and PRISM PLUS used tirofiban and reported beneficial results (62). Whether abciximab adds to the benefits of direct angioplasty for treatment of acute myocardial infarction is being investigated in a trial known as RAPPORT, the results of which will also be known in 1997.

SUMMARY AND RECOMMENDATIONS FOR CLINICAL PRACTICE (TABLE 34.3)

In patients undergoing percutaneous interventional procedures without coronary stenting, the following antithrombotic strategy is recommended:

1. All patients should receive 325 mg aspirin daily before the procedure and indefinitely after it.
2. Consideration should be given to treating all

patients with abciximab bolus plus a 12-hour infusion at the time of the procedure. Appropriate platelet count monitoring should be done after the procedure.
3. All patients should receive heparin intravenously during the procedure to maintain an ACT between approximately 300 and 350 seconds in the absence of abciximab and between approximately 200 and 300 seconds when administering concomitant abciximab therapy.
4. No indication is found for the routine use of postprocedural heparin therapy, although a course of 12–24 hours following a complicated procedure (e.g., residual thrombus, dissection, and so forth) may be appropriate.
5. Ticlopidine given at 250 mg twice daily is an appropriate antiplatelet alternative for the aspirin-allergic patient. It should be started 2–3 days in advance of the procedure if possible. Monitoring of white blood cell counts may be indicated in the patient receiving chronic therapy beyond 2 weeks.

In patients receiving coronary stents, additional recommendations for antithrombotic therapy include:

1. Abciximab use should be considered in bailout situations and probably other clinical high-risk situations such as acute unstable angina and acute myocardial infarction. More data are needed before recommending the widespread concomitant use of abciximab and coronary stenting.
2. All patients should receive 325 mg aspirin daily indefinitely and concomitant 250 mg ticlopidine twice daily for 1 month. Alternative length-of-therapy strategies have not been tested.

References

1. de Feyter PJ, de Jaegere PP, Serruys PW. Incidence, predictors, and management of acute coronary occlusion after coronary angioplasty. Am Heart J 1994;127:643–651.
2. Califf RM, Fortin DF, Frid DJ, et al. Restenosis after coronary angioplasty: an overview. J Am Coll Cardiol 1991;17:2B–13B.
3. Mark DB, Talley JD, Topol EJ, et al. Economic assessment of platelet glycoprotein IIb/IIIa inhibition for prevention of ischemic complications of high-risk coronary angioplasty. Circulation 1996; 94:629–635.
4. Hillegass WB, Peterson ED, Jollis JG. What cost of therapies to reduce restenosis is justified [Abstract]. Circulation 1993;88 (Suppl I):I-145.
5. Gruentzig AR, Senning A, Siegenthaler WE. Non-

operative dilatation of coronary artery stenosis: percutaneous transluminal coronary angioplasty. N Engl J Med 1979;301:61–68.

6. Bull BS, Korpman RA, Huse WM, et al. Heparin therapy during extracorporeal circulation. J Thorac Cardiovasc Surg 1975;69:674–684.

7. Ferguson JJ, Dougherty KG, Gaos CM, et al. Relation between procedural activated coagulation time and outcome after percutaneous transluminal coronary angioplasty. J Am Coll Cardiol 1994; 23: 1061–1065.

8. Narins CR, Hillegass WB, Nelson CL, et al. Activated clotting time predicts abrupt closure risk during angioplasty. Circulation 1996;93:667–671.

9. Antiplatelet Trialists' Collaboration. Collaborative overview of randomised trials of antiplatelet therapy. I. Prevention of death, myocardial infarction, and stroke by prolonged antiplatelet therapy in various categories of patients. Br Med J 1994;308: 81–106.

10. EPIC Investigators. Use of a monoclonal antibody directed against the platelet glycoprotein IIb/IIIa receptor in high-risk coronary angioplasty. N Engl J Med 1994;330:956–961.

11. Platelet glycoprotein IIb/IIIa receptor blockade and low-dose heparin drug percutaneous coronary revascularization. N Engl J Med 1997;336: 1689–1696.

12. The RESTORE Investigators. Effects of platelet glycoprotein IIb/IIIa blockade with tirofiban on adverse cardiac events in patients with unstable angina or acute myocardial infarction undergoing coronary angioplasty. Circulation 1997;96: 1445–1453.

13. The IMPACT-II Investigators. Effects of competitive platelet glycoprotein IIb/IIIa inhibition with Integrilin in reducing complications of percutaneous coronary intervention. Lancet 1997;349: 1422–1428.

14. Lefkovits J, Plow EF, Topol EJ. Platelet glycoprotein IIb/IIIa receptors in cardiovascular medicine. N Engl J Med 1995;332:1553–1559.

15. Popma JJ, Coller BS, Ohman EM, et al. Antithrombotic therapy in patients undergoing coronary angioplasty. Chest 1995;108 (Suppl):4865–5015.

16. Waller BF, Gorfinkel HJ, Rogers FJ, et al. Early and late morphologic changes in major epicardial coronary arteries after percutaneous transluminal coronary angioplasty. Am J Cardiol 1984;53:42C–47C.

17. Honye J, Mahon DJ, Jain A, et al. Morphological effects of coronary balloon angioplasty in vivo assessed by intravascular ultrasound imaging. Circulation 1992;85:1012–1025.

18. Solymoss BC, Cote G, Leung TK, et al. Pathology of PTCA complications. Circulation 1988;78 (Suppl II):II-449.

19. Manolis AS, Melita-Manolis H, Stefanadis C, et al. Plasma level changes of fibrinopeptide A after uncomplicated coronary angioplasty. Clin Cardiol 1993;16:548–552.

20. Vaitkus PT, Watkins MW, Witmer WT, et al. Characterization of platelet activation and thrombin generation accompanying percutaneous transluminal coronary angioplasty. Coron Artery Dis 1995;6:587–592.

21. Shammas NW, Cunningham MJ, Pomerantz RM, et al. Markers of hemostatic activation in affected coronary arteries during angioplasty. Thromb Haemost 1994;72:672–675.

22. Smith AJ, Holt RE, Fitzpatrick JB, et al. Transient thrombotic state after abrupt discontinuation of heparin in percutaneous coronary angioplasty. Am Heart J 1996;131:434–439.

23. McGarry TF Jr, Gottlieb RS, Morganroth J, et al. The relationship of anticoagulation level and complications after successful percutaneous transluminal coronary angioplasty. Am Heart J 1992;23: 1445–1451.

24. Ferguson JJ. All ACTs are not created equal. Texas Heart Inst J 1992;19:1–3.

25. Ellis SG, Roubin GS, Wilentz J, et al. Effect of 18- to 24-hour heparin administration for prevention of restenosis after uncomplicated coronary angioplasty Am Heart J 1989;117:777–782.

26. Friedman HZ, Cragg DR, Glazier SM, et al. Randomized prospective evaluation of prolonged versus abbreviated intravenous heparin therapy after coronary angioplasty. J Am Coll Cardiol 1994; 24: 1214–1219.

27. Lincoff AM, Tcheng JE, Bass TA, et al.; for the PROLOG investigators. A multicenter-randomized, double-blind pilot trial of standard versus low dose weight-adjusted heparin in patients treated with the platelet GP IIb/IIIa receptor antibody c7E3 during percutaneous coronary revascularization [Abstract]. Am J Cardiol 1997;79:286–291.

28. Moliterno DJ, Califf RM, Aguirre FV, et al. Effect of platelet glycoprotein IIb/IIIa integrin blockade on activated clotting time during percutaneous transluminal coronary angioplasty or directional atherectomy (the EPIC trial). Am J Cardiol 1995; 75:559–562.

29. Colombo A, Hall P, Nakamura S, et al. Intracoronary stenting without anticoagulation accomplished with intravascular ultrasound guidance. Circulation 1995;91:1676–1688.

30. Schomig A, Neumann FJ, Kastrati A, et al. A randomized comparison of antiplatelet and anticoagulant therapy after the placement of coronary-artery stents. N Engl J Med 1996;334:1084–1089.

31. Pepine CJ, Holmes DR Jr. Coronary artery stents. J Am Coll Cardiol 1996;28:782–794.

32. Hirsch J. Heparin. N Engl J Med 1991;324: 1565–1574.

33. Weitz JI, Hudoba M, Massel D, et al.. Clot-bound thrombin is protected from inhibition by heparin-anti-thrombin III but is susceptible to inactivation by antithrombin III-independent inhibitors. J Clin Invest 1990;86:385–391.

34. Topol EJ, Bonan R, Jewitt D, et al. Use of a direct antithrombin, hirulog, in place of heparin during coronary angioplasty. Circulation 1993;87: 1622–1629.

35. Bittl JA, Strony J, Brinker JA, et al. Treatment with bivalirudin (Hirulog) as compared with heparin during coronary angioplasty for unstable or post-infarction angina. Hirulog Angioplasty Study Investigators. N Engl J Med 1995;333:764–769.

36. van den Bos AA, Deckers JW, Heyndrickx GR, et al. Safety and efficacy of recombinant hirudin (CGP 39 393) versus heparin in patients with stable angina

undergoing coronary angioplasty. Circulation 1993;88:2058–2066.

37. Serruys PW, Herrman JP, Simon R, et al. A comparison of hirudin with heparin in the prevention of restenosis after coronary angioplasty. Helvetica Investigators. N Engl J Med 1995;333:757–763.

38. Granger CB, Becker R, Tracy RP, et al. Thrombin generation, inhibition and clinical outcomes in patients with acute myocardial infarction treated with thrombolytic therapy and heparin: results from the GUSTO trial. J Am Coll Cardiol; in revision, 1997.

39. Kottke-Marchant K, Zoldhelyi P, Zaramo C, et al. The effect of desirudin vs heparin on hemostatic parameters in acute coronary syndromes: the GUSTO IIb hemostasis substudy [Abstract]. Circulation 1996;94 (Suppl I):I-72.

40. Cohen M, Demers C, Gurfinkel E, et al., for the ESSENCE group. Primary end point analysis from the ESSENCE trial: enoxaparin vs unfractionated heparin in unstable angina and non-q wave infarction. Circulation 1996;94 (Suppl I):I-554.

41. Kruse KR, Greenberg CS, Tanguay J-F, et al. Thrombin and fibrin activity in patients treated with enoxaparin, ticlopidine and aspirin versus the conventional coumadin regimen after elective stenting: the ENTICES trial [Abstract]. J Am Coll Cardiol 1997; February:334A.

42. Harrington RA. Antithrombotic therapy during percutaneous coronary intervention. J Thomb Thrombol 1995;2:21–28.

43. Steele PM, Chesebro JH, Stanson AW, et al. Balloon angioplasty. Natural history of the pathophysiological response to injury in a pig model. Circ Res 1985;57:105–112.

44. Reverter JC, Beguin S, Kessels H, et al. Inhibition of platelet-mediated, tissue factor-induced thrombin generation by the mouse/human chimeric 7E3 antibody: potential implications for the effect of c7E3 treatment on acute thrombosis and clinical restenosis. J Clin Invest 1996;98:863–874.

45. Defreyn G, Bernat A, Delebassee D, et al. Pharmacology of ticlopidine: a review. Semin Thromb Hemost 1989;15:159–166.

46. Hass Wk, Easton JD, Adams HP, et al. A randomized trial comparing ticlopidine hydrochloride with aspirin for the prevention of stroke in high-risk patients. Ticlopidine Aspirin Stroke Study Group. N Engl J Med 1990;322:404–405.

47. Fitzgerald GA. Ticlopidine in unstable angina: a more expensive aspirin? Circulation 1990;82:17–26.

48. Balsano F, Rizzon P, Violi F, et al. Antiplatelet treatment with ticlopidine in unstable angina: a controlled multicenter clinical trial. Circulation 1990;82:296–298.

49. Coller BS. Blockade of platelet GPIIb/IIIa receptors as an antithrombotic strategy. Circulation 1995;92:2373–2380.

50. Tcheng JE, Ellis SG, George BS, et al. Pharmacodynamics of chimeric glycoprotein IIb/IIIa integrin antiplatelet antibody fab 7E3 in high-risk coronary angioplasty. Circulation 1994;90:1757–1764.

51. Ellis SG, Tcheng JE, Navetta FI, et al. Safety and antiplatelet effect of murine monoclonal antibody 7E3 Fab directed against platelet glycoprotein IIb/IIIa in patients undergoing elective coronary angioplasty. Coron Artery Dis 1993;4:167–175.

52. Lincoff AM, Califf RM, Anderson K, et al; for the EPIC Investigators. Striking clinical benefit with platelet GP IIb/IIIa inhibition by c7E3 among patients with unstable angina: outcome in the EPIC trial [Abstract]. J Am Coll Cardiol 1997;30:149–156.

53. Lefkovits J, Ivanhoe RJ, Califf RM, et al. Effects of platelet glycoprotein IIb/IIIa receptor blockade by a chimeric monoclonal antibody (abciximab) on acute and six-month outcomes after percutaneous transluminal coronary angioplasty for acute myocardial infarction. Am J Cardiol 1996;77:1045–1051.

54. Aguirre FV, Topol EJ, Ferguson JJ, et al. Bleeding complications with the chimeric antibody to platelet glycoprotein IIb/IIIa integrin in patients undergoing percutaneous coronary intervention. Circulation 1995;91:2882–2890.

55. Topol EJ, Califf RM, Weisman HF, et al. Randomised trial of coronary intervention with antibody against platelet IIb/IIIa integrin for reduction of clinical restenosis: results at six months. Lancet 1994;343:881–886.

56. Tcheng JE, Harrington RA, Kottke-Marchant K, et al. Multicenter, randomized, double-blind, placebo-controlled trial of the platelet integrin glycoprotein IIb/IIIa blocker integrelin in elective coronary intervention. Circulation 1995;91:2151–2157.

57. Harrington RA, Kleiman NS, Kottke-Marchant K, et al. Immediate and reversible platelet inhibition after intravenous administration of a peptide glycoprotein IIb/IIIa inhibitor during percutaneous coronary intervention. Am J Cardiol 1995;76:1222–1227.

58. Berkowitz SD, Harrington RA, Rund MM, et al. Acute profound thrombocytopenia after c7E3 fab (abciximab) therapy. Circulation 1997;95:809–813.

59. Zidar JP, Kruse KR, Thel MC, et al, for the IMPACT II Investigators. Integrelin for emergency coronary artery stenting [Abstract]. J Am Coll Cardiol 1996;27(Suppl A):138A.

60. Serruys PW, de Jaegere P, Kiemeneij F, et al. A comparison of balloon-expandable-stent implantation with balloon angioplasty in patients with coronary artery disease. N Engl J Med 1994;331:489–495.

61. Fischman DL, Leon MB, Baim DS, et al, for the Stent Restenosis Study Investigators. A randomized comparison of coronary-stent placement and balloon angioplasty in the treatment of coronary artery disease. N Engl J Med 1994;331:496–501.

62. Cody RJ. Results from late breaking clinical trials sessions at ACC '97. J Am Coll Cardiol 1997;30:1–7.

35

Balloon Valvuloplasty: Indications, Techniques, and Results

Howard C. Herrmann, MD

INTRODUCTION: HISTORY

The first successful report of the therapeutic use of a balloon for stenotic valvular heart disease was by Kan et al., in 1982, in a child with pulmonic valve stenosis (1). Subsequently, Lababidi applied the procedure to congenital aortic stenosis (2). In adults, Pepine et al. performed the first balloon pulmonic valvuloplasty in 1982 (3). In 1984, Inoue et al. used a uniquely designed balloon to report the first successful percutaneous mitral commissurotomies in patients with rheumatic mitral stenosis (4). Shortly thereafter, Lock et al. reported on a series of children with rheumatic mitral stenosis using the more widely available pulmonary balloon (5). In 1986, Cribier et al. extended balloon aortic valvuloplasty to adults with calcific aortic stenosis (6). The potential of valvuloplasty in patients with calcific mitral stenosis was also demonstrated in 1986 (7, 8).

For many reasons, over the past 5 years, percutaneous balloon valvuloplasty has begun to be more widely applied. National and geographic registries of both children and adults with congenital and acquired stenotic valvular heart disease have been reported (9–12). It has been estimated that more than 5000 valvuloplasty procedures are performed annually, most in the United States (13). As experience with percutaneous valvuloplasty procedures has in-

creased, so has the evolution of its application and understanding of its limitations. For example, the number of mitral valve procedures performed has steadily increased, whereas aortic valve dilations, particularly in adults, have decreased. This chapter discusses indications, technical aspects, results, and complications of balloon valvuloplasty in the most commonly stenosed valves in adults followed by a brief discussion of other large balloon applications.

AORTIC STENOSIS

Assessment of the patient with valvular aortic stenosis is reviewed in Chapters 25 and 40. Congenital aortic stenosis is caused by fusion of the valve leaflet apparatus, thus providing only a small orifice for blood ejection. In adults, aortic stenosis can occur as a result of rheumatic fever. In the United States, aortic stenosis more commonly results from calcium deposition on a congenitally bicuspid valve or a normal valve in the elderly.

Surgical valve replacement has been shown to reduce the symptoms associated with aortic stenosis and to improve patient survival (14, 15). This is the standard therapy to which any new treatment, such as valvuloplasty, must be compared and judged. Unfortunately, as will be discussed subsequently, percutaneous balloon valvuloplasty has not been demonstrated to markedly improve the survival of these patients, because of the limited improvement that is achieved in aortic valve area and a high rate of restenosis (9, 16, 17). However, despite these limitations, balloon aortic valvuloplasty is still applied in certain subsets of patients where the surgical risk may be high or short-term symptom palliation is all that is required.

Techniques

Retrograde Femoral

The most commonly used technique for balloon aortic valvuloplasty involves retrograde placement of the balloon across the aortic valve over a guidewire introduced from the femoral artery (6) (Fig. 35.1). A large lumen introducer sheath (10–14 F) is placed in the femoral artery in standard fashion. The necessary size varies for each individual balloon and has to be large enough to accommodate the balloon after an inflation-deflation cycle, which may be larger than its preinflation wrapped diameter. Some operators prefer not to use a sheath, and progressively dilate the soft tissues and femoral artery prior to balloon insertion. The stenotic aortic valve can be crossed with a 7 or 8 F pigtail catheter and a straight guidewire. It is important to position the pigtail catheter in the left ventricle

without traversing any of the chordae tendinea, which is best accomplished by advancing the pigtail catheter with fluoroscopic monitoring done in a right anterior oblique projection.

Once the gradient and cardiac output are measured, a guidewire is inserted and curled in the left ventricular apex. Generally, a 260 cm 0.038-inch guidewire provides adequate stiffness, but extra-stiff wires may be helpful in some cases. The tip is curved into an exaggerated 'J' shape, conforming to the apex, to minimize ventricular ectopy and the chance of ventricular perforation. It is important to include the core of the wire in the shaped portion or this protection may not be provided. The pigtail catheter can then be removed and a balloon inserted over the wire and positioned across the stenotic valve for inflation (Fig. 35.1, 1–2). Balloon valvuloplasty catheters (Mansfield Scientific Co., Watertown, MA) have an inflated diameter between 15 mm and 25 mm and vary in length from 3 to 5.5 cm (Fig. 35.1, 1–3). They are made of polyethylene and can be hand inflated using a 60 mL syringe with pressures less than 4 atm. Custom devices have been designed to facilitate balloon inflation and deflation, but these are not commercially available.

No optimal number and duration of inflation is known, but because blood pressure usually falls during inflation, the inflations should be kept brief. After the balloon is deflated, it can be pulled back into the aorta between inflations to allow the blood pressure to recover.

After three to four inflations or elimina-

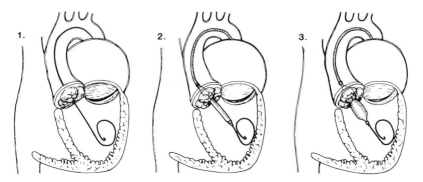

Figure 35.1. Retrograde femoral artery technique of percutaneous balloon aortic valvuloplasty.

tion of the "waist" in the inflated balloon, it should be removed. This is best achieved by maintaining negative pressure on the balloon and rotating it as it is removed through the sheath. The guidewire remains in the ventricle to facilitate recrossing the valve and reassessing the hemodynamics. Based on these measurements, a larger or longer balloon can be inserted and the process repeated until the desired results are achieved. In the authors' experience, the longer balloons "fix" better in the valve, but care must be taken to avoid trapping the balloon within the ventricle, which can lead to catastrophic ventricular perforation (9). Most valves can be dilated with a 20 mm diameter balloon, and the initial balloon size should be less than the diameter of the aortic annulus as measured with echocardiography or angiography. Smaller balloons can be used first in smaller patients and those with large gradients; larger balloons may occasionally be necessary to achieve an adequate hemodynamic effect, but balloons larger than 23 mm diameter have been associated with rupture of the aortic annulus and are not recommended (18).

Several balloon modifications are being evaluated that may improve the ease or safety of this technique. Lower profile balloons that will fit through smaller sheaths are being developed. Catheters with several tandem-mounted balloons to allow stepped sequential inflations with a single catheter and catheters with a curved pigtail-type end to guard against ventricular trauma have also been designed. Finally, catheters with multiple, side-by-side balloons or with multiple lumens to facilitate pressure recordings may be useful (19, 20). The availability of these devices may be limited as the frequency of aortic valvuloplasty procedures continues to decline.

The pharmacologic management of patients undergoing balloon aortic valvuloplasty involves several modifications to standard catheterization laboratory protocol. In addition to local anesthesia, mild sedation, and systemic anticoagulation with heparin, patients should receive a single dose of periprocedural antibiotic prophylaxis to avoid the rare complications of access site infection and endocarditis (21, 22). This can be accomplished with a cephalo-sporin or vancomycin (1 g) administered intravenously 1 hour before the procedure. All patients should have blood typed and cross-matched to minimize transfusion delays in the event of a vascular complication. A vasopressor and inotropic agent should be readily available should hypotension occur during or after balloon inflation. For this, we have found dobutamine to be particularly useful in patients with severely depressed left ventricular function (see *Results* later in this section). Finally, several general measures should be employed during valvuloplasty. These include right-side heart catheterization to measure cardiac output and pulmonary artery pressure, systemic blood pressure monitoring, usually from a contralateral femoral sheath, and pacing capability readily available, particularly for patients with pre-existing conduction abnormalities.

Alternate Techniques

Several alternative techniques for aortic valvuloplasty have been described, which may be useful in special situations. In the patient with peripheral vascular disease, the balloon can be introduced from either brachial artery via surgical cutdown. Similarly, the balloon can be inserted trans-septally in an antegrade fashion from the femoral vein after placing a guidewire across both the mitral and aortic valves (23). Finally, a bifoil balloon or two balloons can be simultaneously introduced from two arterial access sites (24, 25). This technique may minimize the fall in blood pressure during inflation by providing a potential space around the balloons for ejection, but it increases both the procedure complexity and the potential for complications (26, 27). In our experience, more than 95% of procedures can be accomplished with the retrograde femoral technique; alternative techniques offer few advantages and should be reserved for situations where the femoral technique is not applicable.

Results

The hemodynamic results of balloon aortic valvuloplasty in several large series of pa-

Table 35.1.
Hemodynamic Results of Percutaneous Balloon Valvuloplasty in Adult Patients with Aortic Stenosis

Author (reference)	Patients (n)	Age (yr)	Mean Gradient (mm Hg)		Cardiac Output (1/min)		Aortic Valve Area (cm²)	
			Pre	Post	Pre	Post	Pre	Post
Cribier et al. (28)	92	75	75	30	—	—	0.5	0.9
Block and Palacios (29)	90	79	61	30	3.6	3.9	0.4	0.8
Brady et al. (21)	26	86	59	31	3.6	3.6	0.5	0.7
Lewin (131)	125	76	70	30	4.3	4.6	0.6	1.0
NHLBI Registry (9)	674	78	55	29	4.0	4.1	0.5	0.8
Kuntz et al. (17)	205	78	67	33	4.4	4.8	0.6	0.9
Weighted means	—	78	61	30	3.8	3.9	0.5	0.8

NHLBI, National Heart, Lung, and Blood Institute.

tients are summarized in Table 35.1. In general, the results of valvuloplasty are remarkably similar in all of these studies, with an approximately 50% reduction in mean transaortic gradient and greater than a 50% increase in calculated aortic valve area. Although a residual gradient of 30 mm Hg and a postprocedure valve area less than 1.0 cm² initially appear disappointing when compared with the results of surgery, this small hemodynamic improvement may result in a marked improvement in patient symptoms (9, 21, 28, 29). For example, Brady et al. reported on an elderly cohort of patients (mean age of 86 years) in which improved symptoms of heart failure and angina were demonstrated in most patients (21). Similarly, in the National Heart, Lung and Blood Institute (NHLBI) registry (9), most patients (75%) experienced at least one functional class improvement in heart failure.

Unfortunately, despite the symptomatic improvement that most patients experience shortly after aortic valvuloplasty, the natural history of this illness is not greatly altered (9, 132). Kuntz et al. (17) examined the long-term outcome of 205 patients and demonstrated that death, recurrent symptoms, or need for repeat valvuloplasty or surgery occurred in 50% of the patients by 1 year and in 75% within 2 years of the initial procedure (Fig. 35.2). This poor long-term outcome is caused by restenosis, which occurs in most patients within 2 years (16, 17). In one study with repeat catheterization, restenosis was documented by hemodynamic

criteria in 48% of patients 7 months postprocedure (16). Repeat balloon aortic valvuloplasty has been advocated by some investigators to treat restenosis (30); however, the results achieved with the second procedure are often not as good as achieved with the first (31). We advocate repeat valvuloplasty only in patients who have a marked and sustained symptomatic improvement with their first procedure and remain poor surgical candidates (see selection criteria later in this section).

Lack of sustained benefit with aortic valvuloplasty probably reflects the pathology of the stenotic lesion and the mechanism by which balloon valvuloplasty alters it. In congenital and acquired rheumatic aortic stenosis, balloon dilation improves valve function by separating fused commissures. However, the relief of calcific aortic stenosis in adults by balloon dilation involves additional mechanisms. Postmortem and intraoperative studies by McKay et al. suggest that fracture of nodular calcium deposits, resulting in improved leaflet mobility, may also contribute to the effects of balloon dilatation (32, 33). Some of the immediate hemodynamic improvement noted may also be due to leaflet or annular stretching, which may not result in long-term benefit (32). The results of aortic valvuloplasty could potentially be improved if patients with the specific pathologic characteristics most amenable to balloon dilation could be selected for this procedure, but this hypothesis has never been tested.

The effect of balloon aortic valvu-

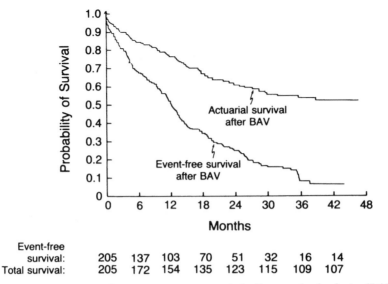

Event-free
survival: 205   137   103   70   51   32   16   14
Total survival: 205   172   154   135 123 115 109 107

Figure 35.2. Long-term outcome after percutaneous aortic balloon valvuloplasty (*BAV*). Actuarial survival and survival without need for repeat valvuloplasty or surgery are shown. (Reprinted with permission from Kuntz RE, Tosteson ANA, Berman AD, et al. Predictors of event-free survival after balloon aortic valvuloplasty. N Engl J Med 1991;325:17–23, with permission.)

loplasty on left ventricular function requires separate comment. Several investigators have demonstrated that left ventricular function improves following valvuloplasty, with the greatest improvement apparent in patients with the most depressed initial systolic function (34–36). These changes appear to result from improvement in left ventricular loading conditions (37). However, depressed left ventricular function may not improve, despite a reduction in afterload, provided by either valvuloplasty or surgery, if irreversible myocardial damage caused by fibrosis is present. These patients have a poor prognosis (38) and may be at high risk for complications during balloon valvuloplasty, which may further increase left ventricular afterload. In these patients, we recommend a dobutamine infusion during the procedure to improve left ventricular contractility and provide greater cardiac reserve during balloon inflations. Dobutamine is titrated to increase cardiac output 50 to 100% (5–10 µg/kg/min). Using this technique in patients with low-flow, low-gradient critical aortic stenosis and depressed left ventricular function (mean ejection fraction = 0.18), we accomplished balloon valvuloplasty without complica-

tions and increased the aortic valve area by 80% (38A).

Complications

A number of complications can occur as a consequence of aortic balloon valvuloplasty. Procedural mortality has been surprisingly low (< 5%), and usually it results from ventricular perforation or annulus rupture (9, 17, 18). This low mortality reflects, in part, the small effect balloon dilation has on calcific valves. With the advent of longer balloons, procedural mortality can be kept close to, or below, 1% with careful attention to guidewire position and avoiding balloons more than 23 mm diameter. In addition, the mortality rate remains low even in elderly patients with coexisting medical problems in whom the surgical risk may be markedly higher (21, 39).

The most frequent (5 to 10%) complications of aortic valvuloplasty are vascular access problems resulting from the introduction of large caliber balloons and sheaths in the femoral arteries of elderly patients, who often with peripheral vascular disease (9,

21). These complications include hematoma, hemorrhage, groin infection, pseudoaneurysm, and arterial-venous fistula formation, which may require surgical repair or blood transfusion (9). It is our practice to always reverse heparin with protamine sulfate prior to sheath removal, and to have a low threshold for early transfusion in patients developing a hematoma or hemorrhage because of the poor tolerance of hypovolemia by patients with severe aortic stenosis.

Other complications that can develop include arrhythmias (5 to 10%), such as transient left bundle branch block and ventricular ectopy, systemic emboli (1 to 5%) resulting in stroke, myocardial infarction, or peripheral damage, and severe aortic insufficiency (1%) (9, 17, 21, 39). The relatively low frequency of aortic regurgitation after balloon valvuloplasty again emphasizes the lack of a major effect of the balloon on the calcific pathology.

Selection and Indications

Aortic valve replacement carries a perioperative mortality of rate of approximately 5% in adult patients (14, 40), and it should be the procedure of choice in most adults with aortic stenosis. However, the risks of surgery increase with age and coexisting medical conditions (40–42). In one study of unselected octogenarians, the mortality rate for aortic valve surgery was 28%, and it may be as high as 50% in patients with cachexia, depressed left ventricular function, previous myocardial infarction, or hemodynamic compromise (43). Selection of elderly patients without these risk factors may allow aortic valve replacement with a lower mortality rate (41).

The major reason that valvuloplasty has a role in the management of elderly patients with calcific aortic stenosis is that valvuloplasty frequently improves patient symptoms in the short term with less risk than surgery, despite a high restenosis rate and little survival benefit. This risk:benefit analysis would suggest that valvuloplasty offers the most benefit, despite its limitations, to patients with the highest surgical risks.

Thus, aortic valvuloplasty should not be viewed as a competing alternative to aortic valve replacement, which can offer much greater long-term benefit, but as a lower-risk and lower-benefit alternative in patients at greatest surgical risk.

Balloon valvuloplasty appears to have a substantially lower procedural mortality rate in several surgically high-risk subgroups. Studies have demonstrated low procedural mortality rates in octogenarians undergoing balloon valvuloplasty, although later mortality during follow-up was high (21, 39). This underscores the need for good communication between the patient and physician to allow the patient to adequately balance the potentially higher early risk of surgery against the lower risk and lower long-term benefit of balloon valvuloplasty. Similarly, patients with severely depressed left ventricular function and those in cardiogenic shock may benefit from valvuloplasty (35, 44). Some practitioners, including cardiac surgeons, have advocated valvuloplasty in this setting to stabilize the patient and allow improvement in nutritional status or treatment of infection to reduce the risk of planned aortic valve surgery—the so-called bridge-to-surgery indication.

Lastly, several investigators have demonstrated good results with noncardiac surgery in patients with critical aortic stenosis treated by valvuloplasty before their operations (45, 46). Although the need for valvuloplasty in this setting has not been tested in a randomized fashion, the higher risk of noncardiac surgery in such patients suggests that attempts to lower this risk with valvuloplasty are reasonable (47). Similarly, the results of valvuloplasty may offer information about the eventual cardiac surgical risk in patients with depressed left ventricular function. If the left ventricular ejection fraction improves after valvuloplasty, it can be inferred that the original depression was caused more by afterload mismatch than by irreversibly impaired myocardial function, making surgery somewhat less risky (15). However, in our experience, it may be difficult to demonstrate the small improvement produced by valvuloplasty in patients with severely depressed left ventricular function.

On the basis of this discussion, we

would recommend balloon valvuloplasty as treatment in the following patient groups: (*a*) as palliative therapy to improve symptoms in patients at high surgical risk for cardiac or noncardiac reasons, including advanced age (usually > 80 years), coexisting cardiac problems (severe coronary artery disease, severe pulmonary hypertension, extremely poor left ventricular function), coexisting medical illness (renal, hepatic, or obstructive lung diseases); (*b*) in patients in whom the life-prolonging benefits of aortic valve replacement may be limited, as in the case of a malignancy or other severe debilitating or terminal disease; (*c*) to attempt to lessen the risk of an urgent noncardiac procedure; and (*d*) to temporarily improve aortic valve obstruction to stabilize an unstable state, often as a bridge to surgery.

In all of these circumstances, it is important that cardiac surgical input be obtained to fully inform the patient regarding treatment options. Age alone should not be used to deny a patient surgery, but it should be considered along with the other factors mentioned to arrive at a risk assessment for surgery. In this regard, we have found the Parsonnet et al. model especially useful to predict the eventual results of surgery in high-risk patients (48). Patients should be followed carefully after valvuloplasty for improvement in left ventricular function and evidence of restenosis and recurrent symptoms.

MITRAL STENOSIS

The pathophysiology of mitral valve stenosis is discussed in Chapters 25 and 40. Percutaneous balloon valvuloplasty has been used primarily in the treatment of rheumatic mitral stenosis, since the first descriptions of the technique by Inoue et al. (4) and Lock et al. (5), but it may also be effective in some types of congenital mitral stenosis (49). Although the incidence of rheumatic fever has been declining since the middle of the 1900s (50), isolated outbreaks have recently been reported in the United States (51), and it continues to be a common malady in many developing countries. It is likely that many patients with rheumatic

mitral stenosis will continue to require treatment during the coming decades.

Techniques

Double-Balloon Antegrade

The double-balloon technique and the Inoue technique (described later in this section) are the most commonly used techniques for percutaneous balloon mitral valvuloplasty. It became apparent early in the valvuloplasty experience that single polyethylene balloons, manufactured in sizes up to 25 mm diameter, were not sufficiently large enough to dilate most adult mitral valves (52). Larger polyethylene balloons (up to 30 mm diameter) produced adequate results, but resulted in larger atrial septal defects when passed across the atrial septum (53). Thus, in the double-balloon antegrade technique, as originally described by Al Zaibag et al. (54), and modified by Palacios et al. (55), two balloons (each < 20 mm diameter) are introduced across the mitral valve and simultaneously inflated (Fig. 35.3).

With the double-balloon antegrade, the left atrium is accessed through the interatrial septum (antegrade) from the right femoral vein using standard trans-septal catheterization equipment (56). A Mullen's sheath is in-

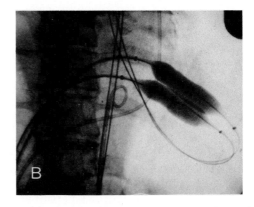

Figure 35.3. Double balloon antegrade technique of percutaneous balloon mitral valvuloplasty.

serted into the left atrium, through which an end-hole balloon-tipped catheter can be floated across the mitral valve, avoiding the chordae tendinea. It is then turned in the left ventricular apex using a curved-tipped guidewire and advanced out the aortic valve (5). A long guidewire (260 cm) is then introduced through this catheter from the femoral vein, across the atrial septum and the mitral and aortic valves, terminating in the descending aorta. This procedure can then be repeated (54), or a special double-lumen catheter used (55) to place a second guidewire adjacent to the first one. Some operators pass both guidewires through the Mullen's sheath without using a second catheter. Two polyethylene balloons are then introduced, one over each guidewire, and simultaneously inflated to dilate the stenotic valve (Fig. 35.3). Advancing the guidewires into the aorta can be technically difficult and time consuming, and some operators prefer to leave them curled in the left ventricle, as with the retrograde aortic technique. In our experience, this is more likely to cause arrhythmias, provide a less stable position during balloon insertion, and it may increase the risk of left ventricular perforation.

When both balloons are introduced through the same septal puncture, the interatrial septum is first dilated with a 6–8 mm diameter balloon to facilitate passage of the larger balloons. In most adults, two 20 mm diameter polyethylene balloons give good results (12, 52, 57). In some cases, a combination of smaller balloons may be preferable to avoid overdilating the valve and producing regurgitation (12, 58, 59). Some practitioners advocate single catheters used with combinations of balloons in bifoil or trefoil configurations (57, 60). Finally, retrograde techniques that do not require septal dilation (61) or that avoid the need for trans-septal catheterization altogether (62, 63) have been described. Although those techniques can reduce the size of the atrial septal defect, they increase the potential for arterial and aortic valve trauma.

Inoue Technique

The Inoue antegrade technique was first performed by Kanji Inoue in 1982 (4), intro-

duced into clinical investigation in the United States in 1989, and approved for use in 1994. It has become the most widely applied technique worldwide (63A). In this technique, the Inoue balloon is introduced trans-septally into the left atrium from the femoral vein after dilating the interatrial septum. It is then advanced across the mitral valve with the aid of an internal steering stylet. With initial inflation, only the distal segment of the balloon enlarges, allowing it to be pulled back against the valve and away from the ventricular apex. With further inflation, the proximal and middle sections are also inflated, thus fixing the balloon in position and dilating the valve (Fig. 35.4).

The device itself is a latex and nylon mesh balloon with several unique features. The segmental hourglass inflation profile aids positioning and fixation in the stenotic valve and reduces the risk of ventricular perforation. Because it can be stretched and slenderized, the balloon's profile is reduced when entering the femoral vein and crossing the interatrial septum and the ability to steer the tip assists in crossing the valve. Balloon compliance allows progressively larger balloon inflations with a single device, and a rapid inflation-deflation cycle, which minimizes hypotension. Left atrial pressure can be measured through the central lumen after each inflation. Finally, no guidewire is required in the left ventricle, thus reducing the frequency of arrhythmias. These characteristics have allowed the performance of simpler and faster procedures (64).

Echocardiography can be useful during balloon mitral valvuloplasty for several reasons. With the Inoue technique, progressively larger balloon inflations can be performed with a single device. Evaluation of the valve opening with two-dimensional and Doppler echocardiography, and assessment of mitral regurgitation by color-flow imaging, is helpful in deciding when sufficient valve dilation has been achieved (65). Recently transesophageal echocardiography has also been used during mitral valvuloplasty (66). Potential advantages of this technique include superior ability to (a) exclude intra-atrial thrombus, (b) guide and localize the fossa ovalis during trans-septal

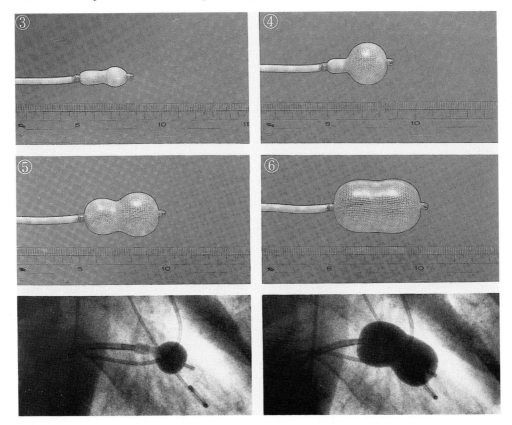

Figure 35.4. Stages of balloon inflation for percutaneous balloon mitral valvuloplasty using the Inoue technique are illustrated (*upper four panels*) and by fluoroscopy (*lower two panels*).

puncture, (*c*) aid in balloon positioning, (*d*) assess results, and (*e*) reduce fluoroscopic time.

Results

Postmortem and in vitro studies of the mechanism of successful balloon mitral valvuloplasty have demonstrated that separation of fused commissures is the major effect of balloon dilation (67, 68). **Commissural splitting can occur even with moderate valvular calcification and is analogous to the effects of surgical commissurotomy** (68). Stretching the mitral annulus and fracturing nodular calcium, which improves leaflet mobility, may also contribute to the effects of balloon dilation in some patients (69).

Hemodynamic results of balloon valvuloplasty in a patient with rheumatic mitral stenosis are shown in Figure 35.5. The results of several large series utilizing multiple techniques are summarized in Table 35.2. As can be seen from this table, the initial hemodynamic results are similar, despite different techniques, with a greater than 50% reduction in mean transmitral gradient and an approximate doubling in calculated mitral valve area. Elevated pulmonary artery pressures tend to fall immediately, and may continue to fall for several months after valvuloplasty, although they may remain elevated in patients with long-standing mitral stenosis and pathologic obliterative vascular changes (70). Cardiac surgery should be considered in patients with persistent pulmonary hypertension and residual mitral valve disease (70A).

Several studies have compared the double-balloon and Inoue techniques. Because the mechanism of successful balloon valvuloplasty requires splitting fused commissures, it has been suggested that the double-balloon, rather than single circular balloon, technique can achieve superior results by exerting maximal force laterally toward the commissures. In fact, retrospective comparisons of the hemodynamic results have

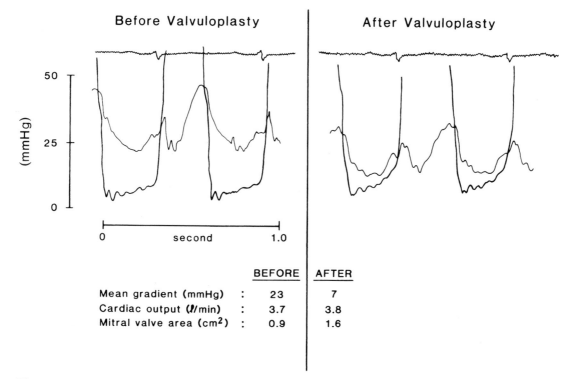

	BEFORE	AFTER
Mean gradient (mmHg) :	23	7
Cardiac output (*l*/min) :	3.7	3.8
Mitral valve area (cm^2) :	0.9	1.6

Figure 35.5. Hemodynamic findings before and after percutaneous balloon mitral valvuloplasty in a 78-year old woman with severe, symptomatic mitral stenosis. Valvular total echocardiographic score was 9. Dilation performed with an Inoue balloon inserted trans-septally, inflated in stepwise fashion to maximal diameter of 25 mm.

Table 35.2.
Hemodynamic Results of Percutaneous Balloon Valvuloplasty in Large Series of Adult Patients with Mitral Stenosis

Author (reference)	Techniques[a]	Patients (n)	Age (yr)	Mean Gradient (mm Hg)		Cardiac Ouput (1/min)		Mitral Valve Area (cm^2)	
				Pre	Post	Pre	Post	Pre	Post
Babic (61)	R	54	39	18	9	5.1	6.1	1.2	2.3
Vahanian (57)	D, S (trefoil)	200	43	16	6	2.6	3.1	1.1	2.2
Herrmann (12)	D, S	67	53	15	7	4.2	4.8	1.0	2.0
Ruiz (79)	D	285	44	17	5	3.8	5.4	0.9	2.4
Hung (78)	I	219	43	13	6	4.4	4.7	1.0	2.0
Herrmann (80)	I	200	53	14	6	4.2	4.6	1.0	1.8
Weighted means			46	15	6	3.2	3.9	1.0	2.1

[a] I, Inoue; D, double balloon antegrade; S, single balloon; R, retrograde.

demonstrated greater increases in valve area with the double-balloon technique (134). However, the increased incidence of small atrial septal defects produced by the double-balloon technique and the inclusion of shunt flow in the cardiac output determination may have contributed to this finding (135). In two small randomized trials comparing these techniques, no significant difference in mitral valve area after valvuloplasty was found (71, 136).

Balloon valvuloplasty and surgery have also been compared. Retrospective and nonrandomized comparisons are difficult because of differences in baseline characteristics and selection bias. Two prospective, randomized trials compared balloon valvuloplasty with closed surgical commissurotomy (137, 138). In both trials, no deaths occurred and similar hemodynamic results were found. At long-term follow-up, the hemodynamic results were maintained equally in both groups with similar restenosis rates and functional status (137).

Open surgical commissurotomy has been compared with balloon valvuloplasty in three randomized trials (139–141). The results of Reyes et al. are typical (139). In this study, 60 Indian patients with favorable anatomy for balloon valvuloplasty were randomized to the Inoue balloon technique or surgery. Mitral valve area increased to about 2.0 cm^2 in both groups, but was better maintained at 3 years in the balloon valvuloplasty patients. Functional capacity and event-free survival at 3 years were similar (139). Although the similar safety and efficacy with lower cost and greater patient comfort would seem to favor balloon valvuloplasty over surgery, it should be emphasized that these results were obtained in ideal balloon valvuloplasty candidates and may not apply to patients with suboptimal valve morphology. Similarly, no comparison has been done of less ideal patients with mitral valve replacement surgery.

Few studies have examined the long-term follow-up hemodynamics after balloon valvuloplasty. Clinical and hemodynamic studies have suggested that approximately 20% of patients with an initially successful procedure will develop recurrent symptoms within 1 year (12, 74, 80, 90, 142). However, these studies used a heterogeneous popula-

tion of patients undergoing dilation with a variety of techniques. Other studies have identified echocardiographic features that increase the likelihood of restenosis (74, 78). In the Palacios et al. study, the restenosis rate (loss of 50% of the initial gain in mitral valve area) was 42% in patients with, and 4% in patients without, these echocardiographic characteristics (74). Early symptom recurrence likely may be caused by mitral regurgitation or inadequate initial dilation rather than by restenosis. Furthermore, restenosis rates based on the final immediate catheterization-determined valve area may overestimate the true restenosis rate because of valve stretching (69).

In longer term follow-up, the absence of need for mitral valve replacement or repeat valvuloplasty is the most objective measure of a successful procedure. Cohen et al. reported on 146 patients in the United States who underwent single and double-balloon valvuloplasty with a 5-year actuarial event-free survival rate of 51% (142). The event-free survival was as high as 84% in a subset with lower echocardiographic scores and fewer symptoms. Similar rates of event-free survival, ranging from 65 to 76% at 4–5 years, have been reported by others with even better survival rates in optimal candidates (143, 144).

Most patients report dramatic improvements in dyspnea and functional capacity after balloon valvuloplasty (57, 12, 74). In the M-HEART multicenter balloon valvuloplasty registry, 69% of the patients experienced clinical improvement as a result of valvuloplasty 15 months after the procedure, and mean functional class improved from 2.9 to 1.4 (12). However, objective improvement in exercise capacity shortly after valvuloplasty has not been demonstrated by all investigators (75, 76), which suggests that exercise training may be necessary to reverse the peripheral effects of deconditioning that is associated with chronic mitral stenosis (75). Left ventricular systolic function may also improve after successful valvuloplasty, probably as a result of improved filling and increased preload (77).

Complications

Procedure-related mortality, the most serious complication of balloon mitral valvuloplasty, occurs in 0.5 to 3% of cases, usually the result of cardiac perforation (11, 12, 58, 78, 79). Perforation and tamponade can occur in up to 7% of procedures in multicenter studies (11, 12) and is lowest in single centers with a large experience (58, 78, 79). In the M-HEART multihospital study, cardiac perforation occurred in seven patients, resulted in tamponade in five patients, and required emergency surgery in four of these patients, two of whom subsequently died (12). For this reason, mitral valvuloplasty should be performed only in centers with facilities for cardiac surgery and by operators experienced in trans-septal catheterization techniques. The Inoue balloon technique may offer some advantages in this regard, because it does not require a left ventricular guidewire and it is pulled away from the ventricular apex during inflation (78). However, perforation during the trans-septal procedure can still occur (80). Finally, some investigators have demonstrated improved results, and fewer complications, with increased experience (58).

Other complications include systemic embolism (1 to 4%); arrhythmias, including complete heart block (81); vascular injury and hemorrhage; atrial septal defects; and mitral regurgitation (12, 57, 78, 79, 81). Systemic embolism can result from disruption of left atrial thrombus, valvular debris, or balloon rupture with introduction of air; cerebral vascular accidents, myocardial infarction (often inferior due to right coronary artery embolization), or peripheral arterial problems affecting the leg or kidney can also occur (12, 57, 78, 79).

The incidence of iatrogenic atrial septal defects caused by balloon passage through the interatrial septum depends on the method of assessment. Left-to-right intracardiac shunts can be measured by oximetry, in up to 25% of procedures, immediately after valvuloplasty, with any of the antegrade techniques (12, 57, 74, 79, 80, 82). With more sensitive techniques, such as color-flow and transesophageal echocardiography, atrial shunting is detectable after most such procedures (83, 84). Although retrograde valvuloplasty techniques can reduce the incidence of shunts (61, 63), most of the septal defects appear to close during short-term follow-up (74, 82, 83). Factors affecting atrial septal defects development include balloon size, the location of the trans-septal puncture in muscular or membranous septum, and the amount of wire and balloon manipulation required to dilate the valve (85, 86).

Small increases in the grade of mitral regurgitation are common after balloon valvuloplasty, occurring in up to 50% of patients; however, moderate and severe regurgitation with an increase of two or more angiographic grades is less common (5 to 10%) (11, 12, 57, 87, 145). Increased regurgitation correlates with balloon size (12), but it also depends on valve morphology. Severe mitral regurgitation may result from valvular disruption or wide splitting of the commissures. In one series of patients undergoing Inoue balloon valvuloplasty, the incidence of severe regurgitation was 7.5%, most often (43%) caused by rupture of the chordae tendinae to the anterior or posterior mitral leaflet (145). Other causes as assessed by echocardiography included tearing of the leaflet (usually the posterior one) and wide splitting of the commissures with a central regurgitant jet (145).

Severe mitral regurgitation incidence does not appear to be significantly different with the double-balloon technique compared with the Inoue technique (146, 147). However, the mechanism seems to involve leaflet tears more commonly than chordal rupture (88, 89). Factors associated with the development of severe regurgitation include balloon size (12, 148), calcified valves (57, 145), and pre-existing mitral regurgitation (145). Unfortunately, no variables have been reliable predictors of this complication. The Massachusetts General Hospital (MGH) group has recently attempted to develop an echocardiographic score based on a retrospective analysis of patients who develop severe regurgitation after double-balloon valvuloplasty (149). This study suggests that leaflet tears are more likely if the leaflets have inhomogeneous thickening in the presence of commissural and subvalvular calcification (149).

During Inoue balloon valvuloplasty, a stepwise technique of repeated inflations with increasing balloon diameters maximizes the increase in valve area while avoiding the creation of severe mitral regurgitation (65). Most patients with new mitral regurgitation after valvuloplasty can be managed medically (12, 89); however, valve replacement is eventually required in most patients developing severe regurgitation (80, 145).

Selection and Indications

In screening potential candidates for balloon mitral valvuloplasty, two-dimensional echocardiography is a valuable tool. Specific features of valvular morphology can be assessed, including leaflet thickening and mobility, valvular calcification, and subvalvular disease (59, 91). **Several studies have demonstrated better results in patients with pliable valves and a minimum of leaflet thickening, immobility, calcification, and subvalvular involvement** (52, 59, 78, 91). Individual factors that have been reported to adversely influence the immedi-

ate results of valvuloplasty include valvular thickening (59), leaflet immobility (91), and subvalvular disease (80). In one widely used system, a score is assigned to each of four factors to provide a total score ranging from 4–16 (Table 35.3) (87, 92). Patients with scores of ≤8 have been shown to have the best immediate (52, 87, 92) and long-term (74) results. Although these investigations were done in patients undergoing double-balloon procedures, similar results have been demonstrated with the Inoue balloon technique (151). In patients with severe valvular and subvalvular deformity, (MGH echocardiographic score ≤10), actuarial 3-year event-free survival was 42% compared with 77% in all patients (151). Balloon valvuloplasty may be a reasonable palliative therapeutic option for some patients with severe valvular deformity and at high surgical risk.

Echocardiography is also useful to screen patients for left atrial thrombus, a

Table 35.3.
The Massachusetts General Hospital Echocardiographic Scoring System for Mitral Valve Morphology[a]

Leaflet Mobility	Subvalvular Thickening
Grade 1: Highly mobile valve with restriction of only the leaflet tips	Grade 1: Minimal thickening of chordal structures just below the valve
Grade 2: Midportion and base of leaflets have reduced mobility	Grade 2: Thickening of chordae extending up to one third of chordal length
Grade 3: Valve leaflets move forward in diastole mainly at the base	Grade 3: Thickening extending to the distal third of the chordae
Grade 4: No or minimal forward movement of the leaflets in diastole	Grade 4: Extensive thickening and shortening of all chordae extending down to the papillary muscle

Valvular Thickening	Valvular Calcification
Grade 1: Leaders near normal (4–5 mm)	Grade 1: A single area of increased echo brightness
Grade 2: Midleaflet thickening, marked thickening of the margins	Grade 2: Scattered areas of brightness confined to leaflet margins
Grade 3: Thickening extends through the entire leaflets (5–8 mm)	Grade 3: Brightness extending into the midportion of leaflets
Grade 4: Marked thickening of all leaflet tissue (> 8–10 mm)	Grade 4: Extensive brightness through most of the leaflet tissue

Reprinted with permission from Abascal VM, Wilkins GT, O'Shea JP, et al. Prediction of successful outcome in 130 patients undergoing percutaneous balloon mitral valvotomy. Circulation 1990;82:448–456; with the permission of the American Heart Association.
[a] Echocardiographic scores were derived from the analysis of leaflet mobility, valvular and subvalvular thickening, and valvular calcification, and graded from 1 to 4 according to the above criteria. The total score was the sum of each of these echocardiographic features (maximum 16).

relative contraindication to balloon valvuloplasty. In this regard, transesophageal echocardiography may be especially helpful in examining the left atrium, atrial appendage, and interatrial septum (93, 150). In our center, transesophageal echocardiography is routinely performed before all balloon valvuloplasty procedures to exclude left atrial thrombus and to further assess valve morphology and the grade of mitral regurgitation. Although some have also advocated transesophageal echocardiographic monitoring during the procedure, we use transthoracic echocardiography to assess the results of each balloon inflation (150).

Other factors influencing the immediate results of mitral valvuloplasty with the single or double-balloon technique include the total effective balloon dilating area (52, 57, 91), age (74, 78), atrial fibrillation (52, 78), fluoroscopic valvular calcium (74, 78), and left atrial enlargement (52, 78, 94). The Inoue technique appears to be less sensitive to overall echocardiographic score (65, 80), but this may reflect, in part, a greater variability in subjective scoring by multiple investigators. In multivariate analysis, the absence of prior surgical commissurotomy and younger age were identified as significant predictors of the gain in mitral valve area (80). Previous surgical commissurotomy reduced the mean percentage increase in valve area from 94 to 55%, but a successful procedure was still achieved in 78% of patients without an increased risk of complications (80). Therefore, it seems reasonable to treat these patients with balloon valvuloplasty before recommending repeat surgery. Similarly, many elderly patients have an increased risk at surgery and may derive substantial benefit from valvuloplasty (95). Finally, successful valvuloplasty for symptomatic patients during pregnancy has also been reported (96).

Mitral valve area alone should not be used to select patients for balloon valvuloplasty. Pan et al. demonstrated excellent results with valvuloplasty in 21 patients with valve areas $\geq 1.5 \, cm^2$ (97). In our experience, symptomatic patients with mild and moderate stenosis tend to have more pliable valves; thus, larger valve areas and improvement in symptoms are obtained following balloon valvuloplasty (152). Finally, the Gorlin formula may underestimate the severity of mitral stenosis in some patients because of large body size or high cardiac output (152).

On the basis of the factors discussed, we recommend percutaneous balloon mitral valvuloplasty to patients with mitral stenosis who are symptomatic and to those with pulmonary hypertension, unless they have a severely calcified or immobile valve (echo-score ≥ 12), left atrial thrombus on echocardiogram, or severe mitral regurgitation. Patients with recent embolic events, left atrial thrombus, or atrial fibrillation should be treated with warfarin for several months and then undergo reassessment, preferably with transesophageal echocardiography. During the procedure, patients should receive systemic anticoagulation with heparin and antibiotic prophylaxis. Finally, it is essential that the operator have experience with trans-septal catheterization and know how to manage its complications. Emergency cardiac surgical support must be available. Currently both the double-balloon and Inoue antegrade techniques offer satisfactory results, but both require experience and demonstrate a learning curve for results and complications.

In general, one can expect that 70 to 80% of selected patients will obtain a long-term improvement (at least 2–3 years) with mitral valvuloplasty. In 10 to 20% of patients, the hemodynamic result will be inadequate, and 5 to 10% will suffer a complication, including mitral regurgitation; many of these patients will require early mitral valve replacement. All patients should be carefully followed clinically, and with echocardiography, for evidence of worsening regurgitation and development of recurrent symptoms.

PULMONIC STENOSIS

Percutaneous balloon valvuloplasty had its origin in the treatment of congenital pulmonic valve stenosis in an 8-year-old child by Kan et al. and in an adult by Pepine et al. in 1982 (1, 3). It has subsequently become the **procedure of choice in infants and children** (98). Although valvuloplasty has also been applied in adult pulmonic stenosis (3, 99, 100, 154), fewer data are available because of the relatively low incidence of this problem. Because pulmonic stenosis is usually congenital, patients surviving without treatment to adulthood are often asymptomatic or have hemodynamically insignificant stenosis.

Technique, Results, and Complications

Pulmonic valvuloplasty resembles the technique employed in other valve lesions. The balloon is introduced from the femoral vein over a guidewire that has been placed in the pulmonary artery, positioned across the stenotic valve, and inflated. Single polyethylene balloons are most commonly applied, but the Inoue balloon and double balloons can also be used for this procedure. Optimal dilation appears to be achieved with a balloon diameter 20 to 50% larger than the valve annulus in pediatric patients (101),

but the balloon may not need to be larger than the annulus in adult patients (154).

The hemodynamic results of valvuloplasty have been best studied in children. In the large multicenter valvuloplasty and angioplasty of congenital anomalies registry of almost 800 children, mean gradient decreased from 71 to 28 mm Hg after valvuloplasty (102). In adults, Fawzy et al. described 22 patients with severe congenital pulmonic stenosis in whom the peak gradient was reduced by valvuloplasty from 111 to 38 mm Hg (100). Herrmann et al. recently described a series of patients in the United States with congenital and acquired pulmonic stenosis, and demonstrated a reduction in peak transpulmonic gradient from 62 to 22 mm Hg (Fig. 35.6) (99).

Major complications of this procedure, reported by the congenital registry, include death (0.2%), cardiac perforation (0.1%), and tricuspid insufficiency (0.2%), as well as other minor complications (1 to 3%) (102). One death was reported in the Herrmann et al. series of adults as a result of sepsis after the procedure (99). Mild pulmonary valve incompetence can occur after the pro-

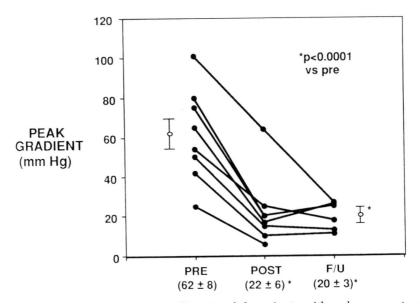

Figure 35.6. Peak transpulmonic valve gradient in adult patients with pulmonary stenosis treated with balloon valvuloplasty (*F/U* = follow-up assessed by Doppler echocardiography). Note further improvement in one patient during follow-up due to regression of infundibular hypertrophy. (Reprinted with permission from Herrmann HC, Hill JA, Krol J, et al. Effectiveness of percutaneous balloon valvuloplasty in adults with pulmonic valve stenosis. Am J Cardiol 1991;68:1111–1113.)

cedure, but it usually resolves during follow-up (154). Patients with severe pulmonic stenosis can also develop right ventricular outflow tract (infundibular) hypertrophy or spasm, which can cause a significant gradient after relief of the valvular obstruction (103). For this reason, calcium antagonists and β-blocking agents should be administered to such patients acutely, and until infundibular gradient regression has been documented (99, 100, 102, 154).

Pediatric patient follow-up has demonstrated sustained improvement up to 4 years after successful balloon dilation (104). Similarly, a sustained decrease in peak gradient has been demonstrated in adults up to 7 years after valvuloplasty (99, 100, 154). All of these patients also had marked improvement in symptoms of fatigue and chest discomfort (99). The results of valvuloplasty in dysplastic pulmonic valves have been more variable, with higher residual gradients (102) and possibly more restenosis (105); technique use in this setting should be considered investigational.

Selection and Recommendations

In adults with congenital and acquired pulmonic stenosis, balloon valvuloplasty offers safe and effective treatment, and the results appear to be sustained for several years. Patients should be considered for this technique if they are symptomatic or have high right ventricular systolic pressures (usually > 70 mm Hg). Follow-up evaluation by echocardiography and right side heart catheterization should be performed, if necessary, to document regression of infundibular hypertrophy and sustained valvular improvement.

OTHER LARGE BALLOON TECHNIQUES

Tricuspid Valve and Bioprostheses

Percutaneous balloon valvuloplasty has been successfully applied to rheumatic tricuspid stenosis. With double-balloon techniques, the effective valve area can be increased more than twofold, resulting in improved cardiac output and patient symptoms in intermediate term follow-up (106, 158). However, because severe tricuspid stenosis is a rare sequela of rheumatic fever, and it is often associated with regurgitation, the applications of this technique may be limited.

Balloon valvuloplasty of bioprostheses must be undertaken with caution because of the nature of the valvular degeneration. Valvular dysfunction may be caused by leaflet rigidity as a consequence of collagen degeneration and calcium deposition, as well as fibrous pannus ingrowth or thrombus formation (107, 108). Case reports of successful dilations of bioprostheses in all four cardiac valves have been reported (109–112), but complications can include cuspal tears or avulsions, and the potential for dislodgement of thrombus, vegetations, or valvular debris seems high (110). Furthermore, short-term follow-up (< 1 year) of bioprosthetic dilations suggests that progressive regurgitation and restenosis may limit this procedure to patients considered at too high a risk for surgery (113).

Coarctation

Aortic coarctation was one of the first nonvalvular conditions treated by balloon dilation. Short- and long-term results are now available in several series of both children and adults (114, 115, 157). In general, single balloons with diameters several times larger than the narrowing and slightly smaller (1–2 mm) than the adjacent normal aorta, are used for dilation (114). The immediate results have included reduction of the peak systolic gradient to less than 20 mm Hg and an increase in coarctation diameter in most patients (114, 115). Complications are infrequent, but they can include femoral artery thrombosis and death caused by aortic tear or catheter-induced rupture (115).

Longer-term results of coarctation dilation have been worrisome because of late aneurysm formation at the dilation site (114, 116). The reported incidence of aneurysms has varied and may be as high as 30 to 50% (116, 117) and it appears to be caused by medial necrosis and thinning with an intact adventitia at the site of an aortic tear (117, 118). Restenosis may also occur after successful dilation in up to one third of patients, and it can be treated by repeat dilation (114). The mechanism of successful dilation involves intima and media tearing, and restenosis occurs because of neointimal hyperplasia (119).

Several uncontrolled studies have suggested better results with balloon dilation in recurrent coarctation after surgical repair compared with native unoperated coarctation (117, 120–122). Recoarctation after surgery can occur in up to 40% of patients; it carries a higher risk for repeat surgery and is often caused by fibrosis and scar formation (117, 120, 122). Endovascular balloon-expandable stents have recently been used for both native and recurrent coarctation with good short-term results (156). However, because of the paucity of late follow-up data, **balloon dilation and stent placement for coarctation must be considered promising, but investigational, techniques.**

Other Techniques

As the successful results of balloon valvuloplasty became widely known, large balloons were applied to a number of other nonvalvular conditions. Successful dilation of congenital pulmonary artery branch stenosis has been reported (123), but it has been limited by elastic recoil and prompted alternate therapies, including the use of balloon-expandable stents (124). Large balloons have been used in superior vena caval obstruction either after Mustard procedures or when caused by tumor encasement (125), and also for a variety of stenotic postsurgical systemic-to-pulmonary conduits with mixed results (126, 127). Several investigators have attempted to alleviate membranous subaortic stenosis by balloon dilation. The results have been variable, with acute reductions in gradient, but with reports of restenosis and the potential for disruption of the aortic valve leading to regurgitation (128). Finally, valvuloplasty balloons have recently been used to make a large opening in the parietal pericardium in patients undergoing pericardiocentesis for cardiac tamponade (129). This procedure of balloon pericardial "windowing" has the potential to reduce the frequency of recurrent pericardial effusions in patients with malignancy (130) (see Chapter 42).

SUMMARY

Balloon valvuloplasty provides an alternative to surgery for paliation of many patients with valve stenosis.

References

1. Kan JS, White RI, Mitchell SE, et al. Percutaneous balloon valvuloplasty: a new method for treating congenital pulmonary valve stenosis. N Engl J Med 1982;307:540–542.
2. Lababidi Z. Aortic balloon valvuloplasty. Am Heart J 1983;106:751–755.
3. Pepine CJ, Gessner IH, Feldman RL. Percutaneous balloon valvuloplasty for pulmonic valve stenosis in the adult. Am J Cardiol 1982;50:1442–1445.
4. Inoue K, Owaki T, Nakamura T, et al. Clinical application of transvenous mitral commissurotomy by a new balloon catheter. J Thorac Cardiovasc Surg 1984;87:394–402.
5. Lock JE, Khalilullah M, Shrivastava S, et al. Percutaneous catheter commissurotomy in rheumatic mitral stenosis. N Engl J Med 1985;313:1515–1518.
6. Cribier A, Saoudi N, Berland J, et al. Percutaneous transluminal valvuloplasty of acquired aortic stenosis in elderly patients: an alternative to valve replacement? Lancet 1986;1:63–67.
7. Palacios IF, Lock JE, Keane JF, et al. Percutaneous transvenous balloon valvotomy in a patient with severe calcific mitral stenosis. J Am Coll Cardiol 1986;7:1416–1419.
8. McKay RG, Lock JE, Keane JF, et al. Percutaneous mitral valvuloplasty in an adult patient with calcific rheumatic mitral stenosis. J Am Coll Cardiol 1986;7:1410–1415.
9. NHLBI Balloon Valvuloplasty Registry Participants. Percutaneous balloon aortic valvuloplasty. Circulation 1991;84:2383–2397.
10. Rocchini AP, Beekman RH, Shachar GB, et al. Balloon aortic valvuloplasty: results of the valvuloplasty and angioplasty of congenital anomalies registry. Am J Cardiol 1990;65:784–789.
11. Block PC. Early results of mitral balloon valvuloplasty (MBV) for mitral stenosis: report from the NHLBI registry. Circulation 1988;78(Suppl II):II-489.

12. Herrmann HC, Kleaveland P, Hill JA, et al. The M-HEART percutaneous balloon mitral valvuloplasty registry: initial results and early follow-up. J Am Coll Cardiol 1990;15:1221–1226.

13. Swan TD. Percutaneous balloon valvuloplasty. New York: Wilkerson Group, Inc., 1988;2A:1–30.

14. Rahimtoola SH. Perspective on valvular heart disease: an update. J Am Coll Cardiol 1989;14(1):1–23.

15. Carabello BA. Do all patients with aortic stenosis and left ventricular dysfunction benefit from aortic valve replacement? Cathet Cardiovasc Diagn 1989;17:131–132.

16. Letac B, Cribier A, Eltchaninoff H, et al. Evaluation of restenosis after balloon dilatation in adult aortic stenosis by repeat catheterization. Am Heart J 1991;122:55–60.

17. Kuntz RE, Tosteson ANA, Berman AD, et al. Predictors of event-free survival after balloon aortic valvuloplasty. N Engl J Med 1991;325:17–23.

18. Lembo NJ, King SB, Roubin GS, et al. Fatal aortic rupture during percutaneous balloon valvuloplasty for valvular aortic stenosis. Am J Cardiol 1987;60:733–736.

19. Meier B, Friedli B, Oberhaensli I, et al. Trefoil balloon for percutaneous valvuloplasty. Cathet Cardiovasc Diagn 1986;12:277–281.

20. van den Berg EJM, Niemeyer MG, Plokker TWM, et al. New triple-lumen balloon catheter for percutaneous (pulmonary) valvuloplasty. Cathet Cardiovasc Diagn 1986;12:352–356.

21. Brady ST, Davis CA, Kussmaul WG, et al. Percutaneous aortic balloon valvuloplasty in octogenarians: morbidity and mortality. Ann Intern Med 1989;110:761–766.

22. Cujec B, McMeekin J, Lopez J. Bacterial endocarditis after percutaneous aortic valvuloplasty. Am Heart J 1988;115:178–179.

23. Block PC, Palacios IF. Comparison of hemodynamic results of anterograde versus retrograde percutaneous balloon aortic valvuloplasty. Am J Cardiol 1987;60:659–662.

24. Voudris V, Drobinski G, L'Epine Y, et al. Results of percutaneous valvuloplasty for calcific aortic stenosis with different balloon catheters. Cathet Cardiovasc Diagn 1989;17:80–83.

25. Isner JM, Salem DN, Desnoyers MR, et al. Dual balloon technique for valvuloplasty of aortic stenosis in adults. Am J Cardiol 1988;61:583–589.

26. Lewin RF, Dorros G, King JF, et al. Aortic annular tear after valvuloplasty: the role of aortic annulus echocardiographic measurement. Cathet Cardiovasc Diagn 1989;16:123–129.

27. Orme EC, Wray RB, Barry WH, et al. Comparison of three techniques for percutaneous balloon aortic valvuloplasty of aortic stenosis in adults. Am Heart J 1989;117:11–17.

28. Cribier A, Savin T, Berland J, et al. Percutaneous transluminal balloon valvuloplasty of adult aortic stenosis: report of 29 cases. J Am Coll Cardiol 1987;9:381–386.

29. Block PC, Palacios IF. Clinical and hemodynamic follow-up after percutaneous aortic valvuloplasty in the elderly. Am J Cardiol 1988;62:760–763.

30. Kuntz RE, Tosteson ANA, Maitland LA, et al. Immediate results and long-term follow-up after repeat balloon aortic valvuloplasty. Cathet Cardiovasc Diagn 1992;25:4–9.

31. Ross TC, Banks AK, Collins TJ, et al. Repeat balloon aortic valvuloplasty for aortic valve restenosis. Cathet Cardiovasc Diagn 1989;18:96–98.

32. McKay RG, Safian RD, Lock JE, et al. Balloon dilatation of calcific aortic stenosis in elderly patients: postmortem, intraoperative, and percutaneous valvuloplasty studies. Circulation 1986;74:119–125.

33. Safian RD, Mandell VS, Thurer RE, et al. Postmortem and intraoperative balloon valvuloplasty of calcific aortic stenosis in elderly patients: mechanisms of successful dilation. J Am Coll Cardiol 1987;9:655–660.

34. Harrison JK, Davidson CJ, Leithe ME, et al. Serial left ventricular performance evaluated by cardiac catheterization before, immediately after, and at 6 months after balloon aortic valvuloplasty. J Am Coll Cardiol 1990;16:1351–1358.

35. Berland J, Cribier A, Savin T, et al. Percutaneous balloon valvuloplasty in patients with severe aortic stenosis and low ejection fraction. Circulation 1989;79:1189–1196.

36. Safian RD, Warren SE, Berman AD, et al. Improvement in symptoms and left ventricular performance after balloon aortic valvuloplasty in patients with aortic stenosis and depressed left ventricular ejection fraction. Circulation 1988;78:1181–1191.

37. Harpole DH, Davidson CJ, Skelton TN, et al. Early and late changes in left ventricular systolic performance after percutaneous balloon aortic valvuloplasty. Am J Cardiol 1990;66:327–332.

38. Davidson CJ, Harrison JK, Pieper KS, et al. Determinants of one-year outcome from balloon aortic valvuloplasty. Am J Cardiol 1991;68:75–80.

38a.Blitz LR, Herrmann HC. Hemodynamic assessment of patients with low-flow, low-gradient valvular aortic stenosis. Am J Cardiol 1996;78:657–661.

39. Letac B, Cribier A, Koning R, et al. Aortic stenosis in elderly patients aged 80 or older. Treatment by percutaneous balloon valvuloplasty in a series of 92 cases. Circulation 1989;80:1514–1520.

40. Craver JM, Weintraub WS, Jones EL, et al. Predictors of mortality, complications, and length of stay in aortic valve replacement for aortic stenosis. Circulation 1988;78(Suppl I):I-85–I-90.

41. Freeman WK, Schaff HV, O'Brien PC, et al. Cardiac surgery in the octogenarian: perioperative outcome and clinical follow-up. J Am Coll Cardiol 1991;18:29–35.

42. Magovern JA, Pennock JL, Campbell DB, et al. Aortic valve replacement and combined aortic valve replacement and coronary artery bypass grafting: predicting high risk groups. J Am Coll Cardiol 1987;9:38–43.

43. Edmunds LH, Stephenson LW, Edie RN, et al. Open-heart surgery in octogenarians. N Engl J Med 1988;319:131–136.

44. DesNoyers MR, Salem DN, Rosenfield K, et al. Treatment of cardiogenic shock by emergency aortic balloon valvuloplasty. Ann Intern Med 1988;108:833–835.

45. Roth RB, Palacios IF, Block PC. Percutaneous aor-

tic balloon valvuloplasty: its role in the management of patients with aortic stenosis requiring major noncardiac surgery. J Am Coll Cardiol 1989;13:1039–1041.

46. Levine MJ, Berman AD, Safian RD, et al. Palliation of valvular aortic stenosis by balloon valvuloplasty as preoperative preparation for noncardiac surgery. Am J Cardiol 1988;62:1309–1310.

47. Powers ER. Percutaneous balloon valvuloplasty for critical aortic stenosis: a bridge to safer noncardiac surgical procedures. Mayo Clin Proc 1989; 64:871–873.

48. Parsonnet V, Dean D, Bernstein AD. A method of uniform stratification of risk for evaluating the results of surgery in acquired heart disease. Circulation 1989;79(Suppl I):I-3–I-12.

49. Grifka RG, O'Laughlin MP, Nihill MR, et al. Double-trans-septal, double-balloon valvuloplasty for congenital mitral stenosis. Circulation 1992; 85:123–129.

50. Massell BF, Chute CG, Walker AM, et al. Penicillin and the marked decrease in morbidity and mortality from rheumatic fever in the United States. N Engl J Med 1988;318(5):280–286.

51. Veasy LG, Wiedmeier SE, Orsmond GS, et al. Resurgence of acute rheumatic fever in the intermountain area of the United States. N Engl J Med 1987;316(8):421–427.

52. Herrmann HC, Wilkins GT, Abascal VM, et al. Percutaneous balloon mitral valvotomy for patients with mitral stenosis. J Thorac Cardiovasc Surg 1988;96:33–38.

53. Herrmann HC, Kussmaul WG, Hirshfeld JW. Single large-balloon percutaneous mitral valvuloplasty. Cathet Cardiovasc Diagn 1989;17:59–61.

54. Al Zaibag M, Al Kasab S, Ribeiro PA, et al. Percutaneous double-balloon mitral valvotomy for rheumatic mitral valve stenosis. Lancet 1986; 1:757–761.

55. Palacios I, Block PC, Brandi S, et al. Percutaneous balloon valvotomy for patients with severe mitral stenosis. Circulation 1987;75:778–784.

56. Weiner RI, Maranho V. Development and application of trans-septal left heart catheterization. Cathet Cardiovasc Diagn 1988;15:112–120.

57. Vahanian A, Michel PL, Cormier B, et al. Results of percutaneous mitral commissurotomy in 200 patients. Am J Cardiol 1989;63:847–852.

58. Tuzcu EM, Block PC, Palacios IF. Comparison of early versus late experience with percutaneous mitral balloon valvuloplasty. J Am Coll Cardiol 1991;17:1121–1124.

59. Abascal VM, Wilkins GT, O'Shea JP, et al. Prediction of successful outcome in 130 patients undergoing percutaneous balloon mitral valvotomy. Circulation 1990;82:448–456.

60. Patel JJ, Mitha AS, Hassen F, et al. Balloon mitral valvuloplasty: single catheter technique comparing bifoil/trefoil and Inoue balloons. J Am Coll Cardiol 1991;17(2):82A.

61. Babic UU, Dorros G, Pejcic P, et al. Percutaneous mitral valvuloplasty: retrograde, transarterial double-balloon technique utilizing the trans-septal approach. Cathet Cardiovasc Diagn 1988; 14:229–237.

62. Stefanadis C, Kourouklis C, Stratos C. Percutane-

ous balloon mitral valvuloplasty by retrograde left atrial catheterization. Am J Cardiol 1990; 65:650–654.

63. Orme EC, Wray RB, Mason JW. Balloon mitral valvuloplasty via retrograde left atrial catheterization. Am Heart J 1989;117(3):680–683.

63a. Vahanian A, Cormier B, Iung B. Percutaneous transvenous mitral commissurotomy using the Inoue balloon: international experience. Cathet Cardiovasc Diag 1994;(Suppl 2):8–15.

64. Herrmann HC. Top 10 reasons to use the Inoue balloon. Cathet Cardiovasc Diagn 1996;38:15.

65. Feldman T, Carroll JD, Isner MJ, et al. Effect of valve deformity on results and mitral regurgitation after Inoue balloon commissurotomy. Circulation 1992;85:180–187.

66. Kronzon I, Tunick PA, Schwinger ME, et al. Transesophageal echocardiography during percutaneous mitral valvuloplasty. J Am Soc Echocardiogr 1989;2:380–385.

67. McKay RG, Lock JE, Safian RD, et al. Balloon dilation of mitral stenosis in adult patients: postmortem and percutaneous mitral valvuloplasty studies. J Am Coll Cardiol 1987;9:723–731.

68. Kaplan JD, Isner JM, Karas RH, et al. In vitro analysis of mechanisms of balloon valvuloplasty of stenotic mitral valves. Am J Cardiol 1987; 59:318–323.

69. Nakatani S, Nagata S, Beppu S, et al. Acute reduction of mitral valve area after percutaneous balloon mitral valvuloplasty: assessment with Doppler continuity equation method. Am Heart J 1991; 121:770–775.

70. Levine MJ, Weinstein JS, Diver DJ, et al. Progressive improvement in pulmonary vascular resistance after percutaneous mitral valvuloplasty. Circulation 1989;79:1061–1067.

70a. Vincens JJ, Temizer D, Post JR, et al. Long-term outcome of cardiac surgery in patients with mitral stenosis and severe pulmonary hypertension. Circulation 1995;92(Suppl II): II-137–II-142.

71. Ribeiro PA, Fawzy ME, Arafat MA, et al. Comparison of mitral valve area results of balloon mitral valvotomy using the Inoue and double balloon techniques. Am J Cardiol 1991;68:687–688.

72. Turi ZG, Reyes VP, Raju S, et al. Percutaneous balloon versus surgical closed commissurotomy for mitral stenosis. Circulation 1991; 83:1179–1185.

73. Patel JJ, Shama D, Mitha AS, et al. Balloon valvuloplasty versus closed commissurotomy for pliable mitral stenosis: a prospective hemodynamic study. J Am Coll Cardiol 1991;18:1318–1322.

74. Palacios IF, Block PC, Wilkins GT, et al. Follow-up of patients undergoing percutaneous mitral balloon valvotomy. Circulation 1989;79:573–579.

75. Marzo KM, Herrmann HC, Mancini D. Effect of balloon mitral valvuloplasty on exercise capacity, ventilation, and skeletal muscle oxygenation. J Am Coll Cardiol 1993;21:856–865.

76. McKay CR, Kawanishi DT, Kotlewski A, et al. Improvement in exercise capacity and exercise hemodynamics 3 months after double-balloon, catheter balloon valvuloplasty treatment of patients with symptomatic mitral stenosis. Circulation 1988;77(5):1013–1021.

77. Goto S, Handa S, Akaishi M, et al. Left ventricular ejection performance in mitral stenosis, and effects of successful percutaneous transvenous mitral commissurotomy. Am J Cardiol 1992; 69:233–237.

78. Hung JS, Chern MS, Wu JJ, et al. Short- and long-term results of catheter balloon percutaneous transvenous mitral commissurotomy. Am J Cardiol 1991;67:854–862.

79. Ruiz CE, Allen JW, Lau FYK. Percutaneous double balloon valvotomy for severe rheumatic mitral stenosis. Am J Cardiol 1990;65:473–477.

80. Herrmann HC, Ramaswamy K, Isner JM, et al. Factors influencing immediate results, complications, and short-term follow-up status after Inoue balloon mitral valvotomy: a North American multicenter study. Am Heart J 1992; 124:160–166.

81. Carlson MD, Palacios I, Thomas JD, et al. Cardiac conduction abnormalities during percutaneous balloon mitral or aortic valvotomy. Circulation 1989;79:1197–1203.

82. Cequier A, Bonan R, Serra A, et al. Left-to-right atrial shunting after percutaneous mitral valvuloplasty. Incidence and long-term hemodynamic follow-up. Circulation 1990;81:1190–1197.

83. Parro A, Helmcke F, Mahan EF, et al. Value and limitations of color Doppler echocardiography in the evaluation of percutaneous balloon mitral valvuloplasty for isolated mitral stenosis. Am J Cardiol 1991;67:1261–1267.

84. Yoshida K, Yoshikawa J, Akasaka T, et al. Assessment of left-to-right atrial shunting after percutaneous mitral valvuloplasty by transesophageal color Doppler flow-mapping. Circulation 1989; 80:1521–1526.

85. Ishikura F, Kagata S, Yasuda S, et al. Residual atrial septal perforation after percutaneous transvenous mitral commissurotomy with Inoue balloon catheter. Am Heart J 1990;120:873–878.

86. Fields CD, Slovenkai GA, Isner JM. Atrial septal defect resulting from mitral balloon valvuloplasty: relation of defect morphology to transseptal balloon catheter delivery. Am Heart J 1990; 119:568–576.

87. Abascal VM, Wilkins GT, Choong CY, et al. Mitral regurgitation after percutaneous balloon mitral valvuloplasty in adults: evaluation by pulsed Doppler echocardiography. J Am Coll Cardiol 1988;11:257–263.

88. Essop MR, Wisenbaugh T, Skoulargis J, et al. Mitral regurgitation following mitral balloon valvotomy. Circulation 1991;84:1669–1679.

89. O'Shea JP, Abascal VM, Wilkins GT, et al. Unusual sequelae after percutaneous mitral valvuloplasty: a Doppler echocardiographic study. J Am Coll Cardiol 1992;19:186–191.

90. Block PC, Palacios IF, Block EH, et al. Late (two-year) follow-up after percutaneous balloon mitral valvotomy. Am J Cardiol 1992;69:537–541.

91. Reid CL, Chandraratna AN, Kawanishi DT, et al. Influence of mitral valve morphology on double-balloon catheter balloon valvuloplasty in patients with mitral stenosis. Analysis of factors predicting immediate and 3-month results. Circulation 1989;80:515–524.

92. Wilkins GT, Weyman AE, Abascal VM, et al. Percutaneous balloon dilatation of the mitral valve: an analysis of echocardiographic variables related to outcome and the mechanism of dilatation. Br Heart J 1988;60:299–308.

93. Kronzon I, Tunick PA, Glassman E, et al. Transesophageal echocardiography to detect atrial clots in candidates for percutaneous trans-septal mitral balloon valvuloplasty. J Am Coll Cardiol 1990; 16:1320–1322.

94. Alfonso F, Macaya C, Iniguez A, et al. Comparison of results of percutaneous mitral valvuloplasty in patients with large (6 cm) versus those with smaller left atria. Am J Cardiol 1992; 69:355–360.

95. Tuzcu EM, Block PC, Griffin BP, et al. Immediate and long-term outcome of percutaneous mitral valvotomy in patients 65 years and older. Circulation 1992;85:963–971.

96. Safian RD, Berman AD, Sachs B, et al. Percutaneous balloon mitral valvuloplasty in a pregnant woman with mitral stenosis. Cathet Cardiovasc Diag 1988;15:103–108.

97. Pan M, Medina A, Suarez de lezo J, et al. Balloon valvuloplasty for mild mitral stenosis. Cathet Cardiovasc Diag 1991;24:1–5.

98. Rao PS. Indications for balloon pulmonary valvuloplasty. Am Heart J 1988;1661–1662.

99. Herrmann HC, Hill JA, Krol J, et al. Effectiveness of percutaneous balloon valvuloplasty in adults with pulmonic valve stenosis. Am J Cardiol 1991; 68:1111–1113.

100. Fawzy ME, Gala O, Dunn B, et al. Regression of infundibular pulmonary stenosis after successful balloon pulmonary valvuloplasty in adults. Cathet Cardiovasc Diagn 1990;21:77–81.

101. Rao PS. How big a balloon and how many balloons for pulmonary valvuloplasty? Am Heart J 1988;116:577–580.

102. Stanger P, Cassidy SC, Girod DA, et al. Balloon pulmonary valvuloplasty: results of the valvuloplasty and angioplasty of congenital anomalies registry. Am J Cardiol 1990;65:775–783.

103. Ben-Shachar G, Cohen MH, Sivakoff MC, et al. Development of infundibular obstruction after percutaneous pulmonary balloon valvuloplasty. J Am Coll Cardiol 1985;5:754–756.

104. McCrindle BW, Kan JS. Long-term results after balloon pulmonary valvuloplasty. Circulation 1991;83:1915–1922.

105. Kan JS, White RI, Mitchell SE, et al. Percutaneous transluminal balloon valvuloplasty for pulmonary valve stenosis. Circulation 1984;69:554–560.

106. Ribeiro PA, Al Zaibag M, Al Kasab S, et al. Percutaneous double balloon valvotomy for rheumatic tricuspid stenosis. Am J Cardiol 1988;61:660–662.

107. Lamberti JJ, Wainer BH, Fisher KA, et al. Calcific stenosis of the porcine heterograft. Ann Thorac Surg 1979;28:28–32.

108. Hetzer R, Hill D, Kerth WJ, et al. Thrombosis and degeneration of Hancock valves: clinical and pathological findings. Ann Thorac Surg 1978; 26:317–322.

109. Calvo OL, Sobrino N, Gamallo C, et al. Balloon percutaneous valvuloplasty for stenotic bioprosthetic valves in the mitral position. Am J Cardiol 1987;60:736–737.

110. McKay CR, Waller BF, Hong H, et al. Problems encountered with catheter balloon valvuloplasty of bioprosthetic aortic valves. Am Heart J 1988; 115:463–465.

111. Waldman JD, Schoen FJ, Kirkpatrick SE, et al. Balloon dilatation of porcine bioprosthetic valves in the pulmonary position. Circulation 1987; 76:109–114.

112. Feit F, Stecy PJ, Nachamie MS. Percutaneous balloon valvuloplasty for stenosis of a porcine bioprosthesis in the tricuspid valve position. Am J Cardiol 1988;58:363–364.

113. Orbe LC, Sobrino N, Mate I, et al. Effectiveness of balloon percutaneous valvuloplasty for stenotic bioprosthetic valves in different positions. Am J Cardiol 1991;68:1719–1721.

114. Rao PS, Thapar MK, Kutayli F, et al. Causes of recoarctation after balloon angioplasty of unoperated aortic coarctation. J Am Coll Cardiol 1989; 13:109–115.

115. Tynan M, Finley JP, Fontes V, et al. Balloon angioplasty for the treatment of native coarctation: results of valvuloplasty and angioplasty of congenital anomalies registry. Am J Cardiol 1990; 65:790–792.

116. Cooper RS, Ritter SB, Rothe WB, et al. Angioplasty for coarctation of the aorta: long-term results. Circulation 1987;75:600–604.

117. Ritter SB. Coarctation and balloons: inflated or realistic? J Am Coll Cardiol 1989;13:696–699.

118. Isner JM, Donaldson RF, Fulton D, et al. Cystic medial necrosis in coarctation of the aorta: a potential factor contributing to adverse consequences observed after percutaneous balloon angioplasty of coarctation sites. Circulation 1987; 75:689–695.

119. Lock JE, Niemi T, Burke BA, et al. Transcutaneous angioplasty of experimental aortic coarctation. Circulation 1982;66:1280–1286.

120. Hellenbrand WE, Allen HD, Golinko RJ, et al. Balloon angioplasty for aortic recoarctation: results of valvuloplasty and angioplasty of congenital anomalies registry. Am J Cardiol 1990; 65:793–797.

121. Cooper SG, Sullivan ID, Wren C. Treatment of recoarctation: balloon dilation angioplasty. J Am Coll Cardiol 1989;14:413–419.

122. Huhta JC. Angioplasty for recoarctation. J Am Coll Cardiol 1989;14:420–421.

123. Ring JC, Bass JL, Marvin W, et al. Management of congenital stenosis of a branch pulmonary artery with balloon dilation angioplasty. J Thorac Cardiovasc Surg 1985;90:35–44.

124. O'Laughlin MP, Perry SB, Lock JE, et al. Use of endovascular stents in congenital heart disease. Circulation 1991;83:1923–1939.

125. Ali MK, Ewer MS, Balakrishnan PV, et al. Balloon angioplasty for superior vena cava obstruction. Ann Intern Med 1987;107:856–857.

126. Ensing GJ, Hagler DJ, Seward JB, et al. Caveats of balloon dilation of conduits and conduit valves. J Am Coll Cardiol 1989;14:397–400.

127. Ritter, SB. Balloon dilation: recession or Inflation? J Amer Coll Cardiol 1989;14:409–412.

128. De Lezo JS, Pan M, Sancho M, et al. Percutaneous

129. Palacios IF, Tuzcu EM, Ziskind AA, et al. Percutaneous balloon pericardial window for patients with malignant pericardial effusion and tamponade. Cathet Cardiovasc Diagn 1991;22:244–249.

130. Ziskind AA, Pearce AC, Lemmon CC, et al. Percutaneous balloon pericardial windowing for the treatment of cardiac tamponade and large pericardial effusions. J Am Coll Cardiol 1993;21:1–5.

131. Lewin RF, Dorros G, King JF, et al. Percutaneous transluminal aortic valvuloplasty: acute outcome and follow-up of 125 patients. J Am Coll Cardiol 1989;14:1210–1217.

132. Bernard Y, Etievent J, Mourand JL, et al. Longterm results of percutaneous aortic valvuloplasty compared with aortic valve replacement in patients more than 75 years old. J Am Coll Cardiol 1992:20:796–801.

133. Deleted in proof.

134. Rihal CS, Holmes DR. Percutaneous balloon mitral valvuloplasty: issues involved in comparing techniques. Cathet Cardiovasc Diag 1994;(Suppl 2):35–41.

135. Marga P, Singh S, Brandis S, et al. Mitral valve area calculations immediately after percutaneous balloon mitral valvuloplasty: effect of atrial septal defect. J Am Coll Cardiol 1993;21:1568–1573.

136. Park SJ, Kim JJ, Park SW, et al. Immediate and one-year results of percutaneous mitral balloon valvuloplasty using Inoue and double-balloon techniques. Am J Cardiol 1993;71:938–943.

137. Turi ZG, Reyes VP, Rajo S, et al. Percutaneous balloon versus surgical closed commissurotomy for mitral stenosis: a prospective, randomized trial. Circulation 1991;83:1179–1185.

138. Patal JJ, Shama D, Mitha AS. Balloon valvuloplasty versus closed commissurotomy for pliable mitral stenosis: a prospective hemodynamic study. J Am Coll Cardiol 1991;18:1318.

139. Reyes VP, Raju S, Wynne J, et al. Percutaneous balloon valvuloplasty compared with open surgical commissurotomy for mitral stenosis. N Engl J Med 1994;331:961–967.

140. Bueno R, Andrade P, Nercolini D, et al. Percutaneous mitral valvuloplasty versus open mitral valve commissurotomy: results of a randomized clinical trial [Abstract]. J Am Coll Cardiol 1993;21:429A.

141. Farhat MB, Ayari M, Bethout F, et al. Percutaneous balloon versus surgical closed and open mitral commissurotomy: short and long-term results [Abstract]. J Am Coll Cardiol 1993;21:428A.

142. Cohen DJ, Kuntz RE, Gordon SPF, et al. Predictors of long-term outcome after percutaneous balloon mitral valvuloplasty. N Engl J Med 1992; 327:1329–1335.

143. Palacios IF. Balloon mitral valvuloplasty: what are the long-term outcomes? Choices in Cardiology 1993;7:398–406.

144. Iung B, Cormier B, Ducimetiere P, et al. Functional results 5 years after successful percutaneous mitral commissurotomy in a series of 528 patients and analysis of predictive factors. J Am Coll Cardiol 1996;27:407–414.

145. Herrmann HC, Lima JAC, Feldman T, et al. Mechanisms and outcome of severe mitral regurgita-

tion after Inoue balloon valvuloplasty. J Am Coll Cardiol 1993;22:783–789.

146. Ruiz CE, Zhang HP, Macaya C, et al. Comparison of Inoue single-balloon versus double-balloon technique for percutaneous mitral valvotomy. Am Heart J 1992;123:942–947.

147. Abdullah M, Halim M, Rajendran V, et al. Comparison between single (Inoue) and double-balloon mitral valvuloplasty: immediate and short-term results. Am Heart J 1992;123:1581–1588.

148. Roth RB, Block PC, Palacios IF. Predictors of increased mitral regurgitation after percutaneous mitral balloon valvotomy. Cathet Cardiovasc Diag 1990;20:17–21.

149. Padial LR, Freitas N, Sagie A, et al. Echocardiography can predict which patients will develop severe mitral regurgitation after percutaneous mitral valvulotomy. J Am Coll Cardiol 1996;27:1225–1231.

150. Roberts JW, Lima JAO. Role of echocardiography in mitral commissurotomy with the Inoue balloon. Cathet Cardiovasc Diag 1994;(Suppl 2):69–75.

151. Post JR, Feldman T, Isner J, et al. Inoue balloon

mitral valvotomy in patients with severe valvular and subvalvular deformity. J Am Coll Cardiol 1995;25:1129–1136.

152. Herrmann HC, Feldman T, Isner JM, et al. Comparison of results of percutaneous balloon valvuloplasty in patients with mild and moderate mitral stenosis to those with severe mitral stenosis. Am J Cardiol 1993;71:1300–1303.

153. Deleted in proof.

154. Chen CR, Cheng TO, Huang T, et al. Percutaneous balloon valvuloplasty for pulmonic stenosis in adolescents and adults. N Engl J Med 1996;335:21–25.

155. Deleted in proof.

156. Bulbul ZR, Bruckheimer E, Love JC, et al. Implantation of balloon-expandable stents for coarctation of the aorta. Cathet Cardiovasc Diag 1996;39:36–42.

157. DeGiovanni JV, Lip GYH, Osman K, et al. Percutaneous balloon dilatation of aortic coarctation in adults. Am J Cardiol 1996;77:435–439.

158. Ribeiro PA, Al Zaibag M, Idris MT. Percutaneous double balloon tricuspid valvotomy: three-year follow-up study. Eur Heart J 1990;11:1109–1113.

SPECIFIC CLINICAL STATES AND THEIR ASSESSMENT AND INTERVENTION BY CATHETER TECHNIQUES

36

The Patient with Known or Suspected Coronary Heart Disease: Stable Ischemic Syndromes

Carl J. Pepine, MD
Mark H. Mines, MD
James A. Hill, MD
Charles R. Lambert, MD, PhD

INTRODUCTION

Patients with known or suspected stable ischemic heart disease comprise a large proportion of those undergoing cardiac catheterization studies. Stable ischemic syndromes, caused by transient cardiac ischemia, are a result of variable contributions made by processes acting to limit or reduce myocardial blood supply and increase oxygen demand. "Fixed" atherosclerotic and dynamic coronary artery narrowings may act alone or in combination transiently to reduce coronary blood flow. Increases in heart rate, blood pressure, contractility, and ventricular size, may act alone or in combination to increase myocardial oxygen demands. **What is needed from cardiac catheterization studies to assess adequately these patients with known or suspected coronary artery disease (CAD) who are clinically stable?** How does one integrate the clinical, noninvasive, and catheterization data obtained in these patients to formulate direction for management?

Numerous studies have shown that the extent and severity of CAD are important predictors of outcome in these patients with stable syndromes. Status of left ventricular function clearly interacts with CAD severity to determine outcome. Coronary angiography with left ventriculography provides an estimate of CAD severity and left ventricular function status. Noninvasively obtained functional assessment of indicators of cardiac ischemia (ECG ST segment, thallium[201] and sestimibi scans, or stress left ventricular wall motion imaging) is most important (1). Other variables important to both outcome and quality of life can also be identified and quantified at cardiac catheterization. They include, for example, mitral insufficiency, pulmonary hypertension, and ventricular aneurysm. Once this information is obtained, the optimal role for catheterization-based or directed therapy, such as percutaneous transluminal coronary angioplasty (PTCA), stenting, or bypass surgery (coronary artery bypass graft [CABG]), can be addressed. This chapter provides a synthesis of these topics relative to specific clinical states associated with stable ischemic syndromes. To do this, we integrate selected data from controlled clinical trials with other evidence-based data (e.g., registries, observational data) when available. From this information the practitioner should be better equipped to recommend and use cardiac catheterization in the management of these patients.

Patients with stable ischemic heart disease will be considered according to the following groups: (*a*) those who have stable symptoms suggesting CAD, (*b*) those who are symptomatic without important angiographic coronary artery stenosis, (*c*) those who have survived myocardial infarction, and (*d*) those who have been asymptomatic but have other findings suggesting that they may be at high risk for CAD.

CHRONIC STABLE ANGINA PECTORIS

Decision for Coronary Angiography

General Considerations Relating to Prognosis

It is important to review briefly some of the factors that are important determinants of prognosis in chronic stable angina patients. These include the anatomic and functional severity of coronary artery disease and a number of patient characteristics (e.g., age, gender, race, and coexisting illness such as diabetes). The practitioner should be aware that as a group, patients with chronic stable angina have low adverse outcomes (e.g., approximately 2% per year for the combined outcome of death or nonfatal myocardial infarction). Thus, it is important to attempt to risk stratify these patients so that diagnostic testing and therapy can be directed to the subgroup at highest risk. Otherwise, little evidence is found that benefit will follow in terms of adverse outcomes with any specific type of treatment. For example, in one recent study, the presence of ischemia during stress testing and daily life identified a subgroup with a 2-year risk for death or nonfatal infarction that exceeded 12% (1A). This study did not include those with left main coronary artery obstruction or severe

multivessel disease with reduced left ventricular function. Nevertheless, revascularization was associated with significant reduction in adverse outcome.

Anatomic

The extent of CAD and severity of left ventricular dysfunction have been repeatedly documented as two important predictors of outcome in patients with chronic stable angina pectoris (Figs. 36.1 and 36.2) (2, 3). As currently performed, however, coronary angiography alone provides mostly anatomic data, but functional data are also important.

Considerable evidence supports the concept that the development of acute ischemia-related events (myocardial infarction and death) relates to plaque rupture involving a coronary lesion that in itself was not severely obstructive in most cases (1B). Severe stenosis account for a minority of such cases. On the other hand, the "vulnerable" (not severely obstructive) lesion usually coexists in a setting of severe obstructive lesions at other sites as evidenced by the findings that most patients dying suddenly have severe disease. This also explains why it has been difficult to show that catheter-based revascularizations focused on severe stenoses prevent death and myocardial infarction.

Functional

As noted above, an increased risk is found for cardiac events, including death, in angina patients who develop objective evidence for transient myocardial ischemia during stress testing (4). A number of **exercise stress test findings may be used to identify those patients at "high risk" for adverse outcomes,** as outlined in Chapter 15. The exercise test also yields other important functional parameters that help predict outcome among patients with comparable coronary anatomic disease (1). Therefore, exercise testing is useful in patients with chronic stable angina. Exercise testing may

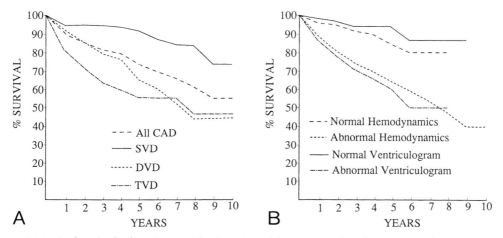

Figure 36.1. A. Survival of patients with chronic stable angina related to extent of coronary artery disease (CAD). *DVD,* double-vessel disease; *SVD,* single-vessel disease; *TVD,* triple-vessel disease. **B.** Survival with coronary artery disease related to hemodynamics and ventriculography. It is apparent that the outcome of patients with stable ischemic syndromes depends directly on the extent of coronary artery disease and abnormal ventricular function. (Reprinted with permission from Burggraf GW, Parker JO. Prognosis in coronary artery disease: angiographic, hemodynamic and clinical factors. Circulation 1975;51:146–156.)

even be done after coronary angiography has defined the anatomic pattern. Stress radionuclide perfusion imaging and dobutamine stress echocardiography are also useful for selected patients (5). These tests can be performed when physical limitation, ECG abnormality that interferes with ST segments, and so forth, precludes other forms of stress testing.

Demographic

Other factors that interact with the severity of CAD, such as age, gender, hypertension, and diabetes, are also important determinants of morbidity and mortality among patients with various anatomic patterns of coronary artery disease. Recent data from our institution suggest that the cohort of patients with chronic stable angina seen in the 1990s is primarily elderly patients, most of whom are female (6). These patients also have a high frequency of associated illnesses such as hypertension and heart failure. Furthermore, almost one half of this cohort considered to have chronic stable angina also reported angina occurring at

rest. Many had frequent angina and angina frequency was closely linked with quality of life. These considerations suggest that the patients seen with chronic stable angina in this decade are more likely to be at higher risk for adverse outcome than those patients from previously reported studies who were predominantly men and younger. Also, because age and gender as well as comorbidity (e.g., as diabetes) influence revascularization risks (6A), these considerations are more important in the decision for coronary angiography.

Thus, coronary angiography provides an estimate of anatomic data that interacts with functional and demographic data to yield information important for management.

Patients Receiving "Optimal" Therapy who have Disabling Symptoms

General agreement is found that coronary angiography to identify patients for revascularization is of proven value in patients with disabling symptoms, caused by transient myocardial ischemia, that recur with

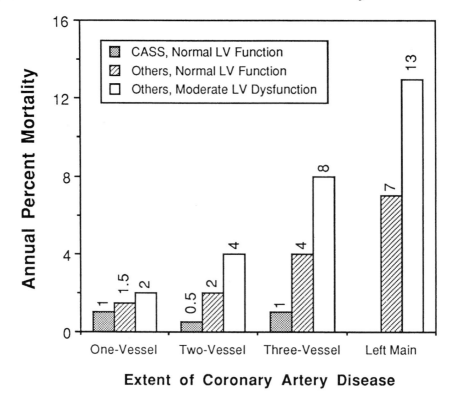

Figure 36.2. Expected annual mortality rate among medically treated patients with coronary artery disease and chronic angina pectoris. Percentages (rounded off) are either from the CASS, or are estimates from other studies, and are presented according to number of diseased vessels and extent of left ventricular (*LV*) dysfunction. Patients with left main coronary disease were excluded from the CASS. (Adapted with permission of the New England Journal of Medicine from Silverman KJ, Grossman W. Current concepts. Angina pectoris: natural history and strategies for evaluation and management. N Engl J Med 1984;310:1712–1717.)

optimal medical therapy (7). Optimal medical therapy is expected to vary from patient to patient and is meant to be individualized. Optimal medical therapy should include lifestyle modification and modification of aggravating factors such as obesity, hypertension, anemia, and smoking, in addition to dose titration of anti-ischemic medications, such as nitrates, calcium antagonists, and β-blockers. Considerable evidence now indicates that HMG-CoA reductase inhibitors are also anti-ischemic, and they reduce need for angiography and revascularization (7A, 7B, 7C). Thus, these agents need to be considered for every patient with known or suspected atherosclerotic disease. Failure of optimal therapy, then, implies that symptoms caused by either myocardial ischemia

or side effects of medications result in a lifestyle that is unacceptable to the patient. In patients meeting this definition, the decision for catheterization and possible revascularization therapy is usually not difficult (see Chapter 15). Most of these patients with chronic stable symptoms will have multivessel CAD and relatively well-preserved left ventricular function. Only about 3 to 5% will have important left main coronary artery obstruction. In about 85 to 90% of the patients with CAD, symptoms will be markedly improved with a revascularization procedure.

Interestingly, approximately 10% will have no important large vessel coronary artery stenosis and no evidence for coronary spasm. Although this excludes obstructive atherosclerotic CAD, some will have transient ischemia caused by microvascular dysfunction as the basis for their symptoms. These latter patients can be reassured that their long-term outcome in terms of freedom from death or myocardial infarction is excellent (8), but disability may be a serious problem.

Patients Without Disabling Symptoms

The more difficult decision is when to recommend angiography and revascularization in patients who are less symptomatic. In such patients, the justification for catheterization is to confirm the diagnosis, predict long-term prognosis, and attempt to improve the predicted long-term prognosis. This course, termed "invasive-directed" management, is considered the more aggressive approach, as opposed to the "noninvasive or conservative" course. The latter management course is to assume that the diagnosis is accurate and use medical therapy alone until the patient develops disabling symptoms. Some balance between these two courses is likely to use catheterization most optimally. It is appropriate to review results that can be obtained with revascularization procedures that are based on management directed by specific catheterization findings.

Management Decisions Based on Angiographic Findings

Left Main Coronary Artery Obstruction

Three multicenter randomized trials have addressed results of bypass surgery in chronic effort angina. The VA Cooperative Study randomized patients to either surgical (286 patients) or medical (310 patients) treatment (9). Despite criticisms regarding high surgical mortality and graft occlusion rates, this study clearly demonstrated im-

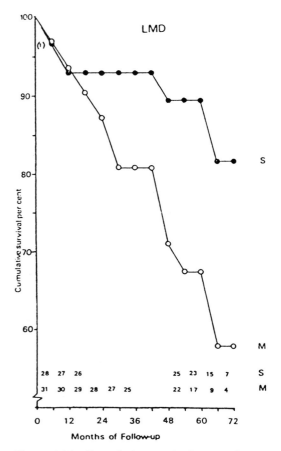

Figure 36.3. Cumulative survival curves for patients with left main disease (*LMD*). *M*, medical group; *S*, surgical group. (Reprinted with permission from European Coronary Surgery Study Group. Prospective randomized study of coronary artery bypass surgery in stable angina pectoris: a progress report on survival. Circulation 1982;65:II-67–71.)

proved survival in the subgroup of patients with left main coronary artery obstruction randomized to initial surgery. These results were confirmed by the European Coronary Surgery Study Group (ECSSG) (10, 11) (Fig. 36.3). As a result, the Coronary Artery Surgery Study (CASS) excluded patients with left main coronary artery obstruction from randomization (12). Data from several observational studies also support the beneficial effect of surgery on survival in patients with left main coronary artery obstruction (13). Surgery is the currently preferred revascularization approach in these patients.

On the other hand, patients with "protected" left main coronary artery obstruction, where at least one patent bypass graft supplies a left coronary artery branch, may be acceptable candidates for catheter-based intervention.

Single-Vessel Coronary Artery Obstruction

Because it was observed from nonrandomized trials that, as a group, chronic stable angina patients with only single-vessel obstruction had relatively low mortality over 5–10 years of follow-up (e.g., 2 to 3% per year), the ECSSG excluded these patients. The other two randomized trials (Veterans Administration (VA) and CASS) found similar 5- to 7-year survival rates in patients with single-vessel obstruction when comparing patients assigned initial medical and surgical treatments. Because such patients (recent onset angina and single-vessel disease) usually do well with medical therapy, and surgery has not been shown to reduce mortality or myocardial infarction rates in such patients, PTCA was initially reserved for those with unsatisfactory symptom responses to medical therapy. As primary success rates with PTCA improved ($\geq 90\%$) and the need for emergency CABG declined ($\leq 3\%$), PTCA emerged as an alternative treatment to chronic drug therapy. The question remained whether PTCA, as an alternative form of revascularization, offers results different from CABG surgery or even medical therapy. The question of PTCA versus CABG in single-vessel obstruction was addressed in several trials (e.g., RITA). In patients with single-vessel obstruction and mild to moderate symptoms, however, a more appropriate comparison is that between PTCA and medical therapy. Given the fact that survival is excellent in this group of patients, the important questions are whether PTCA improves quality of life (specifically, provides freedom from angina and need for medical therapy, and increases exercise tolerance), and whether it does so at an acceptable cost compared with medical therapy.

The ACME (Angioplasty Compared to Medicine) trial investigated these questions (14). In this study, nearly 10,000 patients at eight participating Veterans Affairs medical centers were screened over a 3-year period; 371 patients (4%) were identified who had mild angina or recent myocardial infarction and single-vessel coronary obstruction suitable for PTCA. A total of 212 of these patients, with 70 to 99% diameter stenosis and treadmill exercise-induced ischemia, were then randomly assigned to receive either conventional medical therapy for angina or PTCA and were followed monthly. The proportion of patients who were angina free at each monthly follow-up visit, for each treatment group is shown in Figure 36.4. Patients who had PTCA were urged to undergo repeat PTCA if they had symptoms suggestive of restenosis. After 6 months, patients returned for exercise testing and coronary angiography. Of these, 107 patients were randomized to medical therapy and 105 to PTCA. PTCA was clinically successful in 80 to 100% of patients, with an initial reduction in average percent stenosis from 76 to 36%. Two patients required emergency surgery. By 6 months, symptomatic recurrence necessitated repeat PTCA in 16 patients. Five patients assigned to PTCA and two patients assigned to medical therapy had a myocardial infarction. At 6 months, 64% (61 of 96) of PTCA patients, compared with 46% (47 of 102) of medically treated patients, were free of angina ($P < .01$). The patients in the PTCA group also had a greater increase in the total duration of exercise (2.1 minutes) than did the medical patients (0.5 minute, $P < .0001$) and had longer angina-free time on the treadmill ($P < .01$). The PTCA patients, however, spent more time in the hospital than did the medical treatment group (324 versus 191 days). These results suggest that, as an initial treatment in single-vessel obstruction, PTCA offers earlier and more complete relief of angina than does medical therapy, and it is associated with better exercise performance at 6 months at a cost of more days in the hospital. These PTCA results are similar to the uncontrolled observations reported from the 1985–1986 PTCA registry of the National Heart, Lung, and Blood Institute (NHLBI) (15). Both studies, however, suggest somewhat less complete

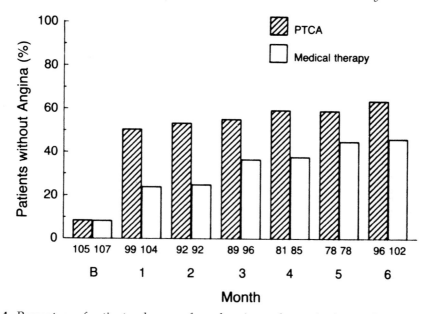

Figure 36.4. Percentage of patients who were free of angina each month after randomization. Horizontal axis shows the month before randomization (*B*, baseline) and clinic visits at months 1 through 6 for each treatment group. Numbers below the bars indicate the numbers of patients evaluated. Note that the difference between percutaneous transluminal coronary angioplasty (PTCA) and medical therapy, in terms of percent of patients without angina, decreases progressively as duration of follow-up increases. (Reprinted with permission from Parisi AF, Folland ED, Hartigan P. A comparison of angioplasty with medical therapy in the treatment of single-vessel coronary artery disease. N Engl J Med 1992;326:10–16.)

relief of angina after PTCA than anticipated after bypass surgery (16), but these results were obtained prior to coronary artery stenting (Chapters 31–33). Decision analysis (17) suggests that PTCA is preferable to both medical and surgical therapy in patients with severe angina and single-vessel or double-vessel lesions amenable to treatment with PTCA, but that PTCA may actually be less cost effective than medical therapy in patients with mild angina. It is likely, however, that no trial currently underway or planned will yield information on PTCA and mortality in this subgroup of patients as compared with surgery or drugs, because the adverse outcome rate is low. PTCA currently has some favorable cost and logistic advantages at 6 months over CABG surgery, but longer term data and data with stenting are needed. However, until results of additional controlled trials are available, clinical judgment must be used to select candidates. Some arbitrary guidelines based on the coronary angiogram are in

order. Presently, in patients with single-vessel obstruction, PTCA, when feasible, appears more clearly indicated than continued medical therapy for those whose lifestyles are limited by symptoms or drug therapy, or who have ischemic responses to stress suggesting high risk (18).

Multivessel Coronary Artery Obstruction

Medical Therapy Versus CABG

Despite general agreement in the aforementioned groups, disagreement results when assessing stable patients with mutivessel coronary disease. In patients with multivessel disease and preserved left ventricular function, both the CASS and VA studies demonstrated similar survival rates for those assigned to either medical or surgical

(CABG) treatment. However, the ECSSG study found significantly increased survival in patients with triple-vessel disease when treated surgically, compared with those assigned medical treatment (94 versus 80.4%, 6-year survival rate). The reason for this difference is probably related to the severity of ischemia in patients in the ECSSG.

Evidence to support this suggestion is provided by the fact that 42% of ECSSG patients had either Canadian Cardiac Society class III or IV angina, whereas CASS excluded patients with severe angina from randomization and a functional test was mandated to document ischemia objectively (19). An observational study of patients with severe angina from the nonrandomized CASS registry did demonstrate improved survival in surgically treated patients who had multivessel CAD (20). It seems reasonable to conclude that patients with multivessel disease, and either signs or symptoms suggesting severe ischemia, may have improved survival with CABG surgery, compared with medical therapy. Because 5-year survival rates in surgically treated patients are similar in both CASS and ECSSG, some of the disparity may be attributed to higher mortality in medically assigned patients. In a group of 117 patients with mild angina or who were asymptomatic and prospectively followed for 4 years after referral, it has been suggested that a subgroup of patients with triple-vessel CAD and preserved left ventricular function who are at high risk for death when treated medically may be identified by exercise testing (21). Forty-three patients with triple-vessel CAD had a 4-year survival of 88%. No deaths occurred in the 12 patients without exercise-induced ST shifts, whereas 31 patients with ischemic ST segment response during exercise had a 4-year survival of 82% (annual mortality 4.5%). Data from the CASS registry on 5302 patients who underwent treadmill testing at the time of catheterization, showed surgical treatment to be more beneficial in patients exhibiting 1 mm of ischemic type ST segment depression than in those without this level of ST segment depression. Surgery was also more beneficial in those who could exercise only to stage I or less of the Bruce protocol, compared with those who exer-

cised longer (22). Seven-year survival of patients in this subgroup was 58% when treated medically, compared with 81% when treated surgically.

The ECSSG patients with two-vessel CAD who had one stenosis involving the proximal left anterior descending artery (LAD), also had improved survival after surgery (Fig. 36.5). Several nonrandomized observational studies provide further support for the prognostic importance of proximal LAD stenosis (23) A report from the CASS registry data suggested that patients with proximal stenoses in any vessel had a poorer prognosis than patients with the same number of obstructed vessels but with distal disease (24). Review of data from 903 patients with combined proximal LAD and left circumflex (most not meeting randomization criteria) demonstrated improved 5-year survival in those surgically versus medically treated (85 versus 55%) (25).

Reduced Left Ventricular Function and Completeness of Revascularization

When comparing patients who had both multivessel disease and poor left ventricular function, defined as an ejection fraction of less than 50%, long-term follow-up from both the VA and CASS studies suggests that surgery improves survival (26–29). Patients with an ejection fraction of less than 50% were excluded from ECSSG. The importance of complete revascularization for relief of angina with CABG has been emphasized (30). One study followed consecutive patients undergoing CABG surgery, with repeat angiography 1 year after operation (31). Complete revascularization was defined as all major vessels greater than 1.5 mm in diameter with stenosis of more than 50% being bypassed. When correlating symptoms with both graft patency and completeness of revascularization, asymptomatic patients had 91% graft patency, as compared with only 27% graft patency in patients whose symptoms were unimproved. Likewise, 87% of patients who had complete revascularization with all grafts patent were asymptomatic. Only 42% of

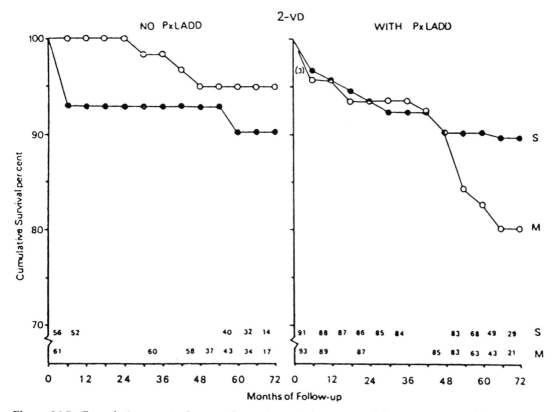

Figure 36.5. Cumulative survival curves for patients with two-vessel disease (*2-VD*) subdivided into two subsets according to absence (*NO*) and presence (*WITH*) of proximal left anterior descending disease (*PxLADD*). *M*, medical group; *S*, surgical group. (Reprinted with permission from European Coronary Surgery Study Group. Prospective randomized study of coronary artery bypass surgery in stable angina pectoris: a progress report on survival. Circulation 1982;65:II-67–71.)

those patients who had incomplete revascularization were asymptomatic (32). From these findings after surgery, one would expect that complete revascularization should be important after PTCA in patients with multivessel disease.

Mabin et al. addressed "completeness of revascularization" in an experience with 229 patients undergoing PTCA, 86 of whom had multivessel disease (33). Of the 153 patients in whom PTCA was initially successful, revascularization was considered complete (no residual diameter stenosis > 70%) in 61% (87 of 143) of patients with single-vessel disease and in 36% (31 of 86) of patients with multivessel disease. The chance of event-free survival (e.g., no angina recurrence, myocardial infarction, death, repeat PTCA, or CABG surgery) was directly influenced by completeness of revascularization.

All patients with multivessel disease, obtaining complete revascularization, had no angina on follow-up, whereas 57% of those patients with partial revascularization were asymptomatic. At 6 months, 79% of patients with complete revascularization had event-free survival compared with only 43% of those who had a residual stenosis (Fig. 36.6).

A subsequent study suggested that despite high primary success rates, defined as dilation of the critical or "culprit" lesion, complete revascularization was obtained in only 46% of patients with multivessel disease (34). As with the Mabin et al. study, cardiac events, need for repeat revascularization procedures, and evidence of residual myocardial ischemia by exercise testing were more frequent in the incompletely revascularized group, despite initial clinical improvement.

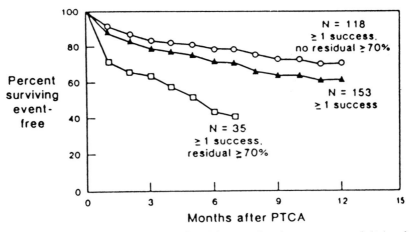

Figure 36.6. Event-free survival after successful dilation of at least one-vessel (*triangles*, n = 153) and in subgroups: with complete revascularization (no residual stenosis, *circles*, n = 118) and with incomplete revascularization (one or more residual stenoses 70% or greater, *squares*, n = 35). The difference between results in the two subgroups is significant (*P* < .001). (Reprinted with permission from Mabin TA, Holmes DR, Smith HC, et al. Follow-up clinical results in patients undergoing percutaneous transluminal coronary angioplasty. Circulation 1985;71:75–760.)

Multivessel PTCA Versus CABG

Given the proved efficacy of PTCA in the patient with single-vessel CAD, frequently the question arises whether patients with multivessel disease, who would be good candidates for CABG, should be given the option for revascularization by PTCA. The concerns about PTCA in this population are related to primary success rates, completeness of revascularization, and the possibility of increased rates of procedural complications and restenosis.

A number of randomized trials addressing this issue have been performed and are summarized in Table 36.1 (35–41). The largest of these is the BARI (Bypass Angioplasty Revascularization Investigation) trial (41). This was a multicenter, prospective, randomized trial initiated by the National Heart, Lung, and Blood Institute (NHLBI) in 1987. Patients with multivessel CAD who met enrollment criteria (e.g., could be revascularized in an equivalent manner by either CABG or PTCA) were randomly assigned to either CABG (914 patients) or PTCA (915 patients). They were then followed for an average of 5.4 years. The in-hospital death rate was 1.3% and 1.1%; Q-wave myocardial infarction rate was 4.6% and 2.1% and

stroke rate was 0.8% and 0.2% (for CABG and PTCA, respectively). The 5-year survival rates for those randomized to CABG was 89.3%, for those randomized to PTCA 86.3% (*P* = .19). The 5-year event rates for freedom from Q-wave myocardial infarction were also similar (80.4 versus 78.7%). However, at 5 years the need for further revascularization procedures was significantly higher in patients randomized to PTCA. Only 8% of patients assigned to CABG required additional revascularization procedures, whereas 54% of the PTCA group needed additional revascularization.

A number of other comparative revascularization studies have been summarized in a recently published meta-analysis. This study combined the results from 3371 patients (1710 PTCA, 1661 CABG) from 9 randomized studies with a mean follow-up of 2.7 years. As with the BARI trial, the outcomes of cardiac death and myocardial infarction were similar with the two therapies (Fig. 36.7) (41A). Again, the rate of repeat revascularization was markedly higher in the PTCA group than the CABG group (33.7 versus 3.3%). Relief of angina was similar at 3 years.

Other nonrandomized studies assessing the feasibility of multivessel PTCA have

Table 36.1.
Summary of Randomized Clinical Trials Comparing PTCA with CABG

Study	Patients (n)	Angiographic Entry Criteria	Follow-up Duration (yr)	Primary Outcome	Secondary Outcomes
BARI	1829	2, 3 vessels > 50% stenosis	5	Death	Repeat revascularization, ETT, angiography, LV function, angina severity, and MI
CABRI	1054	2, 3 vessels > 50% stenosis	5	Angina and functional capacity	Repeat revascularization, angiography, LV function, MI, and death
EAST	392	2, 3 vessels > 50% stenosis	3	Death, MI, ischemia by thallium	Repeat revascularization, angiography, angina severity
GABI	359	2, 3 vessels > 70% stenosis	1	Freedom from angina	Repeat revascularization, MI, and death
RITA	1011	1–3 vessels > 50% stenosis	5	Death and MI	Repeat revascularization, ETT, angina severity, LV function, employment status
ERACI	127	2, 3 vessels	5	Death, MI, angina, repeat revascularization	Complications—in-hospital, completeness of revascularization

BARI, bypass angioplasty revascularization investigation; CABRI, coronary angioplasty bypass revascularization investigation; EAST, Emory angioplasty surgery trial; GABI, German angioplasty bypass trial; RITA, randomized interventional treatment of angina; ERACI, Argentine randomized trial of PTCA versus CABG in multivessel disease; CABG, coronary artery bypass graft surgery; PTCA, percutaneous transluminal coronary angioplasty; ETT, exercise tolerance testing; LV, left ventricular; MI, myocardial infarction.

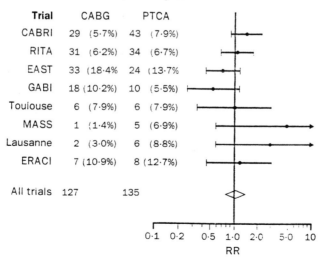

Figure 36.7. Cardiac death and myocardial infarction for PTCA group compared with CABG group in first year since randomization. (Reprinted with permission from Pocock SJ, Henderson RA, Rickards AF, et al. Meta-analysis of randomised trials comparing coronary angioplasty with bypass surgery. Lancet 1995;346:1184–1189.)

also been reported. Dorros et al. reported results of multivessel PTCA in a series of 309 patients (42). Initial angiographic success was achieved in 87% of lesions and in 285 (92%) patients. The complication rate was similar to that of PTCA performed in patients with single-vessel disease. Follow-up studies showed that only 20% had clinical evidence of lesion recurrence, including those who underwent repeat PTCA. On long-term follow-up, 85% of patients had sustained clinical improvement. Cowley et al. reported results of PTCA on 84 patients with two-vessel disease, 14 with triple-vessel disease, and 2 with four-vessel disease (43). In all, 273 lesions were attempted in these 100 patients, with an angiographic success rate of 90% and clinical improvement in 95%. These investigators reported the clinical success rate to be higher than in their total PTCA population (including patients with single-vessel disease) for the same time period. It should be noted that case selection in all nonrandomized trials may have biased the results, as revascularization by PTCA was recommended when lesions were felt amenable to such therapy. Most importantly, in this report the incidence of complications was not appreciably different from that of PTCA done in patients with single-vessel disease. Sustained clinical improvement was noted in many patients, as 64% were event free and 50% were asymptomatic after a mean follow-up of approximately 2 years. No statistically significant difference was found in recurrence rate comparing patients with multivessel PTCA (34%) and patients with single-vessel PTCA (28%) who had PTCA performed during the same time period at that institution.

Special Considerations

Repeat Revascularization

It must be recognized that occlusion after coronary revascularization by CABG or PTCA is an important factor leading to recurrent ischemia and associated morbidity and mortality (44). Follow-up angiographic studies have shown that 15 to 20% of saphenous vein CABGs are occluded by 1 year, and that only about 60% remain patent at 11 years (45). Even the grafts remaining patent often have evidence of important stenosis. Increased progression of native CAD may occur in vessels that have been bypassed. Thus, as a consequence of graft occlusion, stenosis, or progression of native CAD, disabling angina recurs at a rate of up to 5% per year following initially successful CABG surgery, and asymptomatic ischemia may recur at a higher rate. Thus, many patients will become candidates for reoperation with fewer options for conduits, increased risk of complications, and possibly increased mortality (46). Long-term relief of angina is not as effective with repeat surgery (31, 47). For example, in one series of 1000 patients undergoing reoperation from 1969–1982, angina was completely relieved in about 70% of patients 5 years after initial CABG surgery, whereas only 50% were angina free 5 years after reoperation. Internal mammary arteries are increasingly used as conduits, because patency rates appear higher than in veins, averaging about 90% at 10 years in uncontrolled series (48–50). Nonrandomized studies suggest that this improved patency may be translated to improved survival, compared with saphenous vein CABGs (51–53).

Although reoperation can be performed successfully with only a small increase in mortality and complications, **PTCA is an attractive alternative form of therapy for patients with signs or symptoms of recurrent ischemia caused by bypass graft occlusion.** PTCA can be performed on either grafted native vessels or bypass grafts (54–57). In reports evaluating restenosis with respect to the site of PTCA, the distal graft native artery anastomosis seems to behave similarly to a native coronary artery, whereas the aortosaphenous vein graft anastomosis and vein graft body are associated with high rates of restenosis. Also, the risk of infarction is higher with PTCA of lesions in the body of saphenous vein grafts, presumably because of embolic debris. It is important to recognize that graft occlusion after CABG surgery is not the same as restenosis after PTCA. Restenosis occurs in 30 to 45% of cases undergoing successful PTCA, usually within 4–6 months of dilation. The cause of restenosis remains unclear. This process probably is related to platelet activation, thrombosis, noncellular components, and smooth muscle cell injury and proliferation. This restenosis rate is reduced by coronary stenting. As opposed to reoperation following CABG surgery, repeat PTCA for restenosis can be done with a high success rate and few complications (58, 59). Furthermore, a "conduit" (e.g., vein or internal mammary artery) is not used or damaged by PTCA.

Other Special Risk Groups

Although some report that elderly patients undergoing CABG surgery have similar perioperative mortality when compared with younger individuals, CASS demonstrated a significantly increased risk (60, 61). Part of the reason for this disparity may relate to chronologic versus physiologic age. Early reports on the role of PTCA in the elderly vary. One suggests similar initial success rates, complications, and long-term clinical improvement as compared with younger individuals (62). Another suggests a slightly lower primary success rate and higher complication rate (63). However, in this latter study, the magnitude of difference, although statistically significant, was small and may not be clinically important. Currently, it is widely believed that age is not a major determinant of long-term PTCA success. Thus, both PTCA and CABG surgery are feasible in the elderly. Others considered at high risk for CABG surgery include those with depressed left ventricular function and those with poor general medical condition. In select patients, PTCA may be considered palliative for those at high risk for CABG surgery (64).

Synthesis

Based on a review of results of major trials in patients with chronic stable angina and our knowledge of predictors of high risk from noninvasive testing studies, it would appear that coronary angiography directed toward identifying sites for revascularization should be recommended in all patients with chronic stable angina who have "failed optimal medical therapy," as discussed. In stable angina patients who have not failed medical therapy, coronary angiography is also often useful. Because outcome in chronic stable angina patients in general is good, **we recommend an approach to candidate selection for catheterization based on results of stress testing or other findings suggesting high risk for adverse outcome** (e.g., reduced LV function) rather than on a routine catheterization-directed approach. Important prerequisites in the patient with fewer symptoms seem to be documentation of reversible ischemia and the possibility, from the characteristics of the ischemic response, that a large amount of myocardium may be at risk. Thus, we suggest attempting to separate those chronic stable angina patients who have higher risk factors from those with lower risk factors for adverse outcome before the decision for catheterization is made. Once catheterization data are obtained, the following angiographically defined subgroups should be expected to have improved survival with successful bypass surgery: (*a*) left main coronary artery stenosis; (*b*) triple-vessel obstruction with depressed left ventricular function; (*c*) triple-vessel obstruction with normal left ventricular function in patients with moderate to severe angina; (*d*) double-vessel obstruction with normal left ventricular function when one of the occluded vessels is the proximal left anterior descending artery; and (*e*) patients who appear to be at high risk based on risk stratification by noninvasive tests, such as those with ischemia provokable at low workloads or of severe magnitude. When these findings are documented, a recommendation for revascularization seems warranted.

With single-vessel obstruction, no clear mortality benefit over 5–7 years is found, employing initial surgery compared with initial medical treatment. PTCA has been shown to offer earlier and more complete relief of angina than does medical therapy. It should be emphasized that all of the randomized trials compare initially assigned treatment groups. Hence, those assigned initial medical therapy, who undergo

CABG surgery for whatever reason several months later, continue to remain in the medically assigned group for the purposes of the study. Thus, these results refer only to initial treatment choice, likely biasing those in favor of the less invasive approach. Furthermore, these choices can only be made after coronary angiography has been done. It is apparent that with optimal case selection, based on coronary angiography, initial success rates with PTCA may be similar for patients with single- and multivessel CAD. On long-term follow-up, patients with single-vessel disease are more likely to sustain clinical and angiographic improvement than patients with multivessel CAD. Many patients with multivessel disease, however, also may have sustained long-term benefit after PTCA. In patients who have recurrence of signs or symptoms of ischemia, and in those with angiographically documented restenosis, either repeat PTCA or CABG surgery may be readily done with a high success rate. It is our opinion that PTCA and CABG surgery are complementary revascularization techniques that are best used at different stages in the course of generally progressive coronary obstructive disease. Even when PTCA results in acute occlusion, which is rare when stents are readily available, surgical treatment may be performed with relatively low operative mortality/morbidity rates. For those in whom PTCA is unsuccessful and without complication, CABG surgery may be performed electively (65, 66).

Currently available information suggests that it is possible to identify subgroups of patients with chronic stable angina, based on coronary angiographic findings, in whom CABG surgery improves prognosis. Similar information is not available for PTCA, but may be so in the future, and use of PTCA must be governed by clinical judgment based on coronary angiographic findings and patient-related variables.

CORONARY ARTERY SPASM

General Considerations

Among patients with transient myocardial ischemia, coronary spasm plays a role in at least two subgroups. The smaller of these subgroups is termed "variant angina" and comprises about 3 to 4% of patients undergoing coronary angiography for chest pain. Variant angina refers specifically to individuals who have recurrent episodes of chest pain, primarily at rest, associated with ST segment elevation. In the other subgroup, patients who have coronary spasm during ischemia, a wide variety of ST segment and T-wave changes is present. This subgroup is considerably larger than those with only variant angina. A major portion of both subgroups has atherosclerotic obstruction. In general, these patients with spasm respond well to nitrates and calcium antagonists, and the long-term outcome is excellent provided severe atherosclerotic obstruction is not present (67) (Fig. 36.8).

Decision for Coronary Angiography

Diagnostic Considerations

Although noninvasive tests can document transient myocardial ischemia and are useful to formulate a working diagnosis and follow the response to therapy, visualization of spasm during coronary angiography is the reference standard. Angiographic evidence for coronary spasm must be associated with objective evidence of myocardial ischemia to be differentiated from catheter-related spasm. Catheter-related spasm usually occurs at or within a centimeter of the catheter tip, and usually does not cause transient ischemia. In the ideal situation, when evidence of ischemia occurs spontaneously in the catheterization laboratory and the angiographer documents coronary obstruction and its resolution with intracoronary nitroglycerin, the diagnosis of coronary artery spasm is established. Conversely, when patients complain of typical symptoms but without coronary obstruction or evidence for ischemia, coronary spasm can be excluded as the basis for these symptoms.

When spasm does not occur sponta-

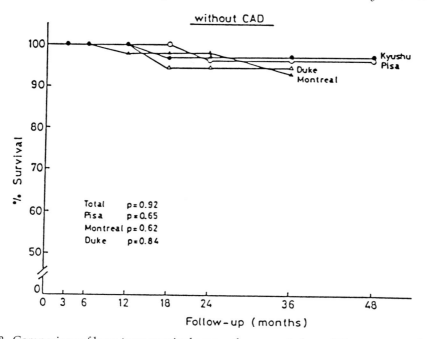

Figure 36.8. Comparison of long-term survival among four reports from different geographic regions: Japan (*Kynshu*), North America (*Montreal* and *Duke*), and Europe (*Pisa*) for variant angina patients without significant coronary artery disease. Survival for this subpopulation is excellent, approximating 95% at 4 years, with no significant differences between reports. (Reprinted with permission from Shimokawa H, Nagasawa K, Irie T, et al. Clinical characteristics and long-term prognosis of patients with variant angina. A comparative study between western and Japanese populations. Int J Cardiol 1988;18:331–349.)

neously during coronary angiography, a provocative test is helpful in those in whom spasm is suspected. In general, ergonovine testing is used for this purpose and the details are provided in Chapter 17. The broad indication for ergonovine testing is the need to know if coronary spasm is contributing to a patient's chest pain syndrome in the absence of contraindications. Some specific clinical situations for testing in patients with coronary angiograms that do not show sufficient obstruction to explain an angina syndrome appear in Table 36.2. Harding et al. (68) reported results of ergonovine testing for coronary spasm in 3447 patients without important ($\leq$ 50% diameter) coronary stenosis. No patients had variant angina. Overall, 4% had a positive test for spasm. Two independent predictors of spasm were identified using multivariate analysis: the amount of visible CAD on the angiograms and a smoking history. Most patients with a positive ergonovine re-

sponse had a coronary stenosis that was between 21 to 51% before the test. Baseline anginal history type (with rest angina excluded) had no predictive value. Using only the two variables, the authors suggest that a subset of patients, comprising approximately 17% of the study group, can be identified with a 10% rate of a positive test result. These considerations should help to reserve testing for the subset of patients most likely to demonstrate spasm during ergonovine administration. These suggestions may also apply to patients with more severe coronary atherosclerosis if suspicion of spasm is high (e.g., rest angina and relatively well-preserved or widely variable effort tolerance). Most recently, considerable attention has been focused on patients with life-threatening ventricular arrhythmias with silent myocardial ischemia caused by coronary spasm (69, 70). Presumably, reperfusion, after a period of spasm-induced ischemia, produced transient prolongation of

Table 36.2.
Specific Clinical Situations Where Provocative Testing for Coronary Spasm May Be Helpful

Rest pain associated with
  No preceding rise in heart rate and/or blood pressure
  Preserved effort tolerance
  Cyclic recurrence often in early AM
  Transient ST segment elevation or ventricular arrhythmias
  Nonspecific or no ECG change
  ECG pattern prohibiting interpretation of ST segment (eg., pacer, left bundle branch block, Wolff-Parkinson-White)
Angina associated with
  Variable exercise threshold
  ST segment elevation during stress testing
  Syncope and/or ventricular dysrhythmias
  Patent coronary bypass grafts
  A $\leq$ 50% coronary stenosis and history of smoking
Assess efficacy of therapy or spontaneous remission

the action potential and Q-T interval, which may be arrhythmogenic (71). Goals of testing are to (*a*) document the presence of spasm; (*b*) define the location and degree of spasm, number of vessels involved, and relationship to atherosclerotic coronary narrowing (e.g., at the site, proximal, distal); and (*c*) provide baseline data for later evaluation of therapy or course of disease (e.g., spontaneous remission). This information is important in terms of prognosis, drug selection, and potential for cardiac surgery (e.g., bypass, plexectomy). Contraindications to ergonovine testing appear in Table 36.3. The first three contraindications are relative because, although risks may increase in some instances, it is necessary to know if spasm is present. The latter five are absolute.

Intracoronary acetylcholine also induces spasm of epicardial coronary arteries in patients with variant angina, when low doses are administered into the coronary artery. In some patients with variant angina, coronary spasm induced by acetylcholine could be suppressed by atropine, a parasympatholytic agent. It is unknown why coronary arteries in patients with variant angina are sensitive to acetylcholine. It might be that

either their coronary vascular endothelium cannot produce sufficient EDRF, or the coronary vascular smooth muscle is hyper-reactive to the direct vasoconstricting effect of acetylcholine, or both. The response seen with this agent is transient and reverses spontaneously within 20–30 seconds. In our laboratory, we infuse intracoronary acetylcholine in graded doses (from 10–8 to 10–4 M). Although intracoronary acetylcholine use has been shown to be reliable and safe (72), ergonovine testing seems to remain a more specific test. The response to acetylcholine may be widely variable even in patients without clinical coronary spasm. Coronary spasm is considered present when a reversible change in coronary artery size is observed to reduce the diameter 50% or greater and is associated with transient ischemia. Objective evidence for myocardial ischemia may include any of the following: (*a*) transient ECG changes, such as ST segment shifts, normalization of previously depressed ST segments, and T-wave peaking; (*b*) exaggerated rise in left ventricular end-diastolic pressure (must be greater than expected from loading effects caused by ergonovine-related increases in aortic pressure and venoconstriction); (*c*) reversible decrease in regional **thallium**[201] uptake or wall motion; and (*d*) abnormal changes in myocardial metabolic indicators.

Once coronary spasm is suggested, a de-

Table 36.3.
Contraindications to Provocative Testing for Coronary Spasm[a]

Relative
  Recent myocardial infarction (within 5 days)
  Uncontrolled angina
  Uncontrolled ventricular arrhythmias
Absolute
  Amenorrhea in a premenopausal woman[b]
  Severe hypertension[c]
  Severe left ventricular dysfunction
  Severe aortic stenosis
  Significant left main coronary stenosis

[a] Adapted from Pepine CJ, Lambert CR. Coronary artery spasm: pathophysiology, natural history, recognition, and treatment. In: Hurst JW, ed. The Heart. 7th ed. New York: McGraw-Hill, 1989.
[b] May use intracoronary acetylcholine.
[c] May use either intracoronary ergonovine or acetylcholine.

finitive diagnosis should be made during coronary angiography, after careful withdrawal of calcium antagonists and long-acting (at least five half-lives) nitrates. Catheterization should be performed in a hospital laboratory with personnel skilled in ergonovine or acetylcholine testing, and should not be performed in a freestanding, nonhospital, outpatient facility. When spasm is suggested in the rare patient who does not show severe atherosclerotic obstruction on a recent angiogram, provocative testing may be done in the coronary care unit with ECG and either nuclear or echocardiographic studies, to detect regional electrocardiographic, perfusion, or wall motion abnormalities. These data, even when suggestive for transient ischemia, do not offer a definitive diagnosis for coronary artery spasm, and we do not recommend this noncatheterization laboratory testing. Although tests for coronary spasm can be performed outside the catheterization laboratory, we believe that the initial test in any patient, and, whenever possible, all tests should be done during catheterization (73). This practice allows hemodynamic, as well as ECG, monitoring and ensures the safest approach to manage potentially serious effects of spasm-related ischemia, such as heart block, ventricular arrhythmias, and hypotension.

Prognostic Considerations

The outcome for patients with spasm and CAD is related to the extent and severity of atherosclerotic CAD and to their left ventricular function (Fig. 36.9). Over 3–5 years, those with variant angina and relatively normal coronary arteries are at low risk (approximately 5%) for events such as death and myocardial infarction. Patients with variant angina, who have only one artery showing 70% or more "fixed" atherosclerotic obstruction, are at low to moderate risk, whereas those with severe multivessel disease are at relatively high (approximately 30%) risk for events. Thus, identification of spasm and CAD are very important in terms of patient management. Again, it is important to emphasize that the defini-

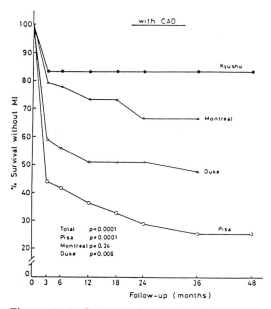

Figure 36.9. Outcome (survival without myocardial infarction [*MI*] from the four reports shown in Figure 36.8 for variant angina patients with significant coronary artery disease. Prognosis is poor in all four studies and depends directly on the severity of coronary disease in the population studied. For example, multivessel coronary artery disease (CAD) was present in 56% of patients in the Pisa study, where outcome was worst, and in only 4% of the Kynshu study, where relative outcome is best. (Reprinted with permission from Shimokawa H, Nagasawa K, Irie T, et al. Clinical characteristics and long-term prognosis of patients with variant angina. A comparative study between western and Japanese populations. Int J Cardiol 1988;18:331–349.)

tive diagnosis of coronary spasm can be made only during coronary angiography.

Management Decisions Based on Angiographic Findings

Currently no published controlled studies are comparing medical with revascularization therapy in coronary spasm patients. David et al. reported results of PTCA in 11 patients with variant angina who had coexisting atherosclerotic coronary stenosis (74). Despite initial success, symptoms persisted that required calcium antagonists, and a high restenosis rate was noted. Corcos et al. also demonstrated a high restenosis rate in a series of 21 patients (75). After repeat angioplasty, however, 75% of patients were asymptomatic, requiring no medical therapy, which suggests that PTCA may play a role in management when spasm was superimposed on organic stenosis (75). More recently, Bertrand et al. suggested a high incidence of restenosis when PTCA was performed in patients with dynamic narrowing (76). Leisch et al. reported that, although PTCA may initially be effective in patients with variant angina, a higher restenosis rate occurs (77), which has also been our experience. Because of the frequently diffuse nature of spasm, stenting is also not useful.

Results of surgical treatment of patients with proved or suspected coronary spasm since calcium antagonists and intravenous nitrates have become available are limited. It is apparent, however, that CABG surgery can be done in patients with spasm superimposed on atherosclerotic obstruction, but results are not as favorable as those found when CABG surgery is done in patients without spasm (78). Perioperative death, myocardial infarction, and recurrent angina are frequent. Likewise, isolated case reports suggest that CABG surgery is not useful in patients with coronary spasm who do not have important atherosclerotic obstruction. Plexectomy combined with CABG surgery has been suggested, but these results are not very encouraging.

Synthesis

It would appear that patients with suspected coronary spasm should have coronary angiography and ergonovine testing, if necessary, in an attempt to identify spasm and associated CAD. Medical therapy (nitrates plus calcium antagonists) should be used in patients with documented coronary spasm. If symptoms or signs of ischemia recur and can be documented as caused by spasm, PTCA may be an appropriate consideration for a few carefully selected patients who also have localized severe atherosclerotic obstruction. Because of the

reported high restenosis rate, the procedure may have to be done several times. CABG surgery may be a consideration in a few patients with severe associated CAD. These few patients probably should have multivessel disease and evidence suggesting that spasm is not diffuse along the course of any vessel. Because of the possibility of recurrent spasm, patients undergoing either PTCA or CABG surgery should continue to receive intravenous nitroglycerin and calcium antagonists during and following the procedure.

These revascularized patients, as well as those treated without revascularization, should continue nitrates and calcium antagonists for at least a year. Judicious withdrawal of antispasm therapy should be contemplated only after an appropriate asymptomatic interval, and with proof (i.e., ambulatory monitoring) that ischemia does not reoccur in either a painful or silent form. In many of these patients, remission will have occurred, and medication will no longer be required.

POSTMYOCARDIAL INFARCTION

General Considerations

The postmyocardial infarction period is known to be associated with substantial morbidity and mortality. Risks for reinfarction and death, however, decrease throughout the first year. Accordingly, identification of those at high risk is standard medical practice in the early postinfarction period. In addition to the status of left ventricular function, other factors have been identified as important in predicting prognosis during this period (79, 80). It has long been known that the presence of postinfarction angina or ischemia detected by stress testing appear to significantly alter prognosis in patients with similar degrees of left ventricular function. Schuster and Bulkley followed 70 patients with early postinfarction angina with either "ischemia at a distance" or ischemia in the infarct zone, and noted a 56% mortality at 6 months (81). Ischemia at a distance was associated with a particularly high mortality rate of 72%.

Ischemia interacts with left ventricular dysfunction to increase risks for adverse outcome. For example, De Feyter et al. noted increased mortality in patients with either ejection fractions less than 30% or with triple-vessel CAD, compared with patients with either ejection fractions greater than 30% or single- or double-vessel CAD (82). On the other hand, patients who could complete 10 minutes of exercise had a much lower reinfarction rate as compared with those who did not complete 10 minutes. Thus, among patients with postinfarction angina, those with left ventricular dysfunction and ischemia, as well as those with triple-vessel CAD, might be expected to have an improved prognosis if these findings were identified at catheterization and if revascularization were performed.

Management Decisions (Conservative Versus Aggressive)

In patients who were asymptomatic or mildly symptomatic postinfarction, three randomized controlled trials of CABG surgery versus medical therapy have shown no distinct benefit in favor of surgery. Norris et al. addressed this issue in 100 consecutive patients believed to be at high risk because they had second or third infarctions (83). Most had triple-vessel CAD and depressed left ventricular function (ejection fraction less than 50%). Those with left main CAD and severe symptoms were not included. All were either asymptomatic or only minimally symptomatic, and they were randomized to receive either CABG or medical therapy. No difference in mortality was found in follow-up to 4.5 years (mean). These same investigators also terminated a similar randomized trial in patients following first infarction, when no trends were observed in favor of surgery (84). Likewise, group C of the CASS report (i.e., those asymptomatic for more than 3 weeks after documented infarction) included 160 postmyocardial infarction patients randomized to either CABG or medical therapy. Again, no signif-

icant improvement was seen after CABG surgery compared with medical therapy (24).

Coronary Artery Bypass Graft Surgery

One might expect that CABG surgery in the postinfarction period would be associated with improved survival. In an observational study, Akhras et al. followed 119 patients with relatively uncomplicated myocardial infarction, and performed exercise testing 2 weeks postinfarction (85). The patients who had positive treadmill tests underwent coronary angiography at 6 weeks. Those patients with triple-vessel CAD, those with critical proximal left anterior descending stenosis as a component of double- or triple-vessel disease, and those with refractory angina despite optimal medical therapy underwent CABG surgery within 3 months of infarction. Most of these patients had triple-vessel disease, and their exercise time averaged only 5.5 minutes; thus, they would be considered high risk. Yet, CABG surgery resulted in a 1-year mortality rate of only 2%. Singh et al., in a study of 108 consecutive patients with angina within 30 days of infarction, undergoing CABG surgery, found 5-year actuarial survival rate to be 87% (86). Although the limitations associated with this type of analysis are numerous, one might infer that CABG surgery may be associated with reduced mortality when done in selected patients with postinfarction angina.

Percutaneous Transluminal Coronary Angioplasty

De Feyter et al. performed PTCA between 48 hours and 30 days after acute myocardial infarction in 53 patients with angina (87). PTCA was initially successful in 89%, and four of the six patients with unsuccessful PTCA had reinfarctions. The procedure-related myocardial infarction rate was somewhat higher than that expected for elective

PTCA done for chronic stable angina. Most patients in this study had single-vessel disease, as patients with multivessel disease were often offered CABG surgery. Angina recurred more frequently in patients with multivessel disease, who had undergone PTCA of only the "ischemia-related vessel" (8 of 17, 47%), than in patients with single-vessel disease (6 of 30, 20%). This difference, however, apparently was not statistically significant. During 6 months of follow-up, no late cardiac deaths occurred, but recurrent myocardial infarction developed in two patients.

Since thrombolytic therapy became a routine treatment for acute infarction, uncontrolled reports suggested that PTCA could enhance revascularization after infarction. It was well known that in a significant minority of patients, thrombolytic therapy either fails to reperfuse the infarct-related artery or leaves behind a severe residual stenosis. Awareness of this problem led some to return to routine angiography; i.e., all patients who received thrombolysis were taken to the catheterization laboratory early after infarction to determine whether reperfusion had occurred. Patients who showed a closed infarct-related artery or a high degree of residual stenosis could then be considered for early, emergent PTCA or bypass surgery. Three trials, phase IIA of the Thrombolysis in Myocardial Infarction (TIMI) trial (88), the Thrombolysis and Angioplasty in Myocardial Infarction (TAMI) trial (89), and the European Cooperative Study (90), assessed this approach. All three found that the mortality rate was higher with emergent, compared with elective, PTCA following thrombolysis.

An early (< 48 hours) catheterization after thrombolysis, with the intent of enhancing revascularization with PTCA, cannot be justified as a routine approach to uncomplicated postinfarction patients. Also, five trials compared the benefits of a routine invasive versus conservative management strategy after thrombolytic therapy: the TIMI IIB trial (91), the TAMI-5 trial (92), the Should We Intervene Following Thrombolysis? (SWIFT) trial (93), the Streptokinase in Acute Myocardial Infarction (SIAM) trial (94), and a study conducted in Israel by Barbash et al. (95). None of these trials demonstrated benefits of sufficient magnitude to justify a routine invasive approach. In fact, if one carefully analyzes the data from these studies, all five show a small, albeit nonsignificant, trend toward an increase in mortality, and the majority rates show a trend toward an increase in nonfatal reinfarction in aggressively managed patients. When these data are pooled (Fig. 36.10), the risks for death and adverse outcome (death and nonfatal myocardial infarction) appear to be significantly higher with the routine invasive strategy (96). It should be emphasized, however, that treatment of myocardial infarction continues to evolve rapidly. We are reaching mortality rate levels that are low where further improvement will be difficult. Other more sensitive measures need to be evaluated as stents and more advanced medical therapies, such as IIb/IIIa receptor antagonists, are incorporated into treatment regimens.

Synthesis

In the postmyocardial infarction period, coronary angiography and revascularization are clearly indicated in patients who have signs or symptoms of recurrent myocardial ischemia or cardiogenic shock. Recurrence of ischemia in this setting is, in itself, indicative of high risk. Successful CABG surgery will prevent recurrent ischemia, and it has the potential to improve survival. Other indications in the early postinfarction period, including cardiogenic shock, are addressed in Chapter 37. For postinfarction patients who do not have ischemia, risk stratification is in order. Many, including ourselves, consider patients with non–Q-wave infarction to be at high risk. For those with either clinical or noninvasively detected indicators of high risk, coronary angiography is indicated. If high-risk anatomy is found—for example, left main coronary artery or three-vessel obstruction, or severe ventricular dysfunction (i.e., ejection fraction 40% or more)—strong consideration should be given to recommend CABG surgery. It should be emphasized that this recommendation relates to potential for

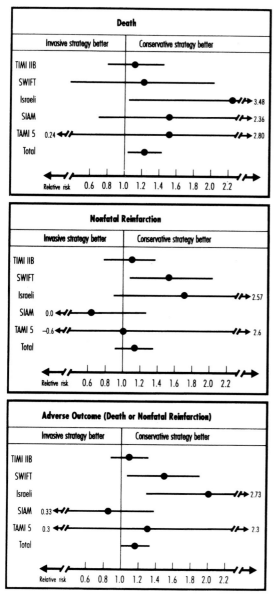

Figure 36.10. Conservative versus invasive strategy for myocardial infarction: relative risk (with 95% confidence limits) of death, nonfatal reinfarction, and adverse outcome (death or nonfatal reinfarction). *SIAM,* Streptokinase in Acute Myocardial Infarction; *SWIFT,* Should We Intervene Following Thrombolysis?; *TAMI,* Thrombolysis and Angioplasty in Myocardial Infarction; *TIMI,* Thrombolysis in Myocardial Infarction.

modifying risk and has not been tested in controlled trials.

It would appear that postmyocardial infarction patients with severe left ventricular dysfunction, recurrent signs or symptoms of ischemia, or multivessel disease are at increased risk for further events. Revascularization with PTCA can be offered in certain settings as an alternative to CABG surgery. As discussed, it would appear at present that patients with single-vessel CAD, excluding those with left main coronary artery stenosis, may be better PTCA candidates, whereas most of those with multivessel CAD may be better CABG surgery candidates.

These data strongly suggest that stable postinfarction patients treated with thrombolytic therapy without demonstrable ischemia should not undergo routine angiographic-directed management.

ASYMPTOMATIC MYOCARDIAL ISCHEMIA

Decision for Coronary Angiography

Diagnostic Considerations

The definition of asymptomatic is not clear in many circumstances. Individuals who were never symptomatic but at high risk for CAD constitute a large subgroup. Included are those who have evidence for silent myocardial ischemia documented by noninvasive testing, those who have ECG changes suggesting silent or unrecognized myocardial infarction, and those without noninvasive test findings suggestive of CAD but who are at extreme high risk because of other factors. Although subjects in these three subsets are all totally asymptomatic, concern arises because the initial clinical manifestation of CAD may be sudden death or acute myocardial infarction. Rates for these events determine the level of concern and ultimately play an important role in weighing the potential risks and benefits to be derived from coronary angiography directed toward CAD diagnosis and identifying candidates for revascularization. Although specific CAD event rates for these patients are not known with certainty, some data are available to help in management. Rather than never symptomatic, recent trends have applied arbitrary time limits on this definition (e.g., without symptoms in preceding 6 weeks was used in ACIP and also the recent American College of Cardiology/American Heart Association (ACC/AHA) coronary angiography guidelines) (1A, 7).

Prognostic Considerations

Ellestad and Wan were among the first to suggest that treadmill tests demonstrating ischemic ST segment responses appear to have the same prognostic significance regardless of whether the ST segment changes are accompanied by symptoms (97). Falcone et al. examined the clinical significance of exercise-induced silent myocardial ischemia in patients with CAD documented by angiography (98). Patients with chest pain and ischemic ST segment changes were compared with patients who had exercise-induced ischemic ST segment changes but no chest pain. The two groups had similar left ventricular function and severity of coronary artery disease. CABG surgery was performed in approximately one half of those with symptoms and one quarter of those without symptoms. After 3 years' follow-up, survival rates of medically treated patients with exercise-induced symptoms and medically treated patients without exercise-induced symptoms were not statistically different, even when patients were classified according to the number of diseased vessels.

Weiner et al. reported on a large group of patients from the CASS registry, who underwent coronary angiography and treadmill testing at approximately the same time and were then followed for 7 years (99). The patients were divided into four groups. Group 1 (Fig. 36.11) consisted of 424 patients who had exercise-induced ST segment depression without angina during exercise testing (i.e., silent ischemia). Of these, 35% were asymptomatic (class I) and another 44% had only mild angina (class II) during other activities. Group 2 had 232 patients, all of whom had angina during exercise testing without clearly ischemic ST segment changes. Group 3 was comprised of 456 patients who had both ischemic ST segment depression and angina during exercise. Group 4 patients had no ST segment depression or symptoms during exercise. All groups had similar frequencies of single- and multivessel CAD, left ventricular

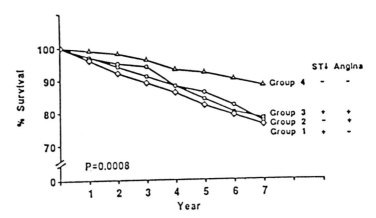

Figure 36.11. Cumulative survival for patients with and without exercise-induced silent ischemia. The 7-year survival rate was similar for patients in *Group 1* (silent ischemia) compared with *Group 2* and *Group 3* (painful ischemia). *Group 4* patients had a substantially better 7-year survival. (Reprinted with permission from Weiner DA, Ryan TJ, McCabe C, et al. Significance of silent myocardial ischemia during exercise testing in patients with coronary artery disease. Am J Cardiol 1987;59:725–729.)

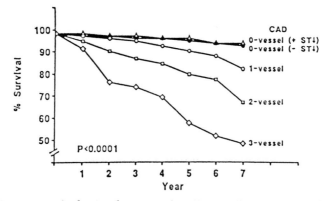

Figure 36.12. Seven-year survival rates for group 1 patients (silent ischemia) based on the severity of coronary artery disease (CAD): a separate group of 282 patients without CAD who had ischemic ST segment depression without angina during exercise testing, and a control group of 1117 patients without CAD and either ischemic ST depression or angina during exercise testing. (Reprinted with permission from Weiner DA, Ryan TJ, McCabe C, et al. Significance of silent myocardial ischemia during exercise testing in patients with coronary artery disease. Am J Cardiol 1987;59:725–729.)

function, and exercise tolerance. The 7-year survival rates from the first three groups with signs or symptoms of ischemia were similar (approximately 78%). Survival of these patients was significantly different compared with group 4 patients who had no signs or symptoms of ischemia during exercise testing. These findings suggest that patients with silent myocardial ischemia, detected by treadmill testing, may have a long-term prognosis that is not different from patients who experience angina. Also, those without signs or symptoms of ischemia during exercise testing have a significantly better prognosis than those with ischemia, despite similar degrees of CAD and left ventricular dysfunction. Further analysis of survival according to severity of CAD of those patients in group 1, who had silent ischemia during exercise, was particularly impressive (Fig. 36.12). Those with two-vessel CAD had a 7-year survival of approximately 70%, and those with three-vessel CAD had a 7-year survival of only 50%. Weiner et al. also compared survival rates of group 1 silent ischemia patients (e.g., exercise-induced ST segment depression and no angina) with a group of 282 patients without CAD who had ischemic-type ST segment depression during exercise, and also with 1117 patients with neither CAD nor ST segment depression. Both of these latter groups showed 7-year survival rates

of greater than 95%, illustrating the lack of prognostic importance of ST segment depression during exercise when CAD is not present.

The frequency of such false-positive responses depends on the prevalence of CAD in the group being tested. Middle-aged, asymptomatic men with multiple risk factors and abnormal exercise ECGs suggesting silent ischemia, have an approximately fourfold increase in CAD mortality over 7 years, compared with patients who have normal exercise ECG responses (100). Considering that perhaps 25% or more of patients, with exercise-induced ECG changes suggesting ischemia, probably have false-positive ECG responses (i.e., ST segment depression but no CAD), these mortality rates underestimate the true prognostic importance of silent ischemia associated with CAD in high-risk, asymptomatic middle-aged men. Finally, Framingham study data documented that approximately 25% of the men and 30% of the women who had myocardial infarction, documented by new Q-waves on a biannual ECG, had unrecognized, frequently silent, myocardial infarctions (101). Ten-year follow-up of these patients indicates that the frequencies of death, recurrent myocardial infarction, and most other CAD end points were essentially the same as those of patients who had painful myocardial infarction. It is well known that postmortem studies often identify a substantial amount of severe coronary atherosclerosis and myocardial scarring in many patients who were thought to be completely asymptomatic.

Recently, reports have emerged dealing with the risk of adverse outcome and ambulant ischemia in patients with clinically stable chest pain syndromes. In one study (102), ambulant ischemia was associated with a twofold to fourfold increase in risk of death. The risk of nonfatal infarction death was increased approximately 14 times in one study (103). Because outcome in coronary artery disease patients is multifactorial, multivariate analysis was used in three studies (102–104). In each study, silent ischemia was the best independent predictor of outcome, among a number of factors that included coronary angiography and exercise test results. It should be emphasized that all these studies are of patients with CAD. Recently, completed controlled trials (ACIP) identified relatively high risk for adverse-outcome patients with stress-induced ischemia and ischemia during daily life (1A). About one third of ACIP patients were "asymptomatic." Revascularization was superior to medical therapy as an initial treatment option in ACIP (1A).

Management Decisions Based on Angiographic Findings

We believe that strong consideration should be given to treating asymptomatic patients with coronary angiographic findings suggesting high risk (e.g., left main and three-vessel CAD or ejection fraction 40% or less) with revascularization therapy. Although not yet definitely proved, this approach is a rational attempt to prevent myocardial infarction, death, and need for subsequent hospitalization in such patients. Currently the only controlled study of patients with definite asymptomatic ischemia, comparing revascularization with medical therapy, is the ACIP (1A). Although this study was designed as a pilot, an impressive difference was found in adverse outcome comparing

revascularization with medical therapy at both 1 and 2 years. Patients who are asymptomatic postinfarction were discussed earlier in this chapter.

It seems reasonable to conclude that certain asymptomatic patients should be approached for cardiac catheterization in a manner similar to patients who have symptoms. Presently, no studies are available randomizing only patients with no symptoms to either PTCA versus CABG surgery or PTCA versus medical therapy. It is uncertain which asymptomatic patients with silent ischemia should be referred for revascularization. Based on results of exercise testing demonstrating that patients have similar prognoses regardless of whether symptoms are present, patients with silent ischemia and stress tests suggesting high risk should undergo coronary angiography. If high-risk anatomy (left main stenosis or three-vessel disease with poor left ventricular function) is present, either CABG surgery (for left main coronary artery) or PTCA (dependent on anatomy) should be considered. Asymptomatic coronary artery disease patients with high-risk radionuclide studies or ischemia during daily life despite medical therapy also should be considered for revascularization.

Several recent observational reports suggest that angioplasty can be safely performed in patients with silent ischemia. Bergin et al. (105) performed angioplasty on 54 asymptomatic patients with reversible ischemia by exercise thallium testing. Initial success was achieved in 48 patients (89%). Of the 48 patients with primary success, 12 developed positive exercise stress tests during follow-up. Ten successfully underwent repeat angioplasty, and the other two required coronary artery bypass. Therefore, in the 46 patients (85%) in whom initial or repeat angioplasty was successful, angioplasty was definitive therapy for silent ischemia. No deaths had occurred after 2 years of follow-up. Stone et al. (106) performed angioplasty on 45 CAD patients with minimal or no symptoms and positive exercise stress tests. Follow-up exercise stress tests or exercise thallium tests documented only 3 of 45 (7%) patients with evidence for recurrent ischemia. At a mean follow-up of 3 years, one patient died and three had nonfatal myocardial infarctions. Five patients underwent late bypass surgery, and 14 required repeat angioplasty. Therefore, the event-free survival at 3 years was 78%. Similar results were also reported in a smaller group of patients from the Cleveland Clinic (107). Thirty-four patients who had documented coronary artery disease without symptoms underwent angioplasty. Thirty-three had ischemia during exercise stress tests before the angioplasty. The procedure was successful in 31 patients (91%) and 1 patient required emergency bypass surgery. Four of the 31 patients with successful angioplasty had evidence of recurrent ischemia during a follow-up exercise stress test. Over a 3-year follow-up, six patients required repeat angioplasty, two required coronary artery bypass grafting, and one had a myocardial infarction. Therefore, the event-free survival was 87%. Anderson et al. (108) performed angioplasty on 114 asymptomatic patients with CAD, 94% of whom had documented silent ischemia. Over a 3.5-year follow-up, 4 patients had myocardial infarctions, 7 underwent CABG, and 30 had repeat angioplasty. No deaths occurred; the event-free survival for those patients having a successful angioplasty was 61%.

Synthesis

Although the mechanism by which such patients have important CAD and episodes of myocardial ischemia and necrosis without warning is unclear, this is not a rare finding. Although family history and other risk factors (e.g., smoking, hypercholesterolemia) predispose patients to CAD, it is clear that many of these asymptomatic patients with abnormal stress responses, and so forth, will not have important CAD. The question of when and for whom should coronary angiography be recommended is asked with increasing frequency. Clinical risk factors alone are not as useful as predictors of CAD when applied to the general asymptomatic population where the likelihood of CAD is low, as they are when applied to selected symptomatic populations where it is higher. Furthermore, when exercise testing

is applied to a population where CAD probability is low, even 1.0 mm or more of ST segment depression is associated with a low adverse event rate of approximately 2 to 4% per year. Even when applied to middle-aged patients with chest pain (e.g., high pretest CAD probability), the sensitivity and specificity for CAD of 1.0 mm or more of ST segment depression on exercise testing range between 60% and 80%. Thus, some decision-making schema to guide recommendations for coronary angiography is required in the evaluation of these asymptomatic patients.

We suggest the schema represented in Figure 36.13. It is similar to that recommended by others (109). Patients aged more than 35 years who have more than one risk factor (e.g., male, hypertensive, smoke cigarettes, or have a family history) should undergo exercise stress testing. If ischemic responses are found suggesting high risk for adverse outcome, coronary angiography is indicated. If ST segment depression suggesting ischemia is present, without evidence for high risk, radionuclide testing is suggested to define further the likelihood of CAD and risk of events. When the likelihood is high, coronary angiography is recommended. In the absence of these high-risk noninvasive findings, it is appropriate to examine the exercise workload achieved to provide more information relative to risk. If a high level was achieved, then the risk of CAD events is too low to recommend coronary angiography. If a high level workload was not reached during exercise testing, however, it is appropriate to also recommend a radionuclide test and, possibly, coronary angiography based on the results of the radionuclide study.

SUMMARY

Diagnostic and therapeutic cardiac catheterization procedures play a central role in the management of many patients with stable ischemic syndromes. In many subsets of patients with these syndromes, revascularization, directed by integration of clinical and coronary angiographic findings, will result in an improved outcome and even re-

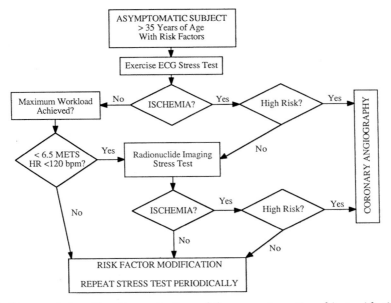

Figure 36.13. Proposed algorithm for evaluation of the asymptomatic subject with risk factors for coronary artery disease. *HR*, heart rate; *METS*, metabolic equivalents.

duced mortality. As more and more patients undergo noninvasive testing and more catheter-based therapeutic techniques are developed, this role will continue to expand.

No single diagnostic test yet yields more diagnostic and prognostic information in patients with CAD than a left side heart catheterization with coronary and left ventricular angiography. However, the question "can they or perhaps can we as a society afford it?" has made this a difficult choice in the 1990s. The data and suggestions reviewed in this chapter should help guide practitioners in their approach to this question.

References

1. Fletcher GF, Balady G, Froelicher F, et al. Exercise standards: a statement for healthcare professionals from the American Heart Association 1995;91:580–615.
1a. Davies RF, Goldberg AD, Forman S, et al., for the ACIP Investigators. Asymptomatic Cardiac Ischemia Pilot (ACIP) study two-year follow-up: outcomes of patients randomized to initial strategies of medical therapy versus revascularization. Circulation 1997;95:2037–2043.
1b. Forrester JS, Shaw PK. Lipid lowering versus revascularization: an idea whose time (for testing) has come. Circulation 1997;96:1360–1362.
2. Silverman KJ, Grossman W. Current concepts. Angina pectoris: natural history and strategies for evaluation and management. N Engl J Med 1984;310:1712–1717.
3. Burggraf, GW, Parker JO. Prognosis in coronary artery disease: angiographic, hemodynamic and 17 clinical factors. Circulation 1975;51:146–156.
4. Schlant RC, Blomqvist CG, Bradenburg RD, et al. A report of the American College of Cardiology/American Heart Association Task Force on Assessment of Cardiovascular Procedures (Subcommittee on Exercise Testing). Guidelines for exercise testing. J Am Coll Cardiol 1986;8:725–738.
5. Ritchie JL, Bateman TM, Bonow RO, et al. Guidelines for clinical use of cardiac radionuclide imaging. Report of the ACC/AHA Task Force on Assessment of Diagnostic and Therapeutic Cardiovascular Procedures. J Am Coll Cardiol 1995;25:521–547.
6. Pepine CJ, Abrams J, Marks RG, et al., for the TIDES Investigators. Characteristics of a contemporary population with angina pectoris. Am J Cardiol 1994;74:226–231.
6a. Writing Group for the Bypass Angioplasty Revascularization Investigation (BARI) Investigators. Five-year clinical and functional outcome comparing bypass surgery and angioplasty in patients with multivessel coronary disease. JAMA 1997;277:715–721.
7. Scanlon P, Faxon DP, Audet AM, et al. ACC/AHA Guidelines for coronary angiography. A report of the American College of Cardiology/American Heart Association Task Force on Prac-

tice Guidelines (Committee on Coronary Angiography). J Am Coll Cardiol 1998, in press.

7a. West of Scotland Coronary Prevention Study. Identification of high-risk groups and comparison with other cardiovascular intervention trials. Lancet 1996;348:1339–1342.

7b. Aengevaeren WRM, Uijen GJH, Jukema W, et al. Functional evaluation of lipid-lowering therapy by pravastatin in the Regression Growth Evaluation Statin Study (REGRESS). Circulation 1997;96:429–435.

7c. Andrews TC, Raby K, Barry J, et al. Effect of cholesterol reduction on myocardial ischemia in patients with coronary disease. Circulation 1997;95:324–328.

8. Bemiller CR, Pepine CJ, Rogers AK. Long-term observations in patients with angina and normal coronary arteriograms. Circulation 1973;47:36–43.

9. Murphy ML, Hultgren HN, Detre K, et al. Treatment of chronic stable angina: a preliminary report of survival data of the Randomized Veterans Administration Cooperative Study. N Engl J Med 1977;297:621–627.

10. Varnaukas E, European Coronary Surgery Study Group. Twelve-year follow-up of survival in the randomized European Coronary Surgery Study. N Engl J Med 1988;319:332–337.

11. European Coronary Surgery Study Group. Prospective randomized study of coronary artery bypass surgery in stable angina pectoris: a progress report on survival. Circulation 1982;65:II-67–71.

12. CASS Principal Investigators and their Associates. Coronary Artery Surgery Study (CASS): a randomized trial of coronary artery bypass surgery (survival data). Circulation 1983;68:939–950.

13. Conti CR, Selby JH, Christie LG, et al. Left main coronary artery stenosis: clinical spectrum, pathophysiology and management. Prog Cardiovasc Dis 1979;22:73–106.

14. Parisi AF, Folland ED, Hartigan P. A comparison of angioplasty with medical therapy in the treatment of single-vessel coronary artery disease. N Engl J Med 1992;326:10–16.

15. Detre K, Holoukov R, Kelsey S, et al. Percutaneous transluminal coronary angioplasty in 1985–1986 and 1977–1981: the National Heart, Lung, and Blood Institute Registry. N Engl J Med 1988;318:265–270.

16. Kirklin JW, Akins CW, Blackstone EH, et al. ACC/AHA guidelines and indications for coronary artery bypass graft surgery: a report of the American College of Cardiology/American Heart Association Task Force on Assessment of Diagnostic and Therapeutic Cardiovascular Procedures (Subcommittee on Coronary Artery Bypass Surgery). Circulation 1991;83:1125–1173.

17. Wong JB, Sonnenberg FA, Salem DN, et al. Myocardial revascularization for chronic stable angina: analysis of the role of percutaneous transluminal coronary angioplasty based on data available in 1989. Ann Intern Med 1990;113:852–871.

18. Ryan TJ, Loop FD, Faxon DP, et al. Guidelines for percutaneous transluminal coronary angioplasty: a report of the American College of Cardiology/ American Heart Association Task Force on Assessment of Diagnostic and Therapeutic Cardiovascular Procedures (Subcommittee on Percutaneous Transluminal Coronary Angioplasty). J Am Coll Cardiol 1988;12:529–545.

19. Bonow RO, Epstein SE. Indications for coronary artery bypass surgery in patients with chronic angina pectoris: implications of the multicenter randomized trials. Circulation 1985;72:V–23–30.

20. Kaiser GC, Davis KB, Fisher LD, et al. Survival following coronary artery bypass grafting in patients with severe angina pectoris (CASS). An observational study. J Thorac Cardiovasc Surg 1985;89:513–524.

21. Bonow RO, Kent KM, Rosing DR, et al. Exercise-induced ischemia in mildly symptomatic patients with coronary artery disease and preserved left ventricular function. N Engl J Med 1984;311:1339–1345.

22. Weiner DA, Ryan TJ, McCabe CH, et al. The role of exercise testing in identifying patients with improved survival after coronary artery bypass surgery. J Am Coll Cardiol 1986;8:741–748.

23. Klein LW, Weintraub WS, Agarwal JB, et al. Prognostic significance of severe narrowing of the proximal portion of the left anterior descending coronary artery. Am J Cardiol 1986;58:42–46.

24. Mock MB, Ringqvist L, Fisher L, et al. The survival of nonoperated patients with ischemic heart disease: the CASS experience [Abstract]. Am J Cardiol 1982;49:1007.

25. Chaitman BR, Davis KB, Kaiser GC, et al., participating CASS Hospitals. The role of coronary bypass surgery for "left main equivalent" coronary disease: the Coronary Artery Surgery Study registry. Circulation 1986;74:III-17–25.

26. Passamani E, Davis KB, Gillespie MJ, et al. A randomized trial of coronary artery bypass surgery: survival of patients with a low ejection fraction. N Engl J Med 1985;312:1665–1671.

27. Killip T, Passamani E, Davis KB. Coronary artery surgery study (CASS): a randomized trial of coronary bypass surgery. Eight years follow-up and survival in patients with reduced ejection fraction. Circulation 1985;72:V-102–109.

28. Detre KM, Takaro T, Hultgren H, et al. Long-term mortality and morbidity results of the Veterans Administration randomized trial of coronary artery bypass surgery. Circulation 1985;72:V-84–89.

29. The Veterans Administration Coronary Artery Bypass Surgery Cooperative Study Group. Eleven year survival in the Veterans Administration Randomized Trial of Coronary Bypass Surgery for Stable Angina. N Engl J Med 1984;311:1333–1339.

30. Cukingnan RA, Carey JS, Wittig JH, et al. Influence of complete coronary revascularization on relief of angina. J Thorac Cardiovasc Surg 1980;79:188–193.

31. Loop FD, Lytle BW, Gill CC, et al. Trends in selection and results of coronary artery reoperations. Ann Thorac Surg 1983;36:380–388.

32. Bell MR, Gersh BJ, Schaff HV, et al., and the investigators of the Coronary Artery Surgery Study. Effects of completeness of revascularization on long-term outcome of patients with three-vessel disease undergoing coronary artery bypass sur-

gery. A report from the Coronary Artery Surgery Study (CASS) registry. Circulation 1992;86: 446–457.

33. Mabin TA, Holmes DR, Smith HC, et al. Follow-up clinical results in patients undergoing percutaneous transluminal coronary angioplasty. Circulation 1985;71:754–760.

34. Vandormael MG, Chaitman BR, Ischinger I, et al. Immediate and short-term benefit of multilesion coronary angioplasty: influence of degree of revascularization. J Am Coll Cardiol 1985;6: 983–991.

35. BARI, CABRI, EAST, GABI, and RITA: coronary angioplasty on trial. Lancet 1990;335:1315–1316.

36. King SB, Lembo NJ, Weintraub WS, et al. A randomized trial comparing coronary angioplasty with coronary bypass surgery. N Engl J Med 1994; 331:1044–1050.

37. Hamm CW, Reimers J, Ischinger T, et al. A randomized study of coronary angioplasty compared with bypass surgery in patients with symptomatic multivessel coronary disease. German Angioplasty Bypass Surgery Investigation (GABI). N Engl J Med 1994;331:1037–1143.

38. CABRI Trial Participants. First year results of CABRI (Coronary Angioplasty versus Bypass Revascularization Investigation). Lancet 1995;346: 1179–1184.

39. RITA Trial Participants. Coronary angioplasty vs coronary artery bypass surgery: the Randomized Intervention Treatment of Angina (RITA) trial. Lancet 1993;341:573–580.

40. Rodriguez A, Boullon F, Perez-Balino N, et al. Argentine randomized trial of percutaneous transluminal coronary angioplasty versus coronary artery bypass surgery in multivessel disease (ERACI): in-hospital results and 1-year follow-up. J AM Coll Cardiol 1993;22:1060–1067.

41. The Bypass Angioplasty Revascularization Investigation (BARI) Investigators. Comparison of coronary bypass surgery with angioplasty in patients with multivessel disease. The Bypass Angioplasty Revascularization Investigation (BARI) Investigators. N Engl J Med 1996;335:217–225.

41a. Pocock SJ, Henderson RA, Rickards AF, et al. Meta-analysis of randomised trials comparing coronary angioplasty with bypass surgery. Lancet 1995;346:1184–1189.

42. Dorros G, Stertzer SH, Cowley MJ, et al. Complex coronary angioplasty: multiple coronary dilatations. Am J Cardiol 1984;53:126C–130C.

43. Cowley MJ, Vetrovec GW, DiSciasco G, et al. Coronary angioplasty of multiple vessels: short-term outcome and long-term results. Circulation 1985; 72:1314–1320.

44. Pepine CJ. Occlusion after coronary revascularization [Editorial]. J Am Coll Cardiol 1990;15: 1259–1260.

45. Bourassa MG, Fisher LD, Campeau L, et al. Long-term fate of bypass grafts: the Coronary Artery Surgery Study (CASS) and Montreal Heart Institute experiences. Circulation 1985;72:V-71–78.

46. Foster ED. Reoperation for coronary artery disease. Circulation 1985;72:V-59–64.

47. Schaff HV, Orszulak TA, Gersh BJ, et al. The morbidity and mortality of reoperation for coronary artery disease and analysis of late results with use of actuarial estimate of event-free interval. J Thorac Cardiovasc Surg 1983;85:508–515.

48. Barner HB, Standeven JW, Reese J. Twelve-year experience with internal mammary artery for coronary artery bypass. J Thorac Cardiovasc Surg 1985;90:668–675.

49. Lewis MR, Dehmer GJ. Coronary bypass using the internal mammary artery. Am J Cardiol 1985; 56:480–482.

50. Bashour TT, Hanna ES, Mason DL. Myocardial revascularization with internal mammary artery bypass: an emerging treatment of choice. Am Heart J 1986;111:143–151.

51. Loop FD, Lytle BW, Cosgrove DM, et al. Influence of the internal mammary artery graft on 10-year survival and other cardiac events. N Engl J Med 1986;314:1–6.

52. Cameron A, Kemp HG, Green GE. Bypass surgery with the internal mammary artery graft: 15 year follow-up. Circulation 1986;74:III-30–36.

53. Akl ES, Ozdogan E, Ohri SK, et al. Early and long-term results of reoperation for coronary artery disease. Br Heart J 1992;68:176–180.

54. Corbelli I, Franco L, Hollman J, et al. Percutaneous transluminal coronary angioplasty after previous coronary artery bypass surgery. Am J Cardiol 1985;56:398–403.

55. Block PC, Cowley MJ, Kaltenbach M, et al. Percutaneous angioplasty of stenoses of bypass grafts or of bypass graft anastomotic sites. Am J Cardiol 1984;53:666–668.

56. Douglas JS, Gruentzig AR, King SB, et al. Percutaneous transluminal coronary angioplasty in patients with prior coronary bypass surgery. J Am Coll Cardiol 1983;2:745–754.

57. El Gamal M, Bonnier H, Michels R, et al. Percutaneous transluminal angioplasty of stenosed aorto-coronary bypass grafts. Br Heart J 1984;52: 617–620.

58. Meier B, King SB, Gruentzig AR, et al. Repeat coronary angioplasty. J Am Coll Cardiol 1984;4: 463–466.

59. Williams DO, Gruentzig AR, Kent KM, et al. Efficacy of repeat percutaneous transluminal coronary angioplasty for coronary restenosis. Am J Cardiol 1984;53:32C–35C.

60. Rahimtoola SH, Grunkemeier GL, Starr A. Ten year survival after coronary artery bypass surgery for angina in patients aged 65 years and older. Circulation 1986;74:509–517.

61. Gersh BI, Kronmal RA, Frye RL, et al. Coronary arteriography and coronary artery bypass surgery: morbidity and mortality in patients ages 65 years or older. A report from the Coronary Artery Surgery Study. Circulation 1983;67:483–491.

62. Raizner AE, Hust RG, Lewis JM, et al. Transluminal coronary angioplasty in the elderly. Am J Cardiol 1986;57:29–32.

63. Mock MB, Homes DR, Vliestra RE, et al. Percutaneous transluminal coronary angioplasty (PTCA) in the elderly patient: experience in the National Heart, Lung, and Blood Institute PTCA Registry. Am J Cardiol 1984;53:89C–91C.

64. Taylor GJ, Rabinovich E, Mikell FL, et al. Percutaneous transluminal coronary angioplasty as pal-

liation for patients considered poor surgical candidates. Am Heart J 1986;111:840–844.

65. Pelletier LC, Pardini A, Renkin J, et al. Myocardial revascularization after failure of percutaneous transluminal coronary angioplasty. J Thorac Cardiovasc Surg 1985;90:265–271.

66. Akins CW, Block PC. Surgical intervention for failed percutaneous transluminal coronary angioplasty. Am J Cardiol 1984;53:108C–111C.

67. Shimokawa H, Nagasawa K, Irie T, et al. Clinical characteristics and long-term prognosis of patients with variant angina. A comparative study between western and Japanese populations. Int J Cardiol 1988;18:331–349.

68. Harding MB, Leithe ME, Mark DB, et al. Ergonovine maleate testing during cardiac catheterization: a 10-year perspective in 3,447 patients without significant coronary artery disease or Prinzmetal's variant angina. J Am Coll Cardiol 1992;20:107–111.

69. Myerburg RJ, Kessler KM, Bassett AL, et al. A biological approach to sudden cardiac death: structure, function and cause. Am J Cardiol 1989; 63:1512–1516.

70. Myerburg RJ, Kessler KM, Malloy S, et al. Life-threatening ventricular arrhythmias in patients with silent myocardial ischemia due to coronary artery spasm. N Engl J Med 1992;326:1451–1455.

71. Myerburg RJ, Kessler KM, Castellanos A. Pathophysiology of sudden cardiac death. Pacing Clin Electrophysiol 1991;14:935–943.

72. Okumura K, Yasu H, Matsuyama K, et al. Sensitivity and specificity of intracoronary injection of acetylcholine for the induction of coronary artery spasm. J Am Coll Cardiol 1988;12:883–888.

73. Pepine CJ, Feldman RL, Conti CR. Recommendations for use of ergonovine to provoke coronary artery spasm. Cathet Cardiovasc Diagn 1980;6: 423–426.

74. David PR, Waters DD, Scholl JM, et al. Percutaneous transluminal coronary angioplasty in patients with variant angina. Circulation 1982;66:695–702.

75. Corcos I, David PR, Bourassa MG, et al. Percutaneous transluminal coronary angioplasty for the treatment of variant angina. J Am Coll Cardiol 1985;5:1046–1054.

76. Bertrand ME, LaBlanche JM, Thieureux F, et al. Comparative results of percutaneous transluminal coronary angioplasty in patients with dynamic versus fixed coronary stenosis. J Am Coll Cardiol 1986;8:504–508.

77. Leisch F, Schutzenberger W, Kerschner K, et al. Influence of variant angina on the results of percutaneous transluminal coronary angioplasty. Br Heart J 1986;56:341–345.

78. Conti CR. Large vessel coronary vasospasm: diagnosis, natural history and treatment. Am J Cardiol 1985;55:41B–49B.

79. Beller GA, Gibson RS. Risk stratification after myocardial infarction. Mod Concepts Cardiovasc Dis 1986;55:5–10.

80. DeBusk RF, Blomqvist CE, Kouchoukos NT, et al. Identification and treatment of low-risk patients after acute myocardial infarction and coronary artery bypass graft surgery. N Engl J Med 1986;314: 161–166.

81. Schuster EH, Bulkley BH. Early postinfarction angina: ischemia at a distance and ischemia in the infarct zone. N Engl J Med 1981;305:1101–1105.

82. De Feyter PJ, van Eenige MJ, Dighton DH, et al. Prognostic value of exercise testing, coronary angiography and left ventriculography 6–8 weeks after myocardial infarction. Circulation 1982;66: 527–536.

83. Norris RM, Agnew TR, Brandt PW, et al. Coronary surgery after recurrent myocardial infarction: progress of a trial comparing surgical with nonsurgical management for asymptomatic patients with advanced coronary disease. Circulation 1981;63:785–792.

84. Norris RM, Barnaby PF, Brandt P, et al. Prognosis after recovery from first acute myocardial infarction: determinants of reinfarction and sudden death. Am J Cardiol 1984;53:408–413.

85. Akhras F, Upward J, Keates J, et al. Early exercise testing and elective coronary artery bypass surgery after complicated myocardial infarction: effect on morbidity and mortality. Br Heart J 1984; 52:413–417.

86. Singh AK, Rivera R, Cooper GN, et al. Early myocardial revascularization for postinfarction angina: results and long-term follow-up. J Am Coll Cardiol 1985;6:1121–1125.

87. De Feyter PJ, Serruys PW, Soward A, et al. Coronary angioplasty for early postinfarction unstable angina. Circulation 1986;74:1365–1370.

88. The TIMI Research Group. Immediate vs. delayed catheterization and angioplasty following thrombolytic therapy for acute myocardial infarction: TIMI IIA results. JAMA 1988;260:2849–2858.

89. Topol FJ, Califf RM, George BS, et al. A randomized trial of immediate versus delayed elective angioplasty after intravenous tissue plasminogen activator in acute myocardial infarction. N Engl J Med 1987;317:581–588.

90. Simoons ML, Arnold AER, Betriu A, et al. Thrombolysis with tissue plasminogen activator in acute myocardial infarction. Lancet 1988;1:197–203.

91. The TIMI Study Group. Comparison of invasive and conservative strategies after treatment with intravenous tissue plasminogen activator. N Engl J Med 1989;320:618–627.

92. Califf RM, Topol EJ, Stack RS, et al. Evaluation of combination thrombolytic therapy and timing of cardiac catheterization in acute myocardial infarction. Circulation 1991;83:1543–1556.

93. SWIFT (Should We Intervene Following Thrombolysis?) Study Group. SWIFT trial of delayed elective intervention vs. conservative treatment after thrombolysis with anistreplase in acute myocardial infarction. Br Med J 1991;302:555–560.

94. Ozbek C, Dyckmans J, Sen S, et al. Comparison of invasive and conservative strategies after treatment with streptokinase in acute myocardial infarction: results of a randomised trial (SIAM) [Abstract]. J Am Coll Cardiol 1990;15(2):63A.

95. Barbash GR, Roth A, Hod H, et al. Randomized controlled trial of late in-hospital angiography and angioplasty versus conservative management after treatment with recombinant tissue-type plasminogen activator in acute myocardial infarction. Am J Cardiol 1990;66(5):538–545.

96. Pepine CJ. Is routine angiography after acute MI still justifiable? [Editorial]. J Myocardial Ischem 1992;4:9–13.

97. Ellestad MH, Wan MK. Predictive implications of stress testing: follow-up of 2700 subjects after maximum treadmill stress testing. Circulation 1975;51:363–369.

98. Falcone C, De Servi S, Poma E, et al. Clinical significance of exercise-induced silent myocardial ischemia in patients with coronary artery disease. J Am Coll Cardiol 1987;9:295–299.

99. Weiner DA, Ryan TJ, McCabe C, et al. Significance of silent myocardial ischemia during exercise testing in patients with coronary artery disease. Am J Cardiol 1987;59:725–729.

100. Multiple Risk Factor Intervention Trial Research Group. Exercise electrocardiogram and coronary heart disease mortality in the Multiple Risk Factor Intervention Trial. Am J Cardiol 1985;55:16–24.

101. Kannel WB, Abbott RD. Incidence and prognosis of unrecognized myocardial infarction: an update on the Framingham Study. N Engl J Med 1984; 311:1144–1147.

102. Deedwania PC, Carbajal EV. Silent ischemia during daily life is an independent predictor of mortality in stable angina. Circulation 1990;81: 748–756.

103. Rocco MB, Nable EG, Campbell S, et al. Prognostic importance of myocardial ischemia detected by ambulatory monitoring in patients with stable coronary artery disease. Circulation 1988;78: 877–884.

104. Gottlieb SO, Weisfeldt ML, Ouvang P, et al. Silent ischemia as a marker for early unfavorable outcomes in patients with unstable angina. N Engl J Med 1986;314:1214–1219.

105. Bergin P, Myler RK, Shaw RE, et al. Transluminal coronary angioplasty in the treatment of silent ischemia. Cathet Cardiovasc Diagn 1988;15: 223–228.

106. Stone GW, Spaude S, Ligon RW, et al. Usefulness of percutaneous transluminal coronary angioplasty in alleviating silent myocardial ischemia in patients with absent or minimal painful myocardial ischemia. Am J Cardiol 1989;64:560–564.

107. Tuzcu EM, Nisanci Y, Simpfendorfer C, et al. Percutaneous transluminal coronary angioplasty in silent ischemia. Am Heart J 1990;119:797–801.

108. Anderson HV, Talley JD, Black AJR, et al. Usefulness of coronary angioplasty in asymptomatic patients Am J Cardiol 1990;165:35–39.

109. Beller GA. Role of nuclear cardiology in evaluating the total ischemic burden in coronary artery disease. Am J Cardiol 1987;59:31C–38C.

37

The Patient with Known or Suspected Coronary Heart Disease: Unstable Ischemic Syndromes

Michael P. Savage, MD
Sheldon Goldberg, MD

INTRODUCTION

The presenting manifestations of coronary artery disease comprise a clinical spectrum ranging from silent ischemia and stable angina to more acute syndromes such as unstable angina, myocardial infarction, and sudden death. The clinical symptoms of an individual patient are largely determined by the underlying coronary pathoanatomy. In patients where an atherosclerotic lesion progressively enlarges over time to obstruct the vessel lumen, coronary blood flow across the lesion may become inadequate during periods of increased myocardial oxygen demand. These patients typically present with signs and symptoms of transient myocardial ischemia that are relatively stable (e.g., exertional angina pectoris). Alternatively, a relatively abrupt change in the biology of an atherosclerotic lesion may occur, leading to an acute reduction in coronary flow. This abrupt reduction in perfusion can be mediated by a variety of intracoronary events including plaque rupture, thrombus formation, and coronary vasospasm (1). Patients with these "complicated" atherosclerotic lesions typically present with one of the unstable ischemic syndromes (e.g., unstable angina, subendo-

cardial infarction, or transmural myocardial infarction). These **acute ischemic events are a major cause of morbidity and mortality in patients with cardiac disease.** This chapter reviews the role of diagnostic and interventional cardiac catheterization in the management of patients with these unstable coronary syndromes.

UNSTABLE ANGINA

General Considerations

Historically, the syndrome of unstable angina pectoris has been described by many names including crescendo angina, accelerated angina, status anginosus, preinfarction angina, and acute coronary insufficiency. The term "intermediate coronary syndrome" has also been used to designate unstable angina pectoris as the clinical and pathoanatomic link between chronic stable angina and acute myocardial infarction (2). Few have improved on Wood's early description of this syndrome (3):

Characteristically . . . the onset of acute coronary insufficiency is sudden, a state of normal health, or of relatively mild angina of effort, with or

Table 37.1.
Braunwald Classification of Unstable Angina

	Clinical Circumstances		
Severity	Class A: Develops in Presence of Extracardiac Condition that Intensifies Myocardial Ischemia (Secondary UA)	Class B: Develops in Absence of Extracardiac Condition (Primary UA)	Class C: Develops Within 2 Weeks of MI (Postinfarction UA)
I. New onset of severe angina or accelerated angina: no rest pain	IA	IB	IC
II. Angina at rest within past month, but not within preceding 48 h (angina at rest, subacute)	IIA	IIB	IIC
III. Angina at rest within 48 h (angina at rest, acute)	IIIA	IIIB	IIIC

MI, myocardial infarction; UA, unstable angina.

without a previous history of cardiac infarction, changing abruptly to one of almost total incapacity. Although the pain is usually provoked by all the familiar triggers, including changes of temperature, a meal, getting into bed at night, or getting up in the morning, as well as by trivial effort and excitement, it may also occur spontaneously when the patient is sitting quietly in a chair reading the paper, or may wake him repeatedly from sleep. An ischemic electrocardiograph taken during an attack of pain confirms the diagnosis of angina pectoris . . . [but] a diagnosis of acute coronary insufficiency denies evidence of cardiac infarction."

Recognizing that **unstable angina pectoris encompasses a heterogenous population of patients,** authors have recently classified patients according to specific subgroups. A commonly used classification identifies three types of unstable angina: (*a*) new onset exertional angina, (*b*) crescendo angina (i.e., prior chronic stable angina with a relatively recent increase in symptom frequency or severity), and (*c*) angina at rest (4). An alternative classification of unstable angina has been proposed by Braunwald (Table 37.1) (5). Class I includes patients with new onset angina or accelerated angina but without rest pain; class II represents angina at rest (subacute) in which there is no history of angina within the preceding 48 hours; class III represents angina

at rest (acute) in which one or more episodes of angina have occurred within the previous 48 hours. According to this scheme, unstable angina class can be further characterized by the patient's specific clinical circumstances: class A refers to secondary unstable angina which is precipitated by coexisting extracardiac conditions (e.g., anemia, fever, arrhythmia, thyrotoxicosis); class B refers to primary unstable angina (i.e., the absence of extraneous conditions present in class A); class C refers to postinfarction angina.

Recognition of the different subsets of patients with unstable angina may be important for clinical decision making, because prognosis is influenced by the initial presentation. **Patients with rest angina have a worse outcome than patients with recent onset or progressive exertional angina** (6, 7). In addition, relatively prolonged (> 15 minutes) angina associated with ST-T wave abnormalities and angina persistence despite intensive medical therapy are associated with a high risk of subsequent myocardial infarction and death (8, 9). The prognostic value of the Braunwald classification of unstable angina has also been demonstrated (10, 11). In one prospective study, data was collected on 417 consecutive patients with unstable angina (10). The angina severity class was predictive of outcome as patients in class III (rest angina within 48 hours) had the highest risk for early myocardial infarction or death and the highest number of revascularization procedures. The clinical class was also predictive because patients in class C (postinfarction angina) had the highest risk of myocardial infarction or death.

Electrocardiograms obtained during a spontaneous episode of angina typically demonstrate transient deviations of the ST segments or T waves. Of 288 patients with unstable angina associated with electrocardiographic changes enrolled prospectively by the National Cooperative Study Group, ST segment elevation was observed in 27%, ST depression in 61%, and T-wave inversion alone in 12% of patients (12). Although ischemic electrocardiographic changes usually normalize shortly after the relief of angina, these abnormalities may persist for several hours or days without enzymatic evidence of myocardial infarction. One study attempted to correlate the direction of ST segment shifts during angina with the extent of coronary artery disease subsequently assessed by coronary angiography (13). No differences were observed in the angiographic extent or disease severity, presence of collaterals, or resting hemodynamics between patients with transient ST segment elevation and patients with transient ST segment depression. However, others have noted that in the presence of critical left main coronary artery stenosis, electrocardiograms during angina typically demonstrate downsloping ST segment depression with negative T waves in the precordial leads (14). The direction of ST segment changes has also been correlated with the location of the angina-producing artery in patients with single vessel disease. Although transient ST segment elevation was frequently observed in unstable angina patients with disease of the right coronary and left anterior descending coronary artery (78 and 48%, respectively), ST segment elevation was uncommon (9%) in patients with disease of the left circumflex coronary artery (15). Studies from our laboratory suggest that regional transmural myocardial ischemia associated with left circumflex occlusion is infrequently accompanied by

ST segment elevation, but it may be associated with ST segment depression alone or no ST segment shift (16). Therefore, the presence or absence of ST segment elevation in association with spontaneous angina is determined not only by the degree of myocardial ischemia, but also by the location of the coronary artery obstruction. The **absence of ECG change during chest pain suggests either that the symptoms are not caused by myocardial ischemia, or that the ischemia involves the true posterior left ventricular wall** as a consequence of left circumflex occlusion.

Another diagnostic technique that may have a useful role in the management of patients with unstable angina is continuous electrocardiographic monitoring. Several groups have now demonstrated that frequent episodes of silent ischemia are common in patients with unstable angina. Furthermore, the persistence of silent ischemia by Holter monitoring, despite therapy that prevents recurrent angina, predicts an increased likelihood of adverse clinical events (17–19). Recently the prognostic value of serum troponin levels has been demonstrated in several studies. In patients with acute coronary syndromes, elevated troponin levels are associated with increased risk of subsequent myocardial infarction and death, even in the absence of creatine kinase elevation (20–22).

In March 1994, a federally sponsored clinical practice guideline was published on the diagnosis and treatment of unstable angina (23). Jointly sponsored by the Agency for Health Care Policy and Research (AHCPR) and the National Heart, Lung, and Blood Institute (NHLBI), this landmark document prepared by an expert interdisciplinary panel represents the first national guideline on the management of ischemic heart disease. In the initial evaluation of patients with unstable angina, the guideline stresses the importance of risk stratification for adverse outcomes (Table 37.2). It suggests that patients in the low-risk category can be managed initially as outpatients with follow-up reassessment within 72 hours. Patients at intermediate or high risk should be admitted to the hospital and receive intensive medical therapy. Routine medications should include aspirin, beta blockers,

Table 37.2.
Short-Term Risk of Death or Nonfatal Myocardial Infarction in Patients with Symptoms Suggesting Unstable Angina

High Risk	Intermediate Risk	Low Risk
At least one of the following features must be present: Prolonged ongoing (> 20 min) rest pain Pulmonary edema Angina with new or worsening mitral regurgitation murmurs Rest angina with dynamic ST changes ≥ 1 mm Angina with S_3 or rales Angina with hypotension	No high-risk feature but must have any of the following: Rest angina now resolved, but not low likelihood of CAD Rest angina (> 20 min or relieved with rest or nitroglycerin) Angina with dynamic T-wave changes Nocturnal angina New-onset CCSC III or IV angina in past 2 weeks, but not low likelihood of CAD Q waves or ST depression ≥ 1 mm in multiple leads Age > 65 years	No high- or intermediate-risk feature but may have any of the following: Increased angina frequency, severity, or duration Angina provoked at a lower threshold New-onset angina within 2 weeks to 2 months Normal or unchanged ECG

Reprinted with permission from Braunwald E, Jones RH, Mark DB, et al. Diagnosing and managing unstable angina. Circulation 1994;90:613–622.
CAD, coronary artery disease; CCSC, Canadian Cardiovascular Society Classification.

and nitrates in combination (23–25). Calcium blockers should not be considered as initial therapy but should be reserved for patients who are unresponsive to beta blockers and nitrates or for patients with variant angina.

We routinely use intravenous heparin in the initial treatment of unstable angina, particularly in patients with symptoms at rest or with ischemic electrocardiographic changes. Several randomized trials demonstrated a significant reduction in the incidence of myocardial infarction with intravenous heparin. Transmural myocardial infarction developed in 15% of 114 patients following a 1-week course without heparin in comparison with an infarction rate of only 3% in 100 patients treated with 5000 U of intravenous heparin every 6 hours (26). Heprin's usefulness (1000 U/hour), aspirin (325 mg, twice daily), and both in combination was examined in a controlled trial involving 479 patients with unstable angina (27). Myocardial infarction incidence was reduced in all treatment groups compared with placebo. Meta-analysis of six randomized studies of unstable angina suggests that **heprin and aspirin use provides a 33% relative reduction in risk of myocardial infarction or death compared with aspirin alone** (28). The benefit of oral aspirin in unstable angina patients during longer-term follow-up of 3 to 24 months has also been demonstrated by several controlled trials (29–31). Preliminary studies also suggest an **important therapeutic role for platelet glycoprotein IIb/IIIa receptor antagonists in patients with unstable angina** (32, 33).

Role of the Cardiac Catheterization Laboratory in Unstable Angina Pectoris

Optimal timing and indications for cardiac catheterization in patients with unstable angina have not been definitively established. The goal of cardiac catheterizaton in patients with unstable angina is to provide detailed anatomic information to aid in determining prognosis and management.

Guidelines for cardiac catheterization and myocardial revascularization recommended by the AHCPR task force are illustrated in Figure 37.1. In patients with recurrent angina on maximal medical therapy, cardiac catheterization should be undertaken promptly to assess the patient for potential revascularization with transcatheter intervention or coronary artery bypass surgery. We also often recommend cardiac catheterization for patients with unstable angina whose symptoms initially improve after intensification of medical therapy. As shown by Gazes' study of the natural history of unstable angina before the era of aspirin and beta-blocker therapy, within 3 months of clinical presentation acute myocardial infarction or death will occur in ap-

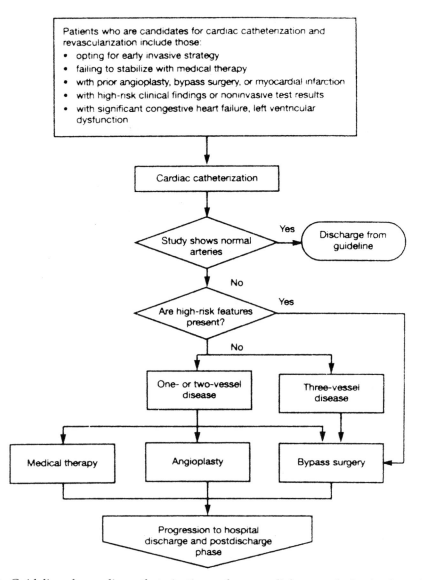

Figure 37.1. Guidelines for cardiac catheterization and myocardial revascularization in patients with unstable angina, from the Agency for Health Care Policy and Research Task Force. (Adapted from Braunwald E, Jones RH, Mark DB, et al. Diagnosing and managing unstable angina. Circulation 1994; 90:613–622.)

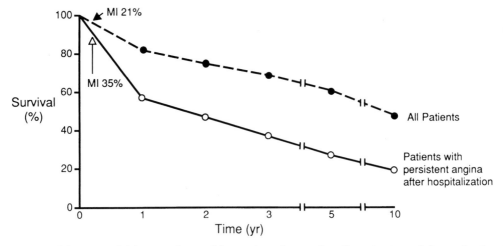

Figure 37.2. The natural history of unstable angina, shown for all patients and for patients with continued anginal symptoms during hospitalization. Within 3 months (*arrows*), acute myocardial infarction occurred in 21% of all patients (with an associated mortality of 41%) and in 35% of the high-risk subgroup with persistent angina (with an associated mortality of 63%). (Adapted from Gazes PC, Mobley ME, Faris HM, et al. Preinfarctional (unstable) angina—a prospective study—ten year follow-up. Circulation 1973;48:331–337.)

proximately 20% of patients (Fig. 37.2) (9). In light of the variable course of the disease in these patients and the high incidence of untoward cardiac events soon after symptom onset, evaluation of coronary anatomy is extremely valuable in patient management. Patients with rest angina associated with ST or T wave changes are at particularly high risk and should undergo early evaluation for revascularization. Patients with a pattern of crescendo angina have a relatively high incidence of left main coronary artery and triple-vessel disease and, therefore, cardiac catheterization should be done to identify these candidates for coronary artery bypass graft surgery (34). In patients with new onset exertional angina, it may be reasonable to defer cardiac catheterization if no ischemic changes are seen on the resting electrocardiogram and if symptoms are controlled after institution of medical therapy. **Exercise testing can be used to assess risk and help guide the need for further invasive testing** (35). Patients with angina at a low exercise workload, marked ischemic changes, or exercise-induced hypotension warrant coronary angiography. On the other hand, exercise stress testing is contraindicated in high-risk patients presenting with rest angina and electrocardio-

graphic evidence of ischemia. Exercise testing in these patients rarely mitigates the need for cardiac catheterization, delays more definitive evaluation, and exposes the patient to additional risk (Fig. 37.3). In such patients, it is preferable to undertake cardiac catheterization after initial intensification of medical therapy.

Approach to the Patient in the Cardiac Catheterization Laboratory

The importance of adequate anti-ischemic medical therapy in preparation for cardiac catheterization cannot be overemphasized. Angiography may precipitate acute ischemia and myocardial dysfunction in these unstable patients. Therefore, meticulous attention must be paid toward optimal stablization of the patient beforehand. Factors that increase myocardial oxygen demand, such as infection, fever, anemia, congestive heart failure, and tachyarrhythmias, should be identified and treated. Multiple antianginal drugs are recommended to minimize myocardial oxygen demand, which can be estimated clinically by the heart rate-blood pressure product. Oral or parenteral beta blockade should be used to achieve a resting heart rate of approximately 60 bpm. This reduces the potential for aggravating myocardial ischemia during the procedure and allows optimal angiographic assessment of coronary anatomy, which is not possible at rapid heart rates.

The clinical status of the patient on entry to the catheterization suite dictates the sequence of the cardiac catheterization procedure and the approach to data acquisition. The most important immediate concern is whether the patient is having ongoing myocardial ischemia. Continuous electrocardiography monitoring should be done to detect arrhythmias or ischemic ST-T wave changes. This is best done by a multichannel recorder with the capability of monitoring several leads simultaneously. We have found it useful to monitor an inferior lead (lead II) and a precordial lead (V_2 or V_4). Al-

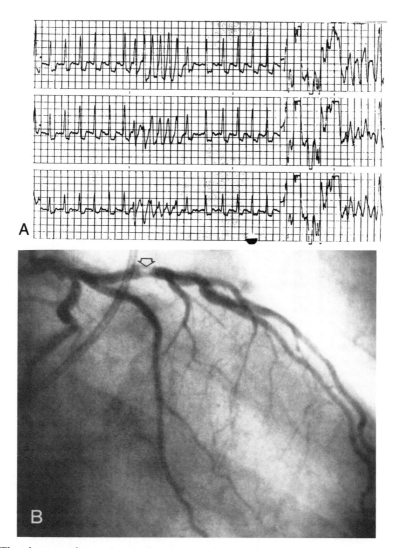

Figure 37.3. The danger of exercise testing in a patient with new onset rest angina. **A.** Treadmill exercise test demonstrating marked ST depression and ventricular fibrillation, which necessitated multiple electrical countershocks. **B.** Left coronary angiogram (right anterior oblique [RAO][1] projection) subsequently showed a critical stenosis of the proximal left anterior descending coronary artery (*arrow*).

ternatively, other leads can be used if they have shown more pronounced changes in a previous 12-lead electrocardiogram.

In patients with persistent angina on entry to the catheterization laboratory, initial attempts at stabilization should include nasal oxygen, intravenous beta-blockade, intravenous nitroglycerin, and adequate analgesia. In patients with ongoing ischemia refractory to these intensive pharmacologic maneuvers, insertion of an intraaortic balloon pump should be considered. Intraaor-

tic balloon counterpulsation should be initiated prior to coronary angiography in patients with ongoing angina associated with hemodynamic compromise (i.e., pulmonary edema or hypotension) or marked ST segment shifts (Fig. 37.4). Obviously, the decision to use the intraaortic balloon pump in this setting must be individualized. For example, if left main or severe multivessel coronary disease is suggested, and the patient is likely to be a candidate for coronary artery bypass surgery, balloon pump inser-

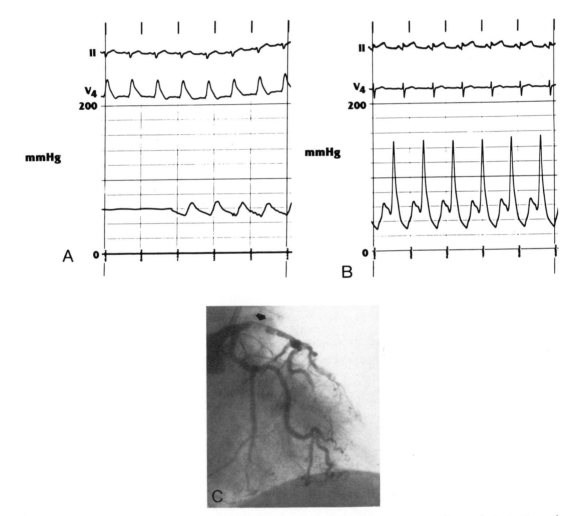

Figure 37.4. Usefulness of the intraaortic balloon pump during emergency cardiac catheterization of a patient with an unstable ischemic syndrome. **A.** Surface electrocardiogram and arterial pressure showing marked ST elevation and profound hypotension. **B.** Relief of acute injury current in lead V_4 and improved arterial pressure by intraaortic balloon counterpulsation. **C.** The coronary angiogram was then safely obtained and demonstrated subtotal occlusion of the proximal left anterior descending artery with preserved, but sluggish, antegrade flow.

tion will be useful to stabilize the patient and allow safe performance of both the diagnostic catheterization procedure and subsequent surgical revascularization. Alternatively, if the patient is hemodynamically stable and single-vessel disease is suggested because of the abrupt onset of symptoms, one can proceed expeditiously with coronary angiography and immediate coronary angioplasty, thus averting the risks associated with the intraaortic balloon pump. Another group of patients in whom coronary angiography should be done first are those with a history of variant angina (see also Chapters 17 and 36). Spontaneous coronary spasm should be suspected in this group of patients. Selective administration of intracoronary nitroglycerin into the involved artery, followed by repeat angiography, will be both diagnostic and therapeutic if spasm is present (36).

Cardiac catheterization in patients with unstable angina can be done by either the brachial or femoral routes (see Chapter 9). The approach used is best determined by the experience of the individual operator. The femoral approach provides a margin of safety in that immediate vascular access for intraaortic balloon counterpulsation is available should hemodynamic deterioration occur during the procedure. The type of angiographic contrast agent must also be individualized. Injection of radiographic contrast during coronary angiography results in important electrical and hemodynamic changes. These include slowing of the heart rate, prolongation of the QT interval, depression of myocardial contractility and systemic arterial pressure, and elevation of left ventricular end-diastolic pressure. These effects may be particularly deleterious in the unstable patient and contribute to the risk of the procedure. Nonionic and low-osmolar contrast agents allow cardiac catheterization in a more physiologic manner in unstable patients (37, 38) (see also Chapter 13). Compared with ionic high-osmolar contrast agents, these agents have significantly less electrical and mechanical depressant effects (39). We use low-osmolar agents routinely in patients with unstable angina and one or more of the following: rest angina within 48 hours of the cardiac catheterization, suspected

critical left main disease, aortic stenosis, congestive heart failure, and bradyarrhythmias. The availability of biplane x-ray equipment has also been useful for unstable angina patients because total contrast volume can be reduced.

We often use a 7 F vascular sheath in the femoral vein, through which a 7 F Baim-Turi catheter is advanced to measure right side heart pressures. The bipolar electrodes at the tip allow this catheter also to function as a temporary pacemaker when positioned within the right ventricle. Right side heart pressures are particularly useful in the setting of hypotension, congestive heart failure, prior myocardial infarction, or pulmonary hypertension. Ability to measure the right side heart and pulmonary vascular pressures also allows assessment of the hemodynamic effects of acute ischemia. An abrupt rise in pulmonary artery and pulmonary-capillary wedge pressures in a patient with transient ischemia implies either acute left ventricular dysfunction or acute mitral insufficiency caused by papillary muscle ischemia (Fig. 37.5). For patients in whom right side heart pressures are not recorded, a 6 F sheath is placed to provide central venous access for medication or a temporary pacing catheter. A 5 or 6 F sheath is then inserted into the femoral artery and 5000 U of intravenous sodium heparin can be administered. In patients with unstable angina and resting ischemic electrocardiographic changes already receiving intravenous heparin, it is not advisable to abruptly discontinue the heparin infusion. We have observed a number of patients who developed acute coronary thrombosis and myocardial infarction before cardiac catheterization when intravenous heparin was discontinued more than 6 hours prior to the planned procedure (Fig. 37.6). A prudent alternative is to reduce the infusion rate by one half 2 to 4 hours beforehand. This approach minimizes the potential for sudden rebound of acute ischemic events known to occur soon after heparin discontinuation in patients with unstable angina (40).

Left ventriculography can be done prior to coronary angiography to assess basal left ventricular hemodynamics, systolic function, and mitral valve competence. This is usually well tolerated in patients who have been stable for 24 to 48 hours prior to the procedure. On the other hand, left ventriculography can precipitate myocardial ischemia. Therefore, left ventriculography should be deferred until after coronary angiography in patients with active myocardial ischemia or if left ventricular end-diastolic pressure is markedly and persistently elevated (> 20 mm Hg) despite nitroglycerin. In patients with ongoing ischemia, it is often best to omit left ventriculography altogether unless the information is essential for planning therapy and cannot be sufficiently assessed by noninvasive methods (e.g., suspected mitral insufficiency or ventricular aneurysm). Again, nonionic or low-osmolar contrast agents are particularly useful in this setting.

The left coronary artery should be routinely visualized first. Attention should be directed initially toward assessing the left main coronary artery because this is the most threatening location for coronary obstruction. Significant left main stenosis will be present in 10 to 15% of patients with unstable angina. Critical stenosis at the left main ostium is often first signaled by dampening of the pressure waveform on catheter tip entry into the ostium (Fig. 37.7). This finding will be observed with preformed end-hole catheters, such as Judkins or Amplatz catheters, but may not be observed with side-hole catheters, such as multipurpose or Sones catheters. When ostial stenosis is suggested, multiple test injections of contrast media should be avoided, as repeated injections are potentially hazardous in this circumstance. Initial injection should be performed with cinefilming so that, if a critical ostial lesion is confirmed, the risk of repeated contrast injections can be averted. The patient with unstable angina and critical left main coronary artery disease is one of the most high-risk combinations encountered in the laboratory. Although diagnostic catheterization is usually done with very low mortality, the risk is substantial in patients with left main coronary stenosis where procedural mortality approaches 1% (41).

When left main coronary stenosis is suggested, it is of utmost importance to take precautions to prevent bradycardia and hypotension that may lead to further hypoperfusion and acute cardiogenic shock. Clinical features that suggest a high likelihood of

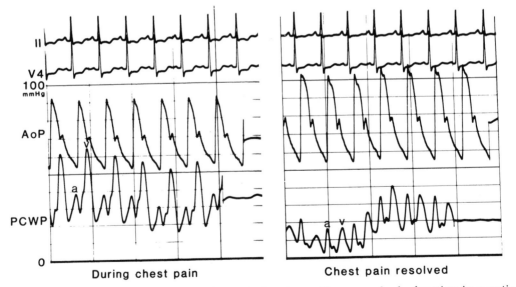

During chest pain   **Chest pain resolved**

Figure 37.5. Acute mitral regurgitation due to ischemic papillary muscle dysfunction in a patient with unstable angina and critical stenosis of the left circumflex coronary artery. During angina (**left**), marked ST segment depression is accompanied by arterial hypotension (*AoP*) and large V waves in the pulmonary-capillary wedge pressure (*PCWP*) tracing. After relief of angina (**right**), improvement is found in the hemodynamics and electrocardiogram.

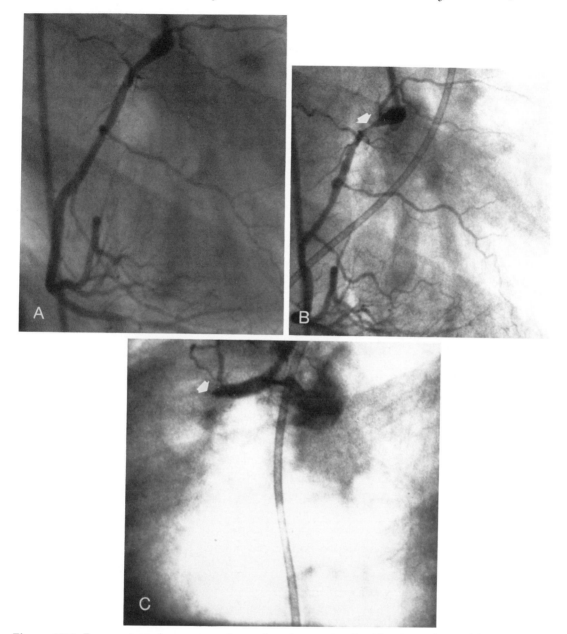

Figure 37.6. Progression of coronary atherosclerosis associated with onset of unstable angina, as shown by serial angiograms over a 3-year period. **A.** Initial right coronary angiogram shows no significant disease. **B.** Repeat angiogram 3 years later, after the development of unstable angina, shows a new severe stenosis of the proximal right coronary artery (*arrow*). **C.** Acute thrombotic occlusion of the right coronary artery occurring hours after discontinuation of intravenous heparin infusion.

left main coronary artery obstruction include any of the following: history of crescendo symptoms superimposed on chronic stable angina, ST segment depression in both inferior and anterior ECG leads simultaneously, and calcification of the left main coronary artery on fluoroscopy (42). In addition, prior exercise stress testing, accom-

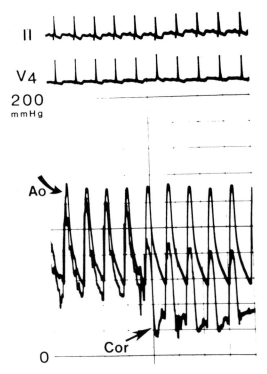

II

V4

200
mmHg

Ao

Cor

0

Figure 37.7. Importance of continuous pressure monitoring during catheter entry into coronary ostium in a patient with unstable angina. Simultaneous pressure recordings from the arterial sheath (*Ao*) and diagnostic catheter are shown during catheter engagement of the left coronary artery (*Cor*). The presence of a critical stenosis of the left main ostium is signaled by the dampening and ventricularization of the pressure waveform on catheter tip entry into the ostium.

panied by marked ST segment depression at a low workload or a fall in blood pressure, is associated with a high incidence of left main coronary artery disease. Under these conditions, several steps should be taken routinely prior to left coronary angiography to maintain hemodynamic stability during the procedure. Selective coronary angiography should be undertaken before ventriculography, and low-osmolar contrast agents should be used. Volume loading with intravenous hydration is used to reduce the potential for hypotension, and a pacing catheter should be considered to prevent bradycardia during coronary angiography. Injections into the left coronary artery should be limited to the minimal number sufficient for diagnostic purposes. In all

cases, the initial angiographic projections should be those that best delineate the left main coronary artery without overlap or foreshortening: the shallow right anterior oblique view (0° to 15°), and the 30° to 45° left anterior oblique view with 30° to 40° of cranial angulation (Fig. 37.8) (see also Chapter 17). If a critical proximal stenosis is present, sufficient diagnostic information should be available for clinical decision-making with these views alone. Unless the severity of a given stenosis is in doubt, additional injections are extraneous and may cause otherwise avoidable complications. If a critical left main coronary artery stenosis is excluded, additional views can then be undertaken to best delineate the remaining coronary anatomy.

Coronary Angiographic Findings

When patients with unstable angina are considered regardless of subgroup, coronary angiography demonstrates a distribution of single, double, and triple vessel disease similar to that seen in patients with chronic stable angina (43). As in the case of chronic stable angina, the left anterior descending coronary artery is the most commonly affected vessel in unstable angina. The 15% incidence of significant left main coronary artery obstruction in patients with unstable angina is higher than that of patients with stable angina (42, 44, 45). Approximately 5 to 10% of patients thought to have unstable angina have normal coronary angiograms. Coronary spasm and microvascular dysfunction are possible causes of angina in many of these patients (43, 46).

As noted, unstable angina encompasses a heterogeneous population of patients with distinctive subgroups. The expected angiographic findings and extent of coronary disease vary depending on the patient's history and presentation. Patients with crescendo angina usually have severe left main or multivessel coronary artery disease. Crescendo angina refers to the development of either rest pain or an increase in the frequency or severity of exertional pain superimposed on previously stable chronic angina. More than one half of patients pre-

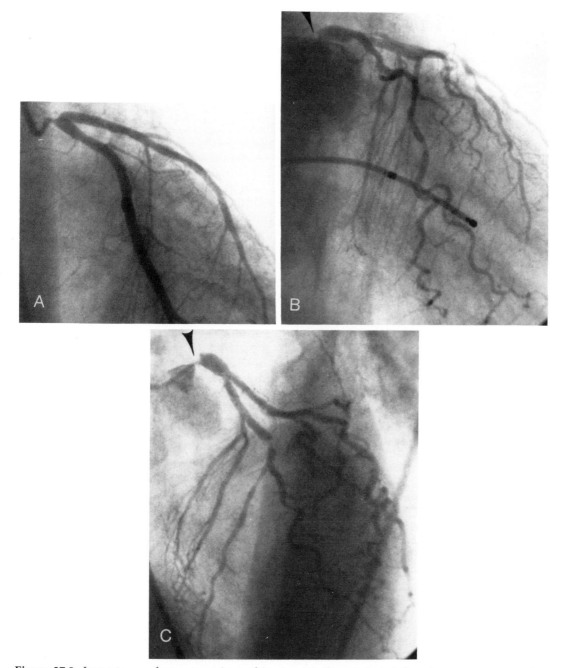

Figure 37.8. Importance of proper angiographic views to demonstrate left main coronary artery disease in unstable patients. **A.** The shallow right anterior oblique (RAO) projection shows severe ostial stenosis. **B.** The shallow RAO angiogram from another patient with critical left main artery disease; the proximal left coronary artery is not well seen because of the contrast in the aortic sinus and superimposed soft tissue densities. **C.** Same patient as in **B,** the shallow left anterior oblique (LAO) projection with cranial angulation demonstrates a severe stenosis of the left main coronary artery (*arrow*), as well as a proximal left anterior descending stenosis.

senting for angiographic evaluation with unstable angina have a crescendo pattern (47). Crescendo angina is associated with significant left main coronary artery disease in more than 20% of patients, and multivessel disease (without critical left main coronary artery obstruction) in more than 60%, whereas single-vessel disease is observed in only 10%. In contrast, single-vessel disease is present in approximately one half of all patients with unstable angina of less than 90 days duration (44). The incidence of significant left main coronary artery and triple-vessel disease is much lower in these patients with unstable angina of recent onset, as compared with those with crescendo angina (47). These observations have important clinical implications in terms of assessing patients as potential candidates for revascularization procedures. Patients with crescendo angina tend to have significant left main or multivessel coronary disease often requiring coronary artery bypass surgery. Patients with new onset angina frequently have single-vessel disease amenable to transcatheter intervention. An additional and important subgroup of patients present with the clinical syndrome of variant angina (i.e., angina occurring exclusively at rest and associated with transient ST segment elevation). Although normal or near normal coronary anatomy is a frequent finding in this population, severe fixed atherosclerotic stenoses are associated with coronary spasm in two thirds of patients with variant angina (43). Moreover, patients with variant angina associated with severe (> 70%) atherosclerotic stenoses have a worse prognosis than those without severe fixed lesions. Coronary angioplasty has been used successfully in those patients with variant angina and severe fixed atherosclerotic lesions (48) (Fig. 37.9). Coronary angiography, therefore, should be routinely performed to define the underlying anatomy and to determine appropriate therapy in patients presenting with this clinical syndrome (49, 50).

The pathogenesis of unstable angina has been the subject of several reviews (1, 51, 52). Evidence indicates that unstable rest angina is a dynamic process associated with abrupt reduction in coronary blood flow. Serial coronary angiographic studies have demonstrated that unstable angina is usually associated with recent worsening of coronary stenosis severity (Fig. 37.6) (50). Development of unstable angina appears invariably associated with an acute change in coronary anatomy caused by one or more of the following mechanisms: plaque rupture, coronary thrombosis, and coronary spasm (53) (Figs. 37.10–37.12). It is important to emphasize that more than one of the above mechanisms may contribute to the development of unstable angina in a given individual patient.

In patients with unstable angina, the morphology of coronary artery lesions has been qualitatively assessed by coronary angiography (Fig. 37.13) (54). The "angina-producing" lesion appears as an eccentric stenosis associated with a sharp overhanging edge or irregular borders in more than 70% of patients. This finding is observed in only 16% of patients with stable angina. These lesions have been characterized as complicated or complex eccentric type II lesions. Histopathologic studies indicate that these complicated stenoses are caused by ruptured atherosclerotic plaques and partially occlusive thrombi (55).

The specific role of thrombus formation in the development of unstable angina has recently been elucidated by biochemical, angiographic, and angioscopic observations. Biochemical studies have demonstrated evidence for enhanced platelet activation and fibrin formation (56–58) and for impaired fibrinolytic activity (59). Furthermore, increased thrombin activity has been identified as a marker of increased risk of early cardiac events (60). Coronary angiography detects intraluminal filling defects consistent with coronary artery thrombus in up to 57% of patients with unstable angina (57–62). The incidence of coronary thrombus during coronary angiography appears to be directly related to the time interval between the last anginal attack and the angiographic study. **Angiographically evident thrombi are particularly common in patients studied within hours of a rest angina** episode (61–66). In one study of 37 patients undergoing coronary angiography during ongoing anginal attacks, 21 (57%) had intracoronary thrombus present, 14 (38%) had fixed stenoses without evidence

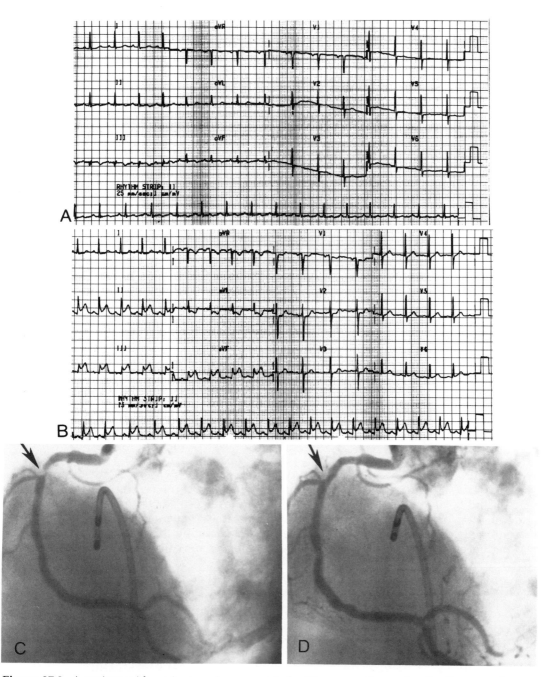

Figure 37.9. A patient with variant angina associated with severe atherosclerotic disease and treatment with percutaneous transluminal coronary angioplasty (PTCA). **A** and **B.** Serial electrocardiograms before and during rest angina. Note the transient ST elevation in inferior leads. **C.** Right coronary angiogram shows a complex lesion of the proximal right coronary artery persisting after nitroglycerin (*arrow*). **D.** Right coronary angiogram after PTCA with good result (*arrow*).

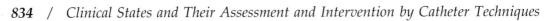

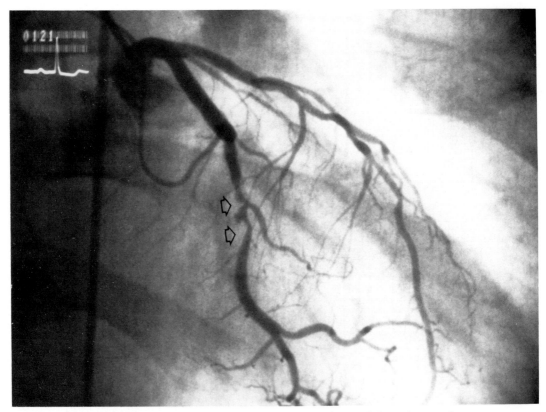

Figure 37.10. Angiographic features of plaque rupture, intraluminal thrombus, and coronary spasm, underlying unstable ischemic syndromes. Ulcerated plaque (*arrows*) in left circumflex coronary artery in a patient with unstable angina.

of thrombus, and 2 (5%) had coronary spasm (64). More recently observations made using flexible fiberoptic angioscopes indicate that coronary mural thrombus is present in nearly all patients with unstable rest angina, even when thrombi are not detected by angiography. Of seven patients with rest angina undergoing intraoperative angioscopy at the time of coronary bypass surgery, thrombus was seen angioscopically in all seven, whereas thrombus was apparent angiographically in only one patient (Fig. 37.14) (67). Similarly, **coronary thrombus was present in 14 of 15 (93%) patients undergoing percutaneous angioscopy within 48 hours of an unstable angina** episode; the thrombi seen in association with unstable angina typically have a grayish-white appearance, which differs from the reddish thrombi seen with acute myocardial infarction (68). Therefore, coro-

nary angioscopy is a more sensitive technique than coronary angiography in detecting intravascular thrombi in patients with unstable ischemic syndromes. Nevertheless, detecting thrombus by coronary angiography remains an important predictive factor associated with adverse clinical events (Fig. 37.15).

Treatment of Unstable Angina with Interventional Cardiac Catheterization

Coronary Angioplasty

Percutaneous transluminal coronary angioplasty is an increasingly important tool in the treatment of unstable angina pectoris (see Chapters 27 and 28). In one report, 44% of 360 consecutive patients hospitalized with unstable angina were candidates for percutaneous transluminal coronary angioplasty (PTCA) (69). Patients with symptoms refractory to maximal medical therapy should be referred for revascularization. PTCA would also be appropriate for patients initially stabilized on medical therapy who have severe stenosis of a proximal vessel, in light of the propensity of such lesions to progress to complete occlusion (70, 71). According to an early report from the original NHLBI registry, results of angioplasty in the treatment of single-vessel coronary artery disease were comparable when either stable or unstable

angina was present (72). Immediate angiographic success rates of PTCA were 63% in 214 patients with stable angina and 61% in 442 patients with unstable angina. In-hospital mortality rates were 0.5 and 0.9% for the two groups, respectively. After 18 months of follow-up in the unstable angina group, the incidence of mortality was 2.6%, and the incidence of myocardial infarction was 9.5%. Procedural success rates subsequently improved with the introduction of steerable guidewire catheter systems. Angioplasty success rates in 952 patients with unstable angina in the 1985–86 NHLBI PTCA registry improved to 84%, which was comparable to an 86% success rate in stable angina patients (73). However, major in-hospital complications occurred

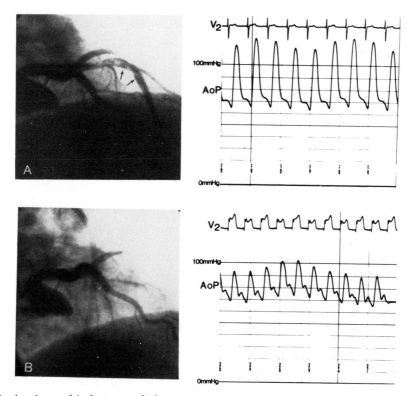

Figure 37.11. Angiographic features of plaque rupture, intraluminal thrombus, and coronary spasm, underlying unstable ischemic syndromes. **A.** Baseline coronary angiogram, electrocardiogram, and aortic pressure (*AoP*) recordings in a patient with unstable angina. Note a large thrombus is present within the proximal left anterior descending artery (*arrows*). **B.** Repeat angiogram and electrocardiogram during chest pain in the same patient, showing total acute occlusion of the left anterior descending coronary artery associated with marked ST segment elevation and hypotension.

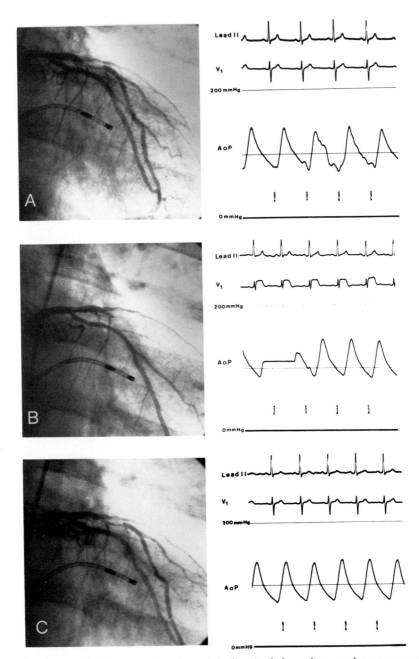

Figure 37.12. Angiographic features of rupture, intraluminal thrombus, and coronary spasm. **A–C.** Coronary spasm (elicited by ergonovine) superimposed on a severe atherosclerotic stenosis in a patient with rest angina. **A.** Control. **B.** Ergonovine. **C.** IC TNG. (Reprinted with permission from Goldberg S. Coronary artery spasm and thrombosis. Philadelphia: FA Davis, 1983.)

CONCENTRIC LESIONS

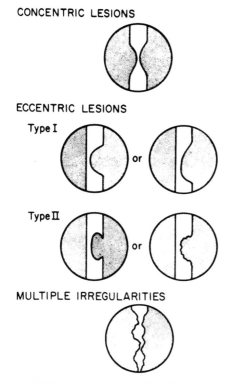

ECCENTRIC LESIONS

Type I

Type II

MULTIPLE IRREGULARITIES

Figure 37.13. Angiographic classification of lesion morphology. In patients with unstable angina, the ischemia-producing artery often has the appearance of an eccentric type II lesion with irregular borders or sharp overhanging edges. Similar findings have been noted in non–Q-wave infarction. (Reprinted with permission from Ambrose JA, Winters SL, Arora RR, et al. Angiographic evolution of coronary morphology in unstable angina. J Am Coll Cardiol 1986; 7:472–478.)

by a near normal exercise capacity and the absence of ischemia by thallium scintigraphy in 80% of patients. Table 37.3 summarizes the acute and long-term outcome of coronary angioplasty in unstable angina pectoris from several large series (72–77).

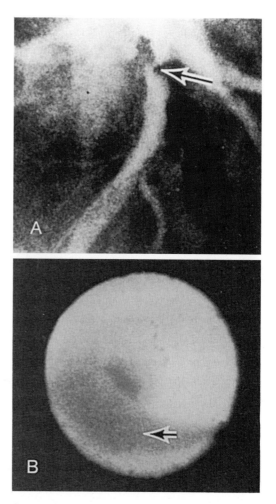

Figure 37.14. Coronary angiographic and angioscopic findings in a patient with unstable rest angina. **A.** Coronary angiography demonstrates a high-grade eccentric stenosis of the left anterior descending coronary artery (*arrow*). **B.** Angioscopy demonstrates a large crescent-shaped thrombus, which is not apparent angiographically. (Reprinted with permission from Sherman CT, Litvack F, Grundfest W, et al. Coronary angioscopy in patients with unstable angina pectoris. N Engl J Med 1986;315:913–919.)

more frequently in unstable angina patients (9.7 versus 6.0%). In another report, emergency PTCA was successful in 56 of 60 patients (93%) with unstable angina pectoris refractory to maximal medical therapy (74). Although no procedural deaths occurred, four patients had acute coronary occlusions (7%), resulting in acute myocardial infarction, despite emergency coronary artery bypass graft surgery. After a minimum follow-up of 6 months, one death occurred, and the restenosis rate was 28%. Improved functional status after sustained successful PTCA was demonstrated

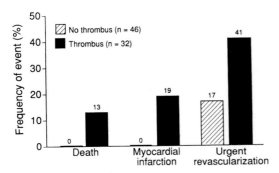

Figure 37.15. Prognostic significance of angiographic thrombus to adverse clinical outcomes in patients with unstable angina. (Reprinted with permission from Freeman MR, Williams AE, Chisholm RJ, et al. Intracoronary thrombus and complex morphology in unstable angina. Relation to timing of angiography and in-hospital cardiac events. Circulation 1989;80:17–23.)

Single-vessel PTCA of the angina-producing artery or "culprit lesion" may be suitable for selected patients with unstable angina and multivessel disease (Fig. 37.16) (79). This approach, however, is limited by the frequent recurrence of angina caused by incomplete revascularization (80, 81). Therefore, PTCA in patients with multivessel disease should ideally achieve revascularization comparable with coronary artery bypass graft surgery (81).

We have also found interventional cardiac catheterization techniques to be useful in the treatment of unstable ischemic syndromes following coronary bypass surgery (82). Myocardial ischemia occurring early after coronary bypass surgery is typically caused by graft thrombosis resulting from a mechanical graft problem, whereas late ischemic events are caused by progressive atherosclerotic lesions with or without plaque rupture (Fig. 37.17). Cardiac catheterization is essential to define the underlying anatomic substrate, which is often complex in the postoperative setting. A variety of interventional catheterization strategies may be useful, depending on the specific angiographic findings. In patients with acute graft thrombosis, reperfusion and amelioration of ischemia can be achieved with selective infusion of thrombolytic drugs into the involved graft. In patients with unstable angina caused by atherosclerotic disease in the bypass graft, transcatheter intervention can be an effective alternative to surgical revascularization. In other patients with bypass graft occlusions not amenable to PTCA, dilation can be undertaken within the diseased native coronary artery.

In general, the procedure in patients with unstable angina is similar to that of elective PTCA undertaken in patients with stable symptoms. However, because these vessels are more reactive in terms of developing coronary spasm and thrombosis, safeguards against these untoward events are especially warranted. **To reduce the po-**

Table 37.3.
Coronary Angioplasty for Unstable Angina

| References | No. | Success (%) | Major Complications (%) | | | Follow-up Events (%) | | | |
			Death	MI	CABG	Mo.	Death	MI	Recurrent Angina
NHLBI (1977–1981) (72)	442	61	0.9	—	—	18	3	9	—
NHLBI (1985–1986) (73)	952	84	1.3	3.3	4.4	24	5	10	42
Plokker (75)	469	88	1.0	4.9	3.0	60	6	—	212
deFeyter (76)	200	89	0.5	8.0	9.0	24	3	12	24
Myler (77)	807	84	0.2	3.6	5.1	37	5	5	30
TIMI IIIB (78)	278	97	0.5	4.3	1.4	—	—	—	—

MI, myocardial infarction; CABG, coronary artery bypass graft; NHLBI, National Heart, Lung, and Blood Institute; TIMI, Thrombolysis in Myocardial Infarction.

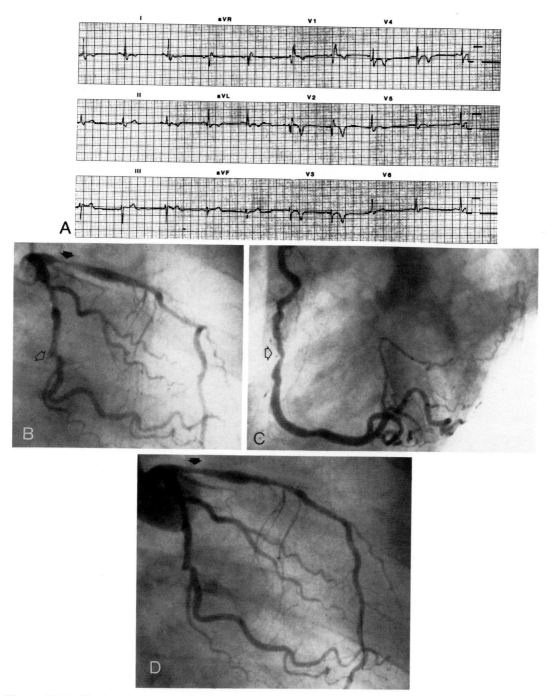

Figure 37.16. Single-vessel angioplasty of the "culprit lesion" in a patient with new onset unstable angina and multivessel disease. **A.** Electrocardiogram shows anterior lead ST wave changes, which implicate the left anterior descending artery as the culprit vessel. **B** and **C.** Left and right coronary angiograms, respectively, demonstrating multivessel involvement (*arrows*). **D.** PTCA (*arrow*) of the proximal left anterior descending coronary artery stenosis was performed with resolution of angina.

tential for coronary spasm during PTCA, patients are pretreated with high doses of calcium antagonists, and intracoronary nitroglycerin is administered immediately prior to dilation. To reduce the potential for thrombotic coronary occlusion during PTCA, all patients should be pretreated with aspirin (83, 84); and, this should be continued after the procedure for at least 6

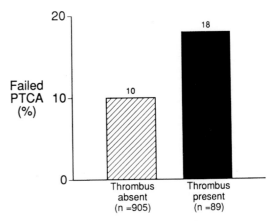

Figure 37.18. Procedural failure of coronary angioplasty as a function of angiographic thrombus. (Reprinted with permission from Savage MP, Goldberg S, Hirshfeld J, et al. Clinical and angiographic determinants of primary angioplasty success. J Am Coll Cardiol 1991;17: 22–28.)

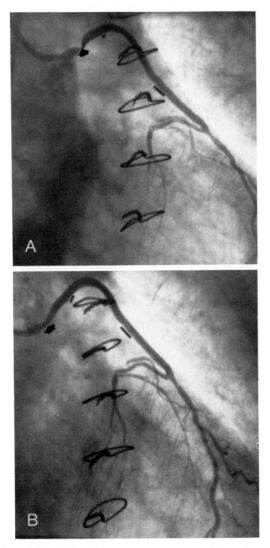

Figure 37.17. Vein graft angiograms in patient with unstable angina developing 8 years after coronary bypass surgery. **A.** Severe stenosis near aortic anastomosis (*arrow*). **B.** Results after percutaneous transluminal coronary angioplasty (PTCA) of stenosis (*arrow*).

months (85). **Platelet glycoprotein IIb/IIIa receptor blockade may provide additional benefit in this setting** (see Chapter 34). In the EPIC Trial, monoclonal antibody c7E3 Fab use resulted in a 35% relative reduction in ischemic complications in patients with either acute ischemic syndromes or high-risk lesions (86).

Selection of contrast agent may also be important to angioplasty outcome. Several investigators have reported a higher incidence of coronary thrombus formation during PTCA associated with nonionic contrast agents (87–89). Therefore, we favor use of the ionic low-osmolar agent, ioxaglate, in these high-risk patients. Patients with unstable angina are at increased risk of abrupt closure during PTCA because of the thrombogenic milieu of the culprit lesion and the high incidence of pre-existent thrombus. Intracoronary thrombus noted by either angiography or angioscopy has been identified as an important risk factor associated with PTCA failure and with acute coronary occlusion during dilation (Fig. 37.18) (90–96). Prolonged heparin infusion prior to PTCA in patients with unstable angina has been reported to improve the immediate outcome of PTCA (from 81 to 91%) and to reduce acute closure rates (from 8 to 1.5%)(97). Optimal duration of anticoagulant therapy and timing of PTCA are uncertain. The potential role of direct thrombin inhibitors as an alternative to heparin also is unclear (98, 99). Where clinical circumstances allow, deferring intervention for several days or even weeks may be prudent to allow thrombus resolution and healing of intimal fissures. A retrospective study of 807 unstable angina patients demonstrated a lower success rate and an increased complication rate of angioplasty when performed early (within 1–2 weeks) after symptom onset (77).

New Interventional Devices

Although the role of the new interventional devices in the treatment of unstable angina is in evolution, device-specific niches based on lesion morphology have emerged (100, 101). Excimer laser and rotational atherectomy can be useful in the treatment of ostial lesions and long stenoses (102–104). Because the culprit lesions responsible for unstable angina characteristically have eccentric type II morphologies, directional atherectomy may have particular applicability in this setting (Fig. 37.19). Directional atherectomy appears well suited to the treatment of these complex eccentric stenoses in large vessels (105). On the other hand, enthusiasm for directional atherectomy has been dampened by the completion of randomized trials that demonstrated an increased risk of complications, including myocardial infarction and distal embolization, compared with balloon angioplasty (106, 107). Preliminary results suggest a potential role for thrombectomy devices, such as the transluminal extraction and rheolytic thrombectomy catheters, in the treatment of clot laden lesions. Preliminary analysis of the TOPIT Trial suggested a reduction in major cardiac complications in patients with acute ischemic syndromes treated with transluminal extraction rather than balloon angioplasty (108).

Metallic intracoronary stents have been effective in improving suboptimal angioplasty results and in managing abrupt closure (109–111) (see Chapters 31–33). **Stents also have been used to treat complex lesions not amenable to conventional PTCA** (Fig. 37.20). The basic mechanism of action appears to be a scaffolding effect, which

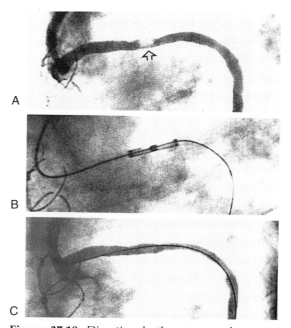

Figure 37.19. Directional atherectomy of coronary bypass graft stenosis in a patient with unstable angina. **A.** Baseline; note that the complex eccentric lesion morphology is not well-suited for conventional balloon dilation. **B.** Atherectomy. **C.** Postatherectomy.

tacks down intimal dissection flaps and resists elastic recoil. The role of stents for thrombotic lesions is uncertain because of the potential increased risk for stent thrombosis (112).

In contrast to other new devices, stent implantation confers a lower restenosis rate than conventional angioplasty (113–115). Restenosis reduction by stents has important implications for the treatment of patients with unstable ischemic syndromes, because unstable angina is associated with an increased risk of restenosis following balloon angioplasty (116). Although patients with unstable angina were excluded from the BENESTENT trial, unstable angina was present in approximately one half of patients enrolled in the STRESS Trial (114, 115). In both studies, stent placement was associated with a relative reduction in restenosis of approximately 30% compared with a strategy of angioplasty with stenting as a bail-out contingency.

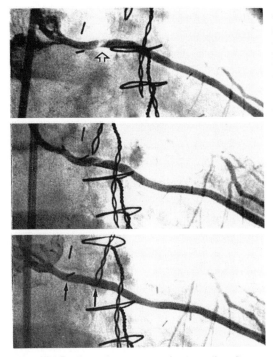

Figure 37.20. Use of coronary stenting for disrupted vein graft stenosis in a patient with medically refractory rest angina. **A.** Baseline. **B.** After balloon angioplasty, minimal improvement is seen. **C.** After stent placement (*arrows* indicate proximal and distal ends of the stent).

Thrombolytic Therapy

Because of the important role of thrombus formation in the pathophysiology of unstable angina, the utility of thrombolytic therapy in this syndrome has generated significant clinical investigation (117). Vetrovec et al. in 1982 (118) reported partial or complete resolution of thrombi in 10 of 13 ischemic-related vessels following infusion of intracoronary streptokinase (mean dose 187,000 IU). Another uncontrolled study (119) demonstrated improvement in coronary flow at 24 hours in 16 of 22 patients with total or subtotal coronary occlusion treated with either intracoronary streptokinase (210,000 IU over 45 minutes) or intravenous tissue plasminogen activator (100 mg over 3 hours). In contrast, Ambrose et al. found no significant change in quantitative coronary angiography after intracoronary streptokinase (mean dose 177,000 IU) in 36 consecutive patients with unstable angina or non–Q-wave infarction (120). The role of prophylactic intracoronary urokinase during angioplasty in patients with unstable angina was prospectively evaluated in the TAUSA trial (121). In this study, 464 patients with rest angina were randomized in double blind fashion to intracoronary urokinase (250,00 or 500,000 U) or to placebo given in divided doses during the procedure. Compared with the control group, patients receiving urokinase experienced significantly greater acute vessel closures (10.2 versus 4.3%) and in-hospital clinical events (12.9 versus 6.3%). The cause for the paradoxical, detrimental effect of urokinase is unknown, but possible mechanisms include intramural hemorrhage and procoagulant effects of the thrombolytic drug caused by platelet activation.

Intravenous thrombolytic therapy has been evaluated in several controlled trials. Although clinical improvement in unstable angina was demonstrated in one small study of intravenous tPA (122), larger trials have failed to show a clinically significant benefit from it (123–125). The UNASEM trial compared intravenous anistreplase (30 mg) with placebo in 159 patients with a clinical history of unstable angina associated with ischemic ECG changes (126). Repeat angiography after 12–28 hours demonstrated a significant mean stenosis reduction by 11% in the anistreplase group versus 3% in the placebo group. However, no difference in adverse cardiac events was found between the two groups. Bleeding complications were more common in patients receiving thrombolytic therapy (26 versus 9%). Another trial involving intravenous urokinase was terminated prematurely after interim analysis suggested more frequent clinical events after thrombolysis (127).

Addressing many of the design limitations of prior studies, the TIMI-3A trial evaluated the angiographic effects of intravenous tPA in 306 patients with acute rest angina or non–Q-wave myocardial infarction (128). Coronary angiography was performed 11 ± 6 hours from the episode of qualifying chest pain after which patients were randomized to either placebo or intravenous tPA (0.8 mg/kg given over 90 minutes). Pretreatment angiography demonstrated definite thrombi in 35% and possible thrombus in 40%. The primary end point, "measurable improvement" in the culprit lesion by repeat angiography at 24 hours ($\geq$ 10% reduction of stenosis, or an increase of two TIMI flow grades) was seen in 25% of tPA and 19% of placebo treated patients (P = ns). "Substantial improvement" ($\geq$ 20% reduction of stenosis) was seen with tPA in 15% of all culprit lesions versus 5% with placebo ($P < .0l$). Non–Q-wave infarction and definite angiographic thrombus were associated with greater benefit from thrombolytic therapy. Substantial improvement after tPA was observed in 33% of lesions associated with non–Q-wave myocardial infarction (versus 8% for placebo), in 36% of lesions with thrombus (versus 15% for placebo), and in 60% of recent total occlusions (versus 30% for placebo). Therefore, although intravenous tPA resulted in improvement in only a minority of lesions associated with these unstable ischemic syndromes, a modest benefit was suggested in specific patient subgroups.

TIMI IIIB Trial

The TIMI IIIB Trial sought to determine the efficacy of both thrombolytic therapy and routine interventional therapy (early catheterization followed by revascularization) in patients with acute ischemic syndromes (129). The trial enrolled 1473 patients within 24 hours of ischemic pain at rest, considered to represent unstable angina or non–Q-wave myocardial infarction. Using a 2 × 2 factorial study design, patients were randomized to (*a*) tPA or placebo and (*b*) an invasive strategy (early catheterization and revascularization) or a conservative strategy (catheterization and revascularization only for recurrent ischemia). All patients were treated with bedrest, anti-ischemic medications, aspirin, and heparin.

The primary outcome for the thrombolysis comparison (death, myocardial infarction, or failure of initial therapy at 6 weeks) occurred in 54.2% of tPA treated patients and 55.5% of placebo treated patients (P = ns). However, myocardial infarction occurred more frequently in the tPA group

(7.4 versus 4.9%, $P = .04$). In addition, four patients developed intracranial hemorrhage after tPA, whereas none occurred after placebo. The primary outcome for the comparison of interventional strategies (death, myocardial infarction, or unsatisfactory stress test at 6 weeks) occurred in 18.1% of patients assigned to a conservative strategy and 16.2% of patients assigned to the invasive strategy (P = ns). However, use of the invasive strategy conferred advantages of a shorter hospitalization, a lower incidence of rehospitalization, and reduced need for antianginal medications.

One year follow-up of patients in this trial has also been reported (Fig. 37.21) (130). In the entire study population of patients with unstable angina or non–Q-wave myocardial infarction, 1-year event rates were relatively low for mortality (4.3%) and nonfatal myocardial infarction (8.8%). The incidence of death or nonfatal infarction for the tPA and placebo groups were similar (12.4 versus 10.6%). The incidence of death or myocardial infarction was also similar for the invasive and conservative strategies (10.8 versus 12.2%). However, after 1 year, use of a myocardial revascularization procedure was frequent in both groups regardless of the initial intention-to-treat strategy: 64% in the invasive strategy group and 58% in the conservative strategy group.

Thus, the TIMI IIIB study suggests that both invasive and conservative approaches are appropriate options for patients with acute ischemic syndromes. The incidence of death and myocardial infarction is comparable for the two strategies. The invasive strategy provides slight advantages in terms of shorter hospital stay and fewer repeat hospitalizations. When an initial conservative approach is taken, most patients ultimately require revascularization because of medical therapy failure. **The addition of an intravenous thrombolytic agent is not beneficial and may be harmful.**

ACUTE MYOCARDIAL INFARCTION

General Considerations

The concept that coronary artery thrombi are involved in the pathogenesis of acute

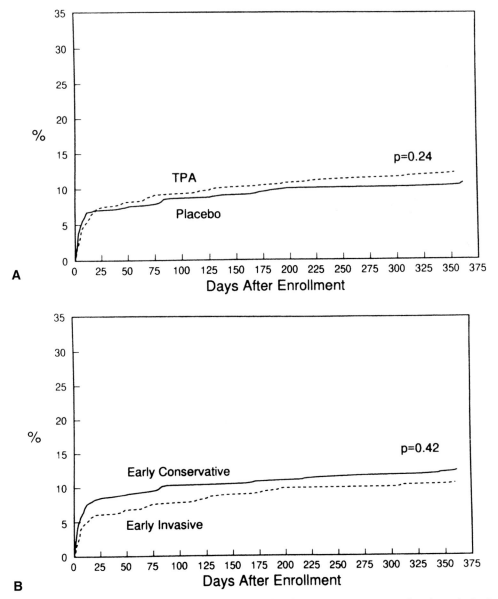

Figure 37.21. Cumulative rates of death or myocardial infarction at 1 year in the thrombolysis in myocardial infarction (TIMI) IIIb trial. **A.** Comparison of tissue plasimogen activator (*TPA*) and placebo. **B.** Comparison of early invasive and early conservative strategies. (Reprinted with permission from Anderson HV, Cannon CP, Stone PH, et al. One-year results of the thrombolysis in myocardial infarction (TIMI) IIIb clinical trial. A randomized comparison of tissue-type plasminogen activator versus placebo and early invasive versus early conservative strategies in unstable angina and non-Q wave myocardial infarction. J Am Coll Cardiol 1995;26:1643–1650.)

myocardial infarction was first suggested by Herrick in 1912 (131). In subsequent decades, the cause of acute myocardial infarction was widely debated until 1980, when DeWood et al. demonstrated conclusively

by early coronary angiography that patients with evolving transmural myocardial infarction had total occlusion of the infarct-related artery caused by coronary thrombus (132) (Fig. 37.22). Acute myocardial infarc-

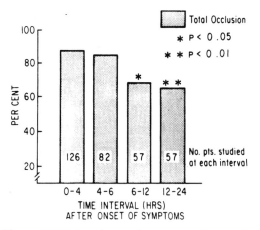

Figure 37.22. Incidence of coronary artery occlusion during the early hours of acute myocardial infarction. (Reprinted with permission from DeWood MA, Spores J, Notske R, et al. Prevalence of total coronary occlusion during the early hours of transmural myocardial infarction. N Engl J Med 1980;303:897–902.)

tion was associated with total occlusion of the infarction-related artery in nearly 90% of patients who underwent coronary angiography within 6 hours of symptom onset. Coronary thrombi were retrieved in 52 of 59 patients who underwent emergency coronary artery bypass graft surgery. In contrast, in patients catheterized more than 12 hours after symptom onset, the incidence of complete coronary artery occlusion decreased to 65%, presumably because of spontaneous clot lysis by the patient's intrinsic fibrinolytic system. Myocardial necrosis is a dynamic process that begins within 20 minutes after occlusion of an epicardial coronary artery and is generally completed by 6 hours after interruption of coronary flow in the experimental setting. Therefore, effective reperfusion treatment of acute myocardial infarction should begin as early as possible.

In 1981, Rentrop et al. reported that intracoronary streptokinase given during evolving transmural infarction was associated with reperfusion of the infarct-related artery in 75% of treated patients (133). Subsequently, the efficacy of intracoronary streptokinase in recanalizing acutely occluded coronary arteries was reported to be between 62 and 85% (134–142). Reperfusion rate was increased in patients with persistent ischemic discomfort and in subgroups of patients who were treated relatively early after symptom onset (142, 143). Reperfusion was usually re-established within 30 minutes of intracoronary drug infusion, with greater efficacy reported by some authors who used subselective techniques (135).

Because the goal of re-establishing antegrade coronary flow during acute myocardial infarction is to salvage myocardium in the region supplied by the affected coronary artery, end points for measuring the efficacy of coronary thrombolysis include changes in left ventricular function, as well as mortality. Assessment of left ventricular function after intracoronary thrombolysis showed only modest improvement (136) or no significant benefit (137–139). These findings were probably because of relatively late drug administration because of logistic constraints involved with intracoronary administration of thrombolytic agents. Effects of intracoronary streptokinase on mortality were reported in the Western Washington Randomized trial (137, 144). When intracoronary streptokinase was administered within 12 hours of symptom onset, the 30-day mortality rate was reduced from 11.2% in patients treated with placebo to 3.7% in patients treated with intracoronary streptokinase. Although this difference in mortality was no longer statistically significant at 1 year, the treated patients had a 44% lower mortality rate when compared with the placebo group. Those whose reperfusion was successful had significant reduction in mortality, as compared with those whose reperfusion was not successful, when the infarction was located in the anterior region.

Because of the delays inherent in transporting patients to the catheterization laboratory to administer intracoronary thrombolysis, the effects of intravenous lytic agents were examined in patients with acute myocardial infarction. This therapy could be started earlier in the course of the infarction. If intravenous treatment proved effective in achieving coronary reperfusion, the overall effects on myocardial salvage and mortality might be expected to be superior to intracoronary drug delivery. The results of various randomized trials with intravenous streptokinase use showed re-

Table 37.4.
Survival Benefit of Intravenous Streptokinase in Acute Myocardial Infarction as a Function of Time From Onset

Hours from Onset	Mortality (%)		Relative Risk	
	Control	Streptokinase	(95% CI)	P
< 1	15.4	8.2	0.49 (0.34–0.69)	0.0001
< 3	12.0	9.2	0.74 (0.63–0.87)	0.0005
> 3–6	14.1	11.7	0.80 (0.66–0.98)	0.03
> 6–9	14.1	12.6	0.87 (0.64–1.19)	NS
> 9–12	13.6	15.8	1.19 (0.75–1.89)	NS

Adapted from the T-3A Investigators. Early effects of tissue plasminogen activator, added to conventional therapy, on the culprit coronary lesion in patients presenting with ischemic cardiac pain at rest. Circulation 1993;87:38–52. CI, confidence interval; NS, not significant.

perfusion rates that were substantially lower than those achieved with intracoronary streptokinase. Early recanalization varied between 31 and 55% (145, 146). Most trials that reported higher reperfusion rates lacked pretreatment angiography and, therefore, included patients with initial subtotal occlusion of the infarction-related artery. Despite the lower rate of acute coronary reperfusion with intravenous streptokinase, an improvement in left ventricular function has been demonstrated when therapy is initiated early (147, 148). An improvement in mortality was also conclusively demonstrated in large randomized trials. The GISSI study (149), which included 11,712 patients randomized to either placebo or intravenous streptokinase (1.5 million units over 1 hour), demonstrated an 18% reduction in in-hospital mortality in the treated group. Of note, the salutary effect of intravenous streptokinase on mortality was more pronounced in patients treated early after symptom onset (Table 37.4). This benefit persisted at 1 year follow-up. A similar benefit was shown by ISIS-2, a randomized trial involving 17,187 patients with suspected acute myocardial infarction (150). In this study, the added benefit of low-dose aspirin (162 mg) given immediately alone or in conjunction with thrombo-

lytic treatment was demonstrated (Fig. 37.23).

Although beneficial, early clot lysis by intravenous thrombolytic agents remained limited by relatively low reperfusion rates reported with intravenous streptokinase. To increase coronary recanalization rates, investigators began using more potent lytic agents, the most notable being recombinant tissue plasminogen activator (rtPA). The results of studies on this fibrin-specific, short half-life thrombolytic agent demonstrated substantially higher early coronary reperfusion rates, as compared with those of intravenous streptokinase. When coronary patency on the 90-minute angiogram was used as the end point, successful reperfusion was present in 62 to 75% of patients treated with intravenous rtPA (145, 146, 151, 152). When "front loaded" 90-minute infusions were used, acute reperfusion rates exceeded 80% (153, 154). Left ventricular function and survival both improved with rtPA therapy (155, 156). However, it remained unclear whether the apparent advantage of intravenous rtPA over streptokinase in terms of acute reperfusion rates translated into lower patient mortality. In the GISSI-2 trial of 12,490 patients treated within 6 hours from symptom onset, no significant difference between rtPA and streptokinase was

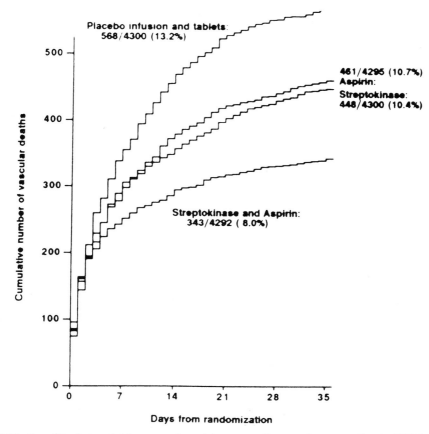

Figure 37.23. Benefit of streptokinase and aspirin on cardiovascular mortality in ISIS-2 (Reprinted with permission from ISIS-2 (Second International Study of Infarct Survival) Collaborative Group. Randomized trial of intravenous streptokinase, oral aspirin, or both or neither among 17,187 cases of suspected acute myocardial infarction. Lancet 1988;2:545–549.)

observed in hospital mortality (157, 158). In the ISIS-3 study, 41,299 patients within 24 hours of the onset of suspected acute myocardial infarction were randomized to treatment with streptokinase, rtPA, or anistreplase; half of all patients were then randomly assigned to subcutaneous heparin (12,500 IU twice daily for 1 week) plus aspirin and half to aspirin alone (159). No significant differences in mortality were seen among the three thrombolytic agents, irrespective of subcutaneous heparin use.

In contrast to these results were the findings of the GUSTO trial, a randomized open-label study involving 41,121 patients enrolled within 6 hours of symptoms onset (160). Mortality at 1 month was significantly lower after a front-loaded regimen of rtPA plus intravenous heparin than after streptokinase (6.3 versus 7.3%, $P = .001$). The survival advantage with rtPA persisted after 1-year follow-up (161). Left ventricular function correlated with the coronary patency rate at 90 minutes into treatment; ventricular function was best in the rtPA treated group and in patients with normal perfusion in the infarct artery, irrespective of treatment (162). Mortality at 30 days was lowest (4.4%) among patients with normal coronary flow and highest (8.9%) among patients with no flow. Patency at 90 minutes was seen in 81% of the rtPA treated group versus 54 to 60% in the streptokinase treated groups; however, at 180 minutes no differences were seen in patency among the treatment groups. These findings are consistent with the concept that the beneficial effects of improved survival and myocardial performance associated with rtPA are because of its ability to achieve more rapid and complete reperfusion of the infarct-related artery.

An important problem that remained following successful coronary thrombolysis was the presence of a high-grade residual coronary stenosis in the infarct-related artery (163). Significant residual coronary stenosis in the infarct-related artery would limit improvement in myocardial function (164). In addition, severe residual stenosis was associated with a significant rate of reocclusion and reinfarction (151, 165–168). This prompted investigators to study the effects of PTCA on the infarct-related artery. Coronary angioplasty could be used either as primary treatment for totally occluded infarct-related arteries (169–172) or in conjunction with thrombolytic agents (149, 152, 167, 169, 173–175). If used in the latter situation, PTCA could be performed immediately after or during thrombolysis, or the procedure could be performed in a delayed elective manner (151, 152). Thus, the optimal timing of PTCA remained an important concern. This issue was addressed in the Thrombolysis and Angioplasty in Myocardial Infarction trial (TAMI), which compared the efficacy of immediate versus delayed elective PTCA after coronary thrombolysis with intravenous rtPA (151). When rtPA was administered approximately 3 hours after symptom onset to 386 patients with acute evolving myocardial infarction, the patency of the infarction-related artery was demonstrated in 288 patients (75%) at 90 minutes. Of these patients, 197 were randomized to either immediate angioplasty or delayed elective PTCA at 7 to 10 days. The 91 patients who could not be randomized were excluded because of predefined angiographic criteria including multivessel and left main coronary artery disease. Of the 197 randomized patients, 99 patients were assigned to immediate angioplasty and 98 patients to delayed angioplasty. The rates of reocclusion were similar in both groups (11 versus 13%), and neither group exhibited a significant improvement in global left ventricular function. A modest improvement in regional wall motion was similar for both treatment groups. However, the rate of emergency coronary angioplasty, because of recurrent ischemia or infarction, was significantly higher for the patients assigned to the delayed PTCA strategy. The crossover rate for emergency PTCA was 16% for the delayed elective angioplasty group, whereas only 5% of the patients assigned to immediate PTCA required repeat emergency angioplasty. Of particular note was substantial interim reduction in stenosis severity prior to intervention in 14% of patients assigned to the elective delayed PTCA strategy; this was most likely because of continued clot lysis, and it obviated the need for angioplasty in this important subgroup of patients. Together, these findings suggest that one suitable treatment strategy for patients with evolving myocardial infarction might be early administration of an intravenous thrombolytic, with delayed elective PTCA if needed. These patients would require close observation for signs of recurrent ischemia with the option for emergent invasive revascularization if necessary.

When PTCA was used as the primary treatment modality without thrombolysis, marked improvement in luminal diameter was accompanied by significant improvement in left ventricular ejection fraction (170). In a randomized trial of PTCA compared directly with intracoronary streptokinase infusion, the rates of coronary recanalization were similar in both treatment groups, as were the times to achieve reperfusion. However, in patients treated with primary PTCA, the residual coronary stenosis was significantly less (43 ± 31%) than in the group treated with intracoronary streptokinase (83 ± 17%). Preservation of ventricular function was superior in the PTCA-treated patients. Serial left ventriculograms revealed that both the change in ejection fraction and regional wall motion at 7 to 10 days showed significantly greater improvement in the group treated with primary PTCA.

The relative efficacy of angioplasty and intravenous thrombolytic therapy has been compared in several prospective, randomized trials (176–180). In these trials, patients with evolving myocardial infarction either underwent emergent angioplasty or received intravenous thrombolytic drugs (rtPA or streptokinase) within 12 to 24 hours of the onset of chest pain. These stud-

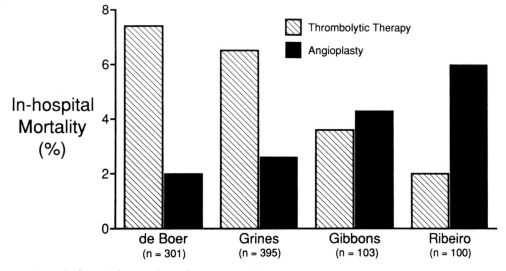

Figure 37.24. In-hospital mortality of patients with acute myocardial infarction in four randomized trials comparing thrombolytic therapy and balloon angioplasty.

ies consistently showed that angioplasty was effective in restoring patency of the infarct-related artery in more than 90% of patients, a rate superior to that achieved by the thrombolytic agents. Patients assigned to angioplasty were less likely to have reocclusion of the infarct-related artery and had a lower incidence of recurrent ischemia and reinfarction. In addition, strokes were less frequent with PTCA than with thrombolytic therapy. Mortality in the four randomized trials are shown in Figure 37.24. Although no statistically significant differences in mortality were demonstrated in any individual trial, a meta-analysis of these trials suggested a significant survival benefit from PTCA with a 44% relative reduction in mortality during hospitalization (181).

Controversy over the relative merits of primary angioplasty and thrombolytic therapy in the treatment of acute myocardial infarction continues to inspire debate (182, 183). Important criticisms of the randomized trials have emphasized the differences in the thrombolytic protocols used. None of the studies used the accelerated or "front-loaded" regimen of rtPA, which had been demonstrated by the GUSTO trial to be a superior mode of thrombolytic therapy. In addition, the benefits of PTCA observed in the relatively small randomized trials could not be replicated in a larger community-

based setting. In the Myocardial Infarction Triage and Intervention (MITI) Project registry, 3145 patients underwent either primary PTCA or received thrombolytic treatment within 6 hours of the onset of acute myocardial infarction (184). In-hospital mortality was similar for patients treated by angioplasty (5.5%) or thrombolysis (5.6%). At 4-year follow-up, mortality remained comparable in both groups. In addition, no significant difference in mortality of high-risk subgroups was observed between the two treatments. The findings of the MITI study supports the view that both options represent acceptable reperfusion therapies that are associated with low mortality rates in patients with acute myocardial infarction.

The relative efficacy of primary PTCA and front-loaded rtPA was prospectively evaluated in a substudy of the GUSTO II trial, the preliminary results of which have been just recently reported (The GUSTO IIb Angioplasty Substudy Investigators, N Engl J Med 1997;336:1621–1628). In this substudy, 1138 thrombolytic eligible patients were randomized within 12 hours of the onset of acute myocardial infarction. At 30 days, PTCA and rtPA were associated with comparable rates of death (5.7 versus 7.0%, $P = 0.37$), reinfarction (4.5 versus 6.5%, $P = 0.13$), and disabling stroke (0.2 versus

0.9%, $P = 0.11$). A composite outcome of death, reinfarction, or stroke was observed in 9.6% of patients in the PTCA group and 13.7% of patients in the rtPA group ($P = 0.033$). However, very recent data indicate that this benefit is lost at 6 months.

Modes of Clinical Presentation

The invasive cardiologist may be asked to evaluate and treat patients who fall into several distinct clinical settings:

1. In the acute phase of evolving myocardial infarction;
2. In a stable state during the first week after the patient has received thrombolytic therapy;
3. During recurrent myocardial ischemia after thrombolytic treatment has already been administered.

Patients Presenting in the First 12 Hours of Acute Myocardial Infarction

A rapid and complete assessment should be made of the hemodynamic status of patients presenting in the first 12 hours after myocardial infarction. Critical historical elements include the patient's age, time from onset of symptoms to presentation, and presence of continued ischemic discomfort. The patient should be screened for specific contraindications to thrombolytic treatment (Table 37.5). In addition, we ascertain whether there is a prior history suggesting coronary artery disease, duration of any prior anginal symptoms, and whether prior

Table 37.5.
Contraindications to Thrombolytic Therapy

History of coagulopathy or bleeding diathesis
Active peptic ulcer disease or internal bleeding
Prior cerebrovascular accident
Intracranial neoplasm or AV malformation
Severe uncontrolled hypertension
Recent surgery, invasive procedure, or trauma
Prolonged cardiopulmonary resuscitation
Left atrial or left ventricular thrombus
Pregnancy
Diabetic hemorrhagic retinopathy

coronary bypass surgery or angioplasty has been performed. On physical examination, blood pressure, heart rate, and status of the neck veins and lungs are quickly assessed, as is the heart for presence of any murmurs, gallops, or rubs. Of particular importance are the peripheral pulses if urgent invasive procedures are contemplated.

The electrocardiogram is scrutinized for rhythm disturbances, repolarization abnormalities, and status of the QRS complex. In addition to ST segment elevation, a common finding that may be present is the acute growth in R wave amplitude in the same leads that demonstrate ST segment elevation. The time course for R wave loss and the development of pathologic Q waves may be variable, and we do not consider the presence of Q waves per se as a contraindication for acute intervention. An additional important finding is the presence of persistent ST segment depression in the precordial leads, which is accompanied by chest pain of longer than 30 minutes. Because most acute myocardial infarction interventional trials have required the presence of ST segment elevation, the distribution of the infarction-related arteries has been divided approximately equally between the left anterior descending and the right coronary arteries, which together account for 85 to 90% of cases. Recent evidence indicates that persistent ST depression in the precordial leads may also be a marker of acute posterior infarction caused by circumflex coronary artery occlusion (16,185). Therefore, patients with ongoing ischemia accompanied by this electrocardiographic finding may represent another important subgroup who may benefit from acute intervention.

The decision to attempt reperfusion by urgent catheterization is made on the basis of a combination of clinical factors, including duration of symptoms, persistent discomfort accompanied by continued injury current, and hemodynamic status of the patient. If the decision it made to attempt coronary reperfusion, the choice must be made quickly among several treatment options:

1. The patient may be taken directly to the catheterization suite for diagnostic study and possible urgent revascularization.
2. Intravenous thrombolytic agents may be administered, and the patient taken for urgent

catheterization to precisely define left ventricular function and coronary anatomy. Decisions regarding the method and timing of PTCA or coronary artery bypass graft surgery are made on the basis of the catheterization findings.

3. Intravenous thrombolytic agents can be administered, followed by a "period of observation" watching for clinical signs of reperfusion.
4. Intravenous thrombolytic agents may be administered; the patient can then be admitted to the coronary care unit, and a decision regarding catheterization can be made electively based on the patient's clinical course.

We favor option 1 when catheterization facilities are immediately available or when specific contraindications to thrombolytic treatment exist. The decision whether to perform revascularization by PTCA or coronary artery bypass graft surgery is made on the basis of specific angiographic criteria. It should be pointed out that emergency PTCA in acute myocardial infarction may have certain advantages in properly equipped tertiary care facilities. For example, in a study performed by Rothbaum et al. (171), 151 patients with evolving acute myocardial infarction (including 18 patients in cardiogenic shock) underwent emergency coronary angioplasty as primary treatment. The population included 18 patients with cardiogenic shock (12%). PTCA was successful in 132 (87%) patients, and the mean residual stenosis severity was 29%. The in-hospital mortality rate for the entire group was 9%, with 7 of 13 deaths occurring in patients presenting with cardiogenic shock or intractable ventricular tachyarrhythmias. The hospital mortality rate was 5% in patients with successful angioplasty versus 37% in those who had unsuccessful attempts. A potential advantage of primary PTCA over systemic thrombolysis is a lower incidence of bleeding complications. In addition, primary PTCA may be associated with a lower incidence of intramyocardial hemorrhage compared with that associated with thrombolytic therapy (186).

Emergent cardiac catheterization, to define the coronary anatomy and to guide reperfusion strategy, may also be appropriate for patients with ongoing pain and with

suggested acute myocardial infarction but who do not have ST segment elevation on the electrocardiogram. Such patients comprise approximately one third of all patients with acute myocardial infarction. We favor anatomy-specific therapy directed by the catheterization findings in these patients, because intravenous thrombolysis has not proved effective in this subgroup (149, 150). When catheterized shortly after symptom onset, most patients with acute myocardial infarction but without ST segment elevation have nonoccluded infarct-related arteries (187). Approximately 40% of patients have occluded infarct-related arteries, typically associated with either nondominant left circumflex involvement or an occluded vessel with collateral flow.

Option 2 has been a common strategy of many hospitals with interventional programs. The reasons for this are several-fold. The information gained from urgent diagnostic catheterization is crucial to identify patients with persistent occlusion of the infarction-related artery. Because up to 20 to 30% of patients receiving rtPA and a greater percentage of those receiving streptokinase do not reperfuse acutely, a substantial number of patients have persistent occlusion of the infarction-related artery, who could possibly benefit from salvage or "rescue" angioplasty (Fig. 37.25). Although rescue angioplasty is associated with higher reocclusion rates and less functional recovery of ventricular function than reperfusion achieved by successful thrombolysis, patients with successful rescue angioplasty have favorably low acute and long-term mortality rates (188) (Fig. 37.26). Acute coronary angiography offers the additional advantage of identifying high-risk patients who would be candidates for urgent coronary artery bypass graft surgery. Another factor favoring immediate angiography is that current noninvasive methods are relatively insensitive to assess reperfusion following thrombolytic therapy (189, 190). As has been pointed out by others, chest pain and ST segment changes accurately predict vessel patency in only 25% of patients and vessel occlusion in only 44% of patients (170).

Despite the potential advantages of urgent catheterization, several prospective studies have failed to demonstrate an overall

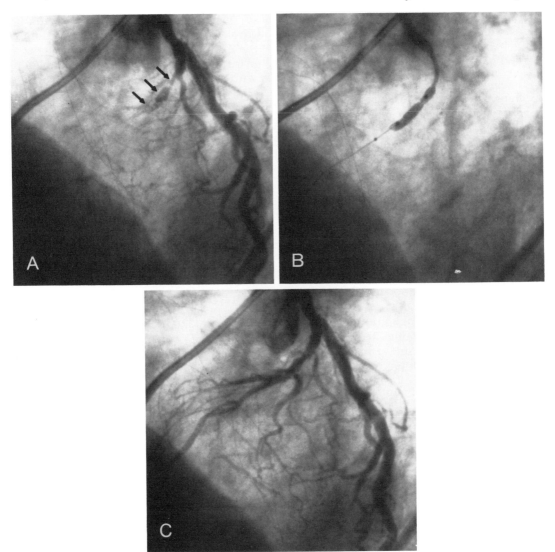

Figure 37.25. Rescue angioplasty following failed thrombolysis in a patient with acute anterior myocardial infarction. **A.** Persistent occlusion of the left anterior descending coronary artery is present (*arrows*) despite a 90-minute infusion of intravenous rtPA. **B.** Balloon inflation in the totally occluded segment. **C.** Restoration of the left anterior descending artery patency following angioplasty.

clinical benefit for the routine use of immediate coronary angiography and angioplasty following intravenous rtPA (Table 37.6). The Thrombolysis in Myocardial Infarction (TIMI) IIA study evaluated whether immediate cardiac catheterization with adjunctive PTCA confers an advantage over the same procedures performed electively 18 to 48 hours after admission (191). All patients were treated with intravenous rtPA within 4 hours of the onset of acute myocardial infarc-

tion. Of 195 patients randomized to the immediate intervention group, PTCA was attempted in 141 patients and was successful in 84%. Of 194 patients randomized to the delayed catheterization group, PTCA was attempted in 107 patients and was successful in 93%. No differences were found between the immediate and delayed intervention groups in predischarge ejection fraction (50.3 versus 49.0%), reinfarction (6.7 versus 4.1%), or early mortality (7.2 versus 5.7%).

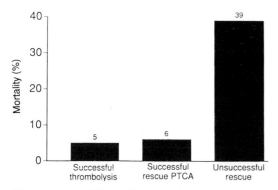

Figure 37.26. Effect of successful rescue angioplasty on in-hospital mortality following intravenous thrombolytic therapy. (Reprinted with permission from Abbottsmith CW, Topol EJ, George BS, et al. Fate of patients with acute myocardial infarction with patency of the infarct-related vessel achieved with successful thrombolysis versus rescue angioplasty. J Am Coll Cardiol 1990;16: 770–778.)

Immediate catheterization was associated with an increased frequency of bleeding requiring transfusion (20.0 versus 7.2%) and coronary artery bypass surgery (16.4 versus 7.7%). A different study design was used by the TAMI investigators (151). In this trial, all patients were emergently catheterized after rtPA infusion; patients with patent infarct artery with residual high-grade stenosis were then randomized to immediate or delayed PTCA. Immediate PTCA conferred no benefit to left ventricular function, coronary reocclusion, or mortality. On the other hand, an increased need for emergency bypass surgery was seen in patients undergoing immediate rather than delayed angioplasty (7 versus 2%, respectively). Thus, acute PTCA for infarct arteries successfully reperfused after thrombolysis cannot be recommended. The European Cooperative Study Group also failed to demonstrate any clinical benefit of immediate PTCA following intravenous rtPA administration (192). In this randomized trial of 367 patients with acute myocardial infarction treated with rtPA, 14-day mortality was higher in the group treated with immediate PTCA (7%) than in the group treated with a conservative strategy (3%).

Based on the results of these studies, **emergency coronary angiography and angioplasty following intravenous thrombolytic therapy appear unwarranted as a rou-**

Table 37.6.
Randomized Trials of Immediate Coronary Angioplasty Versus Delayed Intervention Following Intravenous rtPA

	TAMI		TIMI IIA		ECSG	
	Immediate PTCA	Delayed PTCA	Immediate Delayed	Delayed PTCA	Immediate PTCA	Delayed Catheterization
Patient #	99	98	195	194	183	184
Time of intervention	90 min	7–10 days	120 min	18–48 h	60 min	10–22 days
Patients having PTCA (%)	100%	52%	70%	55%	68%	6%
PTCA success	85%	94%	84%	94%	61%	—
Ejection fraction predischarge	0.53	0.56	0.50	0.49	0.51	0.51
Mortality	4%	1%	7%	6%	7%	3%
Reocclusion	11%	13%	—	—	13%	11%
Emergency CABG	7%	2%	4%	2%	2%	< 1%
Blood transfusion	21%	14%	11%	3%	10%	4%

TAMI, Thrombolysis and Angioplasty in Myocardial Infarction; TIMI, Thrombolysis in Myocardial Infarction; ECSG, European Cooperative Study Group; PTCA, percutaneous transluminal coronary angioplasty; CABG, coronary artery bypass graft.

tine measure and may be associated with a higher rate of complications. On the other hand, emergency interventional catheterization might be beneficial for certain patients (e.g., patients with extensive anterior infarction or cardiogenic shock), and the role of invasive therapies in the management of these high-risk subgroups requires further systematic evaluation. Patients with hemodynamic compromise and ongoing evidence of ischemia despite thrombolytic therapy may benefit from option 2, because it presents many important advantages in managing these critically ill patients: assessment of right heart hemodynamics, adjunctive support with intraaortic balloon counterpulsation, and identification of those with persistent occlusion caused by failed thrombolysis.

The potential role of rescue angioplasty for failed thrombolysis was evaluated in the TAMI-5 study (193). In this trial, 575 patients with acute myocardial infarction of less than 6 hours were randomly assigned, in a 3 × 2 factorial design, to treatment with one of three thrombolytic drug regimens and to one of two catheterization strategies, immediate catheterization with angioplasty for failed thrombolysis or deferred catheterization at 5–10 days. With the aggressive catheterization strategy, acute patency was achieved in 96% of infarction-related arteries. The predischarge patency rate was excellent in both groups: 94% in the aggressive group versus 90% in the conservative group. Although no difference was seen between the two treatment strategies in predischarge ejection fraction (54% in both), a significant 20% improvement in regional wall motion within the infarct region was observed in the group treated with rescue angioplasty. Although in-hospital death and reinfarction were low in both groups, the aggressive treatment group had a significantly less complicated clinical course because of a lower incidence of recurrent ischemia (35 versus 25%). More recent trials have yielded mixed results to the role of rescue angioplasty. In the TIMI I trials, rescue PTCA appeared to offer no significant benefit to patients with thrombolytic failure (194). These results contrast with those of a prospective trial of 151 patients with acute anterior myocardial infarction and persistent occlusion of the left anterior descending artery who were randomly assigned to rescue PTCA or conservative management (195). At 30 days, death or severe heart failure occurred in 6.4% of patients treated with rescue angioplasty compared with 16.6% of patients treated conservatively.

Option 3 seems somewhat problematic in that the various clinical markers of reperfusion (relief of chest pain, rapid devolution of ST segments, reperfusion arrhythmias) are too insensitive to accurately predict the status of the infarction-related artery (189, 190).

Option 4 is most applicable for the community hospital setting when no immediate access to a catheterization facility is available. Thus, intravenous thrombolytic agents can be rapidly administered, and the patient can be evaluated in an elective fashion for diagnostic catheterization and revascularization as necessary. Option 4 is also an acceptable strategy in centers with catheterization laboratories if the patient has no contraindication to thrombolytic therapy and if the hemodynamic status appears stable. When a conservative "wait-and-see" strategy is selected post-thrombolysis, one should anticipate a 15 to 25% rate of intercurrent ischemic events necessitating urgent revascularization (151, 196).

The role of routine cardiac catheterization and elective angioplasty in the clinically stable patient who has received intravenous thrombolytic therapy remains controversial (197–200). Consensus guidelines for invasive evaluation of patients with myocardial infarction, published by the ACC/AHA task force, are presented in Table 37.7 (201). General agreement is found that myocardial revascularization is indicated for patients with objective evidence of ischemia on the predischarge low-level stress test. In the absence of postinfarction angina or a positive predischarge stress test, the results of the TIMI II-B and SWIFT trials indicate that cardiac catheterization and coronary angioplasty may not be necessary as a routine strategy (see Table 37.8) (202, 203). In the TIMI II-B study, 3262 patients treated with rtPA within 4 hours of onset of acute myocardial infarction were randomly assigned to an **invasive** strategy (coronary angiography after 18 to 48 hours

Table 37.7.
ACC/AHA Guidelines for Invasive Evaluation of Patients with Acute Myocardial Infarction[a]

Coronary Angiography and Possible PTCA
Class I
1. Patients with spontaneous episodes of myocardial ischemia or episodes of myocardial ischemia provoked by minimal exertion during recovery from infarction.
2. Before definitive therapy of a mechanical complication of infarction such as acute mitral regurgitation, VSD, pseudoaneurysm, or LV aneurysm.
3. Patients with persistent hemodynamic instability.

Class IIa
1. When MI is suspected to have occurred by a mechanism other than thrombotic occlusion at an atherosclerotic plaque. This would include coronary embolism, certain metabolic or hematologic diseases, or coronary artery spasm.
2. Survivors of acute MI with depressed LV systolic function (LV ejection fraction $\leq$ 40%), congestive heart failure, prior revascularization, or malignant ventricular arrhythmias.
3. Survivors of acute MI who had clinical heart failure during the acute episode, but subsequently demonstrated well-preserved LV function.

Class IIb
1. Coronary angiography performed in all patients after infarction to find persistently occluded infarct-related arteries in an attempt to revascularize the artery or to identify patients with three-vessel disease.
2. All patients after a non–Q-wave MI.
3. Recurrent VT or VF, or both, despite antiarrhythmic therapy in patients without evidence of ongoing myocardial ischemia.

Class III
1. Routine use of coronary angiography and subsequent PTCA of the infarct-related artery within days after receiving thrombolytic therapy.
2. Survivors of MI who are thought not to be candidates for coronary revascularization.

Routine Coronary Angiography and PTCA after successful thrombolytic therapy
Class I
None
Class II
None
Class III
1. Routine PTCA of the stenotic infarct-related artery immediately after thrombolytic therapy.
2. Percutaneous transluminal coronary angioplasty of the stenotic infarct-related artery within 48 hours of receiving a thrombolytic agent in asymptomatic patients without evidence of ischemia.

Reprinted with permission from Ryan TJ, Anderson JL, Antman EM, et al. ACC/AHA Guidelines for the management of patients with acute myocardial infarction: executive summary. Circulation 1996;94:2341–2350.
[a] Explanation of Classes
   Class I: Conditions for which there is evidence for and/or general agreement that a given procedure or treatment is beneficial, useful, and effective.
   Class II: Conditions for which there is conflicting evidence and/or a divergence of opinion about the usefulness or efficacy of a procedure or treatment.
   Class IIa: Weight of evidence or opinion is in favor of usefulness or efficacy.
   Class IIb: Usefulness or efficacy is less well established by evidence or opinion.
   Class III: Conditions for which there is evidence and/or general agreement that a procedure or treatment is not useful or effective and in some cases may be harmful.

followed by prophylactic PTCA of infarct arteries for stenoses (60% but < 100%) or to a **conservative** strategy (angiography and PTCA performed only for spontaneous or exercise-induced ischemia). In the group assigned to the invasive strategy, PTCA was attempted in 54% with complete success in 85% and partial success in 8%. Death or re-infarction within 6 weeks (the primary end point) occurred in 10.9% of the invasive group and in 9.7% of the conservative group (P = ns). At 1 year follow-up, similar results were noted with death or reinfarction in 14.7% of the invasive strategy group and 15.2% in the conservative strategy group (204). It should be noted that cardiac cathe-

Table 37.8.
Comparison of Two Randomized Trials of Delayed, Elective Angioplasty Versus Conservative Management Following Thrombolysis

	TIMI IIB		SWIFT	
	Invasive	Conservative	Invasive	Conservative
Thrombolytic agent	rtPA	rtPA	APSAC	APSAC
Follow-up	6 wk	6 wk	1 yr	1 yr
Patients (No.)	1636	1626	397	463
Angiography (%)	93%	33%	95%	13%
PTCA (%)	57%	16%	43%	3%
PTCA success rate	93%	92%	87%	—
Late ejection fraction	0.51	0.50	0.51	0.52
Mortality	5%	5%	6%	5%
Reinfarction	6%	6%	15%	13%

TIMI, Thrombolysis in Myocardial Infarction; SWIFT, Should We Intervene Following Thrombolysis? APSAC, anisoylated plasminogen streptokinase activator complex.

terization and myocardial revascularization was undertaken in 45% and 36%, respectively, in the group assigned to conservative therapy. In addition, subgroup analysis indicated a survival benefit for those patients with prior myocardial infarction when treated by the interventional approach. One-year mortality in patients with prior myocardial infarction was 17% in the conservative group versus 10% in the invasive group ($P = .03$). Therefore, the TIMI II-B results demonstrate that successful thrombolysis does not invariably dictate a need for additional myocardial revascularization procedures. Rather, a more judicious use of mechanical interventions would be to reserve invasive therapies for patients with recurrent ischemia and for high-risk patients with previous myocardial infarction.

Specific Approach to the Patient

After the diagnosis of acute myocardial infarction has been established, intravenous thrombolytics should be rapidly determined in the emergency department and administered according to recommended dosage schedules. Alternatively, thrombolytic therapy can be deferred and primary angioplasty performed if access to the cardiac catheterization suite is readily available. In patients with major contraindications to thrombolytic therapy, emergency

cardiac catheterization and coronary angioplasty are undertaken, particularly with ongoing symptoms early in the course (< 12 hours) of the acute infarction. Cardiogenic shock represents another important indication for urgent interventional catheterization (see below). Cardiac catheterization immediately after intravenous thrombolytic administration remains controversial. A minority of patients have resolution of chest pain and ST segment elevation shortly after thrombolytic administration. Because the overwhelming majority of these patients will have reperfused (190), a conservative wait-and-see approach is warranted in this patient subset. On the other hand, we perform urgent angiography in patients with persistent evidence of ischemia if evidence of a large risk area is found by electrocardiogram (e.g., extensive anterior infarcts) and provided that the time course is relatively early. The principal aim of catheterization is to provide a rapid "look-see" of the acute coronary anatomy to identify patients with persistent occlusion of the infarct artery who might benefit from rescue PTCA.

After arriving at the cardiac catheterization suite, a 6 F sheath is placed in the patient's femoral vein. A 5 or 6 F sheath is placed in the femoral artery in patients who have received prior intravenous thrombolysis, whereas a 7 or 8 F long sheath is placed when primary PTCA is planned. A pacing catheter may be placed in the right atrium or ventricle, and the patient is maintained on systemic heparin. Arterial pressure is constantly monitored through the sidearm of the arterial sheath. A pigtail catheter is then placed in the left ventricle, taking care to avoid ventricular irritability, which is more pronounced in this setting. Baseline hemodynamic data are recorded. Contrast left ventriculography is performed using low osmolar contrast agents to avoid hemodynamic compromise. We perform ventriculography with injection rates of 12 to 14 mL/second for total volumes of 36 to 42 mL. We usually perform selective cineangiography by visualizing the suspected noninfarction-related vessel first. This approach has the advantage of documenting the presence or absence of collateral flow to the infarction-related artery. We then perform an angiogram of the infarction-related vessel, obtaining paired orthogonal views that best demonstrate the anatomy and the perfusion status of the infarction-related artery.

Angiographic Findings

If a patient is taken directly to the catheterization suite in the first 6 hours of acute myocardial infarction without prior administration of thrombolytic agents, the infarction-related artery will demonstrate total occlusion in approximately 90% of cases. Although coronary spasm may be associated with coronary occlusion in some individuals, intracoronary administration of nitroglycerin only occasionally restores antegrade flow. The electrocardiogram is carefully monitored for changes in the level of ST segment elevation and arrhythmias (we routinely monitor two electrocardiogram leads, one reflecting the infarction zone and the other the contralateral myocardial zone). Both a decrease in the ST segment and an abrupt increase in ST segment elevation have been described in conjunction with reperfusion (173). Dysrhythmias that occur include accelerated idioventricular rhythm (Fig. 37.27), ventricular tachycardia and fibrillation, sinus bradycardia, and asystole. Moreover, hypotension during reperfusion of the inferoposterior left ventricular wall (Bezold-Jarisch reflex) may occur (205). At the time of these events we immediately repeat the coronary angiogram to assess the perfusion status of the infarction-related artery.

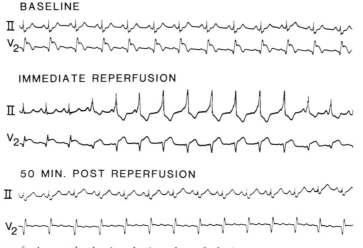

Figure 37.27. Reperfusion arrhythmias during thrombolytic treatment in a patient with evolving myocardial infarction. **Top.** Baseline electrocardiogram tracing showing ST elevation in lead V$_2$. **Middle.** The electrocardiogram following 7 minutes of streptokinase infusion showing accelerated idioventricular rhythm. **Lower.** The electrocardiogram 50 minutes after successful thrombolysis, showing resolution of the ST elevation and arrhythmia. (Reprinted with permission from Goldberg S, Greenspon AJ, Urban PL, et al. Reperfusion arrhythmia: a marker of restoration of antegrade flow during intracoronary thrombolysis for acute myocardial infarction. Am Heart J 1983;105:26–32.)

Table 37.9.
**Definitions of Perfusion Status Used
in the TIMI Trial**

Grade	Definition
0: No perfusion	There is no antegrade flow beyond the point of occlusion.
1: Penetration without perfusion	Contrast material passes beyond area of obstruction, but "hangs up" and fails to opacify, entire coronary bed distal to obstruction for duration of cineangiographic filming sequence.
2: Partial perfusion	Contrast material passes across obstruction and opacified coronary bed distal to obstruction or its rate of clearance from distal bed (or both) are perceptibly slower than its entry into or clearance from comparable areas not perfused by previously occluded vessel (e.g., the opposite coronary artery or coronary bed proximal to obstruction).
3. Complete perfusion	Antegrade flow into bed distal to obstruction occurs as promptly as antegrade flow into bed proximal to obstruction, and clearance of contrast material from the involved bed is as rapid as clearance from an uninvolved bed in same vessel or opposite artery.

Perfusion status of the infarction-related artery is classified according to the TIMI criteria shown in Table 37.9. If TIMI grade 0 or 2 perfusion is present, the cardiologist should consider performing salvage PTCA to acutely restore normal antegrade flow. In patients with occluded infarction-related arteries and severe three-vessel or left main coronary artery disease, a strong case can be made for urgent coronary artery bypass graft surgery. If single-vessel or double-ves-

sel disease is present with lesions deemed suitable for PTCA, urgent PTCA of the infarct-related artery may be undertaken. If TIMI grade 3 perfusion is demonstrated in the infarct-related artery in conjunction with a stenosis greater than 70% and coexistent left main coronary artery or severe triple-vessel disease, we recommend bypass grafting. Usually this procedure can be delayed until the next day. Infarct arteries shown to be patent with TIMI 3 flow in patients with single or double-vessel disease are generally best left untouched in the acute phase. The conservative approach has the advantage of allowing for continued clot lysis as occurs in 10 to 15% of patients. Furthermore, acute PTCA is associated with greater vessel reactivity and a resultant increased need for emergency coronary artery bypass graft surgery. As noted, mortality rates tend to be increased in patients subject to acute PTCA following successful thrombolysis. In patients with early reperfusion, PTCA can be generally reserved for those patients with recurrent anginal symptoms or with evidence of myocardial ischemia by stress testing.

PTCA Procedure

If the patient is a candidate for PTCA, the diagnostic catheter is exchanged for a suitable guide catheter. Heparin is administered to maintain an activated clotting time greater than 300 seconds. As suggested in an EPIC trial substudy of 64 patients with acute myocardial infarction, platelet glycoprotein IIb/IIIa receptor blockade may improve longer term outcomes in this setting (206). A flexible guidewire is carefully passed through the occlusion. At this point, it is not usual for the reperfusion arrhythmias described above to occur, especially in patients with grade 0 to 1 perfusion prior to PTCA. The patient is stabilized and the operator proceeds with the dilation. At this point, a vigorous guide catheter contrast injection is performed in an attempt to outline the course of the distal vessel. The balloon is then carefully placed in the occlusion or stenosis. We perform the first inflation generally for 1 to 2 minutes, slowly increasing the pressure in the balloon until it is 1 to 2 atm above the popping pressure of the stenosis. After balloon deflation, the electrocardiogram and hemodynamics are reassessed, and a test injection is performed. After substantial improvement in flow is noted, a half exchange is then performed (i.e., the balloon dilation catheter is removed from the guide catheter while a 300 cm exchange guidewire is left in place in the distal infarct-related artery). Guide catheter injection is then repeated, which usually results in excellent visualization of the infarct-related artery. If a satisfactory angiographic result is obtained, we observe the vessel for 15 to 30 minutes, specifically watching for signs of abrupt reclosure. If this occurs, we recross the stenosis and perform more prolonged inflations to enhance plaque molding and "tack down" intimal disruptions. Coronary stenting may also be effective both in primary therapy and in patients with suboptimal results from balloon angioplasty (see Chapter 33).

Patients Presenting in a Stable State After Administration of Thrombolytic Agents

With the increasingly widespread use of intravenous thrombolytic agents, a greater percentage of patients are receiving them in the community setting. Subsequent transfer will often then be undertaken so that diagnostic catheterization can be performed. Most such patients will demonstrate pathologic Q waves, along with enzymatic evidence of myocardial necrosis. In review of the clinical history, information regarding chest pain, resolution of ST segment changes, and reperfusion arrhythmias in the post-thrombolysis phase should be ascertained. In addition, we attempt to identify whether serial serum creatine kinase values reflect an early peak and washout (i.e., less than 16 hours after onset of symptoms) suggesting reperfusion.

The catheterization findings in these patients will most often show an akinetic or hypokinetic region of myocardium supplied by the infarction-related artery. The infarction-related artery may be totally occluded, or more likely it will be patent with a high-grade residual stenosis. Patients with left main and triple-vessel coronary artery disease should be referred for coronary artery bypass graft surgery.

We generally perform PTCA on candidates with suitable angiographic anatomy and residual myocardium in jeopardy, realizing that it is often difficult to quantify the amount of salvageable myocardium supplied by the infarct-related artery. At the time of PTCA, we note whether recurrent ischemia and ST segment change occur with balloon dilation. These findings may contribute important markers of myocardial salvage, although direct evidence for this hypothesis is currently lacking. On the other hand, elective PTCA is not recommended as a routine strategy in stable patients with negative stress test findings after thrombolysis (201). In one small randomized trial, patients with residual stenoses after thrombolytic therapy, but without postinfarction angina or ischemia on stress testing, were randomized to PTCA or medical therapy. PTCA conferred no benefit on acute or late clinical outcomes (207).

Role of Late Opening of Infarct-Related Coronary Arteries

Several lines of evidence support the concept that restoring antegrade flow in the infarct-related artery, days or even weeks after the acute infarction, may confer significant survival benefit. A retrospective investigation conducted on 132 men catheterized 4–5 weeks after myocardial infarction and followed for 4 years showed that having a spontaneously patent infarction-related artery was associated with 0 deaths in 44 patients; of the 88 men with occluded infarction-related arteries, 21 deaths (18%) ($P < .001$) occurred (208). It should be noted that these two groups were comparable in terms of age, left ventricular ejection fraction, and extent of coronary artery disease. Further studies suggest that this possible survival benefit may be secondary to a reduced incidence of lethal ventricular arrhythmias, because late potentials were noted less frequently in patients with open infarction-related arteries (209). Furthermore, a preliminary study has demonstrated that PTCA of occluded infarct-related arteries obliterates these late potentials (210). Late reperfusion has also been shown to result in improved ventricular remodeling and reduced infarct expansion (211–212). Therefore, the benefit of opening infarct-related arteries in the days or weeks following an acute myocardial infarction warrants further study in prospective randomized trials.

Patients Presenting with Recurrent Infarction

Patients recently treated with thrombolytic agents who do not undergo cardiac catheterization constitute a group at risk for reocclusion and reinfarction (213). The rate of coronary reocclusion after administration of thrombolytic agents varies from 10 to 40% (151, 166–168, 196), with most reocclusions occurring in the first 48 hours after treatment. Emergency PTCA (either with or without repeat infusion of rtPA) is generally performed in such patients. Once reinfarction has occurred, the prospect for myocardial salvage diminishes significantly and clinical complications become more likely. For this reason, patients receiving thrombolytic therapy in the community hospital setting should be considered for transfer within 24 to 48 hours to a center with capability of providing timely diagnostic and therapeutic cardiac catheterization (214).

Patients with Cardiogenic Shock

Cardiogenic shock can develop if 40% or more of the left ventricular mass is infarcted (215). The **hospital mortality rate of patients with acute myocardial infarction complicated by shock has remained a dismal 80 to 90%** despite modern coronary care units and availability of intraaortic balloon counterpulsation (216–220). The results of thrombolytic therapy alone have been dis-

appointing in this setting. The GISSI trial enrolled 280 Killip class IV patients; no reduction in mortality was seen in the group treated with intravenous streptokinase. The Society of Cardiac Angiography registry reported 45 patients with cardiogenic shock who received intracoronary streptokinse within 4 hours of infarct onset (221). Compared with patients without shock, successful reperfusion of the infarct vessel was significantly lower (43%) and the mortality rate was higher (67%). However, the mortality rate of shock patients who had successful reperfusion was 42%, in contrast to 84% of shock patients without reperfusion.

Although the results of randomized trials are not yet available, data from numerous series indicate that the optimal treatment strategy for patients with cardiogenic shock includes urgent catheterization with myocardial revascularization when anatomically suitable. Adjunctive use of intraaortic balloon counterpulsation is generally useful in maintaining hemodynamic support during these procedures, and a potential role has also been suggested for other circulatory assist devices such as percutaneous cardiopulmonary bypass (222).

Early intervention appears crucial, however, the window of opportunity for beneficial reperfusion may extend beyond the 6 to 12-hour clinical envelope normally applied for myocardial salvage in patients without shock. The progressive nature of cardiogenic shock reflects an inexorable downhill cycle of myocardial injury with deterioration of cardiac function leading to further ischemia and perpetual ongoing myocardial damage (223). Revascularization, when performed within 16–24 hours from the onset of shock, appears to improve the prognosis of these patients. DeWood et al. reported a mortality rate of only 25% when urgent coronary bypass surgery and counterpulsation was performed within 16 hours from the onset of acute infarction complicated by shock; in contrast, mortality exceeded 70% when surgery was undertaken after 18 hours (224). Improved outcomes have been similarly reported with emergent coronary angioplasty (225–229). Successful reperfusion with PTCA can be achieved in 54 to 73% of patients. Although these procedural success rates are lower than those

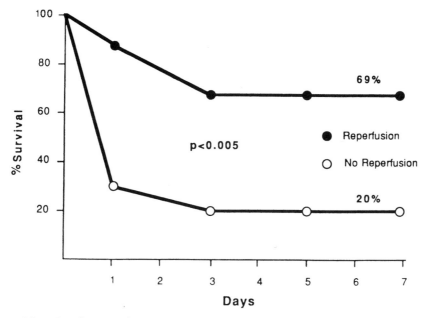

Figure 37.28. Mortality from cardiogenic shock in patients with and without successful reperfusion by coronary angioplasty. (Reprinted with permission from Lee L, Bates ER, Pitt B, et al. Percutaneous transluminal coronary angioplasty improves survival in acute myocardial infarction complicated by cardiogenic shock. Circulation 1988;78:1345–1351.)

seen in patients without shock, mortality appears to be significantly reduced in patients with successful reperfusion (23 to 39%) compared with patients without reperfusion (71 to 93%) (Fig. 37.28).

POSTINFARCTION ANGINA AND NON–Q-WAVE INFARCTION

General Considerations

Angina occurring within the first few days or weeks after myocardial infarction is a disturbing symptom and is common even in patients without prior thrombolytic treatment (230). **Early postinfarction angina often heralds recurrent infarction** and has been associated with a relatively grim prognosis. In one series of 70 consecutive patients with postinfarction angina, a 56% mortality rate was observed after a follow-up period of only 6 months (231). Patients with electrocardiographic evidence of ischemia at a distance from the initial infarct zone were at particularly high risk with a 6-month mortality rate of 72%, as compared

with a 33% mortality in patients with recurrent ischemia within the infarct zone. Patients with early postinfarction angina, therefore, warrant an aggressive management approach with cardiac catheterization to identify potential candidates for transluminal or surgical revascularization.

Patients with subendocardial or non–Q-wave infarction are especially likely to experience recurrent ischemia early on (230, 232). Reinfarction occurred in 43% of 58 patients with non–Q-wave infarction carefully studied by Marmor et al. (230). The high rate of reinfarction in these patients appears to reflect the unique coronary pathoanatomy of non–Q-wave myocardial infarction (233). In contrast to acute Q-wave myocardial infarction, which is associated with occluded infarct vessels, coronary angiography performed within 6 hours of the onset of acute non–Q-wave myocardial infarction usually demonstrates a patent infarct-related artery associated with a complex, high-grade stenosis (Fig. 37.29). In patients presenting with ST segment elevation treated with thrombolytic therapy, non–Q-wave infarction is similarly associated with a higher patency of the infarct-related artery

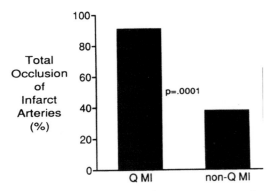

Figure 37.29. Frequency of total coronary occlusion during the first 6 hours of non–Q-wave myocardial infarction compared with Q-wave myocardial infarction. Total occlusion of the infarct-related artery was present in only 39% of patients with acute non–Q-wave infarction versus 91% of patients with acute Q-wave infarction (233). (Reprinted with permission from Keen WD, Savage MP, Fischman DL, et al. Comparison of coronary angiographic findings during the first six hours of non-Q wave and Q wave myocardial infarction. Am J Cardiol 1994;74:324–328.)

and an increased rate of reinfarction (234). Non–Q-wave myocardial infarction is considered a class II indication for cardiac catheterization by the ACC/AHA task force (201). Given the high risk associated with this patient subset, we generally advocate early interventional catheterization on a preemptive basis prior to recurrent angina and infarction. This approach is supported by a small trial of patients with anterior non–Q-wave myocardial infarction. Patients treated by an invasive approach including revascularization had lower mortality and reinfarction rates than patients managed conservatively (235). Other investigators alternatively recommend stress testing to determine the need for invasive studies in these patients (236). This controversy is being addressed in a large randomized controlled trial (VANQWISH) comparing a routine invasive strategy with a conservative noninvasive strategy, and a recent report suggests no benefit and a tendency for harm with the invasive strategy.

Catheterization Laboratory

Coronary angiography in patients with early postinfarction angina caused by is-chemia within the infarction zone typically reveals a high grade but not totally occluded culprit lesion in the infarction-related artery (237). Total occlusion of the infarction vessel is a less common finding and, when present, usually is associated with collateral flow that allows for preserved myocardial viability within the infarct region. Because of the relatively high incidence of single-vessel disease in this setting, recurrent ischemia in the infarction zone can frequently be managed with PTCA. DeFeyter et al. reported a success rate of 89% in 53 patients with postinfarction angina treated by angioplasty (238). However, PTCA was complicated by an 11% rate of myocardial infarction or emergency bypass surgery. We have also reported the effective use of PTCA on the infarction-related artery in 54 patients with ischemia in the zone of prior infarction (237). PTCA was successful in 94% (33/35) of critical stenoses and in 58% (11/19) of total occlusions. Two patients (4%) required emergency surgery, but no new infarctions or deaths occurred. After approximately 1 year of follow-up, only one reinfarction and no deaths occurred. Thus, PTCA was associated with an excellent long-term outcome in this group of unstable patients. Other investigators have reported similar results (239, 240).

In patients with postinfarction angina caused by ischemia at a distance, coronary angiography invariably reveals multivessel disease. Typically, the infarction-related artery is totally occluded whereas one or more contralateral vessels demonstrate a critical stenosis jeopardizing noninfarcted regions of myocardium. Early postinfarction ischemia at a distance from the infarction zone has been attributed to interruption of collateral flow from the occluded infarction-related artery to the territory of another diseased vessel (231). Unstable angina with ischemia at a distance may also develop after a clinically stable interval of several months or years following the initial infarction, because of interim disease progression. PTCA of vessels contralateral to the infarcted region will be undertaken at potentially increased risk to the patient. With a prior infarction, abrupt closure of a contralateral vessel may result in severe left ventricular dysfunction and hemodynamic decompensation (241). Accordingly, patients with postinfarction ischemia at a distance are often treated with coronary bypass surgery. However, our experience has demonstrated that with careful case selection, coronary angioplasty offers an effective therapeutic option for many of these patients (242). Selection criteria for use of PTCA in this high-risk population have been reviewed in detail elsewhere (243). These considerations include the likelihood of primary successful angioplasty based on lesion morphology, expected outcome with alternative therapies, total area of myocardium potentially at risk, and capability of protecting ischemic myocardium potentially at risk (e.g., with intraaortic balloon counterpulsation). The status of the collateral circulation is also an important consideration. If a stenosed contralateral vessel supplies collateral flow to the infarct-related vessel, initial dilation of the infarct-related artery may be performed first to provide reciprocal collaterals during subsequent angioplasty of the contralateral vessel. Widespread application of PTCA in patients with left ventricular dysfunction has been restrained by the potential for unresolved vessel closure and by a limited ability to protect the acutely ischemic myocardium. With the advent of coronary stenting, the clinical outcomes after abrupt closure have improved (244–246). Future technical innovations with the capability of better protecting the ischemic myocardium will further expand the use of interventional catheter techniques in high-risk patients with these acute coronary syndromes (247). For example, cardiopulmonary bypass support provides hemodynamic stability during PTCA in selected patients with advanced left ventricular dysfunction (248, 249), although short-term ischemic complications remain significant in such patients because of the risk of periprocedural reocclusion (250).

SUMMARY

The role of the cardiac catheterization laboratory has radically evolved as we near the new millennium. Less than two decades ago, acute coronary insufficiency and acute myocardial infarction were considered major contraindications to cardiac angiography. Today, cardiac catheterization holds a preeminent place in patient management, by elucidating the pathophysiology of these acute syndromes and by the continuing development of life-saving transcatheter therapies. Future therapeutic innovations, especially those targeted at the unstable plaque and coronary thrombus, will benefit even more patients with unstable ischemic syndromes.

Acknowledgment

We thank Dorothy Lennox and Denise Gidaro for their secretarial assistance in preparing this chapter.

References

1. Gorlin R, Fuster V, Ambrose JA. Anatomic-physiologic links between acute coronary syndromes. Circulation 1986;74:6–9.
2. Scanlon PH. The intermediate coronary syndrome. Prog Cardiovasc Dis 1981;23:351–364.
3. Wood P. Acute and subacute coronary insufficiency. BMJ 1961;1:1779–1782.
4. Conti CR, Brawley RK, Griffith LSC, et al. Unstable angina pectoris: morbidity and mortality in 57 consecutive patients evaluated angiographically. Am J Cardiol 1973;32:745–750.
5. Braunwald E. Unstable angina: a classification. Circulation 1989;80:410–414.
6. Bertolasi CA, Tronge JE, Riccitelli MA, et al. Natural history of unstable angina with medical or surgical therapy. Chest 1976;70:596–605.
7. Rizik D, Healy S, Margulis A, et al. A new clinical classification for hospital prognosis of unstable angina pectoris. Am J Cardiol 1995;75:993–997.
8. Sharma GV, Deupree RH, Luchi RJ, et al. Identification of unstable angina patients who have favorable outcome with medical or surgical therapy (eight-year follow-up of the Veterans Administration Cooperative Study). Am J Cardiol 1994;74(5):454–458.
9. Gazes PC, Mobley ME, Faris HM, et al. Preinfarctional (unstable) angina—a prospective study—ten year follow-up. Circulation 1973;48:331–337.
10. vanMiltenburg-van Zijl AJM, Simoons ML, Veerhoek RJ, et al. Incidence and follow-up of Braunwald subgroups in unstable angina pectoris. J Am Coll Cardiol 1995;25:1286–1292.
11. Calvin JE, Klein LW, VanderBerg BJ, et al. Risk stratification in unstable angina. JAMA 1995;273:136–141.
12. Russell RO, Moraski RE, Kouchoukos N, et al. Un-

stable angina pectoris: national cooperative study group to compare surgical and medical therapy. Am J Cardiol 1978;42:839–848.

13. Plotnick GD, Conti CR. Transient ST segment elevation in unstable angina: prognostic significance. Am J Med 1979;67:800–803.

14. Sclarovsky S, Rechavia E, Strasberg B, et al. Unstable angina: ST segment depression with positive versus negative T wave deflections. Clinical course, ECG evolution, and angiographic correlation. Am Heart J 1988;116:933–941.

15. Papapietro SE, Niess GS, Paine TD, et al. Transient electrocardiographic changes in patients with unstable angina: relation to coronary arterial anatomy. Am J Cardiol 1980;46:28–33.

16. Berry C, Zalewski A, Savage M, et al. Surface electrocardiogram in the detection of transmural myocardial ischemia during coronary artery occlusion. Am J Cardiol 1989;63:21–26.

17. Nademanee K, Intarachot V, Josephson MA, et al. Prognostic significance of silent myocardial ischemia in patients with unstable angina. J Am Coll Cardiol 1987;10:1–9.

18. Gottlieb SO, Weisfeldt ML, Ouyang P, et al. Silent ischemia predicts infarction and death during 2 year follow-up of unstable angina. J Am Coll Cardiol 1987;10:756–760.

19. Langer A, Freeman MR, Armstrong PW. ST segment shift in unstable angina pathophysiology and association with coronary anatomy and hospital outcome. J Am Coll Cardiol 1989;13:1495–1502.

20. Lindahl B, Venge P, Wallentin L. Relation between troponin T and the risk of subsequent cardiac events in unstable coronary artery disease. Circulation 1996;93:1651–1657.

21. Ohman EM, Armstrong PW, Christenson RH, et al. Cardiac troponin T levels for risk stratification in acute myocardial ischemia. N Engl J Med 1996; 335:1333–1341.

22. Antman EM, Tanasijevic MJ, Thompson B, et al. Cardiac-specific troponin I levels to predict the risk of mortality in patients with acute coronary syndromes. N Engl J Med 1996;335:1342–1349.

23. Braunwald E, Jones RH, Mark DB, et al. Diagnosing and managing unstable angina. Circulation 1994;90:613–622.

24. Gottlieb SO, Weisfeldt ML, Ouyang P, et al. Effect of the addition of propranolol to therapy with nifedipine for unstable angina pectoris: a randomized, double-blind, placebo-controlled trial. Circulation 1986;73:331–337.

25. Report of the Holland Interuniversity Nifedipine/Metoprolol Trial (HINT) Reserach Group. Early treatment of unstable angina in the coronary care unit: a randomised, double blind, placebo controlled comparison of recurrent ischaemia in patients treated with nifedipine or metoprolol or both. Br Heart J 1986;56:400–413.

26. Telford AM, Wilson C. Trial of heparin versus atenolol in prevention of myocardial infarction in intermediate coronary syndrome. Lancet 1981;1: 1225–1228.

27. Theroux P, Ouimet H, McCans J, et al. Aspirin, heparin, or both to treat acute unstable angina. N Engl J Med 1988;319:1105–1111.

28. Oler A, Whooley MA, Oler J, et al. Adding heparin to aspirin reduces the incidence of myocardial infarction and death in patients with unstable angina. JAMA 1996;276:811–815.

29. Lewis HD, Davis JW, Archibald DG, et al. Protective effects of aspirin against acute myocardial infarction and death in men with unstable angina. Results of a Veterans Administration cooperative study. N Engl J Med 1983;309:396–403.

30. Cairns JA, Gent M, Singer J, et al. Aspirin, sulfinpyrazone, or both in unstable angina. Results of a Canadian multicenter trial. N Engl J Med 1985; 313:1369–1375.

31. Wallentin LC, and the Research Group on Instability in Coronary Artery Disease in Southeast Sweden. Aspirin (75 mg/day) after an episode of unstable coronary artery disease: long-term effects on the risk for myocardial infarction, occurrence of severe angina and the need for revascularization. J Am Coll Cardiol 1991;18:1587–1593.

32. Theroux P, Kouz S, Roy L, et al. Platelet membrane receptor glycoprotein IIb/IIIa antagonism in unstable angina. Circulation 1996;94:899–905.

33. Schulman SP, Goldschmidt-Clermont PJ, Topol EJ, et al. Effects of Integrelin, a platelet glycoprotein IIb/IIIa receptor antagonist, in unstable angina. Circulation 1996;94:2083–2089.

34. Luchi RJ, Scott SM, Deupree RH, and the Principal Investigators and Their Associates of Veterans Administration Cooperative Study No. 28. Comparison of medical and surgical treatment for unstable angina pectoris. Results of a Veterans Administration cooperative study. N Engl J Med 1987;316:977–984.

35. Butman SM, Olson HG, Gardin JM, et al. Submaximal exercise testing after stabilization of unstable angina pectoris. J Am Coll Cardiol 1984;4: 667–673.

36. Buxton A, Goldberg S, Hirshfeld JW, et al. Refractory ergonovine-induced coronary vasospasm: importance of intracoronary nitroglycerin. Am J Cardiol 1980;46:329–334.

37. Feldman RL, Jalowiec DA, Hill JA, et a. Contrast media-related complications during cardiac catheterization using Hexabrix or Renografin in high-risk patients. Am J Cardiol 1988;61:1334–1337.

38. Steinberg EP, Moore RD, Powe NR. Safety and cost effectiveness of high-osmolality as compared with low-osmolality contrast material in patients undergoing cardiac angiography. N Engl J Med 1992;326:425–430.

39. Gertz EW, Wisneski JA, Chill D, et al. Clinical superiority of a new nonionic contrast agent (iopamidol) for cardiac angiography. J Am Coll Cardiol 1985;5:250–258.

40. Theroux P, Waters D, Lam J, et al. Reactivation of unstable angina after the discontinuation of heparin. N Engl J Med 1992;327:141–145.

41. Davis K, Kennedy JW, Kemp HG, et al. Complications of coronary angiography from the Collaborative Study of Coronary Artery surgery (CASS). Circulation 1979;59:1105–1112.

42. Plotnick GD, Greene HL, Carliner NH, et al. Clinical indicators of left main coronary artery disease in unstable angina. Ann Intern Med 1979;91: 149–153.

43. Rutherford JD, Braunwald E, Cohn PF. Chronic ischemic heart disease. In: Braunwald E, ed. Heart disease. 3rd ed. Philadelphia: WB Saunders, 1988: 1314–1378.

44. Victor MF, Likoff MJ, Mintz GS, et al. Unstable angina pectoris of new onset: a prospective clinical and arteriographic study of 75 patients. Am J Cardiol 1981; 47:228–232.

45. Alison HW, Russell RO, Mantle JA, et al. Coronary anatomy and angiography in patients with unstable angina pectoris. Am J Cardiol 1978;48: 204–209.

46. Diver DJ, Bier JD, Ferreira PE, et al. Clinical and arteriographic characterization of patients with unstable angina without critical coronary arterial narrowing. Am J Cardiol 1994;74:531–537.

47. Plotnick GD, Fisher ML, Carliner-NH, et al. Cardiac catheterization in patients with unstable angina: recent onset vs. crescendo pattern. JAMA 1980;244:574–576.

48. Corcos T, David PR, Bourassa MG, et al. Percutaneous transluminal coronary angioplasty for the treatment of variant angina. J Am Coll Cardiol 1985;5:1046–1054.

49. Bott-Silverman C, Heupler FA, Yiannikas J. Variant angina: comparison of patients with and without fixed severe coronary artery disease. Am J Cardiol 1984;54:1173–1175.

50. Moise A, Theroux P, Taeymans Y, et al. Unstable angina and progression of coronary atherosclerosis. N Engl J Med 1983;309:685–689.

51. Fuster V, Badimon L, Badimon JJ, et al. The pathogenesis of coronary artery disease and the acute coronary syndromes. N Engl J Med (Part 1) 1992; 326:242–250. (Part 2) 1992;326:310–318.

52. Forrester JS, Litvack F, Grundfest W, et al. Perspective of coronary disease seen through the arteries of living man. Circulation 1987;75:505–513.

53. Goldberg S. Coronary artery spasm and thrombosis. Philadelphia: FA Davis, 1983.

54. Ambrose JA, Winters SL, Stern A, et al. Angiographic morphology and the pathogenesis of unstable angina pectoris. J Am Coll Cardiol 1985;5: 609–616.

55. Levin DC, Fallon JU. Significance of the angiographic morphology of localized coronary stenoses: histopathologic correlations. Circulation 1982;66:3316–3320.

56. Fitzgerald DJ, Roy L, Catella F, et al. Platelet activation in unstable coronary disease. N Engl J Med 1986;315:983–989.

57. Kruskal JB, Commerford PJ, Franks JJ, et al. Fibrin and fibrinogen-related antigens in patients with stable and unstable coronary artery disease. N Engl J Med 1987;317:1361–1365.

58. Eisenberg PR, Kenzora JL, Sobel BE, et al. Relation between ST segment shifts during ischemia and thrombin activity in patients with unstable angina. J Am Coll Cardiol 1991;18:898–903.

59. Zalewski A, Shi Y, Nardone D, et al. Evidence for reduced fibrinolytic activity in unstable angina at rest. Clinical, biochemical, and angiographic correlates. Circulation 1991;83:1685–1691.

60. Ardissino D, Merlini PA, Gamba G, et al. Thrombin activity and early outcome in unstable angina pectoris. Circulation 1996;93:1634–1639.

61. Vetrovec GW, Cowley MJ, Overton H, et al. Intracoronary thrombus in syndromes of unstable myocardial ischemia. Am Heart J 1981;102: 1202–1208.

62. Bresnahan DR, Davis JL, Holmes DR, et al. Angiographic occurrence and clinical correlates of intraluminal coronary artery thrombus: role of unstable angina. J Am Coll Cardiol 1985;6:285–289.

63. Capone G, Wolf NM, Meyer B, et al. Frequency of intracoronary filling defects by angiography in angina pectoris at rest. Am J Cardiol 1985;56: 403–406.

64. Gotoh K, Minamino T, Katoh 0. The role of intracoronary thrombus in unstable angina: angiographic assessment and thrombolytic therapy during ongoing anginal attacks. Circulation 1988; 77:526–534.

65. Freeman MR, Williams AE, Chisholm RJ, et al. Intracoronary thrombus and complex morphology in unstable angina. Relation to timing of angiography and in-hospital cardiac events. Circulation 1989;80:17–23.

66. Rehr R, Disciascio G, Vetrovec G, et al. Angiographic morphology of coronary artery stenoses in prolonged rest angina: evidence of intracoronary thrombosis. J Am Coll Cardiol 1989;14: 1429–1437.

67. Sherman CT, Litvack F, Grundfest W, et al. Coronary angioscopy in patients with unstable angina pectoris. N Engl J Med 1986;315:913–919.

68. Mizuno K, Satomura K, Miyamoto A, et al. Angioscopic evaluation of coronary-artery thrombi in acute coronary syndromes. N Engl J Med 1992; 326:287–291.

69. de Feyter PJ, Serruys PW, Suryapranata H, et al. Coronary angioplasty early after diagnosis of unstable angina. Am Heart J 1987;114:48–54.

70. Neill WA, Wharton TP, Fluri-Lundeen J, et al. Acute coronary insufficiency: coronary occlusion after intermittent ischemic attacks. N Engl J Med 1980;302:1157–1162.

71. Rafflenbeul W, Smith LR, Rogers WJ, et al. Quantitative coronary angiography: coronary anatomy of patients with unstable angina pectoris reexamined 1 year after optimal medical therapy. Am J Cardiol 1979;43:699–707.

72. Faxon DP, Detre KM, McCabe CH, et al. Role of percutaneous transluminal coronary angioplasty in the treatment of unstable angina: report from the National Heart, Lung, and Blood Institute Percutaneous Transluminal Coronary Angioplasty and Coronary Artery Surgery Study Registries. Am J Cardiol 1983;53:131C-135C.

73. Bentivoglio LG, Holubkov R, Kelsey SF, et al. Short and long term outcome of percutaneous transluminal coronary angioplasty in unstable versus stable angina pectoris: a report of the 1985–1986 NHLBI PTCA Registry. Cathet Cardiovasc Diagn 1991;23:227–238.

74. de Feyter PJ, Serruys PW, van den Brand, et al. Emergency coronary angioplasty in refractory unstable angina. N Engl J Med 1985;313:342–346.

75. Plokker HWT, Ernst SMPG, Bal ET, et al. Percutaneous transluminal coronary angioplasty in patients with unstable angina pectoris refractory to

medical therapy. Cathet Cardiovasc Diagn 1988; 14:15–18.

76. de Feyter PJ, Suryapranata H, Serruys PW, et al. Coronary angioplasty for unstable angina: immediate and late results in 200 consecutive patients with identification of risk factors. J Am Coll Cardiol 1988;12:324–333.

77. Myler RK, Shaw RE, Stertzer SH, et al. Unstable angina and coronary angioplasty. Circulation 1990;82(Suppl II):II-88—II-95.

78. Williams DO, Braunwald E, Thompson B, et al. Results of percutaneous transluminal coronary angioplasty in unstable angina and non-Q wave myocardial infarction. Circulation 1996;94: 2749–2755.

79. Wohlgelernter D, Cleman M, Highman HA, et al. Percutaneous transluminal coronary angioplasty of the "culprit lesion" for management of unstable angina pectoris in patients with multivessel coronary artery disease. Am J Cardiol 1986;58: 460–464.

80. de Feyter PJ, Serruys PW, Arnold A, et al. Coronary angioplasty of the unstable angina-related vessel in patients with multivessel disease. Eur Heart J 1986;7:460–467.

81. Faxon DP, Ghalilli K, Jacobs AK, et al. The degree of revascularization and outcome after multivessel coronary angioplasty. Am Heart J 1992;123: 854–859.

82. Slysh S, Goldberg S, Dervan JP, et al. Unstable angina and evolving myocardial infarction following coronary bypass surgery: pathogenesis and treatment with interventional catheterization. Am Heart J 1985;109:744–752.

83. Barnathan ES, Schwartz JS, Taylor L, et al. Aspirin and dipyridamole in the prevention of acute coronary thrombosis complicating coronary angioplasty. Circulation 1987;76:125–134.

84. Schwartz L, Bourassa MG, Lesperance J, et al. Aspirin and dipyridamole in the prevention of restenosis after percutaneous transluminal coronary angioplasty. N Engl J Med 1988;318:1714–1719.

85. Savage MP, Goldberg S, Bove AA, et al. Effect of thromboxane A2 blockade on clinical outcome and restenosis after successful coronary angioplasty. Circulation 1995;92:3194–3200.

86. The EPIC Investigators. Use of a monoclonal antibody directed against the platelet glycoprotein IIb/IIIa receptor in high-risk coronary angioplasty. N Engl J Med 1994;330:956–961.

87. Gasperetti CM, Feldman MD, Burwell LR, et al. Influence of contrast media on thrombus formation during coronary angioplasty. J Am Coll Cardiol 1991;18:443–450.

88. Esplugas E, Cequier A, Jara F, et al. Risk of thrombosis during coronary angioplasty with low osmolality contrast media. Am J Cardiol 1991;68: 1020–1024.

89. Piessens JH, Stammen F, Vrolix MC, et al. Effects of ionic versus a nonionic low osmolar contrast agent on the thrombotic complications of coronary angioplasty. Cathet Cardiovas Diagn 1993; 28:99–105.

90. Savage MP,Goldberg S, Hirshfeld J, et al. Clinical and angiographic determinants of primary angioplasty success. J Am Coll Cardiol 1991;17:22–28.

91. Mabin TA Holmes DR, Smith HC, et al. Intracoronary thrombus: role in coronary occlusion complicating percutaneous transluminal coronary angioplasty. J Am Coll Cardiol 1985;5:198–202.

92. Ellis SG, Roubin GS, King III SB, et al. Angiographic and clinical predictors of acute closure after native vessel coronary angioplasty. Circulation 1988;77:372–379.

93. Detre KMl, Holmes DR Jr, Holubkov R. Incidence and consequences of periprocedural occlusion. The 1985–1986 National Heart, Lung, and Blood Institute Percutaneous Transluminal Coronary Angioplasty Registry. Circulation 1990;82: 739–750.

94. Myler RK, Shaw RE, Stertzer SH. Lesion morphology and coronary angioplasty: current experience and analysis. J Am Coll Cardiol 1992;19: 1641–1652.

95. White CJ, Ramee SR, Collins TJ, et al. Coronary thrombi increase PTCA risk. Circulation 1996;93: 253–258.

96. Waxman S, Sassower MA, Mittleman MA, et al. Angioscopic predictors of early adverse outcome after coronary angioplasty in patients with unstable angina and non-Q wave myocardial infarction. Circulation 1996;93:2106–2113.

97. Lukas MA, Deutsch E, Barnathan E, et al. Influence of heparin therapy on percutaneous transluminal coronary angioplasty outcome in unstable angina pectoris. Am J Cardiol 1990;65:1425–1429.

98. Fuchs J, Cannon CP, and the TIMI 7 Investigators. Hirulog in the treatment of unstable angina. Circulation 1995;92:727–733.

99. The GUSTO IIb Investigators. A comparison of recombinant hirudin with heparin for the treatment of acute coronary syndromes. N Engl J Med 1996;335:775–782.

100. Goldberg S. Coronary angioplasty in the 1990s—new tools for old troubles. J Invasive Cardiol 1990;2:211–216.

101. King III SB. Role of new technology in balloon angioplasty. Circulation 1991;84:2574–2579.

102. Cook SL, Eigler NL, Shefer A, et al. Percutaneous excimer laser coronary angioplasty of lesions not ideal for balloon angioplasty. Circulation 1991;84: 632–643.

103. Bittl JA, Sanborn TA. Excimer laser-facilitated coronary angioplasty relative risk analysis of acute and follow-up results in 200 patients. Circulation 1992;86:71–80.

104. Teirstein PS, Warth DC, Haq N. High speed rotational coronary atherectomy for patients with diffuse coronary artery disease. J Am Coll Cardiol 1991;18:1694–1701.

105. Ellis SG, de Cesare NB, Pinkerton CA. Relation of stenosis morphology and clinical presentation to the procedural results of directional coronary atherectomy. Circulation 1991;84:644–653.

106. Topol EJ, Leya F, Pinkerton CA, et al. A comparison of directional atherectomy with coronary angioplasty in patients with coronary artery disease. N Engl J Med 1993;329:221–227.

107. Holmes DR, Topol EJ, Califf RM, et al. A multicenter, randomized trial of coronary angioplasty versus directional atherectomy for patients with sa-

phenous vein bypass graft lesions. Circulation 1995;91:1966–1974.

108. Kaplan BM, Gregory M, Schreiber TL, et al. Transluminal extraction atherectomy versus balloon angioplasty in acute ischemic syndromes: an interim analysis of the TOPIT Trial [Abstract]. Circulation 1996;94:I-317.

109. Sigwart U, Urban P, Golf S. Emergency stenting for acute occlusion after coronary balloon angioplasty. Circulation 1988;78:1121–1127.

110. Fischman DL, Savage MP, Leon MB, et al. Effect of intracoronary stenting on intimal dissection after balloon angioplasty: results of quantitative and qualitative coronary analysis. J Am Coll Cardiol 1991;18:1445–1451.

111. Roubin GS, Cannon AD, Agrawal SK. Intracoronary stenting for acute and threatened closure complicating percutaneous transluminal coronary angioplasty. Circulation 1992;85:916–927.

112. Fischman DL, Savage, MP, Goldberg S. Coronary stent thrombosis. In: Hirshfeld JW, Herrmann HC, eds. Clinical use of the Palmaz-Schatz intracoronary stent. Mount Kisco, New York: Futura Publishing Co., 1993:125–135.

113. Savage MP, Schatz RA, Leon MB, et al. Long-term angiographic and clinical outcome after implantation of a balloon-expandable stent in the native coronary circulation. J Am Coll Cardiol 1994;24:1207–1212.

114. Serruys PW, deJaegere P, Kiemeneij F, et al. A comparison of balloon-expandable-stent implantation with balloon angioplasty in patients with coronary artery disease. N Engl J Med 1994;331:489–495.

115. Fischman DL, Leon MB, Baim DS, et al. A randomized comparison of coronary-stent placement and balloon angioplasty in the treatment of coronary artery disease. N Engl J Med 1994;331:496–501.

116. Leimgruber PP, Roubin GS, Hollman J, et al. Restenosis after successful coronary angioplasty in patients with single-vessel disease. Circulation 1986;73:710–717.

117. Waters D, Lam J, Theroux P. Newer concepts in the treatment of unstable angina pectoris. Am J Cardiol 1991;68:34C-41C.

118. Vetrovec GW, Leinbach RC, Gold HK, et al. Intracoronary thrombolysis in syndromes of unstable ischemia: angiographic and clinical results. Am Heart J 1982;104:946–952.

119. DeZwaan C, Bar FW, Janssen JHA, et al. Effects of thrombolytic therapy in unstable angina: clinical and angiographic results. J Am Coll Cardiol 1988;12:301–309.

120. Ambrose JA, Hjemdah-Monsen C, Borico S, et al. Quantitative and qualitative effects of intracoronary streptokinase in unstable angina and non-Q wave infarction. J Am Coll Cardiol 1987;9:1156–1165.

121. Ambrose JA, Almeida OD, Sharma SK, et al. Adjunctive thrombolytic therapy during angioplasty for ischemic rest angina. Results of the TAUSA Trial. Circulation 1994;90:69–77.

122. Gold HK, Johns JA, Leinbach RC, et al. A randomized, blinded, placebo-controlled trial of recombinant human tissue-type plasminogen activator in patients with unstable angina pectoris. Circulation 1987;75:1192–1199.

123. Williams DO, Topol EJ, Califf RM, et al. Intravenous recombinant tissue-type plasminogen activator in patients with unstable angina pectoris: results of a placebo-controlled, randomized trial. Circulation 1990;82:376–383.

124. Freeman PM, Langer A, Wilson RF, et al. Thrombolysis in unstable angina: randomized double-blind trial of t-PA and placebo. Circulation 1992;85:150–157.

125. Nicklas JM, Topol EJ, Kander N, et al. Randomized, double-blind, placebo-controlled trial of tissue plasminogen activator in unstable angina. Am Coll Cardiol 1989;13:434–441.

126. Bar FW, Verheugt FW, Col J. Thrombolysis in patients with unstable angina improves the angiographic but not the clinical outcome. Results of UNASEM, a multicenter, randomized placebo-controlled, clinical trial with anistreplase. Circulation 1992;86:131–137.

127. Schreiber TL, Rizik D, White C, et al. Randomized trial of thrombolysis versus heparin in unstable angina. Circulation 1993;86:1407–1414.

128. The T-3A Investigators. Early effects of tissue plasminogen activator, added to conventional therapy, on the culprit coronary lesion in patients presenting with ischemic cardiac pain at rest. Circulation 1993;87:38–52.

129. The TIMI IIIb Investigators. Effects of tissue plasminogen activator and a comparison of early invasive and conservative strategies in unstable angina and non-Q wave myocardial infarction. Circulation 1994;89:1545–1556.

130. Anderson HV, Cannon CP, Stone PH, et al. One-year results of the thrombolysis in myocardial infarction (TIMI) IIIb clinical trial. A randomized comparison of tissue-type plasminogen activator versus placebo and early invasive versus early conservative strategies in unstable angina and non-Q wave myocardial infarction. J Am Coll Cardiol 1995;26:1643–1650.

131. Herrick JB. Clinical features of sudden obstruction of the coronary arteries. JAMA 1912;59:2015–2020.

132. DeWood MA, Spores J, Notske R, et al. Prevalence of total coronary occlusion during the early hours of transmural myocardial infarction. N Engl J Med 1980;303:897–902.

133. Rentrop KP, Blanke H, Karoch KR, et al. Selective intracoronary thrombolysis in acute myocardial infarction and unstable angina pectoris. Circulation 1981;63:307–317.

134. Methey DG, Kuck KH, Tilsner V, et al. Nonsurgical coronary artery recanalization in acute transmural myocardial infarction. Circulation 1981;63:489–497.

135. Ganz W, Ninomiya K, Hashida J, et al. Intracoronary thrombolysis in acute myocardial infarction: experimental background and clinical experience. Am Heart J 1981;102:1145–1149.

136. Anderson JL, Marshall HW, Bray BE, et al. A randomized trial of intra-coronary streptokinase in the treatment of acute myocardial infarction. N Engl J Med 1983;308:1312–1318.

137. Kennedy JW, Ritchie JL, Davis KB, et al. Western

Washington randomized trial of intracoronary streptokinase in acute myocardial infarction. N Engl J Med 1983;309:1477–1482.

138. Khaja F, Walton JA, Brymer JF, et al. Intracoronary fibrinolytic therapy on acute myocardial infarction. N Engl J Med 1983;308:1305–1311.

139. Rentrop KP, Feit F, Blanke H, et al. Effects of intracoronary streptokinase and intracoronary nitroglycerin infusion on coronary angiographic patterns and mortality in patients with acute myocardial infarction. N Engl J Med 1984;311:1457–1463.

140. Simoons ML, van de Brand M, DeZwaans C, et al. Improved survival after early thrombolysis in acute myocardial infarction. Lancet 1985;2:578–581.

141. Raizner AE, Tortoledo FA, Verani MS, et al. Intracoronary thrombolytic therapy in acute myocardial infarction: a prospective, randomized, controlled trial. Am J Cardiol 1985;55:301–308.

142. Kennedy JW, Gensini GG, Timmis GC, et al. Acute myocardial infarction treated with intracoronary streptokinase: a report of the Society for Cardiac Angiography. Am J Cardiol 1985;55:871–877.

143. Weinstein J. Treatment of myocardial infarction with intracoronary streptokinase: efficacy and safety data from 209 United States cases in the Hoechst-Roussel Registry. Am Heart J 1982;104:894–898.

144. Kennedy JW, Ritchie JL, Davis KB, et al. Western Washington intracoronary streptokinse trial follow-up. N Engl J Med 1985;312:1073–1078.

145. Verstraete M, Bory M, Collen D, et al. Randomized trial of intravenous recombinant tissue-type plasminogen activator versus intravenous streptokinase myocardial infarction. Lancet 1985;1:842–847.

146. Sheehan FH, Braunwald E, Canner P, et al. The effect of intravenous thrombolytic therapy on left ventricular function: a report on tissue-type plasminogen activator and streptokinase from thrombolysis in myocardial infarction (TIMI Phase I) trial. Circulation 1987;75:817–829.

147. White HD, Norris RM, Bown MA, et al. Effect of intravenous streptokinase on left ventricular function and early survival after acute myocardial infarction. N Engl J Med 1987;317:850–855.

148. ISAM Study Group. A prospective trial of intravenous streptokinase in acute myocardial infarction (ISAM). N Engl J Med 1986;314:1465–1471.

149. Gruppo Italiano Per Lo Studio Della Streptochinasi Nell' infarto Miocardico (GISSI). Effectiveness of intravenous thrombolytic treatment in acute myocardial infarction. Lancet 1986;1:397–401.

150. ISIS-2 (Second International Study of Infarct Survival) Collaborative Group. Randomized trial of intravenous streptokinase, oral aspirin, or both or neither among 17,187 cases of suspected acute myocardial infarction. Lancet 1988;2:545–549.

151. Topol EJ, Califf RM, George BS, et al. A randomized trial of immediate versus delayed elective angioplasty after intravenous tissue plasminogen activator in acute myocardial infarction. N Engl J Med 1987;317–588.

152. Guerci AD, Gerstenblith G, Brinker JA, et al. A randomized trial of intravenous tissue plasminogen activator for acute myocardial infarction with subsequent randomization to elective coronary angioplasty. N Engl J Med 1987;317:1613–1618.

153. Neuhaus K-L, Feuerer W, Jeep-Teebe S, et al. Improved thrombolysis with a modified dose regimen of recombinant tissue-type plasminogen activator. J Am Coll Cardiol 1989; 14:1566–1569.

154. Wall TC, Califf, RM, George BS. Accelerated plasminogen activator dose regimens for coronary thrombolysis. J Am Coll Cardiol 1992;19:482–489.

155. O'Rourke M, Baron D, Keogh A, et al. Limitation of myocardial infarction by early infusion of recombinant tissue-type plasminogen activator. Circulation 1988;77:1311–1315.

156. Wilcox RG, Olsson CG, Skene AM, et al. Trial of tissue plasminogen activator for mortality reduction in acute myocardial infarction. Anglo-Scandinavian study of early thrombolysis (ASSET). Lancet 1988;2:525–530.

157. Gruppo Italiano Per Lo Studio Della Sopravvivenza Nell' Infarto Miocardico. GISSI-2: a factorial randomised trial of alteplase versus streptokinase and heparin versus no heparin among 12,490 patients with acute myocardial infarction. Lancet 1990;336:65–71.

158. The International Study Group. In-hospital mortality and clinical course of 20,891 patients with suspected acute myocardial infarction randomised between alteplase and streptokinase with or without heparin. Lancet 1990;336:71–75.

159. ISIS-3 (Third International Study of Infarct Survival) Collaborative Group. ISIS-3: a randomised comparison of streptokinase vs tissue plasminogen activator vs anistreplase and of aspirin plus heparin vs aspirin alone among 41,299 cases of suspected acute myocardial infarction. Lancet 1992;339:753–770.

160. The GUSTO Investigators. An international randomized trial comparing four thrombolytic strategies for acute myocardial infarction. N Engl J Med 1993;329:673–682.

161. Califf RM, White HD, Van de Werf F, et al. One year results from the global utilization of streptokinase and tPA for occluded coronary arteries (GUSTO-I) trial. Circulation 1996;94:1233–1238.

162. The GUSTO Angiographic Investigators. The effects of tissue plasminogen activator, streptokinase, or both on coronary-artery patency, ventricular function, and survival after acute myocardial infarction. N Engl J Med 1993;329:1615–1622.

163. Satler LF, Pallas RS, Bond OB, et al. Assessment of residual coronary arterial stenosis after thrombolytic therapy during acute myocardial infarction. Am J Cardiol 1987;59:1231–1233.

164. Wyatt HL, Forrester JS, Goldner S, et al. Effect of graded reductions on regional and total cardiac function. Am J Cardiol 1975;36:185–192.

165. Harrison DG, Ferguson DW, Collins SM, et al. Rethrombosis after reperfusion with streptokinase: importance of geometry of residual lesions. Circulation 1984;69:991–999.

166. Gold HK, Leinbach RC, Garabedian HD, et al. Acute coronary reocclusion after thrombolysis with recombinant human tissue-type plasmino-

gen activator: prevention by a maintenance infusion. Circulation 1986;73:347–352.

167. Chesebro JH, Knatterud G, Roberts R, et al. Thrombolysis in myocardial infarction (TIMI) trial. Phase I. A comparison between intravenous tissue plasminogen activator and intravenous streptokinase. Circulation 1987;76:142–154.

168. Topol EJ, O'Neill WW, Langburd AB, et al. A randomized, placebo-controlled trial of intravenous recombinant tissue-type plasminogen activator and emergency coronary angioplasty in patients with acute myocardial infarction. Circulation 1987;75:420–428.

169. Hartzler GO, Rutherford BD, McConahay DR, et al. Percutaneous transluminal coronary angioplasty with and without thrombolytic therapy for treatment of acute myocardial infarction. Am Heart J 1983;106:965–973.

170. O'Neill W, Timmis GC, Bourdillon PD, et al. A prospective randomized clinical trial of intracoronary streptokinase versus coronary angioplasty for acute myocardial infarction. N Engl J Med 1986;314:812–818.

171. Rothbaum DA, Linnemeier TJ, Landin RJ, et al. Emergency percutaneous transluminal coronary angioplasty in acute myocardial infarction: a 3 year experience. J Am Coll Cardiol 1987;10:264–272.

172. O'Keefe JH Jr, Rutherford BD, McConahay DR, et al. Early and late results of coronary angioplasty without antecedent thrombolytic therapy for acute myocardial infarction. Am J Cardiol 1989;64:1221–1230.

173. Meyer J, Merx W, Schmitz H, et al. Percutaneous transluminal coronary angioplasty immediately after intracoronary streptolysis of transmural myocardial infarction. Circulation 1982;66:905–913.

174. Serruys PW, Wijns W, ban den Brand M, et al. Is transluminal coronary angioplasty mandatory after successful thrombosis? Br Heart J 1983;50:257–265.

175. Stack RS, O'Connor CM, Mark DB, et al. Coronary perfusion during acute myocardial infarction with a combined therapy of coronary angioplasty and high-dose intravenous streptokinase. Circulation 1988;77:151–161.

176. Lieu TA, Gurley J, Lundstrom RJ, et al. Primary angioplasty and thrombolysis for acute myocardial infarction: an evidence summary. J Am Coll Cardiol 1996;27:737–750.

177. deBoer MJ, Hoorntje JCA, Ottervanger JP, et al. Immediate coronary angioplasty versus intravenous streptokinase in acute myocardial infarction: left ventricular ejection fraction, hospital mortality and reinfarction. J Am Coll Cardiol 1994;23:1004–1008.

178. Grines CL, Brown KF, Marco J, et al. A comparison of immediate angioplasty with thrombolytic therapy for acute myocardial infarction. N Engl J Med 1993;328:673–679.

179. Gibbons RJ, Holmes DR, Reeder GS, et al. Immediate angioplasty compared with the administration of a thrombolytic agent followed by conservative treatment for myocardial infarction. N Engl J Med. 1993;328:685–691.

180. Ribeiro EE, Silva LA, Carneiro R, et al. Randomized trial of direct coronary angioplasty versus intravenous streptokinase in acute myocardial infarction. J Am Coll Cardiol 1993;22:376–380.

181. Michels KB, Yusuf S. Does PTCA in acute myocardial infarction affect mortality and reinfarction rates? A quantitative overview (meta-analysis) of the randomized clinical trials. Circulation 1995;91:476–485.

182. Lange RA, Hillis LD. Should thrombolysis or primary angioplasty be the treatment of choice for acute myocardial infarction? N Engl J Med 1996;335:1311–1312.

183. Grines CL. Primary angioplasty—the strategy of choice. N Engl J Med 1996;335:1313–1315.

184. Every NR, Parsons LS, Hlatky M, et al. A comparison of thrombolytic therapy with primary coronary angioplasty for acute myocardial infarction. N Engl J Med 1996;335:1253–1260.

185. Boden WE, Kleiger RE, Gibson RS, et al. Electrocardiographic evolution of posterior acute myocardial infarction: importance of early precordial ST segment depression. Am J Cardiol 1987;59:782–787.

186. Waller BF, Rothbaum DA, Pinkerton CA, et al. Status of the myocardium and infarct-related coronary artery in 19 necropsy patients with acute recanalization using pharmacologic (streptokinase, r-tissue plasminogen activator), mechanical (percutaneous transluminal coronary angioplasty) or combined types of reperfusion therapy. J Am Coll Cardiol 1987;9:785–801.

187. Savage MP, Keen W, Fischman D, et al. Early angiography during acute myocardial infarction: correlation of surface electrocardiography with coronary pathoanatomy [Abstract]. J Am Coll Cardiol 1991;17:346A.

188. Abbottsmith CW, Topol EJ, George BS, et al. Fate of patients with acute myocardial infarction with patency of the infarct-related vessel achieved with successful thrombolysis versus rescue angioplasty. J Am Coll Cardiol 1990;16:770–778.

189. Miller FC, Krucoff MW, Satler LF, et al. Ventricular arrhythmias during reperfusion. Am Heart J 1986;112:928–931.

190. Califf RM, O'Neill WW, Stack RS, et al. Failure of simple clinical measurements to predict perfusion status after intravenous thrombolysis. Ann Intern Med 1988;108:658–662.

191. The TIMI Research Group. Immediate vs delayed catheterization and angioplasty following thrombolytic therapy for acute myocardial infarction: TIMI II A results. JAMA 1988;260:2849–2858.

192. Simoons ML, Betriu A, Col J, et al.; for the European Cooperative Study Group for Recombinant Tissue-Type Plasminogen Activator (rtPA). Thrombolysis with tissue plasminogen activator in acute myocardial infarction: no additional benefit from immediate percutaneous coronary angioplasty. Lancet 1988;1:197–202.

193. Califf RM, Topol EJ, Stack RS, et al. Evaluation of combination thrombolytic therapy and timing of cardiac catheterization in acute myocardial infarction. Results of thrombolysis and angioplasty in myocardial infarction—Phase 5 randomized trial. Circulation 1991;83:1543–1556.

194. McKendall GR, Forman S, Sopko G, et al. Value of rescue percutaneous transluminal coronary angioplasty following unsuccessful thrombolytic therapy in patients with acute myocardial infarction. Am J Cardiol 1995;76:1108–1111.

195. Ellis S, Ribeiro-da Silva, Heyndrickx G, et al. Randomized comparison of rescue angioplasty with conservative management of patients with early failure of thrombolysis for acute anterior myocardial infarction. Circulation 1994;90:2280–2284.

196. Ellis SG, Topol EJ, George BS. Recurrent ischemia without warning. Analysis of risk factors for in-hospital ischemic events following successful thrombolysis with intravenous tissue plasminogen activator. Circulation 1989;80:1159–1165.

197. Topol EJ, Holmes DR, Rogers WJ. Coronary angiography after thrombolytic therapy for acute myocardial infarction. Ann Intern Med 1991;114:877–885.

198. Guadagnoli E, Hauptman PJ, Ayanian JZ, et al. Variation in the use of cardiac procedures after acute myocardial infarction. N Engl J Med 1995;333:573–578.

199. Pilote L, Miller DP, Califf RM, et al. Determinants of the use of coronary angiography and revascularization after thrombolysis for acute myocardial infarction. N Engl J Med 1996;335:1198–1205.

200. Selby JV, Fireman BH, Lundstrom RJ, et al. Variation among hospitals in coronary angiography practices and outcomes after myocardial infarction in a large health maintenance organization. N Engl J Med 1996;335:1888–1896.

201. Ryan TJ, Anderson JL, Antman EM, et al. ACC/AHA Guidelines for the management of patients with acute myocardial infarction: executive summary. Circulation 1996;94:2341–2350.

202. TIMI Study Group. Comparison of invasive and conservative strategies following intravenous tissue plasminogen activator in acute myocardial infarction: results of the Thrombolysis in Myocardial Infarction (TIMI) Phase II Trial. N Engl J Med 1989;320:618–627.

203. SWIFT (Should We Intervene Following Thrombolysis?) Trial Study Group. SWIFT trial of delayed elective intervention vs conservative treatment after thrombolysis with anistreplase in acute myocardial infarction. BMJ 1991;302:555–560.

204. Williams DO, Braunwald E, Knatterud G, et al. One-year results of the thrombolysis in myocardial infarction investigation (TIMI) Phase II Trial. Circulation 1992;85:533–542.

205. Goldberg S, Greenspon AJ, Urban PL, et al. Reperfusion arrhythmia: a marker of restoration of antegrade flow during intracoronary thrombolysis for acute myocardial infarction. Am Heart J 1983;105:26–32.

206. Lefkovits J, Ivanhoe RJ, Califf RM, et al. Effects of platelet glycoprotein IIb/IIIa receptor blockade by a chimeric monoclonal antibody (abciximab) on acute and six-month outcomes after percutaneous transluminal coronary angioplasty for acute myocardial infarction. Am J Cardiol 1996;77:1045–1051.

207. Ellis SG, Mooney MR, George BS, et al. Randomized trial of late elective angioplasty versus conservative management for patients with residual stenoses after thrombolytic treatment of myocardial infarction. Circulation 1992;86:1400–1406.

208. Cigarroa RG, Lange RA, Hillis LD. Prognosis after acute myocardial infarction in patients with and without residual anterograde coronary blood flow. Am J Cardiol 1989;64:155–160.

209. Lange RA, Cigarroa RG, Wells PJ, et al. Influence of anterograde flow in the infarct artery on the incidence of late potentials after acute myocardial infarction. Am J Cardiol 1990;65:554–558.

210. Boehrer JD, Glamann B, Lange RA, et al. Effect of coronary angioplasty on late potentials one to two weeks after acute myocardial infarction. Am J Cardiol 1992;70:1515–1519.

211. Pizzetti G, Belotti G, Margonato A, et al. Coronary recanalization by elective angioplasty prevents ventricular dilation after anterior myocardial infarction. J Am Coll Cardiol 1996;28:837–845.

212. Topol EJ, Califf RM, Vandormael M, et al. A randomized trial of late reperfusion therapy for acute myocardial infarction. Circulation 1992;85:2090–2099.

213. Schroder R, Neuhaus KL, Leizorovicz A, et al.; for the ISAM Study Group. A prospective placebo controlled double-blind multicenter trial of intravenous streptokinase in acute myocardial infarction (ISAM): long-term mortality and morbidity. J Am Coll Cardiol 1987;9:197–203.

214. Muller DWM, Ellis SG, Woodlief LH, et al. Determinants of the need for early acute intervention in patients treated conservatively after thrombolytic therapy for acute myocardial infarction. J Am Coll Cardiol 1991;18:1594–1601.

215. Page DL, Caulfield JB, Kastor JA, et al. Myocardial changes associated with cardiogenic shock. N Engl J Med 1971;285:133–137.

216. Killip T, Kimball JT. Treatment of myocardial infarction in a coronary care unit. Am J Cardiol 1967;20:457–464.

217. Scheidt S, Ascheim R, Killip III T. Shock after acute myocardial infarction: a clinical and hemodynamic profile. Am J Cardiol 1970;26:556–564.

218. Goldberg RJ, Gore JM, Alpert JS, et al. Cardiogenic shock after acute myocardial infarction: incidence and mortality from a community-wide perspective, 1975 to 1988. N Engl J Med 1991;325:1117–1122.

219. Scheidt S, Wilner G, Mueller H, et al. Intra-aortic balloon counterpulsation in cardiogenic shock: report of a cooperative clinical trial. N Engl J Med 1973;288:979–984.

220. Califf RM, Bengtson JR. Cardiogenic shock. N Engl J Med 1994;330:1724–1730.

221. Kennedy JW, Gensini GG, Timmis GC, et al. Acute myocardial infarction treated with intracoronary streptokinase: a report of the society for cardiac angiography. Am J Cardiol 1985;55:871–877.

222. Shawl FA, Domanski MJ, Hernandez TJ. Emergency percutaneous cardiopulmonary bypass support in cardiogenic shock from acute myocardial infarction. Am J Cardiol 1989;64:967–970.

223. Gutovitz AL, Sobel BE, Roberts R. Progressive nature of myocardial injury in selected patients with cardiogenic shock. Am J Cardiol 1978;41:469–475.

224. DeWood MA, Notske RN, Hensley GR, et al. In-

traaortic balloon counterpulsation with and without reperfusion for myocardial infarction shock. Circulation 1980;61:1105–1112.

225. Lee L, Bates ER, Pitt B, et al. Percutaneous transluminal coronary angioplasty improves survival in acute myocardial infarction complicated by cardiogenic shock. Circulation 1988;78:1345–1351.

226. Hibbard MD, Holmes DR Jr, Bailey KR. Percutaneous transluminal coronary angioplasty in patients with cardiogenic shock. J Am Coll Cardiol 1992;19:639–646.

227. Moosvi AR, Khaja F, Villanueva L, et al. Early revascularization improves survival in cardiogenic shock complicating acute myocardial infarction. J Am Coll Cardiol 1992;19;907–914.

228. Gacioch GM, Ellis SG, Lee L, et al. Cardiogenic shock complicating acute myocardial infarction: the use of coronary angioplasty and the integration of the new support devices into patient management. J Am Coll Cardiol 1992;19:647–653.

229. Lee L, Erbel R, Brown TM, et al. Multicenter registry of angioplasty therapy of cardiogenic shock: initial and longterm survival. J Am Coll Cardiol 1991;17:599–603.

230. Marmor A, Sobel BE, Roberts R. Factors presaging early recurrent myocardial infarction ("extension"). Am J Cardiol 1981;48:603–610.

231. Schuster EH, Bulkley BH. Early post-infarction angina. Ischemia at a distance and ischemia in the infarct zone. N Engl J Med 1981;305:1101–1105.

232. Gibson RS, Beller GA, Gheorghiade M, et al. The prevalence and clinical significance of residual myocardial ischemia 2 weeks after uncomplicated non-Q wave infarction: a prospective natural history study. Circulation 1986;6:1186–1198.

233. Keen WD, Savage MP, Fischman DL, et al. Comparison of coronary angiographic findings during the first six hours of non-Q wave and Q wave myocardial infarction. Am J Cardiol 1994;74: 324–328.

234. Matetzky S, Barabash GI, Rabinowitz B, et al. Q wave and non-Q wave myocardial infarction after thrombolysis. J Am Coll Cardiol 1995;26: 1445–1451.

235. Lotan CS, Jonas M, Rozenman Y, et al. Comparison of early invasive and conservative treatments in patients with anterior wall non-Q wave acute myocardial infarction. Am J Cardiol 1995;76: 330–336.

236. Gibson RS. Management of acute non-Q-wave myocardial infarction: role of prophylactic pharmacotherapy and indications for predischarge coronary angiography. Clin Cardiol 1989;12:III-26–III-32.

237. Hopkins J, Savage M, Zalewski A, et al. Recurrent ischemia in the zone of prior myocardial infarction: results of coronary angioplasty of the infarct-related artery. Am Heart J 1988;115:14–19.

238. DeFeyter PJ, Serruys PW, Soward A, et al. Coronary angioplasty for early postinfarction unstable angina. Circulation 1986;74:1365–1370.

239. Gottlieb SO, Walford GD, Ouyang P, et al. Initial and late results of coronary angioplasty for early postinfarction unstable angina. Cathet Cardiovasc Diagn 1987;13:93–99.

240. Morrison DA. Coronary angioplasty for medically refractory unstable angina within 30 days of acute myocardial infarction. Am Heart J 1990;120: 256–260.

241. Murphy DA, Craver JM, Jones EL, et al. Hemodynamic deterioration after coronary angioplasty in the presence of previous left ventricular infarction. Am J Cardiol 1984;54:448–450.

242. Savage MP, Dervan JP, Zalewski A, et al. Percutaneous transluminal coronary angioplasty in patients with prior myocardial infarction: angioplasty at a distance from the prior infarct zone. Am Heart J 1987;114:1102–1110.

243. Savage MP, Goldberg S. Coronary angioplasty in the high risk patient. In: Goldberg S, ed. Coronary angioplasty. Philadelphia: FA Davis, 1988: 169–180.

244. Schomig A, Kastrati A, Mudra H, et al. Four-year experience with Palmaz-Schatz stenting in coronary angioplasty complicated by dissection with threatened or present vessel closure. Circulation 1994;90:2716–2724.

245. Altmann DB, Racz M, Battleman DS, et al. Reduction in angioplasty complications after the introduction of coronary stents: results from a consecutive series of 2242 patients. Am Heart J 1996;132: 503–507.

246. Goldberg S, Savage M, Slota P, et al. Coronary artery stents: a new era in interventional cardiology. In: Topol EJ, ed. Textbook of interventional cardiology—update 20. Philadelphia: WB Saunders, 1996:291–302.

247. Zalewski A, Savage M, Goldberg S. Protection of the ischemic myocardium during percutaneous transluminal coronary angioplasty. Am J Cardiol 1988;61:54G–60G.

248. Shawl FA, Domanski MJ, Punja S, et al. Percutaneous cardiopulmonary bypass support in high-risk patients undergoing percutaneous transluminal coronary angioplasty. Am J Cardiol 1989;64: 1258–1263.

249. Shawl FA, Quyyumi AA, Bajaj S, et al. Percutaneous cardiopulmonary bypass-supported coronary angioplasty in patients with unstable angina pectoris or myocardial infarction and a left ventricular ejection fraction ≤ 25%. Am J Cardiol 1996;77:14–19.

250. Vogel RA, Shawl F, Tommaso C, et al. Initial report of the national registry of elective cardiopulmonary bypass supported coronary angioplasty. J Am Coll Cardiol 1990;15:23–29.

38

Microinfarction Associated with Percutaneous Coronary Intervention

Barbara E.Tardiff, MD
Kenneth W. Mahaffey, MD
E. Magnus Ohman, MD
Robert M. Califf, MD

INTRODUCTION

Percutaneous coronary revascularization has become a common and routine procedure, representing a major therapeutic advance in the management of patients with ischemic heart disease. As experience with percutaneous interventions has increased and technical improvements have accrued, the incidence of hemorrhagic and technical complications has decreased (1). However, a persistent and perplexing problem has been the **frequent observation of clinically evident myocardial infarction, as diagnosed by appropriate electrocardiographic criteria or cardiac markers** (typically creatine kinase [CK] MB) in patients undergoing these procedures (2–6). Although enzyme elevations are commonly observed in patients with evolving acute infarctions after procedural complications, **asymptomatic patients with seemingly uncomplicated procedures also account for a high proportion of enzyme elevations.**

Early data suggested that although transient elevations in cardiac markers following interventional procedures occurred relatively often, they were thought to be clinically inconsequential (3). These studies were based on limited, short-term follow-up of small numbers of patients. With examination of greater numbers of patients with extended follow-up, a more worrisome picture has emerged. **In several large databases, patients with transient elevations in cardiac markers have had a higher cardiac mortality rate** during extended follow-up than those without elevations, independent of other predictors of mortality. Other cardiac complications also occur more commonly. A thorough understanding of the incidence and implication of these events is imperative for immediate and long-term clinical management of patients undergoing revascularization procedures and for critically evaluating new interventions. A review of this topic leads to the conclusion that enzyme elevations that reflect myocardial necrosis during revascularization procedures are undesirable clinical outcomes and must be considered both in assessing new drug therapies and in determining which procedures should be used in which patients.

BACKGROUND

Historical Context and Concerns

Initial interest in increased circulating cardiac enzymes following coronary artery bypass grafting (7, 8) was followed by uncertainty about the usefulness of CK-MB as a measure of perioperative injury. Enzyme elevations were often observed in the absence of clinically apparent cardiac damage (8, 9), which prompted controversy about whether common enzymatic markers such as creatine kinase and its MB fraction are specific enough to differentiate between skeletal muscle damage and myocardial injury in cardiac operations.

As percutaneous revascularization procedures became common practice, elevations in enzyme levels in the circulation following these interventions were noted. Although appropriate concern was expressed that the increase in enzyme levels might reflect myocardial cell damage during the procedure, initial small series suggested that no increased risk was seen of late adverse events in patients with such elevations (3, 10, 11). As new drugs and devices have been evaluated prospectively in large numbers of patients undergoing percutaneous interventions over the last several years, however, it has become evident that transient elevations in cardiac enzymes that equal or exceed levels seen in a typical myocardial infarction are common (2, 4–6, 12, 13). In general, new devices have not reduced the observed rate of periprocedural infarction (see Chapters 28–33).

Frequency and magnitude of these enzyme events mandates careful deliberation in two important areas: the clinical practice question of whether a patient should be treated differently after such an episode and the clinical research dilemma as to how to use these enzyme events in assessing the value of a new therapy or procedure. Although a number of unresolved or incompletely resolved issues still exist, recent reports have begun to clarify the relationship between elevations of biochemical markers and subsequent cardiac morbidity and in aggregate provide insight into the rational interpretation of periprocedural infarctions.

Diagnostic Methods and Definitions for Myocardial Infarction

Interpretation of data regarding periprocedural infarction studies is confounded by variations in markers, assays, or criteria for diagnosing myocardial infarction. The clinical definition of myocardial infarction remains variably specified, in part a result of the continuing evolution of diagnostic technology and in part a reflection of the continuum of acute coronary syndromes.

Enzymatic Markers

The historical standard definition of myocardial infarction is based on the evaluation of both CK and CK-MB by an immunoassay—a doubling of total creatine kinase with more than 5% of the total representing the CK-MB considered diagnostic (14). CK-MB assays are now predominantly mass assays, whereas total CK continues to be measured by immunoassay. Interpretation of CK-MB as a proportion of total CK may be misleading when the two assays measure different components (mass and activity), so in current practice an abnormal CK-MB mass level is the primary criterion for diagnosing myocardial infarction.

The definition of myocardial infarction as originally adopted by the World Health Organization evaluated serum enzyme changes occurring in the context of typical or atypical symptoms of myocardial ischemia (14). However, many patients without typical symptoms of acute myocardial ischemia have enzymatic evidence of myocardial necrosis associated with an increased risk of poor clinical outcomes.

Although it is not clear whether elevation of CK-MB is sufficient for diagnosis of myocardial infarction in all situations, **a qualitative relationship between release of CK and CK-MB and poor outcome has been observed** (15–17) for spontaneously occurring infarctions. In the periprocedural and perioperative setting, the situation has been less clear. In surgical patients, because a small pool of CK-MB exists in noncardiac tissues, CK and CK-MB may not be specific enough to differentiate between skeletal muscle damage and myocardial injury. Perhaps some release of CK-MB should be expected as a routine sequela of revascularization, whether it occurs by percutaneous intervention or surgically. However, large elevations of CK-MB postoperatively are associated with evidence of myocardial damage by perfusion imaging and pathologic examination (9, 18–20), and patients with even modest elevations after percutaneous procedures fare less well than those without enzymatic evidence of myocardial necrosis (6, 21). Although the picture is far from complete, most available data and the absence of another validated diagnostic tool support the use of CK-MB as a marker of infarction in the procedural setting.

In most centers, total CK is the primary measurement; CK-MB is quantitated only in those patients with elevated total CK. Total CK is not specific for myocardial necrosis (22), and also it may not be sensitive enough to identify patients with myocardial necrosis occurring in the periprocedural setting. Where both have been measured prospectively in randomized trials in patients undergoing percutaneous interventions, transient elevations of CK-MB have been noted to occur even when the total CK remains within the normal range (3, 21, 23).

Electrocardiographic Criteria

Electrocardiogram (ECG) use in the diagnosis of myocardial infarction in the periprocedural setting also has limitations. The criteria used to determine whether an ECG reflects new myocardial necrosis are not as well defined as generally believed. The specifications that have been used include a new 2-grade Q-wave worsening of the Minnesota code; a new 1-grade worsening of the Minnesota code with major ST-T wave worsening; new 30-msec Q-waves in two contiguous leads; new 30-msec Q-waves in two contiguous leads at least 1 mm deep; new 40-msec Q-waves; pathologic Q waves (24–30). The Minnesota code is one of the few systems that has been validated, and it has received extensive use in epidemiologic studies and clinical trials (24–26). In autopsy series, specificity of major Q-wave codes for myocardial necrosis exceeds 90%, although the code may not be sensitive enough to detect smaller events (31–35). Among patients with autopsy evidence of myocardial infarction, 30 to 40% will have

had major Minnesota code Q waves and 60% major or minor Minnesota code Q waves.

The Selvester QRS score is another method that has been validated for estimating the size of anterior, inferior, and posterolateral infarcts with high specificity in control populations (95%), and moderate sensitivity for identifying anterior (67%), inferior (90%), and posterolateral (45%) infarctions (36, 37). Both the Minnesota and Selvester methods achieve less accuracy in patients with multiple infarcts. The term "new significant Q waves" may be defined variably in definitions of new myocardial infarction but using the Selvester system, would include Q (30 for I, aVL (lateral); (30 for II, aVF (inferior); (30 for V_5, V_6 (apical); and any Q for V_1, V_2, V_3; and (20 for V_4 (anterior) (38).

It is not clear whether either coding system can be applied equally in both chronic and acute heart disease. The Minnesota code was validated in patients with chronic heart disease and in settings where patient position, lead placement, and heart rate were typically consistent and where conduction disturbances and other dynamic changes were uncommon. It has not been studied to the same extent in patients with acute heart disease, and it may be that the specified criteria are less reliable where patient position, lead placement, and heart rate are more variable and conduction disturbances and dynamic changes are common.

Especially in the acute population, the evolution of myocardial ischemia and necrosis can result in significant ECG changes over time, which may further cloud the interpretation of findings. Ascertainment of major ST-T wave abnormalities during acute ischemia is dependent in part on the timing of ECG acquisition. Q-waves can develop instantaneously or over several hours, and changes present at one point may not be evident on subsequent evaluations. In the Program Of Surgical Control of Hyperlipidemia (POSCH), 34% of subjects with codeable Minnesota code Q-wave items lost a codeable Q-QS pattern, on average, after 2.2 years (39).

It is clear that incident rates of Q-wave events can vary considerably depending on the definition used. ECG scoring systems provide insight into the extent of myocardial necrosis and additional incremental information regarding prognosis, but they are not optimal for myocardial infarct detection. Further investigation is needed to assess the usefulness of specific changes in both detecting new events and comparing clinical outcomes as determined by different criteria.

Newer Biochemical Markers

Myocardial tissue contains a variety of molecular species, in addition to CK-MB, that may be markers for myocardial necrosis. Myoglobin, CK isoenzymes, and myosin light chains frequently appear in serum within 1 to 2 hours of the onset of symptoms, and they are useful early indicators of myocardial infarction (22, 40, 41). These assays are valuable as screening tests, but because they lack cardiac specificity they are not useful as diagnostic tests for periprocedural infarction.

Troponin T (TnT), troponin I (TnI), and troponin C (TnC) are proteins that act as a complex to regulate muscle contraction. Troponins found in cardiac and skeletal muscle have different enough protein structures (isoforms) to permit sensitive assays to be developed for the cardiac-specific forms. Cardiac-specific troponin I and T appear to have a high level of sensitivity and specificity for myocardial necrosis (42, 43). They have recently been shown to have prognostic value beyond CK-MB in patients with acute coronary syndromes (44). Although limited information exists related to percutaneous coronary revascularization, mild transient elevations have been noted after uncomplicated percutaneous cardiac procedures (45–47). In the Karim et al. Study, 60% of patients having angioplasty had elevated TnT (>0.04 ng/mL), whereas elevated CK was observed in only 16% (45). Troponin T was elevated in all patients who had a balloon inflated for more than 5 minutes. The long-term implications of these findings are not yet established, but early data indicate that elevations in more specific cardiac markers parallel those seen for CK-MB.

Although these newer markers of myocardial necrosis may have exciting prognostic applications, CK-MB remains the gold standard for diagnosis (42). Importantly, because many interventions are performed for patients with acute coronary syndromes, both TnT and TnI have long circulating half-lives (5–14 days), so new episodes of necrosis cannot easily be discriminated from recent infarctions. Additional studies are needed to define the role of the troponin markers in the evaluation of periprocedural myocardial infarction.

Pathophysiologic Correlates: Relation Between Cardiac Enzymes, Cellular Processes, and Clinical Events

Substantial investigation has been done to identify the pathogenic mechanisms for CK and CK-MB release from the myocardium. Almost all experimental studies in a variety of animal models, isolated heart preparations, and cell cultures have shown that irreversible cellular injury or death is necessary for enzymatic leakage to be detected (48–50). Some controversy remains, however. Heyndrickx et al. have reported that a short period (15 minutes) of coronary artery occlusion in baboons was associated with significant increases in plasma CK and CK-MB enzyme activity in the absence of gross pathologic or histologic evidence of myocardial necrosis (51, 52). Study of rat myocardial cell cultures has demonstrated release of cytosol enzymes during anoxic reversible cell injury (53).

In the clinical setting, **cardiac enzymes are elevated following percutaneous coronary intervention in 5 to 20% of patients.** The factors underlying elevations in cardiac enzymes and the association of these increases with myocardial necrosis after coronary intervention are uncertain. In the 1970s and 1980s, several clinical investigators studied patients undergoing percutaneous coronary intervention to determine relationships among periprocedure symptoms,

ECG evidence of ischemia, and elevated postprocedure enzyme levels. No consensus has been reached about the extent or duration of ischemia that is required for irreversible injury or necrosis to occur during coronary intervention.

Mager et al. studied 357 balloon inflations during successful percutaneous coronary angioplasty in 35 patients (54). Ischemic ECG changes occurred during 324 (91%) balloon inflations at a mean of 20 ± 8 seconds after inflation. Ischemic ECG changes resolved in 313 (97%) of these patients at a mean of 11 ± 5 seconds after balloon deflation. Six patients had elevated CK above the upper limit of normal 12 to 18 hours postprocedure; each of these patients had in-laboratory total occlusion of the artery undergoing intervention, prolonged ischemic ECG changes (at least 7.8 minutes), and ECG evidence of evolving myocardial infarction. Ischemic ECG changes did not exceed 5.4 minutes in any of the patients with CK levels in the normal range postintervention. Twenty-three (66%) patients reported chest pain during balloon inflation including all six patients with elevated CK levels postprocedure. The authors concluded that ischemic ECG changes lasting less than 5.4 minutes are not associated with cardiac enzyme elevation, whereas more prolonged ischemia (more than 7.8 minutes) is associated with abnormal enzyme levels postprocedure. Pauletto et al. studied 24 patients who had percutaneous coronary intervention (11). Mean time of intermittent occlusion was 4.2 ± 2.2 minutes. All but 1 had angina accompanied by ischemic ECG changes during the procedure, whereas 4 of the 24 patients had elevated CK or CK-MB above the upper limit of normal without clinical or electrocardiographic evidence of myocardial infarction. Occlusion times were not reported for patients with and without CK or CK-MB elevations. These findings support the concept that prolonged ischemic symptoms and ECG evidence of ischemia are associated with elevated cardiac enzymes in patients following percutaneous coronary intervention. However, no "cut-off" value has been determined for the duration of ischemia required to produce myocardial necrosis.

Recently, several investigators studied patient clinical characteristics, coronary lesion features, and procedural complications to determine predictors of elevated cardiac enzymes postcoronary intervention (4, 21, 55–61). These studies have demonstrated several characteristics—such as increased age, female gender, unstable coronary syndromes, multivessel disease, use of directional coronary atherectomy (DCA) versus percutaneous transluminal coronary angioplasty (PTCA) or stenting, saphenous vein graft lesions, side branch occlusion, and abrupt closure—that are consistently associated with a risk of increased cardiac enzymes.

Pathogenic mechanisms of CK and CK-MB release in the circulation require continued investigation. Reports demonstrating a lack of necrosis when enzymes are measured raise concern about the adequacy of these specific markers to detect necrosis accurately. However, the well-documented association between elevated enzyme levels postcoronary intervention and worse clinical outcomes supports the importance of these markers (2–5). Further understanding of patient clinical characteristics, lesion features, and procedural complications associated with elevated cardiac enzymes may help elucidate the mechanisms of, factors associated with, and long-term consequence of cardiac enzyme elevations.

REPORTED EXPERIENCE WITH PERCUTANEOUS REVASCULARIZATION

Specific Trial and Observational Data

Abundant evidence from multiple institutions strongly supports a relationship between the appearance of CK-MB in the circulation following percutaneous interventions and a poorer clinical outcome during subsequent clinical evaluations (Table 38.1). Patients who have transient elevations in cardiac markers have a higher cardiac mortality rate during follow-up than those who do not, independent of other predictors of mortality.

Table 38.1.
Prognostic Significance of Periprocedural Cardiac Enzyme Elevations

Investigator/Reference	Number	Follow-up	Diagnostic Criteria	Myocardial Infarction Mortality (%)
Tardiff (23)	2432	30 day	CKMB ≤ 3×	0.3
			CKMB > 3 ×	1.2–4.9
		6 mo	CKMB ≤ 3×	1.4
			CKMB > 3×	2.3–6.5
Harrington (2)	1012	1	CKMB ≤ 3×	1.2
			CKMB > 3× [a]	4.4
Redwood (63)	1897	1	CKMB ≤ 1×	1.1
			CKMB 1 – 4×	3.6
			CKMB > 4×	5.8
Kugelmass (4)	565	2 y ± 1.2	CKMB ≤ 1×	8
			CKMB > 1×	9
Abdelmeguid (62)	4644	mean 36 mo (range 0.08–8.7)	CK ≤ 2×	year 1: 1.8 years 2–5: 1 [b] years 6–10: 0 [b]
			CK > 2×, positive CKMB	year 1: 4.9–8.2 [b] years 2–5: 4% [b] years 6–10: 5 [b]
Kong (64)	373	mean 3.5 y	CKMB ≤ 1.5×	7
			CKMB > 1.5×	15.8

[a] Or new Q or CK > 2× if no CKMB.
[b] Per year.

An early observation by Klein et al. reported that 15% of 249 consecutive patients treated with angioplasty in 1989–1990 had elevations of total CK or CK-MB (3). An apparent clinical event was evident in more than half of the patients whose CK-MB became elevated. In the remainder of cases, transient elevations of cardiac enzymes occurred despite a lack of symptoms indicative of myocardial infarction. Short-term follow-up of the latter patients suggested that in those with successful angioplasty no increased risk was seen of subsequent adverse events despite such elevations. In another study of 558 consecutive patients undergoing successful directional atherectomy or stenting, Kugelmass et al. observed postprocedure elevations of CK-MB above normal in 11.5% (4). No adverse long-term sequelae were detected in follow-up (mean 2 years) of patients with CK-MB elevations up to 50 IU/L (institutional normal 10 IU/L). A trend ($P = .08$) toward decreased late survival was noted in 2.3% of patients who had the highest postprocedure elevations (>50 IU/L). Modest sample size and relative infrequency of death (8 and 9% in pa-

tients with and without CK-MB elevations, respectively) and cardiac events in the follow-up period limited the power of this study to detect a prognostic difference between the two groups.

Abdelmeguid et al. completed a detailed long-term follow-up study of 4863 consecutive patients who underwent percutaneous procedures (5). Patients with unsuccessful procedures were excluded from the analysis. Patients with transient abrupt closure in the laboratory followed by successful opening of the vessel (n = 88) were compared with patients without abrupt closure (n = 4775). The mortality rate of patients with abrupt closure and no increase in CK-MB was no different from patients with successful procedures without abrupt closure. However, patients with elevated CK-MB had significantly decreased survival. A direct relationship between elevation of CK and CK-MB and risk of acute or chronic complications (mean duration of follow-up 41 months) was demonstrated in a multivariable regression analysis. An increase in CK-MB was the most important predictor of cardiac death (risk ratio 1.25; $P < .0001$) in follow-up even after adjusting for clinical, morphologic, and procedural factors that also affect prognosis.

In a subsequent study, these investigators evaluated the baseline characteristics, cardiac enzymes, and clinical outcomes of 4797 patients with successful percutaneous procedures (defined as no death, Q-wave myocardial infarction, or bypass surgery) (62). Excluded were 133 patients because of missing enzyme data (n = 44) or because the CK elevation had a negative MB component (n = 89). Characteristics associated with CK elevation included coronary embolism during the procedure, history of recent myocardial infarction, minor procedural complications (e.g., transient abrupt closure), hypotension, vein-graft procedures,

complex lesions, large dissections, and severe preprocedure stenoses. Morphologic characteristics linked with elevated postprocedure CK were thrombus-associated and complex lesions, saphenous vein graft lesions, and directional atherectomy. In this same group, a continuous relationship was observed between the level of CK-MB elevation and the risk of cardiac death in follow-up (mean 36 months) with no evident threshold (21). No effect on noncardiac death was noted (Fig. 38.1).

Experience of other centers has been reported in recent abstracts. Redwood et al. examined 1897 patients undergoing new device angioplasty (63). A significant number of patients had minor (CK-MB one to four times the upper limit of normal, n =

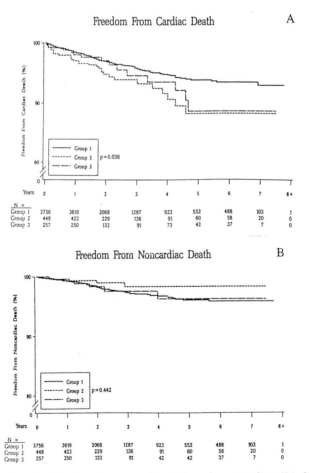

Figure 38.1. Plots showing freedom from cardiac (**A**) and noncardiac (**B**) death according to postprocedure cardiac enzyme level.

499, 26%) or major (CK-MB greater than four times normal, n = 250, 13%) postprocedural elevations. Minor enzyme elevations were associated with a fourfold increase in major in-hospital complications and more than a threefold increase in late mortality (mean follow-up 1 year). A detailed single-center case-control analysis (64) had similar findings, showing a doubling in late mortality rate (mean follow-up 3.5 years) in patients with elevated enzymes (15.8 versus 7%, P = .02). Patients (n = 253) with elevated CK and CK-MB were identified consecutively from a cohort of 2812 patients who underwent percutaneous revascularization at this institution between 1984 and 1993. These cases were matched with 120 control patients who had a procedure during the same month as the case cohort. In a multivariable Cox regression model, the most important predictors of long-term cardiac mortality rate were peak creatine kinase (relative risk 1.05, P < .0001) and ejection fraction (relative risk 0.58, P < .0001).

Examination of several large multicenter data sets reveals similar findings. Harrington et al. reported on 1012 patients enrolled in the CAVEAT trial (comparing excisional atherectomy with angioplasty) (2). A total of 112 patients (11%) met the predefined study criteria for myocardial infarction (increased CK-MB greater than three times the local institutional normal). Myocardial enzyme elevations were associated with higher rates of repeat revascularization, longer hospital stay, greater cost, and, importantly, 1-year mortality. Enzyme elevation was associated with adverse clinical outcomes even after excluding patients with clinically recognized abrupt closure. More recent analyses of the larger Integrelin to Manage Platelet Aggregation to Prevent Coronary Thrombosis (IMPACT II) and GUSTO II data sets have supported these findings even for intermediate follow-up (13, 23). Elevations in CK-MB following even successful percutaneous interventions were associated with increased risk for death and myocardial infarction at 6 months with the degree of risk proportional to the rise in CK-MB.

Most patients studied to date have undergone balloon angioplasty as opposed to treatment with newer devices, such as atherectomy, lasers, and stents. In limited numbers of patients, however, available data indicate that new devices have not reduced the rate of periprocedural infarction and, in the case of atherectomy, devices may be associated with increased release of cardiac enzymes (2, 58). Several investigations reported recently, which demonstrated an association of elevated creatine kinase with higher 1-year mortality, have included or been limited to patients treated with newer devices (2, 4, 21, 63–65). Data are particularly limited for intracoronary stents. Although stents are associated with a significant reduction in repeat revascularization or emergency bypass surgery (66–68), randomized studies have been too small to ascertain whether the periprocedural myocardial infarction rate is favorably affected and to determine if periprocedural infarctions associated with stent placement are prognostically significant.

Percutaneous intervention in patients who have undergone bypass surgery, particularly on lesions in saphenous vein grafts, is also associated with a high rate of periprocedural infarction. As in the case of new devices, data on this specific patient population are limited, but the high reported rates of release of cardiac markers following intervention in these patients should be interpreted as worrisome. Future evaluations of these patients need to include prospective collection of cardiac markers and long-term follow-up.

In aggregate, substantial evidence is now found that changes in cardiac markers following coronary procedures reflect myocardial necrosis occurring at the time of the procedure. Complex relationships surely exist among baseline cardiac risk factors, creatine kinase elevations, and long-term cardiac mortality rate. However, elevated enzymes, independent of other prognostic factors, have been shown to be independently predictive of adverse outcomes, including death, subsequent myocardial infarction, and a need for repeat revascularization procedures. Although risk can be particularly high in patients with abrupt vessel closure or other major procedural complication, risk level appears to increase as a continuous function without an obvious threshold value.

Clinical, Angiographic, and Procedural Characteristics Associated with Elevated Enzymes after Percutaneous Intervention

Published reports identifying specific risk factors associated with elevated cardiac enzymes after coronary intervention have varied substantially in patient populations studied, definition for cardiac enzyme elevation, type of intervention investigated, extent of clinical history available, lesion characteristics collected, identification of periprocedural complications, and statistical analyses performed. A summary of the published reports and the identified univariable predictors of elevated cardiac enzymes postintervention are listed in Table 38.2. Identified multivariable predictors are listed by published report in Table 38.3.

Oh et al. (55) in 1985 published the first

Table 38.2.
Univariable Predictors of Elevated CK/CK-MB After Coronary Intervention

Author/Reference	Clinical Factors	Lesion Factors	Periprocedural Events
Abdelmeguid (21) (n = 4484)	None	Single discrete stenosis[a] Diffuse disease Filling defect Vein graft	Multivessel procedure DCA Higher residual stenosis Transient in-laboratory closure Side branch compromise Major dissection Hypotension requiring vasopressors ≥ 1 minor complication
Hinohara (59) (n = 174)	Age ≥ 70 Unstable angina	Nonrestenotic Acute occlusion Calcification Eccentric Diffuse disease Vessel angulation	Dissection Distal embolization ≥ 2 lesions
Kugelmass (4) (n = 565)	Increased mean age (64 ± 12 vs. 59 ± 12) Female gender	Multivessel disease Thrombus De novo lesion Calcification	DCA vs. stent
Liu (56) (n = 155)	Not analyzed	Diffuse disease of SVG Thrombus Ulceration Increased plaque volume Eccentricity	Not analyzed
Moscucci (60) (n = 664)	Not analyzed	Vein graft Multivessel disease	DCA
Oh (55) (n = 128)	Recent myocardial infarction (< 1 mo)		Chest pain ECG abnormality Side branch occlusion
Popma (58) (n = 1970)	Age Unstable angina	De novo lesion Thrombus	Unsuccessful procedure
Talasz (57) (n = 21)			Side branch occlusion

[a] Negative predictor.
DCA, directional coronary atherectomy.

Table 38.3.
Multivariable Predictors of Elevated CK/CK-MB After Coronary Intervention

Author/Reference	Clinical Factors	Lesion Factors	Periprocedural events
Abdelmeguid (21) (n = 4484)	None	Single discrete stenosis[a]	DCA $\geq$ 1 in-laboratory minor complication Side branch compromise Transient in-lab vessel closure Multivessel procedure Major dissection Residual stenosis
Liu (56) (n = 155)	Not analyzed	Increased plaque volume Diffuse disease	Not analyzed
Tardiff (61) (n = 6348)	Prior CABG Target graft lesion	None examined	None examined

[a] Negative predictor.
CABG, coronary artery bypass graft; DCA, directional coronary atherectomy.

analysis of the association between specific patient or procedural characteristics and elevated cardiac enzymes postprocedure. They followed 128 patients who had successful PTCA for stable or unstable angina. Twenty-five patients had elevated CK-MB following coronary intervention. Univariate analysis of five patient characteristics (age, gender, myocardial infarction within 1 month, prior coronary procedures, and extent of coronary disease) and 10 lesion characteristics and procedural complications (chest pain, ECG abnormalities, branch occlusion, coronary spasm, intimal tear, thrombus, coronary aneurysm, number of vessels treated, residual stenosis, and arrhythmias) showed that patients with recent infarction, chest pain, or ECG abnormalities were at an increased risk for elevation of CK-MB above the normal range following intervention.

More recently, Abdelmeguid et al. (21) published a detailed report of univariable and multivariable predictors for cardiac enzyme elevation following successful PTCA or DCA. They studied 4484 patients with normal (n = 3776) or mild elevations (n = 708) of cardiac enzymes defined as a peak CK level not greater than two times the upper limit of normal following coronary intervention. Patients with normal CK but MB greater than 4% and patients with elevated CK but less than two times normal and MB greater than 4% had significantly

worse clinical outcomes (cardiac death, myocardial infarction, or major ischemic complications) during a mean follow-up of 36 $\pm$ 22 months. They analyzed 14 baseline clinical demographic factors, 8 lesion characteristics, and 13 procedural characteristics and complications to determine predictors of elevated cardiac enzymes. No baseline characteristics differed between the groups with and without elevated CK-MB. However, differences were found in several lesion characteristics and in-laboratory complications. Patients with abnormal postprocedure cardiac enzymes less often had discrete single lesions but more diffuse disease, filling defects, vein graft lesions, or were treated with DCA. In-laboratory complications including side branch compromise, transient vessel occlusion, multivessel procedure, major dissection, transient in-laboratory closure, hypotension requiring vasopressors, or one or more minor complications were statistically more frequent in the group of patients with abnormal CK or CK-MB levels postcoronary intervention. Multivariable regression modeling showed that the independent lesion and procedure **characteristics associated with elevated CK or CK-MB were treatment with DCA, side branch compromise, transient in-laboratory closure, multivessel procedure, major dissection, higher residual stenosis, and one or more in-laboratory minor com-**

plications. Single discrete lesions were a negative predictor for elevated MB.

Liu et al. (56) also reported multivariable predictors of enzyme elevations following coronary intervention. In 155 successful saphenous vein graft balloon angioplasties, 22 procedures were associated with elevations of CK greater than two times the upper limit of normal and elevated CK-MB greater than normal. Of the eight angiographic characteristics analyzed as possible univariable predictors of elevated cardiac enzymes, diffuse disease of the vein graft, thrombus, irregular or ulcerated lesion surface, larger plaque volume, and marked eccentricity were statistically significant predictors. Multivariable regression revealed that increased plaque volume and diffuse disease were significant independent predictors of elevated cardiac enzymes. Tardiff et al. investigated demographic, clinical, and angiographic characteristics to determine preprocedural correlates with myocardial infarction (after percutaneous intervention in 6348 patients from seven clinical trials involving PTCA or DCA) (61). Previous coronary artery bypass grafting (CABG) was the most important preprocedural predictor of myocardial infarction.

Studies by Kugelmass et al. (4) and Talasz et al. (57) also reported univariable factors associated with postprocedural cardiac enzyme elevations. Kugelmass et al. investigated the incidence of CK-MB elevation in 565 consecutive patients with successful DCA. In 11.5% of patients with CK-MB elevation above the institutional upper limit of normal, univariable predictors were increased age, use of DCA compared with intracoronary stents, multivessel disease, treatment of a de novo lesion, and coronary thrombus. In patients with elevated enzymes postprocedure greater than five times the upper limit of normal, female gender and calcified lesions were more often associated with enzyme elevations. These patients were also more likely to have thrombus-containing lesions, multivessel disease, or diabetes.

Talasz et al. studied 21 patients who underwent successful PTCA. Five patients had angiographic evidence of side branch occlusion during the procedure without symptoms or ECG changes, and all five had CK-MB elevation above normal following the intervention. Only 2 of the 16 patients without side branch occlusion had elevated CK-MB.

Several investigators also published abstracts about postprocedural cardiac enzyme elevation. Hinohara et al. (59) evaluated periprocedural CK-MB elevations greater than three times the upper limit of normal in 14.7% of 1749 patients undergoing DCA to identify clinical and angiographic factors associated with these elevations. More patients aged 70 years or more or with unstable angina had increased incidence of elevated enzymes postprocedure. Patients with multiple treated lesions, calcified plaque, lesion eccentricity or angulation, diffuse disease, or non-restenotic lesions also had higher rates of enzyme elevations. Moscucci et al. (60) examined the relationship between CK and CK-MB elevation above normal in 664 nonrandomized patients following successful DCA (n = 326) or Palmaz-Schatz (Johnson and Johnson Interventional Systems, Warren, NJ) stenting (n = 338). Seventy-seven patients had CK or CK-MB elevations postprocedure. CK or CK-MB elevations were more common in patients treated with DCA than with Palmaz-Schatz stenting (17.4% versus 7.9%; $P < .01$), vein graft stenting compared with native coronary stenting (13.1 versus 4.5%; $P < .005$), and multivessel disease compared with single-vessel disease (14.9 versus 9.7%; $P < .05$).

Popma et al. (58) studied the clinical course of 1970 patients undergoing new device angioplasty (directional, rotational, or extraction atherectomy; intracoronary stenting; or excimer laser); 161 patients had postprocedure elevations of CK-MB greater than five times the upper limit of normal. Patients with postprocedure elevations were more likely to be older, have unstable angina, de novo lesions, or visible thrombus, and less likely to have a successful procedure. Patients with and without periprocedural complications (dissection, reduced flow, or abrupt closure) had similar postprocedure cardiac enzyme elevation rates. The report by Popma et al. was the only one to include patients with unsuccessful procedures.

Despite the substantial diversity of these

published reports, several consistent findings are observed. Patients with **unstable angina, female gender,** or **increased age** seem to be at a higher risk for postprocedure cardiac enzyme elevations even with successful procedures. Percutaneous intervention of **de novo or saphenous vein graft lesions** that have associated **thrombus, calcification,** or **eccentricity** are more likely to be associated with enzyme elevation. In addition, patients with **multivessel disease** are at an increased risk. Use of certain interventional devices, specifically **DCA** when compared with balloon angioplasty or intracoronary stents, has an increased incidence of enzyme elevation. Complications during coronary intervention even in asymptomatic patients appear to be associated with increased risk for CK-MB elevation postprocedure; side branch occlusion and transient vessel closure have been most commonly reported.

The patient population undergoing percutaneous intervention is heterogeneous. Identification of these clinical, angiographic, and procedural factors is important in patient risk assessment, in consideration of adjunctive therapies during coronary intervention, or in postprocedure patient management.

Specific Device Issues

Most reported clinical series have involved standard balloon angioplasty. Although a trend has been seen toward increasing the duration of balloon inflation over the last decade, relatively little information is found regarding how long a balloon can be inflated before it leads to sufficient myocardial necrosis to cause CK-MB release. The previously discussed Mager et al. (54) study concluded that balloon inflations of less than 5 minutes are unlikely to give rise to CK leaks.

As noted, the reasons for CK-MB leak after standard balloon angioplasty are related to a multitude of factors. These include side branch occlusion, distal embolization, abrupt closure, and possibly major dissection leading to reduced coronary blood flow. Thrombus appears to be a key factor in the development of distal embolization and CK-MB leak; this is probably the most important factor in elevations in CK-MB after an interventional procedure.

Approximately 20% of patients who undergo standard balloon angioplasty have an elevation in CK-MB (2). Only a small proportion, however, have large myocardial infarctions (CK-MB five or more times the upper limit of normal). That these CK-MB elevations are not isolated findings is further supported by the fact that approximately 15% of patients who undergo balloon angioplasty also develop new ECG changes afterward. The most frequently observed ischemic ECG changes include ST elevation or depression or new symmetric T-wave inversion. New Q-waves are relatively infrequent at about 2% (2).

It has been possible to perform prolonged balloon inflations without giving rise to either ECG changes or CK-MB release by using a perfusion balloon that enables the distal coronary artery bed to be perfused during inflation. Perfusion balloon ability to reduce ischemia detected by ECG changes was documented by a small series of patients who were subjected to both standard balloon angioplasty and perfusion balloon angioplasty using the individual patient as his or her own control (69). In a larger series of approximately 100 patients, all undergoing perfusion balloon angioplasty, no patient was found to have an elevation in CK-MB despite having more than 10 minutes of balloon inflation (70). These findings suggest that prolonged balloon inflation can be performed without giving rise to serious ischemia or CK-MB release if a perfusion balloon is used during the procedure.

Directional Coronary Atherectomy

Directional coronary atherectomy was developed during the late 1980s and evaluated in a number of registries where CK-MBs were not systematically measured. Subsequently, in the CAVEAT trial, patients randomized to directional atherectomy were much more likely to have a CK-MB elevation. Nearly 40% of the patients treated with directional atherectomy in the CAVEAT trial had elevated CK-MB. Of this group, 11% had myocardial infarctions with CK-MB more than five times the upper limit of normal.

Approximately 25% of patients treated with directional atherectomy also had ECG changes postprocedure. At 1-year follow-up, it became apparent that patients who had no elevation in CK-MB had low mortality (1.5%) irrespective of being treated with directional atherectomy or balloon angioplasty (65). Patients who had elevated CK-MB, on the other hand, had twice the 1-year mortality rate at 3.8% ($P < .001$). It is interesting to note that the patients randomized to directional atherectomy showed a trend toward higher mortality at 1 year.

Although subsequent trials (OARS and BOAT) have in general confirmed the presence of mild elevations in CK-MB periprocedurally, the trend toward higher adverse events in patients randomized to atherectomy has not been confirmed (71, 72). The rationale for elevations in CK-MB with atherectomy could be several-fold. First, the atherectomy device is significantly more bulky and takes a minimum of 90 to 180 seconds to make the cuts needed to obtain an enlarged lumen. This process sometimes must be repeated three to four times during the course of the procedure and, thus, the total duration of ischemia may exceed what has previously been associated with elevations in CK-MB. Second, although atherectomy specimens are compressed in the tip of the housing, small amounts of platelet or plaque drifts may escape from the housing by the sheer nature of the cutting device. Distal embolization has been described as a cause for leakage of cardiac markers after percutaneous procedures. The hypothesis of the platelet being a culprit in causing platelet activation with distal platelet emboli occurring is further supported by the finding (in patients who underwent atherectomy in the EPIC trial) that the periprocedural myocardial infarction rate was reduced in patients randomized to abciximab (Reopro Eli Lilly, Indianapolis, IN) versus placebo (73).

In an observational series by Lansky et al. from the Washington Hospital Center, the finding of a high proportion of patients with CK-MB elevation (>2× normal) was confirmed. In their series, as many as 55% of the 102 patients who had directional atherectomy had elevated CK-MB (74). This was significantly greater than among the 174 patients who had balloon angioplasty during the same period (36%, $P < .05$).

Information from the OARS and BOAT trials is important for further understanding the use of atherectomy and the role of periprocedural elevations in cardiac markers (71, 72). It is possible that recent trials have incorporated earlier experiences and that with better understanding of atherectomy device use, the rate of periprocedural myocardial infarction could be reduced. In the meantime, patients undergoing directional atherectomy should receive (Reopro) to prevent periprocedural myocardial infarction, and attention should be paid to the duration of ischemia.

Rotational Atherectomy

The first rotational atherectomy device was the transluminal extraction coronary (TEC) atherectomy device, which was developed to extract the thrombus and plaque material into the catheter by suction. By using the extraction component, it was hoped that distal embolization would be minimized. Initial experience with the device showed that myocardial infarction and CK-MB elevation were rare. More recently, a randomized trial comparing TEC atherectomy versus standard balloon angioplasty in patients with complex vein graft stenosis suggests that this device could reduce the rate of periprocedural myocardial infarction. A nonrandomized series of 124 patients has shown TEC atherectomy to be associated with less CK-MB release (CK-MB > 25 ng/mL) in degenerated saphenous vein grafts than balloon angioplasty (7 versus 22%, $P = .02$). These findings suggest that if distal embolization can be minimized CK-MB release is less likely to occur.

Rotational coronary atherectomy has been studied in one randomized trial that compared it with standard balloon angioplasty and laser angioplasty. The three treatments appeared equivalent in treating complex coronary lesions, but a trend was seen toward a higher rate of periprocedural myocardial infarction in patients treated with lasers and rotational atherectomy. At 6 months, however, less restenosis was found in patients treated with the rotational atherectomy device.

Passing the burr of the rotational atherectomy device has been well documented to be associated with a transient no-reflow phenomenon, which is probably caused by a combination of vasospasm and platelet activation. Interestingly, in the IMPACT-II trial patients who were treated with Integrilin (COR Therapeutics, South San Francisco, CA) had significantly fewer periprocedural myocardial infarctions and other complications than placebo-treated patients (77). Lansky et al. (74) documented similar proportions of patients with elevated CK-MB with rotational atherectomy compared with angioplasty in a series of 183 patients. However, another initial series showed that more than 40% of patients undergoing rotational atherectomy had prolonged episodes of ischemia with significantly higher CK-MB elevations (58). Further work is required to ascertain more clearly the risk of rotational atherectomy and CK-MB elevation.

Stents

Two stents are currently approved for use in the United States. The first was the Gianturco-Rubin stent, which was indicated for bail-out stenting (78). Not surprisingly, given this population, a high proportion of patients have had elevated CK-MB in this cohort. In a small series of 31 patients, 91% of the patients had elevated CK-MB. Unfortunately, as the indication for stent use in most of these patients was a large dissection or abrupt closure prior to stenting, we cannot ascertain the risk of periprocedural myocardial infarction in this group. Furthermore, no randomized trial has been done of this device, although an enhancement of the stent has recently been subjected to a large randomized trial. Pending the results of this study, it is assumed that at least the risk of myocardial infarction

with the Rubin stent is not different from other stents.

The second stent approved for use in the United States, the Palmaz-Schatz (Johnson and Johnson Interventional Systems, Warren, NJ) stent (79), has been evaluated in two large randomized trials (66, 75, 76). Rate of myocardial infarction was similar in patients assigned to either coronary stenting or standard balloon angioplasty. No information from these trials has been published regarding CK-MB release. In a large series from the Washington Hospital Center of 320 patients, those treated with stents had a similar rate of CK-MB release as those treated with standard balloon angioplasty (74).

Several mechanisms possibly release CK-MB after coronary stenting. First is distal embolization of platelets and thrombi such as occurs with standard balloon angioplasty. Currently a randomized trial is evaluating stenting with and without Reopro to determine whether platelet embolization can be reduced by Reopro in this patient population. A second possible mechanism is inadvertent occlusion of side branches by the stent during the procedure. Although many of these occlusions open over time, flow is sluggish for a protracted period. This phenomenon has also been well described in patients undergoing standard coronary angioplasty. Talasz et al. showed that CK-MB elevation was noted in all five patients in this series with side branch occlusion (57).

Miscellaneous Devices

Limited information is found regarding CK-MB release after laser balloon angioplasty. As this device is now mostly indicated for total occlusion, it is particularly difficult to study this phenomenon. Patients with total occlusions require prolonged or multiple ablative procedures to restore vessel flow. No comprehensive analysis has been made of CK-MB release in such a population.

The PASSUS device is an embolectomy device that is being developed for lesions with thrombus in them. The device is currently being compared with urokinase to treat thrombi. Limited data from outside the

United States have indicated that this device can dissolve clots, but some evidence is found of distal embolization. The VeGAS trial is currently being conducted in the United States to further explore the value of this device. Other ablative devices for thrombi include some using ultrasound. The Angiosonics ablative device, for example, has been studied in a small number of patients with acute myocardial infarction in Israel, and further studies are underway in patients with thrombus without myocardial infarction.

To date the only atherectomy device that has been found to reduce the rate of CK-MB release is the extraction catheter that applies vacuum suction in the coronary vessel during the procedure. Other atherectomy devices have been associated with either a further increase in the incidence of CK-MB release or a neutral effect compared with balloon angioplasty. Coronary stents are probably similar in their degree of CK-MB release to standard balloon angioplasty, but more studies are required, particularly with regard to side branch occlusion and its long-term significance. Overall, **when devices have been combined with potent anti-platelet therapies, myocardial infarction rate has been reduced**. This suggests a synergism between these therapies and new devices. Further studies in the future should help to clarify this issue further (74).

POTENTIAL MECHANISMS OF MYOCARDIAL DAMAGE ASSOCIATED WITH CORONARY INTERVENTIONS

The mechanism leading to release of CK-MB and myocardial necrosis after coronary interventions is complex. It involves consideration of the diffuse nature of the disease, clinical instability, and hemodynamic factors during the procedure. The relative merit of these different aspects has not been fully elucidated. It is clear that the clinical instability with thrombus formation and platelet activation is probably one of the key factors, whereas the other two add potential risk to an individual patient but are not the main culprit.

In a study of 102 patients without a history of myocardial infarction and with stable coronary artery disease who were undergoing single vessel angioplasty, the role of cyclic flow variation was studied. A Doppler flow guidewire was inserted distal to the stenosis to monitor flow velocity after PTCA continuously for 15 minutes. In most patients (92%), a stable signal could be recorded for 15 minutes after the procedure. In four patients, however, cyclic flow variation was noted, suggesting microplatelet aggregate formation. Interestingly, in three of these four patients, intracoronary thrombosis or acute occlusion occurred shortly after the end of measurements. These findings point to the central role of platelet aggregation being the main culprit for periprocedural complications and possibly CK-MB elevation after what is felt to be otherwise uncomplicated procedures (80).

Activated platelet hypothesis is furthermore supported by the dramatic fall in periprocedural myocardial infarction rates in the trials that have examined new antiplatelet therapies. The **platelet activation** theory is also one of the main reasons for **distal embolization** that has been well described in saphenous vein grafts (81, 82). An interesting observational series by Muhlestein et al. (70) has suggested that thrombus formation seen in coronary arteries can be reversed by immediate administration of Reopro with clot resolution. This highlights the powerful role of platelet activation in this field.

Although it is poorly understood why CK-MB leaks occur in patients without any obvious signs of embolization or clinical events, patients with diffuse coronary artery disease are probably at higher risk for CK-MB leak. The mechanism for CK-MB release in these patients is probably related to intermittent cessation of flow to watershed areas in which ischemia at the time of the procedure leads to infarction. In the study by Kong et al., ejection fraction was an important predictor of CK-MB release, and it is also a well-established independent predictor of long-term survival (6). The additional insult of further myocardial injury in the watershed area probably heightens or further worsens prognosis in this patient population. In the future, therapies need to be developed that can prevent these infarctions from watershed areas. These findings suggest that careful attention to hemodynamic status is of paramount importance during the procedures. Interestingly, studies examining the rate of periprocedural myocardial infarction after emergency CABG following failed angioplasty have suggested that when the hemodynamic status is optimized by using an intra-aortic balloon pump, the rate of periprocedural myocardial infarction can be reduced (83). These findings indirectly support the **watershed theory** and could serve as an avenue for further research.

THERAPEUTIC APPROACHES TO LIMITING MYONECROSIS

Although the mechanism for myonecrosis following percutaneous intervention has not been definitively established, in-laboratory complications such as side branch occlusion, distal embolization, abrupt closure, and reduced thrombolysis in myocardial infarction (TIMI) grade may be responsible for myocardial damage. Limiting these complications may therefore be of benefit in decreasing postintervention enzyme elevations and the corresponding worse clinical outcomes.

Lefkovitz et al. (73) reported that patients who underwent directional coronary atherectomy and were treated with a bolus and infusion of Reopro had a decreased incidence of postprocedure non–Q-wave myocardial infarction compared with patients treated with placebo (4.5% versus 15.4%; $P < .046$). A similar trend was seen in patients treated with PTCA, but the magnitude of the benefit was less given the lower rates of non–Q-wave infarction following PTCA compared with DCA. Similarly, Blankenship et al. (84) reported that patients treated with Integrilin compared with patients treated with placebo in the IMPACT-II trial had a lower rate of in-laboratory complications (a composite of side branch occlusion, distal embolization, abrupt closure, and coronary flow less than TIMI grade 3) (29.1% versus 34.2%; $P < .05$).

In addition, the incidence of postprocedural CK-MB elevation in patients with periprocedural complications was lower in patients treated with Integrilin than in patients treated with placebo (35.0 versus 42%; $P < .012$).

Rupprecht et al. (85) studied patients with unstable angina undergoing PTCA. Patients were randomized to receive intravenous recombinant hirudin, a direct novel thrombin inhibitor, or heparin immediately prior to the procedure. Patients on intravenous heparin prior to randomization had the infusion discontinued. Troponin T elevation following coronary intervention was lower in patients treated with hirudin than in patients treated with heparin (24 versus 58%; $P = .01$). Another potential approach beyond thrombin and platelet inhibition is one that would improve distal coronary blood flow during intracoronary manipulations. Muhlestein et al. (70) studied the safety of prolonged (mean 14 ± 4 minutes) perfusion balloon inflation in 62 consecutive patients undergoing percutaneous coronary intervention. No patients had elevated enzymes or ECG evidence of infarction or ischemia. New devices may incorporate design features that would allow increased distal perfusion during coronary intervention.

These data suggest that aggressive prevention of platelet aggregation or thrombosis may substantially decrease postprocedural enzyme elevations. As clinical trials of new adjunctive pharmacologic therapies or interventional devices are considered, it is important that measurement of postprocedural cardiac enzymes be prospectively planned.

SUMMARY: IMPLICATIONS IN TERMS OF PATIENT MANAGEMENT AND FUTURE RESEARCH

Even when not associated with procedural complications, periprocedural infarctions entail increased risk and poorer outcome. Multiple studies in varying populations and from different investigative groups have noted a relationship between postprocedural enzyme elevations and risk of adverse outcomes. These abnormal elevations of cardiac-specific enzymes occurring with interventional procedures must be interpreted as microinfarctions and should be further examined as significant events in patients undergoing percutaneous revascularizations.

Unfortunately, no universally accepted and applied diagnostic criterion has been determined to detect infarction at the time of intervention. Substantial variations in the methods used for diagnosing periprocedural infarctions and a lack of uniformity in terms of follow-up leaves many issues unresolved, particularly with respect to the newer biochemical markers.

Relationship between postintervention microinfarctions and adverse subsequent outcomes has not been fully settled. It is not clear whether it is myocardial necrosis or severity of the patient's underlying illness that is responsible for the associated risk. Although several investigators have been unable to demonstrate that the prognostic import of elevated enzymes is explained by greater underlying disease, these analyses may not have included complete consideration of important coronary morphology. A need exists for more data including long-term patient follow-up to clarify this relationship.

Interpretation of periprocedural enzymes is complex for patients with evolving infarctions and elevated enzymes at the time of intervention. A gradient of risk is suggested by current data, with minimal risk for slight elevations and the highest risk and poorest outcomes for events involving injury to a large amount of myocardium as suggested by higher levels of enzyme elevation; but, the explanation may be more complex for patients with recent infarctions.

It is also not entirely clear whether all interventional devices are equal with regard to the interpretation of periprocedural microinfarctions. Although available data suggest that the overall implication of enzyme elevations occurring after procedures is the same regardless of the device used, the relationship between magnitude of elevation and prognostic impact may not be consistent. In any case, it is clear that prospective evaluation of new treatment strategies and new devices should include an assessment of the frequency of periprocedural microinfarction as well as extended follow-up to document the effect on morbidity and mortality.

Despite these limitations and given the consistency of current data, clinical care of patients undergoing intervention should include routine measurement of CK and CK-MB and a preprocedural and postprocedural ECG. A reasonable schedule for the enzymatic assays is baseline and 8 and 16 hours after the procedure (85). Patients who have an elevation in cardiac markers of greater than the upper limit of normal who also have periprocedural complications (such as abrupt closure or distal embolization) should probably be closely observed in an inpatient setting for 2 to 3 days after the procedure, similar to patients with an uncomplicated non–Q-wave myocardial infarction. Standard therapies such as beta-blockers, nitrates, and aspirin should be administered after an infarction. These precautions are particularly indicated in patients with higher elevations, greater than threefold the upper limit of normal. Patients who have a transient elevation of cardiac markers but no defined clinical events and an excellent angiographic result could be discharged 1 to 2 days after the procedure with standard postinfarction therapies. In all patients with peri-interventional infarctions, there should be heightened awareness of the poor long-term prognosis. Careful monitoring during the first few years after the procedure is a prudent approach, although additional studies are necessary to establish whether any specific strategy can alter long-term prognosis.

Prevention of periprocedural myocardial infarctions should be consciously pursued. This includes avoiding use of devices known to cause elevation in cardiac markers except for patients who cannot be treated otherwise. Antiplatelet agents, which have been shown to reduce the incidence of recurrent acute coronary events, including the newer more potent IIb/IIIa inhibitors such as Reopro, should be given to all appropriate patients. Optimization of antithrombotic therapy via careful monitoring of activated clotting time and heparin dosing is critical and may be of benefit with use of the more potent antiplatelet drugs.

Further investigation should focus on the development of new devices and therapies that can reduce the rate of myocardial infarction. Such advances will enhance the options for treating patients with ischemic heart disease and improve their overall outcome.

References

1. Detre KM, Holmes DR Jr., Holubkov R, et al. Incidence and consequences of periprocedural occlusion. The 1985–1986 National Heart, Lung, and Blood Institute Percutaneous Transluminal Coronary Angioplasty Registry. Circulation. 1990;82: 739–750.

2. Harrington RA, Lincoff AM, Califf RM, et al. Characteristics and consequences of myocardial infarction after percutaneous coronary intervention: insights from the Coronary Angioplasty Versus Excisional Atherectomy Trial (CAVEAT). J Am Coll Cardiol 1995;25:1693–1699.

3. Klein LW, Kramer BL, Howard E, et al. Incidence and clinical significance of transient creatine kinase elevations and the diagnosis of non-Q wave myocardial infarction associated with coronary angioplasty. J Am Coll Cardiol 1991;17:621–626.

4. Kugelmass AD, Cohen DJ, Moscucci M, et al. Elevation of the creatine kinase myocardial isoform following otherwise successful directional coronary atherectomy and stenting. Am J Cardiol 1994; 74:748–754.

5. Abdelmeguid AE, Whitlow PL, Sapp SK, et al. Long-term outcome of transient, uncomplicated in-laboratory coronary artery closure. Circulation. 1995;91:2733–2741.

6. Kong TQ, Davidson CJ, Meyers SN, et al. Prognostic implication of creatine kinase elevation following elective coronary artery interventions. JAMA 1997;277(6):461–466.

7. Oldham HN, Kong Y, Bartel AG, et al. Risk factors in coronary artery bypass surgery. Arch Surg 1972; 105:918–923.

8. Warren SG, Wagner GS, Bethea CF, et al. Diagnostic and prognostic significance of electrocardiographic and CPK isoenzyme changes following coronary bypass surgery: correlation with findings at one year. Am Heart J 1977;93:189–196.

9. Rucker CM, Dugall JC, Ganter EL, et al. The detection of perioperative myocardial infarction in aortocoronary bypass surgery. Chest 1979;75:300.

10. Santana JO, Haft JI, LaMarche NS, et al. Coronary angioplasty in patients eighty years of age or older. Am Heart J 1992;124:13–18.

11. Pauletto P, Piccolo D, Scannapieco G, et al. Changes in myoglobin, creatine kinase and creatine kinase-MB after percutaneous transluminal coronary angioplasty for stable angina pectoris. Am J Cardiol 1987;59:999–1000.

12. Redwood SR, Popma JJ, Kent KM, et al. Predictors of late mortality following ablative new-device angioplasty in native coronary arteries [Abstract]. J Am Coll Cardiol 1996;27(Suppl A):167A–168A.

13. Tardiff BE, Granger CB, Woodlief L, et al. Prognostic significance of post-intervention isozyme elevations [Abstract]. Circulation 1995;92(Suppl I):I-544.

14. Joint International Society and Federation of Cardiology/World Health Organization Task Force. Nomenclature and criteria for diagnosis of ischemic heart disease. Circulation 1979;59:607–609.

15. Nicod P, Gilpin E, Dittrich H, et al. Short- and long-term clinical outcome after Q wave and non-Q wave myocardial infarction in a large patient population. Circulation 1989;79:528–536.

16. White RD, Grande P, Califf L, et al. Diagnostic and prognostic significance of minimally elevated creatine kinase-MB in suspected acute myocardial infarction. Am J Cardiol 1985;55:1478–1484.

17. Madias JE, Gorlin R. The myth of acute "mild" myocardial infarction. Ann Intern Med 1977;86: 347–352.

18. Roberts AJ, Combes JR, Jacobstein JG, et al. Perioperative myocardial infarction associated with coronary artery bypass graft surgery: improved sensitivity in the diagnosis within 6 hours after operation with 99m Tc-glucoheptonate myocardial imaging and myocardial-specific isoenzymes. Ann Thorac Surg 1979;27:42–48.

19. McGregor CG, Muir AL, Smith AF, et al. Myocardial infarction related to coronary artery bypass graft surgery. Br Heart J 1984;51:399–406.

20. Van Lente F, Martin A, Ratliff NB, et al. The predictive value of serum enzymes for perioperative myocardial infarction after cardiac operations. An autopsy study. J Thorac Cardiovasc Surg 1989;98: 704–710.

21. Abdelmeguid AE, Topol EJ, Whitlow PL, et al. Significance of mild transient release of creatine kinase-MB fraction after percutaneous coronary interventions. Circulation 1996;94:1528–1536.

22. Jaffe AS, Serota H, Grace A, et al. Diagnostic changes in plasma creatine kinase isoforms early after the onset of acute myocardial infarction. Circulation 1986;74:105–109.

23. Tardiff BE, Califf RM, Tcheng JE, et al. Post-intervention cardiac enzyme elevations: prognostic significance in IMPACT II [Abstract]. J Am Coll Cardiol 1996;27(Suppl A):A-83A.

24. Tunstall-Pedoe H, Kuulasmaa K, Amouyel P, et al. Myocardial infarction and coronary deaths in the world health organization MONICA project: registration procedures, event rates, and case-fatality rates in 38 populations from 21 countries in four continents. Circulation 1994;90:583–612.

25. Rautaharju PM, Calhoun HP, Chaitman BR. NOVACODE serial ECG classification system for clinical trials and epidemiologic studies. J Electrocardiol 1992;24:179–187.

26. Crow RS, Prineas RJ, Jacobs DR, et al. A new epidemiologic classification system for interim myocardial infarction from serial electrocardiographic changes. Am J Cardiol 1989;64:454–461.

27. Chaitman BR, Jaffe AS. What is the true peri-procedure myocardial infarction rate? Does anyone know for sure? The need for clarification. Circulation 1995;91:1609–1610.

28. Ambrose JA, Almeida OD, Sharma SK, et al. Adjunctive thrombolytic therapy during angioplasty for ischemic rest angina: results of the TAUSA trial. Circulation 1994;90:69–77.

29. Sutton JM, Ellis SG, Roubin GS, et al., for the Gianturco-Roubin Intracoronary Stent Investigator Group. Major clinical events after coronary stenting: the multicenter registry of acute and elective Gianturco-Roubin stent placement. Circulation. 1994;89:1126–1137.

30. Bittl JA, Sanborn TA, Tcheng JE, et al., for the Percutaneous Excimer Laser Coronary Angioplasty Registry. Clinical success, complications and restenosis rates with excimer laser coronary angioplasty. Am J Cardiol 1992;70:1533–1539.

31. Kahn JK, Rutherford BD, McConahay DR, et al. Outcome following emergency coronary artery bypass grafting for failed elective balloon coronary angioplasty in patients with prior coronary bypass. Am J Cardiol 1990;66:285–288.

32. Califf RM, Harrell FE, Jr., Lee KL, et al. The evolution of medical and surgical therapy for coronary artery disease. A 15-year perspective. JAMA 1989; 261:2077–2086.

33. Maleki M, Manley JC. Venospastic phenomena of saphenous vein bypass grafts: possible causes for unexplained postoperative recurrence of angina or early or late occlusion of vein bypass grafts. Br Heart J 1989;62:57–60.

34. von Hodenberg E, Kreuzer J, Hautmann M, et al. Effects of lipoprotein (a) on success rate of thrombolytic therapy in acute myocardial infarction. Am J Cardiol 1991;67:1349–1353.

35. Brophy JM, Joseph L. Placing trials in context using bayesian analysis: GUSTO revisited by Reverend Bayes. JAMA 1995;273:871–875.

36. Hiyoshi Y, Omae T, Hirota Y, et al. Clinicopathological study of the heart and coronary arteries of autopsied cases from the community of Hisayama during a 10-year period. Part V. Comparison of autopsy findings with electrocardiograms—Q.QS items of the Minnesota Code. Am J Epidemiol 1985; 121:906–913.

37. Uusitupa M, Pyorala K, Raunio H, et al. Sensitivity and specificity of Minnesota Code Q-QS abnormalities in the diagnosis of myocardial infarction verified at autopsy. Am Heart J 1983;106:753–757.

38. Pahlm US, Chaitman BR, Rautaharaju PM, et al. Comparison of various electrocardiographic methods for estimating myocardial infarct size [Abstract]. Circulation. 1996;94 (Suppl I):I-371.

39. Karnegis JN, Matts J, Tuna N. Development and evolution of electrocardiographic Minnesota Q-QS codes in patients with acute myocardial infarction. Am Heart J 1985;110:452–459.

40. Ohman EM, Casey C, Bengtson JR, et al. Early detection of acute myocardial infarction: additional diagnostic information by serum myoglobin in patients without ST elevation. Br Heart J 1990;63: 335–338.

41. Katus HA, Remppis A, Scheffold T, et al. Intracellular compartmentation of cardiac troponin T and its release kinetics in patients with reperfused and nonreperfused myocardial infarction. Am J Cardiol 1991;67:1360–1367.

42. Adams JE, Abendschein DR, Jaffe AS. Biochemical markers of myocardial injury: is MB creatine kinase the choice for the 1990s. Circulation 1993;88: 750–763.

43. Katus HA, Remppis A, Neumann FJ, et al. Diagnostic efficiency of troponin T measurements in acute myocardial infarction. Circulation 1991;83: 902–912.

44. Ohman EM, Armstrong PW, Christenson RH, et al. Cardiac troponin T levels for risk stratification in acute myocardial ischemia. N Engl J Med 1996; 335:1333–1341.

45. Karim MA, Shinn M, Oskarsson H, et al. Significance of cardiac troponin T release after percutaneous transluminal coronary angioplasty. Am J Cardiol 1995;76:521–523.

46. Hunt AC, Chow SL, Shiu MF, et al. Release of creatine kinase-MB and cardiac specific troponin-I following percutaneous transluminal coronary angioplasty. Eur Heart J 1991;12:690–693.

47. Rupprecht HJ, Terres W, Ozbek C, et al. Recombinant hirudin (HBW 023) prevents troponin-T release after coronary angioplasty. J Am Coll Cardiol 1995;26:1637–1642.

48. Hearse DJ, Humphrey SM. Enzyme release during myocardial anoxia: a study of metabolic protection. J Mol Cell Cardiol 1975;7:463–482.

49. Neubauer S, Hamman BL, Perry SB, et al. Velocity of the creatine kinase reaction decreases in postischemic myocardium: a 31P-NMR magnetization transfer study of the isolated ferret heart. Circ Res 1988;63:1–15.

50. Siegel RJ, Said JW, Shell WE, et al. Identification and localization of creatine kinase B and M in normal, ischemic and necrotic myocardium. An immunohistochemical study. J Mol Cell Cardiol 1984; 16:95–103.

51. Heyndrickx GR, Amano J, Kenna T, et al. Creatine kinase release not associated with myocardial necrosis after short periods of coronary artery occlusion in conscious baboons. J Am Coll Cardiol 1985; 6:1299–1303.

52. Fishbein MC. Creatine kinase release after brief coronary occlusion. J Am Coll Cardiol 1985;6: 1304–1305.

53. Piper HM, Schwartz P, Spahr R, et al. Early enzyme release from myocardial cells is not due to irreversible cell damage. J Mol Cell Cardiol 1984;16: 385–388.

54. Mager A, Sclarovsky S, Wurtzel M, et al. Ischemia and reperfusion during intermittent coronary occlusion in man: studies of electrocardiographic changes and CPK release. Chest 1991;99:386–392.

55. Oh JK, Shub C, Ilstrup DM, et al. Creatine kinase release after successful percutaneous transluminal coronary angioplasty. Am Heart J 1985;109: 1225–1231.

56. Liu MW, Douglas JS, Jr., Lembo NJ, et al. Angiographic predictors of a rise in serum creatine kinase (distal embolization) after balloon angioplasty of saphenous vein coronary artery bypass grafts. Am J Cardiol 1993;72:514–517.

57. Talasz H, Genser N, Mair J, et al. Side-branch occlu-

sion during percutaneous transluminal coronary angioplasty. Lancet 1992;339:1380–1382.

58. Popma JJ, Merritt AJ, Altmann DB, et al. Clinical importance of non-Q-wave myocardial infarction after new device angioplasty [Abstract]. Circulation 1993;88:I-578.

59. Hinohara T, Vetter JW, Robertson GC, et al. CK MB elevation following directional coronary atherectomy [Abstract]. Circulation 1995;92 (Suppl I):I-544–545.

60. Moscucci M, Cohen DJ, Kugelmass AD, et al. Should small (non-Q wave) myocardial infarctions be considered "major" or "minor" complications after otherwise successful stenting or atherectomy [Abstract]. Circulation 1993;88:I-548

61. Tardiff BE, Mabe B, Wildermann N, et al. Predictors of myocardial infarction (MI) with percutaneous revascularization in a large multicenter population [Abstract]. J Am Coll Cardiol 1997;29 (Suppl A):277A–278A.

62. Abdelmeguid AE, Ellis SG, Sapp SK, et al. Defining the appropriate threshold of creatine kinase elevation after percutaneous coronary interventions. Am Heart J 1996;131:1097–1105.

63. Redwood SR, Popma JJ, Kent KM, et al. "Minor" CPK-MB elevations are associated with increased late mortality following ablative new-device angioplasty in native coronary arteries [Abstract]. Circulation 1995;92 (Suppl I):I-544.

64. Kong TQJ, Davidson CJ, Meyers SN, et al. Prognostic implication of creatine kinase elevation following elective coronary artery interventions. JAMA 1997;277:461–466.

65. Elliott JM, Berdan LG, Holmes DR, et al. One-year follow-up in the coronary angioplasty versus excisional atherectomy trial (CAVEAT I). Circulation 1995;91:2158–2166.

66. Serruys PW, de Jaegere P, Kiemeneij F, et al. A comparison of balloon-expandable-stent implantation with balloon angioplasty in patients with coronary artery disease. N Engl J Med 1994;331: 489–495.

67. Cohen DJ, Krumholz HM, Sukin CA, et al. In-hospital and one-year economic outcomes after coronary stenting or balloon angioplasty: results from a randomized clinical trial. Circulation 1995;92: 2480–2487.

68. Roubin GS, Cannon AD, Agrawal SK, et al. Intracoronary stenting for acute and threatened closure complicating percutaneous transluminal coronary angioplasty. Circulation 1992;85:916–927.

69. Quigley PJ, Hinohara T, Phillips HR, et al. Myocardial protection during coronary angioplasty with an autoperfusion balloon catheter in humans. Circulation 1988;78:1128–1134.

70. Muhlestein JB, Quigley PJ, Ohman EM, et al. Prospective analysis of possible myocardial damage or hemolysis occurring as a result of prolonged autoperfusion angioplasty in humans. J Am Coll Cardiol 1992;20:594–598.

71. Baim DS, Cutlip D, Ho KKL, et al. Acute results of directional coronary atherectomy in the balloon versus optimal atherectomy trial (BOAT) pilot phase. Coron Artery Dis 1996;7:290–293.

72. Dussaillant GR, Mintz GS, Popma JJ, et al. Intravascular ultrasound, directional coronary atherectomy, and the Optimal Atherectomy Restenosis Study (OARS). Coronary Artery Dis 1996;7(4): 294–298.

73. Lefkovits J, Blankenship JC, Anderson KM, et al. Increased risk of non-q wave myocardial infarction after directional atherectomy is platelet dependent: evidence from the EPIC trial. J Am Coll Cardiol 1996;28:849–855.

74. Lansky AJ, Popma JJ, Mintz GS, et al. Frequency and prognostic importance of creatine phosphokinase myocardial isoforms after successful balloon and new device coronary angioplasty. J Invas Cardiol 1996;8:3C–9C.

75. Fischmann DL, Leon MB, Baim DS, et al. A randomized comparison of coronary-stent placement and balloon angioplasty in the treatment of coronary artery disease. N Engl J Med 1994;331: 489–495.

76. Macaya C, Serruys PW, Ruygrok P, et al. Continued benefit of coronary stenting versus balloon angioplasty: one year follow-up of BENSTENT trial. J Am Coll Cardiol 1996;27:255–261.

77. Randomised placebo-controlled trial of effect of eptifibatide on complications of percutaneous coronary interventions: IMPACT-II. Integrilin to minimise platelet aggregation and coronary thrombosis-II. Lancet 1997;349(9063):1422–1428.

78. Roubin GS, Robinson KA, King SB, et al. Early and late results of intracoronary arterial stenting after coronary angioplasty in dogs. Circulation 1987;76: 891–897.

79. Schatz RA, Baim DS, Leon M, et al. Clinical experience with the Palmaz-Schatz coronary stent: initial results of a multicenter study. Circulation 1991;83: 148–161.

80. Sunamura M, Di Mario C, Piek JJ, et al. Cyclic flow variations after angioplasty: a rare phenomenon predictive of immediate complications. Am Heart J 1996;131:843–848.

81. Gurbel PA, Davidson CJ, Ohman EM, et al. Selective infusion of thrombolytic therapy in the acute myocardial infarct-related coronary artery as an alternative to rescue percutaneous transluminal coronary angioplasty. Am J Cardiol 1990;66: 1021–1023.

82. Lefkovits J, Holmes DR, Califf RM, et al. Predictors and sequelae of distal embolization during saphenous vein graft intervention from the CAVEAT-II trial. Coronary Angioplasty versus Excisional Atherectomy Trial. Circulation 1995;92(4):734–740.

83. Armstrong B, Zidar JP, Ohman EM. The use of intraaortic balloon counterpulsation in acute myocardial infarction and high risk coronary angioplasty. J Intervent Cardiol 1995;8:185–191.

84. Blankenship JC, Sigmon KN, Tardiff BE, et al., for the IMPACT II E. Investigators. Effect of glycoprotein IIb/IIIa receptor inhibition on specific in-lab complications of coronary intervention and resultant CKMB elevation in the IMPACT II trial [Abstract]. Circulation 1996;94 (Suppl I):I-198.

85. Califf RM, Abdelmeguid AE, Kuntz R, et al. Myonecrosis after revascularization procedures. J Am Coll Cardiol 1998;31.

39

Economic Issues Related to Diagnosis and Therapy in Coronary Heart Disease

Eric L. Eisenstein, DBA
Daniel B. Mark, MD, MPH

INTRODUCTION

When Werner Forssmann performed the first human heart catheterization as a 25-year-old surgical resident, he undoubtedly had little expectation that this self-experiment would spawn a multibillion dollar industry (1). However, by 1993 more than a million diagnostic catheterizations were being performed annually in the United States (2) at an estimated cost of $2.1 billion (3)—nearly 0.5% of all US health care expenditures (4). The greatest growth in diagnostic catheterization use occurred in the decade between 1979 and 1989 as the annual number in the United States grew from 300,000 to 1,000,000 procedures (2), and, although the use of diagnostic catheterization began to level-off in 1990, coronary artery disease (CAD) revascularization increased to nearly 400,000 percutaneous transluminal coronary angioplasty procedures (PTCA) and 500,000 coronary artery bypass graft (CABG) procedures by 1993 (1).

The early growth of invasive cardiology in the 1960s and 1970s was facilitated both by a series of technologic innovations (5–7) and by the enactment of Medicare legislation, which provided medical insurance for the elderly and created a demand for these services. By the early 1980s this highly favorable economic situation began to change. Medicare's annual expenditures grew to $36 billion in 1983 (8) when the federal government implemented its Medicare diagnosis related group (DRG) prospective payment system to contain costs by encouraging hospitals to perform fewer services and to reduce inefficiencies in operations (9). Private insurers also responded to rising health care costs by implementing a variety of containment measures including DRG reimbursement, competitive bidding, and alternate payment mechanisms (e.g., preferred provider organizations [PPOs] and capitation). These **changes in reimbursement continue to shift financial responsibility from payers to providers**, many of whom have found that their reimbursements do not cover their expenses (10, 11). In the 1990s, influential health care policy makers have concluded that interventional cardiology is facing a maturing market for its services in a society overburdened with health care expenses. Thus, they predict that in the future competitive pricing and cost management (rather than technologic innovation) will be the primary determinants of most successful interventional cardiology programs (12).

Given the present cost-conscious health

care environment, it is essential that cardiologists understand the economics of CAD as thoroughly as they understand its pathophysiology. Unfortunately, few cardiology training programs give adequate attention to clinical economics. This chapter provides an overview of clinical economics as applied to diagnostic and interventional cardiology. In particular, we review the major concepts and terminology of clinical economics, describe the different types of economic analyses, and demonstrate how these concepts and methods have been used to assess the costs and cost-effectiveness of the primary CAD interventional procedures (angiography, PTCA, and CABG). We also review recent studies on the costs and cost-effectiveness of newer devices (e.g., stenting and atherectomy) and newer pharmacologic agents (e.g., platelet inhibitors and low molecular weight heparin).

ECONOMIC CONCEPTS

Outcomes

Medical care has both clinical and economic outcomes (13, 14). Clinical outcomes are a measure of the effectiveness of medical care (e.g., lives saved per hundred patients treated), whereas economic outcomes address its value (e.g., cost per year of life saved). These outcomes differ in that clinical outcomes are almost always assessed from the patient's perspective, whereas economic outcomes may be assessed from multiple perspectives (i.e., patient, provider, payer, or society), which often assign different values to the same medical service (15). For example, the wages a patient loses during a hospitalization for diagnostic catheterization are costs for the patient and society but not for the provider or payer.

Costs, Charges, and Reimbursement

The terms "cost" and "charge" are frequently used interchangeably in the medi-

cal literature (16–18); however, each has a distinct meaning (13). Cost is the amount of money a provider expends to provide a good or service to a patient; charge is that good or service's price to a payer; and reimbursement is the amount the provider actually receives from the payer for the good or service. Usually, a product's cost to a provider is less than what will be billed to a payer (which, in turn, may be different from the amount the payer reimburses the provider).

Cost Typologies

Accountants have developed cost classification systems for use in different types of analyses. Marginal analysis studies relationships between changes in patient volume and changes in costs (19). Costs varying in direct proportion with unit changes in patient volume are termed **variable costs** (e.g., contrast medium or catheters), whereas costs not varying with changes in patient volume are termed **fixed costs** (e.g., equipment and facilities). Fixed costs are always defined for a specific capacity (e.g., maximum of four coronary angiography procedures per day in a catheterization laboratory suite) because all costs become variable with extreme changes in patient volume when additional equipment and facilities are required. The two hybrid cost categories are **semivariable** (or **mixed**) **costs,** which have both fixed and variable components (e.g., utilities with a fixed connection fee and a variable fee based on usage volume), and **semifixed** (or **stepfixed**) **costs,** which vary in a stepwise manner as patient volume changes (e.g., nursing unit supervisory time, which varies with the number of nursing units that are open).

A second type of analysis is product costing, which seeks to determine all of the costs involved in producing and distributing a good or service (e.g., coronary angiography, PTCA,, or CABG). In this analysis, **direct costs** (e.g., technician time and contrast medium) are clearly and directly associated with specific patients, whereas **indirect costs** (e.g., clerical time and computer equipment used to schedule procedures) are not (19). Indirect costs may originate within the catheterization laboratory or within other cost centers providing services to the catheterization laboratory (e.g., the hospital laundry, human resources, and hospital administration). Because these costs are not directly traceable to patients, formulas are used to allocate a portion of the indirect costs to specific patients so that unit costs (total cost per patient) can be calculated. In today's catheterization laboratory, indirect costs often constitute 30 to 50% of the total costs of care. Because the accuracy of indirect cost allocation techniques can have a dramatic impact on a catheterization laboratory's profitability, many health care organizations are beginning to implement activity-based cost accounting systems that offer better means for measuring and allocating indirect costs (20–22).

Economists define three types of health care costs: medical, patient, and nonmedical (23). Medical costs are associated with the actions of health care providers, whereas patient and nonmedical costs are incurred by the patient and other nonmedical personnel (e.g., value of a patient's time waiting for and receiving treatment, or family members' time caring for patients recuperating from CABG surgery) (23). Although the recent US Public Health Service standards recommend including all three cost types in a cost-effectiveness analysis (23), patient and nonmedical costs are rarely included in economic analyses of interventional cardiology procedures because they are difficult to identify and measure.

Cost Calculation Methods

The results of an economic analysis are sensitive to the methods used in identifying and measuring costs of care (24). Although short-hand methods to estimate the total costs of care using patient characteristics and DRG payments have been proposed (25), they are not recommended because they estimate generic costs and not the costs of specific providers and patients. The two methods normally recommended for estimating costs are called **"bottom-up"** (or

micro) and **"top-down"** costing. Bottom-up costing uses industrial engineering techniques to estimate the cost of each resource used in treating a patient whereas the top-down method estimates costs from line-item charges on patient bills. An 18-hospital study of 40 DRGs, representing 75% of Medicare charges, found that average case costs calculated using the top-down method were only 4.4% greater than those calculated using the bottom-up method (26). However, variances were greater for specific DRGs with the top-down method overestimating DRG 106 (CABG with cardiac catheterization) costs by 14.7% and underestimating DRG 122 (circulatory disorders, with acute myocardial infarction [AMI] and cardiovascular complication, discharged alive) costs by 8.2%. Another study compared top-down with bottom-up costing for PTCA and CABG patients in a single institution and found that average case costs were approximately the same (27). Because of the small differences reported in both of these studies, **the top-down and bottom-up methods may be considered comparable.**

The top down ratio of cost:charges (RCC) method is preferred for multicenter cost analyses because it is a single methodology that can be used in any non-Veterans Administration or military hospital in the United States (14). The RCC method uses two standardized inputs that have been defined by the Health Care Finance Administration (HCFA): the Medicare Cost Report and the Uniform Billing Form of 1992 (UB-92). Each hospital annually submits a Medicare Cost Report detailing the relationship between its charges and its costs. The departmental RCC in this report may be used to convert line-item charges on the UB-92 bill into line-item cost estimates. Inpatient RCC are in Worksheet C, Part I of the Medicare Cost Report. Unfortunately, no universally applicable top-down methods are found for converting physician fees into costs. Thus, if a bottom-up cost accounting system that uses industrial engineering techniques to estimate physician costs exists in an organization, these estimates should be used in economic analyses. Otherwise, state-specific Medicare Fee Schedules, which use a standardized resource-based costing methodology, can be used as estimates of physician costs.

Marginal and Incremental Costs

The costing methods described compute average costs for patient care. However, decision makers more often want to know the costs for treating a single patient or the costs of moving a group of patients from one management strategy to another. Economists define **marginal cost**, the cost of treating one more (or less) patient, as the variable costs of care plus any fixed costs incurred because equipment and facilities capacities have been exceeded (19). Similarly, economists define **incremental cost**, the cost of shifting a group of patients from one treatment to another, as all costs that would be incurred if the decision were made (28). Because of the difficulties and inaccuracies inherent in estimating marginal and incremental costs, most economic analyses in the medical literature use average costs, which overestimate marginal and incremental costs.

Adjusting for Costs Over Time (Discounting)

Recent clinical trials have determined that the cumulative costs of PTCA and CABG in multivessel CAD patients are approximately equal after 3 to 5 years of follow-up with greater CABG costs occurring during the index hospitalization and greater PTCA costs during the follow-up period (29, 30). **Economists use discounting (the reverse of compound interest) to adjust for cash flows that occur at different times,** such as those in PTCA and CABG. In these calculations, the present value of a follow-up period's costs is calculated as

$$\frac{Amt}{(1 + r)^n}$$

where "Amt" is the amount of follow-up costs in a future time period, "r" is the discount rate, and "n" is the follow-up year. Although discount rates ranging from 0 to 8% are reported in the medical literature, a 3% rate has been recommended by the US Public Health Service's Advisory Board when making comparisons using a societal perspective (23), whereas a 5% discount rate has been recommended by a similar group in Canada (31).

Quality of Life

Quality of life in an economic analysis is used to adjust patient life expectancies (quantity) to account for the relative desirability (quality) of different health states. By convention, health state preferences are scored from zero (death) to one (excellent health) despite findings of health states considered worse than death (32). Researchers assess health state preferences using health utility indices and direct assessment methods (33). Because existing health utility indices are generic (i.e., not disease specific), they are generally insensitive to moderate changes in health status. Thus, many researchers favor the direct assessment methods that are more easily tailored for specific diseases. Time trade-off is the easiest direct assessment method to use and understand. In this method, patients (or proxy) are asked a series of questions to determine how much time they would give up to live their remaining years in a healthy state. Thus, a person willing to give up 4.5 years of an expected 15 life years for 10.5 years of excellent health would have a 0.700 quality of life rating (10.5/15). By convention, future life years are discounted at the same rate as future costs in an economic analysis recognizing that future years saved have less value to the patient than current years saved. This also prevents anomalous situations from occurring when cost and effectiveness measures are discounted at different rates in an analysis (34).

HEALTH CARE ECONOMIC ANALYSIS

Types of Analysis

Health care economic analyses assess the value of two or more patient management strategies (diagnostic or therapeutic) by comparing their incremental costs and effectiveness. Because effectiveness of care is always the primary dimension, an economic analysis is generally of little interest when the proposed strategy is less effective than the current standard of care. When difference is not found in effectiveness between the proposed and standard of care strategies, but a difference in cost is found, a cost-minimization analysis is performed. In this situation, only the costs of the two strategies are compared. When the new patient management strategy is both more effective and more costly than the alternative, a comparison of incremental effectiveness versus incremental cost must be made. Finally, when the new strategy is more effective and costs the same or less than the standard of care, the new strategy is said to dominate the current standard of care.

Techniques that measure incremental cost per incremental unit of effectiveness gained (e.g., cost per year of life saved) are special cases of the following equation with different effectiveness measures:

$$\frac{CA - C_B}{E_A - E_B}$$

The numerator in this equation measures the difference in cumulative discounted cash flows (C) for patient management strategies (A and B) and the denominator measures the difference in cumulative discounted effectiveness (E) for the same strategies. Three forms can be used for these analyses: cost-benefit analysis, cost-effectiveness analysis, and cost-utility analysis (15). **Cost-benefit analysis measures effectiveness in economic terms,** allowing a cost:benefit ratio (dollars of cost per dollar of benefit) or a difference (benefits minus costs) to be calculated. Because placing an economic value on medical outcomes, especially lives saved, is difficult and imprecise, this method is rarely used in health care, despite the advantage of producing a value that is easily compared with other nonmedical expenditures.

Although the term cost-effectiveness is frequently misused in the medical literature to denote any form of economic study (15, 35), within health economics, this term tra-

ditionally has been reserved for studies comparing incremental costs versus incremental effectiveness with effectiveness measured in terms of medical outcomes. Thus, in a clinical trial, the effectiveness measure could be years of life saved and the resulting cost-effectiveness measure would be cost per year of life saved. Cost-utility analysis, which is closely related to cost-effectiveness analysis, measures effectiveness as quality-adjusted medical outcomes such as **quality-adjusted years of life saved (QALY).** Because of the importance of quality of life in patient outcomes, the US Public Health Service's Advisory Board on Economic Analysis Standards combined cost-effectiveness and cost-utility analysis into a single category with effectiveness always measured as quality-adjusted medical outcomes (23). However, until better means for assessing quality of life in all disease states are developed, many health care economic studies will continue to report cost-effectiveness without quality adjusting outcomes.

Cost-Effectiveness Computations

Table 39.1 shows the cost-effectiveness computations used to compare two hypothetical

Table 39.1.
Cost-Effectiveness Computations

	Strategy A	Strategy B
Index costs	$15,000	$10,000
Follow-up costs		
Year 1	$ 0	$ 1,000
Year 2	$ 0	$ 4,000
Cumulative costs	$15,000	$15,000
Discounted costs		
Year 1	$ 0	$ 971
Year 2	$ 0	$ 3,770
Present value	$15,000	$14,741
Quality of life	0.900	0.800
Life expectancy	10 y	10 y
Discounted life expectancy	8.530 LY	8.530 LY
Discounted QOL	7.677 QALY	6.824 QALY
Cost per LY (cost minimization)		($259)
Cost per QALY (cost-utility)	$303.63	

LY, life years; QOL, quality of life; QALY, quality-adjusted years of life saved.

patient management strategies. Strategy B has lower index hospitalization costs ($10,000 versus $15,000), whereas strategy A has lower follow-up costs ($0 versus $5000) and results in a higher quality of life rating for its patients (0.900 versus 0.800). The cumulative, 2-year costs of both strategies are $15,000; however, because follow-up costs are discounted at a rate of 3% per year, the present value of strategy B's costs are $259 less than those for strategy A ($14,741 versus $15,000). Patients under both strategies have a life expectancy of 10 years, equaling 8.530 discounted life years (LY) using a 3% discount rate. However, strategy A's effectiveness measurement, discounted quality-adjusted life expectancy, is higher than strategy B's (7.677 versus 6.824 QALY) because of its higher quality of life rating (0.900 versus 0.800). When quality of life is not considered, both strategies have identical effectiveness (8.530 LY), and our economic comparison reduces to a cost minimization analysis in which strategy B has $259 lower cumulative discounted costs ($15,000 versus $14,741). However, after taking differences in quality of life into account, strategy A has greater effectiveness (7.677 versus 6.824 QALY), yielding a net benefit for strategy A of 0.853 QALY with $259 in higher costs. In this situation, cost-effectiveness analysis (or, strictly speaking, cost-utility analysis) indicates that moving from strategy B to strategy A yields a cost increase of $303.63 per QALY ($259/0.853 QALY). Thus, in this hypothetical example, when quality of life is not considered, strategy B is economically more attractive (same outcomes, lower costs), whereas when quality of life adjustments are made, strategy A appears economically attractive (more benefits at a low cost per unit of extra benefit), assuming that the decision maker in question wishes to spend extra money to improve the health of a given population.

Economic Analysis Standards

The results of cost-effectiveness analyses are frequently compared using league tables that rank health care alternatives by their ascending cost-effectiveness ratios (36). In Table 39.2, all studies measure effectiveness as costs per years of life saved (YOLS) and all costs have been adjusted to 1993 values. Notice that the cost-effectiveness of a technology varies between patient subgroups so that PTCA's value versus medical therapy is $7400 per YOLS in 55-year-old men with severe angina, but it drops to $110,000 per YOLS if these men have mild angina. Although league tables such as this are attractive guides for health care policy makers in resource allocation decisions, such as those recently attempted in Oregon (37, 38), they also have great potential to mislead because of changes in medical practice (in which either the new or comparison strategy becomes obsolete) or to different discount rates, different methods for estimating costs and benefits, and different countries in the studies comprising the league table (39). Because of difficulties such as these, most authorities recommend using league tables only as general guides and caution against using them deterministically (39, 40).

Several researchers have attempted to define a cut-point for cost-effectiveness ratios—limit beyond which a patient management strategy would not be considered "cost-effective" or "worthwhile." In an analysis of 587 life-saving interventions, Tengs et al. found that the median costs per year of life saved for accepted interventions varied by type with medical interventions at $19,000 per YOLS, injury reduction interventions at $48,000 per YOLS, and toxin control interventions at $2,800,000 per YOLS (41). Researchers have concluded that the range of acceptable costs per year of life saved was closely related to the amount of legislation and litigation in an area (41), and that these differences were not related to different values placed on preventing different types of death (42).

Three studies have proposed binary rules of thumb to assess the cost-effectiveness of new medical technologies (43–45). In 1981, Kaplan and Bush (45) suggested that technologies costing less than $20,000 per QALY were cost-effective, whereas a decade later Goldman et al. (43) proposed that the cost-effectiveness threshold had increased to $40,000 per QALY. Weinstein noted that both benchmarks correspond closely to their respective per capita gross

Table 39.2.
League Table

New Technology	Existing Technology	Patient Population	Cost/YOLS	Report
Beta-blockers	No therapy	Myocardial infarction survivors	$ 850	Wilhelmsson (1981)
CABG	Medical therapy	Left main coronary artery disease	$ 5,600	Weinstein (1982)
PTCA	Medical therapy	Men aged 55 with severe angina	$ 7,400	Wong (1990)
Hypertension screening	No screening	Asymptomatic men aged 60	$ 11,000	Littenberg (1990)
Exercise stress test	No testing	Aged 60 with mild pain and no left ventricular dysfunction	$ 13,000	Lee (1988)
Beta-blockers	No therapy	Hypertensive aged 35–64 no heart disease and ≥ 95 mm Hg	$ 14,000	Edelson (1990)
Lovastatin	No therapy	Men aged 55–64 with heart disease and < 250 mg/dL	$ 20,000	Goldman (1991)
Lovastatin	No therapy	Men aged 45–54 with no heart disease and ≥ 300 mg/dL	$ 34,000	Goldman (1991)
CABG	Medical therapy	Two-vessel coronary artery disease	$ 75,000	Weinstein (1982)
Hypertension screening	No screening	Asymptomatic women aged 20	$ 87,000	Littenberg (1990)
Captopril	No therapy	Aged 35–64 with no heart disease and 95 mm Hg	$ 93,000	Edelson (1990)
PTCA	Medical therapy	Men aged 55 with mild angina	$110,000	Wong (1990)

Adapted from Tengs TO, Adams ME, Pliskin JS, et al. Five hundred life-saving interventions and their cost-effectiveness. Risk Anal 1995;15:369–390.
Costs adjusted to 1993 dollars using the general consumer price index.
CABG, coronary artery bypass graft; PTCA, percutaneous coronary angioplasty; YOLS, years of life saved.

domestic product, which was $13,547 in 1981 but had risen to $24,447 in 1992 (46, 47). Although the authors of the US Public Health Service-sponsored Standards for Cost-effectiveness Analysis concluded that because a cost-effectiveness analysis is dependent on its societal context, they could not recommend a set of cost-effectiveness criteria (23), most health care economic analysts generally agree with Goldman's recommendations that technologies costing less than $20,000 per QALY were attractive in 1992 and those costing $20,000 to $40,000 were consistent with other funded programs (43). Because of increases in the consumer price index, this cut-point becomes a moving target that is now nearer to $50,000 per QALY (3). In fact, Kaplan and Bush's 1981 $20,000 cut-point, inflated using the medical care component of the consumer price index, is $45,862 in 1992 dollars and $53,197 in 1995 dollars (47). In addition to the US Public Health Service-sponsored standards (23, 48–50), other guidelines for conducting and reporting health care economic analyses have also been published in recent years, and they should be used as guides for the reader when assessing this literature (51–54).

APPLICATIONS OF ECONOMIC ANALYSIS

When clinicians consider the use of new diagnostic and therapeutic technologies, they typically want to know (*a*) how much the new technology will cost, (*b*) what factors will cause this estimated cost to vary, (*c*) how the new technology's cost compares with the standard of care, and (*d*) how its cost per unit benefit compares with other accepted technologies. The first question addresses the new technology's average cost, the second addresses its cost in specific patient and setting subgroups, the third addresses its incremental costs, and the fourth addresses its cost-effectiveness. Each of these questions measures a different aspect of the technology's value and is thus an appropriate subject for clinical economic analysis. We begin this section by reviewing the average costs (total and component) of diagnostic and therapeutic CAD procedures, and by identifying factors that may cause significant variation in these costs. We then compare the relative costs and cost-effectiveness of these procedures and discuss newer therapies that have the potential to change basic interventional cardiology cost-effectiveness relationships.

Interventional Cardiology Cost Analysis

Various patient, treatment, provider, and geographic characteristics have been investigated as potential cost determinants for patients undergoing invasive CAD procedures (28). Yet, although patient characteristics correlate well with overall patient risk and even 30-day mortality for acute myocardial infarction (MI) patients (55), they are less predictive of costs for specific episodes of care. Increasing age (≥60 years), female gender, comorbidities (e.g., diabetes), and extent of CAD are the patient characteristics most closely associated with increased CAD procedure costs. **Age** and **comorbidities** are associated with **increasing disease progression, female gender** is associated with **smaller vascular structure**, and **extent of CAD** often serves as a marker for the type of therapy (medical, PTCA or CABG) the patient will receive. Treatment characteristics, especially procedure type and length of stay (LOS), both in intensive care unit (ICU)

and routine care room, generally have the greatest influence on CAD costs of care. However, recent studies have shown that the physician performing a procedure also may be an important predictor of PTCA and CABG costs. Other provider characteristics frequently correlated with costs of care include treatment strategy (aggressive versus conservative), postprocedural complications, facility efficiency (on-site procedure rooms, procedure scheduling, and use of clinical pathways) and facility type (teaching versus tertiary care). Economists also identify local laboratory and/or supply costs as potential predictors of regional cost variances; however, little research has been done on their significance in determining CAD procedure costs. To date, most regional CAD economic research has addressed differences in practice patterns that are associated with differences in resource use and, hence, costs of care.

Coronary Angiography

Studies reporting wide variations in coronary angiography use (56–58) with little difference in patient outcomes (57, 59) have led many policy makers and payers to conclude that this procedure is overused in the United States and that utilization rates should be reduced to levels currently seen in Canada and many European countries. Unfortunately, little evidence is found to refute this conclusion as most economic studies of coronary angiography are older and not applicable to most patients seen in today's catheterization laboratory (60, 61). However, several researchers have investigated the influence of provider characteristics and decisions on the costs of this procedure.

Earlier studies estimated that as much as 45% of all inpatient coronary angiography costs could be saved by performing this procedure in an outpatient setting (62, 63); however, recent studies have made more modest estimates. Although no differences are found in procedure costs between settings, inpatient room and ancillary costs are higher and, in the late 1980s, the marginal cost difference between the inpatient and outpatient settings was $218 ($28 laboratory tests, $153 rooms, and $37 other costs) (64). Hospital type and operator experience also have been shown to influence outpatient coronary angiography costs with significant differences in favor of tertiary versus rural hospitals (because of lower supply and medication costs) and experienced versus inexperienced operators (because of lower costs associated with decreased fluoroscopic, procedural, and compression times) (65).

Percutaneous Intervention

Coronary angioplasty remains the primary revascularization alternative to CABG for CAD patients. Total in-hospital costs for single-vessel PTCA procedures at Duke University Medical Center were $10,219 in 1996 (Table 39.3) (66). Assuming an additional $2200 in costs for physician fees (67), the total cost of a PTCA in 1996 dollars

exceeds $12,000 with an approximately equal split between the catheterization laboratory (52%) and noncatheterization laboratory departments (48%). Catheterization laboratory room and personnel costs ("Other Costs" in Table 39.3) were 26% of in-hospital costs, whereas balloons and abciximab were 9.1% and 7.8%, respectively. Rooms were the most costly noncatheterization laboratory components with step-down and ICU rooms contributing 9.7% and routine care rooms 17.3% to in-hospital costs.

Despite traditionally higher in-hospital costs, **stent use has exploded in the past 2 years** and currently equals the volume of PTCA procedures in some centers (68). Peterson et al. recently compared the in-hospital costs of care for CAD patients receiving single-vessel PTCA with patients receiving nonbail-out stents in the warfarin and ticlopidine eras (Table 39.3) (66). Longer length of stay and use of additional balloons per procedure in warfarin era stenting contributed to $5574 higher index hospitalization costs versus PTCA with $2156 in cathe-

Table 39.3.
Percutaneous Transluminal Coronary Intervention Costs of Care

Cost Category[a]	PTCA 9/95–3/96 (n = 109)	Stent-Warfarin 8/93–1/95 (n = 64)	Stent-Ticlid 9/95–3/96 (n = 217)
Catheterization Laboratory			
Balloons	933	1366	1191
Stents	0	2000	2300
Abciximab	795	0	465
Guide catheter/wire	458	678	492
Contrast agent	483	915	565
Other costs	2657	2523	2708
Total	5325	7481	7730
Rooms			
Routine	1763	3373	1716
Stepdown/ICU	994	1366	1374
Pharmacy	269	1436	308
Laboratory	368	833	380
Other tests	334	317	347
Emergency room	661	600	849
Operating room	219	71	187
Miscellaneous	275	415	292
Total costs	10,219	15,793	13,065

[a] All costs in 1996 dollars.
PTCA, percutaneous transluminal coronary angioplasty.

terization laboratory costs and $3418 in rooms and ancillaries. In the ticlopidine era, fewer balloons were used per stent; however, the number of stents per procedure increased as more complex lesions were undertaken. Ticlopidine era costs also were increased by the introduction of abciximab for high-risk patients, resulting in a net increase of $249 in ticlopidine versus warfarin era catheterization laboratory costs. However, a decline in postprocedural length of stay from 6.3 days in the warfarin era to 2.1 days in the ticlopidine era reduced stent room and ancillary costs by $2979 and yielded a total reduction in stent costs of $2728. Thus, the primary cost difference between ticlopidine era stenting and PTCA was the $2300 cost of stents, 81% of the $2846 differences in costs between these procedures.

Several studies have investigated factors associated with differences in the costs of care for patients receiving interventional cardiology procedures. Preprocedural clinical and angiographic variables (e.g., treatment of acute MI, intra-aortic balloon pumping, creatinine (2.0 mg%, or lesion complexity) explain 30% of the variance in costs, and hospital or decision delays between admission and the time of the procedure account for an additional 6% (67). Adding postprocedural variables (e.g., noncardiac death, rise in creatinine level, urgent CABG procedure, blood product transfusion, and Q-wave MI) increases the explained variance to 65% and including LOS further increases it to 82%. Although the individual physician performing the procedure has not been an independent predictor of total interventional procedure costs in high-volume facilities (67), in lower volume facilities significant operator-specific differences not related to experience have been observed in costs (coronary care unit, pharmacy, laboratory, and total in-hospital) and resource use (pacemaker, contrast medium, LOS, and fluoroscopy time) (69). Independent predictors of catheterization laboratory costs include physician performing the procedure, combined angiography and PTCA, and American College of Cardiology/American Heart Association (ACC/AHA) lesion type B2 or C. When procedure success is included as an independent variable, ACC/AHA lesion type B2 or C is no

longer a significant predictor of catheterization laboratory costs.

Balloon catheter reuse is becoming an important economic issue as catheterization laboratories try to reduce their interventional procedure costs. Several North American and European cardiovascular centers have policies to reuse angioplasty balloon catheters that are marked for single use only, an indication not approved in the United States (70, 71). In a Canadian study comparing a reuse and a single-use strategy, catheter costs per lesion were $370 and $644 at reuse and single-use centers, respectively (72). Both centers had identical angiographic success rates (88%); however, the reuse center used more balloon catheters per lesion (2.4 versus 1.2), with a significantly higher rate of initial balloon failure, longer procedure time, increased contrast medium volume, higher adverse event rate, and longer average LOS (5.1 versus 3.4 days). These findings have been controversial in Canada because both centers were small- or medium-volume, performing fewer than 1.5 procedures per day, and because the reuse center exceeded the Council of Health Technologies in Quebec's recommendation not to reuse a catheter more than twice (73). When these results were used in a decision model, the "best case" scenario offered a potential savings of $480 (5.5% of total hospital costs) with reused catheters, whereas the "worst case" scenario resulted in a $1075 (12.2%) increase compared with a single-use strategy (74). Thus, **although the reuse of balloon catheters can reduce total hospital costs, even a modest increase in complication rates eliminates or exceeds any potential savings.**

CABG Surgery

Costs of CABG have been more extensively investigated than other interventional coronary procedures, in part because of the high cost of these procedures and the frequency with which they are performed. The average in-hospital costs of CABG surgery in the United States for Medicare patients in 1990 were approximately $23,000 (75). Assuming an additional $10,000 in CABG physician fees (76), the total costs of an isolated CABG procedure, approximately $30,000 in 1990, typically exceeds $45,000 in 1997 dollars. Of the total in-hospital costs, rooms account for 37% (25% intensive care and 12% regular care), the operating room accounts for 21%, and the remaining 42% comes from laboratory, medical supplies, pharmaceuticals, and other hospital departments (75).

Patient characteristics account for no more than 20 to 25% of the variance in in-hospital costs of care for CABG (75–77) with older age, female gender, black race, lower ejection fraction, prior CABG, prior MI, severity of CAD, emergency procedures, and comorbidities having the most significant impact on cost (75, 77–81). The two procedural factors associated with increased CABG costs are multiple procedures in a single admission (e.g., coronary angiography or concomitant valvular surgery) and the use of internal mammary arteries (78, 82). Cowper et al. found that, after adjusting for patient characteristics and regional factors, the performing hospital accounted for 17% of the total variation in CABG costs of care (75). Other studies have reported regional differences in the use (57) and costs of invasive cardiac procedures (78, 83).

Although total costs of care are important, many CABG cost studies have focused on postoperative costs as these are assumed to be closely related to LOS and potentially controllable by the attending physician. In one model, preoperative factors predicting postoperative costs, in order of significance, were (*a*) surgeon, aged more than 60 years, (*b*) ejection fraction less than 40%, and (*c*) previous CABG surgery (80). Noticeably, the number of diseased vessels had only a modest impact whereas the surgeon performing the procedure, before and after adjusting for patient characteristics, was the most important predictor of post-CABG costs. Another model found a significant relationship between the number of postoperative complications (adult respiratory distress syndrome, intra-aortic balloon pump (IABP) use, pneumonia, septicemia, major arrhythmia, re-exploration for bleeding, wound infection, neurologic event, fluid overload, and absence of pericarditis) and total hospital costs with one complication adding $1018 and five complications adding $33,833 to total hospital costs (77).

Clinical pathways, minimally invasive coronary artery bypass surgery (MICAB), and lipid lowering agents are three newer technologies that have the potential to dramatically decrease CABG costs during both the index hospitalization and follow-up periods. After implementing a CABG care map, one study found that post- versus pre-care map patients had an $1800 decrease in postoperative costs of care with a 0.6 day decrease in ICU LOS (2.6 versus 2.0 days) and a 1.2 day decrease in total LOS (8.4 versus 7.2 days) (84). Similarly, another center found that in patients with isolated left anterior descending (LAD) artery disease whose lesion morphology was not suitable for PTCA, MICAB had significantly lower charges than CABG ($28,260 versus $31,703, respectively), slightly lower LOS (7.7 versus 8.4 days, respectively), and no difference in in-hospital outcomes (85). The Post CABG trial, in an investigation of revascularization in CABG patients, found that aggressive versus moderate cholesterol lowering treatment reduced the rate of revascularization by 29% (6.5% versus 9.2%) (86). Although an earlier study of lovastatin and restenosis prevention with 6 months of follow-up found no clinical or economic benefit (87), it was terminated before the occurrence of late phase saphenous-vein coronary bypass graft disease (occurring more than 1 year after surgery), which is related to lipid-rich atherosclerosis of the graft similar to that found in native coronary arteries (88). Although the Post CABG trial did not report economic results, findings of this significance point to the potential for cost savings through use of lipid lowering agents after revascularization.

CAD Treatment Cost Comparisons

Several studies have compared the costs of care for various CAD diagnostic and treatment options. Although these studies are not considered cost-effectiveness analyses as they only measure costs and do not assess survival differences, they have contributed to our understanding of the economics of these procedures by precisely measuring costs of care and by providing insights into the importance of follow-up costs when assessing competing diagnostic and treatment strategies.

Table 39.4.
Costs of Coronary Artery Disease Treatment Options

Time Interval/Event	Medicine (n = 1570)	PTCA (n = 838)	CABG (n = 1487)
60-day costs of care	$ 5829	$13,578	$22,124
60 days to 1 year			
Cardiac rehospitalization (%)	16	31	10
Hospital costs (mean)	$ 1819	$ 3143	$ 703
Total 1-year costs	$ 7648	$16,991	$22,827
1 year to 2 years			
Cardiac rehospitalization (%)	12	13	9
Hospital costs (mean)	$ 1784	$ 891	$ 731
Total 2-year hospital costs	$ 9432	$17,882	$23,558
2 years to 3 years			
Cardiac rehospitalization (%)	13	16	7
Hospital costs (mean)	$ 1408	$ 1731	$ 530
Total 2-year hospital costs	$10,840	$19,613	$24,088

Adapted from Mark DB. Economics of acute myocardial infarction. In: Coliff RM, ed. Acute myocardial infarction and other acute ischemic syndromes. St. Louis: Mosby-Year Book, 1996;15.1–15.15.

Patients with CAD have three treatment options: medical therapy, CABG, and percutaneous intervention (Table 39.4). Although CABG has significantly higher costs at 60 days than the other two treatment options ($22,124 versus $5829 for medicine and $13,578 for PTCA), by 3 years cumulative costs of medical therapy ($10,840) and PTCA ($19,613) are closer to those for CABG ($24,088) (89, 90). In an examination of patients at Duke University Medical Center with significant CAD (>75% stenosis), no prior revascularizations, and the absence of non-CAD cardiac disease (Table 39.4), 60-day medical therapy costs were 26% of CABG costs whereas PTCA costs were 61% of CABG costs. By 1 year, significantly more rehospitalizations were found in the medical therapy and PTCA groups resulting in greater follow-up costs, but cumulative medical therapy costs were still only 34% of CABG whereas PTCA had reached 74% of CABG costs. As expected, the medical therapy and PTCA groups continued to have significantly higher follow-up costs in years 2 and 3 with year 3 cumulative undiscounted medical therapy costs at 45% of CABG costs and PTCA at 81%. The cumulative undiscounted cost differential between PTCA and CABG was approximately $7000 for single vessel disease, $6000 for two-vessel disease, but only $2000 for three-vessel disease.

These results suggest that the cost differential between PTCA and CABG is dependent on the prevalence of three-vessel disease in the PTCA population. Although this research demonstrated significant differences in CAD treatment costs among the three therapies, significant differences were found in the life expectancies, particularly in patients with multivessel disease who were not included in this analysis (91).

Recent clinical trials have begun to include economic substudies, which have largely been cost comparisons, in their designs. Significant issues for the interventional cardiologist that are addressed by these studies include the incremental costs of medical therapy versus revascularization; PTCA versus CABG; stent and atherectomy versus PTCA; and abciximab and enoxaparin versus placebo. Collectively these **clinical trial economic substudies represent much of the cutting-edge clinical economics research in interventional cardiology.**

Medical Therapy Versus Revascularization Cost Comparison

The Asymptomatic Cardiac Ischemia Pilot (ACIP) clinical trial randomized patients with clinically stable CAD and ischemia to three treatment strategies: angina-guided medical care, ischemia-guided medical care, and revascularization (Pepine CJ, Mark DB, Bourassa MG, Chaitman BR, Davies RF, Knatterud GL, Forman S, Pratt CM, Sopko G, Conti CR. Cost implications for treatment of cardiac ischemia: an ancillary study from Asymptomatic Cardiac Ischemia Pilot [ACIP]. 1997; unpublished). Angina-guided patients received therapy based on symptoms, whereas ischemia-guided patients were monitored using ambulatory electrocardiographic devices. Patients in both of these medical strategies received either atenolol-nifedipine or diltiazem-isosorbide dinitrate, whereas patients in the revascularization strategy received either PTCA or CABG at the site investigator's discretion. Three months after enrollment, average patient costs for the revascularization arm ($13,421) were significantly greater than for either of the medical strategies ($1525 for angina-guided and $889 for ischemia-guided medical care). However, for the time period of 3 months to 2 years following index hospitalization, the costs for the medical strategies ($6277 and $7749, respectively) were significantly greater than those for the revascularization arm ($3397) because of an increased need for revascularization procedures, drugs, and hospitalizations in medically treated patients. Using follow-up cost data in an economic model, these researchers estimated that the cumulative undiscounted costs for the two medical strategies could approximate those for the revascularization strategy within a 10-year period.

PTCA Versus CABG Cost Comparisons

Two recently completed clinical trials, the Emory Angioplasty Surgery Trial (EAST) and the Bypass and Revascularization Investigation (BARI) sought to compare the cumulative costs of PTCA versus CABG in multivessel CAD patients. EAST reported 6.6% higher CABG 3-year cumulative undiscounted procedural costs ($25,310 versus $23,734) (92, 93). Although PTCA patients in EAST had more chest pain and hospitalizations during the follow-up period, these nonprocedural costs were not included in this trial's economic analysis. In contrast, BARI included all hospitalizations (regardless of diagnosis or length of stay), visits to ten types of physicians and other health care providers, and outpatient cardiac tests and procedures (29). These researchers found that after 5 years of follow-up, total discounted costs in the CABG arm were 4.8% greater than those for PTCA ($58,856 versus $56,147). In BARI subgroup analyses, 5-year cumulative costs were lower in PTCA patients with two-vessel disease and nondiabetics, whereas CABG costs were lower in three-vessel disease patients and diabetics (Table 39.5).

Table 39.5.
BARI Cost-Effectiveness Results

	Cumulative 5-Year Costs (Thousands of Dollars)			Effectiveness (Life-Years Saved)			CABG C–E
	CABG	PTCA	Diff	CABG	PTCA	Diff	Ratio
Overall	58.9	56.1	2.8	4.41	4.31	0.10	$26,555
2-vessel	58.4	52.8	5.6	4.43	4.34	0.09	$61,050
3-vessel	59.4	61.0	(1.6)	4.38	4.26	0.12	CABG dominant
Nondiabetic	54.7	51.7	3.0	4.44	4.44	0.00	PTCA less costly
Diabetic	71.8	74.2	2.4	4.32	3.76	0.56	CABG dominant

Adapted from Hlatky MA, Rogers WJ, Johnstone I, et al., for the BARI Investigators. Medical care costs and quality of life after randomization to coronary angioplasty or coronary bypass surgery. N Engl J Med 1997;336:92–99. BARI, Bypass and Revascularization Investigation; CABG, coronary artery bypass graft; PTCA, percutaneous coronary angioplasty.

Newer Interventional Cardiology Techniques Versus PTCA Cost Comparisons

In the past 2 years, the volume of stent procedures in the United States has increased dramatically and is approaching the PTCA volume in many major medical centers. Economically, the trade-off is between PTCA's lower index hospitalization costs and stenting's lower restenosis rate and lower follow-up costs. The Stent Restenosis Study (STRESS) clinical trial enrolled patients requiring revascularization of a single coronary lesion to assess the long-term medical costs of PTCA versus stent (94). During the index hospitalization, patients randomized to PTCA were more likely to require "re-look" angiography or reintervention (8% versus 2%), whereas stent patients were more likely to have vascular complications requiring surgical repair (7% versus 1%). Patients in the stent arm also required more contrast medium and more balloon catheters (excluding stent delivery), resulting in $1186 higher catheterization laboratory costs. Increased LOS (total and postprocedural) also contributed to the $2233 higher index hospitalization cost of stenting. During the 1-year follow-up period, patients in the PTCA arm had more repeat revascularization procedures and rehospitalizations for cardiac reasons, whereas patients in the stent arm had more rehospitalizations for noncardiac reasons, mainly related to bleeding complications caused by a high-dose of oral anticoagulant. Total 1-year follow-up costs were $1441 less for stent than for PTCA, but the cumulative 1-year costs (index hospitalization plus 1-year follow-up) for stent were $791 higher than for PTCA.

Recent studies have demonstrated that the routine use of **optimal stenting techniques** (high-pressure postdilation and intravascular ultrasound) permit reduced anticoagulation regimens, which may lead to lower vascular complication rates and shorter postprocedural LOS. To assess the economic impact of these techniques, the catheterization laboratory costs for a series of single and multilesion (diffuse disease or multiple lesions of a single coronary artery)

optimal stenting patients were compared with those of PTCA and stent patients in the STRESS trial (95). Catheterization laboratory costs for single-lesion optimal stenting patients averaged $590 and $2197 higher than the STRESS stent and PTCA arms respectively, whereas catheterization laboratory costs for multilesion optimal stenting patients averaged $2582 and $4189 more, respectively, because of increased use of stents and balloons in optimal stenting versus traditional stenting and increased costs of coronary stents in 1995 versus 1991 to 1993 (the STRESS study period).

The ACC Expert Consensus Document on Coronary Artery Stents found that no conclusions could be made regarding the economic impact of stenting versus PTCA because of significant changes in stent practice and costs that have occurred since the STRESS trial (68). Five factors were cited to support this position.

1. The Palmaz-Schatz (Johnson and Johnson Interventional Systems, Warren, NJ) stent now costs approximately $400 more than during the STRESS trial.
2. Optimal stenting changes such as intravascular ultrasound (IVUS) have increased stent catheterization laboratory costs by approximately $1500.
3. Use of aspirin-ticlopidine versus aspirin-heparin-warfarin has reduced complication rates and their associated room and nursing costs by approximately $1000.
4. Omission of warfarin will presumably reduce the need for readmissions from hemorrhage and their associated costs by an additional $300 to $500.
5. Improved stent restenosis rates of 15 to 20% versus 31.6% in STRESS may further reduce costs by $600 to $800.

The consensus group concluded that the net effect of all five factors on 1-year costs of stent versus PTCA was imprecise and could range from cost-savings for stent to $3000 in extra costs. Thus, a definitive recommendation could not be made until the results from newer stent trials are available.

Although less frequently than stenting, atherectomy has also been proposed as an alternative to PTCA. The Coronary Angioplasty versus Excisional Atherectomy Trial (CAVEAT) compared the rates of restenosis in directional coronary atherectomy (DCA) and PTCA for coronary revascularization (96). Stenosis was reduced to ≤ 50% in 89% of atherectomy patients and 80% of PTCA patients; however, atherectomy patients had a higher rate of early complications (11 versus 5%) and $1267 greater in-hospital average costs with the largest share in the cardiac catheterization laboratory ($739). These results were confirmed in the recently completed BOAT trial, which found that despite similar LOS, 2.1 days PTCA and 2.3 days DCA, DCA costs of care for the initial hospitalization exceeded those of PTCA by $1640 with catheterization laboratory differences accounting for $1219 (74%) of that amount (97).

Adjunctive Pharmacologic Agent Cost Comparisons

Although intensive research is being conducted on peptide and nonpeptide, small molecule glycoprotein IIb/IIIa inhibitor use, abciximab is the only product currently available for clinical use. The Evaluation of 7E3 for the Prevention of Ischemic Complications (EPIC) multicenter trial randomized high-risk percutaneous intervention patients to a bolus of abciximab, a bolus plus infusion of abciximab, or a placebo (98, 99) and demonstrated that a bolus and 12-hour infusion of abciximab reduced 30-day clinical events related to abrupt closure by 35% and subsequent major ischemic events (death, MI) or the need for revascularization up to 6 months by 23%. The EPIC Economics and Quality of Life (EQOL) substudy demonstrated a 6-month cost savings for the bolus and infusion arm exclusive of drug costs (100). During the initial hospitalization, the potential cost savings of $622 per patient through reduced ischemic events was offset by $521 in costs related to greater bleeding in abciximab-treated patients. At 6 months, a cumulative cost savings of $1114 was found in the bolus and infusion arm versus the placebo ($16,862 and $17,976, respectively) exclusive of the cost of the drug. After adding in the drug cost, the abciximab bolus and infusion strategy had a net incremental cost of more than $293 over placebo.

Subsequent trials of abciximab in PTCA patients, Evaluation of PTCA to Improve Long-term Outcome by c7E3 GP IIb/IIIa Receptor Blockade (EPILOG) and Chimeric 7E3 Antiplatelet Therapy in Unstable Angina Refractory to Standard Treatment (CAPTURE) were stopped after interim analysis because experimental arm efficacies exceeded predetermined stopping levels (101). Both EPILOG and CAPTURE demonstrated greater effectiveness of abciximab than was reported by EPIC with less bleeding, and these trials have the potential to demonstrate cost-effectiveness or even dominance for abciximab-treated PTCA patients.

Low molecular weight heparin is another pharmaceutical that has great economic potential in the treatment of CAD patients. The Efficacy and Safety of Subcutaneous Enoxaparin in Non–Q-Wave Coronary Events (ESSENCE) clinical trial evaluated the effects of enoxaparin (a low molecular weight heparin) versus heparin in an acute ischemic syndrome population. A preliminary analysis of 30-day resource use found enoxaparin drug costs were $144 ($60 per day for 2.4 days), and net 30-day cost savings from this treatment strategy were $1132 (102). Most of these savings were related to reductions in diagnostic catheterization (57% versus 64%), PTCA (18.0% versus 22.3%), CABG (13.5% versus 17.4%), and rehospitalization (14% versus 17%) in the enoxaparin arm. Thus, enoxaparin appears to be one of the few therapies in cardiovascular medicine that improves medical outcomes and saves money (a situation economists refer to as a dominant strategy). The thrombolysis in myocardial infarction (TIMI) group is currently conducting a second trial with enoxaparin to confirm the results of ESSENCE.

Cost-Effectiveness Comparisons

Diagnostic Tests

Cost-effectiveness studies for diagnostic tests (such as diagnostic cardiac catheterization) are more complex than those for treatments. This is because an effective treatment improves patient outcomes versus alternative treatments, and it is a relatively straightforward task to compute the treatment's incremental costs and its incrementally improved outcomes. In contrast, an effective (accurate) diagnostic test only increases the probability of a correct diagnosis and it does not directly improve patient outcomes. Thus, it is more difficult to show that use of a diagnostic test improves outcomes (such as survival) compared with its alternatives at an acceptable cost (40, 103, 104). Performance parameters such as sensitivity, specificity, and the area under a receiver operating characteristics (ROC) curve are commonly used to assess the results of a diagnostic test. However, a more accurate test does not ensure improved patient outcome. Thus, a diagnostic test's accuracy cannot be used as a surrogate measurement for its cost-effectiveness.

Difficulty in assessing the cost-effectiveness of a diagnostic test originates not with the methodology of economic analysis but rather with the clinical side of the equation. Randomized trials of diagnostic technologies are rare and, as a result, most clinical effectiveness data come from observational studies, which normally examine various accuracy parameters of the test in different clinical settings. Few studies have empiric data linking diagnostic performance to clinical management and outcomes. Consequently, **economic studies of diagnostic technologies frequently use decision models to link the test with outcomes** and to fill in the gaps in empiric data with assumptions that are often based primarily on expert opinion.

Some researchers have attempted to gauge the appropriate use of diagnostic tests as an indirect measure of their value. For example, one study demonstrated that stress testing (imaging and nonimaging) in suspected CAD patients is closely related to the subsequent use of interventional CAD procedures (105). However, utilization rates alone neither demonstrate the appropriate use nor the cost-effectiveness of these tests and procedures. For example, a strategy that assigned all patients with suspected CAD to initial nonimaging stress testing might be less costly if only the costs of the

initial diagnostic testing were considered. However, this strategy might be less cost-effective than a strategy that made initial test assignments to nonimaging stress testing, imaging stress testing, or coronary angiography based on clinical risk assessment (low, intermediate, or high) (106). Thus, when assessing the cost-effectiveness of diagnostic tests and procedures, one must consider their entire clinical context and not merely the costs or usage rates of the diagnostic tests themselves. Relatively few formal cost-effectiveness analyses (economic models or clinical trials) have been performed for the primary CAD interventional procedures (coronary angiography, PTCA, and CABG). In the next two sections, we present the results from studies that have assessed the cost-effectiveness of coronary angiography and revascularization.

Coronary Angiography Versus Medical Therapy Cost Effectiveness

Kuntz et al. evaluated routine coronary angiography and treatment guided by angiography results versus initial medical therapy without angiography after acute MI using a decision model that modeled the life expectancies and lifetime costs of care associated with these management strategies (107). This study found that angiography may be indicated more frequently than is generally recommended and that patient subgroups with severe postinfarction angina or strongly positive exercise tests typically have cost-effectiveness ratios for coronary angiography less than $50,000 per QALY. They also found patient subgroups for whom coronary angiography was cost-effective without prior exercise test screening (e.g., men aged 45 to 64 with prior acute MI) and subgroups for whom coronary angiography was never cost-effective (e.g., men ≥75 with congestive heart failure and ejection fractions <50%). In patients with a positive exercise test, mild postinfarction angina, and a prior MI, routine coronary angiography was cost-effective in all subgroups except congestive heart failure

(CHF) patients aged 75 to 84 years with an ejection fraction 20 to 49%, and women aged 35 to 44. Similarly, in patients with a negative exercise test and no prior acute MI, routine coronary angiography was never cost-effective.

PTCA Versus CABG Cost Effectiveness

Early studies comparing CABG with medical therapy found that CABG had an incremental cost per quality-adjusted life year of $6300 to $7000 in left main artery disease, $13,000 to $14,000 in three-vessel disease, and $32,000 to $86,000 in two-vessel disease (108). However, PTCA was not a treatment option in these analyses. Wong et al. developed a decision model to compare the cost-effectiveness of revascularization (CABG and PTCA) for patients with chronic stable angina (109). This model predicted that treatment costs for CABG and PTCA patients would be the same over the typical patient's lifetime and that PTCA was a reasonable alternative to CABG for two-vessel disease, but that CABG was preferred for three-vessel disease and for patients with comorbidities that increase operative risk. These results were confirmed in the BARI economics substudy, which found that the 5-year cost-effectiveness of CABG versus PTCA was $26,555 per YOLS for all multivessel disease patients, but it was $61,050 per YOLS in two-vessel disease patients and dominant (more effective and less costly) in three-vessel disease patients (Table 39.5) (29). Similarly, PTCA was equally effective and less costly than CABG for nondiabetics, whereas CABG was dominant for diabetics. Thus, the cost-effectiveness of revascularization strategies in multivessel disease patients is highly dependent on the extent of CAD (two or three vessel) and the presence of diabetes.

MANAGED CARE

Innovations in both technology and insurance will continue to shape the future of interventional cardiology just as they shaped its early growth in the 1960s and 1970s. However, in the coming decade innovations in insurance will seek to curb rather than expand demand for interventional cardiology services. Many of the significant innovations in technology will be practice management and administrative rather than clinical, and they will seek to re-engineer the delivery of interventional cardiology services to adapt to the constrained financial environment created by managed care.

In 1995, 58 million Americans were enrolled in health maintenance organizations (HMOs) with an additional 91 million enrolled in preferred provider organizations (PPOs)—the other principal form of managed care (110). In that year, a survey of cardiovascular specialists found that 89% were involved with at least one type of managed care organization and that increased involvement was related to younger age, geographic location in the western United States, practicing in a single-specialty cardiovascular group setting, and the physician's specialty (94% cardiovascular surgeons versus 92% pediatric cardiologists versus 88% adult cardiologists) (111). Overall, **managed care accounted for 26% of total practice revenues and 50% of non-Medicare revenues.** However, it is unclear whether these low rates of dependence on managed care revenues represent smaller markets for cardiovascular specialists in managed care versus fee-for-service or a general reduction in utilization and reimbursement under managed care. One study found that hospital expenditures grew 44% more slowly in areas with high HMO penetration versus those with low HMO penetration (112). Of this reduction, 28% was caused by reductions in service volume and mix, 10% to changes in the intensity of services provided, and 6% to reduction in bed capacity.

To adapt to the financial environment created by managed care, cardiovascular specialists have had to make significant changes in the organization and management of their practices. The degree of change appeared to be a function of practice size with large groups (nine or more physicians) being significantly more active than small groups (one or two physicians) in the implementation of clinical pathways, clini-

Table 39.6.
Provider Profitability Equations

General
  NP = TR − TC
  where NP = Net profit,
    TR = Total revenue,
    TR = Total costs
Fee-for-service
  TR = P*Q
  TC = FC + (v*Q)
  where   P = unit prices and
    Q = service units provided
    FC = fixed costs
    v = unit variable costs
Managed care
  TR = R*E
  TC = FC + (v*U*E)
  where   R = premium rate
    E = enrollment
    FC = fixed costs
    v = variable costs
    U = utilization
Net profit per enrollee
  R − FC/E − v*U

cal data collection systems, outcomes monitoring, and continuous quality improvement programs, while increasing group size and number of managed care contracts, and decreasing practice costs. Of those practices with decreasing costs, 73% had experienced either a reduction or leveling off of income. This is in keeping with a recent study finding a 4% decrease in the average physician's income from 1993 to 1994 after continuous earnings increases from 1985 to 1993 (113).

At a fundamental level, managed care, particularly under full capitation, has changed the parameters for successful practice management. Traditional strategies for profit maximization are dysfunctional in an environment where profitability is no longer tied to service volume and where the provider's orientation has changed from revenue-maximization to cost and utilization management (114). Table 39.6 details these changes. In fee-for-service, total revenue (TR) is a function of unit price (P) and the service units provided (Q) whereas total cost (TC) is a function of fixed costs (FC), unit variable costs (v), and the service units provided (Q). Thus, in fee-for-service, total revenue and total cost both relate to the

quantity of service units provided, and net profit is increased by increasing price and/or the quantity of service units sold or by decreasing variable costs. In fully capitated managed care, total cost is still determined by the quantity of service units provided. However, total revenue is now determined by the number of enrollees and is not related to utilization: TR is a function of the premium rate (R) and the enrollment (E); TC is a function of fixed costs (FC), variable costs (v), utilization (U), and enrollment (E). Thus, as utilization increases, enrollment also must increase if a constant net profit is to be maintained. Under fee-for-service, net income increases with increased utilization. In contrast, in capitation, net income increases with either increasing enrollments or decreasing utilization. Thus, to increase net profit in fee-for-service the incentive is toward overutilization, whereas capitation incentives are for underutilization.

Although the United States is aggressively moving from fee-for-service to managed care as the dominant reimbursement strategy for medical care, few studies accurately assess the economic implications of these changes. Some studies have shown that patients in managed-care systems have lower costs with quality equal to or better than that in fee-for-service care (115–117), even when the same doctor cares for HMO and fee-for-service patients (118). In contrast, **in cardiology at least, other studies have found significantly increased mortality rates when the care of high-risk patients is shifted toward generalists** (119) and when the use of invasive procedures is reduced for high-risk patients (both trends being characteristics of managed care) (120).

SUMMARY

With the change from fee-for-service to managed care reimbursement, physicians will increasingly become responsible for the costs of medical care as well as for its quality (121). In this chapter, we have provided a general introduction to clinical economics and its application to interventional cardiology. Although the quantity and quality of interventional cardiology economic analyses are steadily increasing, many areas remain with little published research to inform and guide the clinician. This is in part because older technologies such as coronary angiography and stress exercise testing were introduced and adopted as standard components of care in an era when costs were not considered important. In other cases, newer technologies have been proven to be economically attractive in one population (e.g., abciximab in high-risk PTCA patients); but, through "indication creep," they are being applied to a broader population in which the economic picture is less well defined. Additionally, as newer technologies are introduced, they are routinely layered on existing technologies (e.g., stents with abciximab), making the net economic picture even less certain. Thus, clinicians need to exercise their judgment when applying economic research to medical practice just as they now exercise their judgment when applying the results of clinical research.

References

1. Forrsmann W. Die sondierung des rechten herzens. Klin Wochenschr 1929;8:2085.
2. American Heart Association. 1996 heart and stroke facts: 1996 statistical supplement. American Heart Association 1996.
3. Mark DB, Hlatky MA, Califf RM, et al. Cost effectiveness of thrombolytic therapy with tissue plasminogen activator as compared with streptokinase for acute myocardial infarction. N Engl J Med 1995;332:1418–1424.
4. Congressional Budget Office. Trends in health spending: an update. Washington, DC, 1993.
5. Sones FM, Shirey EK. Cine coronary arteriography. Modern Concepts of Cardiovascular Disease 1962;31:735.
6. Favaloro RG. Saphenous vein autograft replacement of severe segmental coronary artery occlusion: operative technique. Ann Thorac Surg 1968; 5:334–339.
7. Gruentzig AR, Senning A, Siegenthaler WE. Nonoperative dilatation of coronary artery stenosis—percutaneous transluminal coronary angioplasty. N Engl J Med 1979;301:61.
8. Prospective Payment Assessment Commission. Report and recommendation to the Congress. 1991.
9. Greenberg W. Competition, regulation, and rationing in health care. Ann Arbor: Health Administration Press, 1991.
10. Iglehart JK. The American health care system: Medicare. N Engl J Med 1992;327:1467–1472.
11. Iglehart JK. The American health care system: Medicaid. N Engl J Med 1993;328:896–900.
12. The Advisory Board. Cardiology II: forecast of hospital profitability through and beyond the year 2000. The Advisory Board 1992.
13. Califf RM, Woodlief LH. Endpoints for trials of reperfusion in acute myocardial infarction. In: Califf RM, Mark DB, Wagner GS eds. Acute coronary care. St. Louis: Mosby-Year Book, 1995; 149–165.
14. Mark DB. Economic analysis methods and endpoints. In Califf RM, Mark DB, Wagner GS, eds. Acute coronary care in the thrombolytic era. St. Louis: Mosby-Year Book, 1995;167–182.
15. Drummond MF, Stoddart GL, Torrance GW. Methods for the economic evaluation of health care programmes. Oxford, England: Oxford University Press, 1987.
16. Kelly ME, Taylor GJ, Moses W, et al. Comparative cost of myocardial revascularization: percutaneous transluminal angioplasty and coronary artery bypass surgery. J Am Coll Cardiol 1985;5:16–20.
17. Black AJR, Roubin GS, Sutor C, et al. Comparative costs of percutaneous transluminal coronary angioplasty and coronary artery bypass grafting in multivessel coronary artery disease. Am J Cardiol 1988;62:809–811.
18. Finkler SA. The distinction between costs and charges. Ann Intern Med 1982;96:102–109.
19. Finkler SA. Cost accounting for health care organizations. Gaithersburg, MD: Aspen Publishers, 1994.
20. Cooper R, Kaplan RS, Maisel LS, et al. Implementing activity-based cost management: moving from analysis to action. Montvale, NJ: Institute of Management Accountants, 1992.
21. Yee-Ching LC. Improving hospital cost accounting with activity-based costing. Health Care Management Rev 1993;18:71–77.
22. Doyle JJ, Casciano JP, Arikian SR, et al. Full-cost determination of different levels of care in the intensive care unit: an activity-based costing approach. PharmacoEconomics 1996;10:395–408.
23. Gold MR, Siegel JE, Russell LB, et al. Cost-effectiveness in health and medicine. New York: Oxford University Press, 1996.
24. Hlatky MA, Lipscomb J, Nelson C, et al. Resource use and cost of initial coronary revascularization. Coronary angioplasty versus coronary bypass surgery. Circulation 1990;82 (Suppl IV):IV-208–213.
25. Kukull WA, Koepsell TD, Conrad DA, et al. Rapid estimation of hospital charges from a brief medical record review. Med Care 1996;24:961–966.
26. Ashby JL. The accuracy of cost measures derived from Medicare cost report data. In: Finkler SA, ed. Issues in cost accounting for health care organizations. Gaithersburg, MD: Aspen Publishers, 1994;100–106.
27. Lipscomb J, Cowper PA, Mark DB. Comparison of hospital costs with Medicare cost to charge conversions versus a detailed hospital accounting system in patients being treated for ischemic heart

disease. Presentation at the Association for Health Services Research, San Diego, 1994.

28. Mark DB. Economics of acute myocardial infarction. In: Califf RM, ed. Acute myocardial infarction and other acute ischemic syndromes. St. Louis: Mosby-Year Book, 1996;15.1–15.15.

29. Hlatky MA, Rogers WJ, Johnstone I, et al., for the BARI Investigators. Medical care costs and quality of life after randomization to coronary angioplasty or coronary bypass surgery. N Engl J Med 1997;336:92–99.

30. Weintraub WS, Mauldin PD, Becker E, et al. A comparison of the costs of and quality of life after coronary angioplasty or coronary surgery for multivessel coronary disease: results from the Emory Angioplasty Versus Surgery Trial (EAST). Circulation 1995;92:2831–2840.

31. Canadian Coordinating Office for Health Tech Assessment. Guidelines for economic evaluation of pharmaceuticals: Canada. 1994.

32. Patrick DL, Starks HE, Cain KC, et al. Measuring preferences for health states worse than death. Med Decis Making 1994;14:9–18.

33. Mark DB. Quality of life assessment. In: Califf RM, Mark DB, Wagner GS, eds. Acute coronary care. St. Louis: Mosby-Year Book, 1995;183–199.

34. Keeler DB, Cretin S. Discounting of life-savings and other non-monetary effects. Management Science 1983;29:300–306.

35. Eisenberg JM. Clinical economics. A guide to the economic analysis of clinical practices. JAMA 1989;262:2879–2886.

36. Torrance GW, Feeny D. Utilities and quality-adjusted life years. Techn Assess Health Care 1989;5:559–575.

37. Hadorn DC. Setting health care priorities in Oregon: cost-effectiveness meets the rule of rescue. JAMA 1991;265:2218–2225.

38. Eddy DM. Oregon's methods: did cost effectiveness analysis fail? JAMA 1991;266:2135–2141.

39. Mason J, Drummond M, Torrance G. Some guidelines on the use of cost effectiveness league tables. BMJ 1993;306:570–572.

40. Glassman PA, Model KE, Kahan JP, et al. The role of medical necessity and cost-effectiveness in making medical decisions. Ann Intern Med 1997;126:152–156.

41. Tengs TO, Adams ME, Pliskin JS, et al. Five hundred life-saving interventions and their cost-effectiveness. Risk Anal 1995;15:369–390.

42. Mendeloff JM, Kaplan RM. Are large differences in "lifesaving" costs justified? A psychometric study of the relative value placed on preventing deaths. Risk Anal 1989;9:349–363.

43. Goldman L, Gordon DJ, Rifkind BM, et al. Cost and health implications of cholesterol lowering. Circulation 1992;85:1960–1968.

44. Laupacis A, Feeny D, Detsky AS, et al. How attractive does a new technology have to be to warrant adoption and utilization? Tentative guidelines for using clinical and economic evaluations. Can Med Assoc J 1992;146:473–481.

45. Kaplan RM, Bush JW. Health-related quality of life measurement for evaluation research and policy analysis. Health Psychol 1981;1:61–80.

46. Weinstein MC. From cost-effectiveness ratios to resource allocations: where to draw the line? In: Sloan FA, ed. Valuing health care: costs, benefits, and effectiveness of pharmaceuticals and other medical technologies. Cambridge: Cambridge University Press, 1996;77–98.

47. Anonymous. Statistical abstract of the United States. 1996;116.

48. Russell LB, Gold MR, Siegel JE, et al., for the Panel of Cost-Effectiveness in Health and Medicine. The role of cost-effectiveness analysis in health and medicine. JAMA 1996;276:1172–1177.

49. Weinstein MC, Siegel JE, Gold MR, et al., for the Panel on Cost-Effectiveness in Health and Medicine: Recommendations of the panel on cost-effectiveness in health and medicine. JAMA 1996;276:1253–1258.

50. Siegel JE, Weinstein MC, Russell LB, et al., for the Panel on Cost-Effectiveness in Health and Medicine: Recommendations for reporting cost-effectiveness analyses. JAMA 1996;276:1339–1341.

51. Hillman AL, Eisenberg JM, Pauly MV, et al. Avoiding bias in the conduct and reporting of cost-effectiveness research. N Engl J Med 1991;324:1362–1365.

52. Sonnenberg FA, Roberts MS, Tsevat J, et al. Toward a peer review process for medical decision analysis models. Med Care 1994;32:52–64.

53. Kassirer JP, Angell M. The Journal's policy on cost-effectiveness analyses. N Engl J Med 1994;331:669–670.

54. Hlatky MA, Rogers WJ, Johnstone I, et al. Economic analysis of health care technology. A report on principles. Task Force on Principles for Economic Analysis of Health Care Technology. Ann Intern Med 1995;123:61–70.

55. Lee KL, Woodlief LH, Topol EJ, et al., for the GUSTO-I Investigators. Predictors of 30-day mortality in the era of reperfusion for acute myocardial infarction: results from an international trial of 41,021 patients. Circulation 1995;91:1659–1668.

56. Mark DB, Naylor CD, Hlatky MA, et al. Use of medical resources and quality of life after acute myocardial infarction in Canada versus the United States. N Engl J Med 1994;331:1130–1135.

57. Pilote L, Califf RM, Sapp S, et al. for the GUSTO-1 Investigators. Regional variation across the United States in the management of acute myocardial infarction. N Engl J Med 1995;333:565–572.

58. Guadagnoli E, Hauptman PJ, Ayanian JZ, et al. Variation in the use of cardiac procedures after acute myocardial infarction. N Engl J Med 1995;333:573–578.

59. Peterson ED, Mark DB, Armstrong PW, et al. Does a conservative post-MI catheterization strategy miss severe coronary artery disease: comparisons of use and diagnostic yield in Canada and the US? Circulation 1995;92:120A.

60. Doubilet P, McNeil BJ, Weinstein MC. The decision concerning coronary angiography in patients with chest pain: a cost-effectiveness analysis. Med Decis Making 1985;5:293–309.

61. Dittus RS, Roberts SD, Adolph RJ. Cost-effectiveness analysis of patient management alternatives after uncomplicated myocardial infarction: a model. J Am Coll Cardiol 1987;10:869–878.

62. Beauchamp PK. Ambulatory cardiac catheteriza-

tion cuts costs for hospital and patients. Hospitals 1981;16:62–63.

63. Adams PS Jr, Roub LW. Outpatient angiography and interventional radiology: safety and cost benefits. Radiology 1984;151:81–82.

64. Lee JC, Bengtson JR, Lipscomb J, et al. Feasibility and cost saving potential of outpatient cardiac catheterization. J Am Coll Cardiol 1990;15:378–384.

65. Talley JD, Mauldin PD, Kupersmith J. Economic and angiographic factors in determining optimal catheter size in performing outpatient left-sided heart and coronary angiography. Am J of Cardiol 1996;77:374–378.

66. Peterson ED, Cowper PA, Zidar JP, et al. In-hospital costs of coronary stenting (with or without coumadin) compared with angioplasty. Circulation 1996;94:1891A.

67. Ellis SG, Miller DP, Brown KJ, et al. In-hospital costs of percutaneous coronary revascularization: critical determinants and implications. Circulation 1995;92:741–747.

68. Pepine CJ, Holmes DR, Block PC, et al. ACC expert consensus document: coronary artery stents. J Am Coll Cardiol 1996;28:782–794.

69. Heidenreich PA, Chou TM, Amidon TM, et al. Impact of the operating physician on costs of percutaneous transluminal coronary angioplasty. Am J Cardiol 1996;77:1169–1173.

70. Counseil d'evaluation des technologies de la sante de Quebec: The reuse of single-use catheters. 1993.

71. Conseil d'evaluation des technologies de la sante de Quebec: The reuse of single-use catheters: safety, economical, ethical and legal issus. Can J Cardiol 1994;10:413–421.

72. Plante S, Strauss BH, Goulet G, et al. Reuse of balloon catheters for coronary angioplasty: a potential cost-saving strategy. J Am Coll Cardiol 1994;24:1475–1481.

73. Bourassa MG. Is reuse of coronary angioplasty catheters safe and effective? J Am Coll Cardiol 1994;24:1482–1483.

74. Mak KH, Eisenberg MJ, Eccleston DS, et al. Cost-efficacy modeling of catheter reuse for percutaneous transluminal coronary angioplasty. J Am Coll Cardiol 1996;28:106–111.

75. Cowper PA, Delong ER, Peterson ED, et al. Geographic variation in resource use for coronary artery bypass surgery. Med Care 1997;35(4):320–333.

76. Hlatky MA. Analysis of costs associated with CABG and PTCA. Ann Thorac Surg 1996;61:S30–S32.

77. Mauldin PD, Weintraub WS, Becker ER. Predicting hospital costs for first-time coronary artery bypass grafting from preoperative and postoperative variables. Am J Cardiol 1994;74:772–775.

78. Cowper PA, Delong ER, Peterson ED, et al. Potential for cost savings in high cost coronary bypass surgery patients: a New York state analysis. J Am Coll Cardiol 1996;27:317A.

79. Dudley RA, Harrell FE Jr, Smith LR, et al. Comparison of analytic models for estimating the effect of clinical factors on the cost of coronary ar-

tery bypass graft surgery. J Clin Epidemiol 1993;46(3):261–271.

80. Smith LR, Milano CA, Molter BS, et al. Preoperative determinants of postoperative costs associated with coronary artery bypass graft surgery. Circulation 1994;90:II-124–II-128.

81. Weintraub WS, Jones EL, Craver J, et al. Determinants of prolonged length of hospital stay after coronary bypass surgery. Circulation 1989;80:276–284.

82. Azariades M, Fessler CL, Floten HS, et al. Five-year results of coronary bypass grafting for patients older than 70 years: role of internal mammary artery. Ann Thorac Surg 1990;50:940–945.

83. Eisenstein EL, Newby LK, Pilote L, et al. Do regional differences in invasive cardiac procedure rated drive costs of care for the acute myocardial infarction patient? Circulation 1996;94:506A.

84. Johnson SH, Smith LR, Eisenstein EL, et al. Cost reduction in cardiac surgery: results from the Duke Coronary Artery Bypass Grafting Care Map. J Am Coll Cardiol 1996;27:45A.

85. Fry ETA, Hermiller JB, Lips DL, et al. Comparison of stents, bypass surgery (CABG), and minimally invasive bypass (MICAB) for isolated LAD revascularization: patient selection, outcomes, and cost. Circulation 1996;94:324.

86. The Post Coronary Artery Bypass Graft Trial Investigators: The effect of aggressive lowering of low-density lipoprotein cholesterol levels and low-dose anticoagulation on obstructive changes in saphenous vein coronary artery bypass grafts. N Engl J Med 1997;336:153–162.

87. Gilbert SP, Weintraub WS, Talley JD, et al., for the Lovastatin Restenosis Trial Group. Costs of coronary restenosis (lovastatin restenosis trial). Am J of Cardiol 1996;77:196–199.

88. Fuster V, Vorcheimer DA. Prevention of atherosclerosis in coronary-artery bypass grafts. N Engl J Med 1997;336:212–213.

89. Mark DB, Gardner LH, Nelson CL, et al. Long-term costs of therapy for CAD: a prospective comparison of coronary angioplasty, coronary bypass surgery and medical therapy in 2258 patients. Circulation 1993;88 (Part 2):I–480.

90. Mark DB. Implications of cost in treatment selection for patients with coronary heart disease. Ann Thorac Surg 1996;61:S12–S15.

91. Mark DB, Nelson CL, Califf RM, et al. The continuing evolution of therapy for coronary artery disease: initial results from the era of coronary angioplasty. Circulation 1994;89(5):2015–2025.

92. King SB III, Lembo NJ, Weintraub WS, et al., for the Emory Angioplasty versus Surgery Trial. A randomized trial comparing coronary angioplasty with coronary bypass surgery. N Engl J Med 1994;331:1044–1050.

93. Weintraub WS, Mauldin PD, Becker E, et al. A comparison of the costs of and quality of life after coronary angioplasty or coronary surgery for multivessel coronary artery disease. Results from the Emory Angioplasty Versus Surgery Trial (EAST). Circulation 1995;92(10):2831–2840.

94. Cohen DJ, Krumholz HM, Sukin CA, et al., for the Stent Restenosis Study Investigators. In-hospital and one-year economic outcomes after coronary

stenting or balloon angioplasty: results from a randomized clinical trial. Circulation 1995;92: 2480–2487.

95. Sukin CA, Baim DS, Caputo RP, et al. The impact of optimal stenting techniques on cardiac catheterization laboratory resource utilization and costs. Am J Cardiol 1997;79:275–280.

96. Topol EJ, Leya F, Pinkerton CA, et al. A comparison of directional atherectomy with coronary angioplasty in patients with coronary artery disease. N Engl J Med 1993;329:221–227.

97. Cohen DJ, Sukin CA, Berezin RH, et al., for the BOAT Investigators. In-hospital and follow-up costs of balloon angioplasty and directional atherectomy: results from the randomized BOAT trial. Circulation 1996;94:324A.

98. The EPIC Investigators. Use of a monoclonal antibody directed against the platelet glycoprotein IIb/IIIa receptor in high-risk coronary angioplasty. The EPIC Investigation. N Engl J Med 1994;330:956–961.

99. Topol EJ, Califf RM, Weisman HF, et al., on behalf of the EPIC Investigators: Randomised trial of coronary intervention with antibody against platelet IIb/IIIa integrin for reduction of clinical restenosis: results at six months. Lancet 1994;343: 881–886.

100. Mark DB, Talley JD, Topol EJ, et al., for the EPIC investigators: Economic assessment of platelet glycoprotein IIb/IIIa inhibition for prevention of ischemic complications of high risk coronary angioplasty. Circulation 1996;94:629–635.

101. Ferguson JJ. EPILOG and CAPTURE trials halted because of positive interim results. Circulation 1996;93:637.

102. Mark DB. Results from the ESSENCE economic substudy. Presented, Sci. Sess of the AHA, New Orleans, November 1997.

103. McNeil BJ, Varady PD, Burrows BA, et al. Measures of clinical efficacy: cost-effectiveness calculations in the diagnosis and treatment of hypertensive renovascular disease. N Engl J Med 1975; 293:216–221.

104. Fryback DG, Thornbury JR. The efficacy of diagnostic imaging. Med Decis Making 1991;11:88–4.

105. Wennberg DE, Kellett MA, Dickens JD, et al. The association between local diagnostic testing intensity and invasive cardiac procedures. JAMA 1996; 275:1161–1164.

106. Shaw LJ, Kesler KL, Eisenstein EL, et al., for the Economics of Noninvasive Diagnosis (END) Multicenter Study Group: a multicenter study of 11,372 patients to examine cost-effective strategies for diagnosis of coronary artery disease. J Am Coll Cardiol 1996;27:286A.

107. Kuntz KM, Tsevat J, Goldman L, et al. Cost-effectiveness of routine coronary angiography after acute myocardial infarction. Circulation 1996;94: 957–965.

108. Goldman L. Cost-effective strategies in cardiology. In: Braunwald E, ed. Heart disease: a textbook of cardiovascular medicine. Philadelphia: WB Saunders, 1992;1694–1707.

109. Wong JB, Sonnenberg FA, Salem DN, et al. Myocardial revascularization for chronic stable angina: an analysis of the role of percutaneous transluminal coronary angioplasty based on data available in 1989. Ann Intern Med 1990;113: 852–871.

110. American Association of Health Plans. 1995 HMO and PPO trends report. Washington, DC 1995.

111. DeMaria AN, Lee TH, Leon DF, et al. Effect of managed care on cardiovascular specialists: involvement, attitudes and practice adaptation. J Am Coll Cardiol 1996;28:1884–1895.

112. Robinson JC. Decline in hospital utilization and cost inflation under managed care in California. JAMA 1996;276:1060–1064.

113. Simon CJ, Born PH. Physicians earnings in a changing managed care environment. Health Affairs 1996;15:124–133.

114. Boles KE, Fleming ST. Breakeven under capitation: pure and simple. Health Care Manage Rev 1996;21:38–47.

115. Berwick DM. Quality of health care. Part 5: Payment by capitation and the quality of care. N Engl J Med 1996;335:1227–1231.

116. Retchin SM, Brown B. Elderly patients with congestive heart failure under pre-paid care. Am J Med 1991;90:236–242.

117. Carlisle DM, Siu AL, Keeler EB, et al. HMO versus fee-for service care of older persons with acute myocardial infarction. Am J Pub Health 1992;82: 1626–1630.

118. Hillman AL, Pauly MV, Kerstein JJ. How do financial incentives affect physicians' clinical decisions and the financial performance of health maintenance organizations? N Engl J Med 1989; 321:86–92.

119. Jollis JG, Delong ER, Peterson ED, et al. Outcome of acute myocardial infarction according to the specialty of the admitting physician. N Engl J Med 1996;335:1880–1887.

120. Selby JV, Fireman BH, Lundstrom RJ, et al. Variation among hospitals in coronary angiography practices and outcomes after myocardial infarction in a large health maintenance organization. N Engl J Med 1996;335:1888–1896.

121. Loop FD. You are in charge of cost. Ann Thorac Surg 1995;60:1509–1512.

40

The Patient with Valvular Heart Disease

Michael E. Assey, MD
Bruce W. Usher, MD
Blase A. Carabello, MD

INTRODUCTION

For most symptomatic patients with valvular heart disease, cardiac catheterization is critical in clinical decision making. At catheterization, the primary valve lesion is confirmed and quantified, other valve lesions and important changes in the pulmonary vasculature are defined, associated coronary artery disease is demonstrated, and ventricular function is evaluated. Proper patient management requires an understanding of the pathophysiology and natural history of valvular heart disease, and the integration of data generated from both noninvasive techniques and cardiac catheterization.

When the history and physical examination suggest valvular heart disease, the physician must make several decisions. Establishing the proper cause is important in advising the need for bacterial endocarditis or antistreptococcal prophylaxis, as well as the need for cardiac catheterization. Answers to such questions are greatly facilitated by current noninvasive techniques, particularly Doppler echocardiography. These techniques are helpful in confirming the suggested diagnosis, establishing cause in many instances, and allowing repetitive evaluations of **cardiac chamber size, wall**

thickness, valve area, and **ventricular function** (Table 40.1).

When the decision to proceed with cardiac catheterization is made, the noninvasive evaluation provides the operator with valuable information prior to the procedure. This knowledge can reduce both radiation exposure and volume of contrast material administered, which is particularly important in patients with renal insufficiency or decompensated congestive heart failure.

Throughout this chapter, the complementary nature of certain noninvasive techniques and cardiac catheterization is emphasized, providing a realistic and optimal approach to patient management. For each valvular lesion, a similar format is followed. Initially, there is a brief discussion of cause, clinical presentation, and pathophysiology. Following this, a precatheterization noninvasive assessment is presented, emphasizing information that is helpful in deciding when to proceed with cardiac catheterization. The typical catheterization findings are then presented, with a discussion to how these data are used in clinical decision making. All of these data are then integrated and synthesized, culminating in specific recommendations. Approaching the various valvular lesions in isolation may provide clarity at the expense of realism, because

Table 40.1.
Role of Echo/Doppler in the Assessment of Valvular Heart Disease

Diagnosis
Etiology
Chamber size
Ventricular ejection fraction (systolic function)
Ventricular filling parameters (diastolic function)
Ventricular hypertrophy
Estimate pressure gradients across stenotic valves
Estimate valve areas (aortic, mitral, tricuspid)
Estimate intracardiac pressures (LVEDP in aortic insufficiency; RV peak systolic pressure in tricuspid insufficiency)

LVEDP, left ventricular end-diastolic pressure; RV, right ventricular.

combined valvular lesions are often the most problematic ones for the practitioner. Accordingly, a discussion of some of the commonly occurring combined lesions is included at appropriate points in the chapter.

AORTIC STENOSIS

Clinical Presentation and Pathophysiology

Obstruction to left ventricular outflow may be supravalvular, valvular, or subvalvular. Valvular aortic stenosis may be acquired or congenital. The congenitally bicuspid aortic valve is found in up to 2% of all adults, with half of them having some degree of aortic stenosis by age 50 years (1, 2). **Rheumatic aortic stenosis**, characterized by commissural fusion, is often associated with some degree of aortic insufficiency and usually involves the mitral valve as well. In the degenerative form of acquired aortic stenosis, years of wear on an anatomically normal valve results in fibrosis and leaflet immobility. Calcium deposition occurs at the bases of the cusps, but the commissures are spared. This type of aortic stenosis, frequent in the elderly, is not usually associated with significant aortic insufficiency, unless bacte-

rial endocarditis supervenes. Thus, it is particularly amenable to valvuloplasty, a technique whose indications and limitations are discussed in Chapter 35. **Degenerative calcific aortic stenosis** can also be associated with conduction abnormalities (such as right bundle branch block with left anterior fascicular block), calcification of the mitral annulus, and coronary artery calcification.

The fixed obstruction to left ventricular outflow resulting from valvular aortic stenosis increases left ventricular systolic wall stress, causing parallel replication of sarcomeres and concentric left ventricular hypertrophy (3). When such a pressure overload develops gradually, hypertrophy can provide adequate compensation that maintains left ventricular ejection performance (4). Ejection fraction in adults with compensated aortic stenosis is usually normal or only slightly depressed (5, 6). In **congenital aortic stenosis**, hypertrophy, and perhaps hyperplasia as well, results in supernormal cardiac ejection parameters (7, 8). Left ventricular hypertrophy, however, often leads to abnormal diastolic stiffness (9, 10). As a result, left ventricular diastolic filling pressures are usually elevated, even in compensated aortic stenosis. Some chamber stiffness may be secondary to myocardial ischemia. Both chamber stiffness and hypertrophy regress following removal of the pressure overload (11, 12).

In each of the three common forms of acquired aortic valve stenosis, a long latency period is observed prior to the onset of symptoms. Symptoms include those related to congestive heart failure, angina pectoris, and syncope. These generally occur when the valve is narrowed to an area of 0.7 cm^2 or less, although symptoms can occur in patients with somewhat larger valve areas when other valve lesions, ventricular dysfunction, or coronary artery disease are present (13–15). Development of symptoms is an extremely important point in the natural history of valvular aortic stenosis. Mortality rate may reach 50% in the ensuing 4 years, with a particularly poor prognosis for those patients with symptoms of congestive heart failure (16, 17). Patients with aortic stenosis and congestive failure often have left ventricular dilation and a reduced shortening fraction. However, this may be entirely caused by "afterload mismatch," not depressed myocardial contractility (18). On the other hand, Spann et al. found that for any level of afterload (stress), patients with aortic stenosis and congestive heart failure had underlying contractile impairment (6). Ejection fraction has been shown to return to normal following aortic valve replacement, even in the face of severely depressed preoperative ejection fraction (12, 19). Thus, **no symptomatic patient is denied catheterization and treatment (valve replacement or valvuloplasty) because of a low ejection fraction**, although surgical risk increases significantly as the ejection fraction falls. Because left ventricular ejection fraction generally improves following valve replacement or valvuloplasty, asymptomatic patients are not usually treated prophylactically in hopes of preventing irreversible left ventricular dysfunction. (Management of the asymptomatic patient with aortic stenosis is discussed later in this chapter.)

Precardiac Catheterization Noninvasive Assessment

Patients with left ventricular outflow murmurs, particularly those with associated left ventricular hypertrophy on electrocardiogram, are frequently sent to the noninvasive laboratory to exclude or confirm left ventricular outflow tract obstruction. Doppler echocardiography is used to localize the obstruction to supravalvular, valvular, or subvalvular, and to quantitate the severity. Aortic valve abnormalities such as aortic sclerosis, calcific aortic stenosis, and congenital aortic stenosis (Fig. 40.1) can usually be differentiated from the normal aortic valve by two-dimensional echocardiography.

Doppler echocardiography represents a major advance in assessing the severity of the aortic valve gradient, as well as detecting concomitant mitral, pulmonic, and tricuspid involvement. Several studies have demonstrated a good correlation between the transvalvular gradient measured at cardiac catheterization and the estimated gradient calculated in the noninvasive laboratory using the modified Bernoulli equation (20, 21). In our laboratory, we found a fair correlation ($r = 0.86$) between the peak-to-peak gradient obtained at catheterization and the Doppler-derived gradient (Fig. 40.2). One should not really expect the cardiac catheterization peak-to-peak systolic pressure gradient to be the same as the peak instantaneous gradient derived from Doppler echocardiography. As illustrated in Figure 40.3, a clear temporal inequality exists between peak left ventricular and peak aortic pressure.

It should be noted that the Doppler-derived gradient represents the peak instantaneous gradient calculated from the peak instantaneous blood flow velocity across the valve. When we compared the peak instantaneous gradient obtained at catheterization, using high-fidelity micromanometer catheters, with the peak instantaneous Doppler gradient, an excellent correlation was found (Fig. 40.4). Instantaneous gradients are not routinely assessed in most catheterization laboratories. Thus, the Doppler-derived gradient may be significantly higher than the gradient reported from the catheterization laboratory, particularly when peak-to-peak gradients are compared. However, **the mean Doppler gradient is comparable to the mean planimetered gradient determined at catheterization.** Thus, we primarily rely on the mean Doppler gradient in our noninvasive assessment of aortic stenosis severity.

Because the pressure gradient is flow dependent, severity of aortic stenosis is optimally determined by measurement of valve area (see Chapter 25). Aortic valve area can be estimated noninvasively by combining Doppler and imaging echocardiographic techniques using the continuity equation (22). This technique is particularly valuable in assessing the potential significance of aortic stenosis when the transvalvular mean Doppler gradient is less than 50 mm Hg or when the patient has associated aortic insufficiency. A low valve gradient, resulting from decreased cardiac output, may still represent severe aortic stenosis and can be uncovered by this technique. When high-quality studies are obtained, an aortic valve area greater than 0.9 cm^2 is said to exclude

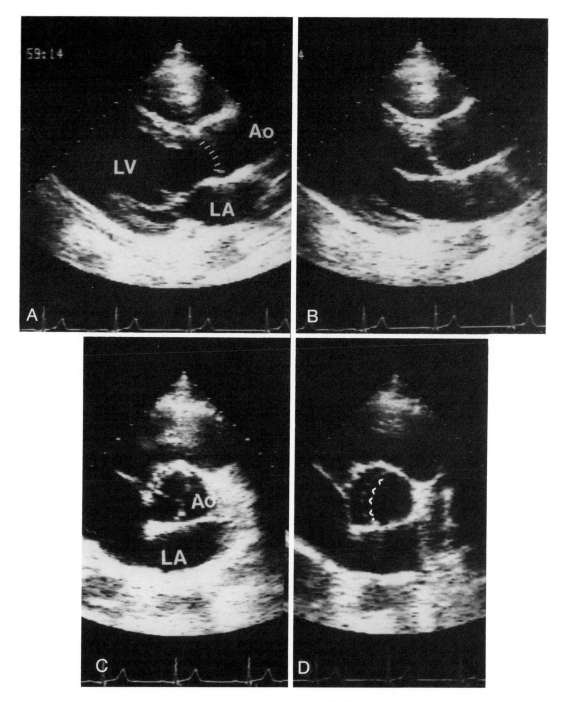

Figure 40.1. Two-dimensional echocardiogram of a congenital bicuspid aortic valve. **A.** Parasternal long-axis view during systole. **B.** Parasternal long-axis view during diastole demonstrates doming of the valve during systole. **C.** Parasternal short-axis view during systole. **D.** Parasternal short-axis view during diastole demonstrates deformity of the valve. *Ao,* aorta; *LA,* left atrium; *LV,* left ventricle.

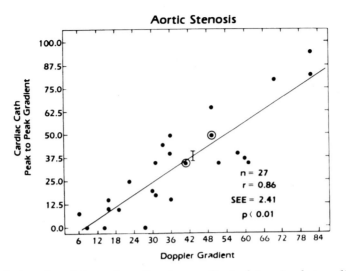

Figure 40.2. Correlation of peak-to-peak aortic valve gradients determined at cardiac catheterization with Doppler-derived peak instantaneous gradients. (Data from the Medical University of South Carolina, Charleston, SC)

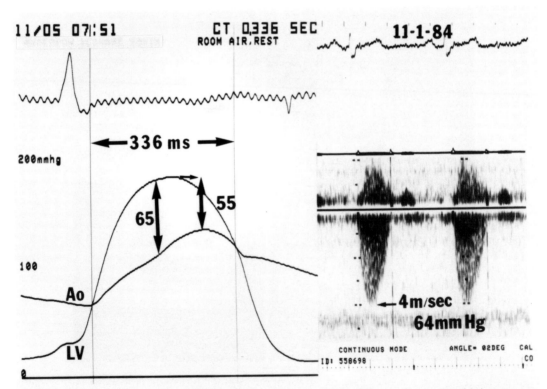

Figure 40.3. Micromanometer recordings of left ventricular (*LV*) and ascending aortic (*Ao*) pressures demonstrating discrepancy between peak-to-peak and peak instantaneous pressures. Doppler velocity envelope demonstrating correlation of Doppler-derived peak instantaneous gradient with peak instantaneous gradient determined by micromanometer catheter measurements.

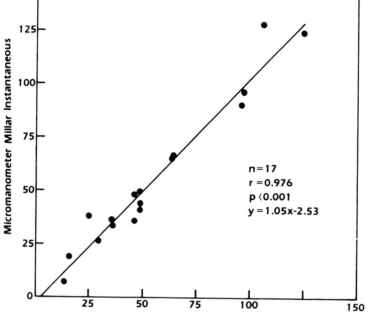

Figure 40.4. Correlation of instantaneous peak aortic valve gradient determined at cardiac catheterization using micromanometer catheter technique (*vertical axis*) with Doppler-derived estimated peak instantaneous gradient (*horizontal axis*). (Data from the Medical University of South Carolina, Charleston, SC.)

severe aortic stenosis (23, 24). An aortic valve area less than 0.60 cm^2 indicates severe aortic stenosis. Many patients, of course, have aortic valve areas between these levels in which case cardiac catheterization is necessary. Catheterization is also needed when high-quality Doppler echocardiographic studies cannot be obtained.

Information obtained in the noninvasive laboratory may have a bearing on the technical aspects of the catheterization procedure. Some may feel a reduced need to enter the left ventricle in cases where severe aortic stenosis is suggested by Doppler study. However, the variability in quality of Doppler studies observed in some patients and some practice settings makes this a suboptimal approach. Should mitral insufficiency be detected by Doppler or physical examination, it is best to enter the left ventricle and perform a ventriculogram to quantify the severity of the mitral insufficiency. Also, physical examination alone may fail to detect the mitral insufficiency murmur

masked by a harsh aortic stenosis murmur. At times, the aortic stenosis murmur has a higher pitch at the cardiac apex, mimicking the murmur of mitral insufficiency (Gallivardin effect).

Availability of nonsurgical valvuloplasty has further expanded the role of Doppler echocardiography in aortic stenosis management. In patients undergoing valvuloplasty, preprocedure and postprocedure gradient measurements allow for serial follow-up with proper identification of restenosis and changes in left ventricular function.

Information Obtained at the Time of Cardiac Catheterization

Cardiac catheterization is performed in a patient with known or suggested valvular aortic stenosis to confirm and quantify the stenosis severity, demonstrate associated valvular lesions, evaluate ventricular function, and define the coronary anatomy. Patients with angina often have coronary artery disease as well. Generally speaking, two thirds of aortic stenosis patients have angina; and, in half of these, obstructive coronary atherosclerosis is demonstrated by coronary angiography (25). Several groups have reported on the accuracy of noninvasive detection of coronary artery disease in patients with aortic stenosis (26, 27). A range of sensitivity and specificity is reported in these studies. We continue to believe that selective coronary angiography is the only safe and reliable means of accurately determining associated coronary artery disease in the patient with aortic stenosis. Consequently, coronary angiography is an important component of the preoperative cardiac catheterization regimen in all aortic stenosis patients at risk for coronary artery disease.

Although somewhat controversial (28–30), when significant coronary artery disease is identified, we generally recommend combined aortic valve replacement and coronary artery bypass surgery. This combined procedure can be performed without increasing the surgical risk, and substantial morbidity may result if significant coronary artery disease is not revascularized.

The catheterization protocol typically begins with obtaining venous access and placement of the right ventricular catheter. When the right atrium is reached, the mean pressure may be normal or elevated with variable types of waveforms. The patient with aortic stenosis and biventricular heart failure may demonstrate an elevated right atrial mean pressure with an abnormally high V-wave secondary to functional tricuspid insufficiency. A prominent A-wave in the right atrial tracing suggests reduced right ventricular compliance secondary to pulmonary hypertension or bulging of the hypertrophied interventricular septum toward the right ventricle. Right ventricular and pulmonary artery pressures are measured in the usual fashion, and the pulmonary artery catheter is left in proper position for later simultaneous determination of cardiac output and transaortic valve gradient.

Left ventricular catheterization is performed from the brachial or femoral artery approaches. Some physicians prefer the trans-septal approach. The left ventricular catheter is advanced to the ascending aorta just above the aortic valve, and central aortic pressure is measured. We generally perform this maneuver with the catheter advanced through a sheath in the femoral artery, allowing for simultaneous evaluation of central aortic and femoral artery pressure curves through a side port in the sheath. The femoral artery pressure curve will be somewhat time delayed and dampened with a systolic pressure over-shoot, although the mean and diastolic pressures are generally similar in the central aorta and femoral artery tracings (Fig. 40.5). If they are not, a transducer malfunction should be suspected. Alternatively, a true biologic gradient may be present, resulting from vascular stenosis between the central aorta and the femoral artery.

Left ventricular catheter is advanced in retrograde fashion across the aortic valve for measurement of left ventricular pressures. Catheter type used is variable and may include a micromanometer single or double-tipped catheter, a pigtail catheter (straightened out and directed with a straight guidewire), a multipurpose catheter, a Sones catheter, or a brachial A-2 catheter. The Sones and brachial A-2 catheters provide a large proximal bore with distal tapering in size and multiple side holes. At times, either a right Judkins or left Amplatz catheter is required to direct the guidewire across a distorted, narrowed valve orifice. Because these coronary catheters are not suitable for left ventriculography, an exchange catheter technique is subsequently required for safe ventriculography. Whenever multiple side holes are present, catheter position is critical as straddling of the valve orifice may produce an erroneous gradient. Indeed, it is important that the catheter be placed as deeply as possible into the body of the left ventricle. Pressure measurement immediately beneath the aortic valve samples the high flow vena contracta, where pressure may be significantly less than in the body of the left ventricle. Left ventricular systolic pressure is measured at fast paper speed, and left ventricular filling pressures are recorded on the appropriate scale.

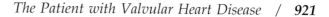

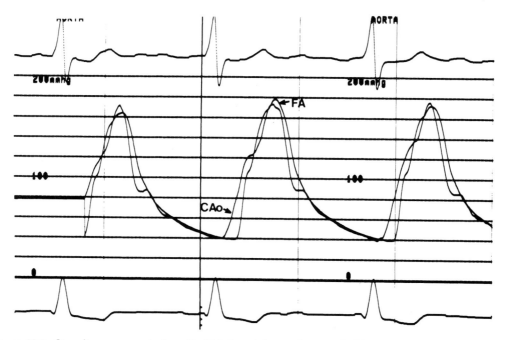

Figure 40.5. Simultaneous central aortic (*CAo*) and femoral artery (*FA*) pressure tracings in a patient with valvular aortic stenosis and chronic atrial fibrillation. The femoral artery pressure overshoots the central aortic systolic pressure, but the diastolic and mean pressures are similar.

The transvalvular gradient can then be measured in a number of ways. Simultaneous left ventricular and femoral artery pressures can be used to determine the aortic valve gradient. Folland, et al. (31) have shown the potential for error when using this technique to measure the aortic valve gradient. As can be seen from Figure 40.6, planimetry of the unaltered left ventricular-femoral artery gradient will overestimate the actual transvalvular gradient. However, temporal alignment of these waveforms, by shifting the femoral artery waveform to the left, will result in an underestimate of the valve gradient. **Averaging the results of the aligned and nonaligned planimetered gradients best approximates the true left ventricular-central aortic (transvalvular) gradient.** Pullback of the ventriculography catheter across the valve sequentially records left ventricular and central aortic pressures. Although not simultaneous, this is generally adequate to determine the gradient in patients with sinus rhythm. Planimetry is performed after superimposing the left ventricular and central aortic pressure

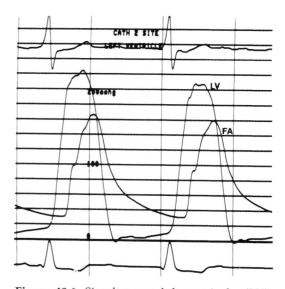

Figure 40.6. Simultaneous left ventricular (*LV*) and femoral artery (*FA*) pressures, the latter measured through the side arm of a femoral sheath. Planimetry of this unaltered left ventricular-femoral artery gradient will overestimate the true transvalvular gradient.

obtained at fast paper speed. An increase in peripheral (brachial or femoral) systolic pressure of 5 mm Hg or more during withdrawal of the catheter across the narrowed orifice indicates severe stenosis. Fifteen of 20 (75%) patients demonstrating this finding had an aortic valve area, calculated by the Gorlin formula, of 6 cm^2 or less; whereas, none of 22 patients with an aortic valve area 0.7 cm^2 or greater demonstrated this sign (32).

Alternatively, high-fidelity, simultaneous left ventricular and central aortic pressures can be recorded through a double-tipped micromanometer catheter (Fig. 40.3). When properly positioned, one transducer is in the left ventricle and the second is in the ascending aorta. Micromanometer catheter use, although somewhat cumbersome, avoids overdamping and catheter whip artifacts, which may be critical when the gradient is small. When the gradient across the aortic valve is low, significant aortic stenosis may still be possible because of a low cardiac output. In this setting, it is best to record simultaneous left ventricular and central aortic pressures, either using a double-tipped micromanometer catheter or by inserting a second catheter through an alternate arterial route.

Catheter position can significantly affect the measured gradient in patients with aortic stenosis (33). Because of intraventricular gradients and the phenomenon of down-stream pressure recovery, measured transvalvular pressure gradient can vary and prevent proper clinical decision making, particularly in patients with moderately severe aortic stenosis. Table 40.2 shows how much gradient can vary depending on the measurement technique. In this patient, a 35 mm planimetered gradient was noted when pressure tracings were obtained from the left ventricle, just below the aortic valve (vena contracta), and the aligned femoral sheath tracing. In contrast, a 71 mm planimetered gradient was noted when the left ventricular pressure tracing was obtained from deep within the ventricle, compared with the unaligned femoral artery sheath pressure curve.

Cardiac output is measured (Fick or thermodilution technique) at the same time that the pressure gradient is recorded. Aortic valve area can then be calculated by the Gorlin formula (Chapter 25). The basic concept of the Gorlin formula is that the pressure gradient across the aortic valve must be viewed in light of the fraction of cardiac output passing through the valve. In essence, it states that if an accurately determined cardiac output is related to an accurately determined gradient by an accurate formula, one can calculate aortic valve area. In 1951, when the Gorlins described their formula (34), they had no data to validate aortic valve calculations or the constants used in the equation, because at that time it

Table 40.2.
Effect of Varying Catheter Positions on Gradient Measurement and Calculated Valve Area in a Single Patient with Aortic Stenosis

Position	Planimetered Gradient (mm Hg)	HR	SEP (secs)	Calculated AA (cm^2)
LV apex-Asc Ao[a]	66	60	0.314	0.72
LV apex-Asc Ao[b]	60	55	0.315	0.83
LV apex-FA unaligned	71	55	0.305	0.78
LV apex-FA aligned	45	55	0.313	1.0
LV subv-Asc Ao[a]	52	60	0.328	0.80
LV subv-Asc Ao[b]	51	55	0.323	0.91
LV subv-FA unaligned	59	62	0.315	0.74
LV subv-FA aligned	35	62	0.322	0.94
Pullback	59	55	0.314	0.85

[a] Asc Ao, ascending aorta at level of coronary arteries.
[b] Asc Ao, ascending aorta above level of coronary arteries.
HR, heart rate; SEP, systolic ejection period; AVA, aortic valve area; LV, left ventricular; FA, femoral artery; Subv, subvalvular.

was considered highly dangerous to cross the aortic valve. Thus, it is not surprising that several limitations of the Gorlin formula in the calculation of aortic valve area have been described. Most importantly, Cannon et al. (35), using valves with fixed orifices, demonstrated that the calculated area increased with cardiac output, although true area did not change. In fact, nearly every investigation in this area has found a direct relationship between valve flow and valve area (valve area increases with valve flow). In some cases, valve area might actually increase because increased flow is associated with increased pressure, which actually opens the valve further; however, such was not true in Cannon's study where the orifice was fixed. Thus, valve area dependence on flow in that study was a mathematical artifact. By knowing actual flow and gradient, Cannon et al. recalculated the constants in the Gorlin equation. They found that the constant K was not a constant at all but varied directly with the square root of the mean pressure gradient. Mathematically, this is described as

$$AVA = \frac{CO}{(KMPG)(MPG)}$$

where AVA = aortic valve area, CO = cardiac output, and MPG = the mean pressure gradient from the original Gorlin formula.

This new equation is then simplified to $AVA = CO/K\ MPG$. Others have also found flow dependence of the Gorlin formula in calculating orifice area (36).

The inverse of Cannon's formula (MPG/CO) is an expression of resistance, a well-established hemodynamic concept. In calculating valve resistance, flow is expressed in milliliters (mL) per beat per systole, yielding the formula:

$R = Gradient\ HR \times SEP\ (sec)$
$\times 1.33\ CO\ L/min$

where HR = heart rate, SEP = systolic ejection period, and CO = cardiac output which expresses resistance in dynes-sec-cm^{-5}.

Currently, the Gorlin formula continues to be used to assess the severity of aortic stenosis. In light of the new revelations about the formula, it must be recognized that at low outputs the Gorlin formula may underestimate aortic valve area. These constraints may seriously hinder its use in accurately assessing the severity of aortic stenosis in humans. The most serious consequence is in the patient with a low transvalvular gradient and a low cardiac output. In such cases, the Gorlin formula is likely to predict that the aortic valve area is "critical" when only moderate aortic stenosis exists. As discussed elsewhere in the chapter, measurement of aortic valve resistance may be useful as an adjunct in assessing stenosis severity. The ultimate decision requires clinical judgment, reflecting the sum of the patient's history, physical examination, Doppler echocardiographic studies, and fluoroscopy (to detect the amount of calcium in the valve). These are all important aids in making the correct clinical decision.

To allow for a quick intraprocedural calculation, Hakki et al. (37) suggested that valve area can be estimated from the cardiac output divided by the square root of the pressure gradient. This ratio ignores the systolic ejection period. It is justifiable, however, because in the resting state, the product of heart rate, ejection or filling period, and Gorlin constant is usually close to 1. However, the systolic ejection period, as with the diastolic filling period, can change significantly when heart rates change, and this has prompted a further modification of the formula by Angel et al. (38). When heart rate exceeds 90 beats per minute (bpm) in aortic stenosis, the derived valve area estimated by the Hakki et al. equation should be further decreased, dividing by 1.35.

In our laboratory, left ventriculography is performed in a modified fashion to optimize patient safety. This includes nonionic contrast agent use, which is less likely to produce potentially deleterious hemodynamic changes. Patients with well-compensated aortic stenosis have small, thick-walled left ventricles that can be adequately opacified without creating ventricular ectopy, with lower than usual contrast volume (approximately 25–30 mL) and injection rate. The patient with high pulmonary-capillary wedge pressure (> 20 mm Hg) can be pretreated with diuretics and other pre-load reducing agents to minimize the risk of precipitating acute pulmonary edema. Ventriculography is necessary if coexistent mitral insufficiency or ventricular aneurysm is suggested. When severe aortic stenosis is found, and aortic insufficiency is neither heard nor demonstrated by Doppler echocardiography, aortography is not essential unless the operating surgeon desired it. **Aortography is performed when supravalvular or subvalvular aortic stenosis is suspected.** In the left anterior oblique view, a jet of negative contrast with domed rigid valve leaflets and poststenotic dilation of the central aorta may be seen in stenotic bicuspid valves.

Data Evaluation and Recommendations

Symptomatic patients with an aortic valve area less than 0.7 cm^2 are offered surgery or valvuloplasty. The decision to when valvuloplasty is used is fully discussed in Chapter 35. At present, we reserve valvuloplasty for the rare symptomatic patient who is not a surgical candidate, because of an unacceptably high surgical risk, excessive non-cardiac morbidity, or patient refusal to undergo surgery. Significant aortic insufficiency or severe coronary atherosclerosis requiring revascularization are general contraindications to valvuloplasty. Because the long-term success rate of aortic valvuloplasty is currently not well-defined, we use frequent (every 3 months) follow-up with Doppler echocardiography as a supplement to our postvalvuloplasty clinical evaluation. It is important to remember that significant restenosis can occur without an increase in postvalvuloplasty gradient if the cardiac output has decreased.

As noted, most patients with aortic stenosis and congestive heart failure will experience significant improvement in left ventricular performance following valve replacement or valvuloplasty (12, 19). No patient is refused surgery (39, 40) or valvuloplasty (41) on the basis of a low ejection fraction. It is hoped that the low ejection fraction is caused by afterload mismatch of aortic stenosis, rather than by depressed

contractility, and that ejection fraction will improve following valvuloplasty or valve replacement. Many patients with low left ventricular ejection fractions and low aortic valve gradients will not improve following surgery or valvuloplasty (42, 43). In such patients, left ventricular wall stress is likely to be low, in which case afterload cannot be significantly reduced by valve replacement or valvuloplasty.

Two approaches are currently under investigation to distinguish which patients with low ejection fractions and low aortic valve gradients will improve. One approach is to administer vasodilators (nitroprusside) or inotropic agents (dobutamine) (44) to increase the cardiac output. In some patients, cardiac output increases sharply without a great increase or even a decrease in gradient (42, 43). In such cases, a much larger calculated valve area will result, indicating only mild aortic stenosis that would not require surgery. In other cases the valve gradient increases in parallel to the cardiac output and the calculated valve area remains in the critical range.

The second approach is calculation of aortic valve resistance. The concept of using valve resistance as an indicator of aortic stenosis severity is appealing, because the formula uses no constants and may be less susceptible to variation in flow across the valve (45).

Cannon et al. (46) recently reported their experience with aortic valve resistance in helping to assess severity of aortic stenosis, particularly in borderline cases. Patients with true aortic stenosis, proven intraoperatively, had a higher aortic valve resistance than those with pseudoaortic stenosis. At present, we consider a valve resistance exceeding 250 dynes-sec-cm^{-5} to indicate significant aortic stenosis. Additional studies, in much greater numbers of patients, are required to prove the ultimate usefulness of this measurement.

Occasionally, noninvasive studies uncover a significant gradient (exceeding 50 mm Hg) in a totally asymptomatic patient. The management of such a patient is controversial. Fifty-one asymptomatic aortic stenosis patients, all with Doppler-derived peak systolic aortic valve gradients exceeding 50 mm Hg (range 50–132 mm Hg), were compared with 39 symptomatic patients

(47). Asymptomatic patients were statistically significantly younger, had higher left ventricular ejection fractions, and were less likely to have a left ventricular strain pattern or left atrial enlargement. During follow-up (17 ± 9 months), 21 of the 51 asymptomatic patients became symptomatic, with dyspnea being the most common initial complaint. Only 2 of the 51 initially asymptomatic patients died. Importantly, both deaths were preceded by the development of angina pectoris or congestive heart failure. Pellikka et al. (48) also examined the natural history of asymptomatic, hemodynamically significant aortic stenosis. In this study, 143 asymptomatic patients were followed for an average of 20 months. In the nonoperative group, only three deaths occurred secondary to aortic stenosis. In all three cases, symptoms of aortic stenosis developed at least 3 months before death. These studies support a conservative approach, albeit with close follow-up, of the asymptomatic adult with hemodynamically significant aortic stenosis.

Currently the recommendation for cardiac catheterization in such asymptomatic patients is controversial. Patients should be carefully instructed concerning bacterial endocarditis prophylaxis and what specific symptoms to watch for in to minimize the chance of unrecognized aortic stenosis symptoms. Serial Doppler studies may be useful in the follow-up of a patient with nonspecific or atypical symptoms. When characteristic symptoms do develop, cardiac catheterization is performed promptly. Inherent in this approach is the risk that an asymptomatic aortic stenosis patient will present with sudden cardiac death. This risk is low, however, and must be weighed against a similar or higher risk for valve replacement.

Aortic stenosis may coexist with mitral stenosis. When the mitral stenosis is severe, the clinical findings of aortic stenosis, particularly the murmur length and intensity, may change. The cardiac output is usually low, resulting in a smaller aortic valve gradient. Precatheterization Doppler echocardiographic studies help prevent an underestimation of aortic stenosis severity in the face of this combined valvular lesion.

When aortic stenosis is accompanied by mitral valve insufficiency, the physical findings expected to be associated with either lesion in isolation may change. For example, the classic carotid upstroke of significant aortic stenosis (pulsus parvus et tardus) may be "normalized" by coexistent mitral valve insufficiency. The relative importance of two systolic murmurs may be difficult to analyze at the bedside. Precatheterization echocardiography with Doppler studies are important in planning catheterization strategy in patients with this mixed lesion. Typically, the left ventricle will be more dilated with the mixed lesion than with isolated aortic stenosis. Indeed, when aortic stenosis is complicated by congestive heart failure, left ventricular dilation is common. In such a case, functional mitral valve insufficiency may be present. Intraoperative transesophageal echocardiography, following aortic valve replacement, is often helpful in deciding if mitral valve surgery is also needed.

In summary, symptomatic patients with aortic stenosis should undergo cardiac catheterization. In asymptomatic patients, a conservative approach is generally recommended even when noninvasive studies (specifically Doppler echocardiography) reveal a significant aortic valve gradient. Obviously, these patients need bacterial endocarditis prophylaxis and close clinical follow-up as previously emphasized. When symptomatic patients are found to have an aortic valve area less than 0.7 cm^2, aortic valve replacement or balloon valvuloplasty is indicated. **Concomitant coronary artery disease or associated valvular lesions may require earlier intervention.**

AORTIC VALVE INSUFFICIENCY

Clinical Presentation and Pathophysiology

Multiple causes are found for aortic insufficiency, including disorders that affect the valve itself (rheumatic heart disease, congenitally bicuspid aortic valve, myxomatous degeneration of the valve, infective endocarditis), as well as those causes that primarily affect the supporting aortic root and annulus (hypertension, trauma, dissection, aortic root aneurysm secondary to cystic medial necrosis). It is important to establish the cause because both the approach to cardiac catheterization and timing of surgical intervention, as well as surgical results, are directly related to the cause of aortic insufficiency. For example, rheumatic aortic insufficiency generally presents as a well-compensated, chronic left ventricular volume overload. Acute aortic insufficiency, secondary to infective endocarditis, may result in major valve disruption and torrential aortic insufficiency, constituting a surgical emergency affecting the timing and type of cardiac catheterization. Indeed, proper identification and management of acute aortic insufficiency is so important that it is discussed separately in this chapter.

As with mitral insufficiency, chronic aortic insufficiency imparts a volume overload on the left ventricle, resulting in increased end-diastolic volume and increased end-diastolic stress, compensated by eccentric left ventricular hypertrophy. However, the higher systemic systolic blood pressure, intraventricular pressures, and ventricular radius, all increase both peak and end-systolic wall stress. This situation mimics the mechanics of a left ventricular pressure overload. In part, this may explain why the natural history of left ventricular function in aortic insufficiency differs from the pure volume overload of mitral insufficiency. Wisenbaugh et al. (49) studied ventricular mechanics in nine patients with severe aortic insufficiency and eight patients with severe mitral insufficiency. Compared with normal subjects, both groups showed reduced ejection performance. Although preload (estimated as end-diastolic stress) was comparably elevated in both groups with regurgitation, afterload (estimated as mean systolic stress) was markedly elevated in aortic insufficiency and normal in mitral insufficiency. In aortic insufficiency, this excessive afterload contributed to poor pump performance, whereas the more favorable loading condition for mitral insufficiency masked underlying contractile dysfunction.

Chronic, slowly progressing, and compensated aortic insufficiency is associated with marked left ventricular dilation and eccentric hypertrophy, resulting in the largest left ventricular mass seen among the valvular lesions. This increased left ventricular size can accommodate the volume overload without increasing intraventricular pressures that would tend to cause an increase in pulmonary venous pressures. The enhanced run-off from the central circulation into the dilated, compliant left ventricle contributes to the widening of aortic pulse pressure and the classic peripheral pulse findings of chronic, compensated aortic insufficiency (50). **When aortic insufficiency decompensates or occurs acutely, these peripheral findings may be absent.**

Precardiac Catheterization Noninvasive Assessment of Chronic Aortic Valve Insufficiency

Echocardiography is useful in establishing the cause of aortic valve insufficiency and assessing aortic root pathology. An estimate of global left ventricular systolic function can be made, and coronary artery disease inferred, by regional wall motion abnormalities. Semiquantification of the severity of aortic insufficiency can be made from the pulsed Doppler interrogation of the left ventricle (Fig. 40.7). With this technique, the depth of the regurgitant jet detected in the left ventricle correlates with the angiographic severity of aortic insufficiency (51). Because the regurgitant jet can be eccentric and/or wide, and affected by varying afterload, Doppler color flow imaging allows a better noninvasive assessment of severity and closer correlation with angiography (52). With this technique, aortic insufficiency severity graded by comparing the area of the regurgitant jet in the short-axis view with the area of the left ventricular outflow tract in that same view (Fig. 40.8). Perry et al. (53) found that the thickness of the regurgitant stream, relative to the area of the left ventricular outflow tract recorded just below the aortic valve, correlated well with angiographic severity (Fig. 40.9).

Continuous wave Doppler flow pattern

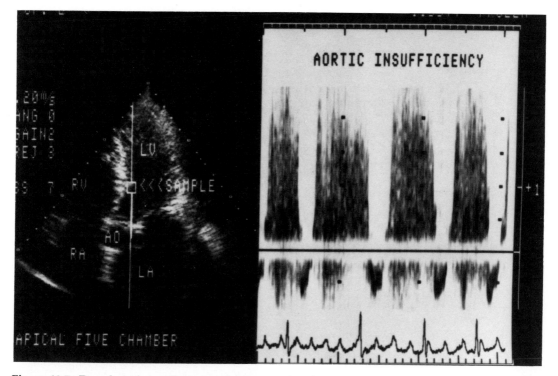

Figure 40.7. Doppler echocardiogram using conventional pulsed wave Doppler to detect aortic insufficiency from apical five-chamber view. *RV,* right ventricle; *RA,* right atrium; *LV,* left ventricle; *LA,* left atrium; *Ao,* aorta.

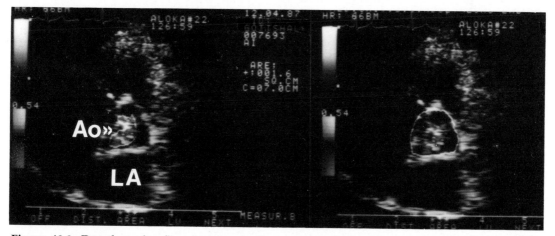

Figure 40.8. Doppler color flow imaging in the parasternal short-axis view demonstrating aortic insufficiency. Severity of insufficiency is estimated by determining the ratio of the area of the Doppler color signal during diastole to the area of the left ventricular outflow. *LA,* left atrium; *Ao,* aorta.

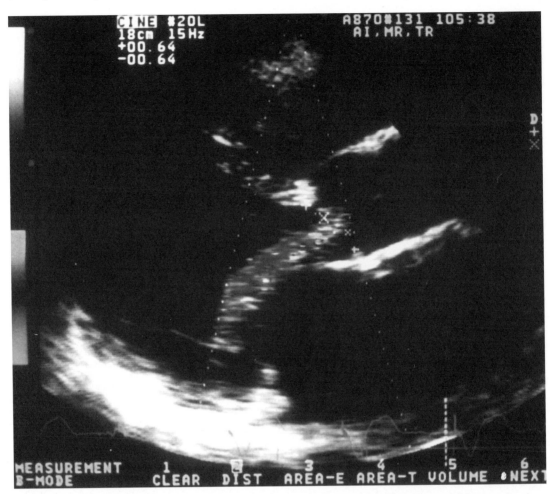

Figure 40.9. Two-dimensional imaging with Doppler color flow in the parasternal long-axis view. The width of the regurgitant jet is 1.1 cm as compared with 2.5 cm width of the outflow tract recorded just below the aortic valve.

of aortic insufficiency allows for an analysis of the decay rate of the velocity profile (pressure or velocity half-time), and gives an indirect assessment of insufficiency severity (54). When aortic insufficiency is severe, the gradient during diastole, between the aorta and the left ventricle, dissipates early in diastole, yielding a more rapid decline in the flow velocity of the aortic insufficiency. This finding may be particularly beneficial when mitral stenosis coexists with aortic insufficiency, because the mitral stenosis itself produces a high-velocity diastolic jet that can complicate mapping during pulsed Doppler evaluation.

When the continuous wave Doppler velocity envelope provides a sharp end-diastolic point, the left ventricular end-diastolic pressure can be estimated if the aortic diastolic pressure (obtained indirectly by cuff) is simultaneously determined (Fig. 40.10).

Information Obtained at Time of Cardiac Catheterization for Chronic Aortic Valve Insufficiency

Right-sided cardiac pressures are generally normal in chronic, compensated aortic insufficiency. Cardiac output measurements are made close to the time of left ventriculography, allowing for calculation of the regurgitant fraction. Regurgitant fraction is the difference between angiographic and forward cardiac output divided by the angiographic cardiac output. Prior to entering the left ventricle, it is important to measure and record central aortic pressure, because the normal discrepancy between central aortic and peripheral systolic pressures (brachial or femoral) is exaggerated in the setting of aortic insufficiency.

Left ventricular end-diastolic pressure varies depending on the severity of aortic insufficiency, compliance of the left ventricle, degree of ventricular hypertrophy, and associated coronary artery disease. The actual degree of aortic insufficiency is determined by the pressure differential between the aortic diastolic and left ventricular diastolic pressure, the length of diastole, and the size of the regurgitant orifice.

The amount of contrast agent entering the left ventricle during aortic root injection allows for a qualitative assessment of severity. Because the left ventricle in aortic insufficiency is often markedly enlarged, failure to inject enough contrast at a rapid enough rate may result in an underestimate of the degree of aortic insufficiency. Although several grading systems have been proposed, we prefer the following. In mild (1+) aortic insufficiency, the contrast from the aortic root fails to reach the left ventricular apex, and the ventricle is cleared of contrast material with each beat. Moderate (2+) aortic insufficiency opacifies the entire left ventricular chamber, but the degree of opacification of the left ventricle is less than the aortic root. Moderately severe (3+) aortic insufficiency occurs when opacification of the entire left ventricle is equal to that of the aorta. Severe (4+) aortic insufficiency indicates total opacification of the left ventricular cavity on the first or second heart

$$LVEDP = DBP - 4(V_{max})^2 \text{ (CW DOPPLER)}$$

AORTIC INSUFFICIENCY

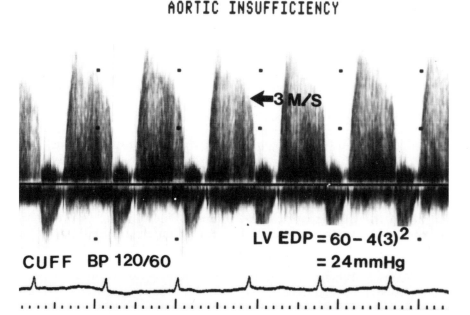

←3 M/S

$$LV\ EDP = 60 - 4(3)^2$$
$$= 24\ mmHg$$

CUFF BP 120/60

Figure 40.10. Doppler estimate of left ventricular end-diastolic pressure (*LVEDP*) in the presence of aortic insufficiency. *DBP*, diastolic blood pressure; *M/S*, meters per second.

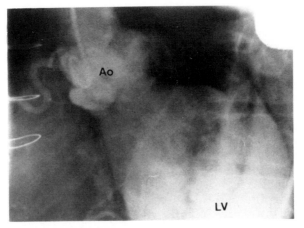

Figure 40.11. Aortogram, performed in the 45° left anterior oblique view in a patient with malfunctioning St. Jude prosthesis. Injection of contrast material through the pigtail catheter resulted in progressive opacification of a dilated left ventricle indicating "4+" aortic insufficiency. *Ao,* ascending aorta; *LV,* left ventricle.

beat following injection of contrast material into the aorta, with progressive opacification during the injection (Fig. 40.11).

Relatively poor correlation is found between noninvasive studies (e.g., pulsed Doppler), qualitative angiographic assessment of contrast reflux, and calculated regurgitant fraction. This discrepancy results from several factors. At least a 10% variation is seen in accuracy when forward cardiac output is computed by the thermodilution method. The amount of contrast material refluxing into the left ventricle varies with catheter position, volume of contrast material injected, and rate of contrast injection. The size of the aortic root (which may be massive in annuloaortic ectasia or ascending aortic aneurysm) and the size of the left ventricular cavity also affect the degree of opacification by a given amount of contrast material. Finally, **the forcefulness of global left ventricular contractility or the presence of associated mitral insufficiency will affect the qualitative assessment by cineangiography.** Left ventricular hypokinesis reduces the rate of contrast clearance, favoring progressive opacification of the left ventricle. When mitral insufficiency is present, contrast material escapes into the left atrium, decreasing the rate and degree of opacification of the left ventricle during aortic injection. Cineangiography in

the 30° right anterior oblique view allows measurement of left ventricular volumes and ejection fraction from an aortic injection when moderately severe or severe aortic insufficiency is present. Our impression is that the degree of regurgitation in the right anterior oblique view appears qualitatively less than a similar degree of regurgitation in the left anterior oblique view.

Data Evaluation and Recommendations for Chronic Aortic Valve Insufficiency

Controversy exists regarding the **appropriate timing of cardiac catheterization** and surgery for patients with chronic aortic insufficiency. Clearly, patients with moderate or severe symptoms caused by this valvular lesion need cardiac catheterization and most likely aortic valve replacement. Asymptomatic or mildly symptomatic patients pose a problem to the timing of catheterization and surgery, because previously reported determinants of a poor surgical outcome appear less reliable in the modern surgical era. Table 40.3 lists many of the frequently quoted noninvasive and invasive indicators of suboptimal surgical outcome

Table 40.3.
**Predictors of a Suboptimal Response to Aortic Valve Replacement
for Chronic Aortic Insufficiency**

	Value	Reference
Echocardiography		
LV shortening fraction	< 0.27	(57)
End-diastolic dimension index	> 38 mm/m^2	(58)
End-systolic dimension	> 55 mm	(55, 57)
End-systolic dimension index	> 26 mm/m^2	(58)
Cardiac Catheterization		
Subnormal left ventricular ejection fraction	< 0.50	(60
Reduced cardiac index	< 2.2 L/m^2	(59)
Elevated pulmonary capillary wedge pressure	> 12 mm Hg	(59)
Large left ventricular end-systolic volume index	> 90 mL/m^2	(61, 62)
Large left ventricular end-diastolic volume index	> 180 mL/m^2	(62)

LV, left ventricular; PCW, pulmonary capillary wedge.

in patients with chronic aortic insufficiency (55–63). Ten of these indicators were applied to 14 patients with isolated aortic insufficiency (3+ or 4+) and an ejection fraction less than 55%. Despite that 82 (58%) of a possible 140 predictors of negative outcome were seen preoperatively, no patient died. All but two patients had a decrease in symptoms and an increase in ejection fraction into the normal range after operation (56). Such results suggest that although these indicators are useful guidelines in the management of chronic aortic insufficiency, they should not, of themselves, supercede clinical judgment in determining the timing of catheterization or surgery. In contrast to mitral insufficiency, patients with aortic insufficiency who have a below normal ejection fraction or increased end-systolic dimensions and volumes may improve following valve replacement in the modern surgical era.

Aortic insufficiency frequently coexists with aortic stenosis and other valvular lesions (64). Severe aortic stenosis and aortic insufficiency cannot, by definition, coexist. However, the combination of a moderate degree of both lesions can cause symptoms and impaired ventricular function. This might require surgery that otherwise would not be needed if lesions of the same severity were present in isolation in different patients. When aortic insufficiency occurs with severe mitral stenosis, the wide pulse pressure responsible for typical peripheral pulse changes of isolated aortic insufficiency is usually absent. Doppler echocardiography will aid the physical examination when this combination is suggested. Hemodynamically, the mitral stenosis will attenuate the left ventricular volume overload expected of isolated aortic insufficiency. End-systolic stress/volume relationships are useful in assessing left ventricular contractility in this setting (65).

When aortic insufficiency coexists with mitral insufficiency, the cause may be rheumatic, combined prolapse of both valves, or dilation of annuli from various types of connective tissue diseases. Mitral insufficiency may also be functional in the setting of aortic insufficiency with left ventricular dilation. Separate contrast material injections into the aorta and the left ventricle are usually needed to assess severity accurately. When this is done, sufficient time should be allowed to elapse between injections for the hemodynamic effects of the initial contrast injection to dissipate.

Many patients have received a porcine heterograft valve replacement for aortic insufficiency and other valvular lesions. In general, patients receiving such a biologic valve are those in whom anticoagulation is contraindicated. Unfortunately, **the natural history of these valves is somewhat unpredictable.** Indeed, the likelihood of leaflet calcification and other types of valvular degeneration is substantial as these valves age. Figure 40.12 shows a degenerated Carpentier-Edwards porcine heterograft taken from the aortic position of a 63-year-old

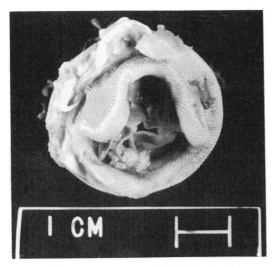

Figure 40.12. Degenerated Carpentier-Edwards porcine heterograft taken from the aortic position 4.5 years following implantation for aortic stenosis. The leaflets are fused and heavy calcification is seen in the sinuses and along the medial aspect of the valve ring.

woman. The valve had been implanted 4.5 years previously for aortic stenosis.

Preclinical deterioration of these valves can sometimes be identified by echocardiography (66). We frequently use echocardiography (specifically transesophageal echocardiography) to identify this early subclinical valvular deterioration. In our experience, sudden valve disruption, caused by a tear or perforation in a calcified or otherwise degenerating leaflet, can cause severe clinical deterioration without premonitory symptoms. Although one must consider many factors in the decision, we tend to replace an aging porcine heterograft with echocardiographic evidence of such degeneration, even in the absence of clinical symptoms.

ACUTE AORTIC VALVE INSUFFICIENCY

Clinical Presentation and Pathophysiology

Acute aortic valve insufficiency represents a true surgical emergency even in a patient with apparently mild congestive heart failure. It generally occurs as a complication of infective endocarditis, aortic root trauma, or dissection; and, it must be promptly identified and appropriately treated if cardiovascular collapse is to be avoided. Unlike chronic aortic valve insufficiency, no dilated left ventricle accommodates the sudden increase in left ventricular diastolic volume. Left ventricular filling pressure rises severely and prematurely during each diastole. As a result, the mitral valve is prematurely closed prior to the onset of left ventricular systole (67). This premature closure of the mitral valve protects the left atrium and pulmonary vascular bed from increased volume and pressure, but it causes a severe increase in left ventricular wall stress. The increased ventricular diastolic wall stress can cause subendocardial ischemia, myocardial infarction, and lethal ventricular arrhythmias. On physical examination, premature closure of the mitral valve diminishes the first heart sound. The combination of tachycardia and a soft first heart sound makes timing of the murmur difficult (Fig. 40.13).

Precardiac Catheterization Noninvasive Assessment of Acute Aortic Valve Insufficiency

The M-mode echocardiogram of a patient with acute aortic insufficiency who developed premature closure of the mitral valve while receiving antibiotics for aortic valve endocarditis appears in Fig. 40.14. Early mitral closure occurred when left ventricular pressure exceeded left atrial (pulmonary-capillary wedge) pressure (Fig. 40.15). Vasodilator therapy with sodium nitroprusside attenuated the hemodynamic abnormality. The fall in peripheral resistance produced by this potent systemic vasodilator reduced aortic diastolic regurgitation volume, decreasing the prematurity of mitral valve closure. Pepine et al. (68) demonstrated similar hemodynamic improvement and loss of premature mitral valve closure when administering nitroprusside in chronic aortic insufficiency.

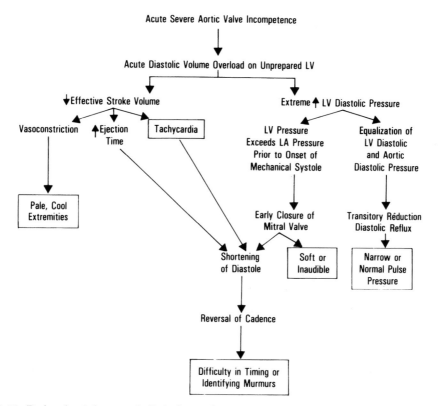

Figure 40.13. Pathophysiology and clinical correlates in acute aortic insufficiency. Note explanations for potential difficulty in timing the murmur of aortic insufficiency. *LA,* left atrial; *LV,* left ventricular.

In acute aortic insufficiency, echocardiographic or angiographic detection of a vegetation on the aortic valve suggests the diagnosis of endocarditis, as does detection of a flail leaflet in the proper clinical setting. In some instances, associated myocardial or annular abscess can be detected. In our view, a suggestion of endocarditis is a strong indication for transesophageal echocardiography and Doppler studies. The transesophageal approach is more sensitive and specific in identifying the vegetation and other complications of endocarditis such as annular abscess and fistulous tracts (Fig. 40.16). Doppler color flow imaging is helpful in establishing the presence or absence of a left to right shunt from a fistula. When the acute aortic insufficiency is caused by dissection of the aorta, two-dimensional echocardiography can be useful in detecting the dissection and determining its extent (Fig. 40.17). Omoto et al. (69) showed the value of biplane transesopha-

geal echocardiography in patients with aortic dissection. Use of both transverse and longitudinal scans allowed correct identification of both the true lumen and the false lumen in all 30 aortic dissections. Longitudinal scanning was slightly better than transverse scanning in detecting the entry sites of types I and III dissections. With the recent availability of omniplane transesophageal echocardiography, the sensitivity and specificity of the technique has been further enhanced (70).

Information Obtained at the Time of Cardiac Catheterization for Acute Aortic Valve Insufficiency

Patients with acute aortic insufficiency may be too ill to undergo emergency catheterization and contrast injection without pretreatment with systemic vasodilator drugs. If aortic valve echocardiography demonstrates large vegetation, particularly with a flail aortic valve, it may be best not to cross the aortic valve at the time of cardiac catheterization because of the risk of embolization. Other laboratories, however, have not found the risk of embolization to be increased by catheterization. When the left ventricle is not entered, but a left ventriculogram is considered necessary, adequate opacification of the left ventricle may be obtained by injection of contrast material into the aortic root in severe aortic insufficiency.

Right ventricular cardiac catheterization is important, particularly if a left to right intracardiac shunt is suspected. Such a shunt may be the result of endocarditis with abscess and fistula formation. In acute aortic insufficiency, the left ventricular pressure tracing shows a high left ventricular end-diastolic pressure. This is the limiting factor to further regurgitation from the central aorta, striking late diastolic rise (earlier diastasis which shortens the acute aortic insufficiency murmur); a left ventricular end-diastolic pressure that exceeds pulmonary-capillary wedge pressure early in diastole; and loss of the usual distinct A-wave seen in chronic ventricular hypertrophy (Fig. 40.15A).

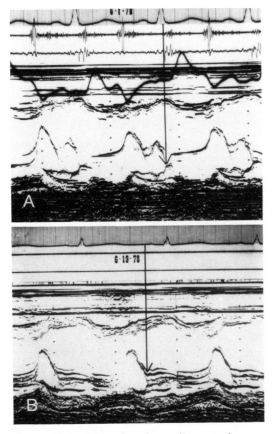

Figure 40.14. M-mode echocardiogram demonstrating mitral valve closure point in a patient with acute aortic insufficiency secondary to bacterial endocarditis. **A.** Mitral valve closure point is normal (*arrow*) on admission. **B.** Early closure of the mitral valve detected 18 days later while receiving antibiotic therapy. (Reprinted with permission from Assey ME. Echocardiography in diagnosis and managing aortic valve endocarditis. South Med J 1981;74:561.)

Data Evaluation and Recommendations for Acute Aortic Valve Insufficiency

Because acute aortic valve insufficiency represents a surgical emergency, immediate cardiothoracic surgical consultation is needed for any patient with this condition. High-quality noninvasive studies, in the proper clinical setting, accurately define the cause and complications of the acute aortic insufficiency, and they may make cardiac catheterization unnecessary. Invasive studies are required if coronary anatomy must be determined. **Catheterization is also needed when noninvasive studies indicate intracardiac abscess formation with possible fistulas, or if need exists to define the anatomy of the aortic root.** Although these patients are critically ill, complete cardiac catheterization while on vasodilators provides detailed information for the surgeon and will maximize the chances of operative success. In fact, because aortic insufficiency is already established noninvasively, catheterization itself should focus on other possible lesions (associated valve lesions, coronary artery disease, and so forth) that might change the surgical approach.

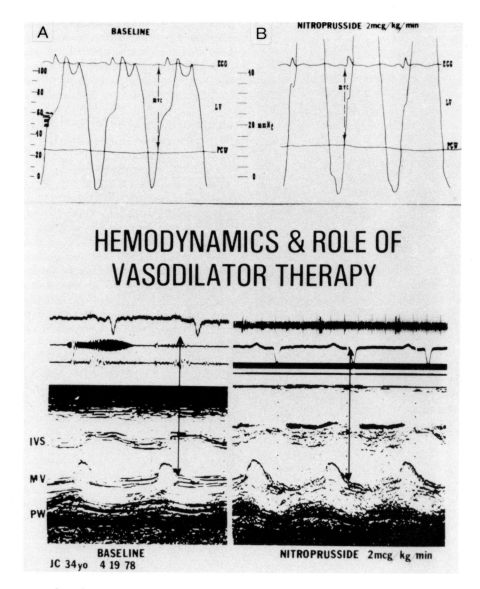

Figure 40.15. Simultaneous intracardiac pressure recordings (**top**) and M-mode echocardiograms (**bottom**) obtained in the cardiac catheterization laboratory in a patient with acute aortic insufficiency. **A.** Left ventricular end-diastolic pressure (LVEDP) is 60 mm Hg with a simultaneous pulmonary-capillary wedge pressure (PCW) of 26 mm Hg. The LVEDP exceeds the PCW in early diastole, well before the onset of the QRS complex of the electrocardiogram (ECG), with resulting early closure of the mitral valve. **B.** During infusion of nitroprusside, the LVEDP decreased to approximately 30 mm Hg and the PCW to 12–14 mm Hg. The LVEDP exceeds the PCW later in diastole, resulting in a shift in the mitral valve closure point to later in diastole at the onset of the QRS complex.

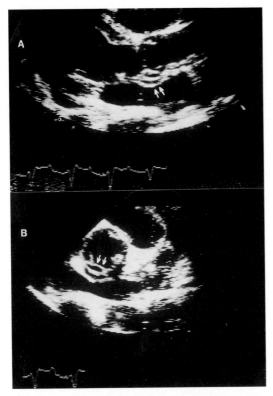

Figure 40.16. Two-dimensional echocardiogram in the parasternal long-axis view (**A**) and the parasternal short-axis view (**B**), demonstrating annular abscess (*double arrows*) in a patient with aortic valve endocarditis.

MITRAL VALVE STENOSIS

Clinical Presentation and Pathophysiology

In most cases, obstruction to left ventricular inflow at the level of the mitral valve results from rheumatic inflammation. As a result, mitral stenosis frequently coexists with mitral insufficiency or rheumatic involvement of other valves. Other rare causes of left ventricular inflow obstruction include congenital mitral stenosis, severe mitral annular calcification, cor triatriatum, and obstruction of the mitral orifice caused by a ball valve thrombus or left atrial myxoma. Although a left atrial to left ventricular gradient may develop when the mitral valve area is reduced to 2 cm², symptoms (dyspnea, he-

moptysis, low output) do not usually develop until the mitral valve area approaches 1 cm², which is 20 to 25% of normal size. At this level of stenosis, when the tachycardia of exercise or rapid atrial fibrillation shortens the diastolic filling period, the obligatory increase in transvalvular gradient frequently produces acute dyspnea.

Precardiac Catheterization Noninvasive Assessment

The patient with a diagnosis suggestive of mitral stenosis should undergo noninvasive study with Doppler echocardiography to confirm the diagnosis and rule out other causes of obstruction at the mitral valve level (myxoma, annular calcification, and so forth). The Doppler echocardiographic evaluation will provide data about the hemodynamic severity of the mitral stenosis, left atrial size, any left atrial masses, mitral insufficiency, and associated involvement of other valves.

Reliability of conventional echocardiography and Doppler echocardiography is now so refined in the case of mitral stenosis that **some patients undergo surgery without a preceding cardiac catheterization.** Generally this applies to patients under the age of 35, particularly women, who do not have signs or symptoms suggesting ischemia. In such patients, however, right ventricular catheterization may still be performed to measure pulmonary artery pressures and calculate pulmonary vascular resistance to aid in risk stratification. As demonstrated in Figure 40.18, planimetry of the mitral valve area from the two-dimensional echocardiographic short-axis view provides excellent correlation with the mitral valve area (Fig. 40.19), calculated from catheterization data by the Gorlin formula. Equally good correlation has been obtained with Doppler-derived mitral valve area using the pressure half-time technique (Fig. 40.20), which we have found to be reliable (Fig. 40.21). It may be superior to the calculation of mitral valve area by planimetry in patients who have undergone prior mitral valve commissurotomy. In such cases, the

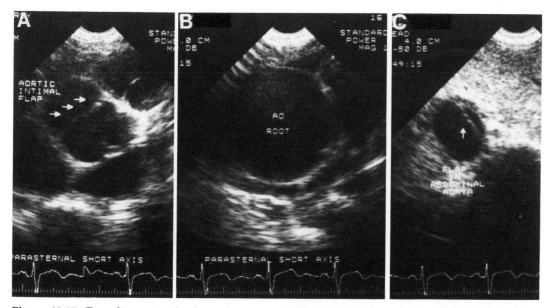

Figure 40.17. Two-dimensional echocardiogram of a patient with an aortic dissection. **A.** Parasternal short-axis view at the level of the aortic valve. **B.** Parasternal short-axis view of the ascending aorta demonstrating dilated aorta. **C.** Short-axis view of abdominal aorta. *Ao,* aorta.

mitral valve orifice is often distorted and difficult to planimeter, and obstruction may be secondary to thickening and fibrosis of the subvalvular apparatus. In patients with associated mitral insufficiency and atrial fibrillation, measurement of mitral valve area by Doppler pressure half-time may be more reliable than the valve area determined at catheterization because of the beat-to-beat variability in diastolic flow.

Optimal noninvasive evaluation requires multiple techniques, particularly when mitral stenosis coexists with other lesions. For example, one study (71) sug-

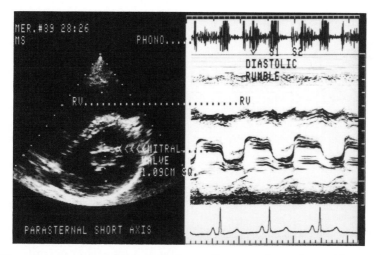

Figure 40.18. M-mode and two-dimensional echocardiogram of a patient with mitral stenosis. The mitral valve area is determined by planimetering the mitral valve orifice in the parasternal short-axis view of the two-dimensional echocardiogram. The mitral valve area is 1.09 cm^2. *RV,* right ventricle.

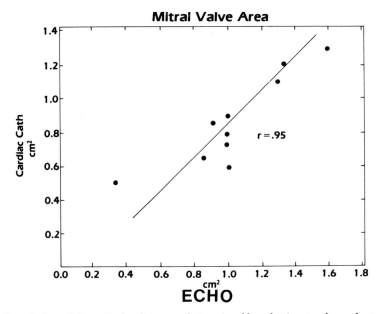

Figure 40.19. Correlation of the mitral valve area determined by planimetry from the two-dimensional echocardiogram with that obtained at cardiac catheterization using the Gorlin formula. (Data from the Medical University of South Carolina, Charleston, SC.)

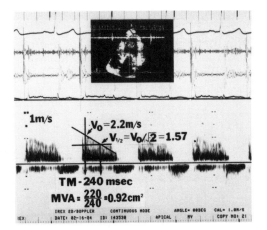

Figure 40.20. Doppler echocardiogram of a patient with mitral stenosis. The mitral valve area is calculated from the Doppler diastolic velocity envelope by the pressure half-time technique. *MVA*, mitral valve area; V_o, peak velocity; $V_{1/2}$, half of the peak velocity; *TM*, time from onset of diastolic Doppler signal to $V_{1/2}$. The known TM for 1 cm^2 valve area is 220 msec.

gested that the estimate of mitral valve area by Doppler pressure half-time was less reliable than the continuity equation when aortic insufficiency was present. However, when mitral stenosis was associated with mitral insufficiency, the continuity equation overestimated the mitral valve area, as compared with cardiac catheterization measurement of it.

In addition to screening patients with rheumatic heart disease, these noninvasive techniques have been useful in predicting which patients can be treated with commissurotomy rather than valve replacement (72). This is an important consideration when timing surgical intervention in mitral stenosis patients with mild or moderate symptoms. An echocardiographic score, developed at the Massachusetts General Hospital, is frequently useful in selecting patients for percutaneous balloon valvuloplasty. Ideal candidates have thin, pliable leaflets with little or no calcification and no significant subvalvular stenosis (73). The noninvasive demonstration of mitral stenosis may also permit valvuloplasty in selected patients without a separate diagnostic cardiac catheterization. Doppler

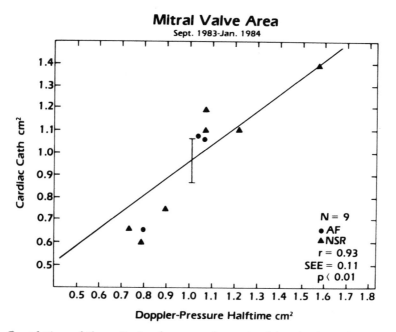

Figure 40.21. Correlation of the mitral valve area determined by the Doppler pressure half-time method with that obtained at cardiac catheterization using the Gorlin formula. *AF*, atrial fibrillation; *NSR*, normal sinus rhythm. (Data from the Medical University of South Carolina, Charleston, SC)

echocardiography is used to follow patients for possible restenosis after balloon valvuloplasty or following surgical commissurotomy.

Pulmonary hypertension may complicate the natural history of mitral stenosis, and with tricuspid insufficiency (Fig. 40.22), Doppler echocardiography can provide an estimate of right ventricular systolic pressure (Fig. 40.23). In the absence of pulmonic stenosis, it will also estimate pulmonary artery systolic pressure. Exercise Doppler echocardiography can be used to uncover pulmonary hypertension not present in the resting state.

Information Obtained at the Time of Cardiac Catheterization

Symptomatic patients with mitral stenosis, in whom noninvasive evaluation confirms significant valvular obstruction, are referred for cardiac catheterization. Mitral stenosis degree can be quantitated, other valvular lesions evaluated, and the pulmonary vascular resistance measured. In addition, fluoroscopic and cineangiographic assessment of the valve aids in deciding whether percutaneous valvuloplasty can be used or, alternatively, whether mitral valve repair, rather than valve replacement, is feasible. Left ventricular function can be evaluated and coronary angiography performed. When high-quality, reliable noninvasive data are available, the major indication for cardiac catheterization of mitral stenosis patients at our institution is the need to demonstrate the coronary anatomy.

The catheterization protocol generally begins with the measurement of right ventricular pressure. If associated tricuspid insufficiency is present, right atrial mean pressure will be elevated and a prominent V-wave may be seen. Alternatively, if obstruction to right ventricular inflow is present secondary to associated tricuspid stenosis, right atrial mean pressure will be elevated, and a prominent right atrial A-wave (larger than the corresponding right ventricular A-wave) will be seen in patients in sinus rhythm. As the catheter is advanced, right ventricular and pulmonary artery pressures are measured and recorded, permitting the diagnosis of associated tricuspid and pulmonic stenosis.

To obtain an accurate transmitral gradient, simultaneous measurement of left atrial (or phasic, nondamped pulmonary-capillary wedge) pressure and left ventricular diastolic pressure are needed. Many laboratories use a balloon-tipped, flow-directed pulmonary artery catheter to estimate pulmonary-capillary wedge pressure from pulmonary artery occlusion pressure. It is important that a true pulmonary-capillary wedge pressure be recorded. **Documentation that the pressure recorded is in fact a true pulmonary-capillary wedge pressure is made by demonstrating high oxygen saturation when blood is drawn from that position (arterial oxygen saturation exceeds 95% or is equal to that of systemic arterial specimen).** Furthermore, the pulmonary-capillary wedge pressure is dis-

tinguished from a damped pulmonary artery pressure by a decrease in mean pressure when the balloon is inflated. Although the normal pulmonary-capillary wedge pressure demonstrates a V-wave greater than the A-wave, this pattern can be reversed in mitral stenosis with sinus rhythm. The pulmonary-capillary A-wave is much larger than the A-wave present on the left ventricular diastolic pressure curve in mitral stenosis.

If the pulmonary-capillary wedge pressure is used as an indirect measure of left atrial pressure, realignment will be required for planimetry of the mitral valve pressure gradient. The pulmonary-capillary wedge pressure is a damped, phase-delayed left atrial pressure, and it should be shifted (to the left) to allow the descent of the V-wave to be superimposed on the descent of the left ventricular diastolic pressure tracing. Pulmonary-capillary wedge pressure may

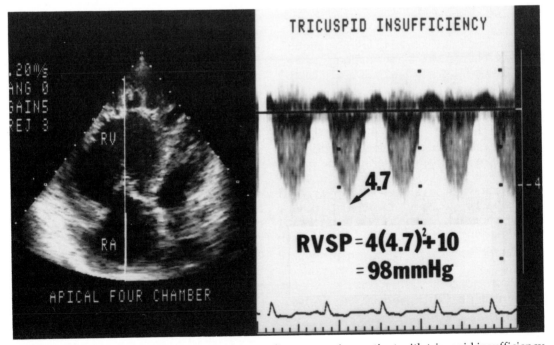

Figure 40.22. Estimation of right ventricular systolic pressure in a patient with tricuspid insufficiency. The *left-hand* panel demonstrates Doppler echocardiogram sampling in the apical four-chamber view. Using this conventional pulsed Doppler and sampling in the right atrium, tricuspid insufficiency is detected. The *right-hand* panel demonstrates continuous wave Doppler echocardiogram in a patient with tricuspid insufficiency. The peak right ventricular pressure (*RVSP*) is estimated from the Doppler-derived pressure gradient across the tricuspid valve in systole added to 10 (an estimate of right atrium [*RA*] pressure). *RV,* right ventricle.

Doppler Estimate of Peak RV Systolic Pressure*

(4 x Vmax²) + 10 = RV systolic pressure

(4 x Vmax²) = Doppler gradient across tricuspid valve

10 = Estimated RA pressure

*Must have tricuspid insufficiency

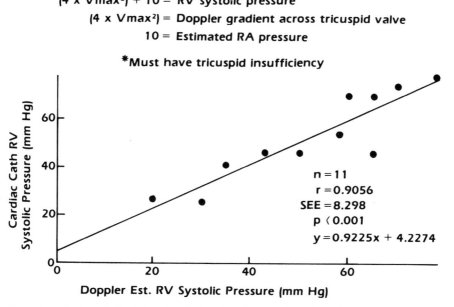

$$(4 \times V_{max}^2) + 10 = \text{RV systolic pressure}$$
$$(4 \times V_{max}^2) = \text{Doppler gradient across tricuspid valve}$$
$$10 = \text{Estimated RA pressure}$$

n = 11
r = 0.9056
SEE = 8.298
p < 0.001
y = 0.9225x + 4.2274

Figure 40.23. Correlation of the Doppler-derived estimate of peak right ventricular (*RV*) pressure with that measured at cardiac catheterization. *Vmax,* maximal Doppler velocity during systole. *RA,* right atrial. (Data from the Medical University of South Carolina, Charleston, SC)

not accurately estimate left atrial mean pressure in the face of associated mitral insufficiency, pulmonary venous obstruction, cor triatriatum, or with a prosthetic mitral valve (74).

For proper calculation of the mitral valve area using the Gorlin equation, cardiac output must be determined while recording the valve gradient. Diastolic filling period and heart rate are also measured, although, as suggested by Hakki et al. (37), and explained earlier, intraprocedural estimation of mitral valve area can be made without exact knowledge of these parameters. This quick calculation is helpful when deciding the need for hemodynamic measurement during exercise. Generally, exercise is performed when a small resting gradient (<5 mm Hg) is seen, but exercise in mitral stenosis has been decreased by the Doppler echocardiographic precatheterization determination of mitral valve area. Invasive exercise study may, however, offer valuable information relating exertional symptoms to hemodynamic abnormalities,

especially in patients with coexistent pulmonary disease or those with histories that are difficult to interpret. Left ventriculography is performed to exclude regional wall motion abnormalities and associated mitral insufficiency. In appropriate age groups, coronary arteriography is necessary to exclude coronary artery disease.

Data Evaluation and Recommendations

Because of excellent noninvasive techniques, it is rare that catheterization provides surprising information in patients with isolated mitral stenosis. In all patients with chest pain or other findings suggesting ischemia, as well as in all men aged more than 35 and women more than 40 years, coronary angiography is recommended. Obviously a review of coronary angiography and a decision regarding need for concomitant coronary artery bypass surgery are important, as is a discussion with the surgeon to whether the patient can be treated with valve repair rather than valve replacement. Percutaneous balloon valvuloplasty has been extensively applied in some centers. Unlike the experience with aortic valvuloplasty, the long-term results of mitral balloon valvuloplasty have been excellent. Technologic advances, as well as operator experience, have contributed to the increased success rate (75). Turi et al. (76) compared percutaneous balloon valvuloplasty with surgical closed commissurotomy in a prospective, randomized trial. In that study, 40 patients were equally randomized to balloon or surgical commissurotomy. Baseline left atrial pressures (26 versus 27 mm Hg), mitral valve gradient (18 versus 19.7 mm Hg), and mitral valve area (1.0 versus 1.0 cm^2) did not differ between the balloon and surgically treated groups. Following percutaneous balloon valvuloplasty, mitral valve area at 1 week was 1.6 $\pm$ 0.6 cm^2 and was the same at 8-month follow-up. For the surgical closed commissurotomy group, mitral valve area 1 week postsurgery was 1.6 $\pm$ 0.7 cm^2 and was unchanged at the 8-month follow-up. No deaths, strokes, or myocardial infarctions were reported, and only a single case of severe mitral regurgitation occurred in each group. Interestingly, because of the cost of disposable equipment, the charge for percutaneous balloon valvuloplasty in India is greater than for the surgical closed commissurotomy. However, the reverse is true in the United States where surgery is more expensive because of physician's fees and operating room charges.

The National Heart, Lung, and Blood Institute (NHLBI) balloon valvuloplasty registry results included 738 patients undergoing percutaneous balloon mitral valvuloplasty in 24 centers (77, 78). In it, 81% of the patients were women, and 25% of all cases had moderate or severe lesions of other valves. Serious complications occurred in 12% of the procedures, including in-laboratory death in eight patients (1%). Within 30 days, 24 cumulative deaths occurred of which 18 were from cardiac cause. Multivariable analysis revealed a smaller valve area and higher echocardiographic score to be strong predictors of early death.

However, the increase in mitral valve area was only weakly related to valve morphology as assessed by echocardiographic score. Thus, the procedure is not done without risks, although if patients are properly selected, hemodynamic and clinical improvement is the rule for most patients. Factors identified as increasing the risks of percutaneous balloon mitral valvuloplasty include: aged more than 70 years, history of cardiac arrest, cerebrovascular disease, dementia, renal insufficiency, cachexia, and class IV congestive heart failure. Other indicators of increased risks include the use of intra-aortic balloon counter pulsation and sympathomimeticamines, as well as a high echocardiographic score ($\geq$13).

Balloon mitral valvuloplasty may be the procedure of choice when mitral restenosis occurs following initially successful surgical commissurotomy. Davidson et al. (79) reported the NHLBI registry experience of 131 (of the 738 total) patients undergoing balloon valvuloplasty following surgical commissurotomy. Whereas hemodynamic changes in those patients were similar to those undergoing balloon mitral valvuloplasty as an initial procedure, symptomatic improvement was slightly less frequent. Those with preserved left ventricular function and lower echocardiographic scores were most likely to improve symptomatically following valvuloplasty for mitral restenosis.

Echocardiography use in patients considered for percutaneous mitral balloon valvuloplasty exemplifies the complementary nature of noninvasive and invasive procedures. Prior to planned valvuloplasty, the echocardiogram provides not only a prognostically useful echocardiographic score, but it may also help avoid complications. Figure 40.24 is an echocardiogram, obtained via the transesophageal approach, prior to planned valvuloplasty for rheumatic mitral stenosis. The study demonstrates a large echogenic mass in the left atrium, with a "swirling" pattern consistent with intra-atrial thrombosis. This clot constitutes a significant procedural risk for systemic embolization and would be a contraindication to the procedure, we believe.

Consideration should be given to the de-

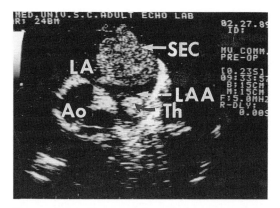

Figure 40.24. Transesophageal echocardiogram performed in a patient prior to planned mitral valvuloplasty. A thrombus (*Th*) is identified in the left atrial appendage and spontaneous echo contrast (*SEC*) is identified in the left atrium (*LA*). *Ao,* aortic valve.

gree of pulmonary hypertension and pulmonary vascular resistance. If they are out of proportion to the degree of mitral obstruction, primary pulmonary vascular disease, chronic lung disease, and recurrent pulmonary emboli (perhaps from a chronically fibrillating right atrium or dilated right ventricle) should be considered. When **marked pulmonary hypertension** and elevated pulmonary vascular resistance are caused by severe mitral stenosis, the pulmonary hemodynamic abnormalities are expected to improve postoperatively (80, 81). However, it may be necessary for the surgeon to decide intraoperatively which patient will require **tricuspid repair,** because the ultimate reduction in pulmonary hypertension may not occur immediately after the mitral obstruction is alleviated. Intraoperative Doppler echocardiography has been used to help decide when to perform tricuspid valvuloplasty (82). Child (83) has offered guidelines for evaluating the tricuspid valve either preoperatively or intraoperatively. Indeed, intraoperative transesophageal echocardiography and Doppler color flow imaging have become routine at most centers including our own.

It has been suggested that a chronically deprived preload or smoldering, subclinical rheumatic myocarditis can cause reduced left ventricular contractility in mitral stenosis. However, left ventricular ejection fraction is usually normal or only slightly reduced. When ejection fraction is decreased, it is often associated with decreased end-systolic wall thickness, as well as with increased peripheral vascular resistance, in which case the resultant increase in afterload may reduce left ventricular systolic performance (84).

Liu et al. (85) recently reported normal systolic function in human mitral stenosis as assessed by end-systolic pressure volume relationships. These investigators did confirm impaired diastolic function, with end-diastolic pressure volume relationships consistently shifted leftward, and with an increased slope. Furthermore, they showed that in human mitral stenosis, the lower compliance of the left ventricle could be acutely reversed by balloon valvuloplasty. Thus, in their study, it appeared that the lower left ventricular compliance was secondary to a functional restriction most likely caused by the left ventricle's attachment to a thickened, immobile valve.

MITRAL VALVE INSUFFICIENCY

Clinical Presentation and Pathophysiology

The mitral valve is anatomically a complex structure with six component parts, including the left atrium, annulus, leaflets, chordae, papillary muscles, and left ventricular free wall (86). Malfunction of any component can result in mitral insufficiency. The left atrial endocardium is continuous with the posterior mitral leaflet. As left atrial size increases, tension is transmitted to this leaflet, producing mitral insufficiency. Accordingly, when mitral insufficiency from any cause results in left atrial enlargement, this will further increase the degree of regurgitation. The mitral annulus is a dynamic structure that can produce mitral insufficiency when it dilates or does not contract adequately during systole. Functional mitral insufficiency can result from left ventricular and annular dilation, or when the annulus calcifies and loses its systolic contraction. Mitral annular calcification occurs most often as an elderly (degenerative) form and in long-standing left ventricular pressure overload (hypertension, aortic stenosis). Mitral annular calcification is also seen in various metabolic disorders, including diabetes, Marfan's syndrome, and chronic renal failure with secondary hyperparathyroidism.

Because of its nearly rectangular shape, the posterior mitral leaflet is subjected to more tension during left ventricular emptying and, therefore, is more often affected by changes in the fibrous skeleton of the heart. The anterior mitral leaflet has no fibrous support, being an extension of the posterior aortic wall. Anterior mitral leaflet proximity to the aortic valve and supporting structures, however, predisposes it to secondary involvement from aortic valve endocarditis.

Rupture of one or more chorda tendineae can cause acute or chronic mitral insufficiency. The chorda can rupture because of chronic degenerative changes in the elderly, fibrocalcific changes secondary to pressure overloads, myxomatous degeneration as part of the mitral valve prolapse syndrome, or as a complication of bacterial endocarditis.

The anterolateral and posteromedial papillary muscles are frequently involved in acute and chronic mitral insufficiency. Each papillary muscle supports both mitral leaflets. If rupture occurs to the belly or the head of either papillary muscle, massive mitral insufficiency is produced causing shock or fulminant pulmonary edema. This condition is usually rapidly fatal without emergency surgical intervention. Rupture of a secondary or tertiary chorda causes subacute mitral insufficiency, which is better tolerated. The base of the papillary muscles is attached to the free wall of the left ventricle, and this connection is frequently affected in ischemic heart disease. This may occur in patients with coronary artery disease who have low ejection fractions and high left ventricular filling pressures. Acute or chronic ischemia of the left ventricular free wall results in regional wall motion abnormalities, preventing proper apposition of the papillary muscles with resultant mitral insufficiency. Primary myocardial dis-

ease, typified by dilated congestive cardiomyopathy, results in a spherically shaped ventricle, causing similar malposition of the papillary muscles, and a varying degree of mitral insufficiency.

Mitral insufficiency is a classic volume overload of the left ventricle. Acutely, this results in increased sarcomere length and left ventricular size (Frank-Starling compensation). Chronically, eccentric left ventricular hypertrophy is an important compensatory mechanism (87–89). The degree of mitral insufficiency depends on the size of the regurgitant orifice, duration of the systolic ejection period, the gradient between the left ventricle and left atrium during ejection, and the relative impedances of the aorta and left atrium (90).

Chronic, compensated mitral insufficiency is not associated with increased left ventricular wall stress. Indeed, it may be reduced because the left ventricular stroke volume can empty into a low pressure left atrium (88). Although this escape valve prevents excessive left ventricular wall stress, it complicates assessment of left ventricular systolic function. Chronic mitral insufficiency affects cardiac pump function in opposing ways. Long-standing volume overload eventually results in reduced myocardial contractile function and cardiac failure. On the other hand, a low pressure left atrium escape valve prevents an increase in left ventricular systolic wall stress or afterload, at least early in the course of this valve lesion. As a result, ejection phase indices of left ventricular systolic function, which are sensitive to changes in afterload such as the ejection fraction, are unreliable in this setting (91, 92). In mitral insufficiency, the ejection fraction is increased or normal until late in the course of the disease. With even a minimal decrease in ejection fraction, extensive reduction may be seen in myocardial contractility (93). The patient with reduced or marginal global left ventricular ejection fraction can significantly worsen after mitral valve replacement as left ventricular wall stress increases (89, 90, 94, 95). Several investigators, however, have reported higher postsurgical left ventricular ejection fractions, reduced mortality, and improved functional status with mitral valve repair (96). This is also true when mitral valve replacement can be altered to maintain intact chordae. Preserving the chordal-papillary muscle attachment allows for preservation of ventricular contractile reserve and, by maintaining smaller ventricular volume, actually reduces postoperative wall stress (97, 98).

Precardiac Catheterization Noninvasive Assessment

Two-dimensional echocardiography allows visual assessment of each of the six components of the mitral valve apparatus, thereby helping establish a cause. Left atrial size can be determined, which aids in establishing whether the mitral insufficiency is acute or chronic. Associated valvular lesions can be identified and overall left ventricular ejection fraction estimated. Regional wall motion abnormalities suggest concomitant coronary artery disease.

Doppler echocardiography is particularly helpful in identifying acute mitral insufficiency, in which case emergent therapy is required even before cardiac catheterization can be performed. Following an acute myocardial infarction, sudden development of pulmonary edema may indicate a mechanical complication, such as rupture of a chorda tendineae. Echocardiography can image the flail mitral leaflet and the paradox of a well-maintained left ventricular ejection fraction despite pulmonary edema or shock. This information may lead to hemodynamic monitoring and vasodilator therapy or intra-aortic balloon counter pulsation prior to cardiac catheterization. Even in the absence of echocardiographically demonstrated flail leaflet, Doppler assessment can provide clues to the acuteness of the mitral insufficiency (Fig. 40.25).

In a more general sense, Doppler echocardiography is useful in semiquantitation of degree of mitral insufficiency. The pulsed Doppler method allows an interrogation of the atrial side of the mitral valve. When a high velocity systolic flow jet is detected, the probe is moved progressively posterior in the left atrium to determine the extent of mitral insufficiency (Fig. 40.26). The further back in the left atrium that the mitral insufficiency jet is detected, the greater the degree

of mitral insufficiency suggested. Multiple views are explored to map the extent of mitral insufficiency in three dimensions. The technique is limited, however, by the eccentricity or broad nature of some regurgitant jets and the varying geometry of the left atrium. For example, if a severe degree of regurgitation is moving in a broad front and into a large left atrium, the degree of mitral insufficiency can be detected much less posteriorly than expected. In general, mitral insufficiency can be accurately classified using this technique, and moderately severe or severe mitral insufficiency is rarely missed (99). The most promising results have come from Doppler color flow imaging by comparing the area of the regurgitant color Doppler signal with the area of the left atrium in orthogonal views (Fig. 40.27). Tribouilloy et al. (100) demonstrated that mitral regurgitation severity can be most accurately assessed by measuring the width of the regurgitant jet during transesophageal Doppler color flow imaging (Fig. 40.28). Correlation with angiographic grading of mitral regurgitation and regurgitant stroke volume was excellent. A jet diameter exceeding 5.5 mm identified severe mitral regurgitation with a sensitivity of 92% and specificity of 92%. Others have found that single-plane transesophageal echocardiography with Doppler color flow mapping correlates best with cardiac catheterization when the maximal regurgitant area is used (101). When the imaged area was less than 3 cm², mild mitral insufficiency was predicted with a sensitivity of 96% and specificity of 100%. In contrast, a maximal regurgitant area exceeding 6 cm² predicted severe mitral insufficiency with a sensitivity of 91% and specificity of 100%. The ratio of regurgitant area to left atrial area also correlated well, but not as closely as that predicted by the measured maximal regurgitant area. Severe mitral insufficiency is also diagnosed when color flow Doppler imaging demonstrates reversal of flow in the pulmonary veins (Fig. 40.29).

Information Obtained at Time of Cardiac Catheterization

An elevation of the mean right atrial pressure suggests right-sided volume overload

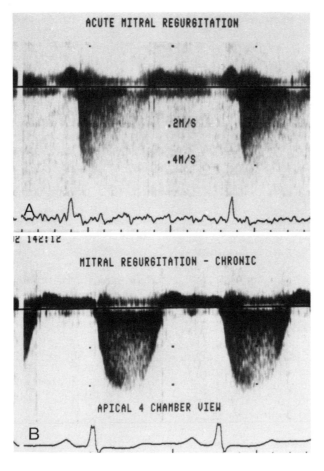

Figure 40.25. Conventional continuous wave, Doppler-obtained velocity envelopes, demonstrating the difference between acute (**A**) and chronic (**B**) mitral insufficiency.

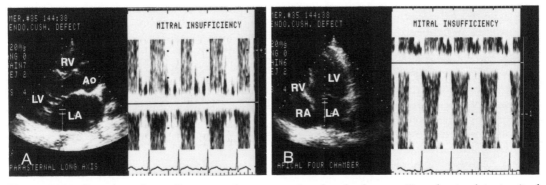

Figure 40.26. Doppler echocardiogram using conventional pulsed wave Doppler to detect mitral insufficiency. **A.** Parasternal long-axis view. **B.** Apical four-chamber view. *Ao*, aorta; *LA*, left atrium; *LV*, left ventricle; *RA*, right atrium; *RV*, right ventricle.

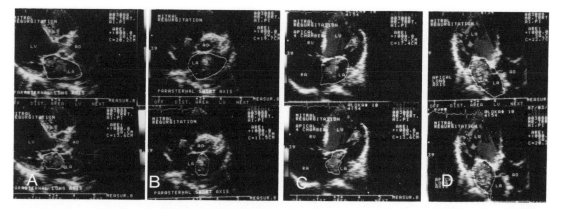

Figure 40.27. Doppler color flow imaging demonstrating mitral insufficiency. Severity of the mitral insufficiency is estimated by determining the ratio of the area of the Doppler signal in the left atrium to the area of the left atrium obtained from four orthogonal views. **A.** Parasternal long-axis view. **B.** Parasternal short-axis view. **C.** Apical four-chamber view. **D.** Apical long-axis view. *Ao,* aorta; *LA,* left atrium; *LV,* left ventricle; *RA,* right atrium; RV, right ventricle.

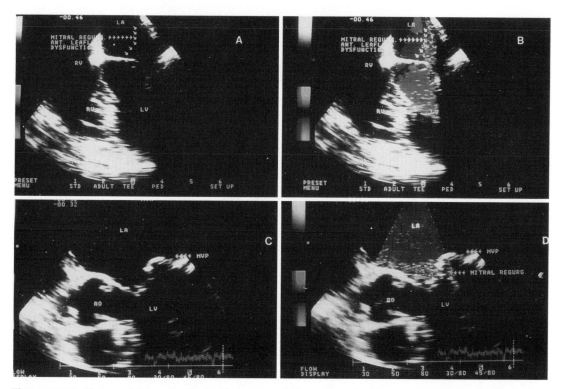

Figure 40.28. Transesophageal echocardiogram with Doppler color flow. **A** and **B.** Mitral regurgitant jet is directed toward the lateral atrial wall, which is consistent with anterior leaflet dysfunction. **C** and **D.** Mitral regurgitant jet is directed medially toward the atrial septum, which is consistent with posterior leaflet dysfunction.

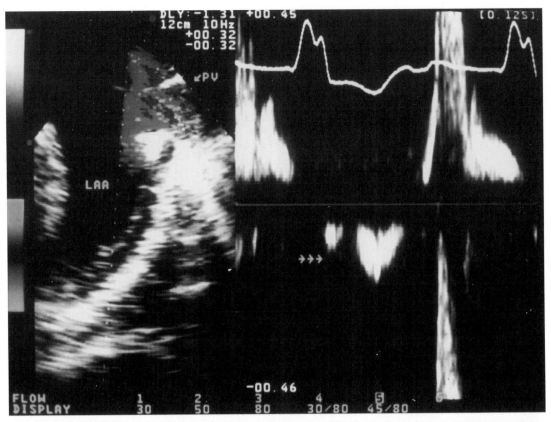

Figure 40.29. Tranesophageal echocardiogram with Doppler color flow and pulsed Doppler of the left superior pulmonary vein demonstrates reversal of flow in the pulmonary vein during systole, which is consistent with severe mitral insufficiency.

from congestive heart failure, tricuspid insufficiency, or, rarely, coincidental pericardial disease. Tricuspid insufficiency may indicate significant pulmonary hypertension from long-standing mitral insufficiency and a need for tricuspid valve replacement or repair at the time of mitral valve surgery. Right atrial mean pressure may also be elevated in tricuspid stenosis, which may accompany rheumatic mitral valve disease. In this setting, the elevated mean pressure will be associated with a large right atrial A-wave in contrast to tricuspid insufficiency, which is associated with a large V-wave or C-V (regurgitant) wave. Right ventricular systolic pressure is measured, and if elevated, pulmonary hypertension or associated pulmonic stenosis is suggested. Advancing the catheter across the pulmonic valve will differentiate these two causes.

Accurate pulmonary artery pressure measurement is important.

If acute mitral insufficiency is present, the regurgitant V-wave may be transmitted back through a small left atrium across the pulmonary vascular bed into the pulmonary arteries. In that situation, the V-wave may be present in the pulmonary artery pressure tracing. The demonstration of such a wave interrupting the normal descent of the pulmonary artery waveform strongly suggests acute and severe mitral insufficiency (102). However, this finding may be absent despite severe mitral insufficiency.

The height of the V-wave in the pulmonary wedge pressure tracing is not always helpful in determining the severity of chronic mitral insufficiency. In this setting, a large, compliant left atrium can absorb a tremendous regurgitant jet without a significant increase in left atrial (pulmonary-capillary wedge) V-wave. In a study of 37 patients with angiographically proved severe mitral insufficiency, 16 (43%) had large V-waves, and in 12 (32%) the V-wave was trivial (103). Pichard et al. (104) evaluated multiple hemodynamic and echocardiographic variables in groups of patients with and without mitral insufficiency, and found that only the ascent slope of the V-wave distinguished the two groups. The size of the V-wave is a function of not only regurgitant volume but also of left atrial size and compliance and the left atrial pressure-volume relationship prior to the onset of systole, among other factors. Other causes of large V-waves in the absence of mitral insufficiency waves include ventricular septal defect, congestive heart failure, and, rarely, mitral obstruction (including mitral stenosis).

With the pulmonary artery catheter in place, systemic arterial pressure is recorded and a ventriculography catheter advanced into the left ventricle. Simultaneous left ventricular and pulmonary-capillary wedge pressures are recorded, looking for a transmitral gradient. With severe mitral insufficiency, transmitral flow is so severely increased that even a normal valve area is relatively stenotic. In contrast to mitral stenosis, no significant mid or late-diastolic gradient is present, and the mean transmitral gradient is trivial. For practical purposes, this should not be a problem of discrimination in the catheterization laboratory because precatheterization echocardiography is accurate in excluding associated mitral stenosis. As soon as the mitral valve gradient is obtained, pulmonary and systemic pressures are again measured and cardiac output determined. Pulmonary and systemic vascular resistances can now be computed and the mitral valve area calculated.

Left ventriculography is performed in a biplane (30° right anterior oblique; 60° left anterior oblique) or monoplane mode (30° right anterior oblique projection). In these views, an accurate estimate can be made of the degree of contrast material regurgitated into the left atrium and ventricular volume measured. Through an appropriate ventriculography catheter, sufficient contrast

agent must be injected to fully opacify the left ventricle at a rate of injection that does not cause significant ventricular ectopy. Ectopic beats should not be used in determining ventricular volumes or qualitative assessment of wall motion to avoid postextrasystolic potentiation of contractility. Also, premature ventricular beats, particularly in runs, can cause reflux of the contrast agent into the left atrium, resulting in pseudomitral insufficiency. They can also increase the degree of mitral insufficiency, causing an overestimate of the actual severity.

Reflux of contrast material into the left atrium that results in faint opacification of the atrium, clearing with each beat, is judged 1+, and correlates roughly with a regurgitant fraction of less than 20%. If cardiac rates are different at the time of ventriculography and forward cardiac output determination, comparative stroke volumes should be used to determine the regurgitant fraction.

When the regurgitant jet opacifies the left atrium and does not clear with each beat, but is less than the opacification of the left ventricle, a grade of 2+ is applied. This generally indicates moderate mitral insufficiency and a regurgitant fraction of 20 to 40%. A designation of 3+ mitral insufficiency indicates that the opacification of the left atrium is equal to that of the left ventricle, and calculated regurgitant fractions typically range from 40 to 60%. Finally, 4+ or severe mitral insufficiency is present when the entire left atrium opacifies with a single beat, progressively opacifies, or when the contrast agent refluxes back into the pulmonary veins (Fig. 40.30). In such cases, a regurgitant fraction of greater than 60% will be calculated.

Several technical factors may cause a discrepancy between the qualitative assessment of the degree of mitral insufficiency and the calculated regurgitant fraction (see Chapter 25). If blood pressure is different at the time of forward cardiac output measurement than at the time of ventriculography, calculation of regurgitant fraction is not reliable. Arrhythmias, such as atrial fibrillation, left atrial dilation, and inaccurate cardiac output determinations, are also sources of discrepancy. The angiographic

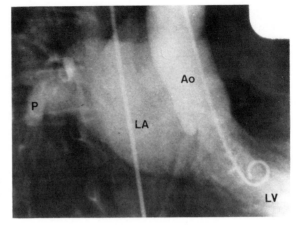

Figure 40.30. Thirty-degree right anterior oblique view of a left ventriculogram shows reflux of contrast material through a dilated left atrium (*LA*) into pulmonary veins (*P*). *Ao*, ascending aorta; *LV*, left ventricle.

cardiac output of the left ventricle may be responsible for the discrepancy if the patient also has associated aortic insufficiency. In this case, total angiographic cardiac output will reflect both aortic and mitral insufficiency, and the calculated regurgitant fraction will be an overestimate of the actual degree of mitral insufficiency. Finally, the inherent errors in valve area calculation and cardiac output computation are potential sources of discrepancy.

Data Evaluation and Recommendations

In chronic mitral insufficiency, patients can be asymptomatic despite a significant reduction in left ventricular contractile function. Noninvasive techniques, including echocardiography, Doppler color flow imaging, and radionuclear studies, are useful adjuncts to patient history and physical diagnosis in assessing left ventricular function. Normalization of what should be supernormal left ventricular systolic function would support cardiac catheterization even in an asymptomatic patient. Exercise treadmill testing is at times useful in convincing a patient who denies symptoms that, in fact, his or her cardiovascular fitness is subnormal. Exercise echocardiography can uncover reduced contractile reserve in chronic mitral insufficiency (105).

Because of low-pressure, low-imped-ance left atrium patients with mitral insufficiency may have normal appearing systolic performance despite reduced myocardial contractility. When the insufficient mitral valve is made competent at the time of surgery, the underlying reduced contractility may be unmasked. Accordingly, considerable research has been aimed at determining at what point patients with mitral insufficiency fail to improve left ventricular function following mitral valve replacement (Table 40.4). A normal or subnormal preoperative global left ventricular ejection fraction usually predicts a suboptimal surgical result (106). In fact, Enriquez-Sarano et al. (107) have shown in a study of more than 400 patients that preoperative ejection fraction should exceed 0.60 to ensure normal postoperative longevity. Likewise Zile et al. found that echocardiographic shortening fraction also had to be super normal to ensure a good outcome (108).

Because increased preload confounds interpretation of ejection phase indexes in mitral regurgitation, end-systolic left ventricular dimension, which is more preload independent, has also been examined as a parameter for timing surgery. The results have been remarkably consistent. Wisenbaugh et al. (109) found an end-systolic dimension of 45 mm (note the contrast to the 55 mm used in aortic insufficiency) separated good from bad outcomes. Zile et al. (108) found an end-systolic dimension index of 2.6 cm/m^2, which when multiplied by the body surface area in that study of

Table 40.4.
Predictors of Suboptimal Response to Mitral Valve Replacement for Chronic Mitral Insufficiency

	Value	Reference
Echocardiography		
LV shortening fraction	< 0.32	(108)
End-diastolic dimension index	> 40 mm/m^2	(108)
End-systolic dimension	> 50 mm	(94)
End-systolic dimension index	> 26 mm/m^2	(108)
Left atrial size	> 50 mm	(110)
Cardiac Catheterization		
Subnormal LV ejection fraction	≤ 0.55	(106)
Elevated LV end-diastolic pressure	> 12 mm Hg	(112)
Large LV end-systolic volume index	> 60 cc/m^2	(62)
Large LV end-diastolic volume index	> 220 mL/m^2	(113)
LV end-systolic stress:volume ratio	< 2.5	(95)

LV, left ventricular.

1.75 cm^2, also equals 45 mm. In turn, this dimension can be converted to an end-systolic volume index of 53 mL/m^2, almost identical to 50 mL/m^2 found to demarcate good from bad outcomes by Crawford et al. (111), and similar to the 60 mL/m^2 found by Borow et al. (62).

End-systolic stress/end-systolic volume ratio use has allowed good discrimination of surgical outcome in patients with chronic mitral insufficiency. This index, which is relatively independent of preload and adjustable for afterload, is a better estimate of myocardial contractility in altered loading states such as mitral insufficiency (91). A ratio of less than 2.5 was associated with a poor surgical result, even in the face of a normal ejection fraction. Mitral valve replacement was successful with a good postoperative functional state when the ratio exceeded 2.5 (95).

Patients with mitral insufficiency who are symptomatic should undergo cardiac catheterization. A recommendation for surgery is based on a full review of all data with major emphasis on left ventricular contractile performance. If associated coronary artery disease is demonstrated, coronary artery bypass surgery should be performed at the time of mitral valve replacement or repair.

Cardiac catheterization is recommended for the asymptomatic patient with significant mitral insufficiency and any evidence of left ventricular systolic dysfunction. Patients in whom serial noninvasive studies indicate decreasing left ventricular systolic function, even in the absence of symptoms, should undergo cardiac catheterization. Noninvasive and cardiac catheterization data, particularly end-systolic parameters of left ventricular function, are useful adjuncts to clinical judgment when recommending mitral valve replacement or repair in such patients (112). **In general, a recommendation for surgery occurs earlier than symptoms might direct**, because of the realization that valve replacement or repair is less successful once myocardial contractility has decreased (113).

TRICUSPID STENOSIS

Obstruction to tricuspid inflow occurs in rheumatic heart disease, virtually always with associated mitral valve involvement and, occasionally, secondary to prosthetic valve dysfunction, in which case the prosthesis has been placed for tricuspid insufficiency. As the frequency of rheumatic heart disease has decreased and surgeons have used tricuspid valvoplasty to repair tricuspid insufficiency, the incidence of tricuspid stenosis has steadily declined.

Elevated right atrial filling pressures and low cardiac output are the hemodynamic hallmarks of tricuspid stenosis. Unlike tricuspid insufficiency, which is characterized by an elevated mean pressure and large V- or regurgitant wave, tricuspid stenosis manifests a large right atrial A-wave, as long as the patient is in sinus rhythm. Atrial fibrillation frequently develops, making exact measurement of transvalvular gradient and tricuspid valve area difficult. The gradient across the tricuspid valve is usually determined at the time of pullback of a catheter from the right ventricle to the right atrium, or by simultaneous measurement of right atrial and right ventricular pressure.

Precatheterization Doppler echocardiographic studies will greatly facilitate catheterization evaluation of patients with suspected rheumatic heart disease by uncovering a lesion such as tricuspid stenosis. At times, the tricuspid valve area can be better estimated noninvasively because of the atrial fibrillation and low holodiastolic gradient discussed. Consequently, a combined noninvasive and invasive evaluation is recommended. When cardiac catheterization and noninvasive data are combined, it is unlikely that the surgeon will be faced with an unexpected finding of significant tricuspid stenosis.

TRICUSPID INSUFFICIENCY

Most tricuspid insufficiency is functional, secondary to dilation of the tricuspid annulus as a result of right ventricular dilation, which, itself, is most often caused by pulmonary hypertension. Any cause of left ventricular failure that results in pulmonary hypertension can cause the right ventricle to dilate with a variable degree of tricuspid insufficiency, even with an anatomically normal valve. Organic tricuspid insufficiency occurs with infective endocarditis or secondary to anterior chest trauma. In the latter case, the tricuspid insufficiency is caused by right ventricular myocardial contusion and disruption of the tricuspid apparatus.

Noninvasive assessment is useful in quantitating the degree of tricuspid insufficiency, perhaps underestimated on physical examination because of more prominent left-side heart murmurs. Echocardiography excludes anatomic disruption of the valve and can demonstrate valvular vegetations. This information is helpful in planning catheterization, because catheter passage through the right ventricle could cause embolization of the vegetation. Pulsed Doppler mapping of the tricuspid insufficiency jet in the right atrium is done in a manner previously described for aortic and mitral insufficiency (Fig. 40.31). As was true with aortic and mitral insufficiency, quantitation of tricuspid insufficiency on the basis of Doppler color flow imaging has yielded generally excellent correlation with angiographic assessment (114). Color flow Doppler detection of systolic reversal of flow in hepatic veins is another useful indicator of severe tricuspid insufficiency.

As mentioned, the velocity shift across the tricuspid valve in tricuspid insufficiency allows an estimate of the right ventricular systolic pressure. The Doppler shift at that level is added to an estimation of right atrial mean pressure, which is made by observing the neck veins (Fig. 40.22).

At the time of cardiac catheterization, tricuspid insufficiency is demonstrated by elevated right atrial mean pressures and a large V-wave in the right atrial pressure tracing. As is true for mitral insufficiency, the height of the V-wave is affected by the patient's rhythm, forcefulness of right ventricular contractility, and, most importantly, size of the right atrium.

When the V-wave is two or three times greater than the right atrial mean pressure, severe tricuspid insufficiency probably exists. In this case, the right atrium is not large enough to accommodate the regurgitant jet without a marked increase in pressure. Absence of a large V-wave, however, does not exclude severe tricuspid insufficiency. Patients with atrial fibrillation and moderate right ventricular volume overload may have a larger than normal V-wave, even without tricuspid insufficiency. This is distinguished from the regurgitant V-wave of tricuspid insufficiency by its timing. The regurgitant wave occurs earlier and blends in with the later occurring antegrade V-wave that is secondary to forward vena caval flow.

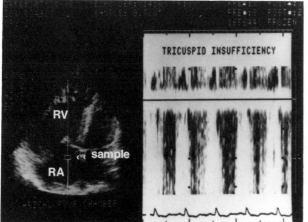

Figure 40.31. Doppler echocardiogram in the apical four-chamber view, using conventional pulsed wave Doppler and sampling in the right atrium, shows tricuspid insufficiency. *RA,* right atrium; *RV,* right ventricle.

As the catheter is passed through the right ventricle and into the pulmonary vascular bed, one would expect to find pulmonary hypertension. When pulmonary hypertension is absent, primary tricuspid valve disease or associated complex congenital disorders, such as Ebstein's anomaly of the tricuspid valve, is suggested. Pericardial disease may cause a similar elevation of right atrial pressure with normal or mildly elevated pulmonary artery pressures. In the case of pericardial disease, however, the characteristic tricuspid insufficiency V-wave would be absent, and left and right ventricular pressures would reveal equalization of diastolic pressures.

Cineangiography is performed in the right anterior oblique view with sufficient volume to opacify the dilated right ventricle chambers, but at a rate of injection that does not cause ventricular ectopy.

With the catheter placed across the tricuspid valve, artifactual tricuspid insufficiency, secondary to a regurgitant orifice created by the catheter itself, will be present. For this reason, right ventricular angiography is not usually performed unless hemodynamic or noninvasive data conflict with the precatheterization clinical impression.

PULMONIC STENOSIS AND PULMONIC INSUFFICIENCY

Pulmonic stenosis and insufficient valvular lesions generally occur as part of complex

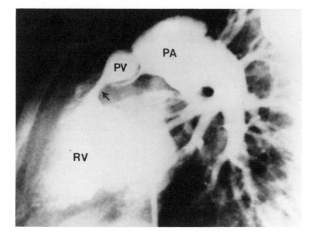

Figure 40.32. Right ventriculogram in a lateral projection of a 20-year-old woman with Noonan's syndrome. *Solid arrow* points to the narrowed right ventricular outflow tract (infundibular stenosis). Superior to the infundibular stenosis, a domed pulmonic valve (*PV*) with marked poststenotic dilation of the pulmonary artery (*PA*) is demonstrated. *RV,* right ventricle.

congenital heart disease (Chapter 43) or, in the case of pulmonary insufficiency, secondary to severe pulmonary hypertension. In the case of pulmonic stenosis, the obstruction may be valvular, subvalvular, or supravalvular, the last of which may be associated with pulmonary artery branch stenosis. It is often difficult to determine the exact position of the pulmonic stenosis at the time of right ventricular catheter pullback; consequently, right ventricular angiography is performed in a view that delineates the right ventricular outflow tract,

pulmonic valve, and (by way of pulmonary angiography) pulmonary branch stenosis. Figure 40.32 demonstrates pulmonic and infundibular stenosis in a 20-year-old patient with Noonan's syndrome. Doming of the pulmonic valve and poststenotic dilation of the pulmonary artery are well demonstrated.

Usually in severe pulmonary stenosis, right atrial filling pressures are elevated with a prominent A-wave, especially when the right ventricular systolic pressure exceeds 60 mm Hg (Fig. 40.33A). An A-wave

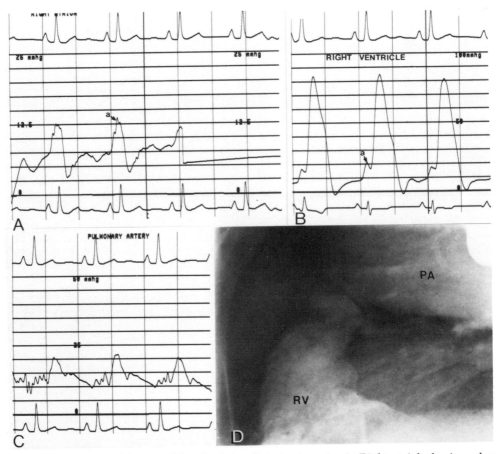

Figure 40.33. A 56-year-old man with valvular pulmonic stenosis. **A.** Right atrial phasic and mean tracing. Although the right atrial mean pressure is normal at 60 mm Hg, a prominent A-wave is present (designated *a* at the arrow). **B.** Right ventricular tracing of the same patient. Right ventricular systolic pressure is markedly elevated at 66 mm Hg, with a prominent A-wave (designated *"a"* at the arrow). **C.** Distal to the pulmonic valve, pulmonary artery pressures are normal (22/10 mm Hg), yielding a peak-to-peak gradient across the pulmonic valve of 45 mm Hg. **D.** Right ventricular angiogram in the lateral projection of the same patient. The infundibulum is not narrowed; however, the valve leaflets are domed, and severe poststenotic dilation of the pulmonary artery is seen. *RV*, right ventricle; *PA*, pulmonary artery.

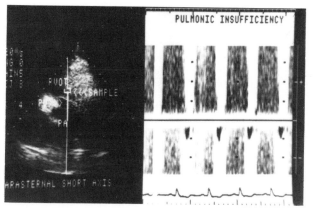

Figure 40.34. Doppler echocardiogram in the parasternal short-axis view. Using conventional pulsed wave Doppler and sampling in the right ventricular outflow tract, pulmonary insufficiency is detected. *PA,* pulmonary artery; *PV,* pulmonary valve; *RVOT,* right ventricular outflow tract.

will not be present, however, if atrial fibrillation has developed. The exact location of right ventricular outflow tract or pulmonary valvular obstruction is demonstrated by a slow pullback of an end-hole catheter with simultaneous fluoroscopy and pressure measurement (Fig. 40.33B and C). Cineangiography is usually performed in the anteroposterior and lateral (Fig. 40.33D) views.

Pulmonary insufficiency is generally secondary to pulmonary hypertension. The right ventricle must absorb the volume overload resulting from blood regurgitated back from the pulmonary vascular bed as well as that entering the right ventricle antegradely across the tricuspid valve. As a result, right ventricular dilation and a varying degree of right ventricular end-diastolic pressure elevation, depending on the compliance of that chamber, will be seen. Because of catheter-produced artifact, cineangiography is generally not useful in pulmonary insufficiency.

Estimation of pulmonary artery systolic pressure, semiquantitative assessment of degree of pulmonary insufficiency, and anatomic evaluation of pulmonic valve are facilitated by Doppler echocardiographic studies (Fig. 40.34). Although pulmonary insufficiency is usually functional, we have seen cases of pulmonic valve endocarditis, secondary to intravenous drug abuse, resulting in significant pulmonic insufficiency.

SUMMARY

Evaluation of a patient with valvular heart disease begins with an accurate history and thorough physical examination. Following this, the physician typically orders one or more noninvasive studies, which usually confirms the diagnosis, and helps answer important management questions, such as the need for bacterial endocarditis prophylaxis and the timing of invasive diagnostic and therapeutic procedures.

Throughout this chapter, we have emphasized that these noninvasive procedures complement and extend the information obtained at the time of cardiac catheterization. In the case of chronic regurgitant lesions, for example, serial measurements of left ventricular systolic performance aid in the proper timing of both cardiac catheterization and valve surgery. In the acutely ill decompensated patient with valvular heart disease, these noninvasive procedures are even more important. Such patients may not tolerate prolonged procedures and injection of large amounts of contrast agents. By appropriately utilizing these noninvasive techniques, the cardiac catheterization protocol can be modified to minimize risks while obtaining all of the information needed to make proper management decisions. Integration of these noninvasive and cardiac catheterization data allows for optimal diagnosis and management of the patient with valvular heart disease.

We close this chapter with a word of caution. Despite impressive technologic advances in both noninvasive and invasive techniques, **clinical judgment remains of paramount importance.** The patient with valvular heart disease is not optimally served by undue reliance on any single noninvasive or invasive measurement. Finally, application of any of these techniques requires confidence in one's own noninvasive and invasive laboratories, emphasizing the need for ongoing quality control in these facilities.

References

1. Roberts WC. The congenitally bicuspid aortic valve—a study of 85 autopsy cases. Am J Cardiol 1970;26:72–79.
2. Finoglio JJ, McAllister HA, DeCastro CM, et al. Congenital bicuspid aortic valve after age 20. Am Cardiol 1977;39:164–172.
3. Grossman W, Jones D, McLaurin LP. Wall stress and patterns of hypertrophy in the human left ventricle. J Clin Invest 1975;56:56–64.
4. Sasayama S, Ross J Jr, Franklin D, et al. Adaptations of the left ventricle to chronic pressure overload. Circ Res 1976;38:172–180.
5. Gunther S, Grossman W. Determinants of ventricular function in pressure-overload hypertrophy in man. Circulation 1979;59:679–688.
6. Spann JF, Bove AA, Natarajan G, et al. Ventricular performance, pump function and compensatory mechanisms in patients with aortic stenosis. Circulation 1980;62:576–584.
7. Donner R, Carabello BA, Black I, et al. Left ventricular wall stress in compensated aortic stenosis in children. Am J Cardiol 1983;51:946–951.
8. Assey ME, Wisenbaugh T, Spann JF Jr, et al. Unexpected persistence into adulthood of low wall stress in congenital aortic stenosis: is there a fundamental difference in hypertrophy response to a pressure overload present from birth rather than acquired? Circulation 1987;75:973–979.
9. Murakami T, Hess OM, Gage JE, et al. Diastolic filling dynamics in patients with aortic stenosis. Circulation 1986;73:1162–1170.
10. Peterson KL, Tauji J, Johnson A, et al. Diastolic left ventricular pressure-volume and stress-strain relationships in patients with valvular aortic stenosis and left ventricular hypertrophy. Circulation 1978;58:77–89.
11. Pantely G, Morton M, Rahimtoola SH. Effects of successful, uncomplicated valve replacement on ventricular hypertrophy, volume and performance in aortic stenosis and in aortic competence. J Thorac Cardiovasc Surg 1978;75:383–391.
12. Kennedy JW, Doces J, Stewart DK. Left ventricular function before and following aortic valve replacement. Circulation 1977;56:944–950.
13. Frank S, Johnson A, Ross J Jr. Natural history of valvular aortic stenosis. Br Heart J 1973;35:41–49.
14. Morrow AG, Roberts WC, Ross J Jr, et al. Clinical staff conference. Obstruction to left ventricular outflow. Current concepts of management and operative treatment. Ann Intern Med 1968;69:1255–1261.
15. Tobin JR, Rahimtoola SH, Blundell PE, et al. Percentage of left ventricular stroke work loss, a simple hemodynamic concept for estimation of severity in valvular aortic stenosis. Circulation 1968;35:868–879.
16. Ross J Jr, Braunwald E. The influence of corrective operations on natural history of aortic stenosis. Circulation 1968;37:V-61–V-66.
17. Chizner MA, Pearle DL, deLeon AC. The natural history of aortic stenosis in adults. Am Heart J 1980;99:419–424.
18. Ross J Jr. Afterload mismatch and preload reserve: a conceptual framework for the analysis of ventricular function. Prog Cardiovasc Dis 1976;18:255–261.
19. Croke RP, Pifane R, Sullivan H, et al. Reversal of advanced left ventricular dysfunction following aortic valve replacement for aortic stenosis. Ann Thorac Surg 1977;24:38–43.
20. Hatle L, Angelsen B. Doppler ultrasound in cardiology—physical principles and clinical applications. 2nd ed. Philadelphia: Lea and Febiger, 1985; 22.
21. Handshoe R, DeMaria AN. Doppler assessment of intracardiac pressures. Echocardiography 1985; 2:127–139.
22. Richards KL, Cannon SR, Miller JF, et al. Calculation of aortic valve area by Doppler echocardiography: a direct application of the continuity equation. Circulation 1986;73:964–969.
23. Oh JK, Taliercio CP, Holmes DR JR, et al. Prediction of the severity of aortic stenosis by Doppler aortic valve area determination: prospective Doppler-catheterization correlation in 100 patients. J Am Coll Cardiol 1988;11(6):1227–1234.
24. Peller OG, Wallerson DC, Devereux RB. Role of Doppler and imaging echocardiography in selection of patients for cardiac valvular surgery. Am Heart J 1987;114:1445–1460.
25. Hakki AH, Kimbiris D, Iskandrian AS, et al. Angina pectoris and coronary artery disease in patients with severe aortic valvular disease. Am Heart J 1980;100:441–449.
26. Kupari M, Virtanen KS, Turto H, et al. Exclusion of coronary artery disease by exercise thallium-201 tomography in patients with aortic stenosis. Am J Cardiol 1992;70:635–640.
27. Samuels B, Kiat H, Friedman JD, et al. Adenosine pharmacologic stress myocardial perfusion tomographic imaging in patients with significant aortic stenosis: diagnostic efficacy and comparison of clinical, hemodynamic and electrocardiographic variable with 100 age-matched control subjects. J Am Coll Cardiol 1995;25:99–106.
28. Richardson JV, Kouchoukos NT, Wright JO, et al. Combined aortic valve replacement and myocardial revascularization: results in 220 patients. Circulation 1979;59:75–83.
29. Kirklin JW, Barratt-Boyes BG. Aortic valve disease: morphology, diagnostic criteria, natural history, techniques, results and indications. Cardiac surgery. New York: John Wiley and Sons, 1986; 374–420.
30. Bonow RO, Kent KM, Rosing DR, et al. Aortic valve replacement without myocardial revascularization in patients with combined aortic valvu-

lar stenosis and coronary artery disease. Circulation 1981;63:243–251.

31. Folland ED, Parisi AF, Carbone C. Is peripheral arterial pressure a reliable substitute for ascending aortic pressure when measuring aortic valve gradients? J Am Coll Cardiol 1984;4:1207–1214.

32. Carabello BA, Barry WH, Grossman W. Changes in arterial pressure during left heart pullback in patients with aortic stenosis: a sign of severe aortic stenosis. Am J Cardiol 1979;44:424–430.

33. Brogan WC III, Lange RA, Hillis LD. Accuracy of various methods of measuring the transvalvular pressure gradient in aortic stenosis. Am Heart J 1992;123:948–953.

34. Gorlin R, Gorlin SG. Hydraulic formula for calculation of stenotic mitral valve, other cardiac valves and central circulatory shunts. Am Heart J 1951; 41:1–19.

35. Cannon SR, Richards KL, Crawford M. Hydraulic estimation of stenotic orifice area: a correction of the Gorlin formula. Circulation 1985;71: 1170–1178.

36. Burwash, IG, Thomas, DD, Sadahiro, M, et al. Dependence of Gorlin formula and continuity equation valve areas on transvalvular volume flow rate in valvular aortic stenosis. Circulation 1994; 89:827–835.

37. Hakki AH, Iskandrian AS, Bemis CE, et al. A simplified valve formula for the calculation of stenotic cardiac valve areas. Circulation 1981;63: 1050–1056.

38. Angel J, Soler-Soler J, Anivarro I, et al. Hemodynamic evaluation of stenotic cardiac valves. II. Modification of the simplified valve formula for mitral and aortic valve areas calculation. Cathet Cardiovasc Diagn 1985;11:127–138.

39. Henry WL, Bonow RO, Borer JS, et al. Evaluation of aortic valve replacement in patients with valvular aortic stenosis. Circulation 1980;61:814–825.

40. Smith N, McAnulty JH, Rahimtoola SH. Severe aortic stenosis with impaired left ventricular function and clinical heart failure: results of valve replacement. Circulation 1978;58:255–264.

41. McKay RG, Safian RD, Lock JE, et al. Assessment of left ventricular and aortic valve function after aortic balloon valvuloplasty in adult patients with critical aortic stenosis. Circulation 1987;75: 192–200.

42. Carabello BA, Green LH, Grossman W, et al. Hemodynamic determinants of prognosis of aortic valve replacement in critical aortic stenosis and advanced congestive heart failure. Circulation 1980;62:42–48.

43. Brogan WC III, Grayburn PA, Lange RA, et al. Prognosis after valve replacement in patients with severe aortic stenosis and a low transvalvular pressure gradient. J Am Coll Cardiol 1993;21: 1657–1660.

44. deFilippi CR, Willett DL, Brickner E, et al. Usefulness of dobutamine echocardiography in distinguishing severe from nonsevere valvular aortic stenosis in patients with depressed left ventricular function and low transvalvular gradients. Am J Cardiol 1995;75:191–194.

45. Ford LE, Felderman T, Chiu YC, et al. Hemodynamic resistance as a measure of functional impairment in aortic valvular stenosis. Circulation 1990;66:1–7.

46. Cannon JD Jr, Zile MR, Crawford FA, et al. Aortic valve resistance as an adjunct to the Gorlin formula in assessing the severity of aortic stenosis in symptomatic patients. J Am Coll Cardiol 1992; 20:1517–1523.

47. Kelly TA, Rothbart RM, Cooper CM, et al. Comparison of outcome of asymptomatic to symptomatic patients older than 20 years of age with valvular aortic stenosis. Am J Cardiol 1988;61:123–130.

48. Pellikka PA, Nishimura RA, Bailey KR, et al. The natural history of adults with asymptomatic hemodynamically significant aortic stenosis. J Am Coll Cardiol 1990;15:1012–1017.

49. Wisenbaugh T, Spann JF, Carabello BA. Differences in myocardial performance and load between patients with similar amounts of chronic aortic versus chronic mitral regurgitation. J Am Coll Cardiol 1984;3:916–923.

50. Sapira JD, Quincke HI, de Musset A, et al. Some aortic regurgitations. South Med J 1981;74: 459–467.

51. Matsuo H, Morita T, Senda S, et al. Noninvasive visualization and estimation of severity of aortic regurgitation by multigated pulsed Doppler technique. In: Spencer MP, ed. Cardiac Doppler diagnosis. Boston: Martinus-Nijhoff, 1983:281.

52. Kitabatake A, Masuyama T, Asao M, et al. Color visualization of two-dimensional distribution of intracardiac flow abnormalities by multigate Doppler technique. In: Spencer MP, ed. Cardiac Doppler diagnosis. Boston: Martinus-Nijhoff, 1983:309.

53. Perry GJ, Helmcke F, Nanda NC, et al. Evaluation of aortic insufficiency by Doppler color flow mapping. J Am Coll Cardiol 1987;9:952–959.

54. Teague SM, Heinsimer JA, Anderson JL, et al. Quantification of aortic regurgitation utilizing continuous wave Doppler ultrasound. J Am Coll Cardiol 1986;8:592–599.

55. Bonow RO, Lakatos E, Maron BJ, et al. Serial long-term assessment of the natural history of asymptomatic patients with chronic aortic regurgitation and normal left ventricular systolic function. Circulation 1991;84:1625–1635.

56. Carabello BA, Usher BW, Hendrix GH, et al. Predictors of outcome for aortic valve replacement in patients with aortic regurgitation and left ventricular dysfunction: a change in the measuring stick. J Am Col Cardiol 1987;10:991–997.

57. Henry WL, Bonow RO, Borer JS, et al. Observations on the optimum time for operative intervention for aortic regurgitation. I. Evaluation of the results of aortic valve replacement in symptomatic patients. Circulation 1980;61:471–483.

58. Gaasch WH, Carroll JD, Levine HJ, et al. Chronic aortic regurgitation: prognostic value of left ventricular end-systolic dimension and end-diastolic radius/thickness ratio. J Am Coll Cardiol 1983;1: 775–782.

59. Samuels DA, Curfman GD, Friedlich AL, et al. Valve replacement for aortic regurgitation: long-term follow-up with factors influencing the results. Circulation 1979;60:647–654.

60. Forman R, Firth BG, Barnard MS. Prognostic sig-

nificance of preoperative left ventricular ejection fraction and valve lesion in patients with aortic valve replacement. Am J Cardiol 1980;45: 1120–1125.

61. Carabello BA, Williams H, Gash AK, et al. Hemodynamic predictors of outcome in patients undergoing valve replacement. Circulation 1986; 74:1309–1316.

62. Borrow KM, Green LH, Mann T, et al. End-systolic volume as a predictor of postoperative left ventricular performance in volume overload from valvular regurgitation. Am J Med 1980;68: 655–663.

63. Levine HJ, Gaasch WH. Ratio of regurgitant volume to end-diastolic volume: a major determinant of ventricular response to surgical correction of chronic volume overload. Am J Cardiol 1983;52: 406–410.

64. Schattenberg TT, Titus JL, Parkin TW. Clinical findings in acquired aortic valve stenosis. Effect of disease of other valves. Am Heart J 1967;73: 322–326.

65. Gash AK, Carabello BA, Kent RL, et al. Left ventricular performance in patients with coexistent mitral stenosis and aortic insufficiency. J Am Coll Cardiol 1984;3:703–705.

66. Herrera CJ, Chaudhry FA, DeFrino PF, et al. Value and limitations of transesophageal echocardiography in evaluating prosthetic or bioprosthetic valve dysfunction. Am J Cardiol 1992;69: 697–699.

67. Botvinick EH, Schiller NB, Wickramasekaran R, et al. Echocardiographic determination of mitral valve closure in severe aortic insufficiency: its clinical implications. Circulation 1975;51:836–847.

68. Pepine CJ, Nichols WW, Curry RC, et al. Reversal of premature mitral valve closure by nitroprusside in severe aortic insufficiency: beat to beat pressure-flow and echocardiographic relationships [Abstract]. Am J Cardiol 1976;37:161A.

69. Omoto R, Kyo S, Matsumura M, et al. Evaluation of biplane color Doppler transesophageal echocardiography in 200 consecutive patients. Circulation 1992;85:1237–1247.

70. Keren A, Kim CB, HU BS, et al. Accuracy of biplane and multiplane transesophageal echocardiography in diagnosis of typical acute aortic dissection and intramural hematoma. J Am Coll Cardiol 1996;28:627–636.

71. Nakatani S, Masuyama T, Kodama K, et al. Value and limitations of Doppler echocardiography in the quantification of stenotic mitral valve area: comparison of the pressure half-time and the continuity equation methods. Circulation 1988;77: 78–85.

72. Erzengin F, Williams G, Rao S, et al. Closed or open mitral valvotomy or valve replacement? J Cardiovas Ultrasonogr 1985;4:253–258.

73. Abascal VM, Wilkins GT, Choong CW, et al. Echocardiographic evaluation of mitral valve structure and function in patients followed for at least 6 months after percutaneous balloon mitral valvuloplasty. J Am Coll Cardiol 1988;12:606–615.

74. Schoenfeld, MH, Palacios IF, Hutter AM Jr, et al. Underestimation of prosthetic mitral valve areas: role of transseptal catheterization in avoiding un-

necessary repeat mitral valve surgery. J Am Coll Cardiol 1985;5:1387–1392.

75. Ruiz, CE, Zhang HP, Macaya C, et al. Comparison of Inoue single-balloon versus double-balloon technique for percutaneous mitral valvotomy. Am Heart J 1992;123:942–948.

76. Turi ZG, Reyes VP, Raju BS, et al. Percutaneous balloon versus surgical closed commissurotomy for mitral stenosis. A prospective, randomized trial. Circulation 1991;83:1179–1185.

77. The National Heart, Lung, and Blood Institute Balloon Valvuloplasty Registry Participants. Multicenter experience with balloon mitral commissurotomy. NHLBI balloon valvuloplasty registry report on immediate and 30-day follow-up results. Circulation 1992;85:448–461.

78. National Heart, Lung, and Blood Institute Balloon Valvuloplasty Registry. Complications and mortality of percutaneous balloon mitral commissurotomy. Circulation 1992;85:2014–2024.

79. Davidson CJ, Bashore TM, Mikel M, et al., for the National Heart, Lung, and Blood Institute Balloon Valvuloplasty Registry Participants. Balloon mitral commissurotomy after previous surgical commissurotomy. Circulation 1992;86:91–99.

80. Dalen JE, Matloff JM, Evans GL, et al. Early reduction of pulmonary vascular resistance after mitral valve replacement. N Engl J Med 1967;277: 387–394.

81. Braunwald E, Braunwald NS, Ross J Jr, et al. Effects of mitral valve replacement on the pulmonary vascular dynamics of patients with pulmonary hypertension. N Engl J Med 1965;273: 509–518.

82. Messina AG, Yao FS, Isom OW, et al. Atrioventricular valve annuloplasty. Assessment by transesophageal echocardiographic Doppler and contrast studies [Abstract]. Clin Res 1987;35:305A.

83. Child JS. Improved guides to tricuspid valve repair: two-dimensional echocardiographic analysis of tricuspid annulus function and color flow imaging of severity of tricuspid regurgitation [Editorial]. J Am Coll Cardiol 1989;4:1217–1222.

84. Gash AK, Carabello BA, Cepin D, et al. Left ventricular ejection performance and systolic muscle function in patients with mitral stenosis. Circulation 1983;67:148–154.

85. Liu CP, Ting CT, Yang TM, et al. Reduced left ventricular compliance in human mitral stenosis. Role of reversible internal constraint. Circulation 1992;85:1447–1456.

86. Roberts WC, Perloff JK. Mitral valve disease: a clinicopathologic survey of the conditions causing the mitral valve to function abnormally. Ann Intern Med 1972;77:939–975.

87. Ross J Jr. Adaptations of the left ventricle to chronic volume overload. Circ Res 1974;35:II-64–II-70.

88. Eckberg DL, Gault JH, Bouchard RL, et al. Mechanics of left ventricular contraction in chronic severe mitral regurgitation. Circulation 1973;47: 1252–1259.

89. Urschel CW, Covell JW, Sonnenblick EH, et al. Myocardial mechanics in aortic and mitral valvular regurgitation. The concept of instantaneous

impedance as a determinant of the performance of the intact heart. J Clin Invest 1968;47:867–872.

90. Yoran C, Yellin EL, Becker RM, et al. Dynamic aspects of acute mitral regurgitation: effects of ventricular volume, pressure and contractility on the effective regurgitant orifice area. Circulation 1979;60:170–176.

91. Carabello BA, Spann JF. The uses and limitations of end systolic indexes of left ventricular function. Circulation 1984;69:1058–1064.

92. Sagawa K. The end systolic pressure volume relation of the ventricle: definition, modifications and clinical use. Circulation 1981;63:1223–1227.

93. Gault JH, Ross J Jr, Braunwald E. Contractile state of the left ventricle in man: instantaneous tension-velocity-length relationships in patients with and without disease of the left ventricular myocardium. Circ Res 1968;22:451–463.

94. Schuler G, Peterson KL, Johnson A, et al. Temporal response of left ventricular performance to mitral valve surgery. Circulation 1979;59:1218–1231.

95. Carabello BA, Nolan SP, McGuire LB. Assessment of preoperative left ventricular function in patients with mitral regurgitation: value of the end systolic wall stress-end systolic volume ratio. Circulation 1981;64:1212–1217.

96. Goldman ME, Mora F, Guarino T, et al. Mitral valvuloplasty is superior to valve replacement for preservation of left ventricular function: an intraoperative two-dimensional echocardiographic study. J Am Coll Cardiol 1987;10:568–575.

97. David TE, Burns RJ, Bacchus CM, et al. Mitral valve replacement for mitral regurgitation with and without preservation of chordae tendineae. J Thorac Cardiovasc Surg 1984;88:718–725.

98. Rozich JD, Carabello BA, Usher BW, et al. Mitral valve replacement with and without chordal preservation in patients with chronic mitral regurgitation: mechanisms for differences in postoperative ejection performance. Circulation 1992;86:1718–1726.

99. Abbasi AS, Allen MW, DeCristofaro D, et al. Detection and estimation of the degree of mitral regurgitation by range-gated pulsed Doppler echocardiography. Circulation 1980;61:143–147.

100. Tribouilloy C, Shen WF, Quere JP, et al. Assessment of severity of mitral regurgitation by measuring regurgitant jet width at its origin with transesophageal Doppler color flow imaging. Circulation 1992;85:1248–1253.

101. Castello R, Lenzen P, Aguirre F, et al. Quantitation of mitral regurgitation by transesophageal echocardiography with Doppler color flow mapping: correlation with cardiac catheterization. J Am Coll Cardiol 1992;19:1516–1521.

102. Carley JE, Wong BYS, Pugh DM, et al. Clinical significance of the V-wave in the main pulmonary artery. Am J Cardiol 1977;39:982–985.

103. Fuchs RM, Heuser RR, Yin FC, et al. Limitations of pulmonary wedge V-waves in diagnosing mitral regurgitation. Am J Cardiol 1982;49:849–853.

104. Pichard AD, Kay R, Smith H, et al. Large V-waves in the pulmonary wedge pressure tracing in the absence of mitral regurgitation. Am J Cardiol 1982;50:1044–1050.

105. Leung DY, Griffin BP, Stewart WJ, et al. Left ventricular function after valve repair for chronic mitral regurgitation: predictive value of preoperative assessment of contractile reserve by exercise echocardiography. J Am Coll Cardiol 1996;28:1198–1205.

106. Gaasch WH, Levine HJ, Zile MR. Chronic aortic and mitral regurgitation: mechanical consequences of the lesion and the results of surgical correction. In: Gaasch WH, Levine HJ, eds. The ventricle: basic and clinical aspects. Boston: Martinus-Nijhoff, 1985;237.

107. Enriquez-Sarano M, Tajik AJ, Schaff HV, et al. Echocardiographic prediction of survival after surgical correction of organic mitral regurgitation. Circulation 1994;90:830–837.

108. Zile MR, Gaasch WH, Carroll JD, et al. Chronic mitral regurgitation: predictive value of preoperative echocardiographic indexes of left ventricular function and wall stress. J Am Coll Cardiol 1984;3:235–242.

109. Wisenbaugh T, Skudicky D, Sareli P. Prediction of outcome after valve replacement for rheumatic mitral regurgitation in the era of chordal preservation. Circulation 1994;89:191–197.

110. Reed D, Abbott RD, Smucker ML, et al. Prediction of outcome after mitral valve replacement in patients with symptomatic chronic mitral regurgitation. The importance of left atrial size. Circulation 1991;84:23–34.

111. Crawford MH, Souchek J, Oprian CA, et al. Determinants of survival and left ventricular performance after mitral valve replacement. Department of Veterans Affairs Cooperative Study on Valvular Heart Disease. Circulation 1990;81:1173–1181.

112. Vokonas PS, Gorlin R, Cohn PF, et al. Dynamic geometry of the left ventricle in mitral regurgitation. Circulation 1973;48:786–796.

113. Salomon NW, Stinson EB, Griepp RB, et al. Surgical treatment of degenerative mitral regurgitation. Am J Cardiol 1976;38:463–468.

114. Suzuki Y, Kambara H, Kadota K, et al. Detection and evaluation of tricuspid regurgitation using a real time, two-dimensional, color coded, Doppler flow imaging system: comparison with contrast two-dimensional echocardiography and right ventriculography. Am J Cardiol 1986;57:811–815.

41

Evaluation for Cardiac Transplantation and Follow-up of the Cardiac Transplant Recipient

Roger M. Mills, Jr, MD
James B. Young, MD

INTRODUCTION

Since the introduction of cyclosporine for immunosupression in the early 1980s, survival after heart transplantation has steadily improved, with 5-year survival rates of approximately 75% now reported from major centers (1). Orthotopic heart transplantation is now accepted therapy for selected patients with end-stage heart failure (2). The catheterization laboratory provides essential data for evaluation of potential heart transplant recipients and for continuing care of patients after transplantation. In this chapter, we address both pre- and post-transplant catheterization procedures with emphasis on preoperative hemodynamic assessment and the postoperative diagnosis and management of cardiac allograft vasculopathy (CAV) in the transplanted heart.

PRETRANSPLANT EVALUATION

Goals of pretransplant cardiac catheterization include:

1. **Safely and completely documenting that the patient has "end-stage" heart disease for** which no other therapy is likely to achieve results comparable to transplantation
2. **Confirming that the patient meets the physiologic requirements for successful transplantation**

Special Preparations for Safe Invasive Studies in Patients with Advanced Heart Failure

Special preparations to minimize procedural risks for pretransplant patients are critical to good outcomes. In patients with advanced heart failure, the potential for contrast media-induced renal dysfunction, management of anticoagulation and arrythmia, and need for optimizing medical therapy, constitute essential precatheterization considerations. (Chapter 13 has dealt with contrast agents in detail.) Advanced heart failure appears to place patients at increased risk for contrast media-associated nephropathy (3). Use of a low osmolality contrast agent in this setting minimizes volume expansion, myocardial depression, and arrythmia; these agents may be less nephrotoxic as well. Careful hydration before and after angiography will ensure adequate urine flow, and it may require administration of both intravenous fluids and supplemental diuretics. Nonsteroidal anti-inflammatory agents and other potentially nephrotoxic drugs (e.g., antibiotics) should be avoided both before and for several days after angiography (3). Warfarin effects can be radically altered by right ventricular failure and hepatic congestion. Advance planning and involvement of home health services may be required to minimize inpatient stay for the catheterization. **Anticoagulation** should be reduced to a level that permits adequate hemostasis after percutaneous vascular catheterization. Endomyocardial biopsy, trans-septal catheterization, or direct left ventricular puncture require normal clotting parameters. Control of arrythmia prior to catheterization is required for optimal hemodynamic and angiographic evaluation. A potential exists, as well, for additional cardiac depression from antiarrythmic therapy. Ravid et al. (4) found antiarrhythmic drug-induced episodes of heart failure in 9% of 167 patients with previous heart failure who were treated with various antiarrhythmics. **Consultation for optimal arrhythmia management should be an integral part of pretransplant care.** Finally, optimal medical therapy including maximal tolerated doses of an angiotensin converting enzyme inhibitor, nontoxic digitalis levels, and possibly 48 to 72 hours of inotropic support to restore good peripheral perfusion and control pulmonary hypertension should be achieved, along with clinical euvolemia, prior to the catheterization.

Planning the Procedure to Confirm "End-Stage" Disease

The catheterization team must review the patient's history and physical findings and carefully plan the evaluation, including any necessary interventions in the laboratory such as exercise or pacing stress, and the infusion of vasoactive drugs to assess pulmonary vascular resistance. Several common situations requiring this meticulous catheterization laboratory technique include assessment of:

1. Valvular heart disease with low cardiac output
2. Coexistent mitral regurgitation and depressed left ventricular systolic function
3. Coronary heart disease with the potential for functional improvement following revascularization
4. Unexplained myocardial dysfunction

Valvular Heart Disease

The role of exercise and pharmacologic interventions to increase cardiac output during hemodynamic assessment of patients with valvular heart disease has been discussed in detail in Chapters 24 and 25. A potential for serious error exists in patients with left ventricular outflow obstruction when forward cardiac output is depressed. Application of the Gorlin valve area formula (5) to small systolic pressure gradients measured across the aortic valve in a low-output state leads to estimation of a significantly reduced valve area. This calculated area may represent a discrepancy between the actual and the effective valve area, as shown in studies of prosthetic valves in vitro (6, 7). Casale et al. (8) have suggested an alternative possibility, flow-dependence of the Gorlin formula determined valve area, after studying 12 patients with aortic stenosis and mean valve gradients less than 45 mm Hg. The investigators compared aortic valve areas calculated by the Gorlin formula at rest and during dobutamine infusion with valve areas calculated by the continuity equation using simultaneous Doppler echo data. During dobutamine infusion, cardiac output increased by 38% and valve area by the Gorlin formula increased in all 12. The valve areas and valve resistance calculated from the continuity equation, however, did not change. The authors concluded that changes in the Gorlin formula valve area reflected flow-dependence of the formula rather than physiologic changes in functional orifice area. For practical purposes, **patients with clinically suspected severe aortic stenosis and depressed forward cardiac output should receive an inotropic intervention to raise the cardiac output, with reassessment of the transvalvular gradient and flow.** Simultaneous determination of Doppler echo data and hemodynamics may also help to identify more accurately those patients who might benefit from surgical intervention.

Mitral Regurgitation

Mitral regurgitation often accompanies left ventricular systolic dysfunction, particularly when ventricular dilation occurs (9). **Hemodynamic assessment of the severity of chronic mitral regurgitation is complicated by left atrial dilation with changes in chamber compliance,** which allow the atrium to act as a pressure-volume "sink". Pulmonary capillary wedge pressure at rest may be only minimally elevated while the left atrium accepts a large portion of the ventricular stroke volume (10). Fuchs et al. (11) reviewed pulmonary capillary wedge pressure tracings obtained from balloon occlusion catheterization of the pulmonary artery in 208 patients, and found that 33% of the individuals with severe mitral regurgitation had only trivial V-waves, whereas 18% of those without mitral regurgitation had prominent V-waves. Figure 41.1 shows

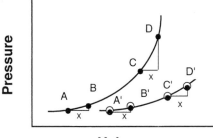

Figure 41.1. Hypothetical left atrial pressure-volume relationships. If the atrium is operating on a relatively flat portion of its pressure-volume relationship, the same regurgitant volume (x) will result in much less pressure elevation (A to B) compared with an atrium operating on a relatively steep portion of its pressure-volume curve C to D). Also, the pressure-volume curve may shift downward and to the right as a result of disease. When this occurs, the same diastolic filling volume (x) evokes a much smaller rise in pressure in both the mildly enlarged atrium (A^1 to B^1) and the markedly enlarged atrium (C^1 to D^1), than in the atrium operating on the pressure-volume curve shown to the left.

Table 41.1.
Angiographic Grading of Mitral Regurgitation from Cine Left

Ventriculography
Grade 0 no reflux into the atrium
Grade 1+ contrast refluxes but does not fill the atrium
Grade 2+ contrast fills the atrium, but less dense than ventricle
Grade 3+ contrast density equal in atrium and ventricle
Grade 4+ atrium completely fills in first cycle, and in late cycles atrium is more densely opacified than ventricle

the hypothesized left atrial pressure-volume relationship that illustrates these findings.

Angiographic assessment of these patients is also difficult. Table 41.1 outlines the angiographic grading scheme usually employed clinically to describe the severity of mitral regurgitation. The highly subjective nature of the assessment is self-evident. In addition, a number of technical factors, including catheter size and position in the ventricle, rate and volume of contrast injection, and the size of the atrium and ventricle, also influence the angiographic grading of mitral regurgitation. Patients with significant regurgitation, however, will demonstrate the severity of their hemodynamic compromise by failing to increase cardiac output normally with exercise (12).

When important mitral regurgitation coexists with impaired left ventricular function, the options either of mitral valve repair or replacement rather than heart transplantation may be considered. Carabello (13) has commented on the lack of firm data on which to base **management decisions** for patients with mitral regurgitation (see also Chapter 40). Veterans Administration survival study data (14) indicate that patients with severe mitral regurgitation and preoperative ejection fraction less that 50% had a poor surgical outcome. In this study, preoperative ejection fraction and end-systolic volume index predicted postoperative end-diastolic volume index. In other words, patients with impaired systolic function before surgery continued to have left ventricular enlargement afterward. Restoration of mitral competence was associated with maintenance of forward output, with a decrease in total stroke volume and ejection fraction. Currently we do not recommend isolated mitral valve repair or replacement for patients with ejection fractions less than 40% (15). The potential for palliation of patients with markedly dilated left ventricles with left ventricular volume reduction procedures combined with surgical restoration of A-V valve competency requires careful clinical investigation. (16)

Coronary Artery Disease

The various options for demonstrating residual left ventricular contractile function, or **viability of noncontractile tissue**, in patients with severe coronary artery disease (CAD) have been extensively reviewed (17). In patients who have not had previous surgery, depressed left ventricular systolic function mandates myocardial viability assessment to identify possible revasularization candidates. The strategy of testing before or after catheterization, and the optimal choice of imaging modality, are beyond the scope of this chapter. However, improvement in systolic function following revascularization by either angioplasty or coronary artery bypass grafting has been well documented (18, 19). For the patient with a left ventricular ejection fraction between 15 and 20% who has not had prior coronary bypass, the risk of revascularization surgery is less than that of transplantation (20). In contrast, the risk of a second or third thoracotomy for coronary artery disease in some cases may not be justified by marked functional improvement (21) even when ischemia can be identified. Transplantation offers an alternative to reoperation for carefully selected individuals with severe left ventricular dysfunction and coronary artery disease. The role of "minimally invasive" reoperation, possibly in combination with advanced catheter-based techniques such as stenting, has not been clearly defined.

Because of the limited availability of suitable donor hearts and the need for careful pretransplant evaluation, patients with acute myocardial infarction complicated by cardiogenic shock were seldom candidates for transplantation in the past. If prompt catheter-based revascularization efforts fail to stabilize a patient who might be an appropriate candidate for transplantation, mechanical circulatory support should now be considered. Patients undergoing staged heart transplantation from total circulatory support have experienced 1 and 2 year survival rates of approximately 65% as compared with more than 80% for isolated orthotopic transplantation (22). Earlier use of recently approved left ventricular support devices (LVADs) may substantially improve these statistics. Patients and their families should be carefully informed about the risks of these dramatic interventions.

Myocardial Dysfunction

Acute myocarditis can mimic myocardial infarction (23–25), and diagnostic catheterization may be required to clarify the clinical situation. However, the diagnosis of myocarditis must be made on clinical criteria. The focal nature of inflammatory cellular infiltrates in most cases of myocarditis, combined with limited tissue sampling available with transvenous right ventricular endomyocardial biopsy, limits the utility of biopsy. Hauck et al. (26) evaluated histologic findings on from one to ten samples obtained using biopsy forceps from postmortem hearts with proven myocarditis. They found false-negative biopsies in 83% of cases if only one specimen was examined, in 55% if five specimens were examined, and in 37% if all ten were reviewed. Further complicating the diagnostic process are occasional false-positive biopsies, which probably occur in at least 3% of patients (27) with even the strictest histologic criteria (28). If clinical evidence strongly suggests acute myocarditis, then consistent myocardial biopsy findings provide additional confirmation. However, negative biopsy findings clearly do *not* exclude a highly suspicious diagnosis. This is clinically important, because 47 of 60 patients reported by Gardiner and Short (23) recovered completely and only 3 of 55 patients followed by Sainani et al. (29) progressed to chronic heart failure after an episode of myocarditis.

In contrast to its limited role in acute myocarditis, myocardial histology aids in the diagnosis of cardiac amyloid, iron overload, or anthracycline toxicity and may help to confirm myocardial involvement in sarcoidosis (27, 30). Biopsy findings can occasionally help differentiate restrictive cardiomyopathy and constrictive pericarditis (see Chapter 42). In summary, with an experienced cardiac pathologist supported by a laboratory prepared to do all clinically required stains, endomyocardial biopsy may offer clinically helpful adjunctive information. Biopsy should not be viewed as a reference standard for most cardiac diagnoses, and it should be used only selectively when strong clinical suspicion indicates one of the previously mentioned conditions.

Confirming the Physiologic Requirements for Successful Heart Transplantation

If orthotopic heart transplantation places an anatomically normal right ventricle in the position of ejecting against significantly elevated pulmonary vascular resistance, acute right ventricular failure and death often result. Potential transplant recipients must have an **initial assessment of pulmonary vascular resistance (PVR)** in the laboratory. Although systemic vascular resistance is usually expressed in metric units (dynessec-cm-5), most transplant cardiologists prefer the simpler "Wood units" for PVR (see Chapter 22), and most adult transplant programs do not index PVR to body surface area.

The importance of assessment of PVR before transplant quickly emerged in the early Stanford experience when three patients with an average PVR of 11.5 Wood units died within 24 hours of transplantation (31). In a series of 107 patients with no attempt to pharmacologically manipulate resistance, operative risk rose continuously with increasing PVR, without a threshold value (32). Assessing long-term survival as opposed to operative risk, Kirklin et al. ana-

lyzed 63 heart transplants and found markedly impaired actuarial survival for patients with PVR of 5 Wood units or greater. In this series, 81% of patients with PVR less than 5 Wood units survived 1 year, compared with only 45% of those with PVR of 5 or greater (20).

In contrast to children with congenital heart disease, adults with marked elevations of PVR caused by acquired heart disease may improve significantly with treatment. Braunwald et al. reported their early experience with mitral valve replacement and document significant falls in PVR from 2 to 12 months postoperatively in 21 of 22 patients (33). Dalen et al. (34) subsequently showed that PVR fell strikingly with the first postoperative day in five patients undergoing mitral valve replacement and concluded that "much of the pulmonary vascular disease . . . may be rapidly reversible."

If pharmacologic intervention reduces PVR, the operative risk for orthotopic heart transplantation falls concomitantly. Costard-Jackle and Fowler (35) reported the Stanford experience with nitroprusside challenge and assessment of PVR in 293 patients. Three-month surgical mortality for those with a PVR less than 2.5 Wood units at baseline was 6.9%. If the baseline PVR exceeded 2.5 Wood units but reduced to 2.5 units or less with a stable arterial blood pressure of 85 mm Hg or greater during graded infusion of nitroprusside, the 3-month mortality rate was 3.8%. In contrast, those patients whose PVR remained above 2.5 units despite nitroprusside had a 3-month mortality rate of 41%, and those who could only achieve a PVR of 2.5 units or less at the expense of systemic hypotension (systolic blood pressure, 85 mm HG) during drug infusion had a 3-month mortality rate of 28%. These dramatic differences make a strong case for careful assessment of PVR with pharmacologic manipulations.

Murali et al. (36) have reviewed the drugs available for acute interventions in the laboratory, and currently available agents are summarized in Table 41.2. Both nitroprusside and prostaglandin E-1 effectively lower PVR (Fig. 41.2). Prostaglandin E-1, however, is expensive and often produces unpleasant nausea and flushing. Epo-

Table 41.2.
Drugs for Intervention in Pulmonary Hypertension

Oxygen: use in all patients
Tolazoline: usually limited to pediatrics
Nitroglycerin: venous capacitance effect predominates
Nitroprusside: systemic arterial effect usually predominates
Adenosine: "pulmonary selective" in low doses; role undefined as yet
PGE-1: expensive, side-effects frequent
Dobutamine: useful in conjunction with nitroprusside
Amrinone: may be helpful for maintenance infusion
Prostacyclin: very potent, not yet approved; systemic and pulmonary effects
Flosequenon: role uncertain; oral available; no intravenous formulation at this time

prostenal (Flolan, Galaxo-Wellcome,) is a stable prostacyclin analog with remarkable pulmonary vasodilating properties approved for use in patients with primary pulmonary hypertension, which may prove useful in highly selected patients for pretransplant evaluation. Adenosine, an extremely potent pulmonary vasodilator, is rapidly metabolized in the lung. Intravenous infusion of low-dose adenosine does not produce significant systemic hypotension or bradycardia (37). Graded infusion of adenosine from 50 to 500 µg/kg/min produced a 37% decrease in PVR at the maximal tolerated dose in 15 patients with pulmonary hypertension (38). Haywood et al. (39) compared adenosine and nitroprusside and found that both agents decreased PVR by approximately 40%, but mean arterial blood pressure fell with nitroprusside and was unchanged with adenosine.

Because patients now wait for months

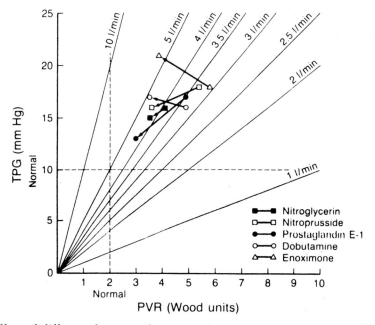

Figure 41.2. Effect of different drugs on the transpulmonary pressure gradient (*TPG*), pulmonary vascular resistance (*PVR*), and cardiac output (*CO*). The observed values of *TPG, PVR,* and *CO* at baseline and after drug intervention for each patient group are plotted against a background of theoretic pressure-resistance lines representing different rates of flow or *CO* as predicted by the hydrodynamic equation for streamlined flow. *Dotted lines* represent normal values for *TPG* (10 mm Hg) and *PVR* (2 Wood units), and they intersect at normal *CO* (5 L/min). All patient groups had a high *TPG* and *PVR* and a low *CO* at baseline. The PVR decreased and *CO* increased with all drugs. Prostaglandin E-1 lowered *TPG* and *PVR* most effectively.

to years for a suitable donor heart, and potent oral agents are available for treatment of heart failure, short-term testing in the laboratory may be less critical than serial determinations of PVR on an outpatient basis. In a series of 102 patients with left ventricular dysfunction, diastolic dysfunction and the degree of functional mitral regurgitation as determined by effective regurgitant orifice size were the strongest predictors of systolic pulmonary artery pressure (40). If effective afterload reduction leads to forward redistribution of left ventricular stroke volume and reduction in functional mitral regurgitation, then elevations in PVR may respond to chronic medical therapy. Little objective data concerning the long-term effects of afterload reduction on PVR and the risk of recurrent elevations of PVR after control are available. In a series of 24 patients referred for transplantation with initial PVR greater than 2.5 Wood units studied at the University of Florida, 10 maintained normal PVR until transplantation with enhanced oral drug therapy alone; 11 required oral afterload reduction with parenteral therapy (inotropes) to support systemic pressure and control PVR, and 3 responded initially to oral agents but subsequently relapsed (Cunningham M, Mills R; unpublished data). In the present transplant environment, elevations of pulmonary vascular resistance refractory to maximal therapy are distinctly unusual.

Recapitulation on the Pretransplant Catheterization

A safe, cost-effective preoperative catheterization in potential candidates for heart transplantation requires clinical acumen, careful planning, and integration of data from many sources, including radionuclide studies, echocardiographic examination, and the exercise laboratory, as well as technical skill. The catheterizing physician should focus on establishing the diagnosis and confirming that transplantation represents an appropriate treatment option. This requires careful assessment of coronary and valvular lesions and it may be particularly difficult when left ventricular outflow obstruction or severe mitral regurgitation coexists with coronary artery disease and depressed left ventricular systolic function. Diagnostic endomyocardial biopsy must be employed selectively with good understanding of the interaction of pretest likelihood of disease and sensitivity-specificity measures. After the decision to consider transplantation, a careful assessment of PVR becomes paramount. A complete catheterization must include **reliable determinations of all parameters of the pulmonary resistance formula, and pharmacologic manipulation if appropriate.**

POST-TRANSPLANT EVALUATION

Optimal management of patients after heart transplantation requires data quantifying rejection severity, graft function, and the state of the coronary circulation. All of these are obtained by cardiac catheterization. Endomyocardial biopsy specimens should be obtained at varying surveillance intervals or whenever acute rejection is suggested. Hemodynamic measurements obtained during right ventricular catheterization at the time of biopsy provide adjunctive data, enhancing analysis of endomyocardial biopsy specimens and influencing the level of treatment. **Long-term prognosis can be established by evaluating coronary artery patency and flow reserve.** In reviewing cardiac catheterization procedures performed in the heart transplant population, we will emphasize differences from the procedures in nontransplant patients (Table 41.3).

Endomyocardial Biopsy

Catheter **right ventricular endomyocardial biopsy** is the most frequent invasive cardiac procedure done after heart transplantation. It is done no differently from endomyocardial biopsy in nontransplant patients (41) (see Chapter 9). The transplant patient, however, presents some unique challenges.

Table 41.3.
Cardiac Catheterization Procedures Used After Heart Transplantation

Endomyocardial biopsy
  Routine surveillance of rejection status
  Ad hoc diagnosis of clinically suspected rejection
  Assessment of cardiac infection (cytomegalovirus, toxoplasmosis, viral genome detection using in vitro hybridization)
Right ventricular catheterization
  Characterization of allograft function
  Correlation of hemodynamic and endomyocardial biopsy information
  Quantification of valvular insufficiency
  Determination of cardiac output
Coronary angiography
  Identify coronary lesions in donor heart
  Characterize transplanted heart's anatomy
  Allows identification of disease progression
  Selects patients for angioplasty, atherectomy, or repeat transplant procedures
Intravascular ultrasound
  Most precise technique to identify allograft arteriopathy
  Doppler assessment of coronary flow reserve
  Determines functional significance of observed allograft arteriopathy

Because routine surveillance of rejection status is required, endomyocardial biopsy is usually performed weekly or bimonthly for the first few months after transplantation, and then annually. This need for multiple sequential biopsies is unusual; in other conditions requiring endomyocardial biopsy, one procedure that procures several good samples usually suffices. Fortunately, most recipients tolerate many repeated internal jugular procedures in the right anterior-lateral cervical region without serious difficulty (see Chapter 9). With slight shifts in needle puncture site, fibrosis does not seem to limit repeated studies (41). If the access puncture site must be rotated, we use the right internal jugular approach first, and move to one of the femoral veins as a second option (42, 43). If necessary, as a third option, we favor the left subclavian approach over either the right subclavian or left internal jugular, because the bioptome assumes a more natural C-shaped curve. This natural curve allows rapid access to the right ventricle. The S-shaped curve required to biopsy the right ventricle from a right subclavian or left internal jugular approach makes bioptome manipulation more difficult.

Many transplant patients gain weight over the years; also after frequent right internal jugular vein punctures, keloidal scars may form in this region. Both of these conditions may make finding the internal jugular vein difficult. We have noted that, in these patients, use of a hand-held, sterilized, Doppler probe designed to detect peripheral pulses is invaluable. We hold the device with the gloved left hand and place it in the right supraclavicular fossa. After detecting the carotid arterial blood flow velocity Doppler signal, the operator angles the probe laterally to identify and localize the softer, more subtle, continuous venous signal produced by blood flow in the internal jugular vein. Needle puncture directly under and in the same direction as the probe uniformly engages the vein.

Four right ventricular biopsy specimens will adequately characterize the rejection process (44). More samples can be obtained for ancillary studies, as necessary. Diffuse sampling of the septal endomyocardium can be ensured by slightly altering bioptome shape or sheath position in between biopsy passes. With multiple prior biopsies, repeated sampling of previous sites will occur. Therefore, every attempt must be made to ensure more widespread sampling. Left ventricular biopsy from a femoral approach, using longer sheaths and bioptomes, may help if clinical suspicion of rejection is high and right ventricular endomyocardial biopsy does not confirm this diagnosis, or if inadequate tissue is obtained because of endocardial fibrosis, or if old sites are repeatedly undergoing biopsy. Occasional use of a different sharper bioptome or moving to another approach to alter bioptome position within the right ventricle may also be useful. The **disposable bioptomes now favored** generally provide adequate samples; however, reusable bioptomes, although stiff and difficult to manipulate, provide larger sample sizes ($6{-}10$ mm^3 versus $2{-}6$ mm^3).

Endomyocardial biopsy of patients with **heterotopic** (as opposed to the usual orthotopic) heart transplants can be a challenging task because of the unusual vascular anastomoses (Fig. 41.4). We use the femoral approach most often for a heterotopic transplant. After venous cannulation, a 0.035-inch J-shaped guidewire is advanced through the native heart right atrium and into the superior vena cava. An 8 F Cook (Bloomington, IN) trans-septal catheter and bioptome sheath is then advanced over the wire into the superior vena cava. This catheter sheath combination is preferable to the 100 cm straight sheath alone (Cordis, Miami, FL), because its curvature facilitates entry into the donor right atrium and the tip usually will float freely into the ventricle. The guidewire is pulled back inside the sheath, and the sheath tip is rotated laterally until it points directly toward the heterotopic right atrium. The guidewire is then readvanced into the atrium, and usually curves without difficulty into the ventricle. If the guidewire does not immediately enter the right ventricle, this catheter-sheath combination can be removed and a pigtail catheter-sheath combination passed over the guidewire and then advanced as a unit into the ventricle. The trans-septal or pigtail catheter is then removed and the biopsy sheath advanced over the wire into the right ventricle. A 104 cm long bioptome is then passed through the sheath (a J-curve 3–4 cm from bioptome tip helps), and multiple sites are biopsied. By changing the degree of J angulations, diffuse sampling of the ventricle can be assured. As with other endomyocardial biopsy procedures, speed and frequent (or continuous) flushing via the sidearm prevent clot formation within the sheath.

Most (approximately 70%) patients with heterotopic heart transplants are, in our experience, biopsied from the femoral approach, but the procedure can be done in some from the right internal jugular approach. After cannulation of the right internal jugular veins and placing a guidewire in the native right atrium, a 23 cm, 8 F introducer sheath (Cordis) is positioned. A 60 cm, 8 F A2 renal angiographic catheter with a bioptome sheath is then placed over the guidewire. The catheter tip is directed laterally toward the heterotopic right atrium and the long guidewire is then advanced into this structure. The A2 catheter follows over the guidewire and, after being placed

in the atrium, the tip is rotated caudally, and then the catheter-guidewire combination is advanced into the heterotopic right ventricle. The bioptome sheath, placed over the A2 catheter at the beginning of the case, can then be positioned in the inflow tract. The guidewire and A2 catheter can be removed, allowing bioptome access to the ventricle. Precautions should be taken to flush frequently to prevent blood from clotting in the bioptome sheath between biopsy passes. We use a continuous flush. Approaching the heterotopic heart from other venous access sites is difficult because of multiple sheath angulations that are required. These approaches to the heterotopic heart yield adequate specimens in approximately 90% of attempts; complications occur rarely. A right ventricular pressure tracing recorded through the sheath gives assurance of appropriate catheter placement.

Specimens must always be placed in appropriate media for each desired analysis. Evaluation of formalin-fixed endomyocardial biopsy specimens relies on hematoxylin and eosin staining to identify and grade lymphocytic infiltration and myocyte damage (45). Masson's trichrome stain helps to detect and quantify fibrosis. Methyl green-pyronin stains may be useful when myocyte depletion is observed in the face of lymphocytic infiltration. Monocytes with a great deal of ribonucleic acid activity stain positive or red, suggesting the inflammatory process is active rather than resolving. Glutaraldehyde fixation for electron microscopy is rarely necessary. Occasionally, immunohistochemical stains can be used to diagnose immunoglobulin deposition along subendocardial vascular structures (46).

Recently, several centers have stressed the importance of "vascular" or **humoral rejection.** This requires that specimens be placed immediately on saline-soaked filter paper and quick-frozen in ornithine carbamoyltransferase. Immunofluorescence studies with fluorescein conjugated antibodies against human IgG, IgM, C3, C1q, fibrinogen, albumen, and mouse immunoglobulin, may demonstrate vascular deposition of immunoglobulin and complement. Patients with humoral rejection have significantly decreased survival compared with those having cellular rejection alone. Saline transport for in vitro hybridization and polymerase chain reaction (PCR) analysis for viral genome segments give insight into complicating infections (47). Occasionally viral cultures are performed on the biopsy sample and the specimen should be placed directly in the culture media bottle.

Complications of endomyocardial biopsy in heart transplant patients do not differ from those detailed in other patients undergoing biopsy except for a greater likelihood of developing a coronary artery-right ventricular fistula of no hemodynamic consequence (48). Because atrial arrhythmias can occur with rejection, atrial flutter, paroxysmal atrial tachycardia, and atrial fibrillation occasionally complicate biopsy procedures. Frequently these arrhythmias can be terminated by gently "tickling" the atrial wall and inducing a premature atrial contraction. Sometimes redoing the biopsy of the ventricle, or inducing a premature ventricular contraction, will terminate the supraventricular arrhythmia. Rapid atrial pacing offers a quick and easy alternative to cardioversion when the arrhythmia is more resistant. Adenosine and verapamil have a propensity to cause complete heart block in the denervated allograft. Rarely, severe tricuspid insufficiency secondary to chordal tear or biopsy is noted. Generally, patients tolerate repeated procedures well. In fact, patients surviving at least 12 months have had a median of eight biopsies in the first post-transplant year, and we have done more than 20 biopsies over a 2 or 3-year period from the same right internal jugular site in many patients without complications or difficulties (41).

Endomyocardial biopsy after heart transplantation in the pediatric population also presents unique challenges, mostly related to performing repeated procedures in small, young patients. In this group, biopsy from the femoral venous approach is much easier and can be performed frequently. The principles of cardiac catheterization in this age group generally apply, as well, to endomyocardial biopsy after heart transplant.

Both the femoral vein and right internal jugular vein approach for pervenous right ventricular biopsy, in adult and pediatric heart transplant patients, allows widespread sampling of ventricular myocardial tissue. The right internal jugular vein approach, however, allows patients to become ambulatory more quickly; and, we believe that, with the exceptions of young patients and heterotopic recipients, this approach is preferable, and patients can undergo the procedure on an outpatient basis.

Hemodynamic Measurements

To understand hemodynamic findings after heart transplantation better, one must realize that these findings change over time (49). Complicating factors, such as rejection and hypertension, affect this change. Because most patients undergoing cardiac transplantation have elevated filling pressures and volume overload, pulmonary hypertension, increased right atrial, right ventricular end-diastolic, and pulmonary capillary wedge pressures will be noted early post-transplant. (See *Physiologic Requirements* section.) A characteristic restrictive hemodynamic pattern emerges when pressure waveforms are carefully scrutinized. Over the first 30 days, these pressures gradually return to normal (Fig. 41.3), and in patients without subsequent rejection, resting hemodynamic data remain normal at 6-month and 12-month follow-up. Hemodynamic changes occur with acute rejection, commonly with elevation of right atrial, pulmonary artery, and pulmonary capillary wedge pressures. In long-term follow-up, a subclinical, latent, restrictive hemodynamic state may persist, but it often requires volume challenge to unmask this state. **Allograft vasculopathy** may also cause myocardial ischemia with systolic and diastolic ventricular dysfunction and abnormal right ventricular diastolic pressure changes. Unexplained **tricuspid insufficiency commonly appears** after cardiac transplantation with characteristic V-waveforms appearing in recordings from the right atrium.

Cardiac output, usually determined by thermodilution, helps to assess overall systolic performance of the graft. Accurate assessment with this technique is impossible in the heterotopic heart transplant patient, however. Cardiac output falls with epi-

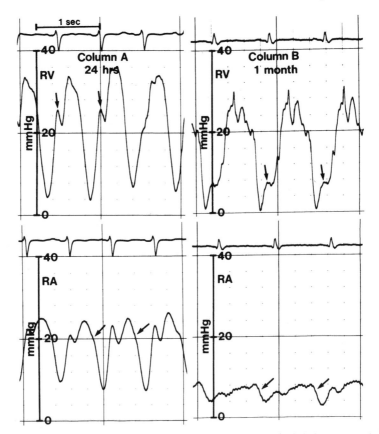

Figure 41.3. Right ventricular (*RV*, **upper tracings**) and right atrial (*RA*, **lower tracings**) obtained in the same patient 24 hours (*Column A*) and 1 month (*Column B*) following heart transplantation. Note the dramatic decrease in RV end-diastolic pressure and A-wave (*arrows*, **top panel**) and decrease in RA V-wave and "Y" descent (*arrows*, **lower panel**). Restrictive hemodynamic findings such as these can generally be made to reappear later during follow-up with rapid volume loading.

sodes of rejection, severe allograft vasculopathy, and chronic diastolic dysfunction. It is critical to relate filling pressures to output and sequentially compare these data in transplant patients to characterize a patient's clinical course and plan treatment protocols. To completely characterize cardiovascular dynamics after heart transplantation, we correlate left and right ventricular ejection fraction (usually done by echocardiography), right ventricular hemodynamic data, and endomyocardial biopsy scores with physical assessment of the patient.

Coronary Angiography in the Heart Transplant Recipient

A form of coronary artery disease after heart transplantation is the limiting factor

in long-term success. Many terms have been used to describe this condition, including spontaneous arteriosclerosis, accelerated graft atherosclerosis, transplant coronary obliterative disease, transplant coronary vasculopathy (with the recent observation of coronary venules involvement), and allograft arteriopathy (50). This latter term seems most appropriate because it describes the same process that can be noted, although with much less frequency, in vessels supplying transplanted kidney, liver, and combined heart-lung grafts. Detection and quantification of severity of allograft arteriopathy is critical in the care of transplant recipients (50). Because initial observations suggested that this problem was prevalent (50–52) and its severity closely linked to long-term survival (53), patients must be

Table 41.4.
Allograft Arteriopathy Characteristics

Concentric subendothelial proliferation
Diffuse coronary vessel involvement
Subendothelial arteries particularly targeted
Elastica intact rather than interrupted
Lesion calcification unusual
Focal lesions less frequently seen
Rapidly developing process
Angina rarely occurs (even when disease severe)
Heart failure is a common presenting condition
Noninvasive diagnosis difficult
Angiographic assessment challenging and comparison to prior angiograms often essential
Intravascular ultrasound promising

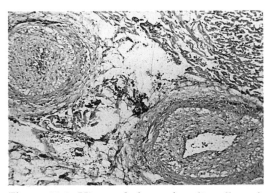

Figure 41.4. Histopathology of cardiac allograft arteriopathy, both diffuse involvement in multiple coronary vessels and intact elastic lamina without calcifications.

periodically reevaluated. The incidence of allograft arteriopathy, determined by coronary angiography, can be as high as 40% at 2 years, and well over 50% at 5 years after heart transplant (50, 51). Autopsy studies have found that the process appears in virtually every cardiac transplant patient, even in those dying only a few months after heart transplant. It seems reasonable to conclude that all heart transplant patients probably have some degree of allograft vasculopathy (54). Most patients studied at 1 or 2 years after heart transplant using **intravascular ultrasound (IVUS)** have evidence of intimal thickening that is not apparent by angiography (55). Unfortunately, little can be done to treat allograft arteriopathy, although one recent report suggests that the calcium antagonist diltiazem may inhibit its progress (56, 57).

The characteristics (Table 41.4) of cardiac allograft arteriopathy that distinguish it from the usual form of CAD seen in nontransplant patients include concentric intimal proliferation, diffuse involvement of multiple coronary vessels (subendocardial vessels, in particular), lack of lesion calcification, rapid development, and an intact elastic lamina (Fig. 41.4) (58, 59). Also, isolated focal epicardial coronary artery lesions are noted less often, associated angina pectoris is rare, and left ventricular systolic dysfunction is often seen late. This diffuse process results in more global patterns of myocardial ischemia than seen with native type coronary atherosclerosis, and graft ar-

teriopathy is difficult to detect with noninvasive procedures that rely on differences in regional myocardial perfusion or function (60). Of course, the concentric and diffuse character of the graft arteriopathy also limits accurate angiographic analysis; however, routine screening and follow-up coronary angiography remains the best method to detect arteriopathy causing significant lumen obstruction and to follow its progression.

Performing the Angiogram

The reasons for performing routine baseline coronary angiography early after heart transplant are summarized in Table 41.5

Table 41.5.
Reasons for Routine Coronary Angiography Early after Heart Transplant

Considerations
Identify donor coronary artery disease
Provide baseline for subsequent angiographic comparison
Significant allograft arteriopathy can appear in first year
Only method to allow identification of diffuse vessel tapering or tertiary vessel cut-off
Allows quantification of dynamics of the process
Prognosis can be more precisely stated
Immunotherapy could be intensified
Traditional risk factors for coronary disease could better be addressed
Retransplantation could be considered

Table 41.6.
Coronary Angiography After Heart Transplant

Considerations
  Perform baseline procedure early after transplant
  Ensure adequate hydration, blood pressure control, and renal function before contrast agent given
  Avoid contrast ventriculography
  Document view angulation, catheter size, and contrast media used
  Analyze serial angiograms quantitatively
  Correlate findings with intravascular ultrasound, function of the allograft, and rejection status

(61). Both visual inspection and quantitative techniques require baseline study to identify accurately angiographic abnormalities in the coronary system of the donor and lesions developing during the first post-transplant year. Between 5 and 10% of donors have some form of CAD (61). Although most have minimal lesions, critical stenosis sometimes appears. Therapeutic intervention, such as angioplasty, might be important in these cases. Furthermore, in a previously abnormal coronary artery, acceleration of allograft arteriopathy might occur because of the combination of endothelial dysfunction and an adverse immunologic milieu. The greatest changes in coronary lumen diameter may occur within the first year after transplant (62, 63). Without early baseline study, this disease would not be apparent. Subsequent coronary angiography should be performed every 1 to 3 years or when confusing clinical situations develop. In patients with unexplained congestive heart failure late (> 3 months) after cardiac transplantation, who have low rejection scores and no evidence of humoral (vascular) rejection, coronary angiography can exclude extensive obstruction causing global ventricular dysfunction. We believe that because angiographic coronary obstruction, particularly when extensive, is associated with an adverse prognosis (53), it is important to characterize allograft arteriopathy accurately.

Table 41.4 lists some unique aspects of the coronary artery examination in heart transplant recipients. Because cardiac trans-

plant patients have hypertension and mild renal insufficiency secondary to chronic cyclosporine administration, one must aggressively address these factors for optimal prevention of contrast-related complications. Transplant patients should be well hydrated with 1–2 L of intravenous isotonic fluid given over a 6 to 12-hour period prior to coronary angiography. Blood pressure can be normalized with calcium antagonists, and contrast agent volumes should be reduced. We use noninvasive methods, rather than contrast ventriculography, to determine ejection fraction and assess ventricular wall motion. We favor 7 or 8 F catheters for maneuverability and image quality to assess graft arteriopathy.

Some anatomic issues are unique to heart transplant patients. Coronary arteries may be very difficult to cannulate with preformed transfemoral catheters because of the aortic arch torque that occurs during surgery. Occasionally, an excessively long

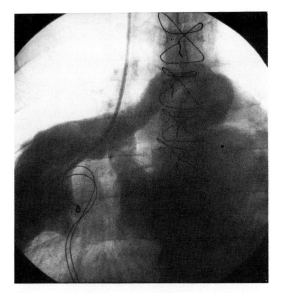

Figure 41.5. Right ventriculogram in patient with heterotopic heart transplant. Catheter has been placed into the right ventricle from the right internal jugular vein. Contrast medium can be seen coursing into the pulmonary artery graft, which is attached (end-to-side) to the main pulmonary artery. Also seen is reflux of contrast into the native right superior vena cava, right atrium, right ventricle, and right ventricular outflow tract.

donor aorta segment is left in place. This, in combination with a small heart placed in a large mediastinal cavity, allows for torsion of the aortic root. Frequently, the left coronary ostium is more posterior and the right more anterior than expected. Although this has little pathologic consequence, manipulation of preformed catheters into coronary ostia can be challenging. A variety of curve dimensions (Amplatz, Judkins, and so forth) or a multipurpose catheter seem most successful. Often, insertion of a guidewire into the catheter assists in cannulation.

For coronary angiography in the heterotopic heart transplant recipient, the unique relationship of the donor aorta to the native heart and native great vessel outflow tracts (Figs. 41.5 and 41.6) requires considerable maneuvering of the catheters. A Judkins right coronary catheter is advanced through a standard sheath into the native aortic arch. The tip is then rotated in the direction of the heterotopic aortic anastomosis, which is end-to-side, and a 0.035-inch J guidewire advanced to the donor heart root with the catheter following. In the left anterior oblique view, the catheter is placed in the

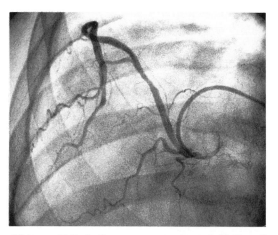

Figure 41.7. Left coronary artery injection 1 month after heterotopic heart transplant. The catheter is a multipurpose (8 F) inserted from the right groin using guidewire assistance as described in the text. Note the unusual torque required to cannulate the left main coronary artery. Also note the unusual course of the artery caused by the rotated, high, heterotopic heart. A type A lesion is observed in the midcircumflex artery, which likely was present in the donor heart prior to transplant. A small and attenuated left anterior descending coronary artery is seen at the bottom of the figure. These observations stress the importance of early angiography. Had this study been performed at 1 year post-transplant without a baseline for comparison, one might have thought that the left anterior descending coronary artery was diffusely diseased with a type B lesion, and a type A lesion in the circumflex artery.

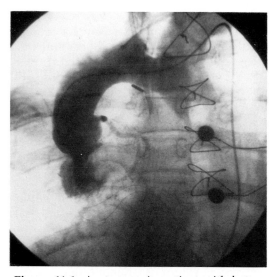

Figure 41.6. Aortogram in patient with heterotopic heart transplant. Catheter passes from the groin to the heterotopic aortic root via the end-to-side anastomosis with the native aortic root. Contrast medium can be seen entering the native aorta as well as refluxing into the right and left donor coronary arteries.

right coronary cusp and rotated counterclockwise until the right coronary ostia is cannulated. The Judkins right coronary catheter may also cannulate the left coronary artery, although sometimes a Judkins left coronary, Amplatz, or multipurpose catheter is required.

The unusual position of a heterotopic transplant causes the left and right anterior oblique views to appear as mirror images of those seen in the native heart, and sometimes long axis clockwise rotation of the implant occurs so that the oblique views are both mirrored and inverse (Fig. 41.7).

All coronary angiography should be performed after nitroglycerin administration, particularly when quantitative measurements are planned. Coronary contrast injections should consist of 8–10 mL boluses, with attempts to limit the total load to preserve renal function. Postprocedure, parenteral hydration continues if filling pressures are normal or low.

Views for post-transplant coronary angiography are no different from those in the nontransplant patient. Views should optimally demonstrate focal epicardial lesions or long lengths of coronary branches. In serial studies, views should be consistent and, if at all possible, patients should be catheterized in the same laboratory using similar sized catheters. Keeping records of the precise angulations used is important for serial evaluation and quantitative analysis.

Appearance of Allograft Arteriopathy

In comparison with patients with native CAD, transplant recipients have fewer proximal epicardial stenoses, and total occlusions occur primarily in the distal vasculature. Furthermore, transplant patients have minimal or no collateral vessels. The Stanford classification of allograft arteriopathy represents the best scheme proposed to date (64). Type A lesions are focal stenoses in epicardial arteries that resemble the typical obstructions in patients with native vessel CAD. Type B lesions are long, tubular, symmetric obstructions in the more distal branches of the epicardial arteries extending into the subendocardial divisions. Type C lesions principally involve more distal vessels, and they are characterized particularly by tertiary branch abrupt cutoff. Patients often exhibit all three classes of allograft arteriopathy during long-term follow-up (Fig. 41.8).

Visual Angiographic Analysis

We assume that all vessels are diseased and our goal is to quantify the severity of allograft arteriopathy. One should have side-by-side projection screens arranged so that comparison of contrast flow and coronary

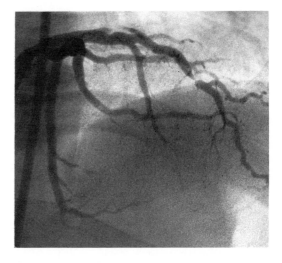

Figure 41.8. Left coronary angiogram (*RAO,* cranial) in a patient 2 years after heart transplant who had an "angiographically normal" study at 1 year. At year 2, "diffuse Type B" narrowing is seen in the left circumflex artery branches. A focal type A lesion is now present in the mid-left anterior descending artery, diffuse type B narrowing in the diagonal branch, distal obtuse marginal branch, and distal circumflex artery, and abrupt "cut-off" type C lesions in the distal branches of both the circumflex and anterior descending arteries.

anatomy can be made with prior studies. Diffuse disease, abrupt vessel cutoff, and progression can then be better interpreted. However, defining the progression of diffuse arteriopathy requires quantitative techniques.

Quantitative Angiography

Quantitative coronary angiography has assumed a prominent role in clinical trials where quantifying progression, regression, and extent of coronary atherosclerosis in epicardial arteries constitutes an end point (65, 66). Furthermore, quantitative analysis of coronary angiograms carries important prognostic implications (67). This technique is particularly suited to analyzing coronary angiograms in the heart transplant patient. At the least, simple, hand-held caliper measurement of predetermined epicardial artery segments should be performed. Obvious epicardial lesions can be quantified. Edge detection or densitometric systems may be more objective. Again, predetermined segments can be analyzed and mean segment diameter determined. Obvious epicardial lesions can be assessed quantitatively in more critical, unbiased fashion. The technical details and pitfalls are provided in Chapters 12, 17, and 21.

Although computer-assisted edge detection or densitometric analysis seems to provide the most reproducible and accurate method for assessing epicardial coronary stenosis severity and vessel mean diameter, none of these techniques are applicable to the type C lesion. Subjective assessment of abrupt vessel cutoff is still necessary and important, but some attempt should be made at quantifying the number of anatomic regions involved with type C lesions.

Angiographic Reporting

Data reported after coronary angiography in heart transplant patients must be standardized. Vessel dominance should be recorded, and the presence of any fistula formation noted. Focal epicardial lesions should be identified, precisely located, and obstruction severity quantified. Quantitative assessment of artery diameter at predetermined segments should be performed. The change in segment diameter from previous studies must be noted (62, 63, 68, 69). The presence, location, and extent of vessel pruning should be detailed, as well as the perception of plaque, and a global assessment of the severity of obstructions. The diameter of any discrete stenosis and area of stenosis can then be calculated. Mean diameter of predetermined coronary segments can be calculated. Assessment of allograft arteriopathy progression can then be made by comparing the mean diameter of all predetermined and abnormal segments in sequential studies.

CORONARY ANGIOPLASTY IN CARDIAC PATIENTS

Because focal and proximal epicardial coronary artery stenosis can occur in the cardiac transplant recipient, and because medical therapy to date has been disappointing in terms of preventing or retarding allograft arteriopathy, palliative therapy with percutaneous transluminal coronary angioplasty (PTCA) has been attempted. In a recent report from 11 cardiac transplant centers (70), 35 patients underwent 51 angioplasty procedures for 95 lesions appearing at a mean of about 4 years after transplant. In most cases, the primary indication for the procedure was the simple appearance of angiographic CAD (43% of the patients); in only 35% of the patients was there noninvasive evidence of ischemia. Success rates in these patients were high (93%), and procedural complications resemble those seen in native vessel angioplasty. In this cooperative report, complications included myocardial infarction with subsequent death in one patient and three significant groin hematomas. Although follow-up is limited, two thirds of the patients had no major adverse outcomes such as death, myocardial infarction, or retransplantation, at a mean of 13 months after angioplasty. However, four patients died less than 6 months after the procedure, and four died more than 6 months after angioplasty (range 6 to 23 months). Two patients required retransplantation 2 months after angioplasty, and one patient had retransplantation 18 months after angioplasty.

In a second, smaller series, heart transplant patients undergoing PTCA at the University of Pittsburgh School of Medicine received no long-term benefit (71). Of eight patients undergoing successful angioplasty, four subsequently died of complications related to allograft arteriopathy.

Other procedures designed to attenuate obliterative processes in the coronary artery, such as directional atherectomy and rotational atherectomy, can also be used; however, again, the likelihood of restenosis or **retarding disease progression** is not known. It is highly unlikely that these specialized procedures would favorably change the prognosis of heart transplant patients because of the diffuse nature of allograft arteriopathy. Recently, the results of a preliminary study of diltiazem in the prevention of heart transplant arteriopathy provided the tantalizing hypothesis that

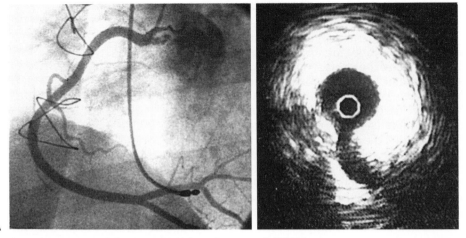

A   B

Figure 41.9. The potential for intravascular ultrasound (IVUS) to assess coronary anatomy. **Right panel** is the IVUS image obtained at the junction of the right coronary artery and the acute marginal branch seen at the distal end of the proximal third of the angiogram in the **left panel.** Note the ability of IVUS to precisely characterize luminal diameter, junctional interfaces, and vessel wall morphology.

this calcium channel blocking agent could be beneficial. **Diltiazem seemed to prevent reduction in coronary artery diameter after heart transplant determined by sequential quantitative angiography** (57). This study also emphasized the importance of quantitative angiographic studies.

Intravascular Ultrasound

Characterization of coronary artery pathology is possible with two-dimensional intravascular ultrasonography (Fig. 41.9 and Table 41.7) (55, 72–74). For the first time, intravascular ultrasound imaging has allowed direct visualization of the coronary lumen, as well as various layers of the coronary artery wall. Because the intima, media, and adventitia of muscular arteries (coronary arteries, in particular) are acoustically distinct, ultrasound imaging can evaluate the shape and size of these structures. Because the media of the coronary artery is less echo dense, intimal and adventitial layer thickness can be determined, as well as medial dimensions. In the normal coronary artery, the internal elastic membrane separating the intima from the media produces a bright inner (luminal) lining of the

image. In vitro and in vivo studies have correlated the ultrasonic appearance of these arterial structures with measurements of normal arteries. St. Goar, et al. (56), compared intracoronary ultrasonography in

Table 41.7.
Intracoronary Ultrasound in the Heart Transplant Patient

Considerations
Precise characterization of vessel wall morphology and luminal characteristics
Calcified versus noncalcified plaque
Presence of thrombus
Concentric versus eccentric
Analysis of all three coronary artery layers
Better quantification of disease extent
Nonobstructive lesions identified and quantified
Better assessment of acute and chronic artery changes after a variety of interventions
Allows analysis of coronary tone after vasoactive drug injection
Allows assessment of therapeutic cardiac catheterization (angioplasty, atherectomy, and so forth)
Limitations of procedure
May cause endothelial injury
Analysis limited to larger epicardial arteries
Requires coronary cannulation to perform
Expensive

heart transplant patients with contrast angiography. In an evaluation of the left anterior descending coronary artery in 80 patients, ultrasound detected allograft arteriopathy more often than angiography. Intimal proliferation was identified early. Studies performed immediately after transplantation served as a reference for coronary anatomy in the donor heart. As expected, some of these hearts had atherosclerotic changes, compatible with early disease already present in the donor. Ultrasound images obtained 1 year or more after transplantation demonstrated a spectrum of abnormalities with a high incidence of clinically silent and angiographically unsuspected intimal thickening.

Intracoronary ultrasonography is currently limited by the size of the coronary probe; small vessel or distal disease will be missed with this procedure. Unfortunately, even small vessel disease in the cardiac transplant patient can account for sudden cardiac death and, when diffuse, significant left ventricular dysfunction. Still, IVUS probably should serve as the reference standard for identification and quantification of cardiac allograft arteriopathy (72).

Assessment of Endothelial Function and Coronary Reserve

Endothelial function has been studied after heart transplantation with both angiography and intravascular ultrasonography. In a recent study, performed 1 year after transplantation, coronary arteries subjected to acetylcholine infusion demonstrated vasoconstriction, suggesting an abnormal endothelial response (74). This was associated with an increase in mean coronary blood flow after acetylcholine measured by intracoronary Doppler flow probe. Coronary blood flow also increased by a factor of five in patients given adenosine. Thus, microvascular function assessed by coronary flow reserve (CFR) in the absence of rejection appeared normal. These data demonstrate not only the utility of IVUS and Doppler assessment of coronary flow in the study of physiologic changes associated with cardiac transplantation, but also demonstrate that endothelial function is abnormal before angiographic disease is present (74, 75). The availability of intracoronary Doppler flow wires for assessment of coronary flow reserve undoubtedly will lead to improved understanding of **CFR in the transplanted heart.**

SUMMARY

The invasive cardiologist and the catheterization laboratory play a major role in long-term care of patients after cardiac transplantation, providing rejection surveillance, determining prognosis in terms of hemodynamic performance of the heart, staging allograft arteriopathy, and offering therapeutic intervention in selected cases with epicardial coronary artery obstruction. Controversial issues, such as the utility of PTCA in these patients, require well-designed clinical trials. Visual interpretation, quantitative angiography, and intravascular ultrasound and Doppler studies, address anatomically different aspects of allograft arteriopathy. A comprehensive post-transplant evaluation requires expertise in biopsy, catheterization, visual and quantitative angiography, and the interventional techniques of angioplasty, intravascular ultrasound, and Doppler. Successfully performing these studies will continually challenge the most expert invasive cardiologist.

References

1. Grattan MT, Moreno-Cabral CE, Starnes VA, et al. Eight-year results of cyclosporine-treated patients with cardiac transplants. J Thorac Cardiovasc Surg 1990;99:500–509.
2. Stevenson LW, Miller LW. Cardiac transplantation as therapy for heart failure. Curr Probl Cardiol 1991;16:219–305.
3. Brezis M, Epstein FH. A closer look at radiocontrast-induced nephropathy. N Engl J Med 1989; 320:179–181.
4. Ravid S, Podrid PJ, Lampert S, et al. Congestive heart failure induced by six of the newer antiar-

rhythmic drugs. J Am Coll Cardiol 1989;14:1326–1330.

5. Gorlin R, Gorlin G. Hydraulic formula for calculation of area of stenotic mitral valve, other cardiac valves, and central circulatory shunts. Am Heart J 1951;41:1–29.

6. Cannon SR, Richards KL, Crawford MH, et al. Inadequacy of the Gorlin formula for predicting prosthetic valve area. Am J Cardiol 1988;62:113–116.

7. Dumesnil JG, Yoganathan AP. Theoretical and practical differences between the Gorlin formula and the continuity equation for calculating aortic and mitral valve areas. Am J Cardiol 1991;67:1268–1272.

8. Casale PN, Palacios IF, Abascal VM, et al. Effects of dobutamine on Gorlin and continuity equation valve areas and valve resistance in valvular aortic stenosis. Am J Cardiol 1992;70:1175–1179.

9. Strauss RH, Stevenson LW, Dadourian BJ, et al. The predictability of mitral regurgitation detected by Doppler echocardiography in patients referred for cardiac transplantation. Am J Cardiol 1987;59:892–894.

10. Braunwald E, Awe WC. The syndrome of severe mitral regurgitation with normal left atrial pressure. Circulation 1963;27:29–35.

11. Fuchs R. Limitations of pulmonary wedge V-waves and diagnosing mitral regurgitation. Am J Cardiol 1982;49:849–854.

12. Haffajee CI. Chronic mitral regurgitation. In: Dalen JE, Alpert JS, eds. Valvular heart disease. Boston: Little Brown, 1981;97–134.

13. Carabello BA. What exactly is 2+ to 3+ mitral regurgitation? J Am Coll Cardiol 1992;19:339–340.

14. Crawford MH, Souche J, Oprian CA, et al., and participants in the Department of Veterans Affairs Cooperative Study of Valvular Heart Disease. Determinants of survival and left ventricular performance after mitral valve replacement. Circulation 1990;81:1173–1181.

15. Bolden JL, Alderman EL. Ventriculographic and hemodynamic features of mitral regurgitation of cardiomyopathic, rheumatic and nonrheumatic etiology. Am J Cardiol 1977;39:177–183.

16. Batista RJ, Santos JL, Takeshita N, et al. Partial left ventriculectomy to improve left ventricular function in end-stage heart disease. J Card Surg 1996;11(2):96–97.

17. Mills RM Jr, Pepine CJ. Heart failure secondary to ischemic heart disease. In: Hosenpud J, Greenberg B, eds. Congestive heart failure. New York: Springer-Verlag; in press.

18. Carlson EB, Cowley MJ, Wolfgang TC, et al. Acute changes in global and regional rest left ventricular function after successful coronary angioplasty: comparative results in stable and unstable angina. J Am Coll Cardiol 1989;13:1262–1269.

19. Topol EJ, Weiss JL, Guzman PA, et al. Immediate improvement of dysfunctional myocardial segments after coronary revascularization: detection by intraoperative transesophageal echocardiography. J Am Coll Cardiol 1984;4:1123–1134.

20. Kirklin JK, Naftel DC, McGiffin DC, et al. Analysis of morbid events and risk factors for death after cardiac transplantation. J Am Coll Cardiol 1988;11;917–924.

21. Mills RM, Kalan JM. Developing a rational management strategy for angina pectoris after coronary bypass surgery: a clinical decision analysis. Clin Cardiol 1991;14:191–197.

22. Oaks TE, Pae WE, Miller CA, et al. Combined registry for the clinical use of mechanical assist pumps and the total artificial heart in conjunction with heart transplantation: fifth official report—1990. J Heart Lung Transplant 1991;10:621–625.

23. Gardiner AJS, Short D. Four faces of acute myopericarditis. Br Heart J 1973;35:433.

24. Costanzo-Nordin MR, O'Connell JB, Subramanian R, et al. Myocarditis confirmed by biopsy presenting as acute myocardial infarction. Br Heart J 1985;53:25–29.

25. Miklozek CL, Crumpacker CS, Royal HD, et al. Myocarditis presenting as acute myocardial infarction. Am Heart J 1988;115:768–776.

26. Hauck AJ, Kearney DL, Edwards WD, et al. Evaluation of postmortem endomyocardial biopsy specimens from 38 patients with lymphocytic myocarditis: implications for the role of sampling error. Mayo Clin Proc 1989;64:1235–1245.

27. Mason JW, O'Connell JB. Clinical merit of endomyocardial biopsy. Circulation 1989;79:971–979.

28. Aretz HT, Billingham ME, Edwards WD, et al. Myocarditis: a histopathologic definition and classification. Am J Cardiovasc Pathol 1987;1:3–14.

29. Sainani GS, et al. Heart disease caused by Coxsackie virus B infection. Br Heart J 1975;37:812.

30. Bristow MR, et al. Efficacy and cost of cardiac monitoring in patients receiving doxorubicin. Cancer 1982;50:32.

31. Griepp RB, Stinson EB, Dong E Jr, et al. Determinants of operative risk in human heart transplantation. Am J Surg 1971;22:192–197.

32. Kirklin JK, Naftel DL, Kirklin JW, et al. Pulmonary vascular resistance and the risk of heart transplantation. J Heart Transplant 1988;7:331–336.

33. Braunwald E, Braunwald NS, Ross J Jr, et al. Effects of mitral valve replacement on the pulmonary vascular dynamics of patients with pulmonary hypertension. N Engl J Med 1965;273:509–514.

34. Dalen JE, Matloff JM, Evans GL, et al. Early reduction of pulmonary vascular resistance after mitral valve replacement. N Engl J Med 1967;277:387–394.

35. Costard-Jackle A, Fowler MB. Influence of preoperative pulmonary artery pressure on mortality after heart transplantation: testing of potential reversibility of pulmonary hypertension with nitroprusside is useful in defining a high risk group. J Am Coll Cardiol 1992;19:48–54.

36. Murali S, Uretsky BF, Reddy PS, et al. Reversibility of pulmonary hypertension in congestive heart failure patients evaluated for cardiac transplantation comparative effects of various pharmacologic agents. Am Heart J 1991;122:1375–1381.

37. Utterback DB, Staples ED, White ED, et al. Basis for the selective reduction of pulmonary vascular

resistance in humans during infusion of adenosine. J Appl Physiol 1994;76(2):724–730.

38. Schrader, BJ, Inbar S, Kaufmann L, et al. Comparison of the effects of adenosine and nifedipine in pulmonary hypertension. J Am Coll Cardiol 1992; 19:1060–1064.

39. Haywood GA, Sneddon, JF, Bashir Y, et al. Adenosine infusion for the reversal of pulmonary vasoconstriction in biventricular failure. Circulation 1992;86:896–902.

40. Enriquez-Sarano M, Rossi A, Seward JB, et al. Determinants of pulmonary hypertension in left ventricular dysfunction. J Am Coll Cardiol 1997; 29:153–159.

41. Young JB, Leon CA, Weilbaecher DA. Endomyocardial biopsy in critically ill patients. The procedure and diagnosis and prognostic potential. Problems in Critical Care 1988;2:433–462.

42. Goy J-J, Gilliard D, Kaufmann U, et al. Endomyocardial biopsy in cardiac transplant recipients using the femoral venous approach. Am J Cardiol 1990;65;822–823.

43. Kern MJ. Endomyocardial biopsy in cardiac transplant recipients using the femoral venous approach. Am J Cardiol 1991;67:342.

44. Sharples LD, Cary NRB, Large SR, et al. Error rates with which endomyocardial biopsy specimens are graded for rejection after cardiac transplantation. Am J Cardiol 1992;70:527–530.

45. Billingham ME, Cary NRB, Hammond ME, et al. A working formulation for the standardization of nomenclature in the diagnosis of heart and lung rejection: heart rejection study group. J Heart Lung Transplant 1990;9:587–593.

46. Hammond EH, Yowell RL, Price GD, et al. Vascular rejection and its relationship to allograft coronary artery disease. J Heart Lung Transplant 1992; 11(Suppl):S111–S119.

47. Lowry R, Adam E, Bitar J, et al. What are the implications of cardiac infection with cytomegalovirus prior to cardiac transplantation? [Abstract]. J Heart Lung Transplant 1993; in press.

48. Fitchett DH, Forbes C, Guerraty AJ. Repeated endomyocardial biopsy causing coronary arterial-right ventricular fistula after cardiac transplantation. Am J Cardiol 1988;62:829–831.

49. Young JB, Leon CA, Short HD, et al. Evolution of hemodynamics after orthotopic heart and heart-lung transplantation: early restrictive patterns persisting in occult fashion. J Heart Transplant 1987;6:34–43.

50. Miller LW. Transplant coronary artery disease [Editorial]. J Heart Lung Transplant 1992;11: S1—S4.

51. Young JB. Cardiac allograft arteriopathy: an ischemic burden of a different sort. Am J Cardiol 1992;70:9F–13F.

52. O'Neill BJ, Pflugfelder PW, Singh NR, et al. Frequency of angiographic detection and quantitative assessment of coronary arterial disease one and three years after cardiac transplantation. Am J Cardiol 1989;63:1221–1226.

53. Gao S-Z, Alderman EL, Schroeder JS, et al. Progressive coronary luminal narrowing after cardiac transplantation. Circulation 1990:82(Suppl IV):IV-269—IV-275.

54. Uretsky BF, Kormos RL, Zerbe TR, et al. Cardiac events after heart transplantation: incidence and predictive value of coronary arteriography. J Heart Lung Transplant 1992;11:S45–S51.

55. Goswitz JJ, Braunlin E, Kub SH, et al. Pathology of heart transplantation: study of autopsied and explanted allografts with emphasis on possible biopsy findings. Clin Transplant 1992;46:450–457.

56. St. Goar FG, Pinto FJ, Alderman EL, et al. Intracoronary ultrasound in cardiac transplant recipients. In vivo evidence of "angiographically silent" intimal thickening. Circulation 1992;85:979–987.

57. Schroeder JS, Gao S-Z, Alderman EL, et al. A preliminary study of diltiazem in the prevention of coronary artery disease in heart-transplant recipients. N Engl J Med 1993;328:164–170.

58. Johnson DE, Gao SZ, Schroeder JS, et al. The spectrum of coronary artery pathologic findings in human cardiac allografts. J Heart Transplant 1989;8:349–359.

59. Johnson DE, Alderman EL, Schroeder JS, et al. Transplant coronary artery disease: histopathologic correlations with angiographic morphology. J Am Coll Cardiol 1991;17:449–457.

60. Smart FW, Ballantyne CM, Cocanougher B, et al. Insensitivity of noninvasive tests to detect coronary artery vasculopathy after heart transplant. Am J Cardiol 1991;67:243–247.

61. Young JB, Smart FM, Lowry RL, et al. Coronary angiography after heart transplantation: should perioperative study be the "gold standard"? J Heart Lung Transplant 1992;11:S65–S68.

62. van der Linden MMJM, Balk AHM, Strikwerda S, et al. Quantitative coronary angiography after cardiac transplantation [Abstract]. Eur Heart J 1992;13(Suppl):70.

63. van der Linden MMJM, Balk AHM, Strikwerda S, et al. Coronary luminal changes in the first year after cardiac transplantation. A quantitative analysis [Abstract]. Eur Heart J 1992;13(Suppl):9.

64. Gao SZ, Alderman EL, Schroeder JS, et al. Accelerated coronary vascular disease in the heart transplant patient: coronary arteriographic findings. J Am Coll Cardiol 1988;12:334–340.

65. de Feyter PJ, Serruys PW, Davies MJ, et al. Quantitative coronary angiography to measure progression and regression of coronary atherosclerosis. Value, limitations, and implications for clinical trials. Circulation 1991;84:412–423.

66. Seiler C, Kirkeeide RL, Gould KL. Basic structure—function relations of the epicardial coronary vascular tree. Basis of quantitative coronary arteriography for diffuse coronary artery disease. Circulation 1992;85:1987–2003.

67. Mancini GBJ, Bourassa MG, Williamson PR, et al. Prognostic importance of quantitative analysis of coronary cineangiograms. Am J Cardiol 1992; 69:1022–1027.

68. Dressler FA, Miller LW. Necropsy versus angiography: how accurate is angiography? J Heart Lung Transplant 1992;11:S56–S59.

69. Mills RM Jr, Hill JA, Theron HDT, et al. Serial quantitative coronary angiography in the assessment of coronary disease in the transplanted heart. J Heart Lung Transplant 1992;11:S52–S55.

70. Halle AA III, Wilson RF, Massin EK, et al. Coro-

nary angioplasty in cardiac transplant patients. Results of a multicenter study. Circulation 1992; 86:458–462.

71. Sandhu JS, Uretsky BF, Reddy S, et al. Potential limitations of percutaneous transluminal coronary angioplasty in heart transplant recipients. Am J Cardiol 1992;69:1234–1237.

72. Waller BF, Pinkerton CA, Slack JD. Intravascular ultrasound: a histological study of vessels during life. The new "gold standard" for vascular imaging. Circulation 1992;85:2305–2310.

73. Valantine H, Pinto FJ, St. Goar FG, et al. Intracoro-
nary ultrasound imaging in heart transplant recipients: the Stanford experience. J Heart Lung Transplant 1992;11:S60–S64.

74. Mills RM Jr, Billett JM, Nichols WW. Endothelial dysfunction early after heart transplantation. Assessment with intravascular ultrasound and Doppler. Circulation 1992;86:1171–1174.

75. Yeung AC, Anderson T, Meredith I, et al. Endothelial dysfunction in the development and detection of transplant coronary artery disease. J Heart Lung Transplant 1992;11:S69–S73.

42
The Patient with Known or Suspected Pericardial Disease

Jamie B. Conti, MD
Jannet F. Lewis, MD
C. Richard Conti, MD

INTRODUCTION

The patient with known or suspected pericardial disease offers a challenge for the clinician, who must be prepared to integrate history and physical examination, as well as invasive and noninvasive data, to obtain a secure diagnosis and initiate treatment. **The pericardium, by virtue of its extravascular location, is poorly visualized with standard angiographic techniques,** and pericardial dysfunction must be surmised from the resulting hemodynamic effects. Sonography (1, 2) or more advanced technology (e.g., computed tomography (CT) scan, magnetic resonance imaging (MRI)) must be used to directly visualize the pericardial structures. These diagnostic procedures, however, only infer hemodynamic significance. Thus, neither approach alone is wholly sufficient to direct effective therapy, and both may need to be repeated during the course of treatment. Symptoms caused by pericardial abnormalities are often masked by more virulent extrapericardial disease processes. Diagnosis requires the recognition that pericardial disease may be associated with a large number of primary disease entities. Physical examination and simple laboratory studies (e.g., chest x-ray and ECG) may be misleading or nonspecific. This chapter provides the reader with a multifaceted and integrated approach to pericardial disease that uses cardiac catheterization in addition to noninvasive studies.

PERICARDIUM: ANATOMY, EMBRYOLOGY, AND PHYSIOLOGY

Pericardium functioning is complex, but it is present in various forms in all vertebrates (3, 4). The adult human pericardium is formed from the embryonic fusion of the mesodermal epimyocardial mantle and the pleuropericardial mantle (5). These mantles join to form a thick fibrous sac that fuses with the adventitia of the great vessels, and it is firmly attached to the diaphragmatic aponeurosis (parietal layer). A more delicate, compliant visceral pericardial layer is directly attached to the epicardium. A space that normally contains a small volume of fluid exists between these two layers. The purpose and origin of the fluid is ill-defined, but it represents more than cardiac lymph fluid (4).

Several functions have been ascribed to the pericardium; however, congenital or acquired absence of the pericardium usually is unnoticed, unless recognized on a chest x-ray done for other reasons. As a membrane, the pericardium behaves similarly to other serosal surfaces. As such, composition and both production and disposition of the fluid are under local cellular and hydrostatic forces. The supportive fibrous pericardium is a rigid constraint that can prevent overdilation of the ventricles during acute stress, and it influences the relationship of filling pressures in all four chambers of the heart. Its thickness acts as a barrier against infection and tumor spread from contiguous structures. The pericardium does elicit systemic responses to pharmacologic and nerve stimulation (e.g., nicotine) (6).

The importance of the pericardium in pathologic states is well appreciated (3, 4) (Table 42.1). As our knowledge of molecular biology, immunology, and virology accumulates, we may be better able to classify pericardial disease (7). Currently pericar-

dial dysfunction is divided into primary disease of the pericardium and secondary processes (e.g., tumor). Most important overall are the hemodynamic effects caused by pericardial disease.

PERICARDIAL EFFUSION

Pericardial effusion is defined as greater than 50 mL of fluid within the pericardial sac. However, accumulation of pericardial fluid does not necessarily imply pericardial disease. Specific disease entities stimulate different morphologic responses from the visceral and parietal pericardia. Thus, pericardial fluid may be composed of fibrin, blood, chyle, inflammatory cells, malignant cells, or a combination of these elements, reflecting the primary disease process. When pericardial disease is present, chest pain may be the most prominent symptom, but pain can be perceived in the middle thorax or shoulders (8). Usually a simple effusion is clinically asymptomatic, and symptoms that are present reflect the primary disease process.

Table 42.1.
Etiology of Pericardial Effusion

Idiopathic
Infectious
    Viral (Coxsackie B, ECHO, human immunodeficiency virus)
    Bacteria (tuberculosis, staphylococcal, gonococcal)
    Fungal (histoplasmosis, *candida*)
Metabolic
    Uremia
    Myxedema
Drug-induced
    Minoxidil
    Hydralazine
    Procainamide
Autoimmune
    Systemic lupus erythematosus
    Scleroderma
    Rheumatoid arthritis
    Rheumatic pancarditis
    Postinfarction (Dressler's syndrome, thrombolysis)
Volume overload (chronic congestive heart failure)
Trauma (penetrating injury, aortic dissection)
Neoplastic
    Pericardial metastasis (melanoma, breast carcinoma)
    Local invasion (lung cancer, lymphoma)

Noninvasive Assessment

Commonly, **enlargement of the cardiac silhouette found on chest x-ray is the first clue to the presence of pericardial effusion.** Electrocardiographic abnormalities consistent with pericarditis and pericardial effusion include PR segment depression, low voltage, ST segment elevation, and electrical alternans. Atrial arrhythmias, especially atrial flutter, are seen in patients with pericarditis, but sinus tachycardia is most frequently observed.

Echocardiography

Echocardiography has become a standard reference for diagnosis of pericardial effusion detected as a posterior echo-free space between the parietal and visceral pericardium. M-mode echocardiography can detect small amounts (15–20 mL) of fluid (9). However, two-dimensional echocardiography more sensitively detects loculated effusion, and it has improved specificity by distinguishing effusion from other posterior echo-free spaces, such as pleural effusion, descending aorta, and marked left atrial enlargement (Figure 42.1). Fluid volume cannot be reliably quantitated, but classification of fluid volume as small (usually confined to the posterior space), moderate, and large (generally surrounding the heart), is reasonably accurate.

Echocardiography has also proved useful in guiding diagnostic or therapeutic pericardiocentesis. Callahan et al. performed echo-guided pericardiocentesis in 117 consecutive patients (10) and reported success in 90% of their patients. No deaths and only one major complication—pneumothorax—occurred. In addition, **serial echocardiographic examination is useful for assessing efficacy of pericardiocentesis or reaccumulation.**

Computerized Tomography and Magnetic Resonance Imaging

Both CT with contrast and MRI are sensitive and specific (11, 12) for detecting thickened pericardium and effusion (13, 14). With both techniques, the pericardium appears as a thick line between the myocardium and pericardial fat. Improved spatial resolution allows the distinction to be made between pleural fluid and pericardial cysts from pericardial effusion (Fig. 42.2). All imaging modalities, with the exception of the chest x-ray, have become more advanced, and each has unique capabilities. For example, CT resolution allows visualization of details not detectable by standard echocardiography and detection of as little as 50 mL of pericardial fluid. Superior tissue characterization, especially with MRI, may provide unique insights into pathologic processes (14). For example, **MRI can accurately define loculated effusion and pericardial thickening, as well as differentiate pericardial from pleural effusions.** MRI also has

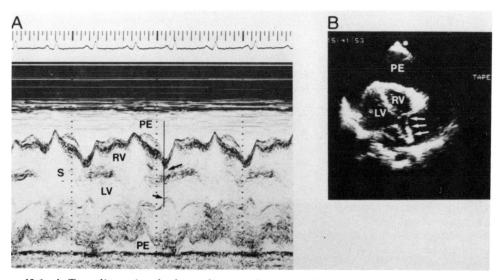

Figure 42.1. A. Two-dimensional echocardiogram demonstrating large anterior and posterior pericardial effusion (*PE*). Note the diastolic collapse of the right ventricular wall (*line*). **B.** A four-chamber view demonstrates collapse of the right atrial wall (*arrows*). *LV,* left ventricle; *S,* septum; *RV,* right ventricle. (Reprinted with permission from Quinones MA. Echocardiography in adult heart disease. Baylor College of Medicine Cardiology Series, 1985;7:4.)

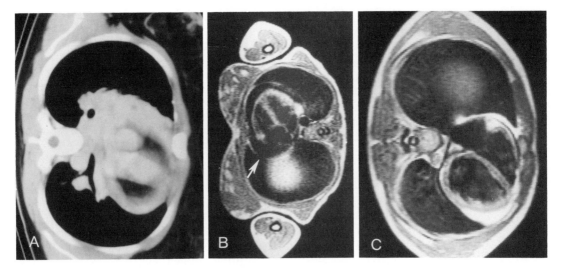

Figure 42.2. A. CT scan of patient with lymphomatous involvement of the pericardium that is noticeably thickened and not clearly separated from the myocardium. **B.** An MRI scan indicating a simple pericardial effusion. Note the thin parietal pericardium (*arrow*) and the normal-sized cardiac chambers. **C.** A magnetic resonance imaging scan of thickened parietal pericardium with associated fluid representing a patient with effusive constrictive pericarditis caused by tuberculosis.

the potential to differentiate hemorrhagic and nonhemorrhagic exudative effusions from transudative effusions (1). Imaging modality choice should be guided by the clinical situation, presence or absence of calcium, an adequate imaging window, and, of course, institutional availability (15).

Invasive Assessment

Pericardiocentesis and Biopsy

Once pericardial effusion is detected, the cardiologist is frequently consulted for further evaluation and management. Usually, pericardial fluid, tissue, or both must be obtained. The possible exception to this practice is in patients with AIDS and a pericardial effusion (see below). Pericardiocentesis and pericardial biopsy are not without potential complications. These risks must be balanced with the benefit, especially in the asymptomatic or only mildly symptomatic patient. Pericardial fluid volume generally follows the course of the primary disease, and pericardiocentesis should be per-

formed only if information derived from the fluid or pericardium would alter therapy, or when tamponade is present. Pericardiocentesis and biopsy techniques are discussed elsewhere (see Chapter 9).

Examination of Pericardial Fluid

Malignancy

No controlled studies conclusively support that acquisition of tissue is superior to fluid analysis alone for diagnosis of malignancy involving the pericardium. We are unaware of a comparison of cell block cytologic analysis with direct tissue biopsy specimen to diagnose malignancy. Nonetheless, data support the value of pericardial cytology as a diagnostic tool (16). One recent report emphasizes that malignant pericardial cytology is a predictor of poor prognosis and, thus, may markedly influence clinical decision making (17). **If pericardial tissue is to be obtained, the subxiphoid pericardiotomy approach is preferred** to the apical approach.

Recently an assay for carcinoembryonic antigen (CEA) in pericardial fluid has been used successfully to differentiate benign from malignant disease (18), with a sensitivity of 75% and a specificity of 100% in the diagnosis of malignant pericarditis.

AIDS

Pericardial effusion is common among patients infected with the human immunodeficiency virus (HIV), particularly those with end-stage disease. A recent study, the Prospective Evaluation of Cardiac Involvement in AIDS (PRECIA), evaluated the prevalence of pericardial effusion and mortality in HIV-infected patients (19). Prevalence of pericardial effusions defined echocardiographically in AIDS patients was 5%, and the incidence 11% per year over a 2-year period. Most effusions were small (80%) and asymptomatic (87%). Survival of AIDS patients with an effusion was markedly decreased when compared with those without effusions, 36 $\pm$ 11% versus 93 $\pm$ 3% at 6 months. No effusions were found in a control group of healthy HIV-negative subjects.

The authors concluded that diagnosis of an asymptomatic pericardial effusion in an HIV-infected individual may signal end-stage disease; and, because most of these effusions are small and commonly are not associated with hemodynamic compromise, an exhaustive search for the cause is usually not indicated.

In a related study, Flum et al. (20) conducted a retrospective review of all patients diagnosed with AIDS who had a pericardial window procedure between 1986 and 1994. In 94% of cases, no change was made in the management of these patients based on the information obtained operatively. Similar to the PRECIA results, they found a high mortality rate at 22 weeks, and concluded that invasive diagnostic procedures provided little practical information and, thus, were not justified.

Tuberculosis

Diagnosis of tuberculous pericarditis may be difficult (21, 22). A relatively new assay, adenosine deaminase (ADA) has been shown useful in this regard (18). Koh et al. (18) measured ADA and CEA in pericardial fluid in 26 patients with moderate to large pericardial effusions and in 19 control patients. With a cutoff value for ADA activity of 40 U/L, sensitivity was 93% and specificity 97% in the diagnosis of tuberculous pericarditis; measurement of ADA was particularly useful in the early diagnosis of tuberculous pericarditis, when other laboratory tests were negative.

Pericardiocentesis can be performed safely and effectively in the catheterization laboratory (see Chapter 9 for a discussion of techniques). As a result of the availability and accuracy of noninvasive studies, neither catheterization nor "blind" pericardiocentesis should be done simply to determine if an effusion is present. Right ventricular cardiac catheterization with pressure recordings can be performed to assess the hemodynamic significance of the effusion; pericardiocentesis can be performed at the same time. Under fluoroscopic guidance, the tip of a right atrial catheter will generally lie some distance from the left border of the cardiac silhouette. If angiography is done, effusion separates the edge of the contrast-filled cardiac chamber or coronary artery from the radiolucency of the lung, and the contour of the right atrial border is straight rather than convex. In addition, techniques such as pericardioscopy can be performed that may be helpful in identifying tumor, foreign bodies, or loculated effusion (23, 24). Flexible fiberoptic pericardioscopy permits visualization of all pericardial surfaces and makes it possible to biopsy selective sites (25). Corticosteroids can be injected into the pericardial space to treat uremic or idiopathic recurrent pericarditis (26, 27). Sclerosing agents (e.g., tetracycline) can also be infused via a small catheter to palliate recurrent malignant pericardial effusions (28, 29). A pigtail catheter can be introduced over a guidewire if chronic infusion or drainage is necessary. In the surgical literature, subxiphoid pericardiotomy has been described in the diagnosis and management of large pericardial effusions associated with malignancy. Although of limited value diagnostically, when compared with examination of pericardial fluid alone, this surgical procedure has a low morbidity and is effective palliative therapy (30).

Pericardiocentesis has also been safely and successfully performed under echocardiographic guidance. In a series of 117 consecutive patients at Mayo Clinic undergoing two-dimensional echo-guided pericardiocentesis, the procedure was effective in all but three performed for therapeutic purpose. In addition, no procedure-related deaths occurred, and the complication rate was low.

Percutaneous balloon catheter pericardiotomy performed in the cardiac catheterization laboratory has been reported with promising initial results and few serious complications (31). Application of this technique at present **should be limited to those patients with serious illness in whom the risk of surgery seems prohibitive.** The percutaneous balloon pericardiotomy registry recently described the following technique: using a subxiphoid approach, a standard pericardial drainage catheter is inserted into the pericardial space and fluid removed (Fig. 42.3). Subsequently, 10–20 mL of contrast material is injected to outline the pericardial space. A 0.038-inch extra stiff guidewire is then advanced into the pericardial space (Fig. 42.4), and the tract through the parietal pericardium is dilated with a 10 F dilator. When this has been accomplished, a 20 × 30 mm dilating balloon is advanced and inflated to further enlarge the tract (Figs. 42.5 and 42.6). Another injection of contrast material is then done to document free flow of contrast material. The registry reports a 93% success rate, with success defined as no requirement for surgical intervention and no recurrence of signs or symptoms of tamponade. The most common complication is fever of unknown cause. Pleural effusions that require chest tube placement are rare and only seen in patients with preexisting pleural effusions. The limitations of this catheter-based therapeutic technique, when compared with surgical pericardiectomy, include lack of direct visualization of the pericardium and inaccessibility of tissue for microscopic examination. With the development of percutaneous fiberoptic catheter pericardioscopy and

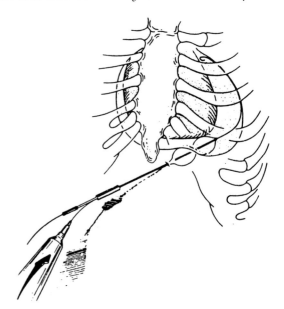

Figure 42.3. Drawing illustrating the percutaneous balloon pericardiotomy technique. The dilating balloon is advanced over a guidewire to straddle the pericardial margin; it is then manually inflated to create the pericardial window. (Reprinted with permission from Ziskind AA, Pearce AC, Lemmon MSN, et al. Percutaneous balloon pericardiotomy for the treatment of cardiac tamponade and large pericardial effusions: description of technique and report of the first 50 cases. J Am Coll Cardiol 1993;21(1):1–5.)

biopsy, these limitations may become less important.

CARDIAC TAMPONADE

Accumulation of pericardial fluid can result in profound hemodynamic effects. These effects depend on the volume of fluid, as well as the rate of accumulation and compliance of pericardium and cardiac chambers impaired. The thick inelastic fibrous pericardium may expand or "creep" over a period of time, accommodating several liters of slowly accumulating pericardial fluid. Alternately, rapid accumulation in the presence of a noncompliant pericardium may cause severe hemodynamic effects. It follows that if noncompressible fluid fills a relatively rigidly encased space shared by a

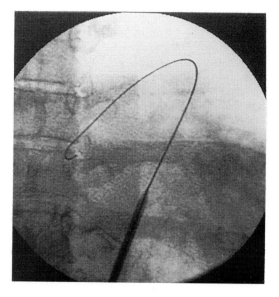

Figure 42.4. Guidewire in pericardial space and dilating sheath in situ. (Reprinted with permission from Ziskind AA, Pearce AC, Lemmon MSN, et al. Percutaneous balloon pericardiotomy for the treatment of cardiac tamponade and large pericardial effusions: description of technique and report of the first 50 cases. J Am Coll Cardiol 1993;21(1):1–5.)

vented, hollow structure, an exponential rise in fluid pressure will cause the pressure to rise in the hollow structure. When the hollow structure is the heart, the distending pressure rise is under physiologic limits, so eventually the hollow viscus will collapse. Many animal and human experiments have documented these findings of cardiac tamponade (3, 4, 32). The essential hemodynamic abnormality of pericardial tamponade is a rise in intrapericardial pressure to equal diastolic pressure in the heart so that diastolic filling is impaired. In cardiac tamponade, ventricular transmural pressure is low. All pericardial effusions can alter cardiac filling. Clinically, patients can be subdivided into two groups.

First are those who develop pericardial effusions rapidly, resulting in Beck's triad of decreasing arterial pressure, increasing jugular venous pressure, and a small quiet heart. This catastrophic event most frequently occurs as a result of traumatic perforation of the heart, postinfarction myocardial rupture, or ascending aortic dissection.

These patients have acute cardiac compression and require diagnosis and therapy promptly and concomitantly.

Second, others may develop effusions gradually. This condition usually allows time for definitive diagnosis and planned treatment. In a report of 56 patients with gradually developing cardiac tamponade, 80% were tachypneic, 77% had tachycardia, 77% had a paradoxical pulse, 64% had a systolic blood pressure less than 100 mm Hg, and only 34% had diminished heart sounds (33). A recent study concluded that a paradoxic pulse greater than 12 mm Hg and a decline of more than 9% in systolic blood pressure during inspiration had an accuracy of 92% and 97%, respectively, in predicting moderate-to-severe tamponade (34). A paradoxic pulse greater than 25 mm Hg was predictive of severe hemodynamic compromise. Of note, neoplastic and uremic diseases accounted for nearly two thirds of the cases. Malignant metastases to the pericardium is reportedly the most com-

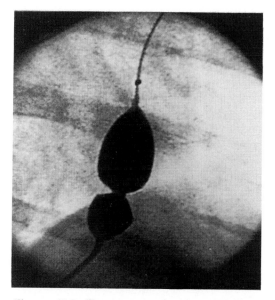

Figure 42.5. Fluoroscopy showing wasting of the balloon by the pericardium. (Reprinted with permission from Ziskind AA, Pearce AC, Lemmon MSN, et al. Percutaneous balloon pericardiotomy for the treatment of cardiac tamponade and large pericardial effusions: description of technique and report of the first 50 cases. J Am Coll Cardiol 1993;21(1):1–5.)

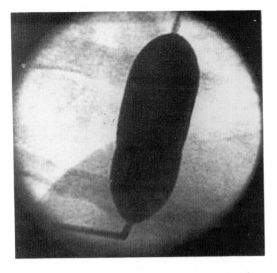

Figure 42.6. Fluoroscopy showing minimal residual wasting of the balloon after full inflation and creation of a window in the pericardium. (Reprinted with permission from Ziskind AA, Pearce AC, Lemmon MSN, et al. Percutaneous balloon pericardiotomy for the treatment of cardiac tamponade and large pericardial effusions: description of technique and report of the first 50 cases. J Am Coll Cardiol 1993;21(1):1–5.)

mon cause of tamponade in hospitalized patients (35). A paradoxic pulse may not develop if left ventricular diastolic pressures exceed the pericardial pressure, as in left ventricular failure. Orthopnea is common in tamponade, and it can reflect transmitted pericardial pressure to the left atrium and elevation of pulmonary venous pressure in the absence of left ventricular systolic dysfunction (4). Jugular venous pressure elevation, with a characteristically prominent *x* descent and absent *y* descent, correlates well with right atrial pressure tracings. **In the setting of hypovolemia, a mismatch may occur in the pericardial pressure and central venous pressure ("low pressure tamponade").**

Noninvasive Assessment

Chest x-ray and fluoroscopy lack sensitivity for assessing pericardial tamponade. Ungated CT scans and MRI also correlate poorly with hemodynamic findings, but they have the advantage of accurately imaging the anterior mediastinum. Newer gated methods promise higher sensitivity because they can detect wall motion abnormalities caused by tamponade. Radionuclide studies have not successfully differentiated hemodynamically important effusions from those that do not impair hemodynamic function. MRI and cardiac ultrasound do help distinguish tamponade from right ventricular infarction and superior vena cava compression that may mimic tamponade. A number of echocardiographic findings have been reported in cardiac tamponade. M-mode studies in patients with tamponade show exaggerated respiratory variations of ventricular filling and cardiac output (36), including greater than normal increase in right ventricular diastolic size, decrease in left ventricular expiratory diastolic dimension (37), and decrease in mitral valve EF slope (38). These changes, although useful, may be difficult to distinguish from normal respiratory variations. The echocardiographic changes that appear to be most helpful in diagnosing cardiac tamponade are collapse of the right cardiac chambers (39–42). Right atrial collapse is uniformly present in patients with tamponade (42). Although sensitive, this sign can be seen with even small effusions, particularly with low right atrial pressure. However, collapse of the right atrium lasting more than one third of the cardiac cycle has a demonstrated sensitivity of 100% and specificity of about 80% (41). Right ventricular diastolic collapse has a reported sensitivity of 92% and specificity of 100% (39, 40). Importantly, right ventricular diastolic collapse may be absent in patients with coexistent pulmonary hypertension (43). Doppler echocardiographic assessment is also useful in documenting the reciprocal respiratory changes in transvalvular flow velocity. Patients with cardiac tamponade show an inspiratory decrease in mitral inflow velocity, left ventricular ejection time, and aortic flow velocity (44, 45). This is accompanied by an increase in tricuspid flow and pulmonic flow velocity. Inferior vena cava plethora and abnormal respiratory changes have also been reported to be sensitive signs of cardiac tamponade (46). A recent report cautions that echocardiographic markers of cardiac tamponade are sensitive and may be present in patients without hemodynamic deterioration (47).

Invasive Assessment

In some cases definitive assessment of the hemodynamic significance of pericardial effusions requires cardiac catheterization. Right atrial catheterization with a stiff catheter can show a discrepancy between the atrial wall marked by the catheter tip and the fluoroscopic border of the heart, confirming the existence of a large effusion. This simple procedure is often overlooked. Pressure tracings reveal the characteristic elevated right atrial pressure with preserved systolic atrial filling or *x* descent. The *y* descent is replaced by a gradually upsloping pressure wave, as diastolic filling is impeded by pericardial pressure. With inspiration, venous pressure usually falls slightly in tamponade but rises in constriction. In tamponade, as opposed to constrictive pericarditis (discussed later in this chapter), increased intrapericardial pressure is exerted on the heart throughout the entire cardiac cycle with only momentary relief during ventricular ejection. In severe acute tamponade, venous return can be completely impeded throughout diastole when cardiac volume and intrapericardial pressure are both maximal. In mild to moderately severe cases of tamponade, right ventricular systolic pressure may rise slightly. With severe compression, right ventricular systolic pressure decreases in proportion to the reduction in stroke volume. However, right ventricular diastolic pressure will be elevated and equal to the right atrial and pericardial pressures. Pulmonary artery diastolic pressure is also elevated to the same level as the right ventricular diastolic pressure with a diminished pulse pressure, and it may be difficult to distinguish pulmonary artery from right ventricular pressure. At times, only catheter tip location by fluoroscopy allows identification of these pressures. Left ventricular systolic pressure is reduced proportionally to the severity of compression, and diastolic pressure is elevated to equal the right ventricular diastolic pressure.

Right ventricular catheterization should be combined with catheterization of the pericardial sac. Pericardial pressure should be measured; it is always elevated in tamponade, and should be within 2 mm Hg of the right atrial and right ventricular diastolic pressures to confirm the diagnosis. Cardiac tamponade occurring in patients with severe left ventricular dysfunction can cause diagnostic problems, as tamponade will occur when intrapericardial pressures equal right atrial pressure. In these cases, right atrial pressure will remain somewhat elevated after pericardiocentesis.

Angiographic studies may show atrial collapse and small hyperactive ventricular chambers. This should reduce stroke volume through the Frank-Starling effect, but activation of the sympathetic nervous system and increased circulating catecholamines also stimulate contraction. Coronary angiography may demonstrate overt coronary artery compression in diastole (48).

Most patients with cardiac tamponade require fluid to be drained. This can be safely accomplished with either fluoroscopic or echocardiographic guidance (10). Volume infusion or inotropic agents may be helpful temporizing therapies until pericardiocentesis is possible. The merits of performing diagnostic pericardiocentesis in the catheterization laboratory have been mentioned. Fluoroscopic documentation of catheter placement is often necessary because of altered pressure tracings.

Data Evaluation, Interpretation, and Decision Making

If tamponade is present, pericardiocentesis can produce striking immediate hemodynamic changes (Fig. 42.7) and may be lifesaving. Both right atrial and pericardial space pressures should fall after pericardiocentesis, and pericardial pressure should be clearly less than atmospheric pressure. The right atrial wave-form returns toward normal with reappearance of a normal diastolic pressure fall or *y* descent. Early diastolic dip

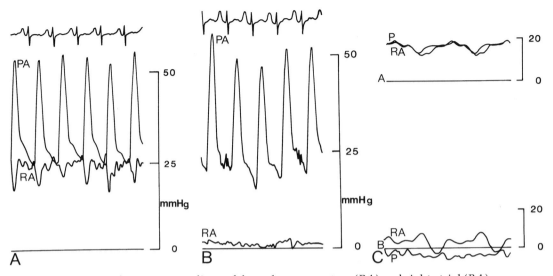

Figure 42.7. A. Simultaneous recordings of the pulmonary artery (*PA*) and right atrial (*RA*) pressures in a patient with scleroderma and pericardial tamponade. Note the elevated PA and RA pressures. **B. After pericardiocentesis, a marked decrease in RA pressure is seen. C. Simultaneous recording of pericardial** (*P*) **and RA pressures.** Note the elevation and equalization of the pressures prior to pericardiocentesis (*top*) and lowering and separation of the pressures postpericardiocentesis (*bottom*).

in ventricular pressures will return toward normal inasmuch as myocardial function permits. Systolic aortic pressure increases, as do pulse pressure and cardiac output. Simultaneous echocardiography will demonstrate rapid normalization of chamber expansion and hemodynamic improvement, coinciding with disappearance of right ventricular diastolic collapse.

The decision to leave the right ventricular and pericardial space catheters in place on leaving the catheterization laboratory is dependent on findings in a given patient. It is imperative to repeat measurements when fluid has been removed to exclude concomitant constrictive physiology (see later in this chapter). Right atrial pressure can be measured serially from a balloon flotation catheter to detect rapid accumulation of pericardial fluid. Serial echocardiograms are probably sufficient for the patient who is unlikely to have fluid reaccumulate quickly. In patients with effusions caused by uremia or neoplastic pericarditis, the pericardial space catheter can be left in place, and therapeutic and sclerosing agents can be instilled. Alternatively, both subxiphoid and transthoracic pericardial drainage procedures have been described (49). Patients who have

recurrent effusions in the absence of uremia or cancer may be considered for either percutaneous catheter balloon pericardiotomy (31) or surgical pericardiectomy, although controversy exists regarding operative intervention (50, 51).

CHRONIC CONSTRICTIVE PERICARDITIS

In constrictive pericarditis, the pericardium restricts diastolic cardiac expansion. Constrictive pericarditis can occur in a variety of diseases. The causes may be similar to those of pericardial effusion with some exceptions (e.g., radiation) (Table 42.1). It is not understood why, with similar diseases, some patients have complete resolution of pericardial effusion and others develop a chronic inflammatory process with pericardial thickening and cardiac compression. Pericardial constriction is commonly seen after tuberculous pericarditis (20, 52). Rheumatoid arthritis is the most commonly associated autoimmune disease (53); constriction is rare with lupuslike drug-induced pleuropericarditis and in rheumatic heart disease (54). It has been described as a late sequela of Dressler's syndrome and hemopericardium of any cause (55, 56). Constrictive pericarditis has also been described as a rare complication of epicardial patch lead placement after cardiodefibrillator implantation (57). Idiopathic disease is now the most common type of constrictive pericarditis. This is a slowly progressive disorder in which signs and symptoms may suggest volume overload.

Once constrictive pericardial disease is established, it does not disappear, even after the primary disease is cured. Because many manifestations are dependent on the blood volume status of the patient, symptoms may wax and wane. Usual clinical presentation to the consultant is refractory edema, often with ascites. The most striking single physical finding in these patients is jugular venous distension. A hypovolemic patient may have a paucity of other physical findings, but jugular venous distension is persistent.

Noninvasive Studies

Chest x-ray may reveal either a slightly enlarged or normal heart size and clear lung fields. Pericardial calcification suggests pericardial constriction, but it is not diagnostic. Electrocardiographic findings are nonspecific (3), but atrial fibrillation is often present. Careful blood pressure measurements may reveal pulsus paradoxus.

As imaging techniques become more advanced, increasingly accurate information can be obtained noninvasively. M-mode and two-dimensional echocardiography is useful to characterize the hemodynamic effects of constriction, but most findings have limited sensitivity and specificity. M-mode echocardiogram may reveal middle and late diastolic flattening of the posterior left ventricular wall (58) and early diastolic notching of the intraventricular septum (59), reflecting the abnormal filling pattern of the left ventricle secondary to restricted free wall motion (60). These abnormalities correlate well with the hemodynamics of restricted cardiac motion. Premature opening

of the pulmonic valve reflects increased right ventricular diastolic pressures (61). On two-dimensional echocardiography, strands of fibrin may be seen coursing from the visceral to the thickened parietal pericardium, suggestive of effusive-constrictive pericarditis. A dilated inferior vena cava without respiratory variation, in conjunction with a normal-sized right atrium and ventricle, supports the diagnosis of constriction. Doppler echocardiography has been shown to be sensitive in demonstrating the hemodynamic effects of constrictive pericarditis (62, 63). For example, in a study of 25 patients with constrictive pericarditis, confirmed at operation, a correct preoperative diagnosis was made in 22 or 88% (64). With expiration, patients demonstrated greater than 25% increase in early mitral flow velocity and increased diastolic flow reversal in the hepatic vein. CT scan and MRI probably offer better diagnostic sensitivity and specificity in detecting a thickened pericardium. CT and MRI may add information about tissue characterization, as well as disclose other mediastinal pathology that may aid diagnosis (14).

Clinical distinction between restrictive cardiomyopathy and constrictive pericarditis is a difficult problem (see Chapter 41). A number of noninvasive diagnostic studies proposed to differentiate constrictive from restrictive pericardial disease assess differences in left ventricular diastolic filling. These include digitized left ventriculograms, digitized M-mode echocardiography, and transesophageal and Doppler echocardiography. Recently, Gasperetti et al. described the use of dynamic hand exercise to develop maximal separation of left and right ventricular pressures at end diastole, thus aiding in differentiation of restrictive cardiomyopathy from constrictive pericardial disease (64). To date, none of these techniques has proved clearly superior in its ability to diagnose one or the other disease process consistently.

Several studies suggest that noninvasive pericardial imaging using CT or MRI can be useful (65–67). Vaitkus et al. reviewed the experience with CT scanning and MRI in differentiating constrictive from restrictive disease (65). In 30 patients studied, all patients with restrictive myocardial disease had a normal pericardium by either CT or MRI; in contrast, those with constrictive disease generally showed pericardial thickening. Data support MRI as the imaging modality of choice for differentiating constrictive pericarditis from restrictive cardiomyopathy (66). Invasive and noninvasive laboratory findings used to distinguish constriction or restriction are summarized in Table 42.2. In addition, patients with long-standing constrictive pericarditis may have myocardial dysfunction caused by the same process that produced pericardial disease or by myocardial atrophy. It has been suggested that the cross-sectional area change of the left ventricle during early diastole, measured by two-dimensional echocardiography, can help distinguish constrictive from restrictive disease (67), corroborating the earlier catheterization study of Tyberg et al. discussed later in this chapter (68). This method makes no correction for heart rate, is labor intensive and, therefore, not practical for routine clinical evaluation. Doppler analysis of mitral valve flow velocity has shown respiratory changes that differ between patients with constrictive pericarditis and restrictive cardiomyopathy, but the reliability of this technique in large numbers of patients has not been established (62).

Invasive Assessment

Catheterization, both left and right ventricle, is usually undertaken to (*a*) evaluate the hemodynamics of constrictive pericarditis to help differentiate it from myocardial disease, and (*b*) assess other problems (e.g., coronary artery disease (CAD), should surgery be required. None of the hemodynamic findings are specific. Certain patients may require volume infusion to elicit so-called "occult" constriction. The characteristic hemodynamic feature of constriction is elevated right atrial pressure associated

Table 42.2.
Laboratory Findings That May Help Differentiate Chronic Pericardial Constriction From Restrictive Cardiomyopathy

Test	Results Suggesting	
	Constriction	Restriction
Chest x-ray	Calcified pericardium	No calcium visible
Echocardiogram	Thickened pericardium; normal systolic wall motion; normal wall thickness	Normal pericardium; wall motion may be reduced; increased LV wall thickening
Computed tomography scan	Thickened pericardium, calcified pericardium	Normal pericardium
Magnetic resonance imaging	Thickened pericardium	Normal pericardium with uniform signal intensity; wall may be thickened
Catheter laboratory: right and left ventricular catheterization	Equilibration of RV and LV diastolic pressures "square root" sign	LVEDP may be > RVEDP
Coronary angiography	Diastolic compression of coronary arteries; coronary artery "crinkling"; increased space between coronary arteries and cardiac silhouette	Normal coronary arteries and normal relationship to epicardial silhouette
Endomyocardial biopsy	Normal	Fibrosis, amyloid, etc.

LV, left ventricular; RV, right ventricular; LVEDP, left ventricular end-diastolic pressure; RVEDP, right ventricular end-diastolic pressure.

with a prominent *y* descent. This finding helps to differentiate constriction, in which limitation to diastolic filling of the ventricle is not present in early diastole (prominent *y* descent), from tamponade, in which limitation occurs in all phases of diastolic filling. Near equalization of right and left ventricular filling pressures is usually recorded from the right atrial and pulmonary artery occlusive pressures. The characteristic "dip and plateau" diastolic filling pressure tracing ("square root sign") may be present (see Fig. 42.8). The "dip" is caused by emptying of the right atrium across a normal tricuspid valve without impaired filling of the ventricle in early diastole. The "plateau" is caused by a rapid rise in right ventricular diastolic pressure, as filling is restricted by the constricting pericardium. Right ventricular diastolic pressure is elevated and systolic pressure is normal to low. Pulmonary hypertension is said not to occur in pure constrictive pericarditis. Wise and Conti demonstrated that a pulmonary artery systolic pressure to right atrial pressure ratio of less than 3.5 correctly differentiated patients with constrictive pericarditis from those with cardiomyopathy (69).

Angiography is an important part of the catheterization procedure. The right atriogram may show straightening of the right atrial border; this is suggestive of constriction. Quantitative analysis of left ventricular angiograms shows that rapid ventricular filling occurs throughout the first half of diastole in patients with constriction (68). In contrast, in restrictive cardiomyopathy, ventricular filling occurs only early in diastole and then slows. Digitized analysis of the left ventricular angiogram is now available in many clinical cardiac catheterization laboratories for this diagnostic test. Coronary angiography is warranted in all patients. An increased distance between the coronary arteries and the cardiac silhouette may confirm the presence of a thick pericardium. A coronary artery segment may be compressed in diastole (70, 71). Decreased crinkling of the coronary arteries has also been described. Identification of coronary artery compression by the pericardium and unsuspected atherosclerotic disease is particularly useful for subsequent operative management (70).

Sometimes, the combination of noninvasive testing, hemodynamic measurements, and angiography will fail to distinguish convincingly whether the process is pericardial or myocardial. Use of right or left ventricle endomyocardial biopsy may be helpful. Nonspecific fibrosis is often found but it does not reliably distinguish constrictive pericarditis from restrictive cardiomyopathy. Myocarditis is also a nonspecific finding, and it should not prevent further evaluation. Specific stains may reveal abnormalities, such as amyloidosis; however, finding of an entirely normal myocardium does not exclude either diagnosis. Unfortunately, in some cases, despite exhaustive evaluation, precise diagnosis may not be apparent prior to thoracotomy.

"Sero-effusive" constrictive pericarditis is a term applied to patients with hemodynamic abnormalities intermediate between constrictive pericarditis and cardiac tamponade. The problem arises when pericardial effusion causes increased intrapericardial pressure in patients with a thickened pericardium. Before removal of pericardial fluid, hemodynamic findings of tamponade predominate with pulsus paradoxes. After removal of fluid, however, right atrial pressure remains abnormally elevated and shows absence of respiratory variation and prominent *y* descent, findings consistent with constriction.

Data Interpretation and Decision Making

Most causes of important constriction can be identified using noninvasive studies and confirmed by cardiac catheterization. Surgery in patients who have occult constriction or who are relatively asymptomatic is usually delayed. **Catheterization may also reveal patients with previously unsuspected myocardial dysfunction or combinations of both constriction and myocardial disease who would be less likely to respond well to surgery.** Following removal of the pericardium, ventricular filling pressures frequently do not return to normal immediately and may take weeks or

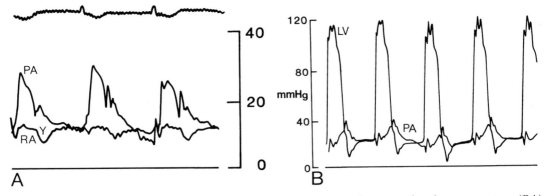

Figure 42.8. Hemodynamics of constrictive pericarditis. **A. Note the normal pulmonary artery** (*PA*) pressure with elevation of the right atrial (*RA*) pressure with a prominent *y* descent. **B. Simultaneous, left ventricular** (*LV*) and pulmonary arterial pressure tracings demonstrating the square root sign ventricular filling pattern.

even months to trend downward. Thus, postoperatively a patient may require diuretics and inotropic support. These observations support the suggestion that some residual myocardial dysfunction is often present with pericardial constriction.

CONGENITAL OR ACQUIRED COMPLETE OR PARTIAL ABSENCE OF THE PERICARDIUM

Congenital defects of the pericardium are not infrequent and they usually are diagnosed at autopsy. Complete absence of the pericardium, an uncommon problem, is characterized on chest x-ray by leftward shift of the cardiac silhouette and a "Snoopy" dog appearance. About 20% of patients with pericardial defects have associated cardiovascular congenital anomalies, including patent ductus arteriosus (67), atrial septal defect (72), mitral stenosis (73), and tetralogy of Fallot (74).

Echocardiography reveals abnormal septal motion, presumably caused by the unrestrained heart (75, 76), increased motion of the posterior wall, and right ventricular enlargement. The pericardial defect is not visualized. CT scanning and MRI are most sensitive in detecting pericardium absence. At cardiac catheterization, no resting

hemodynamic abnormalities are usually found in cases with isolated pericardial absence. Case reports exist of atrial entrapment or compression of coronary arteries; sudden death has occurred in patients with partial absence of pericardium because of strangulation of cardiac structure or compression of the coronary arteries (3, 4). When the pericardium is removed completely to relieve symptoms of partial absence, the patient experiences little residual effect. Surgical removal of the pericardium is usually not associated with any residual problems.

References

1. Hinds, SW, Reisner SA, Amico AF, et al. Diagnosis of pericardial abnormalities by 2D-echo: a pathology-echocardiography correlation in 85 patients. Am Heart J 1992;123(1):143–150.
2. Hoit BD. Imaging the pericardium. Cardiol Clin 1990;8(4):587–600.
3. Fowler NO. The pericardium in health and disease. Mount Kisco, NY: Futura, 1985.
4. Shabetai R. The pericardium. New York: Grune and Stratton, 1981.
5. Sadler RW. Langman's medical embryology. 5th ed. Baltimore: Williams & Wilkins, 1985.
6. Holt JP. The normal pericardium. Am J Cardiol 1970;26:455–465.
7. Maisch B. Myocarditis and pericarditis—old questions and new answers. Herz (Munchen) 1992; 17(2):65–70.
8. Goss CM, ed. Gray's anatomy. 29th ed. Philadelphia: Lea and Febiger, 1973.

9. Horowitz MS, Schultz CS, Clifford S, et al. Sensitivity and specificity of echocardiographic diagnosis of pericardial effusion. Circulation 1974;50: 239–247.

10. Callahan JA, Seward JB, Nishimura RA, et al. Two-dimensional echocardiographically guided pericardiocentesis: experience in 117 consecutive patients. Am J Cardiol 1985;55:476–479.

11. Yousem D, Traill TT, Wheeler PS, et al. Illustrative cases in pericardial effusion misdetection: correlation of echocardiography on CT. Cardiovasc Intervent Radiol 1987;10:162–167.

12. Ansari A, Rholl AO. Pseudopericardial effusions: echocardiographic and computed tomographic correlations. Clin Cardiol 1986;9:551–555.

13. Sechtem U, Tscholakoff D, Higgins CB. MRI of the normal pericardium. AJR 1986;147:239–244.

14. Sechtem U, Tscholakoff D, Higgins CB. MRI of the abnormal pericardium. AJR 1986;147:245–252.

15. Miller, Stephen W. Imaging pericardial disease. Cardiopulmonary imaging. Radiol Clin North Am 1989;27(6):1113–1125.

16. Wiener HG, Kristensen IB, Haubek A, et al. The diagnostic value of pericardial cytology—an analysis of 95 cases. ACTA Cytol 1991;35:149–153.

17. Daley JR, Seward JB, Bailey KR, et al. Malignant pericardial effusion: survival based upon pericardial fluid cytology [Abstract]. J Am Coll Cardiol 1992;19:266A.

18. Koh KK, Kim EJ, Cho CH, et al. Adenosine deaminase and carcinoembryonic antigen in pericardial effusion diagnosis, especially in suspected tuberculosis pericarditis. Circulation 1994;89:2728–2735.

19. Heidenreich PA, Eisenberg MJ, Kee LL, et al. Pericardial effusion in AIDS: incidence and survival. Circulation 1995;92:3229–3234.

20. Flum DR, McGinn JT, Tyras DH. The role of the pericardial window in AIDS. Chest 1995;107: 1522–1525.

21. Hageman JH, Esposo ND, Glenn WW. Tuberculosis of the pericardium, along ROM analysis of forty-four proved cases. N Engl J Med 1964;270: 327–332.

22. Schepers GW. Tuberculous pericarditis. Am J Cardiol 1962;9:248–276.

23. Little AG, Ferguson MK. Pericardioscopy as an adjunct to pericardial window. Chest 1986;89:53–55.

24. Wong KKS. Use of a flexible choledochoscope for pericardioscopy and drainage of a loculated pericardial effusion. Thorax 1986;42:637–638.

25. Kondos GT, Rich S, Levitsky S. Flexible fiberoptic pericardioscopy for the diagnosis of pericardial disease. J Am Coll Cardiol 1986;7:432–434.

26. Fowler NO, Harbin AD. Recurrent acute pericarditis: follow-up study of 31 patients. J Am Coll Cardiol 1986;7:300–305.

27. Rutsky EA, Rostand SG. Treatment of uremic pericarditis and pericardial effusion. Am J Kidney Dis 1987;10:2–8.

28. Sheppard FA, Morgan C, Evans WK, et al. Medical management of malignant pericardial effusion by tetracycline sclerosis. Am J Cardiol 1987;60: 1161–1166.

29. Patel AK, Kosolcharoen PD, Nallasivan M, et al. Catheter drainage of the pericardium. Chest 1987; 92:1018–1021.

30. Campbell PT, Van Trigt P, Wall TC, et al. Subxiphoid pericardiotomy in the diagnosis and management of large pericardial effusions associated with malignancy. Chest 1992;101(4):938–943.

31. Ziskind AA, Pearce AC, Lemmon MSN, et al. Percutaneous balloon pericardiotomy for the treatment of cardiac tamponade and large pericardial effusions: description of technique and report of the first 50 cases. J Am Coll Cardiol 1993;21(1):1–5.

32. Metcalfe J, Woodbury JW, Richards V, et al. Studies in experimental pericardial tamponade. Circulation 1952;5:518–523.

33. Guberman B, Fowler N, Engle P, et al. Cardiac tamponade in medical patients. Circulation 1981;64: 633–640.

34. Curtiss EI, Sudhakar R, Uretsky B, et al. Pulsus paradoxus: definition and relation to the severity of cardiac tamponade. Am Heart J 1988;115: 391–398.

35. Hancock EW. Neoplastic pericardial disease. Cardiol Clin 1990;8(4):673–682.

36. Wayne VS, Bishop RL, Spodick DL. Dynamic effects of pericardial effusion without tamponade. Br Heart J 1983;51:202–204.

37. Feigenbaum H, Zaky A, Waldhunsen JA. Use of ultrasound in the diagnosis of pericardial effusion. Ann Intern Med 1966;65:443–452.

38. Nanda NC, Gramick R, Gross CM. Echocardiography of cardiac valves in pericardial effusion. Circulation 1946;54:500–504.

39. Schiller NB, Botvinick E. Right ventricular compression as a sign of cardiac tamponade: an analysis of echocardiographic ventricular dimensions and their clinical implications. Circulation 1977;56:774–779.

40. Armstrong WF, Shilt BF, Helper D, et al. Diastolic collapse of the right ventricle with tamponade: an echocardiographic study. Circulation 1982;65: 1491–1496.

41. Gillan LD, Guyer D, Gibson TC, et al. Hydrodynamic compression of the right atrium: a new echocardiographic sign of cardiac tamponade. Circulation 1983;68:292–301.

42. Kronzon I, Cohen ML, Winer HE. Diastolic atrial compression: a sensitive echocardiographic sign of cardiac tamponade. J Am Coll Cardiol 1983;2: 770–775.

43. Chandrarana PA. Echocardiography and Doppler ultrasound in the evaluation of pericardial disease. Circulation 1991;84(3):1303–1310.

44. Appleton CP, Hatle LK, Popp RL. Demonstration of restrictive physiology by Doppler echocardiography. J Am Coll Cardiol 1988;11:757–768.

45. Leeman DE, Levine MJ, Come PC. Doppler echocardiography in cardiac tamponade: exaggerated respiratory variation in transvalvular blood flow velocity integrade. J Am Coll Cardiol 1988;11: 572–578.

46. Himelman RB, Kircher B, Rockey DC, et al. Inferior vena cava plethora with blunted respiratory response: a sensitive echocardiographic sign of cardiac tamponade. J Am Coll Cardiol 1988;12: 1470–1477.

47. Levine MJ, Lorell BH, Diver DJ, et al. Implications of echocardiographically assisted diagnosis of pericardial tamponade in contemporary medical pa-

tients: detection before hemodynamic embarrassment. J Am Coll Cardiol 1991;17:59–65.

48. O'Rourke RA, Fischer DP, Escobar EE, et al. Effect of acute pericardial tamponade on coronary blood flow. Am J Physiol 1967;212:549–552.

49. Naunheim KS, Kesler KA, Fiore AC, et al. Pericardial drainage: subxiphoid vs. transthoracic approach. Eur J Cardiothorac Surg 1991;5(2):99–103.

50. Piehler JM, Pluth JR, Schaff HV, et al. Surgical management of effusive pericardial disease. J Thorac Cardiovasc Surg 1985;90:506–516.

51. Jansen EW, Vincent JG, Fost JA, et al. Treatment of pericardial fluid. J Thorac Cardiovasc Surg 1986; 91:795–796.

52. Sagrista-Sauleda J, Permanyer-Miralda G, Soler-Soler J. Tuberculous pericarditis: ten year experience with a prospective protocol for diagnosis and treatment. J Am Coll Cardiol 1988;11:724–728.

53. Thadani U, Iveson J, Wright V. Cardiac tamponade, constrictive pericarditis and pericardial resection in rheumatoid arthritis. Medicine 1975;54: 261–270.

54. Roberts W, Spray T. Pericardial heart disease: a study of its causes, consequences and morphologic features. In: Spodick DH, ed. Cardiovascular clinics. Philadelphia: FA Davis, 1976;7:11–65.

55. Kutcher MA, King SB, Alimuruna BN. Constrictive pericarditis as a complication of cardiac surgery: recognition of an entity. Am J Cardiol 1982;50: 742–748.

56. Cohen MV, Greenberg MA. Constrictive pericarditis: early and late complication of cardiac surgery. Am J Cardiol 1979;43:657–661.

57. Lurie K, Shultz J, Remole S, et al. Constrictive pericardial disease caused by epicardial implantable cardiac defibrillator patches: treatment by pericardial stripping and nonthoracotomy lead system implantation. Am Heart J 1994;128:623–625.

58. Pool PE, Seagren SC, Abassi AS, et al. Echocardiographic manifestations of constrictive pericarditis: abnormal septal motion. Chest 1975;68:684–688.

59. Voelkel AG, Pietro DA, Holland ED, et al. Echocardiographic features of constructive pericarditis. Circulation 1978;58:871–875.

60. Wann LS, Weyman AE, Dillon JC, et al. Premature pulmonary valve opening. Circulation 1977;55: 128–133.

61. Lewis BS. Echocardiography in constrictive pericarditis—another test or diagnostic advance? Journal of Interventional Cardiology 1983;2:532–536.

62. Hatle LK, Appleton CP, Popp RL. Differentiation of constrictive pericarditis and restrictive cardio-

myopathy by Doppler echocardiography. Circulation 1989;79:357–370.

63. Oh JK, Hatle LK, Seward JB, et al. Diagnostic role of Doppler echocardiography in constrictive pericarditis. J Am Coll Cardiol 1994;23:154–162.

64. Gasperetti CM, Sarembock IJ, Feldman MD. Usefulness of dynamic hand exercise for developing maximal separation of left and right ventricular pressures at end-diastole and usefulness in distinguishing restrictive cardiomyopathy from constrictive pericardial disease. Am J Cardiol 1992; 69(17):1508–1511.

65. Vaitkus PT, Kussmaul WG. Constrictive pericarditis versus restrictive cardiomyopathy: a reappraisal and update of diagnostic criteria. Am Heart J 1991;122:1431–1441.

66. Soulen RL. Magnetic resonance imaging of great vessel, myocardial and pericardial disease. Circulation 1991;84(3):1311–1321.

67. Pandian NG, Skorton D, Kieso RA, et al. Diagnosis of constrictive pericarditis by two-dimensional echocardiography: studies in a new experimental model and in patients. J Am Coll Cardiol 1984;4: 1164–1173.

68. Tyberg TI, Goodyer AV, Hurst V, et al. Left ventricular filling in differentiating restrictive amyloid cardiomyopathy and constrictive pericarditis. Am J Cardiol 1981;47:791–796.

69. Wise DE, Conti CR. Constrictive pericarditis. In: Spodick DH, ed. Cardiovascular clinics: pericardial diseases. Philadelphia: FA Davis, 1976;7:197–210.

70. Miller JE, Mansour KA, Hitcher CR. Pericardectomy: current indications, concepts and results in a university center. Ann Thorac Surg 1982;34:40–45.

71. Goldberg E, Stein J, Berger M, et al. Diastolic segmental coronary artery obliteration in constrictive pericarditis. Cathet Cardiovasc Diagn 1981;7: 197–202.

72. Broadbeat JD, Callahan JA, Kincaid OW. Congenital deficiency pericardium. Chest 1966;50:237–241.

73. Fischer JD, Ehrenhaft JL. Congenital pericardial defect. JAMA 1964;133:78–81.

74. Hippona FA, Coumary AB. Congenital pericardial defect associated with tetralogy of Fallot. Circulation 1964;29:132–135.

75. Payvandi MN, Kerber RE. Echocardiography in congenital and acquired absence of the pericardium. Circulation 1976;53:86–92.

76. Ruys F, Paulus W, Stevens C, et al. Expansion of the left atrial appendage is a distinctive cross-sectional echocardiographic feature of congenital defect of the pericardium. Eur Heart J 1983;4:738–741.

43

The Adult with Congenital Heart Disease

F. Jay Fricker, MD

INTRODUCTION

The incidence of congenital heart disease is 8 per 1000 live births. Given the current number of live births in the United States, we would anticipate that nearly 30,000 infants are born yearly with some type of structural congenital heart defect. These defects range from small ventricular septal defects or mild valvular stenosis to lethal forms of congenital heart disease. The most serious forms of congenital heart disease presenting in the first few months of life are the focus of pediatric cardiologists and cardiovascular surgeons. Advancement of surgical techniques have made it possible to repair or palliate nearly all of these infants in the first year of life, resulting in their survival into adolescence and adulthood. **Nearly 85% of infants with congenital heart disease survive to reach adulthood** resulting in nearly one half million adults with congenital heart disease, and this population is growing at 5% per year (1). It has been the prerogative of the pediatric cardiologists to care for young adults because of their experience and interest in congenital heart disease. As this group of young adults with congenital heart disease increase in numbers, the adult cardiology community has developed an appropriate interest in being their primary continuity cardiology consultant.

The adult patient with known or sus-pected congenital heart disease has been the focus of innumerable reviews (1–5). The focus of this chapter is not to be all inclusive, but to review for the adult cardiologist an updated approach to the catheter-based diagnosis and management of the adult patient with known or suspected congenital heart disease.

SPECTRUM OF CONGENITAL HEART DISEASE PRESENTING IN THE ADULT PATIENT

The patient presenting with congenital heart disease usually has:

- Previously undiagnosed congenital heart disease
- Recognized congenital heart defect in childhood, but not repaired
- Adults with surgically repaired or palliated congenital heart defects

PREVIOUSLY UNDIAGNOSED CONGENITAL HEART DISEASE

Undiagnosed congenital heart disease in an adult patient will usually include those defects that have late onset of symptoms or subtle physical findings.

Atrial Septal Defect

The most common congenital heart defect that is diagnosed in an adolescent or adult is **an atrial septal defect.** The clinical findings are often subtle, and they include a soft systolic ejection murmur at the base, a widely split second heart sound, and a low-pitched early diastolic murmur at the low right sternal border. The diagnosis is supported on a chest x-ray with increased heart size involving all of the right heart chambers. Pulmonary vascularity is prominent. Occasionally, a significant atrial septal defect in an adult patient is associated with a normal chest x-ray. The electrocardiogram demonstrates right ventricular hypertrophy with an RSR' in the right precordial leads V_3R and V_1. Anatomically, the most common type of an atrial septal defect is a secundum defect located in the fossa ovalis. The less common defects are an ostium primum atrial septal defect, a sinus venosus defect (often associated with partial anomalous pulmonary venous return), and coronary sinus atrial septal defect. Detailed anatomic location and size can be demonstrated by transthoracic or transesophageal (TEE) echocardiography (Fig. 43.1). No indication is found for heart catheterization unless closure of the atrial septal defect by one of the currently available interventional devices is planned. It would be unusual for children or adolescents to have symptoms from an atrial left-to-right shunt, but adults may become symptomatic because the left-to-right atrial level shunt will increase if left ventricular dysfunction, caused by other generally acquired diseases such as hypertension or coronary artery disease, leads to elevation of left ventricular end-diastolic and left atrial pressure. Controversy exists in regard to the **size of the atrial septal defect** that should be surgically or interventionally closed. In our experience, when a left lower sternal border diastolic murmur and right ventricular hypertrophy are present on the electrocardiogram and the anatomic defect is identified on the echocardiogram, it is recommended to close the atrial septal defect to prevent late dysrhythmia, right ventricular dysfunction, and a paradoxical embolism (6, 7). Atrial septal defect repair in the

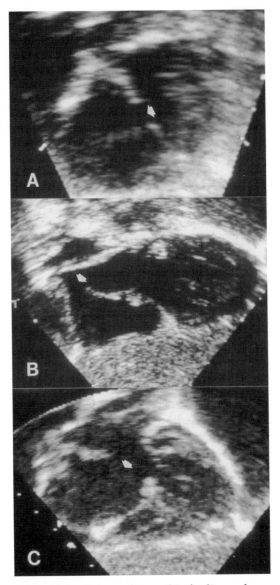

Figure 43.1. Echocardiographic findings of various atrial septal defects in the subcostal views. *Arrows* indicate the defects. **A.** Secundum type. **B.** Sinus venosus type. **C.** Ostium primum defect or partitioned atrioventricular septal defect.

adult has low morbidity and mortality (8). Late atrial flutter or fibrillation occurs in 7 to 10% of patients at follow-up (8). Spontaneous closure incidence in children is 3%, but it is rare in adults (9). Although an atrial septal defect is often present in children and young adults with pulmonary hypertension, we do not believe the left-to-right

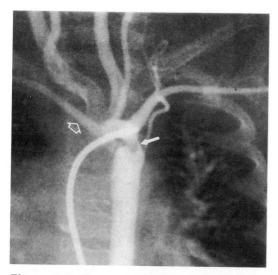

Figure 43.2. Coarctation of the aorta with aberrant subclavian artery. Selective aortogram in the anteroposterior view showing a discrete coarctation at the usual site (*arrow*) and aberrant subclavian artery (*open arrow*).

Although the clinical diagnosis can be made easily, imaging of the aortic arch and great vessels is essential for appropriate intervention. Aortic root angiography is diagnostic (Fig. 43.2), but noninvasive imaging using magnetic resonance imaging (MRI) can give a detailed image of the whole aortic arch and great vessels if done properly (10) (Fig. 43.3). Repair of the native coarctation of the aorta is surgical, although balloon dilation of the coarctation in patients with restenosis is preferred (11) (Fig. 43.4). Postballoon dilation development of aortic aneurysms is reported in a series (12) of native coarctation balloon angioplasty. Late diagnosis and complications of the aorta include aneurysm of the ascending aorta caused by **cystic medial necrosis,** bacterial endocarditis and cerebral vascular accidents (berry aneurysms occur in approximately 4% of adults with coarctation of the aorta).

shunt from an atrial septal defect is a causal factor in the development of pulmonary vascular disease.

Coarctation of the Aorta

Coarctation of the aorta can be missed in childhood and present in adolescence or adulthood. Mechanical obstruction to the aorta should be suggested in any young adult who presents with systemic hypertension. The clinical diagnosis of coarctation of the aorta is easily made if clinically suggested by palpation of the femoral pulses and measurement of blood pressure in the right and left arms and a lower extremity. Other clinical manifestations are the result of **extensive collateral blood flow** around the area of the coarctation through intercostal and internal mammary arteries. Prominent systolic murmurs over the back and anterior precordium indicate this extensive collateralization. The association of a bileaflet aortic valve with coarctation of the aorta is frequent.

Patent Ductus Arteriosus

Patent ductus arteriosus (PDA) can also escape detection in childhood. The most im-

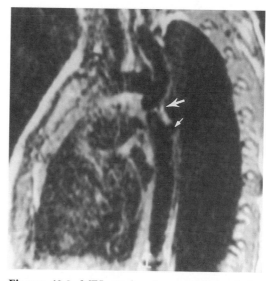

Figure 43.3. MRI study of coarctation of the aorta. This study shows a discrete narrowing (*large arrow*) in the descending aorta and a prominent collateral vessel (*small arrow*).

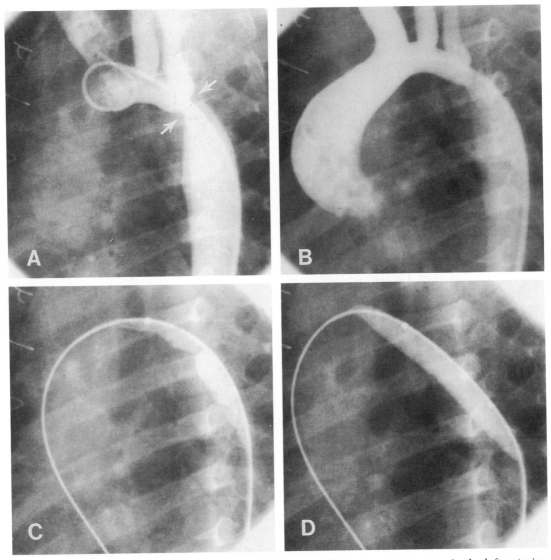

Figure 43.4. Balloon angioplasty for recurrent coarctation of the aorta. Aortogram in the left anterior oblique view of a patient who had undergone surgical repair of coarctation previously demonstrating a discrete narrowing (*arrows*) at the previous site of coarctation (**A**). Following balloon angioplasty, repeat aortogram demonstrating enlargement of the aortic lumen at the previous site of the narrowing (**B**). Significant balloon indentation is noted at the recurrent site of narrowing during initial balloon inflation (**C**) and the indentation was abolished with full balloon inflation (**D**).

portant clinical finding is a continuous murmur under the left clavicle, but this finding may be modified if pulmonary hypertension is present. The diagnosis of PDA can be made echocardiographically without heart catheterization. In the adult patient, aneurysms of the ductus arteriosus have been reported, which complicate surgical repair (13). The recommendation for closure of even a small patent ductus arteriosus is made because of the risk of infective endocarditis. Surgical ligation as well as coil embolization of the ductus has been recommended (14).

Corrected Transposition

Corrected transposition (atrioventricular discordance and ventriculoarterial discordance) if not associated with other structural anomalies can go undetected into adulthood. Associated ventricular septal defect, pulmonic subvalvar stenosis, left atrioventricular valve regurgitation, and heart block are all associated abnormalities. Catheterization approach and angiography have been described (15, 16).

CONGENITAL HEART DEFECTS IN ADULTS RECOGNIZED IN CHILDHOOD NOT REQUIRING SURGICAL INTERVENTION

Many adult patients with congenital heart disease have not required any intervention, but do require ongoing evaluation and assessment. Patients with mild to moderate aortic and pulmonary valvular disease as well as hemodynamically insignificant ventricular septal defects require periodic evaluation.

Aortic Pulmonary Valve Disease

The natural history of **aortic valvular disease** is one of progression, but pulmonary valve disease generally does not increase in severity even as the child grows into adolescence and adulthood. Catheterization for aortic or pulmonary valve stenosis is unnecessary unless balloon valvuloplasty is planned (see Chapters 25, 35, and 40). Balloon dilation of either the aortic or pulmonary valve in the adult patient is now recognized as a patient-preferred initial approach (see Chapter 35). Because of the physical size of an adult patient, often a two-balloon technique is necessary to adequately open up the pulmonary valve (Fig. 43.5).

Ventricular Septal Defect

The natural history of a small to moderate **ventricular septal defect** depends, in large part, on the location of that defect (see Chapter 23). For example, most defects in the perimembranous or muscular septum always decrease in size and many close spontaneously (17, 18). Occasionally, a perimembranous ventricular septal defect is associated with the gradual development of right ventricular outflow tract obstruction from hypertrophy of the moderator band of the right ventricle, creating a double chambered right ventricle with moderate to severe subpulmonic stenosis (19). Perimembranous defect closure can cause a **fibrous subaortic ridge,** which creates an obstruction in the left ventricular outflow tract (20). The subarterial ventricular septal defect, although small and hemodynamically not significant, can create distortion and prolapse of the right or noncoronary leaflet of the aortic valve, causing significant aortic valve regurgitation (Fig. 43.6). The recommendation is surgical closure of the subarterial ventricular septal defects to prevent this complication. In evaluation of patients with suspected or diagnosed small ventricular septal defects, echocardiography should be performed to assess the location of that ventricular septal defect because of this variability in natural history. Catheterization is usually not necessary.

ADULTS WITH SURGICALLY REPAIRED OR PALLIATED CONGENITAL HEART DISEASE

Patients with surgically repaired or palliated congenital heart disease comprise the most complicated group of young adolescents and adults the adult cardiologist encounters. Even congenital heart defects where we would anticipate a complete cure (e.g., atrial septal defect, ventricular septal defect, and coarctation of the aorta) can be complicated by late problems such as atrial dysrhythmias in an atrial septal defect and persistent hypertension or aortic aneurysm after repair of aorta coarctation.

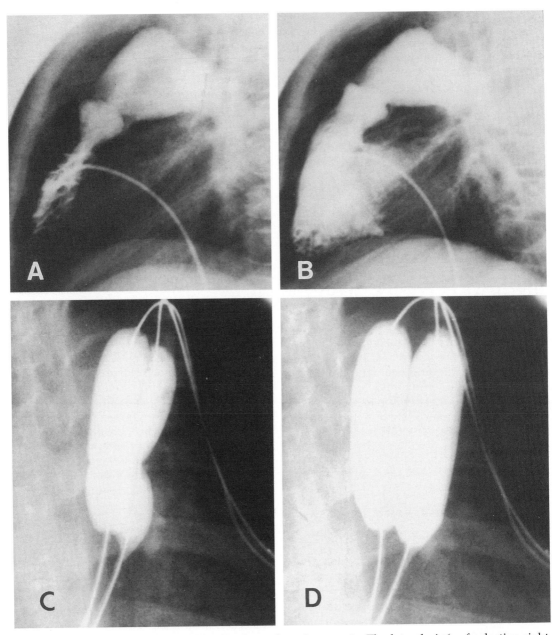

Figure 43.5. Balloon angioplasty for valvular pulmonic stenosis. The lateral view of selective right ventriculogram in a patient with severe valvular pulmonic stenosis showing a thickened and doming pulmonic valve with a narrow jet of contrast (**A**). Following the balloon valvuloplasty, repeat angiogram showing a widely open pulmonic valve orifice (**B**). Two balloons were across the pulmonic valve. Indentations are seen in both balloons at initial inflation (**C**) and abolished completely with further inflation (**D**).

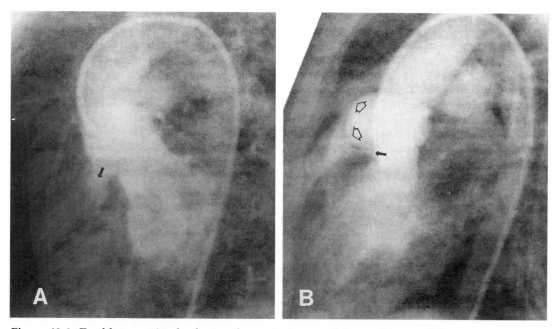

Figure 43.6. Doubly committed subarterial ventricular septal defect. Selective left ventriculogram in the left anterior oblique view showing a subarterial defect (*arrow*) (**A**). Repeat selective angiogram in the same patient in the lateral view showing a narrow jet of the septal defect (*solid arrow*) and marked herniation of the right aortic sinus (*open arrows*) (**B**).

In addition, several complex congenital abnormalities deserve special comments because of their frequency of occurrence and specific problems that the adult cardiologist is likely to encounter in late follow-up.

Tetralogy of Fallot

Tetralogy of Fallot is the most common cyanotic congenital heart malformation. Anatomically it consists of a large malalignment ventricular septal defect and variable degrees of valvular, subvalvar, and branch pulmonary artery stenosis. Surgical repair success depends on the size and arborization pattern of the pulmonary arteries, size of the pulmonary valve annulus, and the presence or absence of associated coronary artery abnormalities (left anterior descending coronary artery from the right coronary artery). Repair of tetralogy of Fallot occurs from infancy to the adult. In some centers palliation with systemic-to-pulmonary artery shunt (e.g., modified H-type shunt for

classic Blalock-Taussig shunt is done for severe right ventricular outflow tract obstruction or hypoxemic spells). Surgical approach for tetralogy of Fallot includes closure of the ventricular septal defect and complete relief of the right ventricular outflow tract obstruction even at the expense of leaving significant pulmonary valve regurgitation. Long-term problems after repair of tetralogy of Fallot include residual right ventricular outflow obstruction and variable degrees of pulmonary valve regurgitation, which cause right ventricular dilation and ventricular dysrhythmias (21). Young adults with **poor hemodynamic result** (i.e., residual right ventricular hypertension or severe pulmonary valve regurgitation) are at high risk for ventricular tachycardia. **Ventricular tachycardia** or bifibrillation is the cause of sudden death in this patient group. The recommendation has been to improve hemodynamic results by relieving right ventricular outflow tract obstruction or replacing the pulmonary valve.

Hemodynamic and angiographic assessment can be helpful in making decisions regarding either pulmonary valve replacement or repeat surgery to relieve right ventricular outflow tract obstruction. In general, right ventricular catheterization with a right ventriculogram in AP projection with cranial angulation and a lateral projection provides sufficient information regarding pulmonary artery anatomy and the site of residual right ventricular outflow tract obstruction. A second injection in the pulmonary artery can angiographically quantitate the degree of pulmonary valve regurgitation. A provocative electrophysiologic study with an intent to induce ventricular tachycardia helps evaluate the potential for ventricular tachycardia and also assess efficacy of antiarrhythmic therapy. A number of authors have addressed treatment of the associated ventricular arrhythmias (22, 23). In patients with tetralogy of Fallot and pulmonary atresia, initial palliation is always done with a systemic-to-pulmonary artery shunt using a modified H-type or classic Blalock-Taussig shunt. Definitive repair is done by closing the ventricular septal defect and placing a homograft conduit between the right ventricle and the pulmonary artery. This **homograft conduit** has a tissue valve, and it is subject to the calcification and degenerative process that has occurred universally in these valves regardless of their preparation.

Transposition of the Great Arteries

In no other congenital heart defect has surgery revolutionized both the early morbidity and long-term outlook than in patients with transposition of the great arteries. Once the technique of coronary artery transfer was mastered, the arterial switch procedure became a reality (24). If coronary artery transfer is successful, the residual problem of supravalvular pulmonary artery stenosis is minimal compared with long-term problems of the Senning or Mustard atrial switch procedures. The initial successful atrial switch procedure was accomplished in the mid-1960s, and now adult patients exist who have survived 30 years since this palliative surgery. The early problems associated with the Mustard and Senning procedures were related to baffle placement and the development of significant systemic and pulmonary venous obstruction (25, 26). If these problems are successfully navigated, late problems can occur with right ventricular (systemic ventricular) dysfunction, tricuspid regurgitation, and conduction systemic disease, including sinus node and AV node dysfunction. **Sinus bradycardia and recurrent supraventricular tachycardia and atrial flutter are common** problems following both atrial switch procedures. Significant right ventricular dysfunction and tricuspid regurgitation are generally dealt with initially by medical management with digoxin and systemic vasodilator therapy. If medical management is not successful, then the surgical options, include transplantation or a complicated attempt at an arterial switch procedure by conditioning the left ventricle to handle systemic afterload. The bradycardia or tachycardia syndrome is managed by a pacemaker with the addition of amiodarone or sotalol as potent antiarrhythmic agents.

If a hemodynamic assessment is required in a patient following a Senning or Mustard procedure, knowledge of the atrial anatomy is essential because the catheter course is modified substantially. If the approach is from the right femoral vein, the catheter course to the superior vena cava needs to be in front of the pulmonary venous atrium into the superior vena cava. The catheter course to the left ventricle and pulmonary artery can be facilitated by a balloon flow directed catheter. If it is necessary to enter the pulmonary venous atrium, a catheter can be passed across the aortic valve and in retrograde fashion from the right ventricle through the tricuspid valve into the pulmonary venous atrium.

In patients with both transposition of the great arteries and a ventricular septal defect, the preferred surgical approach is a Rastelli procedure. This consists of closing the ventricular septal defect by tunneling the left ventricular outflow tract to the aorta. The reconstructed right ventricular outflow tract will be created by a homograft conduit from the right ventricle into the pulmonary artery. Long-term hemodynamic problems associated with this repair would be sub-aortic stenosis because of the tunnel created using the ventricular septal defect patch. In addition, homograft degeneration associated with tissue conduits would be applicable to this situation.

Tricuspid Atresia and Single Ventricle

In 1971, Fontan et al. (27) described a technique for palliation of patients with tricuspid atresia. This technique has now been applied to the treatment of most forms of functional single ventricle. The operation results in separation of systemic pulmonary and venous return by directing systemic venous return into the pulmonary artery without passing through a ventricle. The advantages of this palliative procedure is that it reduces volume overload from the single ventricle and improves systemic oxygenation. A large group of young adults who have been palliated with variations of the Fontan procedure have now reached adulthood. Successful Fontan surgery was once predicated on following the "Ten Commandments of the Fontan Procedure" (28), which are:

1. Pulmonary valve resistance less than 4 U/m^2
2. Pulmonary artery mean pressure less than 15 mm Hg
3. Normal left ventricular function
4. Aged more than 40 years
5. Normal interventricular valve without regurgitation
6. Normal sinus rhythm
7. Normal right atrial size and volume
8. Normal branch pulmonary arteries
9. Normal caval and pulmonary venous return
10. A ratio between the pulmonary artery and aorta diameter greater than 0.75.

These rules have been violated subsequently with successful outcome. Indeed, numerous surgical modifications have been made to the Fontan procedure, but the current one involves anastomosis of the superior vena cava to the pulmonary artery, creating what is termed a "bidirectional cavopulmonary" shunt. Subsequently, the inferior and hepatic venous return is tunneled through the right atrium and the flow-directed **offset anastomosis** is made into the left pulmonary artery (Fig. 43.7).

A detailed analysis of the Mayo Clinic experience with Fontan surgery was reported by Driscoll et al. (29). Long-term survival of these patients is nearly 60%. The factors that have impacted on survival were **diagnosis** other than tricuspid atresia, right atrial isomerism syndromes, early age of operation, increased pulmonary artery pressure, and atrioventricular valve dysfunction. The major problems in the Fontan palliated patient relates to arrhythmias requiring antiarrhythmic medication or pacemaker implantation and complications of high right atrial pressure. The most serious is protein-losing enteropathy and hypoproteinemia. Patients who have had a good hemodynamic result following Fontan surgery often have limited exercise tolerance when compared with their peer group. Other problems include thromboembolic disease and cholestatic liver disease. Current speculation is that a large percentage of patients palliated with Fontan surgery will eventually require orthotopic heart transplantation.

Congenital Heart Disease Associated with Pulmonary Vascular Disease

A significant population remains of adult patients who have pulmonary vascular disease associated with their congenital heart defect. These patients either have had surgical palliation or were inoperable at the time of their initial diagnosis. Progression of pulmonary vascular disease and symptoms related to decreased pulmonary blood flow are variable. Their congenital heart defects are often complicated by symptoms of hyperviscocity (e.g., headaches, extremity pain, and coagulopathy). In addition, bacterial endocarditis and brain abscess can have catastrophic complications. The only option available to this group of patients is lung

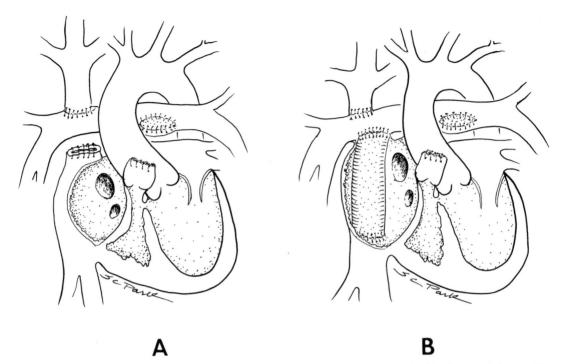

A   **B**

Figure 43.7. A. Bidirectional Glenn anastomosis: The superior vena cava is divided and the cardiac side is oversewn. The cephalic portion of the superior vena cava is sewn to the right pulmonary artery. The main pulmonary artery trunk is divided and the proximal part is oversewn. The distal portion of the pulmonary artery trunk is repaired with a pericardial patch (*dotted*). **B**. Modified Fontan procedure: A lateral baffle is created to direct the inferior vena caval blood flow into the pulmonary artery.

transplantation with repair of their congenital heart defect or heart and lung transplantation.

GENERAL MANAGEMENT OF THE ADULT WITH CONGENITAL HEART DISEASE

It is beyond the scope of this chapter to discuss all the general management problems associated with adults with congenital heart disease. Problems exist that society imposes on this group of patients, and they find it difficult to find employment and obtain life insurance. Even patients with excellent exercise tolerance frequently encounter difficulty obtaining gainful employment because potential employers are reluctant to hire them (fearing their health insurance rates will be high and sick days will be many). These patients need to attain marketable skills to compete in the current employment market. Insurance companies are now reviewing patients with congenital heart disease in regard to their specific lesion and success of their surgical repair. This may not be as much of a critical issue for an adult with congenital heart disease in the future.

Most patients with congenital heart disease can tolerate pregnancy with the one absolute contraindication—advanced pulmonary vascular disease. One of the questions the adult with congenital heart disease frequently asks the physician is what is the risk of congenital heart disease recurring in any offspring. Studies by Whittemore et al. (30) have estimated that the risk of congenital heart defect in the fetus if either parent has congenital heart disease is approximately 10 to 15%.

SUMMARY

In summary, individuals with congenital heart disease are now surviving to adulthood and present special problems for the physicians caring for this group of patients. Care of these patients is complex and should be delivered by a team that includes both adult and pediatric cardiologists, internists, and social workers familiar with the special needs of this group of patients.

Acknowledgment

We thank Sang C. Park, MD, Children's Hospital of Pittsburgh, Division of Pediatric Cardiology, for the illustrations used in this chapter.

References

1. Perloff JK. Longevity in congenital heart disease: A tribute to pediatric cardiology. J Pediatr 1993; 122:549–557.
2. Deanfield JK. Adult congenital heart disease with special reference to the data on long term follow up of patients surviving to adulthood with or without surgical correction. Eur Heart J 1992;13(Suppl II): 111–116.
3. Moller JH, Anderson RC. 1,000 consecutive children with a cardiac malformation with 26 to 37 year follow up. Am J Cardiol 1992;70:661–667.
4. Perloff JK, Child JS, eds. Congenital heart disease in adults. Philadelphia: WB Saunders, 1991.
5. Moodie DS. Adult congenital heart disease. Curr Opin Cardiol 1994;9:137–142.
6. Van Camp G, Schulze D, Cosyns B, et al. Relation between patent foramen ovale and unexplained stroke. Am J Cardiol 1993;71:596–598.
7. Conti CR. Embolic stroke: are we missing the source in many young patients. Clin Cardiol 1993;16:83–84.
8. Horvath KA, Burke RP, Collins JJ, et al. Surgical treatment of adult atrial septal defect: early and long term results. J Am Coll Cardiol 1993;20: 1156–1159.
9. Campbell M. Natural history of atrial septal defect. Br Heart J 1970;32:820–823.
10. Kaemmerer H, Theissen P, Konig U, et al. Follow up using magnetic resonance imaging in adult patients after surgery for aortic coarctation. Thorac Cardiovasc Surg 1993;41:107–111.
11. Wexler L, Higgins CB. The use of magnetic resonance imaging in the adult with congenital heart disease. Am J Card Imaging 1995;9(1):15–28.
12. Lock JE, Bass JL, Amplantz K, et al. Balloon dilatation angioplasty of coarctations in infants and children. Circulation 1983;68:109–116.
13. Coard KC, Martin MP. Ruptured saccular pulmonary artery aneurysm associated with persistent ductus arteriosus. Arch Path Lab Med 1992;116(2): 159–161.
14. Schenck MH, O'Laughlin, MP, Rokey R, et al Transcatheter occlusion of patent ductus arteriosus in adults. Am J Cardiol 1993;72:591–595.
15. Attie F, Soni J, Seyevitz OV, et al. Angiographic studies of atrioventricular discordance. Circulation 1980;62:407–415.
16. Beerman LB. In: Neches WH, Park SC, Zuberbuhler JR, eds. Perspectives in pediatric cardiology of the great arteries. Mt. Kisco, New York: Futura, 1991.
17. Bloomfield DK. The natural history of ventricular septal defect in patients surviving infancy. Circulation 1964;29:914–955.
18. Beeman LB, Park SC, Fischer DR, et al. Ventricular septal defect associated with aneurysm of the membranous septum. J Am Coll Cardiol 1985;5: 118–123.
19. Rowland TW, Rosentahl A, Castaneda AR. Double-chamber right ventricle: experiences with 17 cases. Am Heart J 1975;89:455–462.
20. Anderson RH, Lenox CC, Zuberbuhler JR. Mechanisms of closure of perimembranous ventricular septal defect. Am J Cardiol 1983;52:341–345.
21. Murphy JG, Gerish BJ, Mair DD, et al. Long term outcome in patients undergoing surgical repair of tetralogy of Fallot. N Engl J Med 1993;329:593–599.
22. Deanfield JE, McKenna WJ, Hallidie-Smith KA. Detection of late arrhythmia and conduction disturbances after correction of tetralogy of Fallot. Br Heart J 1980;44:248–253.
23. Garson A, Porter CJ, Gillette PC, et al. Induction of ventricular tachycardia during electrophysiologic study after repair of tetralogy of Fallot. J Am Coll Cardiol 1983;1:1493–1502.
24. Jatene AD, Fontes VF, Paulista PP, et al. Anatomic correction of transposition of the great vessels. J Thorac Cardiovasc Surg 1976;72:364–376.
25. Senning A. Surgical correction of transposition of the great vessels. Surgery 1959;45:966–980.
26. Mustard WT. Successful two stage correction of transposition of the great vessels. Surgery 1964;55: 469–472.
27. Fontan F, Mounicot FB, Baudet E, et al. "Correction" de l'atresie tricuspidienne: rapport de deux cas "corriges" par l'utilisation d'une technique chirurgicale nouvelle. Ann Chir Thorac Cardiovasc 1971;10:39–47.
28. Fontan F, Kirklin, JW, Fernandes G, et al. Outcome after a "perfect" Fontan operation. Circulation 1990;81:1520–1536.
29. Driscoll DJ, Offord KP, Feldt RH, et al. Five to fifteen year follow up after Fontan operation. Circulation 1992;85:469–496.
30. Whittemore R, Hobbins JC, Engle MA. Pregnancy and its outcome in women with and without surgical treatment of congenital heart disease. Am J Card 50:641–651.

44

The Patient with Known or Suspected Disease of the Aorta

Tomas D. Martin, MD
Carl J. Pepine, MD
James A. Hill, MD
Charles R. Lambert, MD, PhD

INTRODUCTION

Patients with known or suspected disease of the aorta in many cases require aortography and often cardiac catheterization studies for optimal management. In this chapter, we review the anatomic and pathophysiologic consequences of these diseases. We integrate information obtained at the bedside with that obtained from the noninvasive laboratory, so that data obtained at the time of catheterization may be more effectively used. A variety of invasive and noninvasive techniques have been used to facilitate the diagnosis of aortic disease, but the standard by which all other diagnostic modalities have been measured has been contrast aortography. Cardiac catheterization with contrast aortography provides clear multiplane visualization of the heart and aorta and all of its branches, and allows assessment of the pathophysiologic consequences of aortic disease (see Chapter 20). Even in the recent past, prior to surgical intervention, all patients with known or suspected disease of the aorta required catheter assessment with contrast aortography whenever possible. **Newer noninvasive tech-** niques, such as transthoracic and, in particular, transesophageal (TEE) echocardiography, high-resolution computed tomography (CT), cine-CT, and, more recently, magnetic resonance imaging (MRI) with its cine and three-dimensional capabilities, have made contrast aortography necessary in only selected cases.**

Diseases of the aorta can be either congenital or acquired. Each of these can be subdivided into several more specific groups. In the congenital category, major abnormalities include coarctation of the aorta, interrupted aortic arch, and supra-valvular aortic stenosis. Acquired diseases of the aorta include four major types: traumatic, aneurysmal (degenerative, atherosclerotic, inflammatory, and mycotic), dissection, and occlusive. **Occlusive disease of the aorta is primarily that of aortoiliac disease.** This spectrum of aortic disease generally falls under the category of peripheral vascular disease and, therefore, will not be discussed in this chapter. Marfan's syndrome will be discussed separately, as it is an inheritable disorder associated with extensive cardiac and aortic manifestations.

CONGENITAL ANOMALIES

Coarctation

Natural History and Pathophysiology

Coarctation of the aorta, defined as a localized narrowing of the aorta usually secondary to a localized thickening of the aortic wall, comprises 5 to 8% of all congenital cardiac anomalies (1, 2). Coarctation most commonly occurs in the preductal or postductal area (Fig. 44.1); however, it has been found in all areas of the aorta, including the abdomen. Pathologically, an abnormal ridge of posterior aortic media protrudes into the lumen to cause an eccentric narrowing just distal to the origin of the left subclavian artery. Isolated coarctation, if left untreated, generally has a poor prognosis, often leading to death before the age of 40. Death is usually secondary to chronic hypertension and its complications (cardiac failure, stroke, and so forth), bacterial endocarditis, or aortic rupture (precoarctation or postcoarctation). For these reasons, precise diagnosis must be pursued in patients with clinical findings suggesting coarctation. **Bicuspid aortic valve, patent ductus arteriosus, ventricular septal defects, and mitral valve abnormalities are frequent associated findings.**

Clinical Findings

Clinical presentation varies. Approximately one half of these patients present in infancy with signs and symptoms of cardiac failure often associated with other cardiac anomalies. In older patients, particularly adults, coarctation is usually asymptomatic. It may be suspected when routine examination or, occasionally, chest x-ray discloses upper extremity hypertension and decreased or absent femoral pulses (3). Sometimes patients complain of claudication. A thrill in the suprasternal notch and systolic ejection murmur may be present. Chest x-rays may reveal cardiomegaly, increased vascular markings, rib notching, and a hypoplastic aortic knob with a dilated poststenotic segment. Electrocardiogram may be normal or show left ventricular hypertrophy in older children. Echocardiography allows evaluation of cardiac chambers and septum along with mitral and aortic valves. Pulsed Doppler echocardiography may localize the coarctation, and continuous wave Doppler can be used to estimate pressure gradient across the coarctation. More recently, CT and MRI have been shown to accurately define the anatomy of coarctation (4) (Fig. 44.2).

Catheterization Findings

Catheter assessment with contrast aortography (Fig. 44.3) and cardiac catheterization remains the definitive diagnostic test in some centers. However, **MRI and TEE have become diagnostic modalities of choice in most institutions.** Catheter assessment may be necessary to provide information relative to the hemodynamic importance of the coarctation. Right and left ventricular catheterization also provides clear delineation of cardiac anatomy and any associated anomalies. In adults aged more than 35 years, coronary angiography may be indicated if a history is found of cardiac disease or ECG abnormalities.

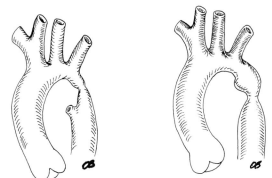

Figure 44.1. Preductal and postductal coarctation.

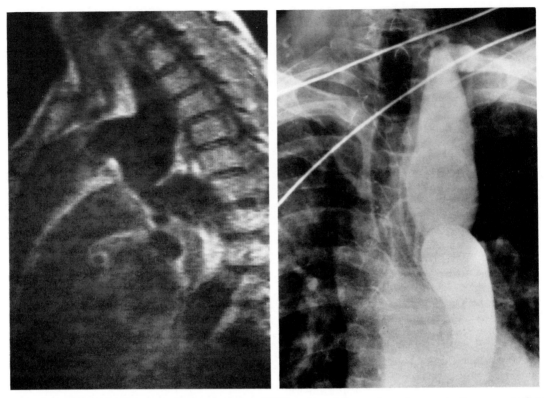

Figure 44.2. Left. Magnetic resonance imaging (MRI) in the oblique plane demonstrating coarctation of the aorta with pre- and poststenotic dilation and aneurysmal dilation of the left subclavian artery. **Right.** Aortogram demonstrating identical findings. (Reprinted with permission from Akins EW, Carmichael MJ, Hill JA, et al. Preoperative evaluation of the thoracic aorta using MRI and angiography. Ann Thorac Surg 1987;44:499–507.)

Data Integration, Decision Making, and Catheter Intervention

Data from noninvasive and invasive tests should provide enough information to make an accurate diagnosis and determine whether other cardiovascular anomalies exist. From these data a treatment plan can be devised. Correction is mandatory in all patients; however, timing of correction varies according to the patient's clinical condition. Patients with severe hypertension or congestive heart failure require correction as early as possible. Those with minimal symptoms can have correction delayed until they are between 4 and 10 years of age. Most coarctations are repaired by one of a variety of surgical procedures, all of which

have good results (5–8). **Percutaneous transluminal balloon angioplasty** is an option that has been reported to provide good early results (see Chapter 35). Balloon angioplasty has also been used for restenosis following surgical correction (9). Briefly, diameters of the coarctation and ascending and descending aorta are measured using catheter diameter as a calibration reference. A 3 cm long balloon angioplasty catheter is chosen so that the balloon outer diameter is approximately 2.5 times the coarctation segment diameter or the maximal ascending or descending aortic diameter, whichever is smallest. The balloon is advanced over a guidewire that is looped in the ascending aorta to help stabilize the balloon. Balloon position is localized using low pressure (about 2 atm) inflation so that the waist caused by the coarctation segment is at mid-

Interrupted Aortic Arch

Natural History and Pathophysiology

Interrupted aortic arch is similar to coarctation of the aorta, except it is a much more severe form with either total disconnection of the ascending and descending aorta or only a fibrous remnant connecting them. Three types have been described (Fig. 44.5): interruption distal to the left subclavian with all the branches of the arch arising from the descending aorta; interruption between the innominate artery and the left common carotid; and the left common carotid and subclavian arising from the descending aorta. The first two types account for most instances of interrupted aortic arch. Ventricular septal defects and a patent

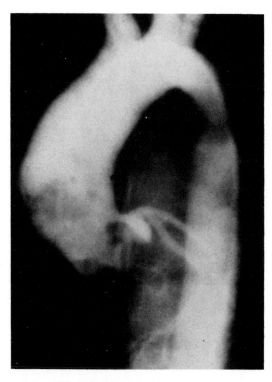

Figure 44.3. Aortogram revealing coarctation of the aorta, dilation of the ascending aorta, domed bicuspid, but competent aortic valve, and normal aortic arch.

balloon (Fig. 44.4). The balloon is inflated until the waist disappears (usually 5–6 atm). A repeat aortogram is recorded. Pressure gradient may not change or even increase for a short period of time after the procedure; but, after several months, it is generally reduced. The coarctation to ascending aortic diameter ratio increases significantly.

Aneurysms have been noted in a significant number of patients several months to years after dilation of native wedge-type coarctation (10, 11). In one report, 43% of patients developed evidence of aneurysm formation at or immediately distal to the balloon dilation site, raising serious concerns about the long-term safety and efficacy of this procedure. The exact role, therefore, for catheter balloon dilation compared with operative correction remains unsettled (12).

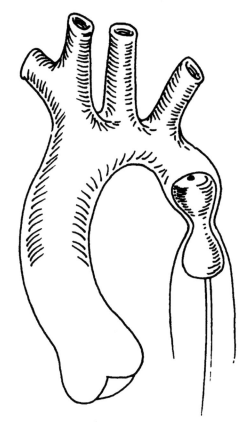

Figure 44.4. Diagram of balloon position for balloon angioplasty of coarctation.

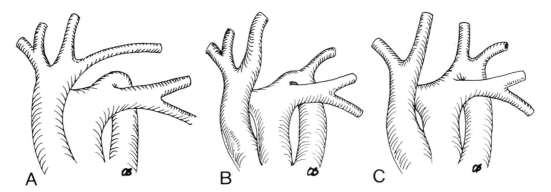

Figure 44.5. Types of interrupted aortic arch. **A.** Interruption distal to the left subclavian artery. **B.** Interruption between the left common carotid and left subclavian arteries. **C.** Interruption between the innominate and left common carotid arteries.

ductus arteriosus are commonly associated, as are other more complex anomalies such as truncus arteriosus or transposition of the great arteries.

In all of these circumstances, the pulmonary artery, via a patent ductus arteriosus, generally provides blood flow to the descending aorta and its branches. Because the right ventricle provides blood to the lower body and the left ventricle provides blood to the upper body, differential cyanosis may be observed. When a ventricular septal defect is present, left-to-right shunting may occur at the ventricular level and right-to-left shunting at the ductus level. How severe this is depends on the resistance in the descending aorta. Occasionally, a patent ductus arteriosus is absent. In this circumstance, blood flow to the lower extremities is dependent on the formation of collaterals via the intercostal and internal mammary arteries, as in severe coarctation.

Clinical Findings

In the most common form, that of a patent ductus and ventricular septal defect in conjunction with an interrupted arch, congestive heart failure occurs early in life, and presentation is in the newborn period. Cyanosis may be observed, depending on the adequacy of mixing in right ventricle and pulmonary artery, but it is variable. Left untreated, survival is limited, with most infants dying within the first several months of life. When this condition is associated with other anatomic abnormalities, the course may be different. In the absence of shunting, cyanosis does not occur and survival may be prolonged well into adulthood.

The ECG generally exhibits right ventricular hypertrophy, particularly in infants, with varying degrees of left ventricular hypertrophy. Chest x-ray will differ depending on presence or absence of intracardiac shunts. When intracardiac shunting exists and the ductus is patent, the cardiac silhouette will be enlarged and the lung fields variably congested depending on how much of the shunted blood preferentially flows into the patent ductus. When no shunts exist, the x-ray will resemble that of coarctation of the aorta. The echocardiogram is helpful to exclude other cardiac abnormalities and to differentiate this condition from aortic atresia. MRI, as in coarctation, provides good visualization of the aorta and may add significantly to noninvasive findings.

Catheterization Findings

As with any catheterization procedure in the patient with congenital heart disease, it is extremely important to completely assess all the abnormalities present. Details of the techniques are discussed in Chapter 43. In the patient with interrupted aortic arch, the descending aorta can be entered either retrogradely through the femoral artery or via the left subclavian if the interruption is proximal to it, or antegradely through a patent ductus, if one is present. The ascending aorta can be entered either retrogradely through the right subclavian (axillary or brachial) artery or antegradely via the inferior vena cava, across the atrial septum, and out the aortic valve. Angiography should be performed in two planes to assess accurately the anatomy of the aortic arch. A steep left anterior oblique or lateral view provides the most information to guide surgical correction.

Data Integration, Decision Making, and Catheter Intervention

Once appropriate diagnosis is made, treatment is surgical correction if possible. A detailed discussion of surgical management of this congenital abnormality is beyond the scope of this chapter. At present no procedure exists for therapeutic catheter intervention.

Supravalvular Aortic Stenosis

Natural History and Pathophysiology

Supravalvular aortic stenosis is generally a congenital aortic defect that is one of three types. The hourglass configuration is most common, and it is associated with thickening of the media and intimal fibrous proliferation. A second type involves formation of a membrane just above the aortic valve with a central orifice; it is associated with a normal size and is the least common type. The final type is tubular hypoplasia of the ascending aorta just above the sinuses of Valsalva. Associated with all of these types is dilation and tortuosity of the coronary arteries presumably because they are exposed to chronic high pressure from the systolic pressure generated in the left ventricle. **Coronary arteries may also be obstructed,** particularly in the ostial region secondary to aortic medial proliferation or adherence of the aortic cusp to the aortic wall near the site of supravalvular stenosis (Figs. 44.6 and 44.7). Premature coronary atherosclerosis is common. This abnormality may also coexist with other congenital abnormalities, commonly pulmonary branch stenosis. Prog-

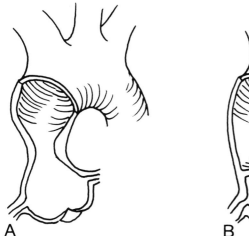
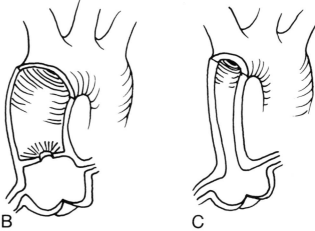

Figure 44.6. Types of supravalvular aortic stenosis. **A.** Hourglass type. **B.** Membranous type. **C.** Hypoplastic type.

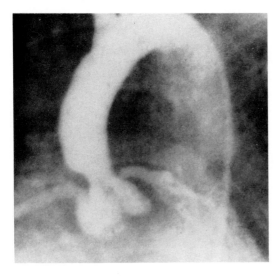

Figure 44.7. Cineangiographic frame of aortogram demonstrating hourglass type of supravalvular aortic stenosis and ostial stenosis of the left coronary artery.

nosis, as in valvular aortic stenosis, is related to degree of stenosis present (13).

Clinical Findings

Supravalvular aortic stenosis frequently has a familial predisposition, and it can be associated with mental retardation and characteristic facial features, including a small chin, wide mouth, malocclusion, wide set eyes, and a broad forehead. Clinically, these patients generally present with the same manifestations as those with valvular aortic stenosis, but earlier in life. Patients with the hypoplastic type are unlikely to reach adulthood because obstruction tends to be more severe. Physical findings are similar to valvular aortic stenosis except for absence of an aortic ejection click and another often well-preserved right carotid pulse.

The ECG in this condition is similar to that in valvular aortic stenosis, with varying degrees of left ventricular hypertrophy. If significant pulmonary stenosis is present, right ventricular hypertrophy may also be present. Chest x-ray in supravalvular aortic stenosis differs from valvular aortic stenosis

in that poststenotic dilation is not present. Doppler echocardiography often demonstrates anatomic abnormality, as well as functional assessment of stenosis severity.

Catheterization Findings

Cardiac catheterization will demonstrate a pressure gradient across the obstruction. Angiography of the aorta or left ventricle will localize the obstruction and guide surgical management (Fig. 44.7). This should be performed using standard views for evaluating the ascending aorta. **Selective coronary angiography may be necessary if a suggestion of myocardial ischemia or coronary obstruction is present** and they cannot be adequately visualized by aortography. It is also necessary to rule out significant pulmonary stenosis with subsequent abnormalities of right ventricular function.

Data Integration, Decision Making, and Catheter Intervention

By integrating results of both noninvasive and invasive examinations, a definitive diagnosis can be made and a therapeutic course chosen. Surgical correction with good results can be accomplished in most cases, except when the ascending aorta is severely hypoplastic or atretic. In these cases, results from correction are poor. Catheter intervention is not recommended.

ACQUIRED DISEASE

Traumatic Aortic Disruption

Etiology, Natural History, and Pathophysiology

Trauma to the aorta can result from blunt or penetrating injury; however, this section is devoted primarily to blunt aortic disruption. Acute transection of the thoracic aorta most commonly occurs at the ligamentum arteriosum or isthmus level, and it is most commonly caused by rapid deceleration. It is suspected that rapid deceleration results in a tearing away of the relatively mobile arch and proximal descending thoracic aorta, from the descending thoracic aorta, which is firmly attached to the paraspinous tissues. This injury causes rapid exsanguination into the free pleural space in most patients. Therefore, acute traumatic disruption of the thoracic aorta should be suspected in any patient who has sustained significant blunt chest trauma, especially those who have undergone rapid deceleration. In one large autopsy series, 85% of patients with blunt aortic injury died before arriving at a hospital. In the small group of patients that survive, injury is initially contained by periaortic tissues; however, rupture into the pleural space can occur at any time. It has been estimated that of those who reach a hospital alive, 10% die within 1 hour, 30% within 6 hours, and 40% within 24 hours (14). Those who survive the early posttraumatic period usually develop aneurysmal dilation of the level of transsection (Fig.

44.8),and they should be treated the same as any other aneurysm, as will be discussed later.

Clinical Findings

The posttraumatic clinical picture seen in patients with aortic tears is extremely variable, ranging from moribund and comatose to virtually asymptomatic. Clinical findings suggestive of a severe chest injury include bruises and/or abrasions to the chest wall, palpable rib and/or sternal fractures, chest wall crepitance, and decreased or absent breath sounds, primarily on the left side, suggestive of a hemothorax. Patients occasionally have decreased femoral pulses and blood pressure, but this is not usual.

Noninvasive evaluation should consist of an upright chest x-ray with a nasogastric tube in place and an ECG. The most common x-ray finding is a widened mediastinum (more than 8 cm at the level of the aortic knob), and the most sensitive is deviation of the esophagus (as seen by the nasogastric tube) to the right. Other findings on the chest x-ray are:

1. Loss of aortic knob
2. Depression of left main stem bronchus greater than 140°
3. Left hemothorax or pneumothorax
4. Rightward deviation of trachea
5. Left apical capping
6. Anterior displacement of trachea (lateral view)
7. Loss of aortopulmonary window (lateral view)
8. Fractured first and/or second rib

The ECG will probably be normal unless the patient has also sustained a cardiac contusion, in which case anterior ST segment or T-wave changes may be present.

Computed tomography scanning with contrast media has been recommended by some surgeons for use in patients suspected of having traumatic aortic disruption; however, this test is not 100% specific. **Because mortality from this injury in the early posttrauma period is so high, we feel no need for further noninvasive studies and contrast aortography should be performed as soon as possible.**

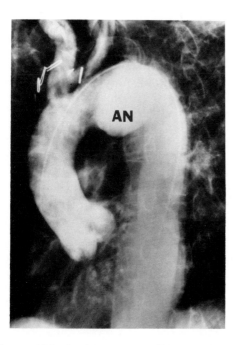

Figure 44.8. Aortogram revealing aneurysmal dilation (*AN*) in the proximal descending thoracic aorta secondary to a chronic transsection.

Catheterization Findings

The best approach is via the femoral artery. The right femoral artery is preferable, as some surgeons will utilize some type of bypass or shunt during the repair, and often the left femoral vessels are used for retrograde perfusion. Passage of the catheter retrograde past the aortic injury is not associated with any increased morbidity. Angiography should be performed in at least two planes (i.e., anterior-posterior, lateral, and/or oblique). Injury to the aorta most commonly occurs at the isthmus; however, injury can occur in any portion. Because all patients with acute traumatic injuries of the aorta have suffered trauma of great force, the incidence of injury to other organs is high. Of special concern are associated abdominal injuries, such as liver, spleen, and kidney, all of which can be easily delineated by abdominal aortography. Therefore, **a total aortogram is necessary in all such patients.**

Data Integration, Decision Making, and Catheter Intervention

Again, if the mechanism of injury and the immediate noninvasive studies are at all suggestive of an aortic injury, immediate angiography is mandatory. Aortography should give precise definition and localization of any aortic injury. Once diagnosis is made, immediate surgical repair should be pursued. No therapeutic catheter intervention is available for this injury.

Aneurysmal Disease

Etiology, Natural History, and Pathophysiology

Aneurysmal disease of the aorta, especially of the abdominal aorta, is common and occurs in more than 6% of patients aged more than 65 years (15). An aneurysm is defined as any dilation of the aorta greater than two times the normal diameter. In most cases, aortic aneurysms are caused by degeneration of vessel wall media, leading to weakening and subsequent dilation. Degenerative diseases of the aorta include cystic medial degeneration, myxomatous degeneration, and atherosclerotic degeneration. Atherosclerosis can produce aneurysmal dilation and occlusive disease.

Mycotic disease and different types of inflammatory disease (Takayasu's arteritis, giant cell, granulomatous, and rheumatoid) also can produce aneurysms of the aorta caused by aortic wall degeneration. Therefore, aneurysmal disease in general will be discussed in this section, as it is beyond the scope of this chapter to discuss each cause in detail. Chronic aortic dissection can also become aneurysmal, and it will be discussed in the section devoted to dissection.

Aortic aneurysms can occur in isolated or multiple segments of the aorta (contiguous or separate) or encompass the entire aorta from the aortic valve to the iliac bifurcation (Fig. 44.9). Aneurysms of the ascending aorta and transverse aortic arch are usually secondary to cystic medial degeneration or myxomatous degeneration. Left untreated, ascending, transverse, and descending thoracic aortic aneurysms will progress, leading to aortic insufficiency (Fig. 44.10), airway, esophagus, pulmonary artery, and great veins compression. They can also rupture into the pericardium, pleura, or mediastinum. **Progression with rupture leads to death in most cases.** It was once thought that thoracic aortic aneurysms rarely ruptured. However, in several studies, the rupture rate of untreated thoracic aneurysms ranged from 46 to 74% with a median interval of only 2 years between detection and rupture (16–18).

Thoracoabdominal aneurysms are defined as aneurysms involving segments of the descending thoracic aorta and abdominal aorta in continuity. These have been divided into four groups or types (19). Type I includes aneurysms that involve the entire descending thoracic aorta and upper abdominal aorta. Type II involves most of the descending aorta and most of the abdominal aorta. Type III involves the distal descending thoracic aorta and most or all of the abdominal aorta. Type IV is confined to

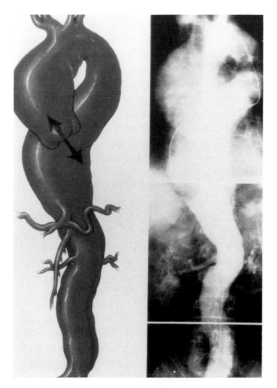

Figure 44.9. Diffuse aortic ectasia or mega-aorta with aneurysmal dilation from the aortic root to the iliac artery origins along with aortic insufficiency. (Reprinted with permission from Crawford ES, Crawford JL. Diseases of the aorta. Baltimore: Williams & Wilkins, 1984:52.)

the abdominal aorta and involves the segment associated with visceral vessels. These aneurysms are included with the thoracoabdominal aortic aneurysms, as the diagnosis, treatment, and associated complications are similar. The most common cause of thoracoabdominal aneurysms is atherosclerotic degeneration, and these aneurysms are commonly associated with hypertension. Natural history of types I and II is similar to that previously discussed for other thoracic aortic aneurysms. Types III and IV are similar to the abdominal aortic aneurysms, as will be discussed. Infrarenal abdominal aortic aneurysms are the most common aneurysms seen and treated (Fig. 44.11). As stated, as many as 6.5% of patients over age 65 will develop an abdominal aortic aneurysm and the frequency is increasing (15). This increased frequency is most likely sec-

ondary to increased awareness of the disease, improved diagnostic modalities, and larger numbers of patients reaching older ages.

Infrarenal abdominal aortic aneurysm repair accounts for 0.8% of general surgical operations and 10% of vascular operations (20). Cause is variable; however, atherosclerotic degeneration is by far the most common. The natural history of all abdominal aneurysms is one of progression, with rupture reported to occur in 50% of patients within 1 year of diagnosis and in more than 90% within 5 years (21). Aneuryms size has been used as a predictor of rupture with an aneurysm more than 6 cm carrying a 43% incidence of rupture and an accompanying mortality rate of 90% (22). Smaller aneurysms, however, are not benign, as those less than 6 cm have been found to have an incidence of rupture of almost 20% with a 55% mortality rate. One autopsy series of patients dying from ruptured abdominal aortic aneurysms found that one third had aneurysms 5 cm or less (23).

Clinical Findings

Clinical presentation of thoracic aortic aneurysms varies and is dependent on site, size, and extent of the aneurysm. Most are asymptomatic until they reach sizable proportion when symptoms occur, such as chest or back pain, stridor, dysphagia or hoarseness. Signs or symptoms of aortic insufficiency can be present if the aneurysm involves the ascending aorta and aortic annulus. Often the first symptoms are those of rupture or impending rupture, and many patients die suddenly with no real symptoms.

Most patients with abdominal aortic aneurysms are asymptomatic at the time of presentation, with one recent series of 666 patients reporting 81% asymptomatic (20). Diagnosis in 70 to 75% of these patients is usually suggested when a pulsating mass in the abdomen is noted by the patient or physician or when calcification shadows are seen on abdominal roentgenograms. When symptoms are present, they usually consist of varying degrees of abdominal, flank, and

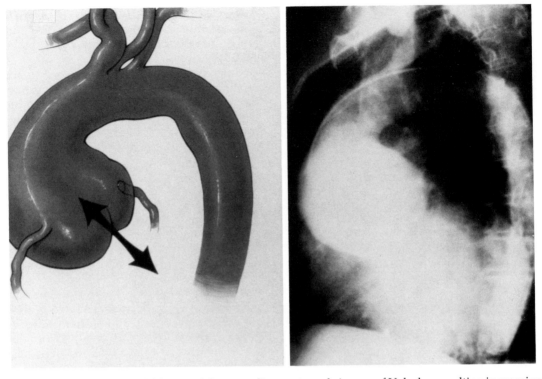

Figure 44.10. Aneurysmal dilation of the ascending aorta and sinuses of Valsalva resulting in massive aortic insufficiency. (Reprinted with permission from Crawford ES, Crawford JL. Diseases of the aorta. Baltimore: Williams & Wilkins, 1984:9.)

back pain. Diagnosis is usually made on physical examination, with an abdominal ultrasound being an easy reliable confirmatory test.

Thoracic aortic aneurysms are often initially suggested in the asymptomatic patient by enlargement of the mediastinal silhouette on plain roentgenograms (Fig. 44.12). When this occurs, noninvasive study of the aorta is indicated. Transthoracic echocardiography is a good initial study to assess the heart and its function, cardiac valves, and aorta root. Transthoracic echocardiography of the distal ascending, transverse arch and descending thoracic aorta, however, is of questionable value because of the technical limitations provided by the intrathoracic structures. **Biplane and multiplane TEE, however, give excellent visualization of the entire intrathoracic aorta.** TEE provides real time visualization, with the ability to evaluate aorta size, and give some hemodynamic measurements and vis-

ualization of previously unrecognized atheromatous debris, acute and chronic dissections, and aortic ulcers (24–26). CT scan of the thorax with contrast has been the definitive noninvasive procedure to evaluate aortic disease (Fig. 44.13); however, more recently, multiple reports have suggested that MRI is as good or better for delineation of aortic abnormalities (27–35). Included in the advantages of MRI are (*a*) excellent soft issue contrast, (*b*) intravascular contrast occurring without need for contrast medium, (*c*) intrinsically three-dimensional view, (*d*) gated images defining cardiac structure and function with excellent resolution, and (*e*) ability to select tomographic planes in virtually any orientation (Fig. 44.14). Akins et al., in a prospective preoperative evaluation of thoracic aortic aneurysms using MRI, found excellent correlation between MRI and angiography (27). In 25% of patients studied, clinically useful information was found that was not available from angiogra-

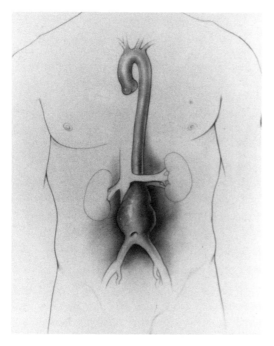

Figure 44.11. Typical appearance of an infrarenal abdominal aortic aneurysm.

phy. MRI limitations include inability to provide definitive hemodynamic and anatomic assessment of the aortic valve, coronary arteries, and arch vessels. Also, severe vessel tortuosity can lead to misinterpretation of the extent of fusiform aneurysms.

Because of the ease and accuracy of abdominal ultrasound and the asymptomatic course, it is reasonable that patients in the susceptible age group (> 50 years) have a yearly screening abdominal ultrasound. If a question is present of extent, either proximal or distal, CT and MRI have proved to be extremely useful.

Catheterization Findings

In patients with aortic aneurysms confirmed by ultrasound, TEE, CT scan, or MRI, and in those who have no history suggestive of cerebral, mesenteric, or peripheral vascular occlusive disease, routine angiography is probably not indicated. If any question arises, however, regarding the

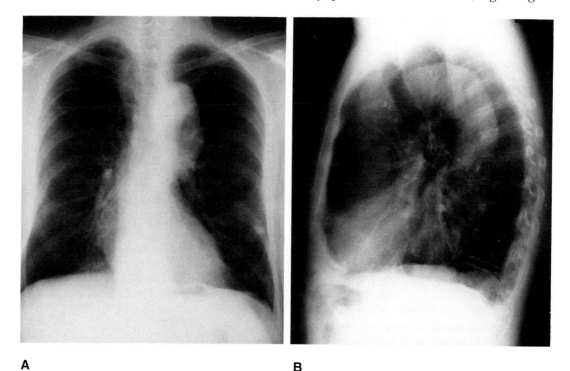

A   B

Figure 44.12. **A** and **B.** Chest x-ray showing widened mediastinal silhouette and enlarged descending thoracic aorta in a patient with a thoracoabdominal aortic aneurysm.

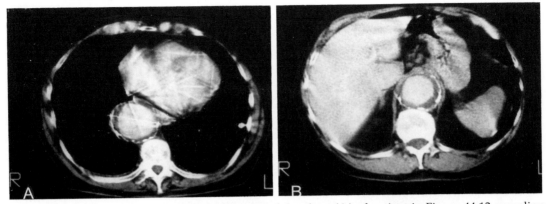

Figure 44.13. Computed tomography (CT) scan of the chest (**A**) of patient in Figure 44.12 revealing extension of the aneurysm into the abdomen (**B**). Note that both the location and the size of the aneurysm are delineated.

aneurysm or the presence of occlusive disease, then angiography should be performed with biplane films of the aortic arch, abdominal aorta, mesenteric and renal vessels, iliacs, and femorals.

Data Integration, Decision Making, and Catheter Intervention

In patients with documented aneurysms of the thoracic aorta, several features must be delineated. First, and foremost, is **the extent of the aneurysm.** In a patient with an ascending aortic aneurysm, it must be determined if the aneurysm is isolated to the ascending aorta or if the aortic arch and coronary ostia and sinuses are involved. If the aneurysm is isolated to the supracoronary aorta and does not involve the arch, repair is relatively simple and involves replacement of that segment alone, using routine cardiopulmonary bypass. If the aneurysm extends into the arch in part or in whole, then a more complicated surgical procedure is necessary. This includes profound hypothermia and circulatory arrest with reimplantation of the great vessels. This procedure is also necessary if the aneurysm is isolated to the aortic arch. If the aneurysm extends proximally to the coronary ostii and sinuses of Valsalva, again, a more complicated procedure is indicated. This requires reattachment of the coronary ostii to the

graft or coronary artery bypass. Extent and severity of associated cardiac disease, primarily aortic valvular disease and coronary artery disease, along with myocardial function must also be determined. Cardiac catheterization is usually necessary in patients with ascending aortic aneurysms, as it provides not only visualization of the aneurysm but also assessment of the aortic valve and coronary arteries. Aortic valvular insufficiency is frequently associated with these aneurysms. When significant aortic valvular disease is present, the valve must be replaced. This can be done separately or with a composite valve graft and reimplantation of the coronary ostia. Associated significant coronary artery disease, if identified, requires coronary artery bypass with the grafts implanted into the aortic graft.

For patients with aneurysms of the descending thoracic aorta, knowledge of the extent of involvement is also extremely important, as it again determines the operative approach. If the aneurysm extends into the distal arch, then cardiopulmonary bypass with profound hypothermia and circulatory arrest, as reported by Crawford, et al. (37), may be necessary. If it extends distally into the distal thorax or upper abdomen, then a thoracoabdominal approach is necessary (Fig. 44.15). Evaluation of the abdominal aorta is extremely important in patients with aneurysms of the descending thoracic aorta, as 25% of these patients have simultaneous abdominal aortic aneurysms (21).

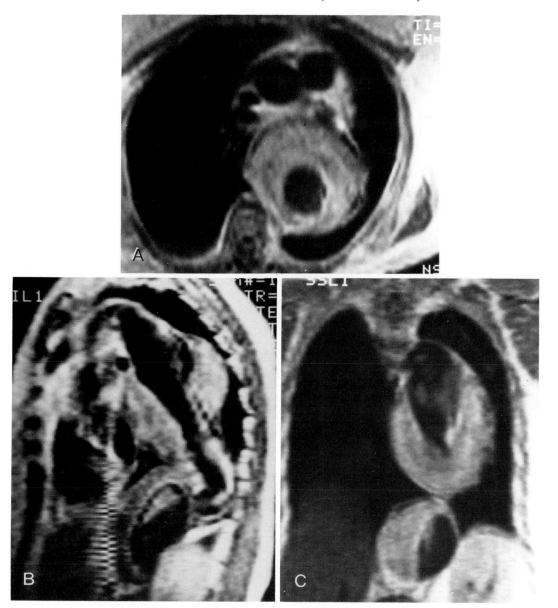

Figure 44.14. Magnetic resonance imaging (MRI) in the axial (**A**), coronal (**B**), and sagittal (**C**) planes accurately defining the full extent and size of a large thoracoabdominal aneurysm. (Reprinted with permission from Akins EW, Carmichael MJ, Hill JA, et al. Preoperative evaluation of the thoracic aorta using MRI and angiography. Ann Thorac Surg 1987;44:499–507.)

Once the diagnosis of a thoracoabdominal aneurysm is suggested, optimal evaluation should include both noninvasive and invasive studies, if indicated. Computed tomography and MRI provide the best information regarding size, extent, and differentiation between dissection and nondissec-

tion (27, 28, 31, 33, 34). However, many authorities still recommend that catheter assessment with biplane aortography is mandatory, as 20% of these patients have been reported to have associated atherosclerotic occlusive disease of visceral vessels, renal arteries, and distal aorta and iliacs. Athero-

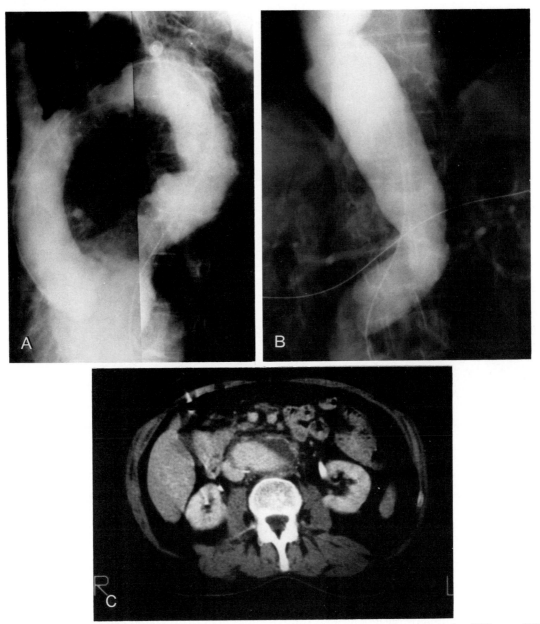

Figure 44.15. Aortogram (thoracic [**A**] and abdominal [**B**]) and computed tomography (CT) scan (**C**) revealing extension of a known descending thoracic aortic aneurysm into the upper abdomen requiring a thoracoabdominal incision for correction.

sclerotic occlusive disease of these vessels may necessitate correction at the time of aneurysm repair (21). In patients with severe mesenteric or renal occlusive disease, bypass or endarterectomy may be considered; if severe peripheral vascular occlusive disease is present, then resection of the aneu-rysm should be coupled with an aorta bi-iliac or bifemoral bypass.

Of particular concern is the high incidence of cardiac disease in these patients. Of the 666 patients reviewed by Johnston and Scobie (20), 45% had a history of myo-cardial infarction, angina, and congestive

Because of this frequency of associated illness, with its related morbidity and mortality in the perioperative period, catheter-directed repair has recently been attempted (34) (Fig. 44.16). The procedure is done by placing a large catheter, "loaded" with a graft and an expandable metallic stent, into the femoral artery via a cutdown. The catheter is advanced in retrograde fashion to position the proximal end of the graft with its associated stent in the descending aorta just before the entry into the aneurysm. The balloon is expanded to fix the proximal part of the graft in place using the stent. An additional stent is used to fix the distal end of

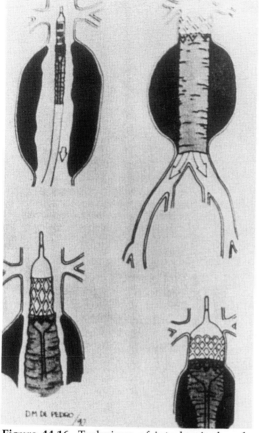

Figure 44.16. Technique of intraluminal exclusion of infrarenal aortic aneurysms using Dacron tube grafts implanted by the transfemoral route. Balloon-expandable stents secure the graft to the aortic wall. (Reprinted with permission from Parodi JC, Palmaz JC, Barone HD. Transfemoral intraluminal graft implantation for abdominal aortic aneurysms. Ann Vasc Surg 1991;5:491. By permission of Blackwell Scientific Publications, Inc.)

heart failure and/or electrocardiographic evidence of ischemia or old infarction, and 6.5% had previous coronary artery bypass. In those who had a myocardial infarction less than 6 months prior to surgery, congestive heart failure (recent or remote), class III or IV angina or unstable angina within the last 6 months, or significant valvular disease (aortic, mitral, or both), a mortality rate of 16% or greater was seen. Therefore, thorough preoperative cardiac evaluation directed at assessing the coronary arteries and left ventricular function should be performed.

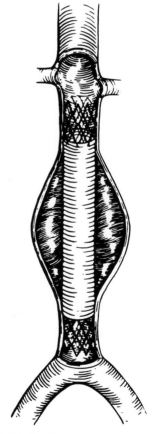

Figure 44.17. Graft-stent combination with both cephalic and caudal stents. (Reprinted with permission from Parodi JC, Palmaz JC, Barone HD. Transfemoral intraluminal graft implantation for abdominal aortic aneurysms. *Ann Vasc Surg* 1991;5:491. By permission of Blackwell Scientific Publications, Inc.)

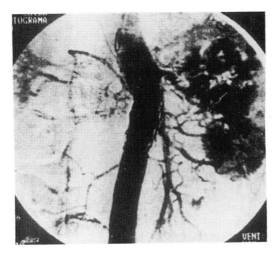

Figure 44.18. Follow-up angiogram of patient in whom a 6 cm infrarenal abdominal aortic aneurysm was treated 53 days previously. (Reprinted with permission from Parodi JC, Palmaz JC, Barone HD. Transfemoral intraluminal graft implantation for abdominal aortic aneurysms. Ann Vasc Surg 1991;5:491. By permission of Blackwell Scientific Publications, Inc.)

the graft (Fig. 44.17). A postprocedure angiogram is shown in Figure 44.18.

Aortic Dissection

Etiology, Natural History, and Pathophysiology

Aortic dissection is one of the most frequent and serious forms of aortic disease. Acute dissection results from a tear in the intima of the aorta that subsequently leads to destruction and separation of the media from the adventitia by an advancing column of blood under high pressure. The cause of the initial intimal tear is variable, usually associated with chronic hypertension and preexisting disease of the aortic wall, such as arteriosclerosis, medial degeneration, aortitis, or trauma. Acute dissections begin in the ascending aorta in 55 to 65% of patients, in the descending aorta in 20 to 30%, in the transverse arch in 10 to 15%, and in the abdominal aorta in less than 2% (38–40).

Two classification systems have been proposed in the past 20 years (Fig. 44.19) (41–45). DeBakey and colleagues first classified aortic dissections into types I, II, and III (41, 42). Type I has the initial intimal tear in the ascending aorta with the dissection continuing through the arch and descending thoracic aorta and into the abdominal aorta (Fig. 44.20). Type II begins in the ascending aorta but ends at the left subclavian artery (Fig. 44.21), and type III begins in the proximal descending thoracic aorta and continues distally. The Stanford classification groups DeBakey type I and II into category A and DeBakey type III into category B (45). This classification is based solely on whether the ascending aorta is involved (category A) or not involved (category B) and does not take into consideration the site of the initial intimal tear.

Dissection can progress proximally, distally, or both; however, the distal dissection is usually much greater. Retrograde dissection rarely occurs when the tear is in the descending thoracic aorta, and virtually never occurs when it begins in the abdominal aorta. Retrograde dissection commonly occurs when the dissection begins on the

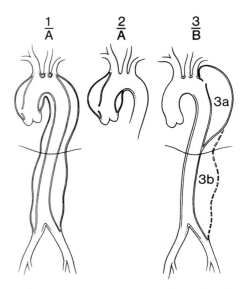

Figure 44.19. Classifications of aortic dissections, DeBakey types 1, 2, and 3, and Stanford types A and B. (See text for discussion.) (Reprinted with permission from Crawford ES, Crawford JL. Disease of the aorta. Baltimore: Williams & Wilkins, 1984;174.)

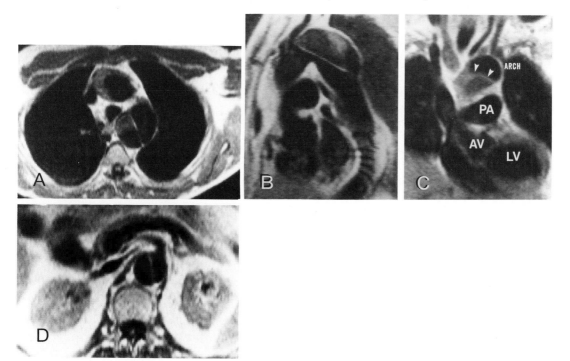

Figure 44.20. Magnetic resonance imaging (MRI) revealing a DeBakey type I dissection with involvement of the ascending aorta (**A**), aortic arch (**B** and **C**) and extension of the dissection into the abdomen (**D**). *ARCH,* aortic arch; *AV,* aortic valve; *LV,* left ventricle; *PA,* pulmonary artery. (Reprinted with permission from Akins EW, Hill JA, Carmichael MJ. MR imaging of blood pool signal variation with cardiac phase in aortic dissection. J Comput Assist Tomogr 1987;11:543–545.)

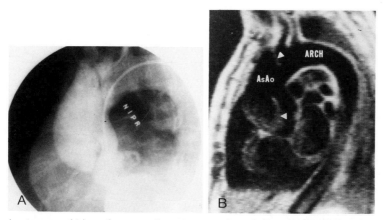

Figure 44.21. Aortogram (**A**) and magnetic resonance imaging scan (MRI) (**B**) sections in a patient with a DeBakey type II aortic dissection where the dissection is limited to the ascending aorta and proximal aortic arch. *AsAo,* ascending aorta; *ARCH,* aortic arch; *NIPR,* nitroprusside. (Reprinted with permission from Hill JA, Lambert CR, Akins EW, et al. Ascending aortic dissection: detection by MRI. Am Heart J 1985;110:894–896.)

inner ascending aortic wall and involves 50% of the circumference. DeBakey type I and II (Stanford type A) dissections start in the ascending aorta or arch, and usually course along the greater curve and upper descending thoracic aorta. Type III (Stanford type B) dissections usually start in the descending thoracic aorta and tear along the left posterior lateral surface. Ninety percent of these, along with the distal extent of DeBakey type I dissections, extend distally along the left posterior lateral surface of the aorta and into the left iliac. This is of particular importance to the angiographer, as the false lumen is commonly entered when catheterization is done via a left femoral approach.

Left untreated, the natural course of aortic dissections is ominous, with a 50 to 90% mortality rate in the acute phase (45). Patients who survive acute dissection are then at a significant risk of developing chronic fusiform aneurysms from dilation of the outer wall of the false lumen. Again, left untreated, 25% of chronic dissections will progress to rupture at the site of the intimal tear. Therefore, in DeBakey types I and II dissections, death is usually secondary to rupture into the pericardium with acute pericardial tamponade, and death from a ruptured type III is most often from exsanguination into the mediastinum or free left pleural space.

Clinical Findings

Classic symptom of an acute dissection is severe, unbearable retrosternal or left-sided chest pain that radiates straight to the back. It is often described as tearing or wrenching in nature and is often associated with diaphoresis, dizziness, and syncope. This pain is not relieved by nitroglycerin and is often refractory to intravenous narcotics. Acute dissections are often associated with sustained or intermittent hypertension or hypotension. Transient or persistent loss of blood pressure or pulses in any aortic branch can occur, and is dependent on the extent and path of the dissection. Clinically, this may present in many forms, including ischemia of one or more extremities (left arm or left leg being the most common). Loss of cerebral blood flow presents as either a transient ischemic attack or a completed stroke, and loss of critical spinal cord blood results in paraplegic or paraparesis. Mesenteric ischemia may also occur and present as abdominal pain with or without distention. This is an ominous sign, as the mortality rate is high if bowel infarction occurs. Again, any of these clinical findings can be transient or permanent, and they are totally dependent on the course of the dissection.

Optimal management of patients with suggested or known dissection requires that the diagnosis be made promptly and that its site of origin and extent be identified as rapidly as possible (43). Also, in this age of thrombolytic therapy of patients with acute myocardial infarction, it is crucial to exclude aortic dissection among patients presenting with acute chest pain syndromes, because giving a thrombolytic agent to a patient with dissection can be catastrophic. Catheterization with aortography and, in many cases, coronary angiography, is considered by many as the reference standard for evaluation of patients with aortic dissection. More recently, noninvasive imagery with CT, MRI, and echocardiography (both TEE and transthoracic TEE) have all been shown useful (44).

Over the last 5 to 10 years CT scan has been considered the most reliable noninvasive modality for assessing aortic dissections. However, multiple reports have shown the efficacy of MRI (27, 28, 31, 33, 35). In one report, MRI supplemented the angiographic assessment of type A aortic involvement when these abnormalities were missed by contrast angiography (27). The high contrast between the signal from the intimal flap and the low signal present in rapidly flowing blood facilitates detection of an aortic dissection. This allows demonstration of false lumen patency, which may be especially important in making the diagnosis. Recently TEE has become the diagnostic modality of choice when acute aortic dissection is suspected (46–51). One of us (Tomas D. Martin) used TEE as the first method of diagnosis in 46 consecutive patients with aortic dissections. No false-positives or false-negatives were documented.

An experienced echocardiographer, however, is mandatory to obtain such results. A recent report comparing these noninvasive strategies found similar sensitivities for detecting dissections using CT (93.8%), MRI (98.3%), and TEE (97.7%), but TTE had a sensitivity of only 59.3% (25). Specificities of both TTE (83%) and TEE (76.9%) were lower than CT (87.1%) and MRI (97.8%), mainly as a result of false-positive findings in the ascending aorta. However, these latter two techniques were not superior to TEE in detecting thrombus, entry site, or aortic insufficiency. These investigators suggested that MRI in stable patients and TEE in unstable patients represented the optimal noninvasive diagnostic strategies.

Catheterization Findings

Disease extent is best determined by aortography in the anterior-posterior, lateral, and oblique projections with injections into both the true and false lumen. The true lumen is best entered from a right brachial artery approach and the false lumen from the left femoral artery. This is especially true in type I and III dissections, as the path of dissection is usually into the left iliac and femoral arteries. It is often difficult to catheterize both the true and false lumen, and it often requires tremendous effort, persistence, and patience from the angiographer. It is likely that both lumens cannot be entered via a single approach, and one should not hesitate to try several catheterization sites. In patients with type I and II dissections, it is extremely important to visualize the coronary arteries and aortic valve, and, if possible, to visualize the tear in the ascending aorta, as the surgical procedure performed is dependent on this information. An example of aortography performed from the right femoral artery with injection into the false lumen of a DeBakey type I aortic dissection is given in Figure 44.22.

Data Integration, Decision Making, and Catheter Intervention

Early in the evaluation of many patients with aortic dissection, the exact diagnosis may not be apparent. Acute myocardial infarction is frequently considered (52). This can be excluded in most patients with the initial ECG; however, as many as 23% will have electrocardiographic abnormalities consistent with myocardial ischemia or infarction. Therefore, in patients with suspected aortic dissection, further evaluation is warranted if their condition permits. If the patient is hemodynamically unstable, however, either from pericardial tamponade or continuing hemorrhage, immediate operative intervention is indicated. Patients who are stable should have pain controlled with intravenous narcotics, and have systolic pressure decreased to 120 mm Hg or less with intravenous nitroprusside and β-blockade. Once stabilized, contrast aortography should be performed, as it is considered the definitive diagnostic test.

Information that must be obtained from aortography and any noninvasive studies include (*a*) site of initial tear; (*b*) extent of the dissection; (*c*) status of all major aortic branches; and (*d*) status of aortic valve and coronary arteries (primarily in type I and II dissections). With this information, an adequate treatment plan can be developed. With type I and II dissections that do not involve the aortic valve or coronary arteries, treatment is supracoronary replacement of the ascending aorta or aortic arch under profound hypothermia and circulatory arrest. If the aortic valve and coronary arteries are involved, then a composite valve graft must be utilized with either reimplantation of the coronary ostia to the graft or ligation of the coronary ostia followed by autologous saphenous vein bypass.

Treatment of acute type III dissections is controversial with operative mortality rate reported to be between 8 and 40%. Therefore, in our opinion, aggressive medical treatment should be instituted. If hypertension can be controlled and no signs present of impending rupture, no surgical intervention may be necessary, as only 15 to 25% will progress to chronic aneurysms or rupture (39, 40, 45). These patients should all be followed closely with CT scan or MRI evaluation at least every 6 months, and subsequent aneurysms should be approached in the same manner as the nondissecting aneurysms.

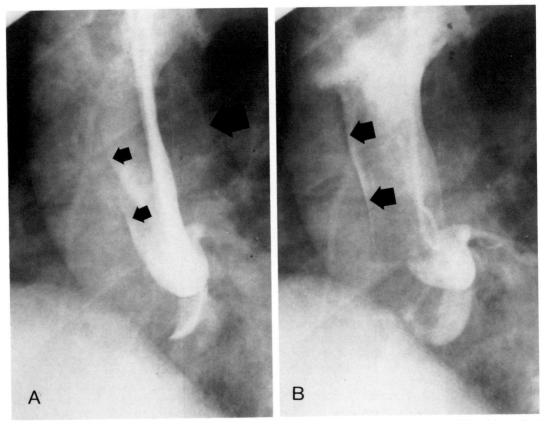

Figure 44.22. Systolic (**A**) and diastolic (**B**) frames during aortography (left anterior oblique) in patient with a DeBakey type I aortic dissection. Injection is into the false lumen and illustrates movement of the intimal flap (*small arrows,* **A** and **B**). Medial extent of the aorta is marked by the *large arrow* in the systolic frame (**A**). The diastolic frame is shown in **B.**

OTHER AORTIC DISEASE

Marfan's Syndrome

Etiology, Natural History, and Pathophysiology

Marfan's syndrome is an inheritable connective tissue disorder with well-known skeletal, ocular, and cardiovascular manifestations (53). Aortic aneurysms and dissections occur as a result of cystic medial necrosis, with these and other cardiovascular manifestations occurring in 98% of patients (54). The natural history of these manifestations is ominous. Ninety-five percent of these patients die of cardiovascular complications, with 50% succumbing at an average age of 32 years (55).

Clinical Findings

Various skeletal manifestations are seen in virtually all patients with Marfan's syndrome, and they include long extremities, fingers, and thumbs; extremely lax joints; sternal and spinal deformities, including pectus excavatum or carinatum and kyphosis or scoliosis; and narrow, highly arched palates (Fig. 44.23). Approximately 70% of these patients will have ocular problems, including myopia and lens subluxation. The most common cardiovascular abnormality is fusiform aortic aneurysm, most fre-

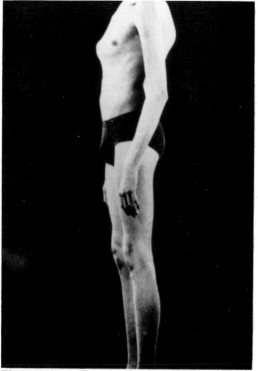

Figure 44.23. The classic physique of a patient with Marfan's syndrome: tall and thin, arm span greater than height, sternal and spine deformities typifying the skeletal manifestations. (Reprinted with permission from Crawford ES, Crawford JL. Diseases of the aorta. Baltimore: Williams & Wilkins, 1984:52:215.)

Catheterization Findings

Catheter findings will vary according to the pathologic manifestation of the disease, and they have been discussed. All patients with Marfan's syndrome, however, should undergo cardiac catheterization for evaluation of coronary anatomy and pathology, as well as valvular disease, if surgical correction is deemed appropriate by noninvasive studies. Many operators prefer to use brachial cutdown allowing direct arterial repair in patients with Marfan's syndrome. An example of aortography in such a patient is given in Figure 44.24, illustrating annuloaortic ectasia commonly seen in Marfan's syndrome.

Data Interpretation, Decision Making, and Catheter Intervention

In Marfan's syndrome, any evidence of aortic or cardiac pathology necessitates careful

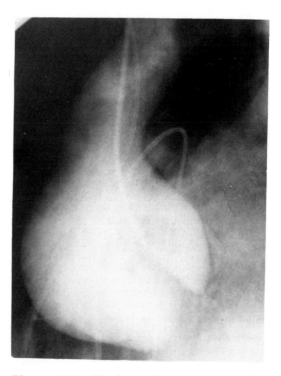

Figure 44.24. Cineframe from aortogram (left anterior oblique) from the right brachial artery in a patient with Marfan's syndrome illustrating annuloaortic ectasia.

quently in the ascending aorta. Others include acute dissections, aortic aneurysms secondary to chronic dissections, cardiac valve abnormalities (most commonly mitral valve prolapse), and occasionally peripheral arterial aneurysms. Clinical findings with each of these have been described.

All patients with known Marfan's syndrome should be followed clinically at frequent regular intervals. Annual chest x-ray should be performed, and if any question is found concerning the aorta, then either a CT scan or MRI should be performed to exclude aneurysm formation or dissection. Echocardiography is also an excellent test for following any known or suspected valvular disease, as well as for following proximal aortic root size.

evaluation and follow-up. This includes complete noninvasive evaluation and catheter assessment if indicated. Early correction of aortic and cardiac abnormalities is mandatory, as mortality rate from these conditions is high. One surgical series reported that 63% of late deaths theoretically could have been prevented had more aggressive treatment been undertaken (54). Data integration, decision making, and catheter intervention techniques for each of the cardiovascular complications of Marfan's syndrome have been discussed in previous chapters. The only difference is to recognize that these patients have multiple systemic manifestations of their disease and that each area must be examined completely.

References

1. Fyler DC, Buckley LP, Hellenbrand WE, et al. Report of the New England regional infarct cardiac program. Pediatrics 1980;65:375–461.
2. Keith JD. Coarctation of the aorta. In: Keith JD, Rower RD, Vlad P, eds. Heart disease in infancy and childhood. 3rd ed. New York: Macmillan, 1978:736–760.
3. Glancy DL, Morrow AG, Simon AL, et al. Juxtaductal aortic coarctation. Analysis of 84 patients studied hemodynamically, angiographically and morphologically after age 1 year. Am J Cardiol 1983;51:537–551.
4. Akins EW, Schuster JD, Victorica BE. Cardiovascular MRI in the pediatric patient [Abstract]. Southeastern Ped Cardiol Soc 1987;September 24–26.
5. Lababidi Z. Neonatal transluminal balloon coarctation angioplasty. Am Heart J 1983;106:752–753.
6. Singer MI, Rowen M, Dorsy TJ. Transluminal aortic balloon angioplasty for coarctation of the aorta in the newborn. Am Heart J 1982;103:131–132.
7. Lock JE, Bass JL, Amplatz K, et al. Balloon dilatation angioplasty of aortic coarctations in infants and children. Circulation 1983;68:109–116.
8. Cooper RS, Ritter SB, Bolinko RJ. Balloon dilatation angioplasty: nonsurgical management of coarctation of the aorta. Circulation 1984;70:903–907.
9. Kan J, White RI, Mitchell SE, et al. Treatment of restenosis of coarctation by percutaneous transluminal angioplasty. Circulation 1983;68:87–94.
10. Brandt B III, Marvin WJ Jr, Rose EF, et al. Surgical treatment of coarctation of the aorta after balloon angioplasty. J Thorac Cardiovasc Surg 1987;94(5):715–719.
11. Pellegrino A, Deverall PB, Anderson RH, et al. Aortic coarctation in the first three months of life: an anatomicopathological study with respect to treatment. J Thorac Cardiovasc Surg 1985;89:121–127.
12. Cooper RS, Ritter SB, Rothe WB, et al. Angioplasty for coarctation of the aorta: long-term results. Circulation 1987;75:600–604.
13. Martin MM, Lammer JH, Shaffer E, et al. Obstruction to left coronary artery blood flow secondary to obliteration of the coronary ostium in supravalvular aortic stenosis. Ann Thorac Surg 1988;45:16–20.
14. Parmley LF, Mattingly TW, Manion WC, et al. Nonpenetrating traumatic injury of the aorta. Circulation 1958;17:1086–1101.
15. Reigel MM, Hollier LH. Surgical repair of abdominal aortic aneurysms. In: Cardiac surgery: state of the art reviews. Surgery of the aorta. Philadelphia: Hanley and Belfas, 1987;1:453.
16. Bickerstaff LK, Pairolero PC, Hollier LH, et al. Thoracic aortic aneurysms: a population based study. Surgery 1982;92:1103–1108.
17. Joyce J, Fairbairn J, Kincaid O, et al. Aneurysms of the thoracic aorta: a clinical study with special reference to prognosis. Circulation 1964;29:176–181.
18. Pressler V, McNamara JJ. Thoracic aortic aneurysm: natural history and treatment. J Thorac Cardiovasc Surg 1980;79:489–498.
19. Crawford ES, Crawford JL, Safi HJ, et al. Thoracoabdominal aortic aneurysms: preoperative and intraoperative factors determining immediate and long-term results of operation in 605 patients. J Vasc Surg 1986;3:389–404.
20. Johnston KW, Scobie TK. Multicenter prospective study of nonruptured abdominal aortic aneurysms. I. Population and operative management. J Vasc Surg 1988;7:69–81.
21. Crawford ES, Crawford JL. Aneurysms of degenerative origin. In: Diseases of the aorta. Baltimore: Williams & Wilkins, 1984;134–166.
22. Szilagyi DE, Smith RF, DeRusso FJ, et al. Contribution of abdominal aortic aneurysmectomy to prolongation of life. Ann Surg 1966;164:678–699.
23. Karmody AM, Leather RP, Goldman M, et al. The current position of nonresective treatment for abdominal aortic aneurysm. Surgery 1983;94:591–597.
24. Oh JK, Seward JB, Khandheria BK, et al. Transesophageal echocardiography in critically ill patients. Am J Card 1990;15:66(20):1492–1495.
25. DeSimone R, Haberbosch W, Iarussi D, et al. Transesophageal echocardiography for the diagnosis of thoracic aorta aneurysms and dissections. Cardiologia 1990;35(5):387–390.
26. Chan KL. Usefulness of transesophageal echocardiography in the diagnosis of conditions mimicking aortic dissection. Am Heart J 1991;122(2):495–504.
27. Akins EW, Carmichael MJ, Hill JA, et al. Preoperative evaluation of the thoracic aorta using MRI and angiography. Ann Thorac Surg 1987;44:499–507.
28. Amparo EG, Higgins CB, Hricak H, et al. Aortic dissection: magnetic resonance imaging. Radiology 1985;155:399–406.
29. Amparo EG, Higgins CB, Shafton EP. Demonstration of coarctation of the aorta by magnetic resonance imaging. AJR 1984;143:1192–1194.
30. Glazer HS, Gutierrez FR, Levitt RG, et al. The tho-

racic aorta studied by MR imaging. Radiology 1985;157:149–155.

31. Geisinger MA, Risius B, O'Donnell JA, et al. Thoracic aortic dissections: magnetic resonance imaging. Radiology 1985;155:407–412.

32. Von Schulthess GK, Higashino SM, Higgins SS, et al. Coarctation of the aorta: MR imaging. Radiology 1986;158:469– 474.

33. Goldman AP, Kotter MN, Scanlon MH, et al. The complementary role of magnetic resonance imaging, Doppler echocardiography, and computed tomography in the diagnosis of dissecting thoracic aneurysms. Am Heart J 1986;111:970–981.

34. Ahn SS, Seeger JM. The surgical clinics of North America. Endovascular Surg 1992;72(4).

35. Hill JA, Lambert CR, Akins EW, et al. Ascending aortic dissection: detection by MRI. Am Heart J 1985;110:894–896.

36. Dinsmore RE, Liberthson RR, Wismer GL, et al. Magnetic resonance imaging of thoracic aortic aneurysms: comparison with other imaging methods. Am J Radiol 1986;146:309–314.

37. Crawford ES, Coseli JS, Safi HJ. Partial cardiopulmonary bypass, hypothermic circulatory arrest, and posterolateral exposure for thoracic aortic aneurysm operation. J Thorac Cardiovasc Surg 1987; 94:824–827.

38. Miller DC, Stinson EB, Oyer PE, et al. Operative treatment of aortic dissections: experience with 125 patients over a sixteen year period. J Thorac Cardiovasc Surg 1979;78:365–382.

39. Crawford ES, Crawford JL. Aortic dissection and dissecting aortic aneurysm. In: Diseases of the aorta. Baltimore: Williams & Wilkins, 1984; 168–214.

40. Ergin MA, Lausman SL, Griepp RB. Acute dissections of the aorta. In: Cardiac surgery: state of the art reviews. Surgery of the aorta. Philadelphia: Hanley and Belfas, 1987;1:337–392.

41. DeBakey ME, Henly WS, Cooley DA, et al. Surgical treatment of dissecting aneurysms of the aorta: analysis of seventy-two cases. Circulation 1961;24: 290–303.

42. DeBakey ME, Henly WS, Cooley DA, et al. Surgical management of dissecting aneurysms of the aorta. J Thorac Cardiovasc Surg 1965;49:130–149.

43. Cigarroa JE, Isselbacher EM, DeSanctis RW, et al. Diagnostic imaging in the evaluation of suspected aortic dissection. N Engl J Med 1993;7:328(1):35–44.

44. Niennaber CA, von Kodolitsch Y, Volkmar N. The diagnosis of thoracic aortic dissection by noninvasive imaging procedures. N Engl J Med 1993;328(1): 1–10.

45. Daily PO, Trueblood HW, Stinson EB, et al. Management of acute aortic dissections. Ann Thorac Surg 1970;10:237–247.

46. Simon P, Owen AN, Havel M, et al. Transesophageal echocardiography in the emergency surgical management of patients with aortic dissection. J Thorac Cardiovasc Surg 1992;103(6):1113–1117.

47. Omoto R, Kyo S, Matsumura M, et al. Evaluation of biplane color Doppler transesophageal echocardiography in 200 consecutive patients. Circulation 1992;85(4):1237–1247.

48. Chan KL. Impact of transesophageal echocardiography on the treatment of patients with aortic dissection. Chest 1992;101(2):406–410.

49. Nienaber CA, Spielmann RP, von Kodolitsch Y, et al. Diagnosis of thoracic aortic dissection. Magnetic resonance imaging versus transesophageal echocardiography. Circulation 1992; 85(2):434–447.

50. Adachi H, Omoto R, Kyo S, et al. Emergency surgical intervention of acute aortic dissection with the rapid diagnosis by transesophageal echocardiography. Circulation 1991;84(5) (Suppl III):4–9.

51. Ballal RS, Nanda NC, Gatewood R. Usefulness of transesophageal echocardiography in assessment of aortic dissection. Circulation 1991;84(5): 1903–1914.

52. Levinson DC, Edmeades DT, Griffith GC. Dissecting aneurysm of the aorta—its clinical, electrocardiographic, and laboratory features: report of 58 autopsied cases. Circulation 1950;1:360–387.

53. Marfan AB. Un cas de deformation congenitale des quartres membres, plus pronouncee aux extremities, caracterisee par l'allongement des os avec un certain degre d'amincussement. Bull Sox Chir Paris 1896;13:220–225.

54. Crawford ES, Crawford JL. Marfan's syndrome. In: Diseases of the aorta. Baltimore: Williams & Wilkins, 1984;215–248.

55. Murdock JL, Walker BA, Halperin BL, et al. Life expectancy and causes of death in the Marfan's syndrome. N Engl J Med 1972;286:804–808.

Appendix: Useful Cardiovascular Equations, Physical Quantities, and Nomograms

Wilmer W. Nichols, PhD

Francesca A. Nicolini, MD

... [W]hen you can measure what you are speaking about, and express it in numbers, you know something about it; but when you cannot measure it, when you cannot express it in numbers, your knowledge is of a meager and unsatisfactory kind; it may be the beginning of knowledge, but you have scarcely, in your thoughts, advanced to the stage of science whatever the matter may be.—Kelvin

Cardiovascular catheterization is concerned with collecting information using hemodynamic, angiographic, and electrophysiologic procedures for diagnostic and therapeutic purposes. Raw data are usually collected in analog form on a strip chart recorder or in angiographic form on digital medium or cine film. To be useful for diagnostic purposes, these raw data must be elaborated into meaningful graphical or numerical information. This Appendix presents some physical quantities, equations (or formulas), definitions, and nomograms that should make interpretation of raw data collected in the cardiac catheterization laboratory relatively easy.

UNITS AND DIMENSIONS

Measuring a physical quantity (or variable) eans comparing it with some standard alled a unit. The numerical ratio of the varile measured and the unit with which it is compared is called the **numerical measure**, or **magnitude**, of the variable. Some variables are measured **directly** with a transducer (e.g., intra-arterial blood pressure), whereas others are **derived** from directly measured variables (e.g., vascular resistance = [mean blood pressure gradient]/ [mean blood flow]).

Variables are defined in terms of three fundamental quantities. The three commonly used quantities in physics (and physiology) are length (L), mass (M), and time (T); in the cgs system the units of measurement of these three quantities are the centimeter (cm), gram (gm), and second (sec), respectively. For example, the speed (or velocity) of travel of the pressure (or flow) pulse along an artery is defined as the distance the pulse moves per unit time. Expressed in dimensional analysis velocity is L/T or LT^{-1} and the unit of measurement is cm/sec. Some commonly used cardiovascular variables are given in Table A.1.

An **equation** in a two-dimensional Cartesian coordinate system is expressed as a function by writing y in terms of x [i.e., $y = f(x)$]. x is the **independent** variable and because the value of y depends on the value of x, y is the **dependent** variable (Fig. A.1). The graphic presentation of these variables is often interchanged in scientific publications, therefore, making the results difficult to interpret. All equations (or functions) must form an **identity** (i.e., both sides of the equation must be the same) not only in numerical value, but also in dimension. For example, vascular resistance (R) is

$$R = (mean\ pressure\ gradient)/(mean\ blood\ flow) \tag{1}$$

The cgs unit for resistance is (see Table A.1)

$$dyne\ sec/cm^5 = (dyne/cm^2)/(cm^3/sec)$$
$$= dyne\ sec/cm^5 \tag{2}$$

TABLE A.1.
Some Commonly Used Cardiovascular Variables

Variable	Common cgs Unit	Abbreviations
Mass	gram (g)	M
Length (diameter)	centimeter (cm)	L
Time	second (sec)	T
Area	cm^2	L^2
Volume	cm^3	L^3
Velocity	$cm\ sec^{-1}$	LT^{-1}
Flow	$cm^3\ sec^{-1}$	L^3T^{-1}
Acceleration	$cm\ sec^{-2}$	LT^{-2}
Force	g cm sec^{-2} (or dyne)	MLT^{-2}
Pressure	dyne cm^{-2}	$ML^{-1}T^{-2}$
Resistance	dyne sec cm^{-5}	$ML^{-4}T^{-1}$
Impedance	dyne sec cm^{-5}	$ML^{-4}T^{-1}$
Work[a]	dyne cm (or erg)	ML^2T^{-2}
Power[b]	dyne cm sec^{-1}	ML^2T^{-3}

[a] Mks unit of work = joule.
[b] Mks unit of power = joule sec^{-1} or watt.
cgs, centimeter, gram, second; m, mass; L, length; T, times.

In dimensional analysis, because a *dyne* = *gm cm/sec²* we have by substitution into equation 2

$$(gm\ cm/sec^2)\ (sec/cm^5)$$

$$= [(gm\ cm/sec^2)/cm^2]/(cm^3/sec)$$

$$gm/(cm^4\ sec) = gm\ cm^{-4}\ sec^{-1}$$

therefore,

$$ML^{-4}T^{-1} = ML^{-4}T^{-1} \qquad (3)$$

which is an identity.

USEFUL DEFINITIONS

Velocity (or Speed)

The velocity of a moving object is the distance (s) it moves per unit of time (t). The defining equation for instantaneous velocity is

$$velocity\ (cm/sec) = \frac{ds}{dt}\ (cm/sec) \qquad (4)$$

whereas average velocity is

$$c_0\ (cm/sec) = \frac{\Delta s}{\Delta t}\ (cm/sec) \qquad (5)$$

Therefore, pulse (pressure or blood flow velocity) wave velocity (or propagation velocity) can be obtained by recording pressure (or blood flow velocity) at two sites a known distance (δs) apart along an artery, and measuring the time delay (δt) between the two signals. Pulse wave velocity should not be confused with blood flow velocity. Blood flow velocity (v) is related to the volume (V) of blood that passes a point in the vascular system in a given period of time, i.e.,

$$v\ (cm/sec) = \frac{1}{\pi r^2} \times \frac{dV}{dt} \qquad (6)$$

where r is the internal radius of the vessel.

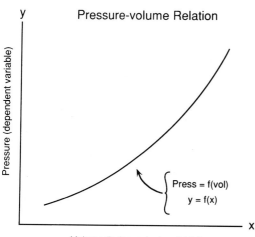

Pressure-volume Relation

Pressure (dependent variable) — y

Volume (independent variable) — x

Press = f(vol)
y = f(x)

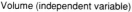

Figure A.1. In this isolated arterial segment preparation, intraluminal pressure is plotted as a function of intraluminal fluid volume. Volume is the independent variable plotted on the x-axis and pressure is the dependent variable plotted on the y-axis. A change in pressure, therefore, is dependent upon the change in intraluminal fluid volume. The converse, however, is not true.

Acceleration

Objects seldom move with constant velocity. In almost all cases, the velocity of an object is continually changing in magnitude. Therefore, the time rate of change of velocity is called instantaneous acceleration (a) such that

$$[A]\ a\ (cm/sec^2) = \frac{dv}{dt} = \frac{d}{dt}\left(\frac{ds}{dt}\right) \qquad (7)$$

Instantaneous blood flow acceleration can be obtained by continuous differentiation of blood flow velocity signal. Maximal blood flow acceleration measured in the ascending aorta has been used as an index of left ventricular contractility (1).

Volumetric Flow

All flowmeters (electromagnetic and ultrasonic) commonly in use today measure velocity (cm/sec) of liquid flow. If rigid flow probes are used with the flowmeters, the system (flowmeter plus probe) can be calibrated to give volumetric flow (cm^3/sec) (F), because the cross-sectional area of the vessel is kept constant by the probe and volumetric flow is linearly related to blood flow velocity (2) (see equation 6), i.e.,

$$F(cm^3/sec) = v\ \pi r^2 \qquad (8)$$

Momentum

The momentum of a particle is the product of its mass (m) and its velocity (v).

$$Momentum = mv \qquad (9)$$

Force

Newton's second law of motion states that the force acting on an object is equal to the rate of change of momentum (mv) of the object, i.e.,

$$Force\ (dyne) = \frac{d}{dt}\ (mv)\ m = \frac{dv}{dt} = ma \qquad (10)$$

Pressure

A force can be applied to a single point of a solid and be sustained by it; but, a force can only be applied to and sustained by a surface of an enclosed liquid. It is convenient, therefore, to describe the force acting on a liquid by specifying the pressure (P), which is defined as the magnitude of a normal force per unit surface area (**Force/Area**). In hemodynamics, pressure is usually expressed in terms of the height (h) of a column of reference liquid (usually mercury or water) with which it is in equilibrium, i.e.

$$P\ (dyne/cm^2) = \rho gh \qquad (11)$$

where p is the density of the liquid in equilibrium with the pressure ($cgs\ unit\ gm/cm^3$) and g is the acceleration caused by gravity (980.67 cm/sec^2 see Table A.2 for some commonly used constants). Intravascular pressure, which is usually expressed in $mm\ Hg$, is converted to cgs units using equation 11 as follows (some useful conversion factors are given in Table A.3):

$$
\begin{aligned}
P\ (mm\ Hg) &= 13.6\ gm/cm^3 \times 980.67\ cm/sec^2 \\
&\quad \times 0.1\ cm \\
&= 1333.7\ gm/cm^3 \times cm/sec^2 \times cm \\
&= 1333.7\ (gm/cm)/sec^2 \\
&= 1333.7\ (gm\ cm/sec^2)/cm^2 \\
&= 1333.7\ dyne/cm^2 \qquad (12)
\end{aligned}
$$

When arterial systolic (SP) and diastolic (DP) blood pressures are measured noninvasively (e.g., with a sphygmomameter),

TABLE A2.
Some Commonly Used Constants

Constant	Common cgs Unit	Value
π	—	3.1416
ϵ	—	2.72
Acceleration caused by gravity	cm sec^{-2}	980.67
Standard atmospheric pressure	mm Hg millibars dyne cm^{-2}	760 1013.3 1.013 × 10^6
Density of mercury	g cm^{-3}	13.6
Density of blood	g cm^{-3}	1.055
Viscosity of blood	dyne sec cm^{-2} (or poise)	0.04
Poisson's ratio for arteries	—	0.05
Velocity of sound in blood	cm sec^{-1}	1500

cgs, centimeter, gram, seconds

TABLE A.3.
Useful Conversion Factors

Meter	= 1.0 m	= 39.37 in
Decimeter	= 0.1 m	= 3.937 in
Centimeter	= 0.01 m	= 0.3937 in
Millimeter	= 0.001 m	= 0.0394 in
Micrometer	= 0.000001 m	= 0.0000394 in
Milliliter	= 0.001 L	= 1 cm^3
Liter	= 1.0567 q	
Kilogram	= 1000 g	= 2.205 l
Gram	= 15.432 grains	= 0.035 oz
Milligram	= 0.001 g	
Radian	= 57°17′44.8″	= 180°/π
Degree	= 0.0174533 radian	
Millimeter Hg of mercury	= 1333.7 dyne cm^{-2}	
Torr	= 1.0 mm Hg	= 13.6 mm H$_2$O
Pascal	= 1.0 Newton/m^2	
KiloPascal	= 7.547 mm Hg	
Pound	= 0.454 Kg	
Pound per square inch (PSI)	= 5.17 mm Hg	

mean arterial blood pressure (*MAP*) can be estimated using the formula:

$$MAP = \frac{(SP - DP)}{3} + DP \qquad (13)$$

Some normal values of blood pressures and blood flows are given in Table A.4.

Vascular Resistance

Resistance is opposition to steady flow of a liquid in a hydraulic system and is defined as the ratio of pressure drop (or gradient) $(P_1 - P_2)$ across the system and flow (F) of liquid through it. In the circulatory system this ratio is called the **vascular resistance**, and it is usually confined to the microcirculation (see Chapter 22).

$$
\begin{aligned}
&Resistance\ (dyne\ sec/cm^5) \\
&= \frac{(P_1 - P_2)(dyne/cm^2)}{F(cm^3/sec)} \\
&= \frac{(P_1 - P_2)(mm\ Hg)}{F(L/min)} \times 80
\end{aligned} \qquad (14)
$$

P_1 and P_2 are the pressures at the proximal and distal ends, respectively, of the sys-

TABLE A.4.
Normal Values of Pressures and Flows

Variable	Unit	Average	Range
Pressures	mm Hg		
Systemic arterial			
Peak systolic		125	100–140
End diastolic		84	60–90
Mean		100	70–105
Left ventricle			
Peak systolic		125	100–140
End diastolic		9	5–12
Left atrium (or pulmonary capillary wedge)			
Mean		7	2–12
"a" wave		10	3–15
"z" point		12	4–18
"v" wave		8	2–12
Pulmonary artery			
Peak systolic		25	17–32
End diastolic		9	4–13
Mean		15	9–19
Right ventricle			
Peak systolic		25	17–32
End diastolic		4	1–7
Right atrium			
Mean		3	1–5
"a" wave		6	3–7
"z" point		3	1–5
"c" wave		4	2–6
"x" wave		2	0–5
"v" wave		5	2–8
"y" wave		2	0–6
Flows			
Ascending aorta			
Peak	$cm^2 sec^{-1}$	520	460–620
Mean (cardiac output)	liters min^{-1}	6	5.2–7.4
Stoke volume	cm^3	82	70–94
Cardiac index	liters $min^{-2} m^{-2}$	3.2	2.6–4.2
Stoke index	$cm^3 m^{-2}$	49	30–65

tem. In the systemic circulation, P_1 is mean arterial pressure and P_2 is mean right atrial pressure. P_2 can usually be disregarded in resistance calculations in the systemic circulation because it is small compared with arterial pressure. In the pulmonary circulation, however, P_2 should be included in the resistance (**pulmonary arteriolar resistance**) calculation. P_2 is usually taken as mean pulmonary capillary wedge pressure or mean left arterial pressure. If P_2 is not used in the calculation, the measurement is defined as total **pulmonary vascular resistance**. Normal values for resistance (and some other useful variables) are given in

Table A.5, and a nomogram for easy estimation of resistance is given in Figure A.2. (Also see Chapter 22.)

Ventricular Work

In physics, work (W) is defined as the product of force and displacement (or distance) in the direction of the force, that is,

$$W \ (dyne \ cm) = Force \times distance \quad (15)$$

TABLE A.5.
Other Normal Values of Cardiovascular Variables

Variable	Unit	Average	Range
Resistance	dyne sec cm^{-5}		
Systemic total		1130	900–1460
Pulmonary total		205	100–300
Arteriolar		67	50–128
Left ventricle			
Volumes	cm^3 m^{-2}		
End systolic		26	20–33
End diastolic		74	60–88
Ejection fraction		0.67	0.58–0.73
Wall thickness	mm	9.2	8.2–10.4
Mass	gm	166	130–190
Maximum dP/dt	mm Hg sec^{-1}	1640	1320–1880
Heart Rate	beats min^{-1}	73	68–78
Stroke work	mjoules	21	16–26
External power	mwatts	1500	1300–1700
Time intervals	sec		
Ejection period		0.27	0.22–0.32
Diastolic filling period		0.44	0.38–0.50
Ascending aortic characteristic			
Impedance	dyne sec cm^{-5}	56	40–74
Oxygen consumption	liters min^{-2} m^{-2}	134	113–148
Arteriovenous oxygen difference	cm^3 liter^{-1}	39	31–49

The *cgs* unit of work is the *erg (dyne cm)*; but, because this unit is small, the *joule (mks unit)* is commonly used (1 joule = 10^7 ergs). In the cardiovascular system, we can only measure "external work" (internal work can be estimated) (3) of the ventricle, which is primarily potential, or pressure energy. Because force is the product of pressure (P) and cross-sectional area (A), we have, by substitution of equations 4 and 8 into equation 15,

$$W \; (dyne \; cm) \; (PA) \; (vt) = (PA) \; (F/A)t = PFt \tag{16}$$

Integration of equation 16 over one cardiac cycle gives stroke work (2–4), i.e.,

$$[B] \; W \; (stroke) = \int_{t_1}^{t_2} PF dt \tag{17}$$

where t_1 and t_2 are the times at which the cardiac cycle begins and ends, respectively.

Ventricular Power

In physics, power is defined as the time rate of doing work, i.e.,

$$
\begin{aligned}
Power \; (dyne \; cm/sec) &= W/t \\
&= (PA) \; (vt)/t \\
&= (PA) \; (v) \\
&= PF
\end{aligned}
\tag{18}
$$

Therefore, total left ventricular (LV) external hydraulic power can be obtained by continuous multiplication of pulsatile ascending aortic blood pressure (P) and flow (F) (LV pressure can also be used instead of aortic pressure). Right ventricular power can be obtained in a similar manner. The cgs unit of power is the erg/sec; but, because this is an inconveniently small unit, the joule/sec, also called the watt (mks unit), is commonly used. Ventricular external power can be separated into two components, one associated with steady blood

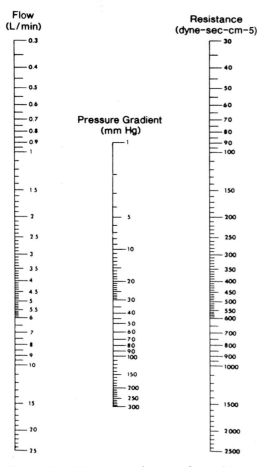

Figure A.2. Nomogram for vascular resistance. To obtain resistance in cgs resistance units, a straight line joining *Flow* (in L/min) and *Pressure Gradient* (in mm Hg) is extended to the *Resistance* axis.

flow and the other with vascular pulsations caused by intermittent ventricular contraction. The steady power component is determined as mean aortic (or mean pulmonary artery) pressure times mean blood flow (or cardiac output); the other (oscillatory or pulsatile power) is determined as the difference between average power (mean of pulsatile pressure times pulsatile flow) and steady power (2, 3).

Density

Mass per unit volume of a substance is called its density (2). The cgs unit of density is *gm/cm³*. Blood density is 1.055 gm/cm³ (2).

Viscosity

Viscosity is that property of a liquid, its internal friction, which causes it to resist liquid flow. The cgs unit of viscosity is the poise, in recognition of the work of Poiseuille. *Poise = dyne sec cm²*. Blood viscosity 0.04 poise (2).

Stress

Stress is the force per unit area that produces a deformation in a material (2, 3). Stress is commonly expressed in cgs units (*dynes/ cm²*) and its fundamental dimension is $ML^{-1}T^{-2}$

$$Stress\ (dyne/cm^2) = \frac{Force}{\pi r^2} \qquad (19)$$

STRAIN

Strain is the ratio of change in a given dimension, such as length (*L*), of a stressed material to its original value in the unstressed state (5). Strain is, therefore, dimensionless.

$$Strain = \Delta L/L \qquad (20)$$

Young's (or Elastic) Modulus

A modulus of elasticity (*E*) is defined as the ratio of a stress to the corresponding strain. This ratio is a constant, characteristic of the material.

$$E\ (dyne/cm^2) = \frac{Stress}{Strain}$$
$$= \frac{Force/\pi r^2}{\Delta L/L} = \frac{Force \times L}{\Delta L \times \pi r^2} \qquad (21)$$

Young's modulus (named for Thomas Young) is commonly expressed in dynes/cm^2 (cgs unit).

Pressure-Strain Elastic Modulus

A direct comparison of the values for the elastic modulus of arteries from all published accounts is not possible because in many cases the wall thickness was not recorded, so that the 'pressure-strain' elastic modulus, E$_p$, introduced by Peterson et al. (6) has been substituted:

$$E_p = D_d \frac{(P_s - P_d)}{(D_s - D_d)} \tag{22}$$

where $(P_s - P_d)$ and $(D_s - D_d)$ are pulse pressure and pulse diameter, respectively, and D$_d$ is the end-diastolic diameter. If static values are desired, $(P_s - P_d)$ and $(D_s - D_d)$ are quasistatic changes in pressure and diameter, respectively, and D$_d$ is the mean diameter corresponding to the mean pressure. Another equation for calculating a pressure-strain elastic modulus (β) was introduced by Kawasaki et al. (7); it has been used in humans by several investigators, including Lanne et al. (8, 9) and Sonesson et al. (10).

$$\beta = \frac{[D_d \ln (P_s/P_d)]}{(D_s - D_d)} \tag{23}$$

Elastic Material

When a material changes shape under an applied force but returns to its initial shape when the force is removed, the material is said to be **perfectly elastic** (2, 3, 5).

Plastic Material

A material that does not return to its initial shape when an applied force is removed is considered **plastic**.

Isotropic

Material with mechanical properties that are independent of the direction of the force applied (i.e., the material has the same elastic properties in all directions) is isotropic; a block of steel is isotropic.

Anisotropic

Material with mechanical properties that are dependent on the direction of the force applied (i.e., the material does not have the same elastic properties in all directions), it is anisotropic; biologic materials are anisotropic.

Viscoelastic

Viscoelastic is time dependence of response to a stress or strain; an important property of biologic materials.

Compliance (Distensibility)

Compliance is a measure of the ability of a hollow structure to change its volume, generally the ratio of volume change to internal pressure change (*dV/dP*). The inverse of compliance is elastance (or stiffness) (i.e., *dP/dV*, the slope of the pressure-volume curve in Fig. A.1).

Ventricular Preload

Ventricular preload is the stretching force to which the myocardial muscle is subjected in its relaxed state just prior to ventricular contraction (4). In the intact heart, this is taken as ventricular end-diastolic volume or pressure.

Ventricular Afterload

Ventricular afterload is the external hydraulic load opposing ventricular ejection. The measurement that best defines afterload is the (aortic or pulmonary) input impedance spectra (2, 3) (i.e., resistance, elastance, and reflectance).

Myocardial Contractility

Myocardial contractility is the change in force of myocardial contraction from the same fiber length.

SOME USEFUL EQUATIONS

Moens-Korteweg and Bramwell-Hill Equations

For large arteries, pulse wave velocity (c_o) is related to physical properties of the vessel wall by the **Moens-Korteweg equation** (2),

$$c_o \ (cm/\sec) = \sqrt{(Eh/\rho 2r}$$ (24)

where

E = Young's modulus of the vessel wall (dyne/cm^2)

h = wall thickness (cm)

r = internal radius of vessel (cm)

ρ = blood desnity (gm/cm^3)

A closely related equation that expresses pulse wave velocity in terms of volume distensibility was first derived by Frank (11) but is commonly referred to as the *Bramwell-Hill equation* (12),

$$[C] \ c_o \ (cm/\sec) = \sqrt{\frac{V}{P} \times \frac{dP}{dV}}$$ (25)

where

v = arterial blood volume (cm^3)

dP = pulse pressure (dyne/cm^2)

dV = increase in arterial blood volume (cm^3) per stroke

In a system with minimal or no reflections, arterial elastance or stiffness (inverse of compliance and distensibility) is related to the pulse wave velocity by the following equation (2)

$$Z_o \ (dyne \ \sec/cm^5) = \frac{\rho c_o}{\pi r^2}$$ (26)

Z_o is called the **characteristic impedance**, and it is the ratio of pulsatile pressure and flow when no reflections are present. The cgs unit of Z_o is the **dyne sec/cm^5**. The effects of age on Z_o and some other cardiovascular variables are given in Table A.6.

Laplace Equation

Increase in length of an elastic homogenous structure is proportional to the tension (or force) applied to it, i.e.,

$$[D] \ P \ (dyne/cm^2) = T\left(\frac{1}{r_1} + \frac{1}{r_2}\right)$$ (27)

where

P = distending pressure (dyne/cm^2)

T = tension (dyne/cm)

r_1, r_2 = principal radii of curvature of the structure (cm)

In the case of a tube (e.g., an artery) of cylindrical cross-section, one radius of curvature (i.e., in the longitudinal plane) is infinite and the other is cylinder radius; the equation thus becomes (13)

TABLE A.6.
Effects of Age on Some Cardiovascular Variables[a]

Variable	Unit	Slope	Intercept
Mean ascending aortic radius	cm	0.0097	0.98
Heart rate	beats/min	0.0486	73.64
Systolic aortic pressure	mm Hg	0.6852	95.00
Diastolic aortic pressure	mm Hg	0.0702	76.12
Mean aortic pressure	mm Hg	0.1911	90.27
Aortic pulse pressure	mm Hg	0.615	18.89
Cardiac output	liters/min	−0.0365	7.85
Stroke volume	mL	−0.5605	109.3
Characteristic ascending aortic impedance	dyne sec cm^{-5}	1.2135	10.3
Peripheral resistance	dyne sec cm^{-5}	9.74	853.97

[a] Variable = Slope × Age + Intercept (Adapted from Nichols WW, O'Rourke MF, Avolino AP, et al. Effects of age on ventricular-vascular coupling. Am J Cardiol 1985;55:1179.)

$$P \ (dyne/cm^2) \ = \ T/r \qquad (28)$$

or

$$T \ (dyne/cm) \ = \ Pr \qquad (29)$$

For a sphere, $r_1 = r_2$ and

$$T(dyne/cm) \ = \ Pr/2 \qquad (30)$$

If the wall has a thickness (h) then the circumferential tension (or stress) (S_c) is given by

$$S_c \ (dyne/cm^2) \ = \ Pr/2h \qquad (31)$$

POISEUILLE'S EQUATION

Experiments dealing with liquid flow (F) in cylindrical tubes were performed by Poiseuille in the mid-1840s. He used glass capillary tubes and steady flow of a Newtonian liquid. The form of Poiseuille's equation with which we are familiar is

$$F \ (cm^3/sec) \ = \ \frac{\pi r^4 (P_1 - P_2)}{8\mu L} \qquad (32)$$

where

r = internal tube radius (cm)

$(P_1 - P_2)$ = mean pressure drop
(or gradient) along tube (dyne/cm^2)

L = length of tube (cm)

μ = viscosity of the contained liquid
(dyne sec/cm^2)

We have for resistance (R) from the Poiseuille equation

$$R \ (dyne \ sec/cm^5) \ = \ \frac{(P_1 - P_2)}{F} \ = \ \frac{8\mu L}{\pi r^4} \qquad (33)$$

Reynolds Equation (Number)

Reynolds number (R_e) is a dimensionless quantity often used to describe the characteristics of steady liquid flow through a straight tube at which transition from laminar to turbulent flow would occur. R_e is defined as

$$R_e \ = \ \frac{2r\rho v}{\mu} \qquad (34)$$

Transition from laminar to turbulent flow of a liquid during steady flow in a tube typically occurs at a Reynolds number of about 2300 (14). This variable is defined as the critical Reynolds number.

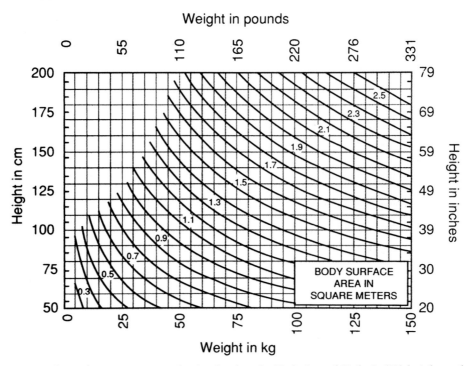

Weight in pounds

Figure A.3. Body surface area curves obtained using the Dubois and Dubois (17) height and weight equation (equation 40). A subject weighing 165 lbs. and 69 inches tall has a body surface area of 1.9 square meters. (Reprinted with permission from Gravenstein and Paulus. Monitoring practice in clinical anesthesia. Philadelphia: JB Lippincott, 1982.)

Orifice Area Equation

(See Chapter 25) Equations used to calculate area of stenotic cardiac valves and central circulatory shunts were derived by Gorlin and Gorlin (15) using Torricelli's Law, which describes blood flow velocity (v) through a round orifice of cross-sectional area (A):

$$[E] \quad v = \sqrt{2g(P_1 - P_2)} \qquad (35)$$

where ($P_1 - P_2$) is pressure gradient (*mm Hg*) across the orifice and g is acceleration caused by gravity (Table A.2). Because F (cm^3/sec) = vA (equation 8), equation 35 can be written as

$$[F] \quad A \ (cm^2) = \frac{F}{\sqrt{2g(P_1 - P_2)}} \\ = \frac{F}{44.3 \sqrt{(P_1 - P_2)}} \qquad (36)$$

Experiments have shown that actual velocity is somewhat smaller than theoretic velocity owing to the effects of liquid viscosity. This can be accounted for by introducing an empiric correction factor (C) called the discharge coefficient (2)

$$[G] \quad A \ (cm^2) = \frac{F}{44.3C \ \sqrt{(P_1 - P_2)}} \qquad (37)$$

When using equation 37, it must be kept in mind that flow across the atrioventricular valves occurs during diastole (diastolic filling period) and flow across the semilunar valves occurs during systole (systolic ejection period). Empiric constant (C) for the tricuspid, pulmonic, and aortic valves, as well as for a patent ductus or ventricular septal defect, is assumed to be 1.0; for the mitral valve it is assumed to be 0.90 (16) (Chapter 25, equations 8 and 9).

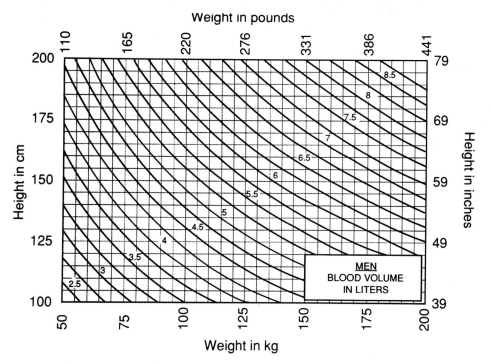

Figure A.4. Total intravascular blood volume curves in men obtained using the Hidalgo, et al. (19), height and weight equation (equation 41). A subject weighing 165 lbs. and 69 inches tall has an intravascular blood volume of 5.0 liters. (Reprinted with permission from Gravenstein and Paulus. Monitoring practice in clinical anesthesia. Philadelphia: JB Lippincott, 1982.)

Cardiac Output Equations

(See Chapter 21) The amount of blood ejected by the ventricle (right or left) per unit time is called the cardiac output and is usually expressed in liters per minute (the cgs unit is cm^3/sec). In general, cardiac index (i.e., cardiac output per square meter of body surface area; see Fig. A.3) is used on the premise that cardiac output is proportional to body surface area.

Of the various methods presently available, direct Fick and the indicator (Indocyanine green or Thermal) dilution methods are most commonly used because of their accuracy, safety, reproducibility, and relative simplicity. Various equations used to calculate cardiac output using these methods are given in Chapter 21.

Temperature Equations

Sometimes it is necessary to convert from degrees Fahrenheit (°F) to degrees Centigade (°C) and vice versa.

$$°F = 1.8 \, °C + 32 \tag{38}$$

and

$$°C = 0.556 \, (°F - 32) \tag{39}$$

USEFUL NOMOGRAMS

Body Surface Area

To obtain cardiac index and stroke index from cardiac output and stroke volume,

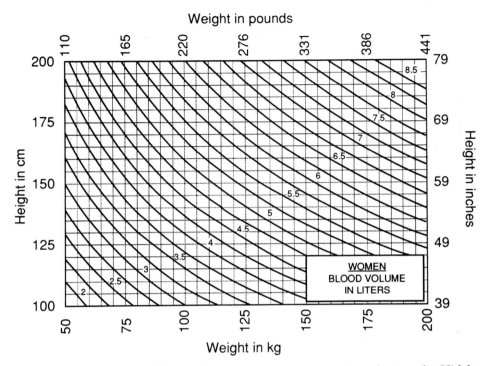

Figure A.5. Total intravascular blood volume curves in women obtained using the Hidalgo et al. (19), height and weight equation (equation 42). (Reprinted with permission from Gravenstein JS, Paulus DA. Monitoring practice in clinical anesthesia. Philadelphia: JB Lippincott, 1982.)

body surface area (*BSA*) is needed. This quantity is usually estimated from a nomogram devised using the Dubosis and Dubosis (17) height (*H*)-weight (*W*) equations:

$$BSA\ (m^2) = 71.84\ H^{0.725} \times W^{0.425} \times 10^{-4} \tag{40}$$

A family of graphs, prepared by Gravenstein and Paulus (18) using the above equation, is shown in Figure A.3.

Total Blood Volume

Total blood volume (*TBV*) is approximately 8% of body weight, and it can be estimated from a patient's height (*H*) and weight (*W*) using equations developed by Hidalog et al. (19). For men:

$$TBC\ (liters) = 0.0236 \times H^{0.725} \times W^{0.425} - 1.229 \tag{41}$$

For women:

$$TBV\ (liters) = 0.0248 \times H^{0.725} \times W^{0.425} - 1.954 \tag{42}$$

These equations were plotted as nomograms (18) and are shown in Figures A.4 and A.5.

References

1. Noble MIM, Trenchard D, Guz A. Left ventricular ejection in conscious dogs: measurement and significance of the maximum acceleration of blood from the left ventricle. Circ Res 1966; 19:139–147
2. Nichols WW, O'Rourke MF. McDonald's blood flow in arteries. 4th ed. Edward Arnold: London; 1997.
3. Milnor WR. Hemodynamics. 2nd ed. Baltimore: Williams and Wilkins, 1989.

4. Berne RM, Levy MN. Cardiovascular Physiology. 7th ed. Mosby: New York; 1997.

5. Lee RT. Vascular Mechanics for the Cardiologist. J Am Col Cardiol 1994; 23: 1289–1295.

6. Peterson LH, Jensen, RE, Parnell J. Mechanical properties of arteries in vivo. Circ Res 1960; 8: 622–639.

7. Kawasaki, T. Sasayama, S., Yagi, S., Asakawa, T., Hirai, T. (1987). Non-invasive assessment of the age related changes in stiffness of major branches of the human arteries. Cardiovasc Res 21: 678–687.

8. Länne T, Stale H, Bengtsson H, et al. Noninvasive measurement of diameter changes in the distal abdominal aorta in man. Ultrasound in Medicine and Biology 1992a:18(5):451–457.

9. Länne T, Sonesson B, Bergqvist D, et al. Diameter and compliance in the male human abdominal aorta: influence of age and aortic aneurysm. Eur J Vasc Surg 1992b;6:178–184.

10. Sonesson B, Hansen F, Stale H, et al. Compliance and diameter in the human abdominal aorta-the influence of age and sex. Eur J Vasc Surg 1993;7: 690–697.

11. Frank O. Die theorie der pulswellen. Z Biol 1920; 85:91–130.

12. Bramwell JC, Hill AV. The velocity of the pulse wave in man. Proc R Soc Land [Biol] 1922; 93: 298–306.

13. Burton AC. Relation of structure to function of the tissues of the walls of blood vessels. Physiol Rev 1954;34:619–642.

14. Schlichting H. Boundary layer theory. 6th edition New York: McGraw-Hill, 1968.

15. Gorlin R, Gorlin, G. Hydraulic formula for calculation of area of stenotic mitral valve, other cardiac valves and central circulatory shunts. Am Heart J 1951;41:1–29.

16. Cohen MV, Gorlin R. Modified orifice equation for calculation of mitral valve area. Am Heart J 1972; 84:839–840.

17. Dubois D, Dubois EF. A height-weight formula to estimate the surface area of man. Proc Soc Exp Biol NY 1916;77.

18. Gravenstein JS, Paulus DA. Monitoring practice in clinical anesthesia. Philadelphia: JB Lippincott, 1982.

19. Hidalgo JV, Nadler SB, Bloch T. The use of the electronic digital computer to determine best fit of blood volume formulas. J Nucl Med 1962;94.

20. Nichols WW, O'Rourke MF, Avolio AP, et al. Effects of age on ventricular-vascular coupling. Am J Cardiol 1985;55:1179–1184.

Index

Page numbers in *italics* denote figures; those followed by a "t" denote tables.